THE OXFORD HANDBOOK OF

PUBLIC HEALTH ETHICS

THE OXFORD HANDBOOK OF

PUBLIC HEALTH ETHICS

Edited by

ANNA C. MASTROIANNI,

JEFFREY P. KAHN,

and

NANCY E. KASS

OXFORD

UNIVERSITY PRESS

OXFORD
UNIVERSITY PRESS

Oxford University Press is a department of the University of Oxford.
It furthers the University's objective of excellence in research, scholarship,
and education by publishing worldwide. Oxford is a registered trade mark of
Oxford University Press in the UK and certain other countries.

Published in the United States of America by Oxford University Press
198 Madison Avenue, New York, NY 10016, United States of America.

Library of Congress Cataloging-in-Publication Data
Data available
Library of Congress Control Number: 2019943545

ISBN: 978-0-19-024519-1

1 3 5 7 9 8 6 4 2
Printed by Sheridan Books, Inc., United States of America

To Ruth Faden, who helped launch the field of public health ethics, and with gratitude for helping to launch each of the three of us.

Acknowledgments

Any project of this scope relies on many people for its success, and we are indebted to what grew into a small army of colleagues. At the University of Washington School of Law, Omar Contreras and Andrea Frey aided us in the early stages of this book's development. Also at the UW School of Law, the indispensable Jaclyn Greenberg provided immense help with organization, communications, and tracking of chapter drafts. Graduate students at Johns Hopkins worked closely with us as well, and include Christian Morales, who provided editorial assistance and formatting of chapters, and Lelia Chaisson and Kristina Hallez, who helped to manage the flow of chapters from final manuscript through the copyediting process and into final publication.

We truly appreciate the 56 peer reviewers who volunteered their time to ensure excellence in the final product: Soji Adeyi, The World Bank Group; Gerald Anderson, Johns Hopkins University; Freida Behets, University of North Carolina, Chapel Hill; Sara Bennett, Johns Hopkins University; David Bishai, Johns Hopkins University; Richard Bonnie, University of Virginia; Kathleen M. Boozang, Seton Hall University; Richard Chaisson, Johns Hopkins University; Joanna Cohen, Johns Hopkins University; Steven Coughlin, Augusta University; Susan Davercamp, Ohio State University; Janet L. Dolgin, Ohio State University; Shauna Downs, Johns Hopkins University; Jonathan Ellen, Johns Hopkins University; Kevin Elliott, Michigan State University; Aaron Goldenberg, Case Western Reserve University; Ken Goodman, University of Miami; Leslie Meltzer Henry, University of Maryland and Johns Hopkins University; Dan Hicks, American Association for the Advancement of Science; Martha Hijar, Entornos Foundation; Michelle J. Hindin, The Population Council; Jessica Holzer, Hofstra University; Jeffrey Kahn, Johns Hopkins University; Nancy E. Kass, Johns Hopkins University; Maureen Kelley, Oxford University; Bartha Knoppers, McGill University; Michiel Korthals, Wageningen University; Carleigh Krubiner, Johns Hopkins University; Keren Ladin, Tufts University; Cheryl Cox Macpherson, St. Georges University; Anna Mastroianni, University of Washington; Sassy Molyneux, Oxford University and Kenya Medical Research Institute; Tanvi Nagpal, Johns Hopkins University; David Pena-Guzman, Johns Hopkins University; Govind Persad, University of Denver; Keshia Pollack, Johns Hopkins University; Stuart Rennie, University of North Carolina, Chapel Hill; Lainie Rutkow, Johns Hopkins University; Daniel Salmon, Johns Hopkins University; Harald Schmidt, University of Pennsylvania; Amy Sepinwall, University of Pennsylvania; Josh Sharfstein, Johns Hopkins University; Jeremy Shiffman, American University; Andrew Siegel, Johns Hopkins University; Colin Soskolne, University of Alberta; Devi Sridhar, University of Edinburgh; Kenneth Stoller, John Hopkins University; Jeff Swanson, Duke

University; John Tasioulas, King's College London; Holly Taylor, Johns Hopkins University; Alison Thompson, University of Toronto; Sean Valles, Michigan State University; Stephen Wilkinson, Lancaster University; Leslie Wolf, Georgia State University; Matthew Wynia, University of Colorado; Jonathan Zenilman, Johns Hopkins University.

To the 11 dedicated colleagues who performed above and beyond our expectations as section editors and the 103 colleagues from around the globe who contributed as authors—we are proud to have worked closely with you all. At Oxford University Press, thanks to Hannah Doyle for support in creating the final book, and Lucy Randall and Peter Ohlin for seeing the value of the work and having the long view in supporting a multi-year project. Your help and support were truly invaluable.

ACM
JPK
NEK

Contents

SECTION SEVEN: SEXUAL AND REPRODUCTIVE HEALTH

SECTION EIGHT: COMMUNICABLE DISEASES

SECTION ELEVEN: INJURIES

SECTION TWELVE: GENETICS

SECTION THIRTEEN: ENVIRONMENTAL HEALTH

Volume Editors

Anna C. Mastroianni, JD, MPH, is Professor of Law at the University of Washington School of Law and Associate Director of the university's Institute for Public Health Genetics. She has additional faculty appointments in the university's School of Public Health (Health Services) and School of Medicine (Bioethics & Humanities; Pediatrics). She is Affiliate Faculty at the Treuman Katz Center for Pediatric Bioethics at Seattle Children's Hospital and Research Institute. Her scholarly work examines the intersection of law, bioethics, and health policy, with a special emphasis on the legal and ethical challenges arising in public health, research, and reproduction. Professor Mastroianni teaches health law, bioethics, and family law in the School of Law and other units throughout the university. Professor Mastroianni's education includes a JD, BA, and BS from the University of Pennsylvania and an MPH from the University of Washington. Before joining the university faculty, she was a practicing attorney and subsequently worked in a number of legal and governmental policy positions, including Staff Director of the President's Advisory Committee on Human Radiation Experiments and Study Director of the National Academy of Medicine of the National Academies of Sciences, Engineering, and Medicine. She serves on international and US advisory committees, most recently for the Wellcome Trust, the Population Council, and the National Academy of Medicine. She is an elected Fellow of the American Association for the Advancement of Science, recognized for her contributions to health policy, law, and bioethics.

Jeffrey P. Kahn, PhD, MPH, is the Andreas C. Dracopoulos Director of the Johns Hopkins Berman Institute of Bioethics, and the Levi Professor of Bioethics and Public Policy. He is also Professor in the Department of Health Policy and Management in the Johns Hopkins Bloomberg School of Public Health. His research interests include the ethics of research, ethics and public health, and ethics and emerging biomedical technologies. He speaks widely in the United States and abroad, has published four books and over 125 articles, and leads or participates in numerous grant-funded research projects. Dr. Kahn is an elected member of the National Academy of Medicine and an elected Fellow of the Hastings Center, and has chaired or served on committees and panels for the National Institutes of Health, the Centers for Disease Control and Prevention, and the Institute of Medicine/National Academy of Medicine, where he is currently Chair of the Board on Health Sciences Policy and the Committee on Aerospace Medicine and Medicine of Extreme Environments. His education includes a BA in microbiology from UCLA, MPH from Johns Hopkins University, and PhD in philosophy from Georgetown University. Prior to joining the faculty at Johns Hopkins, he held the Maas Family Chair in Bioethics and was Director of the Center for Bioethics at the University of Minnesota, and also served as Staff Director for the President's Advisory Committee on Human Radiation Experiments.

Nancy E. Kass, ScD, is Vice Provost for Graduate and Professional Education at Johns Hopkins University, and Phoebe R. Berman Professor of Bioethics and Public Health in the Johns Hopkins Berman Institute of Bioethics and the Johns Hopkins Bloomberg School of Public Health, where she is also Professor of Health Policy and Management. Dr. Kass received her BA from Stanford University, completed doctoral training in health policy from the Johns Hopkins School of Public Health and postdoctoral training at the Kennedy Institute of Ethics, Georgetown University. As Vice Provost, Dr. Kass focuses on issues related to the quality of PhD education, promoting transparency about PhD programs, diversity of the student body, career preparedness, research and professional experiences for students, and mentoring. In her faculty role, Dr. Kass conducts empirical work in bioethics, public health, and human research. Her publications are in the field of US and international research ethics, public health ethics, and ethics and the learning healthcare system. She spent a year on assignment as an expert at the World Health Organization in Geneva and has served as a consultant to the President's Advisory Committee on Human Radiation Experiments, the National Bioethics Advisory Commission, and the National Academy of Sciences, Engineering, and Medicine. Dr. Kass is Chair of the US National Institutes of Health Precision Medicine Initiative Central IRB, previously co-chaired the National Cancer Institute (NCI) Committee to Develop Recommendations for Informed Consent Documents, and served on the NCI's central IRB. Dr. Kass is an elected member of the National Academy of Medicine and an elected Fellow of the Hastings Center.

Section Editors

Ruth Gaare Bernheim, JD, MPH, is the William Hobson Professor and Chair of the Department of Public Health Sciences and the Director of the Institute for Practical Ethics and Public Life at the University of Virginia. Her research interests include ethics, law and public health policy, health disparities, and public-health community needs assessment.

Jessica Fanzo, PhD, is Bloomberg Distinguished Associate Professor of Food Policy and Ethics in the Johns Hopkins Nitze School of Advanced International Studies and Johns Hopkins Berman Institute of Bioethics. Her research interests include international nutrition and food policy and ethics. Her work focuses on developing economies of the Southern Hemisphere.

Elizabeth Fenton, PhD, MPH, is Lecturer in the Bioethics Centre at the University of Otago in Dunedin, New Zealand. She previously served as a Senior Policy and Research Analyst at the US Presidential Commission for the Study of Bioethical Issues. Her research interests include public health emergency ethics, prioritization and resource allocation, and health policy.

Adnan A. Hyder, MD, MPH, PhD, is Senior Associate Dean for Research and Professor of Global Health at the Milken Institute School of Public Health, George Washington University. Part of his work on this volume was conducted during his tenure at the Bloomberg School of Public Health and Berman Institute of Bioethics at Johns Hopkins University. His research interests include research ethics, injury prevention, strengthening health systems and research capacity-building in low- and middle-income countries.

Debra J. H. Mathews, PhD, MA, is Associate Professor in the Department of Pediatrics, School of Medicine, and Core Faculty and Assistant Director for Science Programs for the Johns Hopkins Berman Institute of Bioethics. Her research interests include ethics and policy issues raised by emerging biomedical technologies, within fields such as genetics, stem cell science, and neuroscience.

Leslie Meltzer Henry, JD, PhD, MSc, is Professor of Law at the University of Maryland Francis King Carey School of Law, and Core Faculty in the Johns Hopkins Berman Institute of Bioethics. Her research and scholarship focus on ethical, legal, and policy challenges that arise in the contexts of public health, sexuality and reproduction, and biomedical research.

Maria W. Merritt, PhD, is Core Faculty in the Berman Institute of Bioethics and Associate Professor in the Department of International Health at the Bloomberg School of Public Health, Johns Hopkins University. Her main research interests are in public health ethics, and her work focuses on relating considerations of social justice to economic evaluation.

David B. Resnik, JD, PhD, is Bioethicist and Chair of the Institutional Review Board at the National Institute of Environmental Health Sciences, National Institutes of Health. His research examines ethical, philosophical, and legal issues in science, technology, and medicine.

Brendan Saloner, PhD, is Assistant Professor in the Department of Health Policy and Management at the Johns Hopkins Bloomberg School of Public Health. He holds a joint appointment in the Department of Mental Health at the Johns Hopkins Bloomberg School of Public Health and is Affiliate Faculty in the Johns Hopkins Berman Institute of Bioethics. His research focuses on ethical issues in resource allocation and the delivery of services for people with behavioral health disorders in the United States.

Andrew W. Siegel, JD, PhD, is a Research Scholar in the Johns Hopkins Berman Institute of Bioethics and Affiliate Faculty at the Kennedy Institute of Ethics at Georgetown University. His current research focuses on ethical and legal issues in human stem cell research, exploitation in international research, and privacy.

Holly A. Taylor, PhD, MPH, is Associate Professor in the Department of Health Policy and Management at the Johns Hopkins Bloomberg School of Public Health and Core Faculty in the Johns Hopkins Berman Institute of Bioethics. She uses empirical methods to explore the ethics of human subjects research and ethics and infectious disease.

Contributors

Shanthi Ameratunga, MD, MPH
Professor, School of Population Health
Faculty of Medical & Health Sciences
University of Auckland
St. Johns, Auckland, New Zealand

Gerard Anderson, PhD
Professor, Department of Health Policy and Management
Bloomberg School of Public Health
Johns Hopkins University
Baltimore, Maryland

Daniel Arias, BA
Senior Program Associate
Results for Development Institute
Washington, DC

Yukiko Asada, PhD, MSc
Associate Professor, Department of Community Health and Epidemiology
Faculty of Medicine
Dalhousie University
Halifax, Nova Scotia, Canada

Jeromie M. Ballreich, PhD, MHS
Assistant Scientist, Department of Health Policy and Management
Bloomberg School of Public Health
Johns Hopkins University
Baltimore, Maryland

Mark Barnes, LLM, JD
Ropes and Gray LLP
Boston, Massachusetts

Anne Barnhill, PhD, MA
Research Scholar
Berman Institute of Bioethics
Johns Hopkins University
Baltimore, Maryland

Michele Barry, MD
Senior Associate Dean of Global Health
Director, Global Health Initiatives in Medicine
Director, Center for Innovation in Global Health
Stanford University
Stanford, California

Ruth Gaare Bernheim, JD, MPH
Chair, Department of Public Health Sciences
School of Medicine
Co-Director, Institute for Practical Ethics and Public Life
University of Virginia
Charlottesville, Virginia

Chris Beyrer, MD, MPH
Desmond M. Tutu Professor of Public Health and Human Rights
Director, Center for Health and Human Rights
Bloomberg School of Public Health
Johns Hopkins University
Baltimore, Maryland

Afsan Bhadelia, PhD, MS
Research Associate
Department of Global Health and Population
T.H. Chan School of Public Health
Harvard University
Boston, Massachusetts

David M. Bishai, MD, PhD, MPH
Professor
Department of Population, Family, and Reproductive Health
Bloomberg School of Public Health
Johns Hopkins University
Baltimore, Maryland

Danilo Blank, MD, PhD
Professor of Pediatrics
Faculty of Medicine
Universidade Federal do Rio Grande do Sul
Porto Alegre, Brazil

Gerald Bloom, MDCM
Research Fellow
Institute of Development Studies
Brighton, United Kingdom

Richard J. Bonnie, LLB
Harrison Foundation Professor of Law and Medicine
School of Law
Director, Institute of Law, Psychiatry, and Public Policy
University of Virginia
Charlottesville, Virginia

Jeffrey R. Botkin, MD, MPH
Professor of Pediatrics and Chief of the Division of Medical Ethics and Humanities
School of Medicine
University of Utah
Salt Lake City, Utah

Otis W. Brawley, MD
Chief Medical and Scientific Officer
American Cancer Society
Atlanta, Georgia

David R. Buchanan, PhD, MPH
Professor and Chair, Department of Health Promotion and Policy
School of Public Health and Health Sciences
University of Massachusetts
Amherst, Massachusetts

R. Jean Cadigan, PhD, MA
Associate Professor, Department of Social Medicine
University of North Carolina School of Medicine
Chapel Hill, North Carolina

Devin Alexander Cohen, JD
Ropes and Gray LLP
Boston, Massachusetts

James Colgrove, PhD, MPH
Professor, Department of Sociomedical Sciences
Mailman School of Public Health
Columbia University
New York, New York

Norman Daniels, PhD, MA
Mary B. Saltonstall Professor of Population Ethics
Emeritus Professor of Ethics and Population Health
Department of Global Health and Population
T.H. Chan School of Public Health
Harvard University
Boston, Massachusetts

Claire Davis, MA
Research Program Coordinator
Berman Institute of Bioethics
Johns Hopkins University
Baltimore, Maryland

Debra DeBruin, PhD
Maas Family Chair in Bioethics
Center for Bioethics
University of Minnesota
Minneapolis, Minnesota

Michael J. DiStefano, MBE
PhD student
Bloomberg School of Public Health and
Berman Institute of Bioethics
Johns Hopkins University
Baltimore, Maryland

Priya Duggal, PhD, MPH
Associate Professor
Department of International Health
Bloomberg School of Public Health
Johns Hopkins University
Baltimore, Maryland

James Dwyer, PhD
Professor
Center for Bioethics and Humanities
State University of New York Upstate Medical University
Syracuse, New York

Nicholas Evans, PhD, MS
Assistant Professor
College of Fine Arts, Humanities and Social Sciences
University of Massachusetts
Lowell, Massachusetts

Rachel E. Fabi, PhD
Assistant Professor
Department of Public Health and Preventive Medicine and
Center for Bioethics and Humanities
State University of New York
Upstate Medical University
Syracuse, New York

Ruth R. Faden, PhD, MPH
Philip Franklin Wagley Professor
Berman Institute of Bioethics
Johns Hopkins University
Baltimore, Maryland

Jessica Fanzo, PhD
Bloomberg Distinguished Associate Professor of Global Food & Agricultural Policy and Ethics
Nitze School of Advanced International Studies (SAIS) and
Berman Institute of Bioethics
Johns Hopkins University
Baltimore, Maryland

Mahmoud F. Fathalla, MD, PhD
Professor, Department of Obstetrics and Gynecology
Assiut University School of Medicine
Assiut, Egypt

Elizabeth Fenton, PhD, MPH
Lecturer, Bioethics Centre
University of Otago
Dunedin, New Zealand

Gail Geller, ScD, MHS
Professor
Department of Medicine, School of Medicine
Berman Institute of Bioethics
Johns Hopkins University
Baltimore, Maryland

Laura Greisman, MD
Assistant Professor of Clinical Medicine
Weill Cornell Medical College
Cornell University
New York, New York

Dan Hanfling, MD
Contributing Scholar
Center for Health Security
Bloomberg School of Public Health
Johns Hopkins University;
Clinical Professor
Department of Emergency Medicine
George Washington University
Washington, DC

Robert Hecht, PhD
Founder and President
Pharos Global Health Advisors
Boston, Massachusetts

Gail E. Henderson, PhD, MA
Professor
Department of Social Medicine
University of North Carolina School of Medicine
Chapel Hill, North Carolina

Leslie Meltzer Henry, JD, PhD
Professor
University of Maryland Francis King Carey School of Law;
Core Faculty
Johns Hopkins Berman Institute of Bioethics
Baltimore, Maryland

Adnan A. Hyder, MD, PhD, MPH
Senior Associate Dean for Research and Professor of Global Health
Milken Institute School of Public Health
George Washington University
Washington, DC

Myra F. Hyder, MS
IRB Analyst
Icahn School of Medicine at Mount Sinai
New York, New York

Thomas Inglesby, MD
Director and Professor
Center for Health Security
Bloomberg School of Public Health
School of Medicine
Johns Hopkins University
Baltimore, Maryland

Elana Jaffe, BA
Research Project Manager
Center for Bioethics
University of North Carolina School of Medicine
Chapel Hill, North Carolina

Monique Jonas, PhD
Professor
School of Population Health
University of Auckland
Auckland, New Zealand

Eric T. Juengst, PhD, MA
Director Center for Bioethics
Professor, Department of Social Medicine and Department of Genetics
University of North Carolina School of Medicine
Chapel Hill, North Carolina

Jeffrey P. Kahn, PhD, MPH
Andreas C. Dracopoulos Director and Levi Professor of Bioethics and Public Policy
Berman Institute of Bioethics and
Professor, Department of Health Policy and Management
Bloomberg School of Public Health
Johns Hopkins University
Baltimore, Maryland

Nancy E. Kass, ScD
Vice Provost, Graduate and Professional Education
Phoebe R. Berman Professor of Bioethics and Public Health
Berman Institute of Bioethics and Bloomberg School of Public Health
Johns Hopkins University
Baltimore, Maryland

Stacie P. Kershner, JD
Associate Director
Center for Law, Health & Society
College of Law
Georgia State University
Atlanta, Georgia

Barbara Koenig, PhD
Professor and Director
Program in Bioethics
University of California San Francisco
San Francisco, California

Carleigh Krubiner, PhD
Policy Fellow, Center for Global Development
Washington, DC;
Affiliate Faculty, Berman Institute of Bioethics
Johns Hopkins University
Baltimore, Maryland

Lisa M. Lee, PhD, MA, MS
Associate Vice President for Scholarly Integrity and Research Compliance
Research Professor, Department of Population Health Sciences
Virginia Polytechnic and State University
Blacksburg, Virginia

Jonathon P. Leider, PhD
Independent Consultant
JP Leider Research and Consulting, LLC
Minneapolis, Minnesota

Michelle Huckaby Lewis, MD, JD
Research Scholar
Berman Institute of Bioethics
Johns Hopkins University
Baltimore, Maryland

S. Matthew Liao, PhD
Arthur Zitrin Professor and Director
Center for Bioethics
New York University
New York, New York

Margaret Olivia Little, PhD, BPhil
Director and Senior Research Scholar
Kennedy Institute of Ethics
Professor of Philosophy
Georgetown University
Washington, DC

Tonya Littlejohn, MBBS
Affiliated Scholar, Center for Health and Human Rights
Bloomberg School of Public Health
Johns Hopkins University
Baltimore, Maryland

Paul Lombardo, JD, PhD, MA
Regents' Professor and Bobby Lee Cook Professor of Law
College of Law
Georgia State University
Atlanta, Georgia

Linda Long-Bellil, JD, PhD
Assistant Professor
Department of Family Medicine and Community Health
University of Massachusetts Medical School
Worcester, Massachusetts

Henry Lucas, MSc
Emeritus Research Fellow
Institute of Development Studies
Brighton, United Kingdom

Anne Drapkin Lyerly, MD, MA
Professor of Social Medicine and Associate Director
Center for Bioethics
University of North Carolina School of Medicine
Chapel Hill, North Carolina

Hayley MacGregor, MBChB, PhD, MPhil
Research Fellow
Institute of Development Studies
Brighton, United Kingdom

Cheryl C. Macpherson, PhD
Professor and Chair
Bioethics Department
St. George's University School of Medicine
Grenada, West Indies
Great River, New York

Lawrence Madoff, MD
Director
Division of Epidemiology and Immunization
Massachusetts Department of Public Health
Bureau of Infectious Disease and Laboratory Science
Jamaica Plain, Massachusetts

Anna C. Mastroianni, JD, MPH
Professor, School of Law
Associate Director, Institute for Public Health Genetics
University of Washington
Seattle, Washington

Debra J. H. Mathews, PhD, MA
Associate Professor
Department of Pediatrics
School of Medicine and
Berman Institute of Bioethics
Johns Hopkins University
Baltimore, Maryland

Karen M. Meagher, PhD
Postdoctoral Research Fellow
Center for Genomics and Society
Department of Social Medicine
University of North Carolina School of Medicine
Chapel Hill, North Carolina

Maria W. Merritt, PhD
Associate Professor
Department of International Health
Bloomberg School of Public Health and
Berman Institute of Bioethics
Johns Hopkins University
Baltimore, Maryland

Mark F. Miller, PhD, MBA, MS
Chief of Staff
National Institute of Environmental Health Sciences
Research Triangle Park, North Carolina

Monika Mitra, PhD, MA, MSc
Associate Professor
Lurie Institute for Disability Policy
Heller School for Social Policy and Management
Brandeis University
Waltham, Massachusetts

Margaret Moon, MD, MPH
Associate Professor
Department of Pediatrics
School of Medicine and
Berman Institute of Bioethics
Johns Hopkins University
Baltimore, Maryland

Stephanie Morain, PhD, MPH
Assistant Professor
Center for Medical Ethics and Health Policy
Baylor College of Medicine
Houston, Texas

Mary A. Ott, MD, MA
Professor
Department of Pediatrics
Indiana University School of Medicine
Indianapolis, Indiana

George W. Pariyo, PhD
Senior Scientist
Department of International Health
Bloomberg School of Public Health
Johns Hopkins University
Baltimore, Maryland

Omrana Pasha, MD, MSPH
Senior Scientist
Department of International Health
Bloomberg School of Public Health
Johns Hopkins University
Baltimore, Maryland

Govind Persad, JD, PhD
Assistant Professor
Sturm College of Law
University of Denver
Denver, Colorado

Tonia Poteat, PhD, MPH, MMSc
Assistant Professor
Department of Epidemiology
Bloomberg School of Public Health
Johns Hopkins University
Baltimore, Maryland

Robyn Powell, JD
Research Associate
Lurie Institute for Disability Policy
Heller School for Social Policy and Management
Brandeis University
Waltham, Massachusetts

Madison Powers, JD, MA, DPhil
Professor of Philosophy, Francis J. McNamara, Jr. Chair, and Senior Research Scholar
Kennedy Institute of Ethics
Georgetown University
Washington, District of Columbia

Bridget Pratt, PhD, MIH
Research Fellow
School of Population and Global Health
University of Melbourne
Melbourne, Victoria, Australia

Saumya RamaRao, PhD
Senior Associate
Population Council
New York, New York

David B. Resnik, JD, PhD
Bioethicist
National Institute of Environmental Health Sciences
Research Triangle Park, North Carolina

Yonaira M. Rivera, MPH
PhD candidate
Department of Health, Behavior and Society
Bloomberg School of Public Health
Johns Hopkins University
Baltimore, Maryland

Jennifer Prah Ruger, MA, MSc, PhD, MSL
Amartya Sen Professor of Health Equity, Economics, and Policy
School of Social Policy and Practice
University of Pennsylvania
Philadelphia, Pennsylvania

Brendan Saloner, PhD
Assistant Professor
Department of Health Policy and Management
Bloomberg School of Public Health and
Berman Institute of Bioethics
Johns Hopkins University
Baltimore, Maryland

John Santelli, MD, MPH
Professor
Department of Population and Family Health
Mailman School of Public Health
Columbia University
New York, New York

Ted Schrecker, MA
Professor
Institute of Health and Society
Newcastle University
Newcastle upon Tyne, England

Michael J. Selgelid, PhD
Professor of Bioethics and Director
Monash Bioethics Centre
Monash University
Melbourne, Australia

Sirine Shebaya, JD, PhD
Senior Staff Attorney
Muslim Advocates (affiliation listed for identification purposes only)
Washington, DC

Lois Shepherd, JD
Professor
Center for Biomedical Ethics and Humanities
School of Medicine
University of Virginia
Charlottesville, Virginia

Andrew W. Siegel, JD, PhD
Research Scholar
Berman Institute of Bioethics
Johns Hopkins University
Baltimore, Maryland

Diego S. Silva, PhD, MA
Assistant Professor
Faculty of Health Sciences
Simon Fraser University
Burnaby, British Columbia, Canada

Elise M. R. Smith, PhD
Postdoctoral Fellow
National Institute of Environmental Health Sciences
Research Triangle Park, North Carolina

Maxwell Smith, PhD, MSc
Assistant Professor
School of Health Studies
Western University
London, Ontario, Canada

Andrea Sutherland, MD, MSc, MPH
Director
Public Health Partnerships
Merck
Washington, DC

Holly A. Taylor, PhD, MPH
Associate Professor
Department of Health Policy and Management
Bloomberg School of Public Health and
Berman Institute of Bioethics
Johns Hopkins University
Baltimore, Maryland

Stephen B. Thomas, PhD, MS
Professor, Health Services Administration
Director, Maryland Center for Health Equity
University of Maryland School of Public Health
College Park, Maryland

John Townsend, PhD
Director of Country Strategy
Acting Senegal Country Director
Population Council
New York, New York

Ross Upshur, MD, MSc, MA
Professor and Division Head
Clinical Public Health
Dalla Lana School of Public Health
University of Toronto
Toronto, Ontario, Canada

Effy Vayena, PhD
Professor of Bioethics
Health Ethics and Policy Lab
Department of Health Sciences and Technology
Swiss Federal Institute of Technology
Zurich, Switzerland

Sridhar Venkatapuram, PhD, MPhil, MSc
Senior Lecturer in Global Health and Philosophy
Department of Global Health & Social Medicine
King's College London
London, United Kingdom

Kristin Voigt, DPhil
Assistant Professor
Institute for Health and Social Policy;
Department of Philosophy
McGill University
Montreal, Quebec, Canada

Leslie E. Wolf, JD, MPH
Distinguished University Professor of Law
Director, Center for Law, Health & Society
College of Law
Georgia State University
Atlanta, Georgia

Heather Zelle, PhD, JD, MS
Assistant Professor of Research
Department of Public Health Sciences
School of Medicine and
Institute of Law, Psychiatry, and Public Policy
University of Virginia
Charlottesville, Virginia

Public Health Ethics: An Introduction and Overview

Anna C. Mastroianni, Jeffrey P. Kahn, and Nancy E. Kass

Natural disasters and cholera outbreaks. Ebola, SARS, and concerns over pandemic flu. HIV and AIDS. *E. coli* outbreaks from contaminated produce and fast foods. Threats of bioterrorism. Contamination of compounded drugs. Vaccination refusals and outbreaks of preventable diseases. These are just some of the headlines from the last thirty-plus years highlighting the essential roles and responsibilities of public health, all of which come with ethical issues and the responsibilities they create.

Public health has achieved extraordinary successes. Life-threatening diseases that were once scourges—smallpox and diphtheria, for example—are either non-existent or far less prevalent (CDC, 1999), particularly in wealthier countries, and infant mortality rates are vastly lower in most parts of the world. Motor vehicles, workplaces, and the food supply are all considerably safer than they once were (Berkeley Wellness, 2017). And yet these successes also bring with them ethical tension. Not all public health successes are equally distributed in the population, and extraordinary health disparities between rich and poor still exist. The most successful public health programs sometimes rely on policies that, while improving public health conditions, also limit individual rights. Moreover, the work of public health is always challenged by inadequate resources, raising the question of how best to allocate limited resources.

Resources, financial and otherwise, may only be available to support programs that benefit a particular population or neighborhood, or that reflect a higher public health priority. Which community should receive an asthma prevention program? How should we weigh the interests of programs targeted to children against those targeted for older persons? Which health systems and what types of structures most equitably improve the public's health in low-income countries? Should public resources be dedicated to bioterrorism preparedness or obesity prevention programs? How should vaccines, antivirals, and other life-saving resources be allocated during a global pandemic? Public health practitioners and policymakers face these and other questions of ethics routinely in their work, and they must navigate their sometimes competing responsibilities to the health of the public with other important societal values, such as privacy, autonomy, and prevailing cultural norms.

Whereas medical ethics has a rich history dating back thousands of years, scholarly interest in public health ethics dates only to more recent decades (Kass, 2001; Childress et al., 2002). While overarching ethical commitments of public health are similar to those of medicine, the emphasis is quite different. Public health focuses its attention primarily on population and community health, often engaging in collective action or targeting societal conditions that contribute to better or worse health. This shift in emphasis inevitably leads public health to give moral priority to utility and to equity in ways that medical ethics need not.

A number of years ago, we realized that while there are volumes in the Oxford Handbook series devoted to a range of areas in bioethics, including the Handbooks of Bioethics, Clinical Research Ethics, Reproductive Ethics, Psychiatric Ethics, and Animal Ethics, none are devoted to public health ethics. The time has come. We are pleased to bring together a collection of some of the world's and countries' leaders in public health and ethics to put forward a handbook on a wide range of key issues in public health ethics today.

The 15 sections of the volume begin with 2 sections that discuss the conceptual foundations, ethical tensions, and ethical frameworks of and for public health and how public health does its work. The following 13 sections examine the application of public health ethics considerations and approaches across a broad scope of public health topics. While chapters are arranged into topical sections, each chapter is designed to serve as a stand-alone contribution. This approach makes the book, its sections, and individual chapters useful in a range of applications as part of course materials, or as a reference for students, scholars, and public health professionals.

For this volume, we recruited 11 section editors, primarily from among our talented colleagues at the Johns Hopkins Berman Institute of Bioethics. Together, we identified the most important and pressing topics to be covered in a comprehensive handbook and potential authors who could contribute their expertise to this effort, including leading scholars working in public health ethics and authorities working in relevant areas of public health. The section editors then recruited and worked with chapter authors to identify central issues and ethical challenges within distinct areas in our field. Authors were given substantial freedom in approach and were expected to share their perspectives on their assigned topics.

The resulting volume includes 73 chapters covering many topics from varying perspectives. We recognize that there may be some omitted areas—an acknowledgment of the breadth of activities and areas that define public health in the United States and globally, and the important diversity of ethics issues that occur within them. Indeed, we encourage others to contribute to what this project has begun.

References

Berkeley Wellness. 2017. "CDC: The Top 10 Public Health Achievements in the 20th Century." http://www.berkeleywellness.com/healthy-community/health-care-policy/article/cdcs-top-10-public-health-achievements-20th-century.

CDC (US Centers for Disease Control and Prevention). 1999. "Achievements in Public Health, 1900–1999 Impact of Vaccines Universally Recommended for Children—United States, 1990–1998." *Morbidity and Mortality Weekly Report* 48(12): 243–248.

Childress, J. F., Faden, R. R., Gaare, R. D., Gostin, L. O., Kahn, J., Bonnie, R. J., et al. 2002. "Public Health Ethics: Mapping the Terrain." *Journal of Law, Medicine and Ethics* 30(2): 170–178.

Kass, N. E. 2001. "An Ethics Framework for Public Health." *American Journal of Public Health* 91(11): 1776–1782. doi:10.2105/AJPH.91.11.1776.

PART ONE

FOUNDATIONS

SECTION ONE

CONCEPTUAL FOUNDATIONS, ETHICAL TENSIONS, AND ETHICAL FRAMEWORKS

CHAPTER 1

AN OVERVIEW OF CONCEPTUAL FOUNDATIONS, ETHICAL TENSIONS, AND ETHICAL FRAMEWORKS IN PUBLIC HEALTH

ANDREW W. SIEGEL AND MARIA W. MERRITT

Introduction

Public health is fundamentally concerned with promoting the health of populations through the prevention of disease and injury. It is, at its core, a moral endeavor, because the end it seeks is the advancement of human well-being. Health has intrinsic value inasmuch as it is partly constitutive of individual flourishing. It also has instrumental value in providing some of the conditions necessary for the proper functioning of populations. As Lawrence Gostin (2004, 511) notes, "Without minimum levels of health, people cannot engage in social interactions, participate in the political process, exercise rights of citizenship, generate wealth, create art, and provide for common security."

But while the pursuit of public health is motivated by the aspiration to improve human welfare, there are several different normative lenses through which we can understand the moral foundation of the public health enterprise. These alternative understandings of the foundational values of public health in turn bear on how we articulate and address the ethical challenges that arise in public health.

Consequentialism and Public Health

According to consequentialist ethical theories, the sole justification for an act is the state of affairs it brings about, and the right action or policy is the one that maximizes the particular good (e.g., pleasure, happiness, or welfare) that is sought. Consequentialism might appear to be well suited to public health, given that the goal of public health is to enhance the welfare of populations. And, indeed, the consequentialist perspective does inform some approaches to public health policy. For example, it underlies a cost-effectiveness approach to resource allocation that is embraced by many health economists, and it seeks to maximize the number of healthy life years in the population as a whole through a distribution of resources that results in the most "quality-adjusted life years" (QALYs).

A standard form of moral objection against consequentialism, however, is that a strict adherence to it would, in principle, permit acts that are reasonably considered to be violations of distributive justice and personal autonomy. With respect to concerns about distributive justice, consider the possible use of QALYs as the sole metric to guide health resource allocation, combined with a strictly consequentialist distributive principle of maximizing the number of QALYs gained. QALYs assign a quality-weighted value between 0 and 1 to each year of life under particular health conditions. If, for example, people would accept a 20 percent risk of death to be cured of blindness, one year of life with blindness would be worth 0.8. Allocations based on a strictly consequentialist objective of maximizing the number of QALYs gained would thus give priority to a program that saves the lives of ten sighted persons rather than ten blind persons. But while this distribution might produce the greater overall number of QALYs, there is good reason to consider it grossly unjust, on the grounds that each person's life has equal moral worth. As to concerns about personal autonomy, some examples of public health policies that a consequentialist outlook could warrant, but that many would deem violations of individual rights, include quarantine regulations that offer little due process in public health emergencies, policies that interfere with risky but voluntary and exclusively self-regarding lifestyle choices, and public health surveillance that invades people's privacy.

Deontology and Public Health

One way of overcoming the moral concerns associated with consequentialism is to recognize deontological constraints on the pursuit of a good. On deontological ethical theories, what makes an act right are the intrinsic features of the act rather than the state of affairs that it produces. On deontological approaches (sometimes called duty-based approaches), we have duties toward others (and ourselves) that prohibit certain acts regardless of the good consequences those acts may yield. These duties are often taken to include, among other things, acting in a manner that conforms to norms of fairness and that manifests respect for personal autonomy. Thus, a deontological approach to public health ethics would reject policies that violate obligations grounded in autonomy or distributive justice, even if those policies would maximize population health.

The most prominent frameworks for public health ethics incorporate both consequentialist and deontological considerations; that is, they recognize both that the general justification for the public health enterprise is to produce good health outcomes, and that the demands of justice and respect for individual liberty and privacy rights place limits on the kinds of public health policies that are permissible (Childress et al., 2002; Kass, 2001; Marckmann et al., 2015). These pluralist accounts of the foundational values of public health avoid standard moral objections against consequentialism but give rise to continuing challenges about what weight to attach to each of the values when they come into conflict.

Social Justice and Public Health

While public health ethics frameworks frequently appeal to justice as a principle that operates as a side constraint on the goal of maximizing good health outcomes, some theorists view justice as the moral foundation of public health. One such account posits that health is one of several "essential dimensions of well-being" (which also include respect, self-determination, attachment, personal security, and reasoning) that justice aims to secure (Powers and Faden, 2008). On this view, justice requires that everyone have a sufficient amount of each of the essential dimensions of well-being. This entails both that public health is a direct requirement of justice and that particular attention be given to the most disadvantaged members of society.

Human Rights and Public Health

Human rights comprise, in concept, a high-priority set of moral claims said to be universally held by all people (Nickel, 2017). International documents such as the Universal Declaration of Human Rights (1948) and the International Covenant on Economic, Social and Cultural Rights (1966) recognize a human right to health. Other internationally recognized human rights are focused on societal goods that are determinants of health, such as personal security and education. Advocates for human rights to health and to the determinants of health characterize such rights as morally foundational to public health (Gruskin and Dickens, 2006; Mann, 1997). Moreover, some human rights, such as the right to freedom from discrimination recognized in the Universal Declaration of Human Rights and related documents, can be framed as moral constraints on public health activities (Mann et al., 1994).

The normative accounts outlined above represent some of the major approaches to understanding the moral foundations of public health ethics. Other accounts appeal to, among other things, civic virtue and the promotion of the common good (Jennings, 2007), an ethics of care (Roberts and Reich, 2002), and obligations grounded in a conception of persons as interrelated social beings (Kenny, Sherwin, and Baylis, 2010).

Whatever position one adopts about the moral foundations of public health, many questions remain regarding the specification and application of its foundational values. What are the boundaries of the population whose health we should promote? What principles of distributive justice should govern resource allocation and prioritization? Under what conditions are public health measures that interfere with liberty justified? What is the basis for asserting a human right to health, and what demands does such a right make on public health institutions, policies, and practices? This section of *The Oxford Handbook of Public Health Ethics* explores these and related issues through four chapters, introduced below.

Chapter Overviews

In "Public Health Programs and Policies: Ethical Justifications Distinctive Challenges of Public Health Ethics," Ruth R. Faden, Sirine Shebaya, and Andrew W. Siegel provide an overview of the challenges of public health ethics. They begin by identifying four distinctive characteristics of public health: (1) its focus on the health of populations rather than individuals; (2) its particular commitment to the prevention of disease and injury, rather than with their diagnosis and treatment; (3) its intrinsic orientation toward outcomes; and (4) its reliance on government action for its promotion.

The authors describe how each of these features of public health gives rise to important ethical issues. First, the focus on populations raises issues about the object of public health, especially the question of how broadly we understand the population that public health serves. Often, the relevant "public" is understood in terms of the population of a particular nation-state. But Faden, Shebaya, and Siegel note that this may be problematic, both because diseases cross borders and because there may be moral obligations to promote health that transcend the boundaries of nation-states. Second, the public health focus on prevention raises issues about how future health gains should be weighed against current health gains. Third, the orientation toward outcomes prompts some of the questions about the moral foundations of public health ethics discussed above in the section on "Human Rights and Public Health"—in particular, whether the general justification for public health is consequentialist, or whether we pursue good public health outcomes to fulfill the demands of social justice. Finally, the reliance on government action supported by the force of law raises questions about the justification for the use of state coercion to advance public health, especially where it involves measures that interfere with individual liberty.

In "Public Health Programs and Policies: Ethical Justifications," Faden and Shebaya examine the kinds of moral justification that may be marshaled in support of specific public health interventions. They identify five such justifications:

1. The overall benefit a public health measure produces.
2. The collective efficiency an intervention provides by coordinating action to ensure population-wide compliance.
3. Fairness in the distribution of the burdens of disease and disability.
4. The "harm principle," according to which the only justification for limiting a person's liberty is the prevention of harm to other persons.
5. Paternalism, which is the thesis that a restriction on individual liberty is acceptable if it is necessary to prevent harm or produce a benefit to the agent involved.

The first three justifications concern the justification of public health policies that do not directly benefit all members of the population, while the last two concern the justification of public health measures that interfere with individual liberty. Faden and Shebaya note that there will often be more than one justification of a policy, and they critique frameworks that place a disproportionate emphasis on the liberty-limiting aspects of policies.

These two chapters examine in detail concepts of central moral importance for public health ethics: justice and human rights. As noted above, considerations of both justice and human rights may operate as either side constraints or as moral foundations in frameworks of public health ethics.

In "Justice and Public Health," Govind Persad maps the landscape of justice as applied to public health. He first describes three prominent metrics regarding what to measure in assessing the justice of states of affairs and policy choices; he then describes seven distinct principles regarding who gets what under just distributions of what is measured. The chapter illustrates the overarching point that any metric may be combined with any distributive principle. The example of QALY-oriented strict consequentialism sketched above in the section on "Consequentialism and Public Health" combines a species of "welfarist" metric—purporting to quantify and compare how people experience various health states–with the distributive principle of maximization. By contrast, Powers and Faden's (2008) theory combines a metric of well-being achieved in multiple core dimensions (health being one) with a "sufficientarian" distributive principle aiming for universal achievement of well-being above a certain threshold in all dimensions. Persad also discusses the intersection of justice with individual rights; the geographical, temporal, and biological scope of justice; whether justice applies to individual as well as institutional choices; and strategies for resolving disagreements about justice.

In "Human Rights and Public Health Ethics," S. Matthew Liao offers an account of what human rights are, how they can be morally justified, and how they correspond to moral obligations in public health practice and policymaking, with special attention to the idea of a human right to health. Liao's chapter outlines the "fundamental conditions approach," which holds that "human rights protect the fundamental conditions for pursuing a good life. The fundamental conditions comprise various goods, capacities, and options that human beings qua human beings need, whatever else they might need, in order to pursue certain basic activities" (Liao, this volume). The chapter uses the fundamental conditions approach (Liao, 2015) to develop a conception of "basic health" as the object of the human right to health (which also entails rights to "adequate nutrition, basic health care, and basic education"), and argues that corresponding duties to support effective public health measures are held by everyone, not only governments.

Conclusion

The field of public health ethics has plural foundations in major normative ethical theories, principally consequentialism and deontology, and in ethical concepts such as social justice and human rights. This overview provides some basic background on ethical theory and introduces chapters in the related section of *The Oxford Handbook of Public Health Ethics*. Those chapters together elucidate the moral foundations of public health ethics that are essential in any approach to ethical issues arising in the diversity of public health topic areas.

References

Childress, J. F., Faden, R. R., Gaare, R. D., Gostin, L. O., Kahn, J., Bonnie, R. J., et al. 2002. "Public Health Ethics: Mapping the Terrain." *Journal of Law, Medicine & Ethics* 30(2): 170–178.

Gostin, L. O. 2004. "Health of the People: The Highest Law?" *Journal of Law, Medicine & Ethics* 32(3): 509–515.

Gruskin, S., and Dickens, B. 2006. *Human Rights and Ethics in Public Health* (Washington, D.C.: American Public Health Association).

Jennings, B. 2007. "Public Health and Civic Republicanism: Toward an Alternative Framework for Public Health Ethics." In *Ethics, Prevention, and Public Health*, edited by A. Dawson and M. Verweij, 30–58 (New York: Oxford University Press).

Kass, N. E. 2001. "An Ethics Framework for Public Health." *American Journal of Public Health* 91(11): 1776–1782.

Kenny, N. P., Sherwin, S. B., and Baylis, F. E. 2010. "Re-Visioning Public Health Ethics: A Relational Perspective." *Canadian Journal of Public Health/Revue Canadienne de Santé Publique* 101(1): 9–11.

Liao, S. M. 2015. "Human Rights as Fundamental Conditions for a Good Life." In *Philosophical Foundations of Human Rights*, edited by R. Cruft, S. M. Liao, and M. Renzo, 79–100 (Oxford: Oxford University Press).

Mann, J. 1997. "Medicine and Public Health, Ethics and Human Rights." *Hastings Center Report* 27(3): 6–13.

Mann, J., Gostin, L., Gruskin, S., Brennan, T., Lazzarini, Z., and Fineberg, H. V. 1994. "Health and Human Rights." *Health and Human Rights* 1(1): 6–24.

Marckmann, G., Schmidt, H., Sofaer, N., and Strech, D. 2015. "Putting Public Health Ethics into Practice: A Systematic Framework." *Frontiers in Public Health* 3(23). https://www.frontiersin.org/articles/10.3389/fpubh.2015.00023/full.

Nickel, J. 2017. "Human Rights." In *The Stanford Encyclopedia of Philosophy*, edited by E. N. Zalta (Stanford, Calif.: Stanford University). https://plato.stanford.edu/entries/rights-human/.

Powers, M., and Faden, R. 2008. *Social Justice: The Moral Foundations of Public Health and Health Policy* (Oxford: Oxford University Press).

Roberts, M. J., and Reich, M. R. 2002. "Ethical Analysis in Public Health." *The Lancet* 359(9311): 1055–1059.

CHAPTER 2

DISTINCTIVE CHALLENGES OF PUBLIC HEALTH ETHICS

RUTH R. FADEN, SIRINE SHEBAYA, AND ANDREW W. SIEGEL

Introduction

There is no standard way of organizing the ethics of public health, clinical practice, and biomedical science. These distinctive fields are often presented as focal areas that fall under the broader umbrella term *bioethics*, but sometimes bioethics is presented as the equivalent of medical ethics, or in contrast to public health and population-level bioethics. Whichever approach is preferred, a key question remains: What distinguishes public health ethics from the ethics of clinical practice or the ethics of biomedical science? The answer lies in the distinctive nature of public health. Public health has four characteristics that provide much of the subject matter for public health ethics: (1) it is a public or collective good, (2) its promotion involves a particular focus on prevention, (3) its promotion often entails government action, and (4) it involves an intrinsic outcome orientation. This chapter offers an overview of these characteristics of public health in order to identify the distinctive challenges of public health ethics. It then examines some broader conceptual questions that bear on these challenges.

The Four Characteristics of Public Health and Their Related Ethical Challenges

The first characteristic of public health is that the object of concern in public health is populations, not individuals. Public health is, by its very nature, a public, communal good, where the benefits to one person cannot readily be individuated from those to another, though its burdens and benefits often appear to fall unevenly on different subgroups of the population. This raises a particular set of justificatory challenges that public health ethics has to address: Who is public health good for? Whose health are we concerned with, and what sacrifices is it acceptable to ask of individuals in order to achieve it? Is there a difference between public health and population health? And why is public health a good worth promoting? Any answer to these questions has to take account of the fact that public health measures are often based on *prospective* benefits, not immediately securable benefits.

Second, promoting public health involves a high degree of commitment to the prevention of disease and injury. However, although much of the discussion surrounding public health focuses primarily on this preventive aspect, public health agencies and services also engage in diagnosing and treating illnesses, with all the attendant clinical services that these activities require. Indeed, national health systems are increasingly understood to encompass both preventive functions and the delivery of personal medical services. Often, these functions and services are integrated under a common political or administrative structure. Depending on the specific context in which population health is to be improved, separating public health services and functions from personal medical care services and functions may or may not make sense. That said, policies and programs whose aim is to prevent illness and injury are paradigmatically the territory of public health. Certainly no other social institution is generally recognized as so clearly having this remit.

Public health's commitment to prevention carries with it particular moral challenges. Eliminating or mitigating a harm that already exists is sometimes viewed as being of greater moral importance—or simply as more immediately motivating action—than long-term strategies to prevent a harm from materializing. Although in recent years there has arguably been more emphasis on prevention in health policy, preventive public health interventions continue to receive less funding and public support than medical treatments. For example, despite the increasing focus on wellness in public policy and the workplace, both policymakers and the public still tend to place a higher priority on ensuring that heart patients have access to surgery and medications than on programs to prevent heart disease through diet and exercise. Another factor that can result in prioritizing cures over prevention is that although the costs and burdens of preventive interventions occur largely in the present, the benefits of successful preventive interventions often occur in the future, and usually only to some members of the population, whose identities cannot be predicted in advance and whose numbers can only be estimated probabilistically. Thus, prevention policies and programs raise questions about how we should think about statistical and unidentified lives and persons, and whether health gains in the future should be treated as worth less than health gains in the present. In some cases, the beneficiaries of preventive interventions are members of future generations, complicating the moral picture even further.

Third, achieving good public health results frequently requires government action backed by the force of law. In the United States, the Centers for Disease Control and Prevention (CDC), the Food and Drug Administration (FDA), and the Environmental Protection Agency (EPA) are in part or in whole public health agencies. All nations, and most states or provinces and municipalities, have health departments whose functions include everything from the inspection of commercial food service to the collection and use of epidemiological data for population surveillance of disease. Public health is focused on regulation and public policy, relying less often on individual actions and services. In this, as in all other areas of official state action, we therefore have to address tensions among justice, security, and the scope of legal restrictions and regulations. This is particularly so where the state exercises its coercive powers to advance public health through measures that curtail individual liberties or seek to promote behavioral changes. The role of government power adds to the peculiarity of the justificatory questions surrounding public health, as the exercise of public authority and the imposition of public sanctions and penalties in an area as deeply personal as an individual's health choices require strong justification. Thus, the same questions of a trade-off between personal freedom and collective action that arise in the political arena generally also arise in the public health arena. It is in this context that concerns about paternalism typically emerge.

Fourth, public health has an intrinsic outcome orientation. Promoting public health means seeking to avoid bad health outcomes and to advance good ones. In some discussions of public health ethics, this outcome orientation is viewed as the moral justification and foundation of public health, and, as with many consequentialist schemes, it is presented as needing to be constrained by attention to deontological concerns such as rights and justice-related concerns such as the fair distribution of burdens (Childress et al., 2002; Kass, 2001). This view of public health ethics regards the moral foundation of public health as an injunction to maximize welfare, and therefore regards health as a component of welfare (Powers and Faden, 2006). It frames the core moral challenge of public health as balancing individual liberties with the advancement of good health outcomes. Consider, for example, how liberties are treated in government policies to fluoridate municipal drinking water or compel people with active, infectious tuberculosis to be treated.

An alternative view of public health ethics characterizes the moral foundation of public health as social justice. While balancing individuals' liberties with promoting social goods is one area of concern, it is embedded within a broader commitment to secure a sufficient level of health for all and to narrow unjust inequalities (Powers and Faden, 2006). Thus, another important area of concern is the balancing of this commitment with the injunction to maximize good aggregate or collective health outcomes. Understood this way, public health ethics has deep moral connections to broader questions of social justice, poverty, and systematic disadvantage.

These four distinctive features provide public health ethics with its basic structure and orientation. While each of the four features gives rise its own set of ethical issues, there are some broader conceptual and moral challenges that bear on how the ethical issues described above are addressed. One challenge—related in particular to the first characteristic of public health, but that ramifies across the others—concerns the scope of public health: Whose health does public health seek to protect and promote? Another challenge concerns the boundaries of public health: how broadly or narrowly should we understand what public health entails? These challenges are addressed in turn below.

The Scope of Public Health

An important question arises with regard to the scope of public health: Who is the "public?" The usual assumption is that the public is a discrete unit that corresponds with state boundaries: a single country's population. But in the realm of health, this assumption does not always apply. Communicable diseases have a way of ignoring national boundaries, and preventive measures in one country may be futile if other countries do not follow suit. Moreover, the statist focus is not always readily justifiable: So far as diseases cross borders, should public health interventions do the same? Further questions about justice and equity across borders also arise. For example, do wealthier countries and wealthier individuals have obligations to attend to the public health of less fortunate others?

Depending on the particular health challenge involved, the public in question can be more local or more global than a single country's population. National boundaries are relevant because policies and regulations are usually set by individual countries, and they vary from country to country. They are also relevant for reasons having to do with government control. Countries report their data about communicable disease outbreaks, burden of disease, and other health indicators to global institutions such as the World Health Organization (WHO) on a voluntary basis. Although the International Health Regulations (IHR) to which 196 countries are signatories (WHO, 2018) provide an international structure for global public health, as with much international law and regulation, enforcement mechanisms are weak.

It is not clear what the moral implications of these practical limitations should be for public health. The structure of the problem is similar to environmental challenges such as air pollution and climate change. Determinants of ill health are not restricted by national boundaries, and we are all ultimately connected to each other's health status, at least in some ways. But more importantly, citizens in the developed world are arguably causally connected to some health deprivations in the developing world, for example by upholding restrictions on the production and distribution of generic medications that hinder the containment of easily treatable diseases in resource-poor countries (Pogge, 2002; Grover et al., 2012). This puts public health, and therefore public health ethics, in a special and very interesting position vis-à-vis discussions of global justice, our duties to the distant poor, and the need for global cooperation to address common problems (Holland, 2007).

Another issue that comes up in this connection is whether "public" and "population" are interchangeable terms to designate the entity whose health we are concerned with. Is there a significant conceptual difference, a difference in moral valence, or a difference in attitude and orientation between public health ethics, on the one hand, and population-level health ethics, on the other? The literature presents three general ways of denoting the object of public health: community, the public, and populations. In one sense, the most morally laden manner of designating those who are subject to, and benefit from, public health measures is to think about them as a community (Beauchamp and Steinbock, 1999). Reference to "community" implies a cohesive group, usually with a shared language, culture, history, and geographical location. Characterizing the concern of public health as being the health of the community renders the appeal to the common good as a way of justifying public health interventions more natural (and possibly more plausible).

Reference to "the public" shares some of these same features but tends to be less morally laden. This is in part because "the public" is somewhat more anonymous than "the community" and does not necessarily signal a tight cultural connection. Rather, it connotes a relatively discrete unit with some common institutions and usually a shared political life. Thus, references to the public as well as to the community may encourage the perception that the good we are seeking to advance is that of a geographically bounded unit, with "community" connoting stronger cultural associations, and "public" connoting some kind of official political unit such as a state or a country.

Characterizing the health we are trying to advance as that of populations, by contrast, may minimize the implication that special shared features or characteristics are needed in order for a group of individuals to constitute a collective unit whose health can be of concern. Because of this, it may lend itself more readily to an internationalist, less inward-looking orientation. That is, any population, regardless of nationality or geographic location, has health interests that ought to be attended to and advanced (Wikler and Brock, 2007). Populations can be more local or more global than a community or the public. This way of speaking may also dilute the emphasis on national borders as a way of delineating the scope of concern, and provides more flexibility in the object of concern for public health. In much the same way, discussion of global health, as opposed to international health, is seen as helpful in emphasizing a focus on the health needs of all, as opposed to a focus on international cooperation and the health needs of peoples in countries other than one's own.

This is not to say, of course, that those who prefer the term "public health" to "population health" do not share a global orientation. Indeed, the WHO is generally referred to as a global public health institution, and those who work to promote health transnationally are referred to as public health and not population health professionals. Indeed, although some see a substantive conceptual divergence in ways of thinking about whose health is to be protected and promoted, others see no conflict, at least between the concepts of public health and population health. For example, the Nuffield Council on Bioethics (2007, xv) uses the term "population health" to refer to the collective state of health of members of a population, and "public health" to refer to efforts made to improve the political, regulatory, and economic environments that affect prospects for health. Thus understood, the object of public health is the improvement of population health.

A related challenge central to public health ethics is how to think about public health or population health as a public good. Is the health of the public or of a population a good in its own right, or can it meaningfully be understood only as an aggregation of the welfare interests secured for each individual within that population? Is public health a good that nations and global institutions can rightly seek with the same justificatory structures and limitations with which they seek national security and world peace, or is it somehow a more limited or different kind of political construct?

The Boundaries of Public Health

Given a widening understanding of health and the factors affecting prospects for population health, public health can be viewed as being so expansive as to have no meaningful institutional, disciplinary, or social boundaries. Everything from crime, war, and natural disasters; to population genetics, environmental hazards, marketing, and other corporate practices; to political oppression, income inequality, and individual behavior has been claimed under the rubric of public health. Part of what makes each of these diverse things of concern is their impact on health, and in that sense they are all public health problems. A central role of public health, grounded in social justice, is to bring attention to all aspects of the social or natural world that exert a significant impact on the preservation or promotion of health, and not only to those that can be addressed through traditional public health measures or means.

At the same time, however, health is only one dimension of human well-being. Calling attention to the devastating impact of Taliban rule on the health of women is important, but it should not be confused with reducing the injustices of the oppression of women to its health effects. The assault of such oppression on personal security, self-determination, and respect is of independent moral concern. Similarly, while reducing violence is critical to population health, that does not mean that law enforcement, the criminal justice system, diplomacy, and international relations should be considered tools of public health. Whether and under what conditions it is advantageous to frame or reframe a social problem in public health terms is morally complex. For example, taking a public health rather than criminal justice orientation to gun violence or drug abuse can sometimes contribute to defusing tensions, decreasing negative impacts on racial or other minority groups, and improving overall outcomes (Dorfman and Wallack, 2009).

Because so many of the determinants of the different dimensions of well-being overlap and reinforce one another, it is not surprising that different social institutions and professional communities share common concerns and priorities, nor should it be expected that public policies rest on only one moral consideration such as health or security.

The flip side of this observation is that public health has an obligation to evaluate the impact of its policies and practices on human well-being broadly, and not only on health. Guaranteed access to basic health services can improve health, but, just as importantly, it can also provide people with a sense of social worth and eliminate the insecurity of being unable to provide for loved ones in times of crisis. Similarly, screening programs for sexually transmitted infections may improve health, but, depending on the features of the programs and the contexts in which they are implemented, they may also result in social disrespect, decreased personal security, and unduly burdensome constraints on personal behavior.

The overlapping of effects and justifications is particularly clear in prevention. Immunization, water fluoridation, anti-smoking campaigns, and motorcycle helmet laws are all paradigmatic preventive public health interventions. At the same time, however, interventions that are generally outside the purview of public health institutions and professionals, such as early childhood education, income supports, literacy initiatives for girls, and safe housing programs, can all be effective in preventing illness and injury. In some cases, such interventions may be more effective and efficient in achieving health gains than paradigmatic public health programs. Morally responsible public health policy requires attentiveness to the multiple determinants of health. This requirement does not signal that public health has no boundaries. Rather, public health has a unique relationship of stewardship to one dimension of well-being—health—and to the particular determinants that have a special strategic significance for health. Some of those determinants are the classic focus of public health, such as infectious disease control and the securing of safe food, water, and essential medications. However, exercising that stewardship requires responsiveness to the best available evidence about all the determinants, across the landscape of an interconnected social structure, that have a special strategic relation to health, including those outside the conventional remits of public health agencies and authorities. Policies governing education, foreign assistance, agriculture, and the environment can all have a significant impact on health, just as health policies can have an impact on international relations and national and global economies. Providing public health arguments in defense of particular environmental or educational policies, and recognizing that such policies can have profound effects on health, simply recognizes the complex interweaving of the multiple dimensions of human welfare.

One worry raised by this interconnectedness across spheres of social life and policy is that classifying something as a public health matter could be an effective way of taking it out of the realm of legitimate discussion. If the goal of protecting health is seen as clearly good, then government actions aimed at securing health may be less scrutinized than actions aimed at more controversial ends, leaving public health officials with too much power and too little democratic accountability. As a practical matter, however, these concerns may not be realistic. Although data on this point are hard to come by, it is likely that the reverse is true, that public health agencies and workers are more likely to have insufficient political power, authority, and resources at their disposal to achieve important and pressing goals than to wield too much. It is not usually individuals' civil rights to which public health interventions stand in opposition, but rather private, corporate economic interests such as the tobacco industry, the meat and dairy industries, and so on. Nonetheless, it is worth raising these worries, at least to keep them in view as a possible issue for public health ethics to address.

Even if the worry that expanding the classification of something as a public health matter in some way threatens civil liberties is nothing more than fearmongering, the breadth of what falls under the purview of public health may raise concerns about democratic legitimacy. Insofar as health authorities have a public mandate to advance health, is it therefore appropriate for them to hew to strict guidelines as to what they can undertake in the name of public health, based, at least in part, on the expressed or revealed preferences or values of those within their reach? Under what conditions are measures such as public health surveillance and the banning of certain food materials properly considered to be overreaching by public health authorities, and therefore to constitute a lack of adherence to their democratically given mandate? Public health ethics has to give serious consideration to the question of how exactly the mandate of public health authorities should be specified such that they do not run afoul of the requirements of legitimacy in a democratic political system.

Particularly when government institutions are charged with promoting population health, one task of public health ethics is determining self-imposed limitations and restrictions on what can reasonably come under the auspices of public health authorities. Concerns about individual liberty, about privacy and paternalism, about democratic process, and about the place of health in relation to other aspects of human well-being all come into play here. Thus, public health ethics also has to engage more traditional philosophical questions about the scope of privacy, the reach of public policy, and the limits and legitimacy of government intervention for the public good. Moreover, scarcity and priority-setting always loom large in the context of public health, giving rise to a number of equity, justice, and fairness concerns. As already noted, these issues are especially acute with regard to global health.

Conclusion

Public health is (1) a collective good, (2) focused especially on prevention, (3) reliant on government action supported by the force of law, and (4) intrinsically outcome-oriented. These characteristics of public health give rise to a wide range of ethical issues, such as the balancing of future health gains against current ones, the justification for the state's use of coercive powers to advance health, and the moral foundation of public health. In addition, how many of these issues are framed will depend on how we understand who it is that public health protects and the boundaries of what public health addresses. Together, these moral and conceptual questions form the distinctive challenges of public health ethics.

Acknowledgments

This chapter is in part adapted from "Public Health Ethics" (Faden and Shebaya, 2016).

References

Beauchamp, D. E., and Steinbock, B., eds. 1999. *New Ethics for the Public's Health* (New York: Oxford University Press).

Childress, J. F., Faden, R. R., Gaare, R. D., Gostin, L. O., Kahn, J., Bonnie, et al. 2002. "Public Health Ethics: Mapping the Terrain." *Journal of Law, Medicine and Ethics* 30(2): 170–178.

Dorfman, L., and Wallack, L. 2009. *Moving from Them to Us: Challenges in Reframing Violence among Youth* (Oakland, Calif.: Prevention Institute). https://www.preventioninstitute.org/publications/moving-from-them-to-us-challenges-in-reframing-violence-among-youth.

Faden, R., and Shebaya, S. 2016. "Public Health Ethics." In *The Stanford Encyclopedia of Philosophy*, edited by E. N. Zalta (Stanford, Calif.:, Stanford University). https://plato.stanford.edu/archives/win2016/entries/publichealth-ethics/.

Grover, A., Citro, B., Mankad, M., and Lander, F. 2012. "Pharmaceutical Companies and Global Lack of Access to Medicines: Strengthening Accountability under the Right to Health." *Journal of Law, Medicine, and Ethics* 40(2): 234–250. doi:10.1111/j.1748-720X.2012.00661.x.

Holland, S. 2007. *Public Health Ethics* (Cambridge: Polity Press).

Kass, N. E. 2001. "An Ethics Framework for Public Health." *American Journal of Public Health* 91(11): 1776–1782. doi:10.2105/AJPH.91.11.1776.

Nuffield Council on Bioethics. 2007. *Public Health: Ethical Issues* (London: Nuffield Council on Bioethics). http://nuffieldbioethics.org/wp-content/uploads/2014/07/Public-health-ethical-issues.pdf.

Pogge, T. W. 2002. "Responsibilities for Poverty-Related Ill Health." *Ethics and International Affairs* 16(2): 71–79. doi:10.1111/j.1747–7093.2002.tb00398.x.

Powers, M., and Faden, R. R. 2006. *Social Justice: The Moral Foundations of Public Health and Health Policy* (New York: Oxford University Press).

Wikler, D., and Brock, D. W. 2007. "Population-Level Bioethics: Mapping a New Agenda." In *Ethics, Prevention, and Public Health*, edited by A. Dawson and M. Verweij, 78–94 (Oxford: Clarendon Press).

WHO (World Health Organization). 2018. "International Health Regulations (IHR)." http://www.who.int/topics/international_health_regulations/en/.

CHAPTER 3

PUBLIC HEALTH PROGRAMS AND POLICIES: ETHICAL JUSTIFICATIONS

RUTH R. FADEN AND SIRINE SHEBAYA

Introduction

Public health as a social institution draws its foundational moral legitimacy from the essential and direct role that health plays in human flourishing, whether that role is ultimately understood in terms of maximizing health or of promoting health in order to advance a broad conception of social justice. As powerful as this general justification is, however, it is often too broad to provide sufficient moral warrant for specific public health policies and programs. In this chapter, we put forward five justifications for public health interventions, each of which speaks to a different set of reasons why any particular policy or program might be ethically appropriate: (1) overall benefit, (2) collective action and efficiency, (3) fairness in the distribution of burdens, (4) prevention of harm (the harm principle), and (5) paternalism.

Two observations are worth making at the outset. First, public health policies are rarely defended by only one justification. Usually a mixed set of justifications can plausibly be provided. For example, tax policies intended to decrease cigarette consumption can be defended both by appeal to paternalism and by appeal to reducing the harms of second-hand smoke to children in the home and in automobiles. Second, the impact of a public health policy is often not uniform across all the individuals affected by the policy, and thus different justifications are sometimes put forward specific to these different people. This complexity is unavoidable, since it results from the nature of public health. The focus of public health is population health, but populations are rarely internally uniform with regard to all features that are morally relevant to any particular policy. Some people may stand to benefit from the policy, while others may not. Moreover, in line with concerns about democratic legitimacy and state overreaching, some members of the population may support the policy, while others may object. Consider, for example, a New York City policy prohibiting restaurants from serving sugar-sweetened beverages in containers holding over sixteen ounces, which was eventually struck down by the courts. Public opinion polling suggests that while more New Yorkers opposed the policy than supported it, the level of opposition varied from one borough of the city to another (Grynbaum and Connelly, 2012).

The first three justifications for public health policies—overall benefit, collective action and efficiency, and fairness—speak specifically to the context in which some members of the affected population do not directly benefit from a policy or object to it. The next two justifications appeal to the significance of harm, both to others and to oneself. They apply more specifically to traditional concerns about balancing respect for liberty with advancing health, and are more prevalent in the public health ethics literature than the previous three. In the fourth justification, the argument is from a relatively uncontroversial Millian harm principle (Mill and Gray, 1998), while the fifth justification is from somewhat more tendentious paternalistic principles.

Depending on the specifics of a public health policy, any number of these justifications may be applicable, and they are generally used to best effect in combination. The chapter closes with a look at the limits of frameworks that focus disproportionately on liberty considerations and at the importance of considering the range of possible moral justifications in analyzing public health policies.

Overall Benefit

Ultimately, all people benefit from public health interventions, and from having trusted regulatory agencies such as the US Centers for Disease Control and Prevention (CDC) or the Food and Drug Administration (FDA) make decisions about such interventions and their reach. All things considered, having public health regulation is better than not having it. Public health decisions made on the basis of overall statistics and demographic trends are ultimately better for each one of us, even if particular interventions may not directly benefit some of us. Thus, the task of public health ethics is not necessarily to justify each particular intervention directly. Rather, public health interventions in general, as long as they stay within certain pre-established parameters, can be justified in the same way a market economy, the institution of private property, or other similarly broad and useful conventions that involve some coercive action but also enable individuals to access greater benefits can be justified: when properly regulated and managed, their existence is by and large better than their absence for everyone.

So structured, the justification for particular public health interventions, requirements, or restrictions is derivative of or parasitic on a higher-level justification. This argumentative strategy has a lot of appeal, particularly as a way of justifying the existence of regulatory government agencies such as the FDA or CDC. However, it is ultimately insufficient on its own and needs to be supplemented by other kinds of ethical arguments, since it does not provide a basis for the parameters themselves, or for ethical oversight or scrutiny with regard to the particular decisions such agencies take. This is similar to the case of the free market, in which it is by and large preferable to have free markets than to not have them, but this does not render specific aspects of the operations of markets immune to criticism and reform from an ethical point of view.

Collective Action and Efficiency

A related justification views health as a public good, the pursuit of which is not possible without ground rules for coordinated action and near-universal participation. Thus, public health is viewed as having the structure of a coordination or collective efficiency problem. If one person (or at least, a sufficient number of such persons) decides to go when the traffic light is red and stop when the traffic light is green, it does not matter that everyone else is following the rules: this person will disrupt the smooth functioning of the system, with potentially dangerous results. Similarly, if one person (or a sufficient critical mass of such persons) decides not to abide by a public health regulation because the regulation does not directly benefit that person, or because the person otherwise objects, the ramifications will likely be felt by others in her or his environment and beyond. A classic example is when an outbreak of measles can be traced to the intentional undervaccination of children by their parents (Omer et al., 2009; Sugerman et al., 2010; Thompson et al., 2007). Everybody has to participate because, failing their involvement, neither they nor anyone else can reap the benefit of a healthy society.

In many public health contexts, the only feasible or acceptably efficient way to implement a policy affects the entire population, leaving no option, or only very burdensome options, open to individual noncooperation. Perhaps the most celebrated such example is water fluoridation, but all safety regulations affecting the food and drug supply and consumer products share this character, as do many environmental and occupational health standards. Here, collective efficiency considerations loom large. Although people want healthy environments and products, individuals are simply not positioned to make independent decisions about the impact on health and safety of their environment and of the hundreds of thousands of products available in the modern marketplace. Ceding this function to government institutions staffed with health experts is prudent and essential to the general welfare and social justice in the same respect as ceding protection of our interests in personal physical security to government institutions staffed with law enforcement and national defense experts is prudent and essential to the general welfare (Mill and Gray, 1998).

Collective efficiency arguments rely on claims about the sheer number and technical complexity of the decisions that need to be made to protect health in the environment and in the marketplace, as well as the indivisible character of responses to some health threats. These arguments are buttressed by claims about the cognitive limitations and bounded rationality of individual human decision-makers, and by the disproportionate political power of corporate interests and the practices they use to manipulate and exploit our cognitive weaknesses against our health interests (Ubel, 1999).

Fairness in the Distribution of Burdens

Yet another appeal that can be used to defend certain public health interventions that impose unequal burdens on different members of a population relies on considerations of fairness. The basic premise of this line of argument would be that burdens should be roughly equivalent for everyone. This view justifies taxing different income brackets at different rates. The same could be said for certain public health "burdens," understood as both the burdens of disease and disability and the burdens of public health interventions. Based on considerations such as a particular group's likelihood to contract a certain disease or overall health status, other parts of the population can legitimately be asked to "contribute," as it were, in order to make the distribution of disease burdens more equitable. For example, part of the rationale for requiring child immunization prior to enrollment in school is that this is a way to ensure that low-income children, who are generally less healthy than other children, have access to the needed vaccines (Feudtner and Marcuse, 2001; Orenstein and Hinman, 1999).

Perhaps a more pertinent example is Japan's seasonal influenza immunization policy between 1962 and 1994, where children were immunized against influenza explicitly in order to protect the elderly, for whom contracting seasonal flu is more likely to be fatal, and immunization more likely to be burdensome (Reichert et al., 2001; Sugaya, 2014). Yet another example of public health interventions that appear to be guided by this justification is rubella vaccination of children for the sake of pregnant women and their offspring (Marin et al., 2010; Miller et al., 1997). This reasoning can help explain why individuals are sometimes asked to bear public health burdens that do not directly benefit them. However, as with the tax example, the question of how far we can go in redistributing health-related burdens will likely continue to plague any proponent of this justificatory strategy. Moreover, questions about the plausibility of viewing health-related burdens as subject to distribution in this manner may also arise.

The Harm Principle

It is likely that no classic philosophical work is cited more often in the public health ethics literature than John Stuart Mill's essay "On Liberty" (Mill and Gray, 1998). In that essay, Mill defends what has come to be called the "harm principle," which has been interpreted as holding that the only justification for interfering with the liberty of an individual, against his or her will, is to prevent harm to others. The harm principle is relied upon to justify various infectious disease control interventions, including quarantine, isolation, and compulsory treatment. In liberal democracies, the harm principle is often viewed as the most compelling justification for public health policies that interfere with individual liberty. For example, a prominent view in the United States is that it was not until the public became persuaded of the harmful effects of second-hand smoke that the first significant intrusion into smoking practices—the banning of smoking in public places—became politically feasible. Perhaps because of the principle's broad persuasiveness, it is not uncommon to see appeals made about harm to others in less than obvious contexts. Defenders of compulsory motorcycle helmet laws, for example, argued that the serious head injuries sustained by unprotected cyclists diverted emergency room personnel and resources, thus harming other patients (Jones and Bayer, 2007).

The harm principle has been interpreted to include credible threats of significant economic harm to others as well as physical harm. Returning again to smoking policy, various restrictions on the behavior of smokers have been justified by appeal to the financial burden on the health care system of caring for smoking-related illnesses. The claim that smokers impose economic harms on the rest of us, and thus that reducing smoking saves society money, is empirically questionable. Within the health care system there may be some cost savings, but people who would have died in late middle age of smoking-related illnesses are now likely to live into their seventies and beyond, with ailments that will continue to impose costs on the health care system—perhaps exceeding the costs of what would have been their smoking-related causes of death. Similarly, costs to the social security system increase (because nonsmokers live longer), while revenues from taxes on smoking products decrease (Cohen, Neumann, and Weinstein, 2008; Russell, 1986, 2009).

As with all such principles, questions remain about its specification. How significant must the threat of harm be, with regard to both its likelihood and its magnitude? Consider, for example, the debate in the United States about the appropriateness and necessity of isolating asymptomatic health professionals returning from providing care to Ebola patients in West Africa. Are physical harms to the health of others to be weighted more than economic harms or setbacks to other interests? Whether interpreted narrowly or broadly, there are limits to the public health cases that can plausibly be addressed by the harm principle. Moreover, in the context of commitments to social justice and general welfare, and the other justifications described above, too exclusive a focus on the harm principle can undermine otherwise justifiable government mandates and regulation. It is undeniable that individuals have much broader and more multidimensional interests than narrowly self-directed physical ones, and in that sense it is not unreasonable to have a fairly expansive understanding of "harm" in a public health context. However, adherence to the—admittedly somewhat artificial—heuristic of construing individuals' interests as exclusively their self-regarding ones for purposes of determining what sacrifices they may be asked to make is an important way of ensuring checks on potential abuses.

Because the impact of J. S. Mill on public health ethics cannot be overstated, it is important to recognize that Mill does not hold that in the formulation of public policies all liberty interests enjoy an equal presumption in their favor. Mill draws a distinction between interests that are so important that they are immune from state interference, interests that enjoy a presumption in favor of liberty, and interests that enjoy no such presumption. It is presumably the second kind of liberty interest where the harm principle figures prominently (Powers, Faden, and Saghai, 2012). Moreover, what many understand to be core to Mill's view—that individuals are generally best positioned to know what is in their own best interests—is increasingly being challenged (Conly, 2014; Sunstein, 2012).

Paternalism

Not surprisingly, paternalism—understood classically as interfering with the liberty of action of persons, against their will, to protect or promote their welfare—is as controversial in public health policy as the harm principle is uncontroversial (Dworkin, 2005; Feinberg, 1989). Few public health interventions are justified exclusively or even primarily on unmediated, classic paternalistic grounds, although many more public health programs may have paternalistic effects. By contrast, other classes of arguments that are sometimes described as paternalistic, including soft paternalism, weak paternalism, and libertarian paternalism, are evoked more frequently.

Soft and weak paternalism are usually interpreted as interchangeable, though they have sometimes been taken to denote different concepts (Dworkin, 2005). A common interpretation defines this kind of paternalism as interference with choices that are compromised with regard to voluntariness or autonomy. Though people might voice or hold preferences different from the ones that is sought for them, their preferences are not entitled to robust respect if they are formed under conditions that significantly compromise their autonomy or voluntariness, such as cognitive disability or immaturity and, in very limited cases, ignorance or false beliefs. Ignorance and false beliefs are not usually sufficient to make a preference subject to interference, and they generally require being supplemented by stronger considerations such as age, cognitive disability, or harm to others (e.g., one's child). In the normal course of things, we all have at least some preferences based on ignorance and false beliefs that proponents of soft paternalism nonetheless do not think can legitimately be interfered with, unless there is some compelling reason to impute impairment of rationality beyond, say, weakness of will. Adaptive preferences are also considered compromised with regard to autonomy: individuals sometimes modify their preferences in order to be able to adapt to difficult, unjust, or undesirable circumstances. The real significance of adaptive preferences is when they are formed in tragic circumstances of poverty and discrimination, where individuals convince themselves that they do not want the benefits of health, education, equal treatment, and so on because of the excruciating difficulty of continuing to prefer what is out of one's reach. Thus, individuals modify their preferences to their circumstances. In such cases, one arguably cannot take those preferences to indicate underlying values or decisions that ought not be interfered with. Such preferences also do not have the same standing as preferences formed under just or normal background conditions, and are therefore viewed as subject to interference.

It is important to note that in all these cases, justified interference would be based on a finding of significant compromise of autonomy or rationality in the formation or continued holding of particular preferences. This should not be confused with interference based on the content of the preferences. Only the former would be justifiable under weak or soft paternalism, whereas the latter would constitute true or strong paternalism. As always, the demarcations are not as clear in practice as they are in theory—the content of preferences is often precisely what is appealed to in illustrating that a particular preference is compromised—but, by and large, what distinguishes soft paternalism from strong paternalism is the requirement that the decision or preference be fundamentally compromised, and not simply that it be mistaken or ignorant. This principled distinction remains important not least because it reflects a difference in approach or attitude. In the case of strong paternalism, the interference is based on the content of a preference not reflecting what is ostensibly in the preference holder's interest. This is often accompanied by a much stronger view of the legitimacy of external judgments about what is really in a person's interest, and by a stronger likelihood to question individuals' own assessment of their best interests than alternative, softer versions of paternalism. In the case of weak or soft paternalism, persons might hold all manner of preferences not in their best interests that are nonetheless not justifiably interfered with because the relevant compromising conditions do not obtain. In public health policy, soft paternalism has been evoked to justify interventions that limit the ability of adolescents to act on preferences for alcohol, drugs, sexual activity, and driving.

In recent years, public health policy and liberal governments have increasingly looked to interventions called "nudges" to influence health behaviors in desirable directions. Nudges, typically understood as interventions in choice architecture, are the focus of libertarian paternalism. Libertarian paternalism defends interventions by planners (such as public health authorities) in the environmental architecture in which individuals decide and act in order to make it easier for people to behave in ways that are in their best interests (including their health), provided two conditions are satisfied (Thaler and Sunstein, 2003, 2008). First, individuals are steered by these interventions in ways that make them better off, as judged by themselves. Thus, in libertarian paternalism there is no attempt to contravene the will of individuals, in contrast to what some hold to be a necessary feature of paternalism. Second, the interventions must not overly burden individuals who want to exercise their freedom in ways that run counter to their welfare. In this sense, libertarian paternalism claims to be liberty-preserving, and hence libertarian.

A key conceptual question about paternalism is whether the interference with individual liberty must be against the person's will (Beauchamp, 2010). If this feature is a necessary condition of paternalism, then libertarian paternalism is inappropriately titled.

From the standpoint of public health ethics, however, whether libertarian paternalism is appropriately titled is less important than any moral issues it raises and how it is justified. There is a growing literature on the ethics of nudges, much of it focusing on health (Hollands et al., 2013; Quigley, 2013; Saghai, 2013a, 2013b).

Libertarian paternalism is grounded in the extensive empirical literature in cognitive psychology and the decision sciences that supports claims about people's cognitive limitations, bounded rationality, and weakness of will. Although it raises challenging epistemic and political questions about how planners know what individuals judge is in their interests in specific policy contexts, libertarian paternalism may be well suited to public health contexts in which there is broad public consensus in favor of health-promoting behaviors such as eating more fruits and vegetables or getting more exercise, and a general recognition that it is difficult for people to act as prudentially as they would like. Thaler and Sunstein (2008) suggest, for example, that salads rather than French fries could be made the default "side" on restaurant menus, with diners free to request fries if that remains their preference. At the same time, libertarian paternalism has been criticized for failing to take account of the manipulative effects on choice of some marketplace forces. It has also been seen as too restrictive in its conditions (and therefore too weak) to be applicable or adequate for many public health contexts (Nuffield Council on Bioethics, 2007; Ubel, 1999).

A Central Task of Public Health Ethics: Providing a Complete Moral Picture of What Is at Stake

Part of the appeal of libertarian paternalism in public health policy is that, at least in certain contexts, it appears to sidestep, or in some cases resolve, the tension between liberty and health. This tension takes center stage in some analyses of the ethics of public health, such as when public health policies are placed on autonomy-limiting continua and the fourth and fifth justifications dominate the analysis. One such influential continuum is the Nuffield Council's "intervention ladder" (Nuffield Council on Bioethics, 2007), which is presented as a way of thinking about the acceptability and justification of public health policies. The ladder is anchored at one end by what is presented as the least intrusive option, doing nothing, and at the other end by the what is presented as the most intrusive option, eliminating choice altogether (as in compulsory isolation). The council makes plain that all rungs on the ladder, including doing nothing, require justification, and that the ladder is to be taken only as a tool in the moral analysis of public health policies. However, the structure of the ladder and its attendant imagery reinforce the misleading view that balancing individual liberties with achieving health benefits is the primary moral challenge of public health, while at the same time appearing to emphasize ethical concerns about overreaching the mission of public health over ethical concerns about underserving it.

Continua of this sort also oversimplify the complex impact of interventions on choice and liberty, and on relations between citizens and the state. Incentives are not always less restrictive of choice than disincentives, and health promotion campaigns, which are generally ranked at or near the least intrusive end of the continuum, are not always without significant moral concern. Ad campaigns that are transparently sponsored by public health agencies to prevent transmission of influenza by promoting personal infection-control practices, or to reduce obesity by encouraging exercise and healthy eating, do not raise the same moral issues as the embedding of anti-drug or abstinence messages in the storylines of entertainment television programming by these same authorities (FCC, 2000; Forbes, 2000; Goodman, 2006; Krauthammer, 2000; Kurtz and Waxman, 2000). While the latter poses important questions about respect for liberty, government overreaching, and democratic legitimacy, the limited effectiveness of many ad campaigns raises important questions about whether the state is underserving its public health mission. Moreover, in the case of public health problems such as obesity, a reliance on health promotion campaigns and other strategies focused on influencing the behavior of individuals may both inappropriately stigmatize persons who are viewed as obese and fail to place an appropriate burden on the corporate interests and structural social inequalities that arguably account for much of the problem. Thus, depending on the circumstances, health promotion campaigns may be unjust as well as ineffective (Buchanan, 2008; Crawford, 1977; Faden, 1987; McLeroy et al., 1988).

An important task of public health ethics is not only to provide different moral justifications for policies and programs. It is also to critically examine their relationship to one another in the context of particular public health issues and activities so as to ensure a more complete moral picture of what is at stake, and to point out where no sufficient justification exists. In this way, public health ethics can play a more immediate practical role in public life. By raising challenges to and providing moral scrutiny of public health policies, it can contribute to creating an environment of accountability where both abuses and deficiencies are less likely. Thus, in addition to its intellectual significance, public health ethics can be an important element in the scheme of checks and balances that help keep public health authorities from overreaching or underserving their mission.

Acknowledgments

This chapter is a modified version of section 2 of "Public Health Ethics" (Faden and Shebaya, 2016).

References

Beauchamp, T. L. 2010. *Standing on Principles: Collected Essays* (New York: Oxford University Press).

Buchanan, D. R. 2008. "Autonomy, Paternalism, and Justice: Ethical Priorities in Public Health." *American Journal of Public Health* 98(1): 15–21.

Cohen, J. T., Neumann, P. J., and Weinstein, M. C. 2008. "Does Preventive Care Save Money? Health Economics and the Presidential Candidates." *New England Journal of Medicine* 358(7): 661–663.

Conly, S. 2014. "Against Autonomy: Justifying Coercive Paternalism." *Journal of Medical Ethics* 40(5): 349. doi:10.1136/medethics-2013-101444.

Crawford, R. 1977. "You Are Dangerous to Your Health: The Ideology and Politics of Victim Blaming." *International Journal of Health Services* 7(4): 663–680.

Dworkin, G. 2005. "Paternalism." In *The Stanford Encyclopedia of Philosophy*, edited by E. N. Zalta (Stanford, Calif.: Stanford University). http://plato.stanford.edu/archives/win2005/entries/paternalism/.

Faden, R. 1987. "Ethical Issues in Government Sponsored Public Health Campaigns." *Health Education and Behavior* 14(1): 27–37.

Faden, R., and Shebaya, S. 2016. "Public Health Ethics." In *The Stanford Encyclopedia of Philosophy*, edited by E. N. Zalta (Stanford, Calif.: Stanford University). https://plato.stanford.edu/archives/win2016/entries/publichealth-ethics/.

FCC (Federal Communications Commission). 2000. Letter to NORML Foundation Regarding the Investigation into NORML Foundation's Complaint against ABC, CBS, NBC, Fox, and WB. December 22, EB-00-IH-0078. https://transition.fcc.gov/eb/Orders/da002873.txt.

Feinberg, J. 1989. *The Moral Limits of the Criminal Law: Harm to Self* (New York: Oxford University Press).

Feudtner, C., and Marcuse, E. K. 2001. "Ethics and Immunization Policy: Promoting Dialogue to Sustain Consensus." *Pediatrics* 107(5): 1158–1164.

Forbes, D. 2000. "Prime-Time Propaganda: How the White House Secretly Hooked Network TV on Its Anti-Drug Message: A Salon Special Report." In *Salon*, January 13. https://www.salon.com/2000/01/13/drugs_6/.

Goodman, E. P. 2006. "Stealth Marketing and Editorial Integrity." *Texas Law Review* 85: 83.

Grynbaum, M. M. and Connelly, M. 2012. "60% in City Oppose Bloomberg's Soda Ban, Poll Finds." *New York Times*, August 22, 2012.

Hollands, G. J., Shemilt, I., Marteau, T. M., Jebb, S. A., Kelly, M. P., Nakamura, R., et al. 2013. "Altering Micro-Environments to Change Population Health Behaviour: Towards an Evidence Base for Choice Architecture Interventions." *BMC Public Health* 13: 1218. https://bmcpublichealth.biomedcentral.com/articles/10.1186/1471-2458-13-1218.

Jones, M. M., and Bayer, R. 2007. "Paternalism and Its Discontents: Motorcycle Helmet Laws, Libertarian Values, and Public Health." *American Journal of Public Health* 97(2): 208–217.

Krauthammer, C. 2000. "A Network Sellout." *Washington Post*, January 21, A29.

Kurtz, H., and Waxman, S. 2000. "White House Cut Anti-Drug Deal with TV." *Washington Post*, January 14, A1.

Marin, M., Broder, K. R., Temte, J. L., Snider, D. E., Seward, J.F., and Centers for Disease Control and Prevention. 2010. "Use of Combination Measles, Mumps, Rubella, and Varicella Vaccine: Recommendations of the Advisory Committee on Immunization Practices (ACIP)." *Morbidity and Mortality Weekly Report* 59(RR03): 1–12. https://www.cdc.gov/mmwr/preview/mmwrhtml/rr5903a1.htm.

McLeroy, K. R., Bibeau, D., Steckler, A., and Glanz, K. 1988. "An Ecological Perspective on Health Promotion Programs." *Health Education and Behavior* 15(4): 351–377.

Mill, J. S., and Gray, J. 1998. *On Liberty and Other Essays* (New York: Oxford University Press).

Miller, E., Waight, P., Gay, N., Ramsay, M., Vurdien, J., Morgan-Capner, P., et al.1997. "The Epidemiology of Rubella in England and Wales before and after the 1994 Measles and

Rubella Vaccination Campaign: Fourth Joint Report from the PHLS and the National Congenital Rubella Surveillance Programme." *Communicable Disease Report* 7(2): R26–32.

Nuffield Council on Bioethics. 2007. *Public Health: Ethical Issues* (London: Nuffield Council on Bioethics).

Omer, S. B., Salmon, D. A., Orenstein, W. A., Dehart, M. P., and Halsey, N. 2009. "Vaccine Refusal, Mandatory Immunization, and the Risks of Vaccine-Preventable Diseases." *New England Journal of Medicine* 360(19): 1981–1988.

Orenstein, W. A., and Hinman, A. R. 1999. "The Immunization System in the United States—the Role of School Immunization Laws." *Vaccine* 17: S19–S24.

Powers, M., Faden, R., and Saghai, Y. 2012. "Liberty, Mill and the Framework of Public Health Ethics." *Public Health Ethics* 5(1): 6–15.

Quigley, M. 2013. "Nudging for Health: On Public Policy and Designing Choice Architecture." *Medical Law Review* 21(4): 588–621.

Reichert, T. A., Sugaya, N., Fedson, D. S., Glezen, W. P., Simonsen, L., and Tashiro, M. 2001. "The Japanese Experience with Vaccinating Schoolchildren against Influenza." *New England Journal of Medicine* 344(12): 889–896.

Russell, L. B. 1986. *Is Prevention Better Than Cure?* (Washington, D.C.: Brookings Institution Press).

Russell, L. B. 2009. "Preventing Chronic Disease: An Important Investment, but Don't Count on Cost Savings." *Health Affairs* 28(1): 42–45.

Saghai, Y. 2013a. "The Concept of Nudge and Its Moral Significance: A Reply to Ashcroft, Bovens, Dworkin, Welch and Wertheimer." *Journal of Medical Ethics* 39(8): 499–501. doi:10.1136/medethics-2012-101112.

Saghai, Y. 2013b. "Salvaging the Concept of Nudge." *Journal of Medical Ethics* 39(8): 487–493. doi:10.1136/medethics-2012-100727.

Sugaya, N. 2014. "A Review of the Indirect Protection of Younger Children and the Elderly through a Mass Influenza Vaccination Program in Japan." *Expert Review of Vaccines* 13(12): 1563–1570.

Sugerman, D. E., Barskey, A. E., Delea, M. G., Ortega-Sanchez, I. R., Bi, D., Ralston, K.J., et al. 2010. "Measles Outbreak in a Highly Vaccinated Population, San Diego, 2008: Role of the Intentionally Undervaccinated." *Pediatrics* 125(4): 747–755.

Sunstein, C. R. 2012. "The Storrs Lectures: Behavioral Economics and Paternalism." *Yale Law Journal* 122: 1826.

Thaler, R. H., and Sunstein, C. R. 2003. "Libertarian Paternalism." *American Economic Review* 93(2): 175–179.

Thaler, R. H., and Sunstein, C. R. 2008. *Nudge: Improving Decisions about Health, Wealth, and Happiness* (New Haven, Conn.: Yale University Press).

Thompson, J. W., Tyson, S., Card-Higginson, P., Jacobs, R. F., Wheeler, J.G., Simpson, P., et al. 2007. "Impact of Addition of Philosophical Exemptions on Childhood Immunization Rates." *American Journal of Preventive Medicine* 32(3): 194–201.

Ubel, P. A. 1999. "How Stable Are People's Preferences for Giving Priority to Severely Ill Patients?" *Social Science and Medicine* 49(7): 895–903.

Further Reading

Barry, B. 1982. "Humanity and Justice in Global Perspective." *Nomos* 24: 219–252.

Hyder, A. A., Pratt, B., Ali, J., Kass, N., and Sewankambo, N. 2014. "The Ethics of Health Systems Research in Low-and Middle Income Countries: A Call to Action." *Global Public Health* 9(9): 1008–1022.

Institute of Medicine. 1988. *The Future of Public Health* (Washington, D.C.: National Academy Press).

Institute of Medicine. 2003. *The Future of the Public's Health in the 21st Century* (Washington, D.C.: National Academy Press).

Kenny, N. P., Sherwin, S. B., and Baylis, F. E. 2010. "Re-visioning Public Health Ethics: A Relational Perspective." *Canadian Journal of Public Health/Revue Canadienne de Santé Publique*: 9–11.

Lee, L. M. 2012. "Public Health Ethics Theory: Review and Path to Convergence." *Journal of Law, Medicine and Ethics* 40(1): 85–98.

Powers, M., and Faden, R. 2008. *Social Justice: The Moral Foundations of Public Health and Health Policy* (New York: Oxford University Press).

CHAPTER 4

JUSTICE AND PUBLIC HEALTH

GOVIND PERSAD

Introduction

Public health is concerned with the health of entire populations and societies. Questions about how societies ought to be shaped by choices, in public health and elsewhere, are the subject matter of justice. To see how justice intersects with public health, imagine an international public health researcher—we'll call her Julie—examining a World Health Organization chart of life expectancy in South America (see Figure 4.1).

As Julie examines the chart, she sees that life expectancy is over eighty years in Chile, but under seventy years in Bolivia and Guyana. These facts present two questions at the heart of justice: (1) What are the criteria for a good society? (2) What are acceptable differences in what people enjoy within and between societies?

At lunch, Julie tells her colleagues about the chart, while they tell her about their public health projects, which include water quality, vaccinations, urban planning, and taxation and economic policy. Their discussion presents a third question at the interface of justice and public health: Which public health interventions will make for a better society? This question has both an empirical component concerning what outcomes public health interventions will produce, and a normative component concerning which outcomes are worth seeking. Julie and her colleagues also discuss organizational priorities. Some advocate funding interventions that are already recognized as cost-effective. Others argue for funding new interventions that promise to narrow gaps in life expectancy. Still others worry that some of the interventions, such as changes in urban design or taxes on unhealthy foods, would unfairly burden some individuals or groups. Although these discussions may never explicitly use the word *justice*, they involve the sorts of questions examined in the remainder of this chapter.

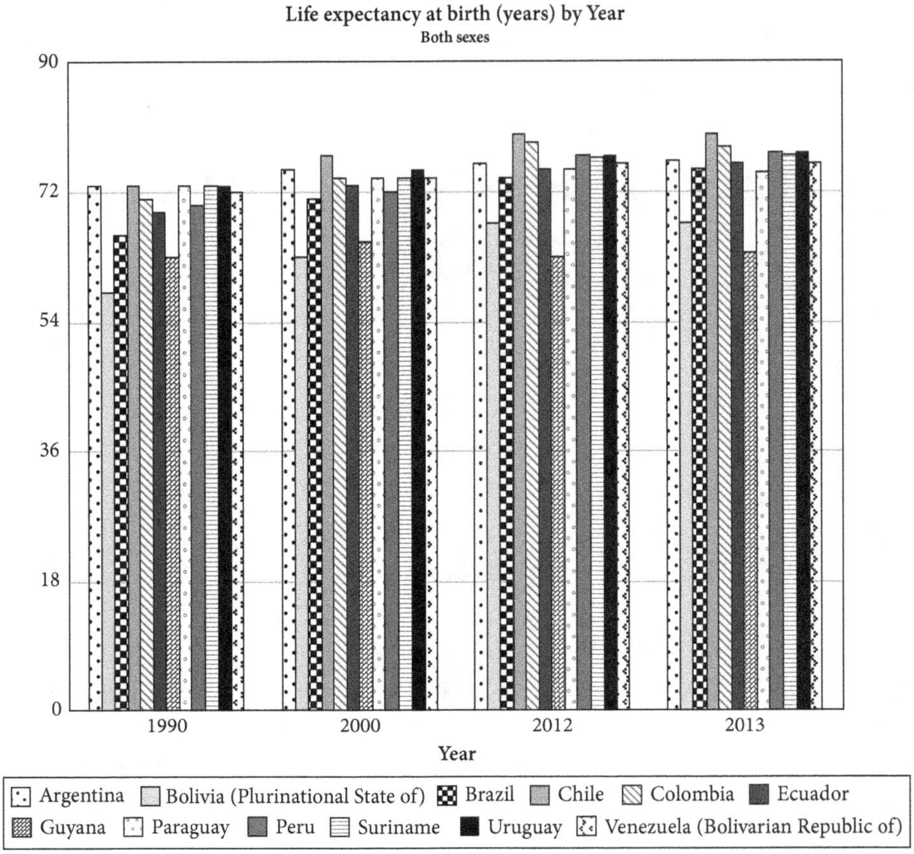

FIGURE 4.1 Life Expectancy at Birth: South America

Source: Reprinted from WHO, 2016. Used with permission of the World Health Organization.

What Should We Measure?: Metrics of Justice

Metrics are methodologies for quantifying and evaluating the contribution of various interventions, including public health interventions, to the achievement of a just society. The three most prominent metrics are those that focus on resources, capabilities, and welfare (Daniels, 1990).

Resources

Resourcist metrics judge the justice of a society by looking at how it distributes resources. John Rawls (1999) proposes a primary goods approach, which has become a prominent resourcist metric. Rawls defines primary goods as including income and wealth, as well as less tangible goods such as rights and social bases of self-respect.

Resourcist metrics make data collection easy and avoid judgments about what a good life is. Some people worry, however, that resourcist metrics are unfair to individuals with disabilities or illnesses who require more resources than others in order to pursue their goals or participate in society (Sen, 1985). Familiar resource metrics for public health audiences include gross domestic product (GDP) and per-capita GDP, which measure a society's total and average economic resources, respectively.

Capabilities

Capability metrics, pioneered by Amartya Sen (1985) and Martha Nussbaum (2003), look at the distribution of capabilities, which are freedoms to engage in various activities. Nussbaum lists ten capabilities with universal importance—life; bodily health; bodily integrity; senses, imagination, and thought; emotions; practical reason; affiliation; interaction with other species; play; and control over one's environment—while Sen (2004) suggests that the list of capabilities can differ between societies and be developed through public discussion.

Capability metrics emphasize active dimensions of human life, such as choice and agency, rather than focusing on passive enjoyment or resource possession. However, critics worry that such metrics underrate the importance of actual outcomes (Arneson, 2010), and that measuring and comparing capabilities may be difficult and intrusive (Freeman, 2006). In light of the former concern, Ruth Faden and Madison Powers (2006) have developed a metric that draws on the capability approach but focuses on actual functionings—the activities individuals engage in—rather than capabilities, and have applied this metric to public health. The Human Development Index, which combines life expectancy, literacy, and income measures, also builds on ideas from the capability approach and is widely used in public health (Fukuda-Parr, 2003).

Welfare

Welfarist accounts assess justice by examining the distribution of welfare. Some welfarist accounts define welfare as a subjective mental state of pleasure, others define it as preference satisfaction, and still others define it using a list of objectively valuable experiences (Parfit, 1984, Appendix I). All of these approaches face problems, which include concerns about repugnant, expensive, and self-sacrificing preferences, as well as concerns that subjective mental states matter far less than the arrangement of external reality (Faden and Powers, 2006; Nozick, 1974). Prominent welfarists include Jeremy Bentham (1843) and Peter Singer (1979), as well as many economists. Welfarist public health metrics include quality-adjusted and disability-adjusted life years (QALYs and DALYs), which are typically generated via surveys of individuals' subjective experiences of different health setbacks (Gold, Stevenson, and Fryback, 2002).

Some public health interventions are similarly attractive regardless of what metric is used. As an example, clean water is likely to improve the resources, capabilities, and welfare of its recipients. For other interventions, however, the choice of metrics matters greatly—alcohol taxes appear less attractive under some welfare-based metrics, which assign weight to drinkers' subjective pleasure, than capability or resource metrics, which assign such pleasure little or no weight.

Who Should Get What? Principles of Distributive Justice

Along with what to measure, we must also consider how to distribute whatever is measured. *Noncorrelative* principles do not try to correlate how much each individual receives with other facts about that individual, whereas *correlative* principles do.

Noncorrelative Principles

Maximization

This principle maximizes what is available, irrespective of distribution. In Julie's example, maximization would favor improving life expectancy by five years in Chile, which has a high life expectancy, over improving it by four years for an equally sized group of individuals in Bolivia, which has a much lower life expectancy. Maximization is often described as *utilitarianism*, though that term is more frequently used to refer specifically to welfare maximization, as opposed to capability or resource maximization. A frequently discussed basis for public health decisions is maximizing the number of QALYs saved or DALYs avoided (Schwappach, 2002).

Maximization becomes more complicated when public health interventions that change the size of the population, such as family planning, are at issue. Applying a maximization approach to interventions that change population size presents a choice between total and average maximization. Maximizing the average favors a smaller population with a lower sum of whatever is valuable, but in which the average individual is better off, whereas maximizing the total favors the opposite. Each view faces problems: the average view is criticized for its unwillingness to add individuals who enjoy a substantial amount of whatever is valuable to a very well-off population when adding these people would fail to maximize the average, while the total view is criticized for favoring policies that produce a vast population in which each individual enjoys little of what is valuable (Parfit, 1984). In an effort to address these concerns, some have attempted to combine elements of both total and average maximization, though no solution appears completely satisfactory (Arrhenius, Ryberg, and Tännsjö 2010).

Prioritarianism: Priority to the Worst Off

Prioritarian approaches assign special importance to helping those at the bottom of a distribution. Strict prioritarian views, such as Rawls's "difference principle" (1999, 67–73), give absolute priority to the worst-off group, while flexible prioritarian views employ a sliding scale of priority, on which priority increases as individuals become worse off (Parfit, 1997, 213). Prioritarian distributive principles have support among health care planners (Ottersen et al., 2008). Incorporating distributional weights into cost-effectiveness analysis, by assigning more importance to QALY increases that go to individuals who are worse off, represents one way of quantifying prioritarian ideas in public health (Ottersen, Mæstad, and Norheim, 2014).

In the WHO example, a flexible prioritarian view might favor a five-year improvement in Guyanese life expectancy over a six-year improvement in Brazil, but not over a ten-year improvement in Brazil. In contrast, a strict prioritarian view will always favor even a minuscule improvement for the worst-off over an enormous one for the better-off. This has prompted criticism of the strict prioritarian view (Arrow, 1973).

Egalitarianism

Egalitarianism aims to reduce inequalities in distribution. In Julie's example, egalitarianism would agree with prioritarianism that extra weight should be given to improving life expectancy in countries with lower life expectancies. Strict egalitarianism aims to achieve complete equality, while looser approaches propose what Elizabeth Anderson (2008) calls "range-constraining rules" that limit the extent of inequality. Many familiar measures of inequality, such as the Gini coefficient (which quantifies the extent to which people's incomes differ), are employed in public health (Wagstaff, Paci, and van Doorslaer, 1991).

Although egalitarian and prioritarian approaches frequently make the same recommendations, prioritarians focus on the absolute position of the worst off, while egalitarians focus on the gap between the worst off and the better off. Therefore, egalitarians, unlike prioritarians, will sometimes advocate "leveling down"; that is, they will sometimes object to an improvement that helps the worst off but increases inequality. Leveling down has been criticized by prioritarians (Parfit, 1997) but defended by some egalitarians (Eyal, 2013).

Sufficientarianism

Sufficientarianism ensures that no one falls below a specified threshold (Shields, 2012). Some define thresholds in absolute terms, while others argue that thresholds of sufficiency must vary with social context (Faden and Powers, 2006). The use of poverty thresholds, such as the $1 per day threshold employed in the Millennium Development Goals (Deaton, 2003), represents the most prominent effort to operationalize a sufficientarian view in a domain relevant to public health. Some human rights documents also define the right to health as a right to adequate or sufficient health (Persad, 2014, 603–604).

As an example, applying a life expectancy threshold of seventy-two years of age to the WHO chart would support public health interventions that increase life expectancy in Bolivia and Guyana, which have life expectancies under seventy-two, but would be neutral between interventions in Paraguay and in Chile, even though Paraguayans live less long on average than Chileans. Sufficientarianism, like prioritarianism, helps those who are worse off while avoiding leveling down. Sufficientarianism has been criticized, however, for ignoring morally relevant differences above or below the selected thresholds (Shields, 2012). Even if improving life expectancy for people in Bolivia and Guyana should be the highest priority, the fact that Paraguayans live less long than Chileans is not obviously irrelevant.

Correlative Principles

Correlative principles aim to correlate what people receive with some other dimension of life in which they differ. Three of the most prominent correlative principles correlate what people receive to (1) their contribution, (2) their effort, and (3) what they have traditionally received.

Contribution

Some theorists have argued that individuals who increase the amount available to be distributed ought to receive more of what is distributed (Miller, 1990). As an example, individuals who have previously donated organs might receive priority for organ transplants in the future (Persad, Wertheimer, and Emanuel, 2009). Even though contribution-based principles will often reach similar conclusions to the noncorrelative maximization principle discussed earlier under the heading "Maximization," contribution-based principles look to past contributions, while maximization looks to future contributions.

Applied to the WHO chart, a contribution-based approach might favor public health efforts that improve life expectancy in Argentina, because the Argentinian economy contributes more to global productivity, over efforts to improve life expectancy in less-developed Guyana. In light of the foundational importance of health to people's lives, however, contribution is arguably an inappropriate basis for distributing health, even if it can be an appropriate basis for distributing other goods (Feiring, 2008).

Effort

Others argue that the distribution of goods should be based on individual effort, with those who put in more effort receiving more. One prominent version of this view is advanced by John Roemer (1993), who argues that we should ensure that people who exercise a "comparable degree of responsibility" do equally well, regardless of their background circumstances. Roemer also proposes a detailed methodology for quantifying effort, though this methodology has not been widely adopted in public health.

As with contribution, there is a worry that an effort-based distribution of health will be unjustly harsh on those who exert little effort (Feiring, 2008). Explaining which kinds of effort should count is also challenging. For instance, even if inefficient farming techniques in Suriname mean that Surinamese farmers exert more effort to produce a given quantity of food than Colombian farmers, rewarding effort that stems from inefficient practices seems like a dubious basis for distributing benefits, including public health benefits. Ultimately, as Susan Hurley (2002) observes, identifying which types of effort matter for distribution seems to require some background account of justice. Once this account has been identified, it is unclear why effort itself matters.

Tradition

A traditionalist view correlates what individuals receive with what they have historically and traditionally received. Applied to Julie's chart, a traditionalist view would attempt to maintain the distribution of life expectancy over time, and so would oppose any proposal that dramatically increases or decreases life expectancy.

Because of their opposition to change and tendency to maintain hierarchy, traditionalist views are often identified with political conservatism and a bias toward the status quo (Brennan and Hamlin, 2004). Such views have also been defended by thinkers such as Jeremy Bentham (1843) and David Hume (1739) on the basis of individuals' psychological attachment to accustomed arrangements. In practice, traditionalism frequently obstructs public health innovations that might improve the lives of some but disrupt the lives of others. For instance, some assert that single-payer health insurance will be difficult to enact in the United States because it would disrupt insurance arrangements to which many have become accustomed (Feder, 2014).

Combining Principles

Any distributive principle can be paired with any metric (see Table 4.1). For instance, while Rawls pairs a resourcist metric with a distributive approach that favors the worst off, it is also possible—as he himself notes—to combine a resourcist metric with a distributive approach that simply maximizes total resources without any special concern for the worst off (Rawls, 1999, 277–285).

Some approaches to distributive justice employ only a single distributive principle, while others include multiple principles, which are weighed against one another.

Table 4.1 Metrics and Principles of Distributive Justice

Metrics	Distributive principles	Prominent approaches
(a) Resources	*Noncorrelative*	Rawlsian: (a) + (2)
(b) Capabilities	(1) Maximization	Utilitarian: (c) + (1)
(c) Welfare	(2) Prioritarianism	Faden and Powers: Modified (b) + (4)
	(3) Egalitarianism	
	(4) Sufficientarianism	
	Correlative	
	(1) Contribution	
	(2) Effort	
	(3) Tradition	

Defenders of multi-principle approaches argue that no single principle adequately captures what is needed for a just society (Persad, Wertheimer, and Emanuel, 2009). However, some worry that multi-principle approaches fail to articulate a principled basis for balancing different principles, such as equality and maximization, against one another (Rawls, 1999, 34–40).

What Else Matters? Individual Rights and Constraints on Distributive Justice

Most accounts of justice recognize certain nondistributive constraints on the pursuit of distributive principles. Rawls (1999), for instance, believes that certain basic liberties, such as freedom of thought and association, political participation, freedom of movement, and the right to hold personal property, must be secured before we begin thinking about the just distribution of resources.

Many public health dilemmas involve conflicts between distributive goals and individuals' basic rights or liberties. Many of these basic rights take the form of *negative rights*, which are rights against intervention. For instance, rights to bodily integrity, freedom of association, or freedom of religion might complicate efforts to require vaccinations against a communicable disease or to quarantine individuals who show signs of infection, even when these public health interventions would improve population health or achieve a better distribution of health. Some libertarian theories (e.g., Nozick, 1974) regard property rights as absolute and prohibit the imposition of taxes, which would have the effect of choking off funding for public health interventions.

Meanwhile, basic *positive rights*, which are rights to receive benefits, can also obstruct public health goals. For instance, recognizing an individual right to lifesaving health care can consume resources that would otherwise be used to promote public health (Persad, 2014; Schmidt, Gostin, and Emanuel, 2015). Other types of rights, such as rights against differential treatment on the basis of race or gender, can also come into conflict with public health initiatives such as targeted screening of poor women of color for human immunodeficiency virus (HIV) infection (Faden and Powers, 2006, vii–viii), or restrictions on the purchase of unhealthy foods (Kass et al., 2014; Barnhill, 2015).

Accounts of justice differ not only in the list of rights they recognize, but also in how they handle conflicts between, on the one hand, distributive aims, such as sufficiency or priority to the worst off, and, on the other hand, basic rights and liberties, such as freedom of association or property rights. Some accounts, like Rawls's, give fundamental liberties absolute priority over distributive aims. Others allow rights to be overridden when doing so can dramatically improve distributive outcomes.

Where Does Justice Apply?: Global Justice and the Scope of Justice

Some accounts of justice give equal weight to all interests that are affected by a given decision. But many others give special weight to some interests. Deciding which interests matter is the question of the *scope* of justice.

The most prominent debates have involved *geographical* scope, which separates theories of justice that give special weight to one's fellow citizens from those that do not. The latter are often termed *cosmopolitan* and the former *statist* or *nationalist* (Emanuel, 2012). This division can be moved further in or further out. For instance, some theories may give special weight to fellow members of one's state or city, or to larger collectivities than the nation-state. Geographical scope has clear implications for public health choices; some interventions, such as vaccinations against communicable diseases, produce great benefits outside a nation's borders, while others have much more local effects.

Other distinctions of scope are also debated. There are, for instance, questions of *temporal* scope (Rawls, 1999; Parfit, 1984): What weight should justice give to the interests of those in the far future or distant past? There are even questions of *biological* scope (Donaldson and Kymlicka, 2013): What weight should be given to the interests of nonhuman animals or of ecosystems? These other forms of scope also bear on public health decision-making. For instance, how we evaluate changes in the design of the built environment that affect carbon emissions will depend on what duties we owe to future generations. Likewise, evaluating the burdens that disease eradication may impose on nonhuman animals who are carriers of disease will implicate questions of biological scope.

What Conduct Does Justice Evaluate?: The Site of Justice

Discussions of the *scope* of justice try to identify the physical or conceptual spaces where justice applies. In contrast, debates regarding the *site* of justice try to identify the actions or interactions that are properly assessed by the standards of justice.

One prominent view on the site of justice, associated with Rawls (1999) and Thomas Nagel (1991), regards distributive justice as applicable to the "basic structure" of society, which comprises institutions such as constitutions or other fundamental legal rules that organize society, as well as the economy, property, and general rules passed by legislatures. So, for example, justice would apply to decisions on whether to impose a tax on unhealthy foods, because these taxes are implemented through binding legislative action. In contrast, distributive justice does not apply to a shopkeeper's decision to sell a large sugary soda to an individual child, because that decision is not part of the basic structure. While there may be good reasons to criticize the shopkeeper, such criticisms are grounded in morality rather than justice, or at least in forms of justice other than distributive justice.

A different perspective on the site of justice is adopted by G. A. Cohen (1997), who frames it in terms of the feminist slogan "the personal is political." In Cohen's view, individual choices, such as selling a sugary soda, must also be evaluated in terms of justice. For Cohen, there is no clear distinction between rules of law, such as taxes or regulations, and individual choices, such as the shopkeeper's choice to sell soda to the child: all are subject to the same form of evaluation.

Debates regarding the site of justice are relevant to the question of how broadly justice applies to public health, and to the question of which actors within public health systems should be concerned about justice. If Cohen's view is correct, then Julie's coworkers who provide direct public health services, such as nurses or epidemiologists in the field, should evaluate their choices in providing care or interviewing people by employing the same principles of justice that apply to structural and legislative decisions. In contrast, if justice applies only to the basic structure of society, then Julie and her colleagues still have reason to care about justice, but providers of direct services can be subject only to norms of professional ethics that are unrelated to, and may deviate from, principles of distributive justice.

Last, many public health interventions, such as anti-smoking or safe-sex campaigns, attempt to shift social norms rather than creating or enforcing binding laws. This raises the question of whether social norms should be evaluated according to principles of justice (Ronzoni, 2008). Social norms are more than purely individual decisions, although norms can be reinforced or threatened by those decisions. However, they are not enforced by the use of binding legal authority. Nonetheless, social norms can have a pervasive influence on individuals' lives.

Who Decides?: Resolving Disagreements about Justice

This discussion has so far illustrated that questions about justice are complex. This complexity produces ample room for disagreement. One place for disagreement concerns choices about how to understand justice, such as which constraints to recognize or which metric to use. Another concerns the resolution of conflicts between different aspects of justice, such as how to weigh constraints against distributive principles. As they try to decide which public health interventions should receive priority for funding and implementation, Julie and her colleagues may face both these types of disagreements.

Disagreements about justice can be resolved in numerous ways. One way is through democracy, where each position is presented to the public, who then determine the best conception of justice. There are two major strands of democracy discussed by political philosophers: aggregative and deliberative. In aggregative democracy, individuals separately evaluate proposals and vote on them; their votes are then aggregated to determine which proposal is selected. In contrast, in deliberative democracy, individuals gather together to discuss and debate the proposals under consideration, with their discussions constrained by certain procedural and substantive norms (Cohen, 2009; Gutmann and Thompson, 2004). After the discussions, individuals either vote independently or reach some sort of communal consensus.

Democracy has the advantage of giving each individual's perspective equal weight, and of ensuring that political decisions are responsive to the public. It faces some challenges, however, in handling certain questions of justice. For instance, determining whose voice counts in democratic decisions requires settling the question of the scope of justice (Goodin, 2007), which makes it difficult to derive an account of the scope of justice from democracy alone. Additionally, if voters are confused or uninterested, they may reach outcomes that are substantively bad, and pure democracy may also reach outcomes that are bad for those in the minority (Arneson, 2009). Finally, real-world decision-making processes, even formally democratic ones, frequently give insufficient weight to the voices of poor or socially excluded groups (Young, 2000).

In public health, democracy frequently plays a role in determining whether a given intervention is implemented or a given consideration is accepted as relevant to justice. For instance, votes about whether to tax sugary drinks or unhealthy foods frequently reflect judgments about the justice of taxation. Similarly, votes on gun control in various states and municipalities raise judgments about the justice of regulation. Norman Daniels and James Sabin (2002) suggest that an approach they call "accountability for reasonableness," which has affinities with deliberative democracy, can be used to set priorities in a variety of health settings, including negotiations between governments and providers of health care services.

Although the most popular way of resolving disagreements rests on some version of democracy, alternatives exist. One prominent alternative to democracy is to appeal to some foundational moral ideal. For instance, Nussbaum (2003) bases her list of capabilities not on democratic, collective judgments, but on an Aristotelian account of what it means for a human being to flourish. Similarly, some utilitarians regard the importance of maximizing overall welfare as a foundational truth to which we can reason by simply reflecting on the nature of human rationality (de Lazari-Radek and Singer, 2014).

Conclusion

Just as medicine's emphasis on individual-level dilemmas connects it with individual morality and ethics, public health's population-level emphasis inevitably connects it with political philosophy and justice. Understanding the landscape of justice will enable actors within public health systems both to evaluate the merits of different public health choices and to compare public health interventions with interventions outside of public health.

References

Anderson, E. 2008. "How Should Egalitarians Cope with Market Risks?" *Theoretical Inquiries in Law* 9(1): 239–270.

Arneson, R. 2009. "The Supposed Right to a Democratic Say." In *Contemporary Debates in Political Philosophy*, edited by Thomas Christiano and John Christman, 197–212 (Oxford: Wiley-Blackwell).

Arneson, R. 2010. "Two Cheers for Capabilities." In *Measuring Justice: Primary Goods and Capabilities*, edited by Harry Brighouse and Ingrid Robeyns, 101–127 (New York: Cambridge University Press).

Arrhenius, G., Ryberg, J., and Tännsjö, T. 2010. "The Repugnant Conclusion." In *The Stanford Encyclopedia of Philosophy*, edited by E. N. Zalta (Stanford, Calif.: Stanford University). http://plato.stanford.edu/archives/spr2014/entries/repugnant-conclusion/.

Arrow, K. 1973. "Some Ordinalist-Utilitarian Notes on Rawls's Theory of Justice." *Journal of Philosophy* 70(9): 245–263.

Barnhill, A. 2015. "Choice, Respect, and Value: The Ethics of Healthy Eating Policy." *Wake Forest Journal of Law and Policy* 5: 1–38.

Bentham, J. 1843. *The Works of Jeremy Bentham, Vol. 1 (Principles of Morals and Legislation, Fragment on Government, Civil Code, Penal Law)* (Edinburgh: William Tait).

Brennan, G., and Hamlin, A. 2004. "Analytic Conservatism." *British Journal of Political Science* 34(4): 675–691.

Cohen, G. A. 1997. "Where the Action Is: On the Site of Distributive Justice." *Philosophy and Public Affairs* 26(1): 3–30.

Cohen, J. 2009. "Reflections on Deliberative Democracy." In *Contemporary Debates in Political Philosophy*, edited by Thomas Christiano and John Christman, 247–265 (Oxford: Wiley-Blackwell).

Daniels, N. 1990. "Equality of What: Welfare, Resources, or Capabilities?" *Philosophy and Phenomenological Research* 50: 273–296.

Daniels, N., and Sabin, J. E. 2002. *Setting Limits Fairly: Can We Learn to Share Medical Resources?* (Oxford: Oxford University Press).

Deaton, A. 2003. "How to Monitor Poverty for the Millennium Development Goals." *Journal of Human Development* 4(3): 353–378.

de Lazari-Radek, K., and Singer, P. 2014. *The Point of View of the Universe: Sidgwick and Contemporary Ethics* (Oxford: Oxford University Press).

Donaldson, S., and Kymlicka, W. 2013. *Zoopolis: A Political Theory of Animal Rights* (New York: Oxford University Press).

Emanuel, E. J. 2012. "Global Justice and the 'Standard of Care' Debates." In *Global Justice and Bioethics*, edited by E. J. Emanuel and J. Millum, 181–212 (New York: Oxford University Press).

Eyal, N. 2013. "Leveling Down Health." In *Inequalities in Health: Concepts, Measures, and Ethics*, edited by N. Eyal, S. Hurst, O. F. Norheim, and D. Wikler, 197–213 (Oxford: Oxford University Press).

Faden, R., and Powers, M. 2006. *Social Justice: The Moral Foundations of Public Health and Health Policy* (Oxford: Oxford University Press).

Feder, J. 2014. "The Inevitability of Disruption in Health Reform." *Timely Analysis of Health Policy Issues* (February). http://www.urban.org/sites/default/files/alfresco/publication-pdfs/413027-The-Inevitability-of-Disruption-in-Health-Reform.PDF.

Feiring, E. 2008. "Lifestyle, Responsibility and Justice." *Journal of Medical Ethics* 34(1): 33–36.

Freeman, S. 2006. "Frontiers of Justice: The Capabilities Approach vs. Contractarianism." *Texas Law Review* 85(2): 385–430.

Fukuda-Parr, S. 2003. "The Human Development Paradigm: Operationalizing Sen's Ideas on Capabilities." *Feminist Economics* 9(2–3): 301–317.

Gold, M. R., Stevenson, D., and Fryback, D. G. 2002. "HALYS and QALYS and DALYS, Oh My: Similarities and Differences in Summary Measures of Population Health." *Annual Review of Public Health* 23(1): 115–134.

Goodin, R. E. 2007. "Enfranchising All Affected Interests, and Its Alternatives." *Philosophy and Public Affairs* 35(1): 40–68.

Gutmann, A., and Thompson, D. 2004. *Why Deliberative Democracy?* (Princeton, N.J.: Princeton University Press).

Hume, D. 1739. *A Treatise of Human Nature* (London: Longman).

Hurley, S. 2002. "Roemer on Responsibility and Equality." *Law and Philosophy* 21(1): 39–64.

Kass, N., Hecht, K., Paul, A., and Birnbach, K. 2014. "Ethics and Obesity Prevention: Ethical Considerations in 3 Approaches to Reducing Consumption of Sugar-Sweetened Beverages." *American Journal of Public Health* 104(5): 787–795.

Miller, D. 1990. "Distributive Justice." In *Market, State, and Community: Theoretical Foundations of Market Socialism*, 151–174 (Oxford: Oxford University Press).

Nagel, T. 1991. *Equality and Partiality* (New York: Oxford University Press).

Nozick, R. 1974. *Anarchy, State, and Utopia* (New York: Basic Books).

Nussbaum, M. 2003. "Capabilities as Fundamental Entitlements: Sen and Social Justice." *Feminist Economics* 9(2–3): 33–59.

Ottersen, T., Mæstad, O., and Norheim, O. F. 2014. "Lifetime QALY Prioritarianism in Priority Setting: Quantification of the Inherent Trade-Off." *Cost Effectiveness and Resource Allocation* 12(1): 1.

Ottersen, T., Mbilinyi, D., Mæstad, O., and Norheim, O. F. 2008. "Distribution Matters: Equity Considerations among Health Planners in Tanzania." *Health Policy* 85(2): 218–227.

Parfit, D. 1984. *Reasons and Persons* (Oxford: Oxford University Press).

Parfit, D. 1997. "Equality and Priority." *Ratio* 10(3): 202–221.

Persad, G. 2014. "The Medical Cost Pandemic: Why Limiting Access to Cost-Effective Treatments Hurts the Global Poor." *Chicago Journal of International Law* 15: 559–611.

Persad, G., Wertheimer, A., and Emanuel, E. J. 2009. "Principles for Allocation of Scarce Medical Interventions." *The Lancet* 373(9661): 423–431.

Rawls, J. 1999. *A Theory of Justice* (Cambridge, Mass.: Harvard University Press).

Roemer, J. E. 1993. "A Pragmatic Theory of Responsibility for the Egalitarian Planner." *Philosophy and Public Affairs* 22(2): 146–166.

Ronzoni, M. 2008. "What Makes a Basic Structure Just?" *Res Publica* 14(3): 203–218.

Schmidt, H., Gostin, L. O., and Emanuel, E. J. 2015. "Public Health, Universal Health Coverage, and Sustainable Development Goals: Can They Coexist?" *The Lancet* 389(9996): 928–930.

Schwappach, D. L. B. 2002. "Resource Allocation, Social Values and the QALY: A Review of the Debate and Empirical Evidence." *Health Expectations* 5(3): 210–222.

Sen, A. 1985. "Well-Being, Agency and Freedom: The Dewey Lectures 1984." *Journal of Philosophy* 82(4): 169–221.
Sen, A. 2004. "Capabilities, Lists, and Public Reason: Continuing the Conversation." *Feminist Economics* 10(3): 77–80.
Shields, L. 2012. "The Prospects for Sufficientarianism." *Utilitas* 24(1): 101–117.
Singer, P. 1979. *Practical Ethics* (New York: Cambridge University Press).
Wagstaff, A., Paci, P., and van Doorslaer, E. 1991. "On the Measurement of Inequalities in Health." *Social Science and Medicine* 33(5): 545–557.
WHO (World Health Organization). 2016. "Life Expectancy at Birth (Years) 2015." http://gamapserver.who.int/gho/interactive_charts/mbd/life_expectancy/atlas.html.
Young, I. M. 2000. *Inclusion and Democracy* (New York: Oxford University Press).

CHAPTER 5

HUMAN RIGHTS AND PUBLIC HEALTH ETHICS

S. MATTHEW LIAO

INTRODUCTION

MANY people who care about public health believe that the human rights framework is and should be an integral part of public health policies (Mann et al., 1994; Mann, 1997; Gruskin and Dickens, 2006). After all, the human right to health is enshrined in the Universal Declaration of Human Rights (UNGA, 1948) and other international documents, such as the International Covenant on Economic, Social and Cultural Rights (UNGA, 1966). In addition, public health policies and human rights interact with one another in myriad ways (Mann, 1997). For instance, public health policies can sometimes "burden" human rights (Mann et al., 1994). Mandatory testing, quarantine, and isolation during pandemic outbreaks require prioritizing public welfare over individual liberty. Human rights violations also often have a negative impact on health. Torture, rape, and other traumatic events are associated with severe psychological trauma in both children and adults (Patel, Kellezi, and Williams, 2014). More positively, protecting human rights often improves health. As an example, helping girls and women to gain access to education, an adequate standard of living, necessary medical care, and safety and security of the person—each of which is identified as the object of a human right by one or more international documents—has significantly improved their ability to protect themselves from diseases such as HIV/AIDS (UNESCO, 2016).

For the human rights framework to be effective at advancing the objectives of public health policies, however, it is important to have an adequate account of the nature and moral justification of human rights generally, and of the right to health in particular. In addition to addressing the skepticism that some people have expressed about whether there is a human right to health (Sreenivasan, 2012, 2016; Buchanan, 2013), it is necessary to delineate who bears the duty (dutybearers) of making real the putative right to health, the scope and limits of moral obligations to promote health, and anything else that is needed to supplement the human rights framework when devising public health policies. The aim of this chapter is to provide an overview of such an account.

The Nature and Grounds of Human Rights

Human rights are, as A. John Simmons (2001, 185) states, "rights possessed by all human beings (at all times and in all places), simply in virtue of their humanity." But which features of humanity ground human rights? According to James Griffin (2008, 2), human rights can be seen as "protections of our normative agency." While such an agency approach has attractive elements, it seems limited in other ways (Liao, 2010a; Tasioulas, 2010). For example, consider the paradigmatic human right not to be tortured. The fact that torture undermines one's agency by undermining one's capacity to decide how to act, and to stick to that decision, is certainly an important factor in justifying the existence of a human right not to be tortured (Griffin, 2008, 52–53). But it seems that the fact that torture causes great pain is also important in justifying a human right not to be tortured. Thus, it counts against the agency approach that it seems to rule out causing great pain as a justification for a human right not to be tortured.

According to Martha Nussbaum (2011, 20–26), capabilities form the basis of human rights. *Capabilities* are an individual's real opportunities to choose and to act to achieve certain functionings, while *functionings* are various states and activities that an individual can undertake. Nussbaum argues that there are ten central human capabilities that are particularly important, as they are "entailed by the idea of a life worthy of human dignity": life; bodily health; bodily integrity; senses, imagination, and thought; emotions; practical reason; affiliation; other species; play; and control over one's environment (33–34). In Nussbaum's view, all human beings are entitled to these capabilities as a matter of human rights (62).

A problem with Nussbaum's capabilities approach is that it seems that a significant number of human rights cannot be adequately explained in terms of capabilities (Liao, 2015a). For example, capabilities do not seem adequate for explaining what might be called status rights, which are rights that protect our moral status as persons. In the Universal Declaration of Human Rights, the right to recognition everywhere as a person before the law (Article 6); the right to equal protection before the law (Article 7); the right against arbitrary arrest, detention, or exile (Article 9); the right to a fair and public hearing (Article 10); and the right to be presumed innocent until proven guilty (Article 11) are all *status rights*, since they protect our moral status as persons. If the capabilities approach were correct, it would imply that one can sometimes choose not to exercise these rights, since capabilities are concerned with real opportunities to choose. But it does not seem that one can sometimes choose whether or not to exercise these rights. For instance, it does not seem that one can sometimes choose not to be recognized everywhere as a person before the law, choose not to have equal protection before the law, choose to be arrested arbitrarily, choose to have an unfair hearing, or choose to be presumed guilty. Hence, capabilities do not seem particularly well suited to explain these rights.

A third answer to the question of which features of humanity ground human rights takes a broader view, according to which human rights are grounded in a plurality of conditions. Liao (2015a) defends the fundamental conditions approach, according to which human rights protect the fundamental conditions for pursuing a good life. The fundamental conditions comprise various goods, capacities, and options that human beings qua human beings need, whatever else they qua individuals might need, in order to pursue certain basic activities, such as deep personal relationships with one's partner, friends, parents, children; knowledge of the workings of the world, of oneself, and of others; active pleasures such as creative work and play; and passive pleasures such as appreciating beauty.

The fundamental goods are resources that human beings qua human beings need in order to sustain themselves corporeally, including food, water, and air. The fundamental capacities are powers and abilities that human beings qua human beings require in order to pursue the basic activities. These capacities include the capacity to think, to be motivated by facts, to know, to choose an act freely (liberty), to appreciate the worth of something, to develop interpersonal relationships, and to have control over the direction of one's life (autonomy). The fundamental options are those social forms and institutions that human beings qua human beings require if they are to be able to exercise their essential capacities to engage in the basic activities. These social forms and institutions include options to have social interaction, to acquire further knowledge, to evaluate and appreciate things, and to determine the direction of one's life. (It may also be possible to use the fundamental conditions approach to justify the rights of some nonhuman animals. For a non-speciesist account of human moral status, see Liao, 2010b.)

The fundamental conditions approach can explain why the fact that torture causes great pain is relevant for the justification of a human right not to be tortured—namely, because freedom from extreme pain is a fundamental condition for pursuing a good life. Likewise, it can explain why there are status rights. When we pursue a good life, conflicts with others are bound to arise. If and when such conflicts arise, we need guarantees that we will be treated fairly and equally. Fair trial, presumption of innocence, equal protection before the law, not being arrested arbitrarily, and similar protections serve to ensure that we will be treated fairly and equally. For this reason, they are things that human beings qua human beings need whatever they might need in order to pursue a good life; that is, they are fundamental conditions for pursuing a good life.

The Nature of Basic Health

Next, let us consider how health should be understood. According to the World Health Organization (WHO), health is "a state of complete physical, mental, and social well-being, and not merely the absence of disease or infirmity." As numerous people have pointed out, this definition seems too broad (Griffin, 2008, 101). Among other things, the WHO's definition seems to imply that if an individual's complete well-being depended on working at one's dream job, then an individual who was not working at her or his dream job would thereby lack health. More charitably interpreted, the WHO may have offered such a broad definition of health because it was motivated to incorporate social determinants of health into the definition of health itself. Researchers have found that health care is only one of many determinants of health; other determinants include nutrition, education, housing, the level of equality in a society, and a clean environment (Wilkinson and Marmot, 2003). One can acknowledge these social determinants of health, however, without defining health in terms of them.

Alternatively, drawing on Christopher Boorse's (1975) work, Norman Daniels (2008, 37) has defined health as "normal functioning for our species." In particular, for Daniels, health is the absence of pathology (diseases, injuries, and disabilities), where pathology is "any deviation from the natural functional organization of a typical member of a species" (37). A problem with this type of definition of health is that it seems to categorize certain health states incorrectly as pathology. For instance, homosexuality interferes with the statistically normal reproductive function of human species, and accordingly, Boorse (1975, 63) has acknowledged that his definition of health implies that homosexuality is a pathology. To make this implication more palatable, Boorse argues that classifying homosexuality as a pathology is a descriptive project and need not carry any normative/practical implications (see also Kingma, 2007; Daniels, 2008, 37–42). Nonetheless, homosexuality does not seem to be a pathology.

To define health in a way that does not invite these objections, let us first distinguish between basic and non-basic health:

> *Basic health* is the adequate functioning of the various parts of our organism that are needed for the development and exercise of the fundamental capacities.
>
> *Non-basic health* pertains to any biological functioning that does not affect the various parts of our organism that are needed for the development and exercise of the fundamental capacities. (Liao, 2016, 263)

Recall that the fundamental capacities are powers and abilities that human beings qua human beings need in order to pursue a good life. Various parts of our organism are needed for the development and exercise of these fundamental capacities. For instance, various life processes (including respiration, digestion, absorption, metabolism, circulation) and various organ systems (including the nervous system, skeletal system, cardiovascular system, digestive system, immune system, and reproductive system) make up, enable, and sustain these fundamental capacities. These parts of our organism need to be adequately functioning in order to support the development and exercise of the fundamental capacities.

Accordingly, an individual has basic health if the various life processes, organ systems, and so on that are needed for the development and exercise of the fundamental capacities in the individual are adequately functioning. An individual does not have basic health if the life processes, organ systems, and so on that are needed for the development and exercise of the fundamental capacities in the individual are not adequately functioning.

Sometimes, parts of our organism can undergo certain developments or experience certain events that do not affect in any way the adequate functioning of the parts needed for the development and exercise of the fundamental capacities. Such developments and events can be classified as non-basic health matters. For instance, one might develop a benign cyst that affects one's singing ability but nothing else. Suppose that the cyst does not affect in any way the adequate functioning of the parts needed for the development and exercise of the fundamental capacities. It would then be classified as a non-basic health matter.

Some of the crucial factors that can affect basic health include diseases, injuries, disabilities, nutrition, behavior, and aspects of the social, political, and economic environment (Liao, 2016). For instance, pathogenic microorganisms such as bacteria and viruses can infect individuals and give them diseases, thereby resulting in the dysfunction of various parts of our organism that are needed for the development and exercise of the fundamental capacities. Or one may behave in a certain way without realizing that a particular action can damage one's basic health. For instance, a man who is heterosexual and does not use intravenous drugs may mistakenly believe that he cannot get HIV, and therefore need not use protection when having sex.

It should be clear that basic health is narrower than the WHO's definition of health. Among other things, the WHO's definition does not distinguish between basic and non-basic health matters. Moreover, one can accept that basic health crucially depends on social determinants of health *and* that health care may be less important than some of these social determinants in promoting basic health, *without* accepting that basic health should be defined or analyzed in terms of these social determinants. Furthermore, this account avoids some of the potential problems that arise with theories that define health in terms of species-typical functioning. For instance, it does not entail that homosexuality is a pathology, since an individual whose sexual orientation is toward members of the same sex can still have basic health.

The Human Right to Basic Health

According to the fundamental conditions approach, there is a human right to basic health because human beings have human rights to the fundamental conditions for pursuing a good life, and basic health is a fundamental condition for pursuing a good life (Liao, 2016). As noted in the section on "The Nature and Grounds of Human Rights," fundamental conditions are fundamental goods, capacities, and options that human beings qua human beings need whatever else they might need in order to pursue a good life. Basic health is a fundamental condition in this sense. Indeed, without the adequate functioning of the various parts of our organism that are needed for the development and exercise of the fundamental capacities, human beings would not possess the requisite fundamental capacities; and without possessing the requisite fundamental capacities, human beings would not be able to pursue a good life. Because basic health is a fundamental condition for pursuing a good life, human beings have a human right to basic health.

A human right to basic health entails, among other things, that we have a right to the essential resources for promoting and maintaining basic health, including adequate nutrition, basic health care, and basic education. Who has the duty to provide these essential resources? On one view, human rights are rights against every able person, in appropriate circumstances, (Cranston, 1973, 69). This view implies that every able person, in appropriate circumstances, has a duty to provide the essential resources for promoting and maintaining basic health to everyone else. But can everyone have such a duty? It might seem that the answer is no. In fact, this is one reason why some people are skeptical that there can be a right to health (Sreenivasan, 2012). Moreover, lest one think that one can avert this concern by designating states as the sole dutybearers of the right to health, it has also been noted that some resource-poor countries, such as Mozambique, do not have sufficient resources to provide basic health for their citizens (Sreenivasan, 2012).

However, two points should make it more plausible that everyone has this duty (Liao, 2015b). First, we can have partial duties. This means that even if one cannot fulfill all that is required of a duty, as long as one is able to fulfill part of what is required, one has a duty to do as much as one can. Second, everyone's having the duty to provide basic health does not mean that everyone has to do the same thing. Thus, the fact that everyone has this duty does not mean that each of us has to provide basic health for everyone else directly. One's duty could instead be to pay taxes in order to support a system that aims to distribute the essential resources for promoting and maintaining basic health to everyone, or at least to as many people as possible. A discussion of how demanding the duty to provide basic health should be, which relates to how demanding morality itself should be (Liao, 2015b), is outside the scope of this chapter, but the present remarks should go some way toward addressing the concern that there cannot be a right to basic health. With respect to resource-poor states like Mozambique, it seems that the appropriate and plausible thing to say is that the rest of us have the responsibility to do as much as we can to help such states acquire the needed resources (Liao, 2016).

As noted above, in addition to basic health care, factors such as nutrition, education, and a clean environment can also affect basic health, and there are corresponding human rights to nutrition, education, and a clean environment. This raises the issue of how much priority should be given to the right to basic health care as opposed to, for example, the right to education. While space constraints prohibit detailed discussion here, it seems that we generally have an obligation to structure our society and political institutions in such a way that every right of every individual is respected and promoted (Liao, 2016). In a world in which this is not possible, we need a theory of distributive justice to determine how resources can be allocated fairly and in such a way as to ensure that as many people's rights are respected and promoted as possible; Govind Persad's chapter in this volume, "Justice and Public Health," provides a helpful overview of theoretical resources.

Addressing Some Skepticisms Regarding the Right to Health

While many people accept that there is a right to health, some are skeptical about the existence of such a right (Sreenivasan, 2012, 2016; Buchanan, 2013). This section will focus on the following argument by Gopal Sreenivasan: The promotion of health, especially public health, often involves providing public goods. Individuals do not have a (claim) right to public goods. Therefore, individuals do not have a right to (the promotion of) health. To support this argument, Sreenivasan gives the example of herd immunity to diphtheria. Herd immunity seems to be a public good in that it is non-rival (its consumption does not diminish the protection available to others); it is non-excludable (if one person can consume it, then no one else in the herd can be excluded without significant cost); and it is indivisible (each person who enjoys it enjoys all of its protection) (Sreenivasan, 2012). At the same time, argues Sreenivasan, it seems that no individual has a right to herd immunity, not just because of the material cost of a vaccination program, but also because of the "moral" cost of compelling people to be vaccinated (257). If promoting health means, among other things, providing public goods such as herd immunity, but if no individual has a right to public goods such as herd immunity, it would seem to follow that individuals do not have a right to (the promotion of) health.

Here is a way to respond to Sreenivasan. Even if, under normal circumstances, there is no right to herd immunity as a specific public good, there may be a defeasible right to some public goods. Under normal circumstances (e.g., there is not a global pandemic outbreak), there is no right to herd immunity, because achieving herd immunity requires compelling people to be vaccinated, and this should not be done, because people have a right to bodily integrity, at least under normal circumstances (Liao, 2015b). However, this does not establish that there could not be rights to public goods, especially in cases where the public goods do not require impinging on an individual's right to bodily integrity. There is not enough space here to offer a detailed defense of a right to a particular public good, but consider the following: Street lighting is a public good. It does not seem implausible that people could have a right to street lighting, especially if traveling on certain streets at night is particularly dangerous. Such a case suggests that there could be a right to public goods, thus calling into question a crucial premise in Sreenivasan's argument against the right to health.

Some Implications for Public Health

These discussions regarding the nature and justification of human rights in general, and the right to health in particular, contribute to the objectives of public health policy in at least two ways.

First, in public health it is common to think that the responsibilities of promoting and enacting public health measures fall on governments, governmental agencies, and large-scale public programs. But if the duty to promote and maintain basic health belongs to everyone, then the responsibilities of promoting and enacting public health measures do not just fall on state actors; they also fall on individuals and nonstate actors such as private philanthropic foundations and transnational corporations. One might ask how individuals can promote and support public health measures. Some possibilities include paying taxes that would help fund public health measures and complying with public health measures themselves. An implication of the latter may be that individuals have the responsibility to have themselves and their children vaccinated against infectious diseases so that they do not place others at risk of such diseases, even granting that compulsory vaccination would violate their right to bodily integrity.

Second, it is worth considering whether human rights concerns exhaust public health policy. John Tasioulas and Effy Vayena (2015) argue that they do not. Suppose that there is an obesity epidemic in a certain population. According to Tasioulas and Vayena, this would be a public health concern, but not a human rights concern, because "[h]uman rights are about how we treat others, not how we treat ourselves. In avoidably neglecting my health, I do not violate my own rights" (e42). However, it is not clear that one could not violate one's own rights. A plausible case can be made that a person would violate his right not to be enslaved if he sold himself into slavery (Arneson, 2010). In addition, basic health is the adequate functioning of the various parts of our organism that are needed for the development and exercise of the fundamental capacities. Obesity threatens to undermine basic health in a number of ways, such as by raising the likelihood of high blood pressure, diabetes, coronary heart disease, stroke, and respiratory problems. Given that there is a human right to the essential resources for promoting and maintaining basic health, it seems that one would have a right to the essential resources for ameliorating obesity. This may include a right to be educated about proper nutrition, a right to have access to nutritious food, and a right to a system of health care that can diagnose, prevent, and treat obesity.

Tasioulas and Vayena (2015, e43) appear to agree, since they say, "Certainly, people have the right to access a healthy diet and also a right to treatment for obesity." They go on to say, however, that "obesity does not necessarily signify a violation of rights, as indicated by the fact that in developing countries this disorder is more prevalent in people of a higher socioeconomic status than in poorer people" (e43). This line of reasoning seems to presuppose that human rights violations could not take place among people of higher socioeconomic status. But consider sexual and racial discrimination, which are arguably human rights violations. Such discrimination can take place among people of higher socioeconomic status. So the fact that obesity may sometimes be more prevalent in a population of a higher socioeconomic status does not by itself mean that there couldn't be human rights violations in such a population.

That said, it seems correct that human rights concerns do not exhaust public health policy. One reason is that there can be conflicts of rights. Conflicts of rights can arise when two people have the same right to the same medical resource, but there is enough for only one of them (same rights conflict); or when one person's or group's right to something (e.g., not to be harmed) requires restricting another person's or group's right to something else (e.g., freedom of movement) (different rights conflict). In cases of conflicts of rights, a theory of how to adjudicate such conflicts (e.g., a theory of distributive justice, as discussed by Persad in this volume) is needed. The need for such a theory suggests that human rights concerns do not exhaust public health policy.

Conclusion

Human rights are an integral part of public health policies. This chapter argues that we can further understand and shape the objectives of these policies by considering the merits and demerits of grounding human rights in terms of agency, capabilities, or fundamental conditions for pursuing a good life, and by recognizing that the proper object of human rights is basic health. Also, these discussions reveal that the duty to promote and maintain public health measures does not fall only on governments, but rather belongs to everyone, and that in cases of conflicts of human rights, we need theoretical resources beyond the human rights framework. Attending to the philosophical nature of human rights and the right to health thereby yields additional insights regarding how public health policies should be understood and devised. Human rights theory deserves to be part of the debate concerning the foundations of public health ethics.

Acknowledgments

Parts of this chapter are drawn from Liao (2015a). The author would like to thank Maria Merritt, Jeff Kahn, Andrew Siegel, and Adam Etinson for their helpful comments regarding earlier versions of this chapter.

References

Arneson, R. J. 2010. "Self-Ownership and World Ownership: Against Left-Libertarianism." *Social Philosophy and Policy* 27: 168–194.
Boorse, C. 1975. "On the Distinction between Disease and Illness." *Philosophy and Public Affairs* 5: 49–68.
Buchanan, A. 2013. *The Heart of Human Rights* (New York: Oxford University Press).
Cranston, M. 1973. *What Are Human Rights?* (London: Bodley Head).
Daniels, N. 2008. *Just Health: Meeting Health Needs Fairly* (Cambridge: Cambridge University Press).
Griffin, J. 2008. *On Human Rights* (Oxford: Oxford University Press).
Gruskin, S., and Dickens, B. 2006. "Human Rights and Ethics in Public Health." *American Journal of Public Health* 96(11): 1903–1905.
Kingma, E. 2007. "What Is It to Be Healthy?" *Analysis* 67(294): 128–133.

Liao, S. M. 2010a. "Agency and Human Rights." *Journal of Applied Philosophy* 27(1): 15–25.

Liao, S. M. 2010b. "The Basis of Human Moral Status." *Journal of Moral Philosophy* 7: 159–179.

Liao, S. M. 2015a. "Human Rights as Fundamental Conditions for a Good Life." In *Philosophical Foundations of Human Rights*, edited by R. Cruft, S. M. Liao, and M. Renzo, 79–100 (Oxford: Oxford University Press).

Liao, S. M. 2015b. *The Right to Be Loved* (New York: Oxford University Press).

Liao, S. M. 2016. "Health (Care) and Human Rights: A Fundamental Conditions Approach." *Theoretical Medicine and Bioethics* 37(4): 259–274.

Mann, J. M. 1997. "Medicine and Public Health, Ethics and Human Rights." *Hastings Center Report* 27(3): 6–13.

Mann, J. M., Gostin, L., Gruskin, S., Brennan, T., Lazzarini, Z., and Fineberg, H. 1994. "Health and Human Rights." *Health and Human Rights* 1(1): 6–23.

Nussbaum, M. C. 2011. *Creating Capabilities: The Human Development Approach* (Cambridge, Mass.: Belknap Press).

Patel, N., Kellezi, B., and Williams, A. C. 2014. "Psychological, Social and Welfare Interventions for Psychological Health and Well-Being of Torture Survivors." *Cochrane Database of Systematic Reviews* 11: CD009317. https://www.cochranelibrary.com/cdsr/doi/10.1002/14651858.CD009317.pub2/full.

Simmons, A. J. 2001. "Human Rights and World Citizenship: The Universality of Human Rights." In *Justification and Legitimacy: Essays on Rights and Obligations*, 179–196 (Cambridge: Cambridge University Press).

Sreenivasan, G. 2012. "A Human Right to Health? Some Inconclusive Scepticism." *Aristotelian Society Supplementary Volume* 86(1): 239–265.

Sreenivasan, G. 2016. "Health Care and Human Rights: Against the Split Duty Gambit." *Theoretical Medicine and Bioethics* 37(4): 343–364.

Tasioulas, J. 2010. "Taking Rights Out of Human Rights." *Ethics* 120(4): 647–678.

Tasioulas, J. and Vayena, E. 2015. "Getting Human Rights Right in Global Health Policy." *Lancet* 385(9978): e42–e44.

UNGA (United Nations General Assembly). 1948. Universal Declaration of Human Rights. Resolution 217 A, December 10. http://www.un.org/en/universal-declaration-human-rights/.

UNGA (United Nations General Assembly). 1966. International Covenant on Economic, Social and Cultural Rights. Resolution 2200 A, December 16. http://www.ohchr.org/EN/ProfessionalInterest/Pages/CESCR.aspx.

UNESCO (United Nations Educational, Scientific and Cultural Organization). 2016. *Education for People and Planet: Creating Sustainable Futures for All—Global Education Monitoring Report* (Paris: UNESCO Publishing). https://en.unesco.org/gem-report/node/1279.

Wilkinson, R., and Marmot, M., eds. 2003. *The Social Determinants of Health: The Solid Facts* (Geneva, Switzerland: World Health Organization).

SECTION TWO

HOW PUBLIC HEALTH DOES ITS WORK

CHAPTER 6

AN OVERVIEW OF ETHICS AND HOW PUBLIC HEALTH DOES ITS WORK

HOLLY A. TAYLOR

INTRODUCTION

MODERN public health in the United States is conducted by a network of private, public, local, state, tribal, and federal organizations, agencies, individuals, and communities. The seeds of this network were planted in the eighteenth century, when local efforts led to the isolation and quarantine of humans and cargo arriving from overseas, with the goal of protecting people from potential disease (IOM, 1988). As science advanced and populations grew, local public health took on the protection of the health and welfare of citizens in additional ways. In general, early American public health efforts were dominated by local- and state-level efforts directed at the needs of local citizens. The role of the federal government in public health began with the establishment of the first marine hospital in 1801 (HHS, 2017). In 1870 the administration of a number of marine hospitals was centralized under the Marine Hospital Service (HHS, 2017). Based in port cities of the United States, the goal of the service was to attend to the health and welfare of merchant seamen. The Marine Hospital Service became the US Public Health Service early in the 20th century (IOM, 1988). Yet, in many ways, states and localities in the United States have maintained considerable responsibility for protecting the public's health.

The ethical mandate of public health has always been to protect and promote the health and well-being of the population. Yet such a goal has sometimes put the practice of public health in direct conflict with the quintessential American value of personal liberty. As such, a recurring ethics question for public health surrounds the degree to which the state can infringe on the autonomous choices of the individual in order to protect or promote the public's health (Bayer and Moreno, 1986; Childress et al., 2002).

The quarantine and isolation of goods and humans centuries ago resulted in questions about the role of public health in regulating commerce and the limits that ought to be placed on infringement of an individual's movements. As populations grew, so did the need for the establishment and upkeep of sewage systems. Identifying who should be responsible for the funding of such infrastructure led to the entanglement of public health with private and commercial interests.

More contemporary perspectives on public health argue that the protection of the public's health ought to be undergirded by a commitment to social justice. In this view, efforts should be made to address health disparities as well as to avoid particular public health efforts that might further disadvantage already disadvantaged groups (Beauchamp, 1976; Powers and Faden, 2008). Today, the US public health system affects every American household and involves activities such as monitoring early warning systems for infectious disease outbreaks and assuring access to childhood vaccination.

Chapter Overviews

The following three chapters in this section of *The Oxford Handbook of Public Health Ethics* examine public health ethics through the lenses of the US public health system, public health interventions, and public health law and regulation, respectively. The chapters are introduced below.

In "The US Public Health System and Ethics," Debra DeBruin and Jonathon P. Leider begin with an introduction to the depth and breadth of the public health system. The authors note that the public health system is generally "invisible" to the general public, at least until something goes wrong, such as an outbreak of disease or the contamination of a water system. They argue that ethical issues pervade the conduct of public health, from the development of national strategies to day-to-day decisions made by local health officers. They conclude with a focus on the ethics of pandemic influenza planning from the perspective of a local health department, emphasizing the challenge of how best to respond to a public health emergency without exacerbating health disparities among the populations affected.

One mechanism by which public health authorities tackle the control and prevention of disease is through the delivery of behavioral interventions. Initially, as outlined above, these interventions targeted the control of communicable disease. While the control and prevention of communicable diseases remains an ongoing focus of public health efforts, the second chapter in this section brings attention to the ethical challenges in the prevention of chronic disease, which presents a growing burden on the health of populations in high-income as well as low- and middle-income settings (NCHS, 2016; Wang et al., 2016).

In "Public Health Interventions: Ethical Implications," David R. Buchanan first distinguishes public health interventions from clinical care delivery. He then argues that there are at least two ways to parse public health interventions. The first is to determine if they are infectious or chronic; the second examines whether interventions are best directed at individuals (e.g., educational) or at the environment (e.g., improving neighborhood safety). Noting that 85 percent of morbidity and mortality in high-income countries is related to chronic disease and its complex web of risk factors, Buchanan focuses most of the chapter on ethics issues related to the prevention and control of chronic disease. He notes that this area raises not only the classic ethical tension between what is best for the community versus what promotes the liberty of the individual, but also more broadly requires attention to social determinants of health. Chronic disease highlights how varying levels of disadvantage can predict the ability of an individual or community to succeed in efforts to prevent or control noncommunicable disease, raising new questions regarding the role of public health in addressing systemic disadvantage.

Buchanan then elaborates on the differences between educational and environmental interventions, highlighting the challenge of understanding the interaction among individual behaviors, social determinants, and the built and natural environment on the health of individuals and the communities in which they live. He delineates three key ethical considerations related to implementing public health interventions directed at chronic disease: the potential individual and community harms to avoid, attention to distributive and social justice, and how to buttress rather than diminish social solidarity.

Public health law has been used as a powerful tool to restrict and promote behaviors of individuals and communities in efforts to enhance the health of the population. The law has been a central tool of public health from the earliest of years of public health in the service of controlling the spread of communicable disease. The landmark US Supreme Court case *Jacobson v. Commonwealth of Massachusetts* (197 U.S. 11 [1905]) concluded that the state could require an individual to be vaccinated against communicable disease despite the informed decision of the individual to refuse. The court ruled that the interests of the state in preventing smallpox outweighed the individual's right to refuse vaccination (Colgrove and Bayer, 2005). Today, public health law, in its many forms, plays a key role in the restriction and regulation of actions taken by individuals, communities, agencies, and organizations to protect and promote health and well-being. The authors of the final chapter in this section knit the two threads of this section—communicable and noncommunicable disease—together by highlighting contemporary examples of the role of law in the age-old challenge of preventing infectious disease and the more modern challenges of obesity and tobacco use.

In "The Intersection of Law, Ethics, and Public Health in the United States," Stacie P. Kershner and Leslie E. Wolf begin by distinguishing health care law from public health law. The former, just as with health care in general, focuses on the relationship between physicians and their patients. The latter focuses on the powers and duties of the state to promote the health of populations. Next, the authors delineate the multiple sources of public health laws: federal and state constitutions, statutes, regulations, court decisions, and executive orders. They introduce the *Jacobson* case as a milestone in public health law that put the court in the position of balancing individual liberty with the health and well-being of the community. The court concluded that individual liberty could be infringed when the proposed measure is necessary to avert a threat to public health, and when the measure is reasonable and proportional given the threat of harm to be averted. The authors note that while public health law often creates limits around potential actions that a public health authority may take, public health ethics can help identify the best options among permissible actions. Kershner and Wolf conclude the chapter with examples of public health law in action in the context of infectious disease prevention, tobacco control, and the prevention of obesity and related chronic diseases.

Conclusion

Over the last two centuries, significant advances have improved population health. Progress has been facilitated through a combination of regulation, public policy, education, and environmental change. Nonetheless, the enterprise of public health has faced, and will continue to face, ethical challenges. Public health must navigate between the promotion of public health and the degree to which the liberty of individuals can be restricted, while also attending to underlying commitments to justice. It also must continue to contend with the extent to which it can regulate the behavior of individuals and communities, or change the environment, to promote the health of populations.

References

Bayer, R., and Moreno, J. 1986. "Health Promotion: Ethical and Social Dilemmas of Government Policy." *Health Affairs* 5(2): 72–85.

Beauchamp, D. 1976. "Public Health as Social Justice." *Inquiry* 13(1): 3–14.

Childress, J., Faden, R., Gaare, R., Gostin, L., Kahn, J., Bonnie, R., et al. 2002. "Public Health Ethics: Mapping the Terrain." *Journal of Law, Medicine & Ethics* 30(2): 170–180.

Colgrove, J., and Bayer, R. 2005. "Manifold Restraints: Liberty, Public Health, and the Legacy of *Jacobson v Massachusetts*." *American Journal of Public Health* 95(4): 571–576.

HHS (US Department of Health and Human Services). 2017. "History." Commissioned Corps of the US Public Health Service. https://www.usphs.gov/aboutus/history.aspx.

IOM (Institute of Medicine). 1988. *The Future of Public Health* (Washington, D.C.: National Academies Press).

NCHS (National Center for Health Statistics). 2016. *Health, United States, 2015: With Special Feature on Racial and Ethnic Health Disparities* (Hyattsville, Md.: National Center for Health Statistics).

Powers, M., and Faden, R. R. 2008. *Social Justice: The Moral Foundations of Public Health and Health Policy* (New York: Oxford University Press).

Wang, H., Naghavi, M., Allen, C., Barber, R. M., Bhutta, Z. A., Carter, A., et al. 2016. "Global, Regional, and National Life Expectancy, All-Cause Mortality, and Cause-Specific Mortality for 249 Causes of Death, 1980–2015: A Systematic Analysis for the Global Burden of Disease Study 2015." *Lancet*. 388(10053): 1459–1544.

CHAPTER 7

THE US PUBLIC HEALTH SYSTEM AND ETHICS

DEBRA DEBRUIN AND JONATHON P. LEIDER

What Governmental Public Health Is and What It Does

Governmental public health is among the least well-known aspects of the broad, complex web of public and private organizations that constitute America's health system (Bradley and Taylor, 2013). The public tends to hear about public health during a disease outbreak, when food safety issues arise, or when questions of government paternalism are topics of conversations in the media (Novick, Morrow, and Mays, 2007). Where health care organizations focus mostly on direct patient care, governmental public health agencies have long been charged with the health of entire communities (CDC, 2010; IOM, 1988). Moreover, while the tools of a clinician might involve a surgical or medicinal intervention, the tools of public health are outbreak investigation, taxation, enforcement, and health education, among other population-oriented activities (Hearne et al., 2015). In some jurisdictions, where populations lack good access to health care, health departments have also long provided direct-care services in addition to population-oriented ones.

This chapter will characterize the mission of public health; describe the governmental public health system infrastructure in the United States and explain how it strives to meet the mission of public health; demonstrate the centrality of ethics to public health systems; outline the types of ethical considerations that arise in the work of public health; and consider a case study to show how ethical concerns arise and may be resolved in the complex, multilevel system of governmental public health.

"Public health" represents the means by which society can protect and promote the health of the population, as well as subpopulations of interest (Faden and Shebaya, 2010; Hardcastle et al., 2011). It focuses on "fulfilling society's interest in assuring conditions in which people can be healthy" (IOM, 1988, 140). Health departments historically provided a small set of services to the populations they served related to surveillance, outbreak investigation, and infectious disease control, as well as some basic safety-net clinical care such as immunizations and clinics (Cutler and Miller, 2005; Nelson and Williams, 2007). There was also a significant emphasis on sanitation to minimize disease incidence and spread. This movement of "public health" began in earnest in the United States in the 1800s in urban areas, eventually working its way to the vast rural and frontier areas of the United States. Formalized public health systems and infrastructure began to arise through the creation of state and local health departments, which quickly became charged with providing additional services and protections, including environmental health, chronic disease control and prevention, and maternal and child health[1] (IOM, 1988).

In the late 1980s, the Institute of Medicine (now the National Academy of Medicine of the National Academies of Sciences, Engineering, and Medicine) recommended that health departments allow private providers and community health centers to provide safety-net clinical services. However, as of 2013, most local health departments (LHDs) have not fully divested their clinical services. LHDs still provide a number of direct clinical services to patients, including vaccinations, clinical screening, and treatment for infectious disease, with some providing primary care directly. Overall, only 5 percent of LHDs provide no clinical services at all (NACCHO, 2014). While LHDs within states have tended to be funded to do similar things (e.g., provide clinical services), intrastate variation was (and is) also substantial (NACCHO, 2014; Parker et al., 2012). The profound variety in the organization and delivery of governmental public health services occurred mainly due to public health's assurance function as a provider of last resort, as well as a lack of other providers—public or private—in many smaller, rural communities (Corso et al., 2000; Handler and Turnock, 1996). Each community had different needs, as well as a different history, legal framework, and funding basis for its LHD. As such, each LHD has come to look a bit different from its neighbor. Moreover, LHD infrastructure has grown in dramatically different directions. Where rural LHDs tend to be smaller and provide more clinical services, a number of the nation's largest LHDs have grown to more closely resemble state health agencies in their size and focus (Harris et al., 2016; Leider, Castrucci, et al., 2015; Meit and Knudson, 2009). Just 5 percent (N=137) of health departments in the United States cover 50 percent of the population. The largest 1 percent covers 15 percent, or over 45 million people (Leider, Castrucci, et al., 2015). The budget of the nation's largest local health department exceeds $1.4 billion—larger than most state health agencies' budgets (ASTHO, 2014; Merrill and Francisco, 2016).

Defining the Terms and the Mission of Public Health

Public health provides a mechanism to protect and promote the health of society. Many modern definitions of public health have been offered, arguably beginning with Charles Winslow's definition, which is both functional and aspirational:

> Public health is the science and the art of preventing disease, prolonging life and promoting physical health and efficiency through organized community efforts for the sanitation of the environment, the control of community infections, the education of the individual in principles of personal hygiene, the organization of medical and nursing service for the early diagnosis and preventive treatment of disease, and the development of social machinery which will ensure to every individual in the community a standard of living adequate for the maintenance of health.
>
> (Winslow, 1920, 30)

Winslow's definition held for over sixty years. Since then, major national and international organizations, such as the Institute of Medicine and the World Health Organization (WHO), have offered their own definitions (IOM, 1988; WHO, 1994). Faden and Shebaya (2010) offer four characteristics that distinguish public health from other public and private entities—characteristics that begin to define the ethical issues faced by public health practitioners: (1) public health is a public or collective good, (2) its promotion involves a particular focus on prevention, (3) its promotion often entails government action, and (4) it involves an intrinsic outcomes-orientation. How health is defined has important implications for the mission (and proper role) of governmental public health (Powers and Faden, 2006). For the WHO, health is "a state of complete physical, mental and social well-being and not merely the absence of disease or infirmity" (WHO, 1994, 1). Since "complete" well-being extends beyond the scope of somatic or behavioral health, adoption of this definition of health broadens the role of governmental public health beyond the primary prevention of disease to addressing all determinants of health and well-being. Other major definitions of health tend to focus more on physical and/or mental status of individuals, as compared to holistic measures of well-being (Kindig and Stoddart, 2003). Governmental public health in the United States tends to focus more on safety and health improvement, although there has been a recent push to incorporate public health systems and systems thinking into nonhealth sectors, such as housing and urban planning, transportation, and education (Wernham and Teutsch, 2015).

Public health concerns not just the health of individuals, but also health within and across groups and communities. As such, scholars have offered a number of definitions of "population health." Kindig and Stoddard (2003, 381) outline the most prominent definition: "the health outcomes of a group of individuals, including the distribution of such outcomes within the group." Beyond a mere aggregation of individuals' health status, Kindig and Stoddard's definition includes a distributional component. Social justice scholars have highlighted this consideration when enumerating ethical issues in public health practice.

Public Health Infrastructure in the United States

Governmental public health in the United States operates within a system of federalism. Practically, this means that while the federal government has broad authority over health issues (especially those with interstate and intercountry ramifications), many public health powers are retained by the states. There is substantial variation in public health infrastructure state to state because of this home rule philosophy.

The United States has a flagship federal public health agency, the Centers for Disease Control and Prevention (CDC). In addition, several agencies conduct public health activities or otherwise influence population health. These include the Health Resources and Services Administration (HRSA), the Food and Drug Administration (FDA), the Environmental Protection Administration (EPA), the Department of Agriculture (USDA), and other agencies within the broad Department of Health and Human Services (HHS) (IOM, 2012). There is one state health agency (SHA) per state, and approximately 2,800 local health departments across the United States (ASTHO, 2014; NACCHO, 2014). There are also territorial and tribal health agencies, which tend to be smaller, integrate health care and public health activities, and emphasize health care services (IOM, 1988; Mays, Halverson, and Scutchfield, 2003).

Public health is financed through a complex web of federal, state, and local funds (Leider, 2016). State funds were once the largest single source of revenue for health departments, but the Great Recession that began in 2007 resulted in cuts in state and local dollars to health departments. Coupled with modest increased federal investment in specific areas like bioterrorism and all-hazards preparedness, federal sources surpassed others in the late 2000s. This has allowed the federal government to significantly dictate the types of programs and services that state and local health departments provide (Leider, 2016). On the one hand, the increased standardization of activities has resulted in access to certain public health protections that is more equal. On the other hand, fewer funds are available to address community-specific needs. It is an open question as to whether this approach is equitable.

The federal government has long had a substantial impact on the nation's health. As Table 7.1 shows, federal policies have addressed both direct care and population-oriented activities for over 200 years, though the United States' public health infrastructure has solidified just in the past 100 years. Historically, the federal government exercised regulatory and enforcement oversight related to public health protections, whether from infectious disease, environmental hazards or pollutants, unsafe working conditions, or hazardous consumer goods. In the mid-twentieth century, the federal government became a large-scale funder of the nation's health, both through health care reforms (e.g., Medicare and Medicaid) and the creation of federal public health infrastructure.

Governmental health departments in the United States perform a variety of services, mostly governed by what is funded and what is required by local, state, or federal law (IOM, 2012). Federal and state agencies tend to conduct high-level regulatory, surveillance, and primary prevention efforts, whereas LHDs tend to be the "boots on the ground," delivering immunizations, doing food safety inspections, conducting health outreach campaigns, and so on (see Table 7.2). National surveys of public health activity largely confirm this theoretical division of labor. In addition to governmental entities, many nongovernmental organizations (NGOs) perform public health activities, especially related to health education and outreach.

Table 7.1 History of Select US Health Policies with Implications for Public Health and Population Health

Direct-care oriented	Population oriented
1798: Federal hospitals for sick/disabled seamen (Marine Hospital Services)	1862: Forerunner to Food and Drug Administration created
1921: Indian Health Services created, first Maternal/Child Health grants	1871: Surgeon General appointed
1924: Veteran's Bureau	1878: National Quarantine Act
1965: Medicare/Medicaid	1891: Marine Hospital Services responsible for screening immigrants
1966: Community Health Centers launched	1930: Forerunner to National Institutes of Health created
1990: Ryan White HIV/AIDS Program funded	1938: Federal Food, Drug, and Cosmetic Act
1997: SCHIP (Children's Health Insurance Program)	1946: Forerunner to Centers for Disease Control and Prevention created
2003: Medicare Modernization Act (Part D—Prescriptions for Seniors)	1971: National Cancer Act
2010: Affordable Care Act	1993: Vaccines for Children Program

Sources: Nelson and Williams, 2007; Patterson, 1986; Harding and Rodgers, 2012.

Table 7.2 Services Most Frequently Provided Directly by US State and Local Health Departments

Local health departments		State health agencies	
91%	Surveillance: Infectious disease	100%	Surveillance: Behavioral risk factors
90%	Adult immunization provision	100%	Surveillance: Infectious disease
90%	Child immunization provision	100%	Surveillance: Reportable disease
83%	Tuberculosis screening	100%	Primary prevention: HIV
78%	Surveillance: Environmental health	100%	Primary prevention: Nutrition
78%	Food establishment inspection	100%	Primary prevention: Tobacco
76%	Tuberculosis treatment	98%	Immunization vaccine order management (Vaccines for Children)
72%	Food safety education	98%	Lab services: Bioterrorism agent testing
69%	Primary prevention: Nutrition	98%	Lab services: Foodborne illness testing
69%	Schools/daycare center inspection	98%	Lab services: Newborn screening
		98%	Surveillance: Vital statistics
		98%	Screening: HIV/AIDS
		98%	Screening: Other STDs
		98%	Childhood immunization registry
		98%	Surveillance: Foodborne illness

Sources: ASTHO, 2016; NACCHO, 2016.

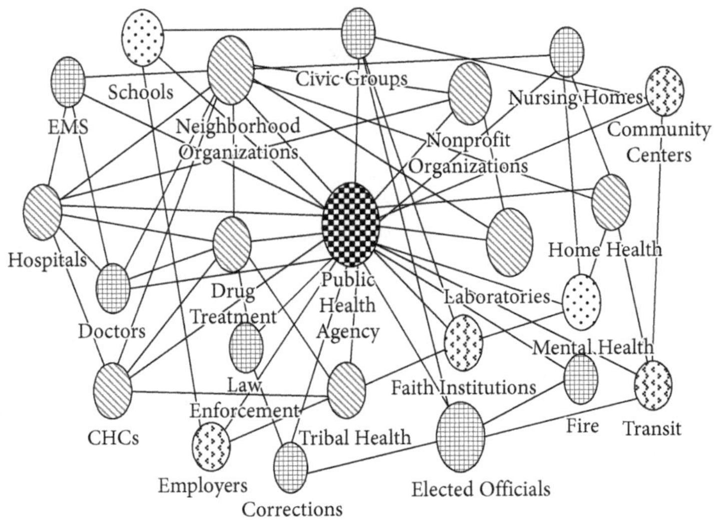

FIGURE 7.1 Actors in the Public Health System

Source: CDC, 2010. Reproduced with permission.

Whereas regulation and enforcement are within the sphere of government, other activities are bolstered by private efforts. Moreover, about three dozen state-level public health institutes and ten public health training centers provide technical assistance to state and local health departments in the United States (Leider, 2016). The institutes and centers are often affiliated with universities (public or private), and they help connect practitioners with evidence-based practices.

Official estimates place the size of the governmental public health workforce at about 300,000 strong across federal, state, and local levels (Beck, Boulton, and Coronado, 2014). However, only about 17 percent of the government workforce has formal training in public health (Leider, Harper, et al., 2015). This has important implications for formal public health education, including ethics. The public health system comprises numerous public and private organizations (see Figure 7.1). Governmental public health is at the center of this system (CDC, 2010). Government action, and inaction, thus creates core challenges for public health ethics.

Ethics and the Public Health System

Professionals working in the public health system routinely confront ethical issues. Indeed,

> [t]he mandate to ensure and protect the health of the public is an inherently moral one. It carries with it an obligation to care for the well-being of communities and it implies the possession of an element of power to carry out that mandate. The need to exercise power to ensure the health of populations and, at the same time, to avoid abuses of such power are at the crux of public health ethics (Thomas et al., 2002, 1057).

Ethical issues pervade all aspects of the work of public health, from the macro level of policy development and large-scale planning to the micro level of day-to-day decision-making.

For example, policies governing disease reporting for public health surveillance must balance protection of the public's health with protections for privacy and confidentiality. Poignant micro-level dilemmas also arise when health department personnel receive reports about, for example, the HIV status of colleagues or friends. In addition, public health interventions routinely limit liberty—consider fluoridation of water, motorcycle helmet laws, and prohibitions on smoking in restaurants. State newborn screening programs engender debates about whether parental consent should be required for screening, not only for research using blood spots. Moreover, social justice issues extend throughout the work of public health, including concerns about reducing health disparities, improving access to health services, reducing the potential stigma of public health campaigns on, for example, tobacco or obesity, and environmental justice issues such as lead in housing or water in low-income communities.

Questions concerning the scope and appropriate boundaries of governmental public health also have ethical significance. How far do the obligations of the public health system extend? As noted above, if health is defined broadly, as the WHO recommends, then the responsibilities of public health encompass the promotion of well-being. Even if health is defined in more limited ways, the scope of public health may extend beyond the common services enumerated in Table 7.2. For example, growing research documents that Americans with lower levels of education face higher levels of risk for chronic illness and premature death (VCU CSH, 2015). Do educational programs fall within the mission of public health? What about jobs programs, affordable and safe housing, or other social programs that may significantly impact health by addressing social determinants of health? An impressive body of research demonstrates the significance of social determinants of health (Marmot, 2005). How does this affect the responsibilities of the public health system? Does it mean the public health system should partner with other governmental systems to implement such programs with an eye toward promoting benefits to health? Should it affect the way public health professionals are trained?

Ethical Issues in Pandemic Influenza Planning

It may be useful to consider how to apply an ethical analysis to a particular topic in terms of how public health systems respond to a particular threat. The example of pandemic influenza planning implicates governmental public health across national, state, local, and tribal systems, and also raises many ethical challenges. Aggressive surveillance and data sharing across governmental agencies can help to protect the public's health, but it can also compromise privacy. Interventions geared toward limiting the spread of infection, such as isolation, quarantine, and other social distancing interventions like closing schools, infringe on personal liberty and can compromise personal well-being by, for example, undermining access to school meals programs. Resources such as vaccines or antiviral medications may be scarce during a pandemic, necessitating ethical guidance for rationing. The ability of health systems to provide care may be dramatically strained, raising questions about the permissibility of compelling health professionals to work, and thus take on potentially significant risk to themselves and their families. These are a few of the many issues that arise due to the complexities of pandemic planning.

One especially pressing challenge for pandemic preparedness concerns health disparities. In particular, socially disadvantaged groups consistently fare worse than more privileged groups in terms of morbidity and mortality during influenza pandemics (see, for example, Blumenshine et al., 2008; Patterson, 1986; Hutchins et al., 2009). Differences across populations in exposure and susceptibility to illness, and in access to care, appear to account for influenza-related health disparities. Members of socially disadvantaged groups tend to be less able to protect themselves from exposure to illness; for example, they may lack resources that would allow them to avoid public transportation, or the employment flexibility to allow telecommuting to work, and they may therefore be unable to adopt recommended social distancing strategies. Socially disadvantaged groups also tend to be more vulnerable to illness, given their higher rates of comorbid chronic conditions that can increase influenza risks. In addition, those who are socially disadvantaged may have poorer access to care (Blumenshine et al., 2008; Quinn et al., 2011). Disparities in influenza morbidity and mortality are thus linked to other health disparities and social inequalities more generally.

Given their persistence—and thus predictability—these disparities in influenza-related morbidity and mortality should be addressed in pandemic plans across public health systems. Indeed, addressing disparities fits centrally with the core mission of public health, given their impact on population health. Moreover, the *Principles of the Ethical Practice of Public Health*, often referred to as the Public Health Code of Ethics, emphasizes that "[p]ublic health should advocate and work for the empowerment of disenfranchised community members, aiming to ensure that the basic resources and conditions necessary for health are accessible to all" (PHLS, 2002, 4). Nevertheless, questions remain about the implications these fundamental commitments have for the particular systems that make up public health. What then must public health professionals do to meet their obligations to address health disparities in the context of pandemic planning?

To begin, public health systems at the state and federal levels need to gather data so that groups who are at higher risk can be identified (Bellagio Meeting, 2006; DeBruin, Liaschenko, and Marshall, 2012). Historical risk-factor data can predict which groups are likely to be at particular risk so that relevant preparations can be made. During a pandemic, event-specific data will be needed to capture the burden of disease associated with the particular strain of pandemic influenza. Public health officials should consider the best approach to gathering data on at-risk populations, as certain sources of data may fail to adequately reflect their situation. For example, hospitalization data may not capture rates of morbidity and mortality in populations lacking adequate access to care. Local and tribal public health systems may be able to provide guidance about approaches to data gathering, given their understanding of their particular communities.

Admittedly, more severe pandemics will impose a greater strain on public health agencies' ability to collect data. Does this potentially limit the obligation to reduce disparities, or does the strength of the obligation demand action in the absence of strong data? Once at-risk groups are identified, further questions arise concerning how to provide services or allocate resources such as vaccines. For example, if members of the public at high risk of death from influenza are prioritized for vaccination, but the vaccine is distributed across geographic areas (e.g., across regions in a given state) in amounts proportional to area population rather than to risk, priority groups may not be reached as needed (DeBruin, Liaschenko, and Marshall, 2012). This further complicates the efforts needed to address disparities, and it heightens questions about the strength of this obligation. Do these difficulties limit, to any extent, the duty to address disparities rather than simply work to reduce morbidity and mortality in the broader population?

Conclusion

As this discussion illustrates, public health professionals must often navigate ethical dilemmas in their work. This means they must be able to identify ethical issues as they arise. The ethical significance of some issues may seem obvious, such as questions about informed consent for newborn screening, or concerns about justice related to health disparities. However, not all ethical issues are so easy to identify. For example, as noted above, questions about the types of data to collect during an influenza pandemic have genuine moral relevance, but recognizing this requires that questions about data collection be explicitly connected to social justice concerns about health disparities. Even when identifying ethical issues seems simple, determining how to resolve these issues is typically far from obvious. Ethical issues tend to be quite complicated and often involve conflicts between values—like those between the value of promoting the public's health, on the one hand, and concerns about privacy, confidentiality, and liberty, on the other.

Given the centrality of ethical challenges to the work of public health, the Council on Linkages Between Academia and Public Health Practice includes ethics among its *Core Competencies for Public Health Professionals* (2014). The Association of Schools and Programs of Public Health includes the ethical dimensions of public health in the critical content for MPH and DrPH degree programs (ASPPH, 2014a, 2014b). Similarly, the Public Health Accreditation Board's latest standards (PHAB, 2013) include a requirement that public health agencies develop and support an infrastructure that promotes ethical decision-making. Thus, these sets of guidelines include explicit expectations concerning ethical practice. They also include responsibilities that are not explicitly framed in terms of ethics but that relate to moral norms, such as cultural competency, consideration of the effect of programs and policies on diverse communities, and solicitation of public input in decision-making (Council on Linkages, 2014; PHAB, 2013).

Given that few who work in governmental public health have formal public health training, it is likely that few have received education in public health ethics, even though ethics is widely recognized as being central to the work of public health. Of course, one does not need formal ethics education to deliberate about moral issues. However, ethics education can support explicit, informed, transparent, and systematic engagement with ethical issues, and thus promote accountability and trustworthiness of decision-making (NACCHO, 2014, Baum et al., 2007, CDC, 2016). To achieve accreditation, public health departments must develop and maintain an ethics infrastructure (PHAB, 2013). This may mean that the department formally adopts the Public Health Code of Ethics as a basis for ethical decision-making, or it may involve the creation of a more substantive ethics infrastructure such as an ethics advisory board (PHAB, 2013). The National Association of County and City Health Officials (NACCHO) recommends that health departments begin to develop their ethics infrastructure by having a leadership model and openly supporting ethical decision-making. Supports include providing training opportunities and other resources for staff (NACCHO, 2015).

It is critical that public health professionals receive the support they need to meet the complex ethical challenges that pervade their work. These challenges arise throughout the work of the governmental public health system, and range from systems issues concerning policy and planning to dilemmas confronting individual public health professionals in their day-to-day work. While it may be laudable for a public health agency to formally adopt the Public Health Code of Ethics as a basis for decision-making, doing so offers little real support for recognizing and resolving ethical challenges as they occur. After all, "[c]odes of ethics are typically relatively brief; they are not designed to provide a means of untangling convoluted ethical issues" (PHLS, 2002, 5). Convoluted ethical issues are not rare in public health. The discussion in this chapter illustrates the sorts of challenges that public health systems routinely encounter as they work to implement ethics guidance, such as the Public Health Code of Ethics, in the messy and detailed context of actual practice. Education programs and ethics advisory boards would provide more robust support than simply adopting the Code of Ethics, but they require political will and dedicated resources. These would be valuable investments in accountability and trustworthiness.

Note

1. By the mid-1990s, federal leaders outlined the ten essential services the public health system must provide: "(1) Monitor health status to identify and solve community health problems. (2) Diagnose and investigate health problems and health hazards in the community. (3) Inform, educate, and empower people about health issues. (4) Mobilize community partnerships and action to identify and solve health problems. (5) Develop policies and plans that support individual and community health efforts. (6) Enforce laws and regulations that protect health and ensure safety. (7) Link people to needed personal health services and assure the provision of health care when otherwise unavailable. (8) Assure competent public and personal health care workforce. (9) Evaluate effectiveness, accessibility, and quality of personal and population-based health services. (10) Research for new insights and innovative solutions to health problems" (CDC, 2010).

References

ASPPH (Association of Schools and Programs of Public Health). 2014a. *DrPH for the Twenty First Century*. http://www.aspph.org/wp-content/uploads/2014/06/DrPH-Report_2014-11-05_FINAL.pdf.

ASPPH (Association of Schools and Programs of Public Health). 2014b. *A Master of Public Health Degree for the Twenty First Century*. http://www.aspph.org/app/uploads/2014/06/MPHPanelReportFINAL_2014-11-03REVISEDfinal1.pdf.

ASTHO (Association of State and Territorial Health Officials). 2014. *ASTHO Profile of Health*, vol. 3. http://www.astho.org/Profile/Volume-Three/.

ASTHO (Association of State and Territorial Health Officials). 2016. *ASTHO Profile of Health*, vol. 4. http://www.astho.org/Profile/Volume-Four/2016-ASTHO-Profile-of-State-and-Territorial-Public-Health/.

Baum, N. M., Gollust, S. E., Goold, S. D., and Jacobson, P. D. 2007. "Looking Ahead: Addressing Ethical Challenges in Public Health Practice." *Journal of Law, Medicine & Ethics* 35(4): 657–667.

Beck, A. J., Boulton, M. L., and Coronado, F. 2014. "Enumeration of the Governmental Public Health Workforce, 2014." *American Journal of Preventive Medicine* 47(5, Suppl. 3), S306–S313.

Bellagio Meeting (Bellagio Meeting on Social Justice and Influenza). 2006. "The Bellagio Statement of Principles." http://www.bioethicsinstitute.org/research/global-bioethics/flu-pandemic-the-bellagio-meeting.

Blumenshine, P., Reingold, A., Egerter, S., Mockenhaupt, R., Braveman, P., and Marks, J. 2008. "Pandemic Influenza Planning in the United States from a Health Disparities Perspective." *Emerging Infectious Disease* 14(5): 709–715.

Bradley, E., and Taylor, L. 2013. *The American Health Care Paradox: Why Spending More Is Getting Us Less* (New York: Public Affairs).

CDC (Centers for Disease Control and Prevention). 2010. "Ten Essential Services of Public Health." http://www.cdc.gov/nphpsp/essentialServices.html.

CDC (Centers for Disease Control and Prevention). 2016. "Public Health Ethics Training Materials." https://www.cdc.gov/od/science/integrity/phethics/trainingmaterials.htm.

Corso, L. C., Wiesner, P. J., Halverson, P. K., and Brown, C. K. 2000. Using the Essential Services as a Foundation for Performance Measurement and Assessment of Local Public Health Systems. *Journal of Public Health Management and Practice* 6(5): 1–18.

Council on Linkages (Council on Linkages Between Academia and Public Health Practice). 2014. *Core Competencies for Public Health Professionals*. http://www.phf.org/resourcestools/Documents/Core_Competencies_for_Public_Health_Professionals_2014June.pdf.

Cutler, D., and Miller, G. 2005. "The Role of Public Health Improvements in Health Advances: The Twentieth-Century United States." *Demography* 42(1): 1–22.

DeBruin, D., Liaschenko, J., and Marshall, M. F. 2012. "Social Justice in Pandemic Preparedness." *American Journal of Public Health* 102(4): 586–591.

Faden, R., and Shebaya, S. 2010. "Public Health Ethics." In *The Stanford Encyclopedia of Philosophy*, edited by E. N. Zalta (Stanford, Calif.: Stanford University). https://plato.stanford.edu/entries/publichealth-ethics/.

Handler, A. S., and Turnock, B. J. 1996. "Local Health Department Effectiveness in Addressing the Core Functions of Public Health: Essential Ingredients." *Journal of Public Health Policy* 17(4): 460–483. http://www.ncbi.nlm.nih.gov/pubmed/9009540.

Hardcastle, L. E., Record, K. L., Jacobson, P. D., Guest, L. O. G., and Leonard, E. W. 2011. "Public Health Reform: Patient Protection and Affordable Care Act Implications for the

Public's Health: Improving the Population's Health: The Affordable Care Act and the Importance of Integration." *Journal of Law, Medicine & Ethics* 39: 317–694.

Harding, D., and Rodgers, R. 2012. *Images from the History of the Public Health Service.* (Bethesda, Md.: National Library of Medicine). https://www.nlm.nih.gov/exhibition/phs_history/.

Harris, J. K., Beatty, K., Leider, J. P., Knudson, A., Anderson, B. L., and Meit, M. 2016. "The Double Disparity Facing Rural Local Health Departments." *Annual Review of Public Health* 37: 167–184.

Hearne, S., Castrucci, B. C., Leider, J. P., Rhoades, E. K., Russo, P., and Bass, V. 2015. "The Future of Urban Health: Needs, Barriers, Opportunities, and Policy Advancement at Large Urban Health Departments." *Journal of Public Health Management and Practice* 21(Suppl. 1): S4–S13. doi:10.1097/PHH.0000000000000166

Hutchins, S. S., Fiscella, K., Levine, R. S., Ompad, D. C., and McDonald, M. 2009. "Protection of Racial/Ethnic Minority Populations during an Influenza Pandemic." *American Journal of Public Health* 99(Suppl. 2): S261–S270.

IOM (Institute of Medicine). 1988. *The Future of Public Health.* A report by the Committee for the Study of the Future of Public Health (Washington, D.C.: National Academy Press).

IOM (Institute of Medicine). 2012. *For the Public's Health: Investing in a Healthier Future.* A report by the Committee on Public Health Strategies to Improve Health (Washington, D.C.: National Academy Press). http://www.nationalacademies.org/hmd/Reports/2012/For-the-Publics-Health-Investing-in-a-Healthier-Future.aspx.

Kindig, D., and Stoddart, G. 2003. "What Is Population Health?" *American Journal of Public Health* 93(3): 380–383. http://www.ncbi.nlm.nih.gov/pmc/articles/PMC1447747/pdf/0930380.pdf.

Leider, J. P. 2016. "The Problem with Estimating Public Health Spending." *Journal of Public Health Management and Practice* 22(2): E1–E11.

Leider, J. P., Castrucci, B. C., Hearne, S., and Russo, P. 2015. "Organizational Characteristics of Large Urban Health Departments." *Journal of Public Health Management and Practice* 21(Suppl. 1): S14–19.

Leider, J. P., Harper, E., Bharthapudi, K., and Castrucci, B. C. 2015. "Educational Attainment of the Public Health Workforce and Its Implications for Workforce Development." *Journal of Public Health Management and Practice* 21(Suppl. 6): S56–S68.

Marmot, M. 2005. "Social Determinants of Health Inequalities." *Lancet* 365(9464): 1099–1104.

Mays, G. P., Halverson, P. K., and Scutchfield, F. D. 2003. "Behind the Curve? What We Know and Need to Learn from Public Health Systems Research." *Journal of Public Health Management and Practice* 9(3): 179–182.

Meit, M., and Knudson, A. 2009. "Why Is Rural Public Health Important? A Look to the Future." *Journal of Public Health Management and Practice* 15(3): 185–190.

Merrill, J., and Francisco, C. 2016. *Report on the Fiscal 2017 Preliminary Budget and the Fiscal 2016 Preliminary Mayor's Management Report* (New York: City Council). https://council.nyc.gov/budget/wp-content/uploads/sites/54/2016/06/816-Public-Health.pdf.

NACCHO (National Association of County and City Health Officials). 2014. *National Profile of Local Health Departments 2014.* http://nacchoprofilestudy.org/.

NACCHO (National Association of County and City Health Officials). 2015. *Building an Ethics Infrastructure in Local Health Departments.* http://eweb.naccho.org/eweb/DynamicPage.aspx?WebCode=proddetailadd&ivd_qty=1&ivd_prc_prd_key=e1e4c80f-569a-4673-a841-56a1ec852d17&Action=Add&site=naccho&ObjectKeyFrom=1A83491A-9853-4C87-86A4-F7D95601C2E2&DoNotSave=yes&ParentObject=CentralizedOrderEntry&ParentDataObject=Invoice%20Detail.

NACCHO (National Association of County and City Health Officials). 2016. *National Profile of Local Health Departments 2016*. http://nacchoprofilestudy.org/.

Nelson, K. E., and Williams, C. M. 2007. "Early History of Infectious Disease: Epidemiology and Control of Infectious Diseases." In *Infectious Disease Epidemiology: Theory and Practice*. 2nd ed. (Burlington, Mass.: Jones & Bartlett).

Novick, L. F., Morrow, C. B., and Mays, G. P. 2007. *Public Health Administration: Principles for Population-Based Management* (Sudbury, Mass.: Jones & Bartlett).

Patterson, K. D. 1986. *Pandemic Influenza 1700–1900: A Study in Historical Epidemiology*. (Totowa, N.J.: Rowan & Littlefield).

Parker, A. M., Shelton, S. R., Morganti, K. G., and Nelson, C. 2012. "Assessing Relationships between State and Local Public Health Organizations: Evidence from the NACCHO 2008 Profile of Local Health Departments." *Journal of Public Health Management and Practice* 18(2): 156–159.

Powers, M., and Faden, R. R. 2006. *Social Justice* (New York: Oxford University Press).

PHAB (Public Health Accreditation Board). 2013. *Standards and Measures*, version 1.5. http://www.phaboard.org/wp-content/uploads/PHABSM_WEB_LR1.pdf.

PHLS (Public Health Leadership Society). 2002. *Principles of the Ethical Practice of Public Health*. https://www.apha.org/-/media/files/pdf/membergroups/ethics/ethics_brochure.ashx.

Quinn, S. C., Kumar S., Freimuth, V. S., Musa, D., Casteneda-Angarita, N., and Kidwell, K. 2011. "Racial Disparities in Exposure, Susceptibility, and Access to Health Care in the US H1N1 Influenza Pandemic." *American Journal of Public Health* 101(2): 285–293.

Thomas, J. C., Sage, M., Dillenberg, J., and Guillory, V. J. 2002. "A Code of Ethics for Public Health." *American Journal of Public Health* 92(7): 1057–1059.

VCU CSH (Virginia Commonwealth University Center on Society and Health). 2015. *Education: It Matters More to Health Than Ever Before*. http://societyhealth.vcu.edu/work/the-projects/education-it-matters-more-to-health-than-ever-before.html.

Wernham, A., and Teutsch, S. M. 2015. "Health in All Policies for Big Cities." *Journal of Public Health Management and Practice* 21(Suppl. 1): S56–S65.

Winslow, C. E. 1920. "The Untilled Fields of Public Health." *Science* 51(1306): 23–33.

WHO (World Health Organization). 1994. "Constitution of the World Health Organization." In *Basic Documents, Fortieth Edition* (Geneva: WHO).

Further Reading

Aragón, T. J. 2013. *The New Population Health Division: Transforming Public Health in San Francisco* (San Francisco: San Francisco Department of Public Health). https://www.sfdph.org/dph/hc/HCAgen/HCAgen2013/March%2019/PHP.pdf.

Buettgens, M., and Holahan, J. 2010. *America under the Affordable Care Act* (New York: Urban Institute). http://www.urban.org/research/publication/america-under-affordable-care-act.

Chen, E. H., and Bodenheimer, T. 2011. "Improving Population Health through Team-Based Panel Management: Comment on 'Electronic Medical Record Reminders and Panel Management to Improve Primary Care of Elderly Patients.'" *Archives of Internal Medicine* 171(17): 1558–1559.

Childress, J. F., Faden, R. R., Gaare, R. D., Gostin, L. O., Kahn, J., Bonnie, R. J., et al. 2002. "Public Health Ethics: Mapping the Terrain." *Journal of Law, Medicine & Ethics* 30(2): 170–178.

DeBruin D. A., Marshall, M. F., Parilla, E., Liaschenko, J., Leider, J. P., Brunquell, D. J., et al., 2010. *Implementing Ethical Frameworks for Rationing Scarce Health Resources in Minnesota during Severe Influenza Pandemic*. http://www.health.state.mn.us/divs/idepc/ethics/implement.pdf.

Flint Water Advisory Task Force. 2016. *Final Report*. https://www.michigan.gov/documents/snyder/FWATF_FINAL_REPORT_21March2016_517805_7.pdf.

Flint Water Study. 2016. *Flint Water Study*. http://flintwaterstudy.org/.

Hacker, K., and Walker, D. K. 2013. "Achieving Population Health in Accountable Care Organizations." *American Journal of Public Health* 103(7): 1163–1167.

Hanna-Attisha, M., LaChance, J., Sadler, R. C., and Champney Schnepp, A., 2016. "Elevated Blood Lead Levels in Children Associated with the Flint Drinking Water Crisis: A Spatial Analysis of Risk and Public Health Response." *American Journal of Public Health* 106(2): 283–290.

Kass, N. 2001. "An Ethics Framework for Public Health." *American Journal of Public Health* 91(11): 1776–1782.

Koh, H. K., and Sebelius, K. G. 2010. "Promoting Prevention through the Affordable Care Act." *New England Journal of Medicine* 363(14), 1296–1299. doi:10.1056/NEJMp1008560.

Lin J., Rutter, J., and Park, H. 2016. "Events That Led to Flint's Water Crisis." *New York Times*, January 21. http://www.nytimes.com/interactive/2016/01/21/us/flint-lead-water-timeline.html.

Marckmann, G., Schmidt, H., Sofaer, N., and Strech, D. 2015. "Putting Public Health Ethics into Practice: A Systematic Framework." *Frontiers in Public Health* 3:23. doi:10.3389/fpubh.2015.00023.

National Center for Education Statistics. 2015. "IPEDS Datacenter." https://nces.ed.gov/ipeds/datacenter/.

Nieburg, P., Bernheim, R. G., and Bonnie, R. 2003. "Ethics and the Practice of Public Health." In *Law in Public Health Practice*, edited by R. Goodman, R. E. Hoffman, W. Lopez, G. W. Matthews, M. Rothstein, and K. Foster (New York: Oxford University Press).

Schoen, C., Doty, M. M., Robertson, R. H., and Collins, S. R. 2011. "Affordable Care Act Reforms Could Reduce the Number of Underinsured US Adults by 70 Percent." *Health Affairs* 30(9): 1762–1771. doi:10.1377/hlthaff.2011.0335.

Sharfstein, J. M. 2014. "The Strange Journey of Population Health." *Milbank Quarterly* 92(4): 640–643.

CHAPTER 8

PUBLIC HEALTH INTERVENTIONS: ETHICAL IMPLICATIONS

DAVID R. BUCHANAN

Definitions and Distinctions

According to a celebrated definition, "[p]ublic health is what we, as a society, do collectively to assure the conditions for people to be healthy" (IOM, 1988, 19). Although medicine and public health share the goal of improving health, they can be distinguished in at least four ways. First, whereas medicine is concerned with individual health, public health seeks to improve the health of the population as a whole. Second, whereas medicine is concerned with treating illness, public health focuses on prevention. Third, whereas physicians focus on internal physiological processes, public health professionals address interactions between people and their environment. Finally, whereas physicians rely on their professional authority to persuade patients to adhere to prescriptions, public health professionals may invoke the police powers of the state to compel compliance, under penalty of law. Each difference holds significant implications for public health ethics.

Public health interventions (PHIs) can be categorized along two axes: infectious versus chronic diseases, and interventions aimed at individuals versus those aimed the environment. Examples of infectious disease interventions that deliver services to individuals include immunizations and directly observed therapy (DOT) to prevent the spread of tuberculosis; infectious disease prevention interventions aimed at the environment range from processes to assure safe water and food supplies to insect vector controls. Chronic disease interventions aimed at individuals include smoking cessation and weight loss programs; chronic disease interventions targeting the environment include strategies such as restricting tobacco advertising or prohibiting indoor smoking.

To introduce one further distinction, infectious diseases are well described by the germ theory of disease, with an intrinsic relationship between exposure to an agent (e.g., a bacterium) and the development of a disease. To explain the onset of chronic diseases, however, epidemiologists had to redefine causality in terms of probabilistic risk factors. After searching in vain for decades for the agent responsible for cancer or heart disease, the now-famous Framingham Heart Study gave rise to a profound paradigm shift in the health sciences (Dawber, Meadors, and Moore, 1951). As the analysis of the data dictated, the "causes" of heart disease had to be redefined in terms of "risk factors." A risk factor is neither necessary nor sufficient to cause disease; it only makes the onset of chronic disease more likely. A person can smoke and not get lung cancer, and people who get lung cancer need not have smoked. The one-to-one relationship between exposure to a specific agent and the onset of a particular disease thus gave way to the complex, multifactorial "neither necessary nor sufficient" risk factor analysis used to explain chronic diseases.

Chronic diseases account for the largest share of the burden of disease today (even in low- and middle-income countries) and they are responsible for more than 85 percent of the disease burden in high-income countries. Although there are important ethical issues in infectious disease control, this chapter focuses on the ethics of chronic disease interventions.

In addition to introducing the concept of risk factors to explain the occurrence of chronic diseases, the Framingham Study highlighted the significant role that human behaviors play in developing chronic diseases. Building on the 1964 report *Smoking and Health* (US Surgeon General, 1964) and the 1975 Lalonde Report, *A New Perspective on the Health of Canadians* (Lalonde, 1975), the 1979 US Surgeon General's *Healthy People* report identified lifestyle behaviors as contributing "as much as half" to rates of morbidity and mortality in the United States, making it the first official statement to indicate that health behaviors are responsible for the greatest part of the disease burden in the country (US Surgeon General, 1979, 9). The role of behaviors in explaining mortality rates was later quantified in a famous article, "Actual Causes of Death in the United States," by J. Michael McGinnis and William H. Foege (1993; updated by Mokdad and colleagues in 2004). Unhealthy behaviors, however, are not randomly distributed, but are instead strongly associated with social position, defined by income, race/ethnicity, and level of education. Thus, one key issue today is how to understand the interaction and relative weight that should be assigned causally to individual behavior choices compared to social structural factors in developing PHIs. For heuristic purposes, the different approaches can be termed "educational" and "environmental" interventions.

Educational and Environmental Interventions

Educational interventions are designed to change the knowledge, beliefs, and predisposing psychological and social factors that lead individuals to engage in unhealthy behaviors (e.g., starting to smoke, overeating). Virtually all current educational interventions acknowledge that information alone is not enough to produce the desired behavior change; to be effective, programs must address the antecedent social and psychological factors associated with initiating unhealthy behaviors. Examples of such factors include self-efficacy, perceived susceptibility, intentions, social support, and social norms (Glanz, Lewis, and Rimer, 1997; Glanz, Rimer, and Viswanath, 2008). The directionality of relationships among the identified factors and whether they are proximal or distal to the behavior of interest (for example, changes in social norms lead to changes in intentions, which in turn lead to changes in behavior) are often schematically depicted in diagrams, referred to as "logic models" in the field, which provide the basic blueprint for designing educational programs (Green and Kreuter, 1991; Funnell and Rogers, 2011).

With growing appreciation of the effects that social context has on the distribution of disease, attention has turned to developing interventions that address the social determinants of health. The "social determinants" of health and disease have been variously identified, but they generally include levels of poverty, racism, education, employment, housing quality, neighborhood environment, inequalities in wealth and status, stigmatization, access to healthy foods, access to medical care and recreational areas, and access to transportation (Wilkinson and Marmot, 2003; Marmot, 2005; Blas and Kurup, 2010). Recognition of the importance of the social determinants is duly credited to the epidemiologist Michael Marmot and his pioneering Whitehall studies dating to the 1970s (Marmot and Winkelstein, 1975; Marmot et al., 1978). Marmot found a highly robust linear relationship between social class (as defined by the British employment classification system) and health status, across virtually all disease categories, despite access to health care through national health coverage. His work was highly influential in informing the British Department of Health and Social Security (DHSS) report *Inequalities in Health* (commonly referred to as the "Black Report"), released in 1980. The Black Report examined four alternative hypotheses and concluded that the cause of health inequalities was differences in material conditions and income (DHSS, 1980; Blane, 1985).

Short of eliminating poverty, a variety of strategies have been developed under the umbrella of environmental interventions. Whether inadvertently, through technological advances such as television and automobiles, or intentionally, through advertising or product placement, physical and social environments have been transformed in ways that are far less conducive to optimal health (for example, such changes have led to people driving instead of walking to work, or children watching TV instead of playing outside). To protect and promote population health, environmental interventions seek to undo or counterbalance these untoward changes in the environment. This approach has gained popular attention in the concept of "nudges," developed by Thaler and Sunstein (2008). One example of the use of nudges is to re-engineer cafeteria lines to feature fresh fruits more prominently, instead of the more typical conspicuous displays of candy and chips.

Key Ethical Concerns in Chronic Disease Control

A number of normative frameworks have been disseminated in recent years to identify, analyze, and weigh different ethical considerations in evaluating PHIs (Kass, 2001; Petrini, 2010; ten Have et al., 2010; Childress et al., 2002; Marckmann et al., 2015). Because of their distinctive characteristics, PHIs raise different and complex trade-offs in balancing key ethical principles than do the ethical challenges raised in medical care. Based on criteria enumerated in these frameworks, PHIs to prevent chronic diseases are liable to raise significant ethical concerns with respect to issues of harm, including threats to individual liberties, justice, and the problem of free riders in relation to social solidarity.

Harms

Three types of harms have been identified in normative analyses of chronic disease control interventions (CDC, 2004). The first pertains to the potential for stigmatizing people who engage in unhealthy behaviors, especially in mass media campaigns. The second pertains to potential opportunity costs, where the implementation of one particular PHI may come at the cost of sacrificing other possibilities. The third, and most common, concern pertains to potential infringements on individual liberties.

Stigma

In developing campaigns that go beyond merely providing factual information, one of the most problematic "educational" interventions involves the use of shame to motivate behavior change. This approach is found in some campaigns against smoking and obesity (Kim and Shanahan, 2003; Brown-Johnson and Prochaska, 2015). For example, Children's Health Care of Atlanta ran a campaign that put up billboards portraying youth with excess weight along with "warning" signs proclaiming "Stocky, Chubby, and Chunky Are Still Fat," or "Fat Kids Become Fat Adults" (Puhl, Peterson, and Luedicke, 2013a, 2013b). The concern is that such campaigns do more harm than good, not only by failing to motivate people to lose weight, but also by actually damaging their mental health. Burris (2008, 475) argues that it is never acceptable to invoke stigma intentionally as a "visceral mode of social control."

However, Bayer (2008, 463) has posed provocative questions about campaigns to "denormalize" tobacco use, asking, "Are there occasions when the mobilization of stigma may effectively reduce the prevalence of behaviors linked to disease and death?" Even more pointedly, he asks if the state can legitimately "engage in efforts that have as their intended goal the stigmatization of such behaviors through campaigns that attempt to tap the power of shame and guilt to affect social norms" (468). There is in fact some evidence indicating that stigma is effective in stimulating individuals to lose and sustain weight loss (Latner et al., 2009).

As the different positions recited here indicate, the line between stigmatization and denormalization is indistinct and contested. Yet the argument seems to rest on a utilitarian calculus: Do the benefits of weight loss outweigh concerns about making people feel bad about themselves? How bad do they have to feel before it becomes unacceptable? In a broader perspective, one must ask whether the goals themselves are being deformed by such methods: Is the goal of public health exhausted by a set of empirical measures of physical fitness, or does the goal necessarily need to incorporate the normative dimensions of justice, respect, and autonomy? To what extent is it appropriate for the field of public health to concern itself with preserving human dignity and self-respect? We return to such deontological considerations in the conclusion.

Opportunity Costs

The issue of opportunity costs arises when an intervention competes against other priorities (Brody, McCullough, and Sharp, 2005). Based on utilitarian calculations of the leading causes of mortality and the most significant behavioral risk factors, government agencies have made major investments in tobacco and obesity prevention programs. But community activists voice concerns that such programs detract attention and resources from other acute problems, such as violence and substance use (Wolff et al., 2003). Similarly, even sympathetic observers have noted that the huge investment in antiretroviral therapies in international settings has diverted resources away from other urgent health problems, such as the dramatically increasing prevalence of diabetes (England, 2008).

Threats to Individual Liberties

Concerns about whether PHIs unduly infringe on individual liberty have been a central theme in public health ethics debates since the landmark 1905 *Jacobson v. Massachusetts* Supreme Court ruling, which found that the state could compel individuals to be vaccinated against smallpox. The historic ruling thus recognized the legal authority and ethical validity of the use of state power to constrain individual liberties to protect the common good (Gostin, 2002).

Calls for new taxes and bans on large soda bottles are only the most recent examples of PHIs to raise questions about potential infringements on individual liberties, provoking charges of paternalism. *Paternalism* is defined as "interference with a person's liberty of action justified by reason referring exclusively to the welfare... of the person being coerced" (Dworkin, 1999, 121).

Environment interventions, in general, pose a greater threat to individual liberties than educational interventions, since persuasive messages to behave prudently are generally considered benign and a legitimate function of government. Interventions designed to abate market-induced incentives or to hinder people from making unhealthy choices by penalizing such choices or imposing environmental constraints present more complex challenges. Moreover, when public health professionals lobby to raise taxes on cigarettes and soda, opponents argue not only that they impinge on personal liberties, but also that the burdens of taxation fall disproportionately on the poor, thus raising issues of fairness and justice (Resnik, 2013; Arno et al., 1996; Hoffman and Tan, 2015; Guindon, 2014; Nestle and Bittman, 2015; Pomeranz, 2012). In light of such concerns, Kass (2001) notes that as the potential burdens of PHIs increase, the value of the goals to be achieved should be proportionately more compelling.

In examining these issues, it is important to note that many alleged infringements on individual liberties rest on the dubious assumption that the government is unduly seeking to alter a pristine environment. Most democratic citizenries, however, have largely passively allowed powerful corporations to shape the environment to advance their interests (e.g., by placing billboards along highways, or placing candy and chips at supermarket checkout counters). While many people appreciate the convenience and affordability that the market provides, others recognize that a collective interest in protecting health often outweighs the modest threats posed by undoing modifications in the environment in order to encourage healthy choices (e.g., by restricting the placement of billboards). Although Sunstein and Thaler's "libertarian paternalism" may sound like a contradiction in terms, it is based on an appreciation that life would simply be too exhausting if people had to deliberate consciously and carefully about every choice they had to make throughout the day (see also Kahneman, 2013). It is in the collective interest of society to think about how to structure the environment to make routine decisions—choices that people do not need, nor want, to rise to the level of conscious deliberation—less hazardous, rather than allowing the choice architecture to be set up solely to serve market interests.

Balancing individual and collective interests raises the issue of respect for the autonomy of the community as a whole. In medicine, individual patients must affirm their voluntary informed consent before undergoing treatment. With PHIs, an equivalent procedure for providing the informed consent of the population affected has not been established. Out of respect for the community's right to self-determination, public health officials have an obligation to assure that there is a high degree of public consensus supporting claims that the health benefits of an action outweigh costs to individual liberties. While it is common for a majority of people to agree to adopt restrictions, it is important to recognize that they are justified only provisionally, by ratification in the court of public opinion, until such time that new evidence leads to reconsideration. Public health advocates can lobby for banning the sale of large sugary drinks, but its ethical warrant lies in convincing a majority of the public that the health benefits outweigh other legitimate moral considerations (Habermas, 1984). Childress et al. (2002) recommend that, other things being equal, public health professionals should opt for the least restrictive approach.

Justice

The ethical justification for PHIs is inextricably intertwined with questions of justice. Although public health is often alleged to be intrinsically utilitarian (the greatest good for the greatest number), there are today prominent calls for social justice in the field. This entreaty was issued in an acclaimed paper by the political scientist Dan Beauchamp, titled "Public Health as Social Justice" (1976). Beauchamp cites the political philosopher John Rawls as his source of inspiration, and many public health professionals today loosely subscribe to a Rawlsian egalitarian theory of justice. The importance of promoting equality was featured in the US Surgeon General's *Healthy People 2000* report, which contained the first official statement that the goal of US Public Health Service was to "reduce health disparities" (US DHHS, 1990). This goal was strengthened to "eliminating" health disparities in *Healthy People 2010*, and reiterated in *Healthy People 2020* (US DHHS 2000, 2010).

Since the original *Healthy People* 2000, there has been growing recognition that one problem with the goal of eliminating health disparities is that differences in health have many causes, only some of which can be considered the result of unjust social arrangements. Genetic diseases, for example, result in significant health disparities, but they are not the result of corrigible social conditions. While the higher prevalence of sickle cell anemia in African American populations is tragic, its distribution is not a matter of the justice of social conditions. As these incongruities have become better appreciated, there has been a shift in terminology toward the use of "health equity," and hence in eliminating health inequities (Baker, Metzler, and Galea, 2005; Braveman and Gruskin, 2003).

In a significant extension of Rawls's work, Norman Daniels (1985, 2001, 2008) argues that if liberal democratic societies have a duty to protect fair equality of opportunity, then they must also have a duty to maintain the normal functioning of human beings. To the extent that disease and disability impair normal functioning, they restrict the range of opportunities open to individuals. It is therefore essential to preserve and restore normal functioning so that people can participate in the social, political, and economic life of society. While the threat to individual liberties must always be kept in mind, public health interventions find justification not only in protecting physical health, but also in enabling people to participate in social and political life without undue impairment, as a matter of justice.

Rawls's theory of justice has been criticized by those who advocate an even stronger egalitarian position, generally referred to the "capabilities approach." Its most prominent exponents are Amartya Sen (1999a, 2009) and Martha Nussbaum (1990, 1993, 2011). From a capabilities perspective, it is insufficient that social institutions be arranged such that they merely provide the *opportunity* for individuals to pursue their life plans, because those opportunities are cruel fictions unless people possess the capability to fulfill their plans successfully. Here, the key question of justice concerns what people are *actually* able to achieve. If people's abilities are so stunted by existing social conditions that the range of opportunities—those that they actually able to pursue—is severely constricted, then one cannot claim to live in a just society, no matter how much people may believe that they have fair opportunity. Rather, a just society is obligated to enable everyone to have the same capacity to pursue the full range of occupations and recreational activities that the most well-off segments of society enjoy, a position that Sen refers to as "substantive freedom" (Sen, 1999b).

Free Riders and the Dilemmas in Social Solidarity

One final topic reflective of key ethical tensions in PHIs lies in the dilemmas of buttressing social solidarity, an issue salient now in the withdrawal of participation from universal immunization protections. The normative issue at stake here is the problem of so-called free riders. The free rider problem refers to the ethical dilemma that arises when some people choose to not contribute an equal or fair share to a given cooperative scheme, but instead count on being able to take advantage of the benefits of the system without doing their part to maintain its overall strength. As the 2015 outbreaks of measles and rubella attest (Clemmons et al., 2015; Majumder et al., 2015), growing numbers of parents are choosing to not get their children vaccinated. Similarly, people know that smoking and obesity raise health insurance premiums, which has triggered fraught public debates about whether or not smokers should be required to pay more. In their analysis of social solidarity, Dawson and Verweij (2012) identify two types, rational and constitutive. They argue that public health has relied on rational solidarity, but it may be better served by promoting constitutive solidarity. Both forms face daunting challenges, albeit with pressures from different directions.

Rational solidarity is realized by means of an implied social contract. People agree to pay taxes and pool resources in order to protect one another from serious and unpredictable health threats, buying in on the tacit assumption that everyone has a rational self-interest in keeping their individual expenditures (whether taxes or health insurance premiums) as low as possible. When people knowingly engage in risky behaviors, however, they break the contract, forcing the rest to have to pay more to cover the additional health care costs incurred. They act like free riders, and thereby undermine rational solidarity.

In contrast, *constitutive solidarity* is forged out of a shared sense of identity. People choose to stand together, not due to some rational cost-benefit analysis for maximizing individual interests, but through positive identification with fellow citizens, based in part on norms of sympathy for the pain and suffering that all must endure. It is a rare person who is not cognizant of the fragility of the human condition and the capriciousness of being stricken by disease. People know that no one has complete control over their health, and so they see each other sharing a common human fate. But where rational solidarity suffers the free rider problem, constitutive solidarity is undermined by social injustices.

There is general public awareness that health risk behaviors are not randomly distributed, but rather are strongly associated with income, race, and level of education. One plausible explanation for these patterns is that they are reflective of the distribution of stress across different social groups (Geronimus et al., 2006). Among other explanations, in one provocative analysis, Factor, Kawachi, and Williams (2011) suggest that members of minority groups react with feelings of frustration and anger at the inequitable distribution of societal benefits and burdens. As a result of their exclusion from a fair share of social benefits, and the disproportionate imposition of its burdens (poverty, unemployment, etc.), some low-income minorities flaunt calls to conform with dominant social norms, taking up drug use, unprotected sex, and other activities, and in the process signaling their resistance and rejection of dominant codes of behavior (Cohen, 2004). When socially identifiable groups are forced to bear an inequitable share of the burden of participating in a particular cooperative scheme, they become alienated and disenfranchised, no longer feeling that the dominant majority identifies with them or sees them as belonging to the same membership group, entitled to the same benefits and protections (Shelby, 2015, 2016). Constitutive solidarity cracks under the strains of social injustice.

The social solidarity necessary for collective action on behalf of the population as a whole is thus being battered on many sides. The broad secular trend toward valuing individual authenticity—of finding one's true and unique self, free from the strictures of social identities and normative demands—feeds the ranks of free riders and reinforces antinomian predilections (Appiah, 2005; Taylor, 1992). The tolerance of poverty and growing social and economic disparities warp the development of the capacity to exercise positive self-determination among those bearing the brunt of those burdens. Never was there a more important time for thinking seriously about the grounds for forging collective action and enacting provisions based on communal identifications and a shared sense of social responsibility.

Conclusion

Public health interventions raise profound questions about individual rights, the obligations of members of collectivities toward one another, and the nature of justice and the just society. As the different issues reviewed here indicate, it is generally not enough to invoke a simple utilitarian calculus in determining whether the overall health benefits of a proposed intervention outweigh the threat of unintended morbidities or deaths. Public health authorities have an obligation to respect both the individual's and the community's right to self-determination. If most chronic diseases these days are strongly associated with individual behaviors, to what extent is it ethically appropriate and justified to shame people or to invoke the police powers of the state to reduce their occurrence?

More poignantly, if such behaviors are in turn strongly associated with income, race, and level of education, to what extent does society have an obligation to improve social conditions for the sake of achieving reductions in morbidity and mortality rates? Further still, are there other more compelling reasons to improve social conditions? Is it possible for modern liberal democracies to tackle questions about human dignity, beyond empirical measures of death, disease, and disability? Does "health" entail an essential ethical dimension (as often implied in the shift to the term "well-being"), where the goal of social interventions is not only to enable people to live longer, but also to enjoy a higher quality of life, one defined by dignity and respect, free from the indignities of feeling inferior? If public health is social justice, then it is incumbent upon the field to implement interventions that create a space in civil society for promoting dialogue and expanding the sphere of consensus around the kind of society we want to live in together (Buchanan, 2008).

References

Appiah, K. A. 2005. *The Ethics of Identity* (Princeton, N.J.: Princeton University Press).

Arno, P. S., Brandt, A. M., Gostin, L. O., and Morgan, J. 1996. "Tobacco Industry Strategies to Oppose Federal Regulation." *JAMA* 275(16): 1258–1262.

Baker, E., Metzler, M., and Galea, S. 2005. "Addressing Social Determinants of Health Inequities: Learning from Doing." *American Journal of Public Health* 95(4): 553–557.

Bayer, R. 2008. "Stigma and the Ethics of Public Health: Not Can We but Should We?" *Social Science & Medicine* 67: 463–466.

Beauchamp, D. 1976. "Public Health as Social Justice." *Inquiry* 13(1): 3–14.

Blane, D. 1985. "An Assessment of the Black Report's Explanation of Health Inequalities." *Sociology of Health and Illness* 7(3): 423–445.

Blas, E., and Kurup, A. S., eds. 2010. *Equity, Social Determinants and Public Health Programmes* (Geneva: World Health Organization).

Braveman, P., and Gruskin, S. 2003. "Defining Equity in Health." *Journal of Epidemiology and Community Health* 57: 254–258.

Brody, B. A., McCullough, L. B., and Sharp R. R. 2005. "Consensus and Controversy in Clinical Research Ethics." *JAMA* 294(11): 1411–1414.

Brown-Johnson, C. G., and Prochaska, J. J. 2015. "Shame-Based Appeals in a Tobacco Control Public Health Campaign: Potential Harms and Benefits." *Tobacco Control* 24(5): 419–420.

Buchanan, D. 2008. "Autonomy, Paternalism, and Justice: Ethical Priorities in Public Health." *American Journal of Public Health* 98: 15–21.

Burris, S. 2008. "Stigma, Ethics and Policy: A Commentary on Bayer's 'Stigma and the Ethics of Public Health: Not Can We but Should We?' " *Social Science & Medicine* 67: 473–475.

CDC (Centers for Disease Control and Prevention). 2004. "Primary Prevention of Type 2 Diabetes Mellitus by Lifestyle Intervention: Implications for Health Policy." *Annals of Internal Medicine* 140: 951–957.

Childress J. R., Faden, R., Gaare, L., Gostin, L.O., Kahn, J., Bonnie, R. J., et al. 2002. "Public Health Ethics: Mapping the Terrain." *Journal of Law, Medicine & Ethics* 30: 170–178.

Clemmons, N. S., Gastanaduy, P. A., Fiebelkorn, A. P., Redd, S. B., and Wallace, G. S. 2015. "Measles—United States, January 4–April 2, 2015." *Morbidity and Mortality Weekly Report* 64(14): 373–376.

Cohen, C. 2004. "Deviance as Resistance: A New Research Agenda for the Study of Black Politics." *DuBois Review* 1: 27–45.

Daniels, N. 1985. *Just Health Care* (New York: Cambridge University Press).

Daniels, N. 2001. "Justice, Health, and Health Care." *American Journal of Bioethics* 1(2): 2–16.

Daniels, N. 2008. *Just Health: Meeting Health Needs Fairly* (Cambridge: Cambridge University Press).

Dawber, T., Meadors, G., and Moore, F. 1951. "Epidemiological Approaches to Heart Disease: The Framingham Study." *American Journal of Public Health* 41: 279–286.

Dawson, A., and Verweij, M. 2012. "Solidarity: A Moral Concept in Need of Clarification." *Public Health Ethics* 5(1): 1–5.

DHSS (UK Department of Health and Social Security). 1980. *Inequalities in Health: Report of a Research Working Group* [Black Report] (London: DHSS).

Dworkin, G. 1999. "Paternalism." In *New Ethics for the Public's Health*, edited by D. Beauchamp and B. Steinbock, 115–130 (New York: Oxford University Press).

England, R. 2008. "The Writing Is on the Wall for UNAIDS." *BMJ* 336: 1072.

Factor, R., Kawachi, I., and Williams, D. R. 2011. "Understanding High-Risk Behavior among Non-dominant Minorities: A Social Resistance Framework." *Social Science & Medicine* 73: 1292–1301.

Funnell, S. C., and Rogers, P. J. 2011. *Purposeful Program Theory: Effective Use of Theories of Change and Logic Models* (San Francisco: Jossey-Bass).

Geronimus, A. T., Hicken, M., Keene, D., and Bound, J. 2006. " 'Weathering' and Age Patterns of Allostatic Load Scores among Blacks and Whites in the United States." *American Journal of Public Health* 96(5): 826–833.

Glanz, K., Lewis, F., and Rimer, B., eds. 1997. *Health Behavior and Health Education: Theory, Research and Practice*. 2nd ed. (San Francisco: Jossey-Bass).

Glanz, K., Rimer, B., and Viswanath K. eds. 2008. *Health Behavior and Health Education: Theory, Research, and Practice*. 4th ed. (San Francisco: Jossey-Bass).

Gostin, L., ed. 2002. *Public Health Law and Ethics: A Reader* (Berkeley: University of California Press).

Green, L., and Kreuter, M. 1991. *Health Promotion Planning: An Educational and Environmental Approach*. 2nd ed. (Mountain View, Calif.: Mayfield).

Guindon, G. E. 2014. "The Impact of Tobacco Prices on Smoking Onset: A Methodological Review." *Tobacco Control* 23(2): e5.

Habermas, J. 1984. *The Theory of Communicative Action* (Boston, Mass.: Beacon Press).

Hoffman S. J., and Tan, C. 2015. "Overview of Systematic Reviews on the Health-Related Effects of Government Tobacco Control Policies." *BMC Public Health* 15: 744.

IOM (Institute of Medicine). 1988. *The Future of Public Health* (Washington, D.C.: National Academy of Sciences Press).

Kahneman, D. 2013. *Thinking, Fast and Slow* (New York: Farrar, Straus and Giroux).

Kass, N. 2001. "An Ethics Framework for Public Health." *American Journal of Public Health* 91(11): 1776–1782.

Kim, S.-H., and Shanahan, J. 2003. "Stigmatizing Smokers: Public Sentiment toward Cigarette Smoking and its Relationship to Smoking Behaviors." *Journal of Health Communication* 8(4): 343–367.

Lalonde, M. 1975. *A New Perspective on the Health of Canadians* (Ottawa: Ministry of National Health and Welfare, Government of Canada).

Latner, J. D., Wilson, G. T., Jackson, M. L., and Stunkard, A. J. 2009. "Greater History of Weight-Related Stigmatizing Experience Is Associated with Greater Weight Loss in Obesity Treatment." *Journal of Health Psychology* 14: 190–199.

Majumder, M. S., Cohn, E. L., Mekaru, S. R., Huston, J. E., and Brownstein, J. S. 2015. "Substandard Vaccination Compliance and the 2015 Measles Outbreak." *JAMA Pediatrics* 69: 494–495.

Marckmann, G., Schmidt, H., Sofaer, N., and Strech, D. 2015. "Putting Public Health Ethics into Practice: A Systematic Framework." *Frontiers in Public Health* 3: 23. http://journal.frontiersin.org/article/10.3389/fpubh.2015.00023/full.

Marmot, M. 2005. "Social Determinants of Health Inequalities." *Lancet* 365: 1099–1104.

Marmot, M., Rose, G., Shipley, M., and Hamilton, P. J. S. 1978. "Employment Grade and Coronary Heart Disease in British Civil Servants." *Journal of Epidemiology and Community Health* 32(4): 244–249.

Marmot, M., and Winkelstein, W. 1975. "Epidemiologic Observations on Intervention Trials for Prevention of Coronary Heart Disease." *American Journal of Epidemiology* 101(3): 177–181.

McGinnis, M., and Foege, W. 1993. "Actual Causes of Death in the United States." *Journal of the American Medical Association* 270(18): 2207–2212.

Mokdad, A., Marks, J., Stroup, D., and Gerberding, J. 2004. "Actual Causes of Death in the United States, 2000." *Journal of the American Medical Association* 291(10): 1238–1243.

Nestle, M., and Bittman, M. 2015. *Soda Politics: Taking on Big Soda (and Winning)* (New York: Oxford University Press).

Nussbaum, M. 1990. "Aristotelian Social Democracy." In *Liberalism and the Good*, edited by R. B. Douglass, G. Mara, and H. Richardson, 203–252 (New York: Routledge).

Nussbaum, M. 1993. "Non-relative Virtues: An Aristotelian Approach." In *The Quality of Life*, edited by M. Nussbaum and A. Sen, 242–269 (Oxford: Clarendon Press).

Nussbaum, M. 2011. *Creating Capabilities: The Human Development Approach* (Cambridge, Mass.: Belknap Press of Harvard University Press).

Petrini, C. 2010. "Theoretical Models and Operational Frameworks in Public Health Ethics." *International Journal of Environmental Research and Public Health* 7(1): 189–202.

Pomeranz, J. L. 2012. "Advanced Policy Options to Regulate Sugar-Sweetened Beverages to Support Public Health." *Journal of Public Health Policy* 33(1): 75–88.

Puhl, R., Peterson, J. L., and Luedicke, J. 2013a. "Fighting Obesity or Obese Persons? Public Reactions to Obesity-Related Health Messages." *International Journal of Obesity* 37(6): 774–782.

Puhl, R., Peterson, J. L., and Luedicke, J. 2013b. "Public Reactions to Obesity-Related Public Health Campaigns: A Randomized Trial." *American Journal of Preventive Medicine* 45: 36–48.

Resnik, D. B. 2013. "Charging Smokers Higher Health Insurance Rates: Is It Ethical?" Hastings Center Bioethics Forum, September 19. http://www.thehastingscenter.org/charging-smokers-higher-health-insurance-rates-is-it-ethical/.

Sen, A. 1999a. *Capabilities and Commodities* (New York: Oxford University Press).

Sen, A. 1999b. *Development as Freedom* (New York: Anchor Books).

Sen, A. 2009. *The Idea of Justice* (Cambridge, Mass.: Belknap Press of Harvard University Press).

Shelby, T. 2015. "Liberalism, Self-Respect and Troubling Cultural Patterns in Ghettos." In *The Cultural Matrix: Understanding Black Youth*, edited by O. Patterson, 498–532 (Cambridge Mass.: Harvard University Press).

Shelby, T. 2016. *Dark Ghettos: Injustice, Dissent, and Reform* (Cambridge, Mass.: Belknap Press of Harvard University Press).

Taylor, C. 1992. *The Ethics of Authenticity* (Cambridge, Mass.: Harvard University Press).

ten Have M., de Beaufort, I. D., Mackenbach, J. P., and van der Heide, A. 2010. "An Overview of Ethical Frameworks in Public Health: Can They Be Supportive in the Evaluation of Programs to Prevent Overweight?" *BMC Public Health* 10: 638. http://bmcpublichealth.biomedcentral.com/articles/10.1186/1471-2458-10-638.

Thaler, R., and Sunstein, C. 2008. *Nudge: Improving Decisions about Health, Wealth and Happiness* (New York: Penguin Books).

US DHHS (Department of Health and Human Services). 1990. *Healthy People 2000: National Health Promotion and Disease Prevention Objectives*. DHHS Publication No. (PHS)90-50212 (Washington, DC: Public Health Service, US Department of Health and Human Services).

US DHHS (Department of Health and Human Services). 2000. *Healthy People 2010: Understanding and Improving Health*. 2nd ed. (Washington, DC: US Government Printing Office).

US DHHS (Department of Health and Human Services). 2010. *Healthy People 2020*. (Washington, DC: US Department of Health and Human Services, Office of Disease Prevention and Health Promotion). https://www.healthypeople.gov/.

US Surgeon General. 1964. *Smoking and Health: Report of the Advisory Committee to the Surgeon General of the Public Health Service*. Public Health Service Publication No. 1103 (Washington, D.C.: Public Health Service, Office of the Surgeon General).

US Surgeon General. 1979. *Healthy People: The Surgeon General's Report on Health Promotion and Disease Prevention*. DHEW Publication No. 79-55071 (Washington, D.C.: General Publications Office, US Department of Health, Education, and Welfare).

Wilkinson, R., and Marmot, M. eds. 2003. *Social Determinants of Health: The Solid Facts*. 2nd ed. (Geneva: World Health Organization).

Wolff, M., Bates, T., Beck, B., Young, S., Ahmed, S., and Maurana, C. 2003. "Cancer Prevention in Underserved African-American Communities: Barriers and Effective Strategies—A Review of the Literature." *Wisconsin Medical Journal* 102(5): 36–40.

CHAPTER 9

THE INTERSECTION OF LAW, ETHICS, AND PUBLIC HEALTH IN THE UNITED STATES

STACIE P. KERSHNER AND LESLIE E. WOLF

An Introduction to Public Health Law

The US Centers for Disease Control and Prevention's list of the "10 Great Public Health Achievements, 1900–1999" highlights the law's role in improving public health (CDC, 1999). Laws that, for example, mandated childhood vaccination, seat belt use, and municipal water fluoridation, and those that regulated workplace safety and inspection, made these achievements realizable (Moulton, Goodman, and Parmet, 2007). As these public health efforts continue and new public health challenges arise, law remains an important public health tool. This chapter explores public health law, including its sources and its limits, as well as its relationship with public health ethics from the US perspective.

Defining Public Health Law

Lawrence Gostin (2008, 4), a leading public health law scholar, defines public health law as "the study of the legal powers and duties of the state, in collaboration with its partners (e.g., health care, business, the community, the media, and academe), to ensure the conditions for people to be healthy (to identify, prevent, and ameliorate risks to health in the population), and of the limitations on the power of the state to constrain for the common good the autonomy, privacy, liberty, proprietary, or other legally protected interests of individuals."

A 2011 Institute of Medicine (IOM) report divides public health law into three categories: (1) laws establishing public health systems' infrastructure and authority, (2) laws designed to improve specific health outcomes, and (3) laws with an incidental public health effect (IOM, 2011; Moulton et al., 2003). The latter two may involve government entities beyond public health departments. For example, public health strongly supports mandatory seat belt use laws because seat belt use demonstrably saves lives in motor vehicle crashes, but authority over those laws may rest with state transportation departments. At the same time, the federal government may influence states' adoption of these laws through the conditions it imposes on highway fund distributions. These three categories are focused on government. While other stakeholders, such as research entities, nonprofits, and grassroots organizations, play important roles in advancing public health, the authority and extent of government action, balanced against individual rights, is the hallmark of public health law.

Health Care Law Compared to Public Health Law

Health care law and public health law are distinct but complementary fields. Legal issues common in health care delivery focus on the individual patient and on physician obligations to their patients; in contrast, public health law emphasizes population health (Tobey, 1926). To illustrate these different perspectives, imagine that an automobile driver is injured in a crash while not wearing a seat belt. Health care law is concerned with treating the driver's injuries. The Emergency Medical Treatment and Active Labor Act (42 U.S.C. § 1395dd) requires the driver be evaluated and provided with emergency medical care, even if uninsured. In contrast, public health law concentrates on avoiding these kinds of injuries through laws that require seat belt use and fining people for failing to comply.

Using Law as a Tool to Improve Health

Public health laws can be directed at individuals, entities, or environments to promote change through education, incentives, or deterrence, or they can alter the physical, informational, or business environment. They can be characterized by the public health framework of primary, secondary, and tertiary interventions.[1] Primary legal interventions include efforts designed to prevent illness or injury, such as mandating vaccination before school entry to control vaccine-preventable diseases (CDC, 2016c; Yang and Silverman, 2015).

Secondary legal interventions are intended to identify public health problems at an early stage to minimize their negative effects. For example, mandatory newborn blood testing seeks to identify infants with rare genetic, endocrine, or metabolic diseases, such as phenylketonuria, and to intervene to prevent death or mitigate disability (Network for Public Health Law, 2016).

Tertiary legal interventions are employed to reduce or remediate harm from illness or injury that has occurred. Examples include state laws that grant immunity from drug charges to opioid users who seek medical assistance for themselves or others experiencing an overdose (Public Health Law Research LawAtlas, 2016a), or laws that authorize first responders to administer naloxone to treat an overdose (Public Health Law Research LawAtlas, 2016b). Neither intervention addresses the underlying addiction, but both may prevent overdose deaths.

Government public health actions may be coercive. The government can mandate behavior that benefits population health, and it can penalize—through fines or imprisonment—individuals not willing to comply voluntarily. Examples include mandatory childhood vaccinations as a condition of school attendance, involuntary detention of people with certain infectious diseases, closure of restaurants with poor sanitation, and destruction of property that poses a toxic hazard. Government action may also incentivize decisions that promote public health. For example, federal and state governments tax cigarettes to discourage smoking. Similarly, the federal government conditions highway funds on states' laws regarding the legal drinking age to prevent injuries from automobile crashes.

Following substantial success with controlling infectious disease, public health began to set loftier goals, as reflected in the IOM's 1988 definition: "Public health is what we, as a society, do collectively to assure the conditions for people to be healthy" (IOM, 1988, 1). There has been a corresponding expansion of public health law to areas such as injury prevention and chronic disease. Moreover, public health law has explicitly embraced social justice as a goal. Gostin's public health law definition reflects this aspect, stating that "the prime objective of public health law is to pursue the highest possible level of physical and mental health in the population, consistent with the values of social justice" (Gostin, 2008, 4). Public health laws that seek to ameliorate inequities include zoning laws that limit the density of fast food restaurants and tax incentives to open grocery stores in low-income neighborhoods to expand healthy food choices for low-income families.

Sources and Scope of Public Health Law in the United States

In the United States, legal authority for public health action is generally derived from the following sources: federal and state constitutions, statutes, regulations, court decisions, and executive orders.

Which government entity has the authority to act depends on the power division between and within the federal and state governments. The federal government is separated into the executive, legislative, and judiciary branches, each with distinct authority and roles. The structure is designed to provide checks and balances among the branches of government. The president and his or her cabinet and agencies make up the executive branch, which enforces the law and further implements it by issuing executive orders and promulgating regulations. Congress (the Senate and House of Representatives) forms the legislative branch, which enacts legislation and authorizes funding. The judicial branch, comprising the Supreme Court and appellate and trial courts, is charged with interpreting the law and resolving disputes. Most states mimic this structure, with a governor leading the executive branch.

The federal government's authority is limited to the "enumerated powers" explicitly granted to it in the US Constitution. The Constitution does not directly reference public health, and the federal government affects public health through its constitutional authority to tax and spend and to regulate interstate commerce (U.S. Const. Art. I, § VIII, Cl. 1.). All powers not explicitly given to the federal government are reserved to the states under the Tenth Amendment. Accordingly, states typically have broader authority to adopt laws to protect their citizen's health, safety, and welfare. These "police powers" permit state governments to restrict liberty to promote the public good.

Preemption also plays an important role in distributing power between governments (Hodge and Corbett, 2016). There are many complexities to preemption law, but, in general, it provides that a higher level of government's law may restrict a lower authority from acting on the same issue. Thus, federal laws can restrict state and local government actions, and state laws can restrict local government action (CDC, 2016b). The higher government may set a minimum standard (e.g., clean air standards) that must be met, but permit lower governments to adopt stricter standards (floor preemption). The higher government may set a standard, but not permit adoption of stricter standards (ceiling preemption). Sometimes a higher level of government does not set a standard but still prevents the lower level of government from acting (null preemption) (ChangeLab Solutions, 2013). Ceiling and null preemption generally take away local control and limit community innovation to address their needs.

Governments' broad power to protect the public health is not unlimited. The US Supreme Court's seminal 1905 decision in *Jacobson v. Massachusetts* (197 U.S. 11 [1905], hereafter *Jacobson*) supports state public health authority, while simultaneously requiring substantial justification to infringe on individual liberty interests. Henning Jacobson refused to be vaccinated against smallpox, as ordered by the Cambridge Board of Health and authorized by Massachusetts law, despite an ongoing epidemic and an effective vaccine (*Jacobson*, 13). The court upheld the state's authority to mandate vaccination because (1) the serious threat of the smallpox epidemic created a public health *necessity*, (2) vaccination was a *reasonable means* to address the public health threat, and (3) the personal risk of vaccination was *proportional* to the threat posed by the disease (*Jacobson*, 27–28, 31, 38–39). The court also required the state to exempt people, such as the very sick or very young, for whom the risks of vaccination could be particularly dangerous (*Jacobson*, 29). The court also affirmed the delegation of state public health authority to local government and deferred to health officials' determinations, a practice that has continued (*Jacobson*, 25, 27).

The principles enunciated in *Jacobson* remain at the heart of many public health law questions (Mariner, Annas, and Glantz, 2005; Gostin, 2005). Public health laws may implicate constitutionally protected interests—from the privacy (bodily integrity) interests at issue in *Jacobson* to First Amendment rights of free speech, freedom of assembly, and religion; to economic interests; to Fifth and Fourteenth Amendment rights to due process and equal protection. At this level, the law reflects the nation's most important values and may draw on ethical principles and theories. Supreme Court Justice Oliver Wendell Holmes Jr. described the law as the "external deposit of our moral life" (Holmes, 1897).[2] Accordingly, as *Jacobson* illustrates, courts will require strong justification when public health laws infringe upon constitutionally protected interests.

The Interplay between Law and Ethics

Law establishes boundaries for what *must* be done (e.g., mandatory disease reporting) and what *cannot* be done (e.g., smoking in public spaces). But often it identifies a range of *permissible* actions, sometimes explicitly and sometimes by interpretation of existing law (CDC and NACCHO, 2012).[3]

When several legal options are permissible, public health ethics can help identify the most appropriate option (CDC and NACCHO, 2012). For example, during an emergency, laws may authorize the distribution of finite resources, but ethics can help determine who receives them first, such as medical professionals, first responders, and those who are most vulnerable.

Ethical and legal analyses are similar, as they both involve a deliberate consideration and articulation of facts, questions, and areas of conflict; an exploration of available options; a decision; and the reasons for the decision. This deliberative process helps in clarifying and justifying decisions, and its transparency can lead to an acceptance of decisions, even when there is disagreement about the outcome. When dilemmas impact constitutionally protected interests, the arguments in law or ethics are likely to be similar, although the specific terms used (e.g., "rights") may differ. But it is also important to remember that law and ethics are different disciplines with different goals (Wolf, 2004).

Although the law can reflect our moral commitments, it may sometimes conflict with them. For example, the US Constitution originally allowed states to count a slave as three-fifths of a person for purposes of representation, and it was many years before blacks and, even later, women were given the right to vote. But even these constitutional rights fell short. During the civil rights movement, many individuals took personal risks to challenge laws that permitted continued legal discrimination against blacks. Their voices and actions served as an impetus for change, both in the law and its enforcement. Accordingly, knowing what the law says is only a starting point. It is important to question the underlying assumptions for any specific law, how it is used and enforced, and whom it impacts, as well as to amend laws, when necessary, to achieve ethical goals.

Public Health Law in Action

This section will illustrate how public health law works in specific examples. The examples of infectious disease, tobacco control, and obesity demonstrate the evolution of public health law and the challenges presented when the traditional justification for public health law—avoiding harm to others—is not clear.

Control of Infectious Diseases

There is a centuries-long history of governments around the world enacting laws to protect their citizenry and their states from infectious diseases such as smallpox, black plague, yellow fever, and cholera (Rothstein, 2015). These laws support quarantine, isolation, limits on travel, and other social distancing measures (CDC and Association of State and Territorial Health Officials, 2010),[4] as well as vaccination and sanitation requirements. These are, as the Supreme Court explained in *Jacobson*, among the "manifold restraints to which every person is necessarily subject for the common good" (*Jacobson*, 26). States traditionally exercise this authority under their police powers, with the federal government having authority for persons entering the United States or crossing state lines.[5]

Tuberculosis (TB), a bacterial disease that usually attacks the lungs, is easily spread to others by air. A person who is infected but not experiencing symptoms has latent TB and is not contagious. However, if not properly treated, latent TB can develop into active TB—especially among those with weaker immune systems—which may be transmitted to other people (CDC, 2015g). Failure to complete treatment can lead to a recurring illness or even drug-resistant TB, which is transmissible. Antibiotic treatment often lasts at least six months and may last up to two years for drug-resistant TB (CDC, 2015h).

The majority of patients diagnosed with TB voluntarily agree to antibiotic treatment. However, some may resist, and some may be unable to comply with treatment. A patient usually has the right to refuse treatment for an illness. However, because TB—particularly drug-resistant TB—presents risks to others, public health officials may order directly observed therapy (DOT), which involves a public health representative or authorized family member observing the patient take the medication so that no dose is missed. Public health authorities may also compel treatment or isolate the patient when a patient fails to complete treatment, as specifically authorized by state statute or presumed under the state's police powers. This power may be delegated to local government (CDC and Centers for Law and the Public's Health, 2009, 16–17, 21–25).

City of Milwaukee v. Washington (304 Wis. 2d 98 [S. Ct. Wisc. 2007], hereafter *Milwaukee*) is illustrative. After Ruby Washington's initial TB diagnosis in June 2005, the city health department assigned her to DOT because she lived in a homeless shelter and had other risk factors for noncompliance. The clinic provided Washington with bus passes to facilitate her travel to the clinic to take her medication under observation; however, she did not comply and could not be located. In August she was held involuntarily for one month for TB treatment after giving birth in a hospital. She was released on condition that she stay at her sister's house and participate in treatment, but again she disappeared. When she was relocated, she was arrested, mistakenly released, and rearrested. At that point the health department ordered her jailed to complete her treatment (*Milwaukee*, 104–109). The court upheld the order because of her repeated failures to complete treatment, which put the community at risk of infection (*Milwaukee*, 117, 134). The court also upheld the decision to confine Washington to jail, rather than a hospital, because both institutions could provide equivalent medical care and enforce the isolation, but the cost to taxpayers for confining her to a hospital room under guard was significantly higher (*Milwaukee*, 131). This last point illustrates that the law does not require the *best* response, merely a *reasonable* one. Thus, what may be legally acceptable may not be ethically preferable.

Although *Milwaukee* may be a more extreme example, courts routinely uphold the use of infectious disease control measures like isolation and quarantine. However, such measures are not appropriate for diseases that are less easily transmitted, like HIV/AIDS, although some called for such restrictions early in the epidemic. Because HIV is not transmitted through casual contact and there were effective means to prevent transmission (e.g., universal precautions and safer sex), quarantine and isolation would infringe too greatly on individual autonomy when balanced against the threat to the public's health, as required by *Jacobson*. However, the HIV/AIDS experience and the more recent Ebola outbreak (WHO, 2015) serve as reminders that misunderstandings and fear can lead to misuses of public health powers (Weiser and Goodman, 2014; Hickox, 2015).

The 2014–2016 outbreak of Ebola in West Africa fanned fears that the fatal disease would spread to the United States. After a Liberian man was diagnosed with the disease upon returning to Dallas, Texas, and died, some states decided to quarantine health care workers and other travelers returning from West Africa. In some places, children of returned workers were required to stay home from school (Gatter, 2014). In most of these cases, these responses were overly restrictive, not based on science, and may have been unconstitutional when applying the balancing test outlined in *Jacobson* and considering principles of due process. They also conflicted with CDC guidance for responding to suspected cases of Ebola (which was modified during the epidemic), but the guidance was not legally binding on states (CDC, 2016a). In contrast, some states used less restrictive options, such as asking returning health care workers to monitor and report their temperatures to public health officials (Hodge, 2015).

Public health officials often have to act with incomplete information. They may come to different conclusions than their counterparts in other states. However, as the Ebola epidemic response suggests, it is critical that government and public health officials exercise their authority wisely and implement restrictions equally and fairly, based on the best available scientific evidence. Inconsistency and overzealous approaches can undermine public trust and ultimately compromise public health efforts.

Tobacco

Whereas a century ago communicable diseases such as influenza and TB were the leading causes of death, chronic diseases, including heart disease and cancer, now account for 48 percent of all US deaths and represent seven of the top ten leading causes of death (CDC, 2015c). Laws responding to these public health threats may require different justifications than those used in the infectious disease context. Legal responses to the public health effects of tobacco use illustrate the challenges faced when the traditional justification of protecting harm to others is more attenuated.

Over fifty years ago, the Surgeon General issued a report confirming that smoking is hazardous to health (US Department of Health, Education, and Welfare, 1964; HHS, 2014). Smoking now accounts for nearly one-fifth of US deaths annually. Lung cancer is the leading cause of US cancer deaths, and yet it is the most preventable, with smoking responsible for 90 percent of lung cancer cases in men and 80 percent in women (CDC, 2015d). Other adverse health effects attributable to smoking include other cancers, stroke, aneurysm, diabetes, and pulmonary diseases (CDC, 2015d). However, until the 2009 enactment of the Family Smoking Prevention and Tobacco Control Act (21 U.S.C. § 387), the federal Food and Drug Administration had no authority to regulate tobacco products. Accordingly, public health authorities have relied on other legal tools to protect the public from the health effects of cigarettes and other tobacco products.

Public health efforts first focused on reducing nonsmokers' exposure to secondhand smoke. Secondhand smoke exposure causes similar negative health effects in nonsmokers as in smokers and accounts for over 41,000 deaths annually from heart disease and lung cancer alone (CDC, 2015d; CDC, 2015e). Beginning in the 1970s, in response to accumulating evidence of these negative health effects, cities (CDC, 2012; Diller, 2014) and states (CDC, 2015f; American Lung Association, 2015) began adopting laws limiting and ultimately prohibiting indoor smoking in public spaces such as schools, health care facilities, restaurants, airports, and government offices, in an effort to protect employees and patrons who could not avoid secondhand smoke. The federal government similarly adopted smoke-free regulations for facilities it controls (41 C.F.R. § 102–74.315 [2008]). Lawsuits arguing for smokers' rights have been unsuccessful, as courts have held that smokers can, for example, eat in a smoke-free restaurant, while nonsmokers cannot eat and avoid secondhand smoke exposure if the restaurant were not smoke-free. As of 2015, twenty-seven states have adopted comprehensive clean indoor air laws, and local ordinances exist in some communities without state laws or where they may adopt stricter laws (Tynan et al., 2016; Tobacco Control Legal Consortium, 2014). However, significant gaps remain: about half the US population is not covered by comprehensive clean air laws, and laws may contain exemptions, such as bars and restaurants serving only adult patrons (Tynan et al., 2016).

More recent efforts seek to prohibit smoking in outdoor public places (CDC and NACCHO, 2012; Americans for Nonsmokers' Rights, 2015). There is some evidence that outdoor secondhand smoke at restaurant patios and porches, public parks, and beaches can negatively impact nonsmokers, but it is weaker than the evidence documenting the health hazards of indoor secondhand smoke exposure (Colgrove, Bayer, and Bachynski, 2011). Accordingly, other arguments, such as the pollution of water and soil and accidental fires caused by cigarette butts, have been used to support these efforts. Nevertheless, without strong evidence that outdoor exposure poses significant harm, there has been resistance to these efforts, which would further restrict individuals' ability to engage in a legal activity. Efforts to prohibit smoking in private spaces, such as apartments and cars with children in them, have similarly met resistance as unduly infringing on individual liberty, despite some evidence that secondhand smoke can affect people in adjacent apartments (King, Peck, and Babb, 2014). In 2015 the US Department of Housing and Urban

Development announced a proposed rule to require all public housing to implement smoke-free policies (Instituting Smoke-Free Public Housing, 80 FR 71762). Such bans could disproportionately affect low-income people who have fewer housing choices.

Other legal tools have been used to address the health effects of smoking. Efforts to prevent children from becoming smokers include conditioning federal funds on the adoption of state laws that prohibit the sale or distribution of products to youth under age eighteen and require inspections of sales outlets for compliance (42 U.S.C.A. § 300x-26 [1992]; SAMHSA, 2015). In addition, states attorneys general brought lawsuits against the major tobacco companies to compensate for Medicaid costs associated with smoking, resulting in the 1998 Master Settlement Agreement, with substantial payments to participating states and limitations on advertising, particularly toward children.[6]

Obesity

Obesity rates more than doubled between 1980 and 2006, and now almost 35 percent of American adults and 17 percent of children are considered obese (Trust for America's Health, 2015). Leading causes of preventable death for adults associated with obesity include heart disease, stroke, type 2 diabetes, and certain cancers (CDC, 2015a). Obese children may experience adult diseases such as type 2 diabetes, heart disease, and sleep apnea; suffer from low self-esteem and depression; and experience difficulty in school (CDC, 2015b).

A number of public health actions have been taken in the fight against obesity. Twenty states impose higher taxes (known as "sin" taxes because of their use to limit tobacco and alcohol consumption) on soda or other sugary drinks than on general groceries; thirty states tax sodas and sugary drinks in vending machines at a rate higher than for general groceries (Bridging the Gap, 2016). The cities of Berkeley, California, and Philadelphia, Pennsylvania, have also imposed additional taxes on sodas (Sahadi and Smith, 2016). Arizona has banned all vending machines from school (Ryan et al., 2006), and federal regulations limit school vending machines to healthy options (7 C.F.R. § 210.11). Some cities and states required calorie counts on menus (Hodge et al., 2011–2012; National Council of State Legislatures, 2016), a local innovation that was incorporated into the federal Patient Protection and Affordable Care Act (Pub. L. No. 111-148, 124 Stat. 119 [2010]), in addition to the menu and labeling requirements of the Food and Drug Administration (FDA, 2016). Recent research demonstrates that the public supports initiatives aimed at obesity that provide information and help promote healthier environments and options, such as menu labeling, but is less supportive of actions that restrict choice (Morain and Mello, 2013).

This resistance was evident in the public reaction to the New York City health department's 2012 "Portion Cap Rule," which the media and public viewed as coercive (Pratt, 2015). The rule limited the size of sodas sold in restaurants, movie theaters, food carts, and stadiums to less than 16 ounces. Negative references to the "nanny state," meaning the state's judgment being substituted for individual choice, were common, although under the law consumers could still purchase multiple drinks, and some locations, like convenient stores, were excluded (Harned, 2013). Despite data showing that sugary drink consumption contributes to being overweight, diabetes, and heart disease, the public reacted negatively to these limits on what they perceived as purely self-regarding behavior (*New York Times*, 2013). In *Matter of New York Statewide Coalition of Hispanic Chamber of Commerce v. New York City Department of Health and Mental Hygiene* (23 N.Y. 3d 681, 690 [2014]), the court reviewing the rule held the department's adoption of the rule overstepped its regulatory authority, because the elected City Council had not addressed the issue. Although in dicta, the court also noted that the law infringed on personal autonomy, had numerous exceptions undermining its potential public health effectiveness, and could negatively impact business.

The New York City ruling highlights the challenges of public health law approaches to preventing obesity and related chronic diseases. Taking a lesson from tobacco, efforts focusing on children, such as promoting nutrition in schools and increasing opportunities for physical activity, may be more successful than limiting adults' choices (Ashe et al., 2009). Laws that change the physical environment to promote physical exercise, provide access to healthy foods, and limit fast foods, such as through zoning, may also receive more support (Ashe et al., 2009). Evidence of economic burden could provide a potential justification for public health law action. In 2008, the medical costs of treating obesity-related diseases were estimated at $147 billion, roughly twice as much as only ten years earlier (Trust for America's Health, 2015). Also, as with tobacco, restrictions may become more acceptable to the public and courts as they become more used to public health efforts at reducing obesity and obesity-related diseases.

Conclusion

As this chapter demonstrates, governments have substantial legal authority to act to improve public health. Traditional powers are coercive and may infringe significantly on individual rights. However, that authority is limited, requires strong justification, and must limit infringement on individual rights. As society confronts public health issues that may not directly harm others, new approaches may be necessary, and public health officials may need to consider the full range of legal options available to them. Public health ethics can be useful in deciding among legal options and whether to exercise legal authority.

Notes

1. The Haddon Matrix, originally used to analyze motor vehicle accidents and now extended to other injury prevention efforts, is another framework that can be used to examine public health problems and make decisions, including law and policy. The matrix looks

at the pre-event, event, and post-event phases and the characteristics of the host (persons involved), vehicle (instrument), physical environment, and social environment (Runyan, 1998).

2. Of course, Justice Holmes also (in)famously upheld Virginia's forced sterilization of Carrie Buck, declaring, "Three generations of imbeciles are enough." The decision, the eugenics principles reflected in it (and in the state's sterilization law), and the assessment of Carrie Buck's mental capacities have since been criticized (Lombardo, 2010).
3. Author Leslie E. Wolf was involved in the development of this resource as a public health law consultant.
4. Social distancing measures vary depending on the severity of the disease and how easily it is spread. They include isolation, quarantine, quarantine of neighborhoods (known as cordon sanitaire), shelter-in-place, closing of schools, canceling of events, prohibiting public gatherings, and closing private businesses. Voluntary measures are preferred; however, mandatory measures may be needed. Note that author Stacie P. Kershner was involved in the editing and implementation of the 2010 version of this resource as an ORISE fellow with the CDC.
5. Federal quarantine and isolation are used sparingly, and there are few cases challenging federal authority. *U.S. ex rel Siegel v. Shinnick*, 219 F. Supp. 789 (E.D.N.Y. 1963) is the most recent case where a federal quarantine or isolation measure was at issue. In *Speaker v. U.S. Department of Health and Human Services Centers for Disease Control and Prevention*, 623 F.3d 1371 (11th Cir. 2010), Andrew Speaker sued the CDC over alleged Privacy Act violations; however, the tuberculosis isolation order was not in question.
6. All states except Mississippi, Florida, Texas, and Minnesota are parties to the Master Settlement Agreement (MSA). These four states had individually settled with the tobacco industry prior to the MSA.

References

Americans for Nonsmokers' Rights. 2015. U.S. Tobacco Control Laws Database. http://www.no-smoke.org/goingsmokefree.php?id=519.

American Lung Association. 2015. "State of Tobacco Control: Did Your State Make the Grade?" Accessed December 26. http://www.stateoftobaccocontrol.org/.

Ashe, M., Bennett, G., Economos, C., Goodman, E., Schilling, J., Quintillani, L., et al. 2009. "Assessing Coordination of Legal-Based Efforts across Jurisdictions and Sectors for Obesity Control." *Journal of Law, Medicine & Ethics* 37(Suppl. 1): 45–54.

Bridging the Gap. 2016. "Beverage and Snack Taxes." http://www.bridgingthegapresearch.org/research/sodasnack_taxes/.

CDC (Centers for Disease Control and Prevention). 1999. "10 Great Public Health Achievements—United States, 1900–1999." *Morbidity and Mortality Weekly Report* 48: 241–243. http://www.cdc.gov/mmwr/preview/mmwrhtml/00056796.htm.

CDC (Centers for Disease Control and Prevention). 2012. "Comprehensive Smoke-Free Laws—50 Largest US Cities, 2000 and 2012." *Morbidity and Mortality Weekly Report* 61: 914–915.

CDC (Centers for Disease Control and Prevention). 2015a. "Adult Obesity Causes and Consequences." https://www.cdc.gov/obesity/adult/causes.html.

CDC (Centers for Disease Control and Prevention). 2015b. "Childhood Obesity Causes and Consequences." http://www.cdc.gov/obesity/childhood/causes.html.

CDC (Centers for Disease Control and Prevention). 2015c. "Chronic Disease Prevention and Health Promotion: Chronic Disease Overview." http://www.cdc.gov/chronicdisease/overview/.

CDC (Centers for Disease Control and Prevention). 2015d. "Smoking and Tobacco Use: Health Effects of Cigarette Smoking." http://www.cdc.gov/tobacco/data_statistics/fact_sheets/health_effects/effects_cig_smoking/.

CDC (Centers for Disease Control and Prevention). 2015e. "Smoking and Tobacco Use: Health Effects of Secondhand Smoke." http://www.cdc.gov/tobacco/data_statistics/fact_sheets/secondhand_smoke/health_effects/.

CDC (Centers for Disease Control and Prevention). 2015f. "State Tobacco Activities Tracking and Evaluation (STATE) System." http://www.cdc.gov/statesystem/.

CDC (Centers for Disease Control and Prevention). 2015g. "Tuberculosis (TB): Basic TB Facts." Accessed December 22. http://www.cdc.gov/tb/topic/basics/default.htm.

CDC (Centers for Disease Control and Prevention). 2015h. "Tuberculosis (TB): Treatment." Accessed December 22. http://www.cdc.gov/tb/topic/treatment/default.htm.

CDC (Centers for Disease Control and Prevention). 2016a. "Notes on the Interim US Guidance for Monitoring and Movement of Persons with Potential Ebola Virus Exposure." http://www.cdc.gov/vhf/ebola/exposure/monitoring-and-movement-of-persons-with-exposure.html.

CDC (Centers for Disease Control and Prevention). 2016b. "Preemption of Local Public Health Laws." https://www.cdc.gov/phlp/docs/preemption-issue-brief.pdf.

CDC (Centers for Disease Control and Prevention). 2016c. "State School and Childcare Vaccination Laws." http://www.cdc.gov/phlp/publications/topic/vaccinations.html.

CDC (Centers for Disease Control and Prevention) and Association of State and Territorial Health Officials. 2010. *Social Distancing Law Assessment Project*. https://www.cdc.gov/phlp/publications/social_distancing.html.

CDC (Centers for Disease Control and Prevention) and Centers for Law and the Public's Health. 2009. *Tuberculosis Control Laws and Policies: A Handbook for Public Health and Legal Practitioners*. http://www.cdc.gov/tb/programs/Laws/default.htm.

CDC (Centers for Disease Control and Prevention) and NACCHO (National Association of County and City Health Officials). 2012. "Facilitator's Manual." In *Good Decision Making in Real Time: Public Health Ethics Training for Local Health Departments*. Facilitator's Manual available upon request, student materials available online. https://www.cdc.gov/od/science/integrity/phethics/trainingmaterials.htm.

ChangeLab Solutions. 2013. "Preemption and Public Health Advocacy: A Frequent Concern with Far-Reaching Consequences." http://www.changelabsolutions.org/sites/default/files/Preemption_PublicHealthAdvocacy_FS_FINAL_20130911.pdf.

Colgrove, J., Bayer, R., and Bachynski, K. E. 2011. "No Where Left to Hide? The Banishment of Smoking from Public Places." *New England Journal of Medicine* 364: 2375–2377.

Diller, P. A. 2014. "Why Do Cities Innovate in Public Health? Implications of Scale and Structure." *Washington University Law Review* 91: 1219–1292.

FDA (Food and Drug Administration). 2016. "Menu and Vending Machines Labeling Requirements." http://www.fda.gov/Food/GuidanceRegulation/GuidanceDocuments RegulatoryInformation/LabelingNutrition/ucm217762.htm.

Gatter, R. 2014. "Science over Fear Is the Lesson of Nurse's Ebola Story." New York: Network for Public Health Law, December 14. Accessed December 23, 2015. https://www.networkforphl.org/the_network_blog/2014/12/10/527/science_over_fear_is_the_lesson_of_nurses_ebola_story.

Gostin, L. O. 2005. "*Jacobson v. Massachusetts* at 100 Years: Police Powers and Civil Liberties in Tension." *American Journal of Public Health* 95: 576–581.

Gostin, L. O. 2008. *Public Health Law: Power, Duty, Restraint* (Berkeley: University of California Press).

Harned, K. 2013. "The Michael Bloomberg Nanny State: A Cautionary Tale." *Forbes*, May 10. http://www.forbes.com/sites/realspin/2013/05/10/the-michael-bloomberg-nanny-state-in-new-york-a-cautionary-tale/#27b3be961c6a.

HHS (US Department of Health and Human Services). 2014. *The Health Consequences of Smoking—50 Years of Progress: A Report of the Surgeon General*. http://www.surgeongeneral.gov/library/reports/50-years-of-progress/full-report.pdf.

Hickox, K. 2015. "Caught between Civil Liberties and Public Safety: Personal Reflections from a Healthcare Provider Treating Ebola." *Journal of Health and Biomedical Law* 11: 9–23.

Hodge, J. G. 2015. "Legal Myths of Ebola Preparedness and Response." *Notre Dame Journal of Law, Ethics and Public Policy* 29: 355–374.

Hodge, J. G., and Corbett, A. 2016. "Legal Preemption and the Prevention of Chronic Conditions." *Preventing Chronic Diseases* 13: 160121.

Hodge, J. G. Orenstein, D. G., Millea C., White L. C., and Sorensen, A. 2011–2012. "Alternative Models to Supplement Menu Labeling." *Nexus: Chapman's Journal of Law and Policy* 17: 79–96.

Holmes, O. W. 1897. "The Path of the Law." *Harvard Law Review* 10: 457–478.

IOM (Institute of Medicine). 1988. *The Future of Public Health* (Washington, D.C.: National Academies Press). http://iom.nationalacademies.org/Reports/1988/The-Future-of-Public-Health.aspx.

IOM (Institute of Medicine). 2011. *For the Public's Health: Revitalizing Law and Policy to Meet New Challenges* (Washington, D.C.: National Academies Press). https://iom.nationalacademies.org/Reports/2011/For-the-Publics-Health-Revitalizing-Law-and-Policy-to-Meet-New-Challenges.aspx.

King, B. A., Peck, R. M., and Babb, S. D. 2014. "National and State Cost Savings Associated with Prohibiting Smoking in Subsidized and Public Housing in the United States." *Preventing Chronic Disease* 11: E171.

Lombardo, P. A. 2010. *Three Generations, No Imbeciles: Eugenics, the Supreme Court, and Buck v. Bell* (Baltimore, Md.: Johns Hopkins University Press).

Mariner, W. K., Annas, G. J., and Glantz, L. H. 2005. "*Jacobson v. Massachusetts*: It's Not Your Great-Great-Grandfather's Public Health Law." *American Journal of Public Health* 95: 581–590.

Master Settlement Agreement. 1998. http://www.naag.org/assets/redesign/files/msa-tobacco/MSA.pdf.

Morain, S., and Mello, M. M. 2013. "Survey Finds Public Support for Legal Intervention Directed at Health Behavior to Fight Noncommunicable Disease." *Health Affairs* 3: 486–96.

Moulton, A. D., Goodman, R. A., and Parmet, W. E. 2007. "Perspective: Law and Great Public Health Achievements." In *Law in Public Health Practice*, edited by Richard A. Goodman (New York: Oxford University Press).

Moulton, A. D., Gottfried R. N., Goodman, R. A., Murphy, A. M., and Rawson, R. D. 2003. "What Is Public Health Legal Preparedness?" *Journal of Law, Medicine & Ethics* 31: 672–83.

National Council of State Legislatures. 2016. "Trans Fat and Menu Labeling Legislation." http://www.ncsl.org/research/health/trans-fat-and-menu-labeling-legislation.aspx.

Network for Public Health Law. 2016. "Legal Toolkit for Newborn Screening DBS." https://www.networkforphl.org/topics__resources/topics__resources/maternal_and_child_health/legal_toolkit_for_newborn_screening_dbs/.

New York Times. "New Yorkers' Views on their Mayor and His Program." 2013. *New York Times*, August 16. http://www.nytimes.com/interactive/2013/08/18/nyregion/new-yorkers-views-on-bloomberg-poll.html.

Pratt, K. 2015. "Lessons from the Demise of the Sugary Drink Portion Cap Rule." *Wake Forest Journal of Law and Policy* 5: 39–104.

Public Health Law Research LawAtlas. 2016a. "Good Samaritan Overdose Prevention Laws." http://lawatlas.org/page/good-samaritan-overdose-prevention-laws.

Public Health Law Research LawAtlas. 2016b. "Naloxone Overdose Prevention Laws." http://lawatlas.org/query?dataset=laws-regulating-administration-of-naloxone.

Rothstein, M. A. 2015. "From SARS to Ebola: Legal and Ethical Considerations for Modern Quarantine." *Indiana Health Law Review* 12: 229–280.

Runyan, C. 1998. "Using the Haddon Matrix: Introducing the Third Dimension." *Injury Prevention* 4: 302–307.

Ryan, K. W., Card-Higginson P., McCarthy S. G., Justus, M. B., and Thompson, J. W. 2006. "Arkansas Fights Fat: Translating Research into Policy to Combat Childhood and Adolescent Obesity." *Health Affairs* 25: 992–1004.

Sahadi, J., and Smith, A. 2016. "Philadelphia Passes a Soda Tax." *CNN Money*, June 16. http://money.cnn.com/2016/06/16/pf/taxes/philadelphia-passes-a-soda-tax/index.html.

SAMHSA (Substance Abuse and Mental Health Services Administration). 2015. "About the Synar Amendment and Program." http://www.samhsa.gov/synar/about.

Tobacco Control Legal Consortium. 2014. "Preemption: The Biggest Challenge to Tobacco Control." http://publichealthlawcenter.org/sites/default/files/resources/tclc-fs-preemption-tobacco-control-challenge-2014.pdf.

Tobey, J. A. 1926. *Public Health Law: A Manual of Law for Sanitarians* (Baltimore, Md.: Williams and Wilkins). http://biotech.law.lsu.edu/cphl/history/books/tobey/tobey-full.pdf.

Trust for America's Health. 2015. *The State of Obesity: Better Policies for a Healthier America 2015*. https://www.tfah.org/report-details/the-state-of-obesity-2015/.

Tynan, M., Holmes, C. B., Promoff, G., Hallett, C., Hopkins, M., and Frick, B. 2016. "State and Local Comprehensive Smoke-Free Laws for Worksites, Restaurants, and Bars—United States, 2015." *Morbidity and Mortality Weekly Report* 65: 623–626.

US Department of Health, Education, and Welfare. 1964. *Smoking and Health: Report of the Advisory Committee to the Surgeon General of the United States*. http://profiles.nlm.nih.gov/ps/access/NNBBMQ.pdf.

US Department of Housing and Urban Development. 2015. Proposed Rule: Instituting Smoke-Free Public Housing, 80 FR 71762. https://www.federalregister.gov/articles/2015/11/17/2015-29346/instituting-smoke-free-public-housing#h-4.

Weiser, B., and Goodman, J. D. 2014. "The Flu, TB and Now Ebola: A Rare Legal Remedy Returns." *New York Times*, October 26. http://mobile.nytimes.com/2014/10/27/nyregion/as-states-look-to-halt-ebola-restrictions-prompt-a-debate.html.

Wolf, S. M. 2004. "Law and Bioethics: From Value to Violence." *Journal of Law, Medicine & Ethics* 32: 293–306.

WHO (World Health Organization). 2015. "Ebola Virus Disease." http://www.who.int/mediacentre/factsheets/fs103/en/.

Yang, Y. T., and Silverman, R. D. 2015. "Legislative Prescriptions for Controlling Nonmedical Vaccine Exemptions." *Journal of the American Medical Association* 313: 247–248.

PART TWO

PUBLIC HEALTH TOPICS

SECTION THREE

HEALTH SYSTEMS AND PUBLIC HEALTH

CHAPTER 10

AN OVERVIEW OF THE ETHICS OF HEALTH SYSTEMS

MARIA W. MERRITT AND ADNAN A. HYDER

Introduction

A health system at the national or subnational level is fundamentally about serving the legitimate health and allied needs of populations, especially those that are vulnerable. As defined by the World Health Organization (WHO), a health system includes "all the activities whose primary purpose is to promote, restore or maintain health" (WHO, 2000, 5). Its fundamental objectives are to improve population health, to respond to people's expectations, and to protect against the financial costs of poor health (WHO, 2000). Also, according to the WHO (2000), four health system functions are critical to the collective achievement of these objectives: stewardship, financing, creating resources, and delivering services. While there are alternate definitions of health systems found in the literature, many of them have these common elements and provide a rationale for investments and actions to achieve good health for all people. It is important at the outset to distinguish "health systems" as characterized by the WHO from "public health systems" as characterized, for instance, by the US Centers for Disease Control and Prevention (CDC), which encompass virtually every sector that touches on health, including law enforcement, arts, recreation, and philanthropy (CDC, 2017). We are concerned here with the narrower subject of "health systems" as a central component of "public health systems."

The application of ethics to health systems has led to the development of specific sets of considerations, often termed "health systems ethics," encompassing a broad range of issues, such as ethics of policy, governance, resource allocation, social justice, and coverage. This chapter provides an overview of the section of *The Oxford Handbook of Public*

Health Ethics dedicated to an examination of some of these issues. Readers wishing to expand their understanding of related topics may also wish to refer to this volume's "Public Health Policy and Politics" section and other resources, such as publications by Bridget Pratt and Adnan A. Hyder (Pratt and Hyder, 2016; Hyder et al., 2014).

That the quality, accessibility, and equitability of health systems is a matter of public health is hard to dispute. Indeed, the two distinctive characteristics of public health most pertinent to health systems are that public health "is a public or collective good" and that "its promotion often entails government action" (see Faden, Shebaya, and Siegel, this volume). First, public health as a collective good is concerned with *populations*: it is "a public, communal good, where the benefits to one person cannot readily be individuated from those to another, though its burdens and benefits often appear to fall unevenly on different sub-groups of the population" (Faden, Shebaya and Siegel, this volume). This characteristic of public health corresponds to the improvement of population health as the first objective of a health system (WHO, 2000). Next, the achievement of this objective and the other objectives of a health system "frequently requires government action backed by the force of law.... In this, as in all other areas of official state action, we therefore have to address tensions among justice, security, and the scope of legal restrictions and regulations" (Faden, Shebaya, and Siegel, this volume). In this overview, we draw on these two ethically relevant characteristics of public health to organize a summary of the key issues addressed in this section, and to identify directions for further explorations of health systems ethics.

Chapter Overviews

In the section's opening chapter, Michael J. DiStefano and Jennifer Prah Ruger examine issues of health systems *stewardship*, *accountability*, and *governance* in public health ethics. Stewardship, as a major health system function, plays a special role because it is the oversight function that regulates all other health system functions (WHO, 2000). The authors argue that stewardship is properly exercised not only through formal structures exclusive to national governments, but also through informal structures that exist in inter- and extragovernmental bodies as well as national governments. All of these institutions engage in *governance*, defined as "the range of both informal *and* formal values, norms, practices, and institutions that provide better order than if we relied purely upon formal regulations and institutions" (Weiss, 2009, 257). The chapter presents stewardship as a form of governance explicitly oriented around normative ethical commitments (Saltman and Ferroussier-Davis, 2000), describes the role of accountability in governance, and identifies issues of public health ethics specific to the accountability of health systems stewards. For all health systems stewards, a central concern of accountability is substantive and procedural clarity regarding systemic objectives and their alignment with the public good. Differentiating among health systems stewards, the authors specify ethical issues in terms of the roles and accountability mechanisms appropriate to states, intergovernmental bodies, and extragovernmental bodies. For instance, issues of enforcement and knowledgeable policy formation pertain to states; issues of international justice pertain to intergovernmental bodies like the WHO and the World Bank; and issues of whether and how to harmonize with governmental activities pertain to extragovernmental bodies like NGOs.

A foundational question in public health ethics is how public health activities are morally justified. Some prominent forms of moral justification appeal to overall benefit, collective efficiency, distributive fairness, and harm prevention (see Faden and Shebaya, this volume). In their chapter, George W. Pariyo and Henry Lucas offer human resources for health as a lens through which to view interactions among these considerations. The efficient and equitable promotion of population health depends upon human resources as one of three principal health system inputs (the other two being physical capital and consumables) under the function of creating resources (WHO, 2000). Because the local and national functioning of the health care workforce is pervasively influenced by global factors, this chapter examines ethical aspects of global human resources for health (HRH). It describes influences on the demand and supply of HRH, highlights aggregate shortfalls and inequitable distribution of HRH as ethical problems, and considers strategies proposed to solve these problems.

The account of national strategies and their associated ethical issues provides a critical perspective on the institutional means by which countries attempt to realize ethical aspirations for HRH. For example, a country's effort to provide equitable access to care of acceptable quality requires consistent monitoring and supervision of both public and private providers. If some services are delegated to lay health workers, they ought to occupy clearly defined roles integrated into a well-supervised workforce where professionals in sufficient numbers remain responsible and accountable for oversight. Conscientious efforts are required to uphold patients' rights to privacy and confidentiality and health workers' rights to a safe, professional environment, with adequate equipment and supplies.

The authors then move to the global level to survey the dynamics of the international market for health personnel and outline parameters for successfully implementing two global conventions codifying relevant rights and obligations: the 1999 Montreal Convention and 2010 WHO Global Code of Practice on International Recruitment of Health Personnel. They conclude with a caution against compromising equity, privacy, confidentiality, and other ethical requirements in the quest to mitigate global HRH shortages.

The remaining chapters each take an overarching perspective on health system performance, presenting two complementary viewpoints on ethical issues at the intersection of health systems and research. Bridget Pratt and Adnan A. Hyder address the ethics of health systems research, understood as knowledge generation in the service of overall health system improvement. Stephanie Morain, Nancy E. Kass, and Ruth R. Faden discuss ethical challenges that arise in efforts to create and maintain "learning" health care systems, which aim to contribute to systemic improvement specifically by integrating knowledge generation into clinical care and implementing clinical care improvements based on the knowledge generated. In keeping with the characteristic concern of public health for populations, both chapters seek to articulate ethical standards for systemic inquiry and research activities typically focused on populations, groups, and facilities rather than individuals as the unit of analysis. An underlying ethical challenge common to both chapters is the need to translate to the collective level certain ethical principles and guidelines that were originally developed with individual protections in the foreground.

Pratt and Hyder note that investment in health systems research (HSR) is increasing as an outgrowth of strong global interest in health system strengthening (Bennett et al., 2008). Accordingly, they identify the characteristic research aims of HSR as describing health system operations, evaluating health system performance, diagnosing the causes of poor performance, and testing remedial interventions, usually at the level of populations or groups served by the system under study. The authors first delineate the application of traditional bioethics principles (respect for persons, beneficence, and justice) distinctively to HSR. They then present the case for supplementing traditional bioethics principles by explicitly extending to health systems *research ethics* several core ethical commitments previously developed for health systems *ethics* as contextual specifications of the traditional principles: citizen engagement, partnership and collaboration, and sustainability. In conclusion, the chapter mentions results from a 2017 review (Pratt et al., 2017) indicating a dearth of formal ethics guidance for the design, conduct, and oversight of HSR, and suggests an agenda for future work to develop comprehensive, useful guidance.

Morain, Kass, and Faden present the concept of a learning health care system (LHCS), whose proponents envision the continuous feedback of findings *from* data collected in conjunction with clinical care *into* the improvement of organizational approaches to subsequent clinical care delivery. This vision is inspired by the need to reduce the incidence of medical errors, curtail the delivery of care that is unnecessary or ineffective, identify which effective treatment strategies work best, and promote the widespread delivery of recommended care. The chapter describes the moral rationale for transitioning to an LHCS in terms of three goals—just health care, high-quality health care, and economic well-being—that societies arguably have an ethical obligation to promote (Faden et al., 2013), with the implication that health care institutions specifically ought to improve justice, safety, and quality in health care (Largent, Joffe, and Miller, 2011; Cuckler et al., 2013). In discussing ethical challenges arising in the transition to and operation of LHCSs, the authors note that long-standing concerns of clinical and research ethics, such as the privacy and confidentiality of patient data, take on a new magnitude and pervasiveness with institutional commitments to the continuous data generation required by LHCSs. Another locus of ethical challenges in LHCSs is both the need to target learning activities disproportionately to areas that reduce disadvantage and the need for responsible adaptation of institutional ethics and regulatory oversight structures, traditionally framed by a sharp distinction between research and practice, to fit with multipurpose systems that aspire to integrate knowledge generation with care delivery (Kass et al., 2013; Lee et al., 2016). Finally, the authors summarize contemporary debates on proposed ethical guidance for the LHCS as a young and still-emerging field (see, for example, Faden et al., 2013; Largent et al., 2011; Platt, Grossman, and Selker, 2013; Fiscella et al., 2015).

Conclusion

Health systems ethics is a key pillar of public health ethics, as the success of public health approaches often lies in the performance of national and state-level health systems. Early explorations of the particularities of health systems ethics reveal the importance of applying health ethics to groups of people, efficiency of systems, transparency of decisions, and responsiveness to people's concerns. Yet while such analysis, as demonstrated by earlier publications and summarized by the chapters in this section, has been critical for the field, much more needs to be done. Future areas of conceptual and empirical work may include determining the specific ethical nuances of successful delivery of health services to remote populations, how the ethics of health policy will affect decisions in health systems, the values espoused by those on the supply-side of health systems, and perceptions of fairness that communities bring to health systems. We encourage readers to address some of these issues and contribute to the field of health systems ethics in the coming years.

References

Bennett, S., Adam, T., Zarowsky, C., Tangcharoensathien, V., Ranson, K., Evans, T., et al. 2008. "From Mexico to Mali: Progress in Health Policy and Systems Research." *Lancet* 372: 1571–1578.

CDC (US Centers for Disease Control and Prevention). 2017. "National Public Health Performance Standards." https://www.cdc.gov/stltpublichealth/nphps/index.html.

Cuckler, G. A., Sisko, A. M., Keehan, S. P., Smith, S. D., Madison, A. J., Poisal, J. A., et al. 2013. "National Health Expenditure Projections, 2012–22: Slow Growth until Coverage Expands and Economy Improves." *Health Affairs* 32(10): 1820–1831.

Faden, R. R., Kass, N. E., Goodman, S. N., Pronovost, P., Tunis, S., and Beauchamp, T. L. 2013. "An Ethics Framework for a Learning Health Care System: A Departure from Traditional Research Ethics and Clinical Ethics." *Hastings Center Report* 43(1): S16–S27.

Fiscella, K., Tobin, J. A., Carroll, J. K., He, H., and Obgedegbe, G. 2015. "Ethical Oversight in Quality Improvement and Quality Improvement Research: New Approaches to Promote a Learning Health Care System." *BMC Medical Ethics* 16(1): 63.

Hyder, A. A., Rattani, A., Krubiner, C., Bachani, A. M., and Tran, N. T. 2014. "Ethical Review of Health Systems Research in Low- and Middle-Income Countries: A Conceptual Exploration." *American Journal of Bioethics* 14(2): 28–37.

Kass, N. E., Faden, R. R., Goodman, S. N., Pronovost, P., Tunis, S., and Beauchamp, T. L. 2013. "The Research-Treatment Distinction: A Problematic Approach for Determining Which Activities Should Have Ethical Oversight." *Hastings Center Report* 43(1): S4–S15.

Largent, E. A., Joffe, S., and Miller, F. G. 2011. "Can Research and Care be Ethically Integrated?" *Hastings Center Report* 41(4): 37–46.

Lee, S. S. J., Kelley, M., Cho, M. K., Kraft, S. A., James, C., Constantine, M., et al. 2016. "Adrift in the Gray Zone: IRB Perspectives on Research in the Learning Health System." *AJOB Empirical Bioethics* 7(2): 125–134.

Platt, R., Grossman, C., and Selker, H. P. 2013. "Evaluation as Part of Operations: Reconciling the Common Rule and Continuous Improvement." *Hastings Center Report* 43(1): S37–S39.

Pratt, B., and Hyder, A. A. 2016. "Governance of Transnational Global Health Research Consortia and Health Equity." *American Journal of Bioethics* 16(10): 29–45.

Pratt, B., Paul, A., Hyder, A. A., and Ali, J. 2017. "Ethics of Health Policy and Systems Research: A Scoping Review of the Literature." *Health Policy and Planning* 32(6): 890–910.

Saltman, R. B., and Ferroussier-Davis, O. 2000. "The Concept of Stewardship in Health Policy." *Bulletin of the World Health Organization* 78(6): 732–739.

Weiss, T. G. 2009. "What Happened to the Idea of World Government?" *International Studies Quarterly* 53: 253–271.

WHO (World Health Organization). 2000. *The World Health Report 2000: Health Systems: Improving Performance* (Geneva: World Health Organization).

CHAPTER 11

HEALTH SYSTEMS STEWARDSHIP, GOVERNANCE, AND ACCOUNTABILITY: ISSUES OF PUBLIC HEALTH ETHICS

MICHAEL J. DISTEFANO AND JENNIFER PRAH RUGER

Stewardship in Relation to Governance and Government

The World Health Organization's *World Health Report 2000* includes *stewardship* among the four major functions of health systems, along with *financing*, *resource generation*, and *service delivery* (WHO, 2000). The WHO characterizes stewardship in terms of the functions undertaken by national governments as guided by health policy objectives; such functions may include crafting and implementing health-related policy and regulating the behaviors of actors like health insurers and providers (WHO, 2016). The WHO and others have envisaged stewardship as a particular form of governance that governments are responsible for carrying out (WHO, 2016; Saltman and Ferroussier-Davis, 2000; Travis et al., 2002).

On closer examination, however, governance includes not only the institutional functions of governments (legislation, regulation, enforcement) as formally constituted political authorities, but also a range of informal "values, norms, practices, and institutions" that are distinct from and complementary to governmental functions, and which, unlike governmental functions, typically exist at the international level as well as the national level (Weiss, 2009, 257). Even though the WHO's explicit characterization of stewardship is limited to government, the *World Health Report 2000* describes several stewardship roles that do not require the formal regulations or political authority of government and could just as well be functions of intergovernmental and extragovernmental bodies, such as "defining the vision and direction of health policy" and "collecting and using information" (WHO, 2000, xiv). Indeed, proliferating entities independently influence global public health primarily through governance—not government—including both intergovernmental bodies (e.g., the WHO and World Bank) and extragovernmental bodies such as civil society organizations (CSOs) and nongovernmental organizations (NGOs) (Ng and Ruger, 2011). These conditions suggest that expanding the explicit scope of stewardship as a form of governance, at least in the health domain, would be plausible. While others have argued that the scope of stewardship ought to include subnational authorities or even professional associations (Travis et al., 2002), defining stewardship only as the role of government or bodies sanctioned by governments obscures the influence of intergovernmental and extragovernmental actors who are not accountable to populations in the same way that governmental actors are.

This chapter conceives of stewardship as a particular form of governance that is the role of both governments and intergovernmental and extragovernmental bodies to carry out. The chapter discusses what stewardship means as a particular form of governance, describes accountability's important role in stewardship, and outlines issues of public health ethics regarding the ways in which specific health systems stewards are held accountable.

Stewardship as Ethically Conscientious Governance

Stewardship can be understood as ethically conscientious governance (Saltman and Ferroussier-Davis, 2000; Kass, 1990; Armstrong, 1997). The obligations of stewardship thus understood present ethical tensions and trade-offs similar to those of public health ethics. As stewards of public health, institutions and organizations face ethical tensions between utilitarian goals of health maximization and deontological goals of protecting autonomy. Ideally, public health stewardship would involve balancing equity and efficiency in promoting health functioning and health agency for all.

Decisions about how to strike an ethically responsible balance, especially when governments employ coercive measures in pursuit of public health goals, must be justifiable. This requirement means that accountability in health systems stewardship is critical. Brinkerhoff (2004, 372) writes that "the essence of accountability is answerability," which he argues entails providing both information and justifications regarding decisions and actions. Because health systems stewardship explicitly engages with ethical tensions and trade-offs regarding public health, strong accountability mechanisms help to ensure that the decisions and actions of the stewards are adequately justified to the public. The next section describes theories and mechanisms of accountability.

Accountability for Governments and Governance

Accountability implies the right of some actors to sanction others when they fail in their responsibilities under an agreed-upon set of standards (Grant and Keohane, 2005). Health systems stewardship requires accountability to justify decisions and behaviors influencing public health. If stewardship is a particular form of governance that both country governments and intergovernmental and extragovernmental bodies are responsible for carrying out, a useful theory of accountability must acknowledge the difference between government and governance and describe accountability mechanisms that can function for these varied actors.

Grant and Keohane (2005) distinguish between two models of accountability, differing primarily by who holds power-wielders (i.e., governments and intergovernmental and extragovernmental bodies) accountable. Under the *participation* model, all those who are affected by the power-wielders' actions are entitled to hold them accountable. For example, in a direct democracy, the people enjoy and are permitted significant influence over individual government decisions through political participation, frequent elections, and substantial congruence on views and goals among representatives and the people. If a power-wielder strays too far from the collective preferences of those affected by its actions, the people are entitled to replace it.

Under the *delegation* model, those who entrust the power-wielders with certain powers hold them accountable, such as when national governments delegate certain health-related work to the WHO. Power-wielders are entrusted with the authority to act within the bounds of some office or to fulfill a general purpose. If power-wielders violate the relevant bounds or purpose, those who originally entrusted them with the power may remove them. Those who delegate to a power-wielder might not always be the same as those affected by the power-wielder's actions. Under the delegation model, a power-wielder's actions do not necessarily have to agree with the collective preferences of those affected, as long as the power-wielder acts according to the arrangement with the delegator.

Several accountability mechanisms—in addition to traditional democratic or electoral mechanisms—arise from these two models (Grant and Keohane, 2005), thus allowing us to make better sense of the ways in which both government and governance bodies may be held accountable. To be sure, nondemocratic mechanisms can operate to hold governments accountable, such as judicial checks on legislative actions, and extragovernmental bodies may incorporate democratic mechanisms, as represented by the WHO's World Health Assembly. However, legal and other nondemocratic mechanisms (e.g., fiscal, market, peer, and public reputational) can also operate to hold intergovernmental and extragovernmental actors accountable. For example, budget restrictions are a form of fiscal mechanism through which individual or institutional donors can hold non-governmental organizations accountable (more below).

Others have also identified nondemocratic mechanisms related to social or community accountability (Paul, 1992). *Voice*, understood as public participation in or protest of power-wielders' decisions and actions, is an example of a peer or public-reputational mechanism. *Exit* is a form of market mechanism whereby consumers of some public service register discontent with one provider by choosing an alternative supplier. When there are no feasible means for exercising voice, exit can also be seen as an accountability mechanism; there have been instances, for example, of individuals refusing free vaccinations from the only possible supplier as a final attempt to protest a government failure to fulfill more basic needs, such as nutrition or education (Rubincam and Naysmith, 2009).

Theories that include multiple factors for accountability include the mutual collective accountability (MCA) framework (Ruger, 2012; Wachira and Ruger, 2011) and the framework presented by Grant and Keohane (2005). MCA calls for all actors working toward a common, specific health goal (e.g., the elimination of an insect vector for Chagas disease) to agree on respective roles and obligations needed to meet this goal. In MCA, institutions and organizations hold each other accountable through clear, transparent, and mutually agreed-upon standards, although transparent agreement regarding who is to do what can also enable those affected by the institutions' work to hold those institutions accountable (Ruger, 2012). For example, an empirical study of MCA in the context of shared health governance evaluated several indicators: (i) goal alignment; (ii) knowledge and mutual understanding of key outcomes and principle indicators for evaluating those outcomes (consensus about the use of indicators and the statistics that measure these indicators and their implications); (iii) adequate levels of resources (human and financial); (iv) effective, efficient resource use for priority areas; (v) meaningful inclusion and participation of key global, national, and subnational groups and institutions; and (vi) special efforts to ensure participation of key vulnerable groups most affected by policy decisions (e.g., the poor, women, youths, persons with disabilities, and the elderly) (Wachira and Ruger, 2011).

Brinkerhoff's work on health systems accountability, while important for its linking of accountability to stewardship and for its identification of linkages between health systems actors, ultimately fails to consider whether and how global organizations are held accountable. Like Travis et al. (2002), Brinkerhoff acknowledges the relevance of nongovernmental actors at a subnational level, but largely excludes intergovernmental and extragovernmental actors that operate globally (see Brinkerhoff, 2004, Figure 1).

Grant and Keohane (2005, 29) offer a framework that outlines several mechanisms through which institutions and those affected by the institutions' work may engage in accountability practices. They argue that "conventional views of accountability"—typically rooted in representative democracy—might be appropriate as an ideal for states, but not for global institutions such as intergovernmental and extragovernmental bodies. Accountability, they state, "implies that some actors have the right to hold other actors to a set of standards, to judge whether they have fulfilled their responsibilities in light of these standards, and to impose sanctions if they determine that these responsibilities have not been met."

Issues of Public Health Ethics in the Accountability of Health Systems Stewards

To promote ethically conscientious governance, health systems stewardship must grapple with the ethical tensions and trade-offs arising from the pursuit of often competing goals. Maximizing health across a population, for example, can conflict with individual agency. Accountability mechanisms can help justify decisions that make trade-offs between these alternative goals. The ethical justification for these decisions is tied to accountability in several ways.

Health systems stewards must be transparent about their ultimate goals and how they align with the public good. How the public good is defined remains an open question in public health ethics, so substantive clarity in goals is integral to the ethical commitment of transparency itself and in holding stewards accountable. A clear sense of what is expected of stewards is essential if they are to be held accountable. However, substantive goals may differ across populations. Thus, the procedure by which health system goals are specified and decided upon—who participates or decides, and by what process—is also of ethical importance.

Accountability mechanisms are such procedures. Given that various accountability mechanisms might allow different populations to hold power-wielders accountable, the substantive goals to which the power-wielders are held accountable might also differ. The question of who ought to decide what counts as the public good should therefore partially prescribe which accountability mechanisms are implemented to hold power-wielders accountable. For example, low-income countries (and the individuals who reside in them) cannot meaningfully participate in the fiscal mechanisms of accountability by which high-income countries wield substantial control over the WHO's direction and decisions (more below). However, so far as the WHO's actions affect low-income countries and their inhabitants, the conviction that these populations ought to exert control over its direction and decisions implies adopting a participation model of accountability and associated accountability mechanisms. Accountability mechanisms are therefore an important procedural link to substantive considerations about the public good in the health sphere.

To be sure, adopting the proper accountability mechanisms might not be sufficient to empower the populations whose conceptions of the public good ought to influence health systems stewards' goals. Accountability, especially when leveraged through civil society organizations with privileged access to disadvantaged populations, can draw attention to existing health inequalities and enable health systems to better meet the demands of social justice. On the other hand, the populations most in need—precisely because of their disadvantage—might be the least likely to participate in even the best-intentioned accountability mechanisms. Relying on accountability mechanisms that ignore this concern might therefore fail to meet the demands of social justice.

Another concern is that the possibility of reaching substantive agreement regarding the public good diminishes as more numerous and diverse populations are invited to join in holding power-wielders accountable. However, adopting the "right" procedures, of which accountability mechanisms are an important part (Daniels, 2000) cannot ensure social justice, since it is imperative to achieve agreement regarding the public good.

Drawing on this overview, we discuss below some specific roles and accountability mechanisms pertaining to states and intergovernmental and extragovernmental bodies engaged in health systems stewardship. These examples are not exhaustive, but they highlight relevant issues of public health ethics related to stewardship and accountability.

States

A common view of determining the public good, including who ought to decide, holds that state boundaries define the "public" (Faden and Shebaya, 2015). *Statists* argue that national boundaries carve out discrete publics, and state health systems may justifiably limit the scope of public health practice to those living within their borders. So far as a state's actions largely affect only its citizens and other residents, a participation model of accountability might not support the consideration of outside populations. Additionally, states are subject to elections or other democratic, legal, or fiscal accountability mechanisms available only to citizens and, sometimes, residents. The delegation model might therefore also justify this limited scope, given that the means of delegation are restricted in this way. However, Thomas Pogge (2002) argues that individuals of the developed world are in fact the cause of many global health inequalities beyond their nations' borders. On this view, adopting the participation model would imply that national health systems ought to be accountable to individuals around the world and could therefore have duties to promote public health globally.

Enforcement Powers

States typically have exclusive power to enforce compliance with regulations at an individual and institutional level. Enforcement powers limit the freedom of individuals and institutions, but they may be justified when the public benefit is large or a specific subgroup is benefited or protected. Accountability is important for ensuring that enforcement powers are tied to such goals.

What mechanisms of accountability are necessary to justify enforcement powers that ostensibly aim at the public good? One answer is that states are democratically accountable to their citizens, and that this accountability mechanism empowers those who ought to have influence over the state's goals and provides the means with which they pursue these goals. However, states differ in the extent to which they are de facto democratically accountable. Some states resemble the participation model of accountability. For example, the Swiss electorate has veto power over federal laws. On the other hand, representative democracies more closely fit the delegation model, giving more influence to representatives than to all those affected by the state's actions. Other countries, such as China, may lack democratic procedures altogether yet still enforce compliance, raising questions about whether these powers are aligned with the public good at all.

Tying the justification of enforcement powers solely to outcomes might be challenging, in that states can struggle to meet health-related goals despite their best efforts. Investigating more comprehensively who has decision-making power and how decisions are made within the state might better identify ethically troubling instances of enforcement. For example, enforcement powers that disproportionately impact disenfranchised populations, such as immigrants, can undermine justice.

The Work of Agencies or Ministries

The crafting and implementation of health-related policy relies on developing expert knowledge and regulations, accomplished largely by executive agencies or ministries. Agencies are typically directly accountable to funders, heads of executive branches, and local boards of health, but only indirectly accountable to communities (IOM, 2011), often through notice and comment periods, which can function as a form of "voice" for the public (Paul, 1992). Many agency or ministry leaders are appointed by executive branch heads and do not require outside approval. The delegation model, therefore, most appropriately describes how agencies or ministries are typically held accountable.

These actors are sometimes criticized for developing regulations that infringe on autonomy. Promoting the public good, however, often requires placing limits on individual autonomy. A lack of participation accountability could be ethically concerning if it prevents agencies or ministries from identifying and acting in the public good as determined by those affected by their actions. The interests of individuals or groups who cannot participate in the available accountability mechanisms might be overlooked, which is concerning from a justice perspective. Still, considering the interests of all individuals and groups might not ensure good outcomes, as a large body of research has demonstrated the many ways individuals fail to think and act rationally. According to this view, it is best to adopt a paternalistic approach and leave decisions about how best to promote public health to expert agencies or ministries.

Intergovernmental Bodies

The WHO

As with other United Nations agencies, the WHO was established by consenting states via a treaty enumerating certain roles it is meant to fulfill. The delegation model of accountability therefore applies to the WHO, meaning the states entrusted the WHO with authority to act within the treaty's bounds, and as delegators they may hold the WHO accountable if it fails to uphold its obligations. Are states the only bodies that should hold the WHO accountable? One objection is that the delegation model leaves the WHO unaccountable to individuals or to nonstate groups (Ruger, 2014). Can the WHO meet the demands of public health ethics without direct accountability to nonstate actors?

Transferred accountability through state members of the World Health Assembly (WHA), the legislative body of the WHO, could be sufficient. Where strong domestic accountability mechanisms exist, states should be best positioned to understand and advocate for their citizens' interests. Unfortunately, many states are not adequately accountable to their citizens. Furthermore, over 75 percent of the 2014–2015 WHO budget consisted of voluntary extrabudgetary donations with donor strings attached (Butler, 2013). Certain states might therefore exercise disproportionate influence in the WHO despite the one-state–one-vote WHA. For example, the United States denied funding after the WHO proposed a new "essential drug program," a move opposed by US pharmaceutical companies (Brown, Cueto, and Fee, 2006). Thus, the WHO might not always act in the best interests of individuals living in less influential countries, raising serious social justice concerns, and inadequate accountability mechanisms might result in greater disadvantages for those already the worst off. The WHO might also fail to maximize the good it achieves if its accountability mechanisms do not incorporate all relevant voices in its decision-making processes.

The World Bank

Representation on the World Bank's Executive Board is unequal, with permanent seats only for large donor countries. Voting share is tied to state contributions, making the United States the only country with effective veto power. Funding for the International Development Association, which provides loans to developing countries, is renegotiated every several years in a process that has historically been co-opted for political ends; for example, the United States secured a World Bank promise during the 1970s that it would not lend to Vietnam (Clinton and Sridhar, 2017). These realities suggest that the World Bank might be primarily accountable to wealthier nations and elite interests through fiscal accountability mechanisms.

The legacy of the Bank's structural adjustment programs, which have been criticized for not only failing to promote health, but also undermining it in some cases (Ruger, 2005; Stuckler and Basu, 2013), ground these concerns. The World Bank has responded to these criticisms. In 2010 the Bank began publishing data about its investment projects. While such reforms have improved decision transparency, they have not done enough to improve decision-making transparency (Clinton and Sridhar, 2017). The former is important for accountability in terms of substantive outcomes and determining if the Bank is effective, but little is known about the Bank's rationale for choosing certain projects over others, or which interests it ultimately privileges. Procedural accountability might still be lacking.

Extragovernmental Bodies

Extragovernmental bodies include civil society organizations (CSOs) and nongovernmental organizations (NGOs), which can operate either within national boundaries or across them as international NGOs (INGOs). CSOs are typically nonprofit organizations established by citizens to promote health. Health-related NGOs typically focus on health services delivery, including preventive services, health education, and advocacy or lobbying.

These organizations have many advantages over states in promoting health. They might be devoted to a particular service (e.g., reproductive services), thereby providing an opportunity for social accountability through market "exit" (Paul, 1992), or to a particular population (e.g., adolescents), and thus have fewer populations to which they are accountable. Often operationally nimble, they can be more flexible and access remote communities. Given their on-the-ground work in communities, they can empower the most vulnerable through education or organization (OECD, 2009); NGOs played an important role in improving access to essential medicines following the implementation of the Agreement on Trade-Related Aspects of Intellectual Property Rights (TRIPS) ('t Hoen, 2002). They can thereby fill a gap in accountability by giving voice to vulnerable individuals seriously affected by the actions of states and intergovernmental bodies, thus serving as "voice surrogates" (Paul, 1992, 1055). Insofar as a participation model of accountability does not obtain among intergovernmental bodies, CSOs may function to correct and check powerful interests and actors. For these reasons, CSOs are often described as more democratic than intergovernmental organizations, and they may help promote justice within health systems.

Of course, CSOs could also fail to check the actions of powerful states and organizations—as well as their own actions. For example, CSOs benefited from increased funding in the 1980s as structural adjustment led to reductions in state public health spending (Doyle and Patel, 2008). With much of this increased funding coming from Western donors, CSOs came to be seen as "passive agents of the neoliberal agenda" (Doyle and Patel, 2008, 1932). CSOs could thus in fact be accountable chiefly to powerful interests. Overall, many interests compete for the attention of CSOs, raising questions about whom these organizations are accountable to in practice, and whether trade-offs in meeting accountability demands are inevitable (Ossewaarde, Nijhof, and Heyse, 2008).

Other criticisms focus specifically on whether CSOs are more democratic than states or intergovernmental organizations. For example, CSO leadership is not typically the result of popular elections. CSOs are usually governed by a board, often composed of friends, with opaque decision-making procedures (Doyle and Patel, 2008). Moreover, CSOs might undermine efforts by states to bolster their own democratic accountability. Insofar as visibly delivering health services to populations in need is one way for states to build democratic accountability, CSOs acting independently of national governments could undermine these efforts.

Conclusion

This chapter argues that stewardship ought to be conceived as a particular form of governance that is the role of both governments and intergovernmental and extragovernmental bodies to carry out. Stewardship as ethically conscientious governance is grounded in an explicit normative commitment to the promotion of justice, including both consequentialist and deontological claims, as part of public health policy and practice. The justification of trade-offs and resolution of tensions among various objectives requires strong accountability mechanisms tied to ethical questions about defining the public good. Other chapters in this volume address related issues. Faden and Shebaya (this volume) ask whether the fundamental moral justification for public health activities is their importance for maximizing good health outcomes or their importance for promoting social justice, or whether it can be both. Achieving either goal is often so complex as to justify tasking expert institutions and organizations with the promotion of public health. Hecht, Arias, and Krubiner (this volume) ask about the relationship between stewardship and governance, stating that "stewardship and governance are separate concepts, though they overlap and entwine substantially."

This chapter has described a theory of accountability that fits the conception of stewardship as ethically conscientious governance, and it has further explored issues of public health ethics in health systems stewardship by discussing specific roles pertaining to states and intergovernmental and extragovernmental bodies. This is not an exhaustive discussion, but it is intended to highlight salient issues and demonstrate how similar analyses might be extended to other health systems actors and functions.

References

Armstrong, J. L. 1997. *Stewardship and Public Service* (Ottawa: Canadian Public Service Commission).

Brinkerhoff, D. W. 2004. "Accountability and Health Systems: Toward Conceptual Clarity and Policy Relevance." *Health Policy and Planning* 19(6): 371–379.

Brown, T. M., Cueto, M., and Fee, E. 2006. "The World Health Organization and the Transition from 'International' to 'Global' Public Health." *American Journal of Public Health* 96: 62–72.

Butler. D. 2013. "Agency Gets a Grip on Budget." *Nature* 498(7452): 18–19.

Clinton, C., and Sridhar, D. 2017. *Governing Global Health: Who Runs the World and Why?* (New York: Oxford University Press).

Daniels, N. 2000. "Accountability for Reasonableness: Establishing a Fair Process for Priority Setting Is Easier Than Agreeing on Principles." *British Medical Journal* 321: 1300–1301.

Doyle, C., and Patel, P. 2008. "Civil Society Organisations and Global Health Initiatives: Problems of Legitimacy." *Social Science and Medicine* 66: 1928–1938.

Faden, R., and Shebaya, S. 2015. "Public Health Ethics." In *The Stanford Encyclopedia of Philosophy*, edited by E. N. Zalta. Stanford, Calif.: Stanford University. https://plato.stanford.edu/entries/publichealth-ethics/#JusFaiPubHea.

Grant, R. W., and Keohane, R. O. 2005. "Accountability and Abuses of Power in World Politics." *American Political Science Review* 99(1): 29–43.

IOM (Institute of Medicine). 2011. "Measurement and Accountability." In *For the Public's Health: The Role of Measurement in Action and Accountability* (Washington, D.C.: National Academies Press).

Kass, H. D. 1990. "Stewardship as a Fundamental Element in Images of Public Administration." In *Images and Identities in Public Administration*, edited by H. D. Kass and B. L. Catron, 113–131 (London: SAGE).

Ng, N., and Ruger, J. P. 2011. "Global Health Governance at a Crossroads." *Global Health Governance* 3(2): 1–37.

OECD (Organisation for Economic Co-operation and Development). 2009. *Society and Aid Effectiveness: Findings, Recommendations, and Good Practice*. Better Aid series (Paris: OECD Publishing).

Ossewaarde, R., Nijhof, A., and Heyse, L. 2008. "Dynamics of NGO Legitimacy: How Organising Betrays Core Missions of INGOs." *Public Administration and Development* 28: 42–53.

Paul, S. 1992. "Accountability in Public Services: Exit, Voice and Control." *World Development* 20(7): 1047–1060.

Pogge, T. W. 2002. "Responsibilities for Poverty-Related Ill Health." *Ethics and International Affairs* 16(2): 71–81.

Rubincam, C., and Naysmith, S. 2009. "Unexpected Agency: Participation as a Bargaining Chip for the Poor." *Health and Human Rights* 11(1): 87–92.

Ruger, J. P. 2005. "The Changing Role of the World Bank in Global Health." *American Journal of Public Health* 95(1): 60–70.

Ruger, J. P. 2012. "Global Health Justice and Governance." *American Journal of Bioethics* 12(12): 35–54.

Ruger, J. P. 2014. "International Institutional Legitimacy and the World Health Organization." *Journal of Epidemiology and Community Health* 68(8): 697–700.

Saltman, R. B., and Ferroussier-Davis, O. 2000. "The Concept of Stewardship in Health Policy." *Bulletin of the World Health Organization* 78(6): 732–739.

Stuckler, D., and Basu, S. 2013. "The Post-Communist Mortality Crisis." In *The Body Economic: Why Austerity Kills* (New York: Basic Books).

't Hoen, E. 2002. "TRIPS, Pharmaceutical Patents, and Access to Essential Medicines: A Long Way from Seattle to Doha." *Chicago Journal of International Law* 3(1): 27–46.

Travis, P., Egger, D., Davis, P., and Mechbal, A. 2002. *Towards Better Stewardship: Concepts and Critical Issues* (Geneva: World Health Organization).

Wachira, C., and Ruger, J. P. 2011. "National Poverty Reduction Strategies and HIV/AIDS Governance in Malawi: A Preliminary Study of Shared Health Governance." *Social Science and Medicine* 72: 1956–1964.

Weiss, T. G. 2009. "What Happened to the Idea of World Government?" *International Studies Quarterly* 53: 253–271.

WHO (World Health Organization). 2000. *The World Health Report 2000: Health Systems: Improving Performance* (Geneva: World Health Organization).

WHO (World Health Organization). 2016. "Stewardship." http://www.who.int/healthsystems/stewardship/en/.

Further Reading

Friedman, A. 2008. "Beyond Accountability for Reasonableness." *Bioethics* 22(2): 101–112.

Packard, R. M. 1997. "Malaria Dreams: Postwar Visions of Health and Development in the Third World." *Medical Anthropology* 17(3): 279–296.

Powers, M., and Faden, R. 2006. *Social Justice* (New York: Oxford University Press).
Rao, M., ed. 1999. *Disinvesting in Health: The World Bank's Prescriptions for Health* (Thousand Oaks, Calif.: SAGE).
Ruger J. P. 2004. "Health and Social Justice." *Lancet* 364(9439): 1075–1080.
Siddiqi, S., Masud, T. I., Nishtar, S., Peters, D. H., Sabri, B., Bile, K. F., et al. 2009. "Framework for Assessing Governance of the Health System in Developing Countries: Gateway to Good Governance." *Health Policy* 90: 13–25.
Yamin, A. E., and Parra-Vera, O. 2009. "How Do Courts Set Health Policy? The Case of the Colombian Constitutional Court." *PLoS Medicine* 6(2). https://doi.org/10.1371/journal.pmed.1000032.

CHAPTER 12

GLOBAL HUMAN RESOURCES FOR HEALTH: ETHICAL ASPECTS

GEORGE W. PARIYO AND HENRY LUCAS

Introduction

The 2006 *World Health Report* focused for the first time on human resources for health (HRH). It identified fifty-seven low- and middle-income countries (LMICs) as being in HRH crisis (WHO, 2006) because their combined number of nurses, midwives, and doctors was less than 23 per 10,000 population, the density associated with coverage of at least 80 percent for skilled birth attendance, infants receiving all vaccines on national schedules, and other essential health interventions (Anand and Bärnighausen, 2004, 2007; Sousa et al., 2006; Dal Poz et al., 2006). In addition to overall HRH shortages, the report also highlighted the inequitable distribution of health workers in many countries (van Rensburg, 2014; Harris et al., 2011; Viscomi, Larkins, and Sen Gupta, 2013).

Increasing Demand for Human Resources for Health

Many LMICs are experiencing the double burden of continued high levels of infectious diseases and increasing prevalence of noncommunicable diseases (Boutayeb, 2006; Omran, 2005; GBD 2013 Mortality and Causes of Death Collaborators, 2014)—the latter partly a consequence of their aging populations (Kuate Defo, 2014; Lesthaeghe, 2014). This combination is seriously challenging weak health systems that have suffered years of underfunding and understaffing (WHO, 2006). In particular, the growing number of patients with chronic conditions has increased pressure on the health workforce (Zaman et al., 2015). Moreover, the diffusion of information and communication technologies has increased access to medical knowledge, leading more people to seek care. While this development is welcome, the increased demand will intensify HRH shortages (Harris et al., 2011; van Rensburg, 2014).

Influences on the Supply of Global Human Resources for Health

Over 100 years ago, the Flexner Report and the Welch-Rose Report prompted, respectively, reform of medical education and the introduction of independent schools of public health in the United States, influencing medical and public health education in newly established schools worldwide (Duffy, 2011; Thomas, 2016). Since then, a rapid growth in enrollment, particularly in the private sector in many countries, has created concerns about the quality of health professionals' education and graduate competencies, especially in LMICs but also in high-income countries (Scheffer and Dal Poz, 2015; Sabde et al., 2014). While regulation of health training institutions is critical to quality assurance, many LMICs lack strong accreditation and certification mechanisms (van Zanten, 2015).

An additional ethical issue concerns the priority given to curative over preventive services (Sengupta, 2013; George, 2015). Typically, both public and private sectors incentivize the provision of care for the sick, marginalizing public health professionals such as epidemiologists, environmental health specialists, nutritionists, and health educators, all of whom could potentially greatly reduce the need for such care. HRH policies also typically focus on the demands of the sick, allocating resources to curative services and medical schools, rather than the often unspoken needs of the much larger population of the not-sick, who might benefit much more if those resources were directed to preventive services and schools of public health (George, 2016).

Midlevel health providers can be empowered through appropriate training and legislation to do more tasks traditionally performed by physicians, and general doctors can be empowered to do some tasks currently undertaken only by specialists, potentially alleviating supply constraints and advancing progress toward universal health coverage (Lassi et al., 2013; Campbell, Buchan, et al., 2013; WHO, 2012). However, this strategy requires clarity as to who has ultimate responsibility for the care delivered.

Strategies Proposed to Improve Global Human Resources for Health

Countries are implementing various strategies to attract and retain health workers in rural and other challenging environments (Dolea, Stormont, and Braichet, 2010). These are to some extent informed by global guidelines and commitments, with some progress reported in implementing World Health Organization (WHO) recommendations on recruiting students from rural backgrounds, locating training institutions in rural areas, and providing financial incentives, scholarships, and other benefits for health workers serving in such areas (Buchan et al., 2013; WHO, 2010a; Campbell, Dussault, et al., 2013).

International action is needed to minimize and mitigate adverse influences of health worker migration on aggregate shortfalls and inequitable distribution of HRH. The Global Health Workforce Alliance (GHWA) convened the first global forum on HRH in 2008 (Global Health Workforce Alliance and WHO, 2018). The resulting Kampala Declaration and Agenda for Global Action outlined interconnected strategies addressing policy, planning, training, recruitment, and retention; the international labor market; and the migration of health workers (WHA, 2006; WHO, 2008). The WHO and GHWA have also developed a global HRH strategy to guide countries in developing and strengthening their health workforces (WHO, 2015a).

A GHWA task force recommended radically scaling up health worker education and training (Global Health Workforce Alliance and WHO, 2008). On the evidence available in 2009, HRH-crisis countries in sub-Saharan Africa would need thirty-six years for physicians and twenty-nine years for nurses and midwives to reach the minimum threshold of 23 per 10,000 population (Kinfu et al., 2009). It is doubtful that this situation can be substantially improved without major investments by external donors.

Reducing attrition is one strategy that can be implemented relatively quickly and need not cost more money. Health workers in service delivery and teachers in health training institutions can be retained through improved recruitment and management practices (Dolea et al., 2010). Students from minority or disadvantaged backgrounds can be retained by providing extra support, for example redirecting tutor assistance toward those who need it most (Pariyo et al., 2009).

Key Ethical Aspects of National HRH Strategies

Key ethical concerns in global HRH relate to equity, workplace and performance ethics, patient rights, and health worker rights.

Equity

The WHO defines *equity* as an "absence of avoidable or remediable differences among groups of people" (WHO, 2016a). Because notions of "avoidable" or "remediable" rely on value judgments, the concept of equity is essentially normative and is among the most debated and contentious in health policy. Whether a given level of inequality is seen as "inequitable" will vary across rival conceptions of equity. Some regard as unacceptable any deviation from the principle that access to health care should be determined only by the "needs" of a given individual, where "need" is another problematic concept (Culyer and Wagstaff, 1992).

Libertarians might insist that health care is simply another commodity, one whose distribution should to a large extent be determined by "market forces," with provisions for the most vulnerable and major catastrophic illnesses (Friedman, 2001). Both extremes may be unrealistic in terms of health policy, given economic, political, and social realities, but they illustrate the wide spectrum of options that would be regarded as ethical by their supporters.

Equity and Human Resources for Health

Here it is most relevant to consider equity in terms of "avoidable or remediable differences" in *access* to HRH between members of different groups, defined in relation to geographical, economic, or institutional factors (O'Neill et al., 2014). One central concern relates to differences of "quality"—qualifications, experience, attitudes to patients—between providers. For example, in rural Bangladesh, "informal health care providers have become the sole provider for poor and underserved people" (Rasu et al., 2014, 515). This will typically result in poorer communities accessing worse care than better-off communities. More problematic are questions relating to provider characteristics such as gender, religion, or race/ethnicity. Should women expect to have access to a female doctor (Nigenda et al., 2003; Zaidi, 1996)? Would this equally apply to men and male doctors (Letshwenyo-Maruatona, 2017)? Should governments attempt to meet the demands of patients for a provider of the same religious faith or ethnic group (Street and Cossman, 2008)?

While public policy can improve equity in terms of access to facilities, equipment, medicines, and other goods by varying the allocation of resources, HRH access raises distinctive ethical issues. Typically, providers can choose which services to offer and where to practice. Governments wishing to improve equity have to use incentives to encourage them to serve disadvantaged groups or offer subsidies to members of such groups for medical bills and/or care-seeking travel (Lu et al., 2013). Both alternatives may require substantial payments to be effective. In particular, it is difficult to persuade well-qualified, experienced doctors with family responsibilities to work in areas with poor-quality medical facilities, limited educational and other services, and minimal opportunities to supplement earnings by private practice (Huicho et al., 2015; Liu et al., 2015). Addressing such concerns may be as important as the provision of financial incentives. A degree of compulsion has been used to increase equitable access in some countries, based on the argument that when public resources are used to subsidize the education of health workers, governments are justified in requiring graduates to serve on a rotational basis in underserved areas (Frehywot et al., 2010). However, this raises additional ethical and practical issues, including the ability of authorities to effectively implement such requirements and implications for the quality of care delivered by health workers deprived of the freedom to practice where they choose. (Cavender and Albán, 1998; Omole, Marincowitz, and Ogunbanjo, 2005).

Equity and Public versus Private Provision

Traditionally, health service provision has been seen as an example of market failure, given the "information asymmetry" allowing providers to influence demand and the "externalities" (third-party impacts) associated with individual decisions, such as the decision to reject immunization (Green, 2007). For that reason, in most countries the state has played a leading role in the financial management and regulation of the health sector, if not in the provision of care (Heath, 2002). In the late 1980s, the International Monetary Fund (IMF) and World Bank promoted a reduced role for the state in many LMICs, along with greater use of private providers (Roehrich, Lewis, and George, 2014; World Bank, 1993). The justification for this included claims that competitive markets would incentivize innovation and efficiency, thus improving services while containing costs (Bennett, McPake, and Mills, 1997; World Bank, 1993).

Even advocates of an increased role for the private sector accept that information asymmetry generates an *incentive* for providers to maximize incomes, for example by limiting consultation time for more indigent clients, prescribing unnecessary treatments, and overcharging, with predictable adverse impacts on accessibility, quality, and cost of services for the least well-off. They would agree on a need for the state to enforce accepted standards of ethical behavior among providers, whether public or private. The behavior of state employees, however, is potentially easier to influence than that of providers employed by a multiplicity of private health care enterprises, and there is ample evidence of the difficulty of designing and implementing effective regulation of the private sector (Sheikh, Saligram, and Hort, 2015; Vora and Mavalankar, 2014).

Ethical Problems of Task-Delegation in Human Resources for Health

Following the Alma Ata Declaration, many countries saw task delegation, in the form of recruiting large numbers of community health workers (CHWs), as a cost-effective way to provide primary care for impoverished rural and urban populations (Cueto, 2004; Newell, 1975). Even though "[m]any countries and many communities can recall a history of training, deployment, and failure" (Tulenko et al., 2013, 847), numerous countries have recently introduced similar policies. It is suggested that by 2015, a million CHWs were involved in the management of diseases such as malaria, pneumonia, malnutrition, and diarrhea in sub-Saharan Africa (Liu et al., 2011; Singh and Sachs, 2013). The coverage, scope, and quality of care provided by such CHW programs need to be carefully evaluated.

Quality of Care

In the 1970s, issues relating to the supervision, regulation, and remuneration of CHWs were often overlooked, resulting in many diversifying into drug-selling or providing services for which they were unqualified (Standing and Chowdhury, 2008). Given that more recent programs address these issues, there would seem to be considerable value in CHWs providing selected services to populations facing limited access to qualified doctors, nurses, and midwives. Even where health worker shortages are not a key issue, CHWs can provide a local interface between communities and the formal health care system, for example by delivering community- or home-based care for patients requiring long-term chronic disease management. However, this could be seen as institutionalizing a downgraded form of health care, delegating providers with rudimentary training, often supported by new technology (Sachs, 2012), to deliver services that had previously been the preserve of highly qualified health professionals.

There is evidence that CHWs can significantly increase access to care for populations not served by professional cadres. Countries such as Ethiopia, Mozambique, and Pakistan appear to have successfully adopted this strategy (Global Health Workforce Alliance and WHO, 2010; Perry, Zulliger, and Rogers, 2014; Lehmann et al., 2009; Haines et al., 2007; Lehmann, Friedman, and Sanders, 2004). Such initiatives have been described as "disruptive innovations" (Christensen et al., 2006, 1–2) and have the explicit aim of providing "good enough" alternatives to underserved populations. However, they may not prove attractive or even acceptable to the more affluent, raising questions about the definition of "good enough." This involves a trade-off confronting all state-supported health systems: ensuring a basic care package for the overall population against providing higher-quality, possibly even "unnecessary," care to a more limited number (New, 1997).

Privacy and Confidentiality

Provider-patient interactions should be private, and any information relating to a patient's condition should not be given to anyone else without the patient's permission. Such information may be extremely sensitive, not only in cases of stigmatizing diseases, such as mental illnesses (Semrau et al., 2015) or those associated with sexual transmission (Liu et al., 2002), but also in many other areas, including reproductive health and heritable conditions. The rapid expansion of computerized information systems has dramatically increased data sharing between providers, threatening confidentiality. This has received limited attention in the design of the many recent mHealth initiatives in LMIC (*mHealth* refers to "medical and public health practice supported by mobile devices . . . and other wireless devices" [mHealth Alliance, 2013, xi]). The difficulty of foreseeing how individual patient data will be stored and used demands reexamination of the familiar issues of privacy, confidentiality, and informed consent.

Fairness to Health Workers

Shortages of qualified providers tend to increase overall workloads, especially for more junior staff, recent graduates, and trainees. Examples reported from Pakistan,

South Africa, and Tanzania include trainees filling staffing gaps (Abbasi, 2014) and overworked interns and community doctors working up to 200 hours overtime per month (Erasmus, 2012). The resulting stress is often exacerbated by difficult working conditions (Mkoka et al., 2015).

Personnel Policies and Practices

A review of motivational factors identified an established career path as a key driver of staff morale (Willis-Shattuck et al., 2008). This was one reason why staff preferred to work in urban environments and to avoid specializations seen as having limited opportunities for advancement, such as mental health (Jack et al., 2013). A study of rural health workers in Tanzania emphasized the role of attractive pension arrangements to offset low salaries; this probably applies in many countries with limited social security schemes (Songstad et al., 2012). Van Lerberghe et al. (2002) discuss common coping strategies (e.g., charging illicit fees, recommending private consultations, and selling notionally free drugs) used by health workers to overcome employment conditions seen as unfair. They emphasize the need to address health workers' underlying concerns and not rely on (often unenforceable) threats of punitive action (Van Lerberghe et al., 2002).

Increasingly, CHWs are performing or enhancing the effectiveness of core public health functions (CDC, 2015a). In many settings, especially in LMICs, they are tasked with frontline delivery of health programs, entailing a time commitment well beyond what one would reasonably expect of a "community volunteer." There are calls for them to be better recognized and supported in terms of training, accreditation, supervision, and remuneration. A number of governments are formalizing CHW activities (Global Health Workforce Alliance and WHO, 2010; Perry, Zulliger, and Rogers, 2014; Lehmann, Friedman, and Sanders, 2004; Singh and Sachs, 2013; Tulenko et al., 2013).

Safe and Professional Environment

The Ebola outbreak in 2013–2016 demonstrated the disproportionate risks health workers often run. "In Liberia and Sierra Leone, the differences are . . . dramatic, with 0.11% and 0.06% of the general population killed by Ebola versus 8.07% of the health-care workers in Liberia, and 6.85% in Sierra Leone" (Evans, Goldstein, and Popova, 2015, e439). Governments and employers have a duty to ensure that health workers receive appropriate protective equipment and training, especially in dealing with highly contagious diseases (CDC, 2015b). Staff may be at risk not only from disease, but also from direct attack, both in conflict situations (Namakula and Witter 2014)—where they are expected to observe the principle of impartiality (UN, 2010)—and when undertaking activities to which sections of the population object, such as family planning or vaccination (Roberts, 2013). In resource-constrained health care systems, it is tempting to give low priority to expenditure on staff protection and personal well-being. Often, the expectation is that health workers will "cope" with unpleasant environments and limited support, especially in neglected areas such as mental health. Poor working environments

(Jack et al., 2013) and lack of support (Mkoka et al., 2015) act as disincentives, often discouraging applications for vacant posts and increasing workloads, adding to staff discontents.

Ethics and the International Market for Health Personnel

The international market for health personnel generates patterns of migration that exacerbate the HRH crisis in LMICs, raising ethical issues concerning the rights and obligations of source countries, transportation carriers, receiving countries, and the migrating health workers themselves. The drivers of health worker migration can be classified as "push factors" that propel them out of source countries and "pull factors" that attract them to receiving countries.

Push Factors

Health workers in LMICs face many challenges (Frenk et al., 2010; Schmidt, 2012; Jack et al., 2013). Poor employment and personnel practices often compel them to undergo lengthy, cumbersome recruitment procedures before being deployed. They may endure low pay and delayed promotions, and are often blamed for health sector deficiencies for which their employers are accountable. Those working in the public sector, often in difficult circumstances, deserve as much support as possible and ought not to be forgotten or subjected to "forced labor" to fulfill the state's objectives (Mkoka et al., 2015; Erasmus, 2012). Strategies to address health worker shortages and reduce migration pressures on health workers must deal specifically with these challenges (Stilwell, Diallo, and Zurn, 2004; Vujicic and Zurn, 2006).

Pull Factors

Underinvestment in training over past decades in some high-income countries, coupled with increasing health care needs because of aging populations, has increased demands for health workers from LMICs. Pay differentials can be significant. For instance, it is estimated based on WHO data (available at http://apps.who.int/nha/database/Regional_Averages/Index/en), that weighted average health expenditure per capita in LMICs was PPP$ 1,255 in 2015 compared to 5,437 in high income countries (PPP$ is Purchasing Power Parity adjusted dollars) (World Health Organization (WHO) n.d.). Policymakers need to acknowledge that health workers will move in response to labor market incentives (Vujicic and Zurn, 2006). For many, it can be irresistible to migrate to settings where incomes are substantially higher and working conditions more amenable than in their home countries.

Global Conventions

Two global conventions codify the rights and obligations of source countries, transportation carriers and receiving countries, and health workers' migration rights: the Convention for the Unification of Certain Rules for International Carriage by Air (the Montreal Convention); and the WHO Global Code of Practice on International Recruitment of Health Personnel (the Code).

The Montreal Convention

The Montreal Convention is a multilateral treaty adopted by the International Civil Aviation Organization (ICAO) in 1999. It lays out the conditions for carriage by air, specifying carriers' and passengers' rights and responsibilities and requiring all carriers to indicate the origin and destination of all passengers (IATA, 1999). The Convention requirements on sharing passenger data, including their occupations, origin, and destination, are potentially a source of minimum data on the international movement of health workers. The extent to which these data should be in the public domain is an area of ethical concern, posing risks to privacy and confidentiality (Cole, 2009; International Organization for Migration, 2016).

The WHO Global Code of Practice on International Recruitment of Health Personnel

The international migration of health personnel poses a challenge to health systems (WHA, 2004). The passing of the Code in 2010 was an important step for the global community in managing the conditions that drive health worker migration. It sets out a common set of principles and recommended practices, and identifies a minimum data set and mechanisms for member states to monitor its implementation (WHO, 2016b, 2010b). A major limitation is that the Code is voluntary and cannot be enforced. Thus, its implementation depends on the goodwill of member states, which will often act in their own self-interest. The Organisation of Economic Co-operation and Development (OECD) requires all OECD members to report on the migration of health workers into and out of their countries (OECD, 2015). A formal review and report to the World Health Assembly in 2015 concluded that while the Code was highly relevant, there were weaknesses and delays in its implementation (WHO, 2013; Siyam et al., 2013; WHA, 2015).

There are country-level challenges in implementing the Code. Some LMICs lack coherent policies on the international migration of health workers. While the health sector is struggling with health worker shortages, some see migration as another source of the much-needed remittances that these workers send back to source countries. Moreover, health workers can reasonably claim to have the basic human right to seek better conditions for themselves and their families and dependents, including through lawful migration within international law and agreements. This presents an ethical dilemma for policymakers. Should they impose restrictions on the migration of health workers without providing better working conditions at home? Can they afford to create the incentives needed for health workers to stay in underserved areas in the context of an increasingly globalized international labor market for skilled health workers? The Code lays out the principles and recommendations for how source and recipient countries can handle these challenges in a transparent and fair way that respects health worker rights to migrate, but without unduly disadvantaging source countries that invest in their professional education.

Some destination countries have increased investment in health worker training and recruitment to meet their own needs. In some cases, through bilateral agreements with source countries, a destination country may provide support to source countries to strengthen HRH training and improve quality. An example is Malawi's Emergency HRH program, implemented with financial support from the United Kingdom (DFID, 2010; Global Health Workforce Alliance and WHO, 2016). Another destination country, Norway, introduced a regulation for its recruiting agencies not to hire health workers from countries designated as being in a state of crisis with respect to HRH (WHO, 2014).

Toward Implementing the Global Conventions

In order for countries to implement the global conventions to which they are signatories, it is necessary to widely disseminate information on the principles, regulations, and provisions that they contain. As a start, all countries ought to be able to collect and share in compiling the data specified in the minimum data set and honor their commitment to report this periodically. After some initial delays, countries have started collecting and reporting basic data for monitoring implementation of the Code (Tangcharoensathien and Travis, 2016).

Another step is to support countries to enact legislation and develop policies that reinforce provisions of these international agreements. For instance, recruiting agencies could be required by law to report a minimum set of data on personnel while also protecting individuals' personal identifying details. Similarly, countries could report on their compliance with existing standards and provisions for the employment and welfare of migratory health workers.

Conclusion

It is clear that without seriously addressing the HRH situation on a global scale as a priority, achieving global aspirational goals such as universal health coverage and sustainable development goals will be much harder. The challenge is that some of the strategies that are being used to mitigate HRH shortages are fraught with compromises of ethical principles of equity, compromises of the right to privacy and confidentiality, and, in some cases, violations of proper ethical conduct or infringement of individual rights to quality care or the right to move in search of a better life. The hope embodied in highlighting these challenges is that affected countries, international agencies, employers, professional associations, and individual health workers themselves may take measures to observe ethical conduct. Above all, they should "do no harm" as they seek to address the global HRH crisis.

References

Abbasi, I. N. 2014. "Protest of Doctors: A Basic Human Right or an Ethical Dilemma." *BMC Medical Ethics* 15: 24.

Anand, S., and Bärnighausen, T. 2004. "Human Resources and Health Outcomes: Cross-Country." *Lancet* 365: 1603–1609.

Anand, S., and Bärnighausen, T. 2007. "Health Workers and Vaccination Coverage in Developing Countries: An Econometric Analysis." *Lancet* 369(9569): 1277–1285.

Bennett, S., McPake, B., and Mills, A. 1997. *Private Health Providers in Developing Countries: Serving the Public Interest?* (London: Zed Books).

Boutayeb, A. 2006. "The Double Burden of Communicable and Non-communicable Diseases in Developing Countries." *Transactions of the Royal Society of Tropical Medicine and Hygiene* 100(3): 191–199.

Buchan, J., Couper, I. D., Tangcharoensathien, V., Thepannya, K., Jaskiewicz, W., Perfilieva, G., et al. 2013. "Early Implementation of WHO Recommendations for the Retention of Health Workers in Remote and Rural Areas." *Bulletin of the World Health Organization* 91(11): 834–840.

Campbell, J., Buchan, J., Cometto, G., David, B., Dussault, G., Fogstad, H., et al. 2013. "Human Resources for Health and Universal Health Coverage: Fostering Equity and Effective Coverage." *Bulletin of the World Health Organization* 91(11): 853–863.

Campbell, J., Dussault, G., Buchan, J., Pozo-Martin, F., Guerra Arias, M., Leone, C., et al. 2013. *A Universal Truth: No Health without a Workforce* (Geneva: World Health Organization). http://cdrwww.who.int/workforcealliance/knowledge/resources/GHWA-a_universal_truth_report.pdf.

Cavender, A., and Albán, M. 1998. "Compulsory Medical Service in Ecuador: The Physician's Perspective." *Social Science and Medicine (1982)* 47(12): 1937–1946.

CDC (US Centers for Disease Control and Prevention). 2015a. "Core Functions of Public Health and How They Relate to the 10 Essential Services." *Leadership Resources*. https://www.cdc.gov/nceh/ehs/ephli/core_ess.htm.

CDC (US Centers for Disease Control and Prevention). 2015b. "Guidance on Personal Protective Equipment (PPE) To Be Used by Healthcare Workers during Management of Patients with Confirmed Ebola or Persons under Investigation (PUIs) for Ebola who are Clinically Unstable or Have Bleeding, Vomiting, or Diarrhea in U.S." http://www.cdc.gov/vhf/ebola/healthcare-us/ppe/guidance.html.

Christensen, C. M., Baumann, H., Ruggles, R., and Sadtler, T. M. 2006. "Disruptive Innovation for Social Change." *Harvard Business Review*, December. https://hbr.org/2006/12/disruptive-innovation-for-social-change.

Cole, P. 2009. "Migration and the Human Right to Health." *Cambridge Quarterly of Healthcare Ethics* 18: 70–77.

Cueto, M. 2004. "The Origins of Primary Health Care and Selective Primary Health Care. *American Journal of Public Health* 94(11): 1864–1874.

Culyer, A. J., and Wagstaff, A. 1992. *Need, Equity and Equality in Health and Health Care* (York, England: University of York Centre for Health Economics). https://www.york.ac.uk/che/pdf/DP95.pdf.

Dal Poz, M. R., Kinfu, Y., Dräger, S., Kunjumen, T., and Diallo, K. 2006. *Counting Health Workers: Definitions, Data, Methods and Global Results*. HRH Discussion Paper (Geneva: World Health Organization). http://www.who.int/hrh/documents/counting_health_workers.pdf.

DFID (Department for International Development). 2010. *Evaluation of Malawi's Emergency Human Resources Programme* (Geneva: World Health Organization). http://www.who.int/workforcealliance/media/news/2010/Malawi_MSH_MSC_EHRP_Final.pdf.

Dolea, C., Stormont, L., and Braichet, J. M. 2010. "Evaluated Strategies to Increase Attraction and Retention of Health Workers in Remote and Rural Areas." *Bulletin of the World Health Organization* 88(5): 379–385.

Duffy, T. P. 2011. "The Flexner Report—100 Years Later." *Yale Journal of Biology and Medicine* 84(3): 269–276.

Erasmus, N. 2012. "Slaves of the State: Medical Internship and Community Service in South Africa." *South African Medical Journal* 102(8): 655–658.

Evans, D. K., Goldstein, M., and Popova, A. 2015. "Health-Care Worker Mortality and the Legacy of the Ebola Epidemic." *Lancet Global Health* 3(8): e439–e440.

Frehywot, S., Mullan, F., Payne, P. W., and Ross, H. 2010. "Compulsory Service Programmes for Recruiting Health Workers in Remote and Rural Areas: Do They Work?" *Bulletin of the World Health Organization* 88(5): 364–370.

Frenk, J., Chen, L., Bhutta, Z. A., Cohen, J., Crisp, N., Evans, T., et al. 2010. "Health Professionals for a New Century: Transforming Education to Strengthen Health Systems in an Interdependent World." *Lancet* 376 (9756): 1923–1958.

Friedman, M. 2001. "How to Cure Health Care." *Hoover Digest* 3. https://www.hoover.org/research/how-cure-health-care-0.

GBD 2013 Mortality and Causes of Death Collaborators. 2014. "Global, Regional, and National Age–Sex Specific All-Cause and Cause-Specific Mortality for 240 Causes of Death, 1990–2013: A Systematic Analysis for the Global Burden of Disease Study 2013." *Lancet* 385(9963): 117–171.

George, M. 2015. "Re-instating a 'Public Health' System under Universal Health Care in India." *Journal of Public Health Policy* 36(1): 15–23.

George, M. 2016. "Being Fair in Universal Health Coverage: Prioritize Public Health Services for Low- and Middle-Income Countries." *American Journal of Public Health* 106(5): 830–831.

Global Health Workforce Alliance and WHO. 2008. *Scaling Up, Saving Lives* (Geneva: World Health Organization).http://www.who.int/workforcealliance/documents/Global_Health%20FINAL%20REPORT.pdf.

Global Health Workforce Alliance and WHO. 2010. *Global Experience of Community Health Workers for Delivery of Health Related Millennium Development Goals: A Systematic Review, Country Case Studies, and Recommendations for Integration into National Health Systems"* Community Health 377 (Geneva: World Health Organization). http://www.who.int/workforcealliance/knowledge/resources/chwreport/en/.

Global Health Workforce Alliance and WHO. 2016. *Country Case Study: Malawi's Emergency Human Resources Programme* (Geneva: World Health Organization). http://www.who.int/workforcealliance/knowledge/case_studies/CS_Malawi_web_En.pdf.

Global Health Workforce Alliance and WHO. 2018. "Global Forums on Human Resources for Health." http://www.who.int/workforcealliance/forum/en/.

Green, A. 2007. *An Introduction to Health Planning for Developing Health Systems* (Oxford: Oxford University Press).

Haines, A., Sanders, D., Lehmann, U., Rowe, A. K., Lawn, J. E., Jan, S., et al. 2007. "Achieving Child Survival Goals: Potential Contribution of Community Health Workers." *Lancet* 369(9579): 2121–2131.

Harris, B., Goudge, J., Ataguba, J. E., McIntyre, D., Nxumalo, N., Jikwana, S., et al. 2011. "Inequities in Access to Health Care in South Africa." *Journal of Public Health Policy* 32(S1): S102–S123.

Heath, J. 2002. *Health Care as a Commodity* (Toronto: University of Toronto). http://homes.chass.utoronto.ca/~jheath/health.pdf.

Huicho, L., Molina, C., Diez-Canseco, F., Lema, C., Miranda, J. J., Huayanay-Espinoza, C. A., et al. 2015. "Factors behind Job Preferences of Peruvian Medical, Nursing and Midwifery Students: A Qualitative Study Focused on Rural Deployment." *Human Resources for Health* 13(1): 90.

IATA (International Air Transport Association). 1999. *Essential Documents on International Air Carrier Liability 1.9: Montreal Convention 1999*. https://www.iata.org/policy/Documents/MC99_en.pdf.

International Organization for Migration. 2016. *Migration and the Right to Health: A Review of International Law*. http://publications.iom.int/system/files/pdf/iml_19.pdf.

Jack, H., Canavan, M., Ofori-Atta, A., Taylor, L., and Bradley, E. 2013. "Recruitment and Retention of Mental Health Workers in Ghana." *PLoS One* 8(2): e57940.

Kinfu, Y., Dal Poz, M. R., Mercer, H., and Evans, D. B. 2009. "The Health Worker Shortage in Africa: Are Enough Physicians and Nurses Being Trained?" *Bulletin of the World Health Organization* 87(3): 225–230.

Kuate Defo, B. 2014. "Demographic, Epidemiological, and Health Transitions: Are They Relevant to Population Health Patterns in Africa?" *Global Health Action* 7: 22443.

Lassi, Z. S., Cometto, G., Huicho, L., and Bhutta, Z. A. 2013. "Quality of Care Provided by Mid-Level Health Workers: Systematic Review and Meta-Analysis." *Bulletin of the World Health Organization* 91(11): 824–833I.

Lehmann, U., Friedman, I., and Sanders, D. 2004. *Review of the Utilisation and Effectiveness of Community-Based Health Workers in Africa*. Working Paper of the Joint Learning Initiative.

Lehmann, U., Van Damme, W., Barten, F., and Sanders, D. 2009. "Task Shifting: The Answer to the Human Resources Crisis in Africa?" *Human Resources for Health* 7: 49.

Lesthaeghe, R. 2014. "The Second Demographic Transition: A Concise Overview of its Development." *Proceedings of the National Academy of Sciences of the United States of America* 111(51): 18112–18115.

Letshwenyo-Maruatona, S. 2017. "Who Do Batswana Men Prefer: Male or Female Health Providers?" *American Journal of Men's Health* 11(6): 1642–1652.

Liu, A., Sullivan, S., Khan, M., Sachs, S., and Singh, P. 2011. "Community Health Workers in Global Health: Scale and Scalability." *Mount Sinai Journal of Medicine: A Journal of Translational and Personalized Medicine* 78(3): 419–435.

Liu, H., Detels, R., Li, X., Ma, E., and Yin, Y. 2002. "Stigma, Delayed Treatment, and Spousal Notification among Male Patients with Sexually Transmitted Disease in China." *Sexually Transmitted Diseases* 29(6): 335–343.

Liu, X., Dou, L., Zhang, H., Sun, Y., and Yuan, B. 2015. "Analysis of Context Factors in Compulsory and Incentive Strategies for Improving Attraction and Retention of Health Workers in Rural and Remote Areas: A Systematic Review." *Human Resources for Health* 13: 61.

Lu, H., Yan, F., Wang, W., Wu, L., Ma, W., Chen, J., et al. 2013. "Do Transportation Subsidies and Living Allowances Improve Tuberculosis Control Outcomes among Internal Migrants in Urban Shanghai, China?" *Western Pacific Surveillance and Response Journal* 4(1): 19–24.

mHealth Alliance. 2013. *Patient Privacy in a Mobile World: A Framework to Address Privacy Law Issues in Mobile Health.* http://www.trust.org/contentAsset/raw-data/03172beb-0f11-438e-94be-e02978de3036/file.

Mkoka, D. A., Mahiti, G. R., Kiwara, A., Mwangu, M., Goicolea, I., and Hurtig, A. K. 2015. "'Once the Government Employs You, It Forgets You': Health Workers' and Managers' Perspectives on Factors Influencing Working Conditions for Provision of Maternal Health Care Services in a Rural District of Tanzania." *Human Resources for Health* 13: 77.

Namakula, J., and Witter, S. 2014. "Living through Conflict and Post-conflict: Experiences of Health Workers in Northern Uganda and Lessons for People-Centred Health Systems." *Health Policy and Planning* 29(Suppl. 2): ii6–ii14.

New, B. 1997. "The Rationing Debate: Defining a Package of Healthcare Services the NHS is Responsible for—The Case for." *BMJ* 314(7079): 498.

Newell, K. W., ed. 1975. *Health by the People* (Geneva: World Health Organization).

Nigenda, G., Langer, A., Kuchaisit, C., Romero, M., Rojas, G., Al-Osimy, M., et al. 2003. "Womens' Opinions on Antenatal Care in Developing Countries: Results of a Study in Cuba, Thailand, Saudi Arabia and Argentina." *BMC Public Health* 3(1): 17.

OECD (Organisation of Economic Co-operation and Development). 2015. *Health Data Governance: Privacy, Monitoring and Research: Privacy, Monitoring and Research* (Paris: OECD Publishing).

Omole, O. B., Marincowitz, G., and Ogunbanjo, G. A. 2005. "Perceptions of Hospital Managers Regarding the Impact of Doctors' Community Service." *South African Family Practice* 47(8): 55–59.

Omran, A. R. 2005. "The Epidemiologic Transition: A Theory of the Epidemiology of Population Change. 1971." *Milbank Quarterly* 83(4): 731–757.

O'Neill, J., Tabish, H., Welch, V., Petticrew, M., Pottie, K., Clarke, M., et al. 2014. "Applying an Equity Lens to Interventions: Using PROGRESS Ensures Consideration of Socially Stratifying Factors to Illuminate Inequities in Health." *Journal of Clinical Epidemiology* 67(1): 56–64.

Pariyo, G. W., Kiwanuka, S. N., Rutebemberwa, E., Okui, O., and Ssengooba, F. 2009. "Effects of Changes in the Pre-licensure Education of Health Workers on Health-Worker Supply." *Cochrane Database of Systematic Reviews* 2: CD007018.

Perry, H. B., Zulliger, R., and Rogers, M. M. 2014. "Community Health Workers in Low-, Middle-, and High-Income Countries: An Overview of Their History, Recent Evolution, and Current Effectiveness." *Annual Review of Public Health* 35: 399–421.

Rasu, R. S., Iqbal, M., Hanifi, S. M. A., Moula, A., Hoque, S., Rasheed, S., et al. 2014. "Level, Pattern, and Determinants of Polypharmacy and Inappropriate Use of Medications by Village Doctors in a Rural Area of Bangladesh." *ClinicoEconomics and Outcomes Research* 6: 515–521.

Roberts, L. 2013. "Disease Eradication: Killings Force Rethinking of Pakistan's Anti-Polio Drive." *Science* 339(6117): 259–260.

Roehrich, J. K., Lewis, M. A., and George, G. 2014. "Are Public-Private Partnerships a Healthy Option? A Systematic Literature Review." *Social Science and Medicine (1982)* 113: 110–119.

Sabde, Y., Diwan, V., De Costa, A., and Mahadik, V. K. 2014. "Mapping the Rapid Expansion of India's Medical Education Sector: Planning for the Future." *BMC Medical Education* 14: 266.

Sachs, J. D. 2012. "Primary Health Care in Low-Income Countries: Building on Recent Achievements." *JAMA* 307(19): 2031–2032.

Scheffer, M. C., and Dal Poz, M. R. 2015. "The Privatization of Medical Education in Brazil: Trends and Challenges." *Human Resources for Health* 13(1): 96.

Schmidt, A. 2012. *Positive Practice Environment Campaigns* (Geneva: World Health Organization). http://www.who.int/workforcealliance/about/initiatives/PPEevaluation_2012.pdf.

Semrau, M., Evans-Lacko, S., Koschorke, M., Ashenafi, L., and Thornicroft, G. 2015. "Stigma and Discrimination Related to Mental Illness in Low- and Middle-Income Countries." *Epidemiology and Psychiatric Sciences* 24(5): 382–394.

Sengupta, A. 2013. *Universal Health Care in India: Making It Public, Making It a Reality.* Occasional Paper 19 (Ontario: Municipal Services Project). https://www.municipalservicesproject.org/sites/municipalservicesproject.org/files/publications/Sengupta_Universal_Health_Care_in_India_Making_it_Public_May2013.pdf.

Sheikh, K., Saligram, P. S., and Hort, K. 2015. "What Explains Regulatory Failure? Analysing the Architecture of Health Care Regulation in Two Indian States." *Health Policy and Planning* 30(1): 39–55.

Singh, P., and Sachs, J. D. 2013. "1 Million Community Health Workers in Sub-Saharan Africa by 2015." *Lancet* 382(9889): 363–365.

Siyam, A., Zurn, P., Gedik, G., Ronquillo, K., Co, C. J., Vaillancourt-Laflamme, C., Perfilieva, G., et al. 2013. "Monitoring the Implementation of the WHO Global Code of Practice on the International Recruitment of Health Personnel." *Bulletin of the World Health Organization* 91(11): 816–823.

Songstad, N. G., Moland, K. M., Massay, D. A., and Blystad, A., 2012. "Why Do Health Workers in Rural Tanzania Prefer Public Sector Employment?" *BMC Health Services Research* 12: 92.

Sousa, A., Tandon, A., Dal Poz, M. R., Prasad, A., and Evans, D. B. 2006. *Measuring the Efficiency of Human Resources for Health for Attaining Health Outcomes across Subnational Units in Brazil* (Geneva: World Health Organization).

Standing, H., and Chowdhury, A. M. R. 2008. "Producing Effective Knowledge Agents in a Pluralistic Environment: What Future for Community Health Workers?" *Social Science and Medicine* 66(10): 2096–2107.

Stilwell, B., Diallo, K., and Zurn, P. 2004. "Migration of Health-Care Workers from Developing Countries: Strategic Approaches to Its Management." *Bulletin of the World Health Organization* 9480(3): 595–600.

Street, D., and Cossman, J. S. 2008. "Perspectives on Mississippi's 21st Century Physician Workforce Supply: Findings from the 2007 MSMD Survey." *Journal of the Mississippi State Medical Association* 49(4): 99–103.

Tangcharoensathien, V., and Travis, P. 2016. "Accelerate Implementation of the WHO Global Code of Practice on International Recruitment of Health Personnel: Experiences From the South East Asia Region." *International Journal of Health Policy and Management* 5(1): 43–46.

Thomas, K. K., 2016. "Cultivating hygiene as a science: The welch-rose report's influence at johns hopkins and beyond." *American Journal of Epidemiology*, 183(5): 345–354. https://academic.oup.com/aje/article-abstract/183/5/345/2196773.

Tulenko, K., Mgedal, S., Afzal, M. M., Frymus, D., Oshin, A., Pate, M., et al. 2013. "Community Health Workers for Universal Health-Care Coverage: From Fragmentation to Synergy." *Bulletin of the World Health Organization* 91(11): 847–852.

UN (United Nations). 2010. *OCHA on Message: Humanitarian Principles* (Geneva: Office for the Co-ordination of Humanitarian Affairs). https://docs.unocha.org/sites/dms/Documents/OOM_HumPrinciple_English.pdf.

Van Lerberghe, W., Conceicaõ, C., Van Damme, W., and Ferrinho, P. 2002. "When Staff Is Underpaid: Dealing with the Individual Coping Strategies of Health Personnel." *Bulletin of the World Health Organization* 80(7): 581–584.

van Rensburg, H. C. J. 2014. "South Africa's Protracted Struggle for Equal Distribution and Equitable Access—Still Not There." *Human Resources for Health* 12(1): 26.

van Zanten, M. 2015. "The Association between Medical Education Accreditation and the Examination Performance of Internationally Educated Physicians Seeking Certification in the United States." *Perspectives on Medical Education* 4(3): 142–145.

Viscomi, M., Larkins, S., and Sen Gupta, T. 2013. "Recruitment and Retention of General Practitioners in Rural Canada and Australia: A Review of the Literature." *Canadian Journal of Rural Medicine* 18(1): 13–24.

Vora, K. S., and Mavalankar, D. V. 2014. "Quality of Reproductive and Child Health Care in the Private Sector in India: Issues and Options." *International Journal of Science and Research* 3(8): 181–186. https://www.ijsr.net/archive/v3i8/MDIwMTUyMTY=.pdf.

Vujicic, M., and Zurn, P. 2006. "The Dynamics of the Health Labour Market." *International Journal of Health Planning and Management* 21(2): 101–115.

WHA (World Health Assembly). 2004. *International Migration of Health Personnel: A Challenge for Health*. WHA59.19. http://apps.who.int/gb/ebwha/pdf_files/WHA57/A57_R19-en.pdf.

WHA (World Health Assembly). 2006. "WHA59.23 Rapid Scaling up of Health Workforce Production." *World Health* 4: 37–38.

WHA (World Health Assembly). 2015. *WHO Global Code of Practice on the International Recruitment of Health Personnel* (Geneva: World Health Organization).

WHO (World Health Organization). 2006. *Working Together for Health: The World Health Report 2006*. (Geneva: World Health Organization).

WHO (World Health Organization). 2008. Health Workers for All and All for Health Workers: The Kampala Declaration and Agenda for Global Action. First Global Forum on Human Resources for Health (Geneva: World Health Organization). http://www.who.int/workforcealliance/forum/2_declaration_final.pdf.

WHO (World Health Organization). 2010a. *Increasing Access to Health Workers in Remote and Rural Areas through Improved Retention* (Geneva: World Health Organization).

WHO (World Health Organization). 2010b. *The WHO Global Code of Practice on the International Recruitment of Health Personnel: Implementation by the Secretariat* (Geneva: World Health Organization).

WHO (World Health Organization). 2012. *Positioning Health in the Post-2015 Development Agenda*. WHO Discussion Paper (Geneva: World Health Organization).

WHO (World Health Organization). 2013. "Monitoring the Implementation of the WHO Global Code of Practice on the International Recruitment of Health Personnel." *Bulletin of the World Health Organization* 91(11): 816–823.

WHO (World Health Organization). 2014. *Migration of Health Workers: The WHO Code of Practice and the Global Economic Crisis* (Geneva: World Health Organization).

WHO (World Health Organization). 2015a. *Global Strategy on Human Resources for Health: Workforce 2030* (Geneva: World Health Organization).

WHO (World Health Organization). 2016a. "Equity." http://www.who.int/healthsystems/topics/equity/en/.

WHO (World Health Organization). 2016b. "*WHO Global Code of Practice on the International Recruitment of Health Personnel* (Geneva: World Health Organization). http://www.who.int/hrh/migration/code/WHO_global_code_of_practice_EN.pdf.

WHO (World Health Organization). n.d., Global Health Expenditure Database. http://apps.who.int/nha/database/Regional_Averages/Index/en.

Willis-Shattuck, M., Bidwell, P., Thomas, S., Wyness, L., Blaauw, D., and Ditlopo, P. 2008. "Motivation and Retention of Health Workers in Developing Countries: A Systematic Review." *BMC Health Services Research* 8: 247.

World Bank. 1993. *World Development Report 1993: Investing in Health* (New York: Oxford University Press).

Zaidi, S. A. 1996. "Gender Perspectives and Quality of Care in Underdeveloped Countries: Disease, Gender and Contextuality." *Social Science and Medicine* 43(5): 721–730.

Zaman, M. M., Bhuiyan, M. R., Karim, M. N., Rahman, M. M., Akanda, A. W., and Fernando, T. 2015. "Clustering of Non-communicable Diseases Risk Factors in Bangladeshi Adults: An Analysis of STEPS Survey 2013." *BMC Public Health* 15: 659.

CHAPTER 13

HEALTH SYSTEMS RESEARCH ETHICS: PUBLIC HEALTH PERSPECTIVES

BRIDGET PRATT AND ADNAN A. HYDER

Introduction

HEALTH systems research (HSR) has been defined as the production of new knowledge to improve the performance of health systems. Health systems are composed of hardware (human resources, service delivery, governance, financing, information technology) and software (norms, values) components (Sheikh et al., 2011). HSR is an evolving field whose boundaries, definitions, and characteristics are still being discussed and debated (Bennett et al., 2011; Sheikh et al., 2011; Gilson, 2012). It is often seen as encompassing or overlapping with a number of other types of research, including health services research, operations research, and implementation research (Gilson, 2012; Hoffman et al., 2012).

HSR is increasingly being funded and conducted as part of health system strengthening efforts worldwide (Bennett et al., 2008). In a global context of persistent disparities in access to high-quality health services, rising health care costs, and lack of financial protection against catastrophic health care expenditures, demand for HSR is rapidly growing (WHO, 2010; WHO, 2013). In recent years, multilateral organizations, bilateral organizations, philanthropic foundations, and national research bodies' investments in HSR in both high-income countries and low- and middle-income countries (LMICs) have risen (Barnett et al., 2015; Bennett et al., 2008; UK Medical Research Council, 2016).

HSR differs from traditional clinical research in several important ways, including its aims, the methods it uses, the nature of interventions under evaluation, and the research participants targeted by studies. HSR seeks to understand health systems in a *real-world* context (as opposed to measuring intervention efficacy under ideal conditions) and is commonly embedded in health care practice; in these respects, HSR studies can be similar to pragmatic clinical trials of health care interventions (Califf and Sugarman, 2015). HSR is characterized by the questions it asks, which typically focus on understanding health system operations, assessing health system performance, exploring the causes of poor performance, or/and developing and evaluating interventions to address particular health system shortcomings. HSR is thus about focusing on problems, and it is often exploratory or descriptive rather than intervention-focused (Gilson, 2012). It is a context-driven field, which means "at all stages of the research endeavor, from prioritization of research questions, to conceptualization and conduct of the research, to interpretation of and communication of findings, [HSR] will benefit from being embedded within a particular context and close engagement with local actors" (Bennett et al., 2011, 1).

The methods used in HSR, in keeping with the nature of the research questions typically under study, include cluster trials, records review, observational studies, participatory action research, case studies, surveys, and economic evaluations. HSR methods and interventions are frequently iterative and dynamic, evolving over the course of a given study. When studied, interventions are generally tested at the population or group level rather than the individual level. Examples of typical interventions under study in HSR include voucher schemes for existing services, community-based health insurance programs, and human resource management strategies for clinics or hospitals—all of which intervene with groups of people rather than targeting individuals (Hyder, Rattani, et al., 2014). In some instances, health system interventions may have a particular disease focus, but they frequently address aspects of the health system, such as human resources or financing, that generate impacts across a broad range of diseases. HSR is a policy-driven field, with a strong emphasis on translating findings into policy and practice (Bennett et al., 2011).

HSR *ethics* is also a relatively new and emerging field. Despite the growth of investment in HSR, particularly in LMICs, there has not been substantial conceptual work done to clarify the field's ethical dimensions (Mills, 2012). Given HSR's distinctive characteristics, it has been suggested that the ethical issues present in the field may be distinctively nuanced relative to the forms of biomedical research that traditional bioethics principles were initially intended to address (Hyder, Rattani, et al., 2014). This chapter will, first, explore the extent to which traditional bioethics principles—respect for persons, beneficence, and justice—are relevant to HSR. To do so, it will draw on a growing body of scholarly work characterizing the various ethical considerations inherent to HSR. It will demonstrate that while traditional bioethics principles are pertinent to HSR, they can be interpreted and applied differently relative to biomedical research.

The chapter will then argue that HSR may further require the application of additional core ethical commitments to consider the full range of ethical issues arising in the field. Ethical commitments to citizen engagement, partnership and collaboration, and sustainability, which are core commitments of the field of health systems ethics, are suggested as necessary for responsible ethical oversight of HSR. These commitments are rooted in or are consistent with one or more of the traditional bioethics principles. For example, the commitment to public engagement has a strong association with respect for persons and a moderate association with justice (Krubiner and Hyder, 2014). The commitments, however, highlight considerations that may not be immediately obvious when considering traditional interpretations of respect for persons, beneficence, and justice. Rather, they provide a more detailed specification of what each principle entails in the context of health systems ethics, which can be applied to HSR (Krubiner and Hyder, 2014). While the ethical issues discussed are globally relevant, the chapter also assumes a deliberate (though not exclusive) focus on LMIC settings.

Application of Traditional Bioethics Principles in HSR

This section will show that the application of the traditional "Belmont" principles, which were originally delineated in the United States for the ethics of research with human subjects (National Commission, 1978), may be applied differently in HSR relative to how they are applied in biomedical research. Upholding respect for persons, beneficence, and justice in HSR involves particularly nuanced considerations due to the field's distinctive features, as described below in relation to each principle. These examples represent a subset of the ethical issues arising in HSR and should not be seen as offering a comprehensive picture.

Respect for Persons

Respect for persons encompasses two moral requirements: "first, that individuals should be treated as autonomous agents, and second, that persons with diminished autonomy are entitled to protection" (National Commission, 1978). In HSR, a concern has been raised that individual autonomy can be particularly difficult to uphold in studies that distribute interventions at the group or population level (such as adjustments to standard services offered at public health facilities). It may be difficult for individuals to avoid being exposed to interventions, and they may be unable to meaningfully refuse to participate, opt out, or withdraw from studies (Hundley et al., 2010; McRae et al., 2011; Gallo et al., 2012). This concern is particularly applicable, for example, where HSR employs cluster trial methodology (Edwards et al., 1999; Gallo et al., 2012; Hutton, 2001; Taljaard et al., 2013; Osrin et al., 2009; Sabin et al., 2008). Cluster trials randomize intact social units, such as households, primary care practices, hospital wards, classrooms, neighborhoods, and entire communities, to differing intervention arms (Weijer et al., 2012). Difficulties in avoiding exposure could arise, for example, where an intervention consists of enacting a new hospital policy for performance-based management of health workers across multiple districts. Short of attending a hospital outside the district, individuals would not be able to avoid being treated by doctors and nurses whose provision of care was guided by the new incentive structure (Pratt et al., 2017). In contrast, in classic biomedical research, individuals can typically avoid exposure to an intervention under study simply by declining to participate in a given trial.

In such cases, it is suggested that "gatekeepers" may play important roles in determining whether it is permissible for researchers to approach participants directly or to enroll a cluster in a study (Edwards et al., 1999; Hutton, 2001; Osrin et al., 2009; Taljaard et al., 2013; Whicher et al., 2015). Gatekeepers may include, among others, locally practicing physicians, a managing partner of a primary care practice, hospital administrative leadership, local religious or cultural leaders, and/or local political leaders (Anderson et al. 2015; Osrin et al. 2009). They may thus be "gatekeepers" of the health system or of the community more broadly. It is likely both may need to be approached for HSR studies to proceed. This recommendation, however, brings with it a range of additional ethical concerns. Gatekeepers may have significant conflicts of interest, and it may be difficult to assess their legitimacy (Anderson et al., 2015; Osrin et al., 2009). Osrin et al. (2009) provide an example in which male gatekeepers' permission is sought for access to prospective female participants within a hierarchical society, which may be seen by some as counterproductive to the main purpose of the research. When an intervention under study aims to change the status quo, which is common in participatory action research, individuals who represent the traditional power structures and authorities within communities or health systems may be a poor choice of gatekeeper.

Being respectful to individuals in HSR may still involve obtaining individual informed consent (unless a waiver of consent is approved in the ethical review process) or informing patients that a study is taking place. It may also mean taking steps to ensure that individuals, particularly members of disadvantaged groups, can opt out or minimize their exposure to the intervention under study (Hyder, Pratt, et al., 2014).

Beyond individual autonomy, where interventions are directed at groups of people, as in cluster-based studies, the emphasis on groups of people as research subjects introduces the ethical challenge of defining the moral status of a group or community. The extension of "respect" from an individual to a population requires further exploration for global health research (Wallwork, 2008). It demands adopting the broader interpretation of respect for *communities* to determine what is ethically required (Weijer and Anderson, 2002). This might entail taking stock of study community priorities and norms and determining appropriate levels of engagement with local leadership, which will present further challenges, particularly in pluralistic communities embodying a range of diverse interests (Hyder, Rattani, et al., 2014).

Beneficence

The ethical principle of beneficence requires protecting persons from harm and making efforts to secure their well-being. It has been interpreted to entail (among other things) minimizing possible harms to research participants, maximizing possible benefits to society, and balancing the risks of harm presented by interventions against possible benefits

Table 13.1 Individual and Collective Risks in HSR

Individual risks in HSR	Collective risks in HSR
Economic/Financial Risks • Time to participate prevents performing daily activities and earning income	*Economic/Financial Risks* • Costs to health system (such as overwhelmed supply side of health system) • Group or health institution finances are harmed • Distortion of local markets
Social Risks • Negative effect on relationships with others (such as doctor-patient relationship) • Privacy (such as improper disclosure of health information) • Reputational harm to health workers where data speaks to poor performance	*Social Risks* • Widening of health inequalities or further marginalization of disadvantaged groups • Lack of intervention sustainability • Group or health institution reputation is harmed
Physical and Psychological Risks • Medical/physical harm • Decreases in intrinsic motivation and well-being • Psychological distress during collection of sensitive information	*Political Risks* • Sociopolitical instability, social discord • External actors push policy measures on LMICs that are ill-suited to their particular context

Source: Adapted from Pratt et al., 2017, 890–910, by permission of Oxford University Press.

(National Commission, 1978). Since HSR is often conducted with groups or populations, it can generate risks and benefits not only for individuals, but also for groups, populations, and health systems. These additional layers of risks and benefits need to be accounted for in HSR studies.

Understanding of the nature, frequency, and severity of risks and potential benefits in HSR is relatively underdeveloped (Fox and Tulsky, 2005). At most, various individual and collective risks for medical, social, economic, and political harms are starting to be described in the literature (see Table 13.1). Specific risks have been linked to particular HSR methods. For example, the following risks are common in HSR using participatory action research methods: social discord, social harms such as stigma (individual or group), and financial harms (Hunt, Gogognon, and Ridde, 2014). These risks differ from those that typically arise in biomedical research, though they can occur in such research. Upholding the principle of beneficence demands employing strategies to minimize such risks, particularly where individuals' ability to opt out of studies cannot be secured. Further work is needed to develop strategies, particularly for minimizing collective risks in HSR.

Justice

Justice demands that the burdens and benefits of research be fairly distributed (National Commission, 1978). This has been interpreted to entail a number of ethical requirements, such as fair selection of research participants, responsiveness, and provision of post-study benefits to participants (CIOMS, 2002; WMA, 2013). While such considerations apply to HSR, interpretation of them may differ. For example, fair subject selection in HSR may demand ensuring that the research population *includes* members of vulnerable groups, or that access to research engagement is equitably distributed (Hunt et al., 2014; Meyers and Andresen, 2000). The evaluation of health system changes often requires the near-universal participation of patients using a service if it is to provide valid information. Additionally, HSR frequently aims to improve health systems for disadvantaged groups (Hyder, Rattani, et al., 2014). Yet, in practice, participants in HSR are likely to represent a limited, better-off subset of the population that will be affected by service changes, because substantial barriers to participation exist for the disadvantaged, including illiteracy, fear of authorities, cost of travel, poorer health, and less secure jobs. According to Cassell and Young (2002, 316), "[w]here [health systems research] contributes to the planning of services and policy making, the voice of the socially excluded may be muffled, and that of the better educated and materially secure, artificially amplified." Here they are discussing the high-income country context, but there is also potential for this to occur in LMIC settings. Exclusion can happen at both the population and individual levels. Entire subpopulations or geographic areas that are vulnerable (e.g., certain districts or groups) can be excluded from the selected research population, and vulnerable individuals and groups within the research population can be excluded from participating. This means studies may prove that interventions are effective for better-off segments of society but fail to determine whether they work for members of disadvantaged groups.

Under the current definitions of "responsiveness" in international research ethics guidelines (CIOMS, 2002; WMA, 2013), research questions ought to address a *health condition or disease* that is present or is a priority in the selected host community or country. So far, the concept has been applied primarily to biomedical needs and outcomes. Because HSR is not a disease-driven field, it has been suggested that responsiveness in HSR should be interpreted in either or both of two ways: (1) as responsiveness to health system needs identified by health system performance assessments, and (2) as responsiveness to health system priorities. The latter entails aligning research with HSR priorities set through country-owned processes involving policymakers from host countries (Pratt and Hyder, 2015c). These priority-setting processes can occur at the national or subnational level (e.g., the district or community level).

HSR and Global Justice

Recent work in bioethics provides moral grounds for the claim that HSR should contribute to the reduction of health disparities between and within countries (Faden et al., 2013; Pratt and Hyder, 2015b). HSR has also been repeatedly identified as an essential means to the goal of achieving global health equity (WHO, 2005; Ministerial Summit on Health Research, 2004). As previously noted, many HSR studies are conducted with the primary aim of enhancing health system performance for disadvantaged and vulnerable populations (Hyder, Rattani, et al., 2014).

Because HSR should play a role, and already has played a role in promoting health equity between and within countries, particularly in LMIC settings, it is appropriate to interpret the principle of justice more expansively for HSR. Upholding justice in HSR requires both achieving a fair balance of burdens and benefits in individual projects and ensuring that the projects advance global health justice. The latter may contribute to achieving the former. However, a fair balance of benefits and burdens may be achieved by providing benefits other than those that advance global health justice. In biomedical research, providing fair benefits is not typically defined or understood as (in part or in sum) providing benefits that advance global health justice.

Ethical Considerations in HSR Relating to Global Justice

If it is accepted that HSR should contribute to reducing global health disparities, then additional ethical concerns can be identified as arising during the conduct of such research. That they are deemed *ethical* considerations stems from their potential to obstruct HSR from advancing global health justice. So far, concerns related to priority-setting and research capacity strengthening have been identified (see Table 13.2). They are described in the HSR literature and, where experienced, they impede projects from furthering a particular concept of global health justice that is articulated in the health capability paradigm (Pratt and Hyder, 2015a). The health capability paradigm defines global health justice as reducing shortfall inequalities in the health of individuals worldwide, with priority going to those who are worst-off in terms of their health. We acknowledge that the concept of global health justice continues to be a matter of debate, and that this is not the only way of defining it. However, the concept used by the health capability paradigm reflects a useful starting point, as it is drawn from one of the

Table 13.2 Ethical Issues in HSR Priority-Setting and Capacity-Building

Priority-Setting

1. Priority-setting for HSR at the global level is often not driven by national or sub-national priorities.
2. Global priorities influence and possibly determine national priorities for HSR in LMICs.
3. Disease-specific health research priority-setting methods that devalue HSR are often employed in global and national research priority-setting.
4. Interpretive priority setting methods for HSR may not utilize an equity criterion.
5. Donors exert substantial control over the selection and implementation of HSR priorities in LMICs.

Capacity-Building

1. Funding for health research capacity-building in LMICs is directed primarily to clinical and epidemiological research at the expense of HSR.
2. Funding for HSR capacity-building in LMICs does not strongly support sustainable and/or long-term capacity development programs, or interventions that build the capacity of research systems.
3. Capacity-building efforts for HSR in LMICs frequently utilize strategies of limited effectiveness.

few political-philosophy theories to address health justice in depth, and its components are consistent with other theories of justice (Pratt, Merritt, and Hyder, 2016).

As an example, the dominant role of donors in priority-setting for HSR in LMICs is inconsistent with global justice for multiple reasons (Pratt and Hyder, 2015a). First, it means that power is concentrated with one type of global actor rather than shared across stakeholders, as required by accounts linking health governance to global health justice (Ruger, 2011, 2012). This makes it less likely that priority-setting for HSR at the global level will reflect the voices of national and subnational actors from LMICs or reach a genuine consensus. Second, donors primarily fund HSR in LMICs on a narrow set of questions related to service delivery and scale up, rather than HSR that is responsive to local needs. While research on service delivery is necessary, it should not be the *only* focus of HSR in LMICs, particularly if it does not emphasize improving service delivery for vulnerable and disadvantaged populations (Pratt and Hyder, 2015a).

A Nuanced Ethical Framework for HSR

Additional core ethical commitments are needed to ensure consideration of the full range of moral issues arising in HSR. Being context-driven and policy-driven means that HSR often has the following features that give rise to particular ethical issues: citizen engagement, collaboration and partnership with research users, and promotion of research translation. Correspondingly, relevant ethical commitments such as public engagement, collaboration, and sustainability can be usefully applied in HSR. These commitments have been identified as core commitments of health systems ethics, though they are not unique to that field (UNAIDS and AVAC, 2011). They highlight ethical considerations that may not be immediately obvious when considering traditional interpretations of respect for persons, beneficence, and justice. Such ethical considerations may also be nuanced for HSR relative to biomedical research (e.g., achieving intervention sustainability across clusters and ensuring meaningful citizen engagement in research priority-setting).

Citizen Engagement

Because health systems vary considerably across different settings, HSR questions must be context-driven (Bennett et al., 2011). Citizen engagement helps to ensure that research questions and intervention design reflect the specific circumstances or problems facing the health system of the host community or country. Engagement is increasingly required when setting research priorities, formulating research questions, and shaping the design, conduct, and dissemination of HSR studies in high-income countries and

LMICs (van Bekkum and Hilton, 2014; Fleurence et al., 2013; Comic Relief, 2013; Doris Duke Foundation, 2018). In the United Kingdom, for example, a requirement of the Department of International Development's Research Programme Consortia funding is that consortia undertake a yearlong "Inception Phase" to further define their research questions and the methodologies to answer them. Engagement with "intended users" of the research must be undertaken during this phase (DFID, 2010).

Yet as individuals are increasingly engaged in research, ethical issues related to their engagement may also occur. Ellis and Kass (2016) note that a set of ethical considerations when engaging patients in health research may also be relevant in the context of HSR, including who is engaged, when they are engaged, and how they are engaged. Citizen roles identified as specifically relevant to engage in health research are patients, families and careers, providers, purchasers, payers, policymakers, and product makers (Concannon et al., 2012). Attention should also be paid to whether the kinds of patients being engaged are representative of the broader population and include members of disadvantaged groups (Ellis and Kass, 2016; Hunt et al., 2014).

At what stages in the research process citizens of different role-types are engaged is another key consideration. As an example from a participatory action HSR project in Burkina Faso, a concern was raised as to whether the most disadvantaged and vulnerable within communities were engaged in both the planning and implementation phases of the project. Where such individuals or groups are excluded, this situation raises concerns related to the absence from these processes of the perspective of those most directly impacted by the project (Hunt et al., 2014).

Finally, whether citizens of different role-types are engaged using collaborative or consultative mechanisms is ethically relevant. Consultation refers to researchers obtaining citizens' input in various ways, but there is no assurance that they will use the information they receive. Collaboration, in contrast, involves shared decision-making between parties (Ellis and Kass, 2016; Pratt, Merritt, and Hyder, 2016).

Collaboration and Partnership with Research Users

HSR is often embedded in practice, which frequently requires conducting studies in partnership with research users such as policymakers, civil society organizations, and health care providers. Like citizen engagement, this also serves to promote context-driven research. Ethical challenges have been identified as arising from the embedded nature of HSR.

Developing respectful, trusting relationships between research teams and national or subnational policymakers and practitioners is challenging, especially when their objectives do not align or there are significant power disparities between partners (Hunt et al., 2014; Krubiner and Hyder, 2016). This power imbalance can obstruct researchers from designing interventions that align with community needs or lead them to test interventions that widen health disparities. It may also mean that researchers sometimes test interventions designed to promote particular political agendas rather than the interests of the public and/or its most disadvantaged members.

Promoting Sustainable Research Translation

Being policy-driven brings an emphasis on translating HSR findings into policy and practice. HSR should lead to sustainable changes that improve health system functioning (Kuruvilla, Mays, and Walt, 2007). Yet a sizeable gap exists in the real world between the evidence generated by HSR and its use in policy and practice (Hyder et al., 2007; El-Jardali et al., 2012). A weak HSR-to-policy interface and its underlying contributing factors are all of ethical concern.

In particular, one component of research translation is ensuring sustainable intervention implementation. Ethical concerns relating to sustainability were raised by a number of health systems researchers in the Krubiner and Hyder (2016) study, often as a criticism of existing pilot studies and programs. Some researchers discussed the fact that the models under investigation were not appropriate for long-term, sustainable solutions, whereas others identified funding and political will as insufficient to support ongoing investment in the test interventions post-study (Krubiner and Hyder, 2016). Similarly, in a cluster trial performed across multiple LMICs, Osrin et al. (2009, 777) reported the following:

> One of the issues for all our trials is the sustainability of the community women's groups after the trial ends. Withdrawal demands extensive discussions with group members. In all cases, we have agreed to give the control clusters the benefits of the intervention if it is shown to be effective. In some cases (Bangladesh, Jharkhand and Orissa, Mumbai), we have assurances of financial support for this from existing funders. In others, we are trying to negotiate a roll-out plan with government representatives.

Issues of sustainability are relevant not only to HSR, but to other types of research as well. Nevertheless, the ethical considerations relating to sustained implementation of HSR interventions across clusters may differ from those relating to ensuring post-trial access to new medicines. This topic requires further investigation.

Additional Ethical Commitments

Given the ethical issues arising in relation to engagement, partnership with research users, and sustainability, the following three core ethical commitments would be appropriate to apply in HSR. These commitments along with others have been proposed by Krubiner and Hyder (2014) for this context.

- *Public engagement* demands active engagement with the public; there should be opportunities for engagement for citizens of multiple role-types, including members of disadvantaged groups.
- *Collaboration* demands collaboration with those within the health system as well as other sectors.

- *Sustainability* demands planning for the long term in order to promote improvements in services being maintained over time. Appropriate transition/exit strategies should be in place for shorter-term projects to minimize the harms of withdrawal.

Future work is needed to operationalize these commitments for HSR practice; that is, to identify what upholding each requires during the conduct of HSR. Doing so calls for exploring what the commitments entail across a diverse body of research—for example, from descriptive studies to intervention-focused studies, from cluster trials to participatory action research, and from national evaluations to community-based research projects. This future work will need to recognize and take account of the practical challenges of upholding commitments to public engagement, collaboration, and sustainability. Beyond these three commitments, other health systems ethics commitments may also be relevant to HSR, and future bioethics scholarship could explore that topic.

Conclusion

Health systems research has distinctive features relative to biomedical research, such as being systems-focused, conducted with groups and populations, context-driven, embedded in health systems operations, and policy-driven. These features (and others) give rise to nuanced ethical considerations at the project level in HSR. More broadly, ethical considerations related to priority-setting and research-capacity strengthening have been identified for HSR that apply at the funder, institutional, national, and global levels (see Table 13.1).

While there is growing scholarship documenting these and other ethical considerations inherent in HSR, guidance on how to address them is lacking. A recent systematic review of the HSR ethics literature found that the majority of existing guidance focuses on obtaining or waiving informed consent and is thus insufficient for HSR (Pratt et al., 2017). The guidance identified comes primarily from the scholarly literature. The review did not identify any formal guidance documents for researchers or research ethics committees on HSR ethics. At most, two relevant guidance/recommendation documents pertaining to cluster trials were identified: "The Ottawa Statement on the Ethical Design and Conduct of Cluster Randomized Trials" (Weijer et al., 2012) and the US Secretary's Advisory Committee on Human Research Protections' *Recommendations on Regulatory Issues in Cluster Studies* (SACHRP, 2014). A report from a NIH Collaboratory Workshop also examines the ethical and regulatory challenges for pragmatic cluster randomized trials (Anderson et al., 2015).

The development of much-needed ethics guidance will, therefore, need to consider ethical issues relating to balancing risks and benefits and justice more comprehensively. It will also need to explore how to apply and operationalize a broader justice principle and additional ethical commitments for HSR. In doing so, it will be important to ask where the responsibilities of individual researchers and projects begin and end in relation to global health justice, public engagement, collaboration, and sustainability. Much policy and practice impact is unpredictable and contingent on many factors coming together at an appropriate time. The extent of researchers' responsibilities as well as the responsibilities of other actors (funders, governments, policymakers) must be appropriately articulated.

References

Anderson, M. L., Califf, R. M., Sugarman, J., and participants in the NIH Health Care Systems Research Collaboratory Cluster Randomized Trial Workshop. 2015. "Ethical and Regulatory Issues of Pragmatic Cluster Randomized Trials in Contemporary Health Systems." *Clinical Trials* 12(3): 276–286.

Barnett, A. G., Herbert, D. L., Campbell, M., Daly, N., Roberts, J. A., Mudge, A., et al. 2015. "Streamlined Research Funding Using Short Proposals and Accelerated Peer Review: An Observational Study." *BMC Health Services Research* 15: 55.

Bennett, S., Adam, T., Zarowsky, C., Tangcharoensathien, V., Ranson, K., Evans, T., et al. 2008. "From Mexico to Mali: Progress in Health Policy and Systems Research." *Lancet* 372: 1571–1578.

Bennett, S., Agyepong, I. A., Sheikh, K., Hanson, K., Ssengooba, F., and Gilson, L. 2011. "Building the Field of Health Policy and Systems Research: An Agenda for Action." *PLoS Medicine* 8: e1001081. https://journals.plos.org/plosmedicine/article?id=10.1371/journal.pmed.1001081.

Califf, R. E., and Sugarman, J. 2015. "Exploring the Ethical and Regulatory Issues in Pragmatic Clinical Trials." *Clinical Trials* 12(5): 436–441.

Cassell, J., and Young, A. 2002. "Why We Should Not Seek Individual Informed Consent for Participation in Health Services Research." *Journal of Medical Ethics* 28: 313–317.

Comic Relief. 2013. *International Grant Strategy* (London: Comic Relief).

Concannon, T. W., Meissner, P., Grunbaum, J. A., McElwee, N., Guise, J. M., Santa, J., et al. 2012. "A New Taxonomy for Stakeholder Engagement in Patient-Centered Outcomes Research." *Journal of General Internal Medicine* 27(8): 985–991.

CIOMS (Council for International Organizations of Medical Sciences). 2002. *International Ethical Guidelines for Biomedical Research Involving Human Subjects* (Geneva: CIOMS). https://cioms.ch/shop/product/international-ethical-guidelines-for-biomedical-research-involving-human-subjects-2/.

DFID (UK Department for International Development). 2010. *Managing the Inception Phase of Research Programme Consortia* (London: Department for International Development).

Doris Duke Foundation.2018. *African Health Initiative Grantmaking Process*. http://www.ddcf.org/what-we-fund/african-health-initiative/.

Edwards, S. J., Braunholtz, D. A., Lilford, R. J., and Stevens, A. J. 1999. "Ethical Issues in the Design and Conduct of Cluster Randomised Controlled Trials." *British Medical Journal* 318: 1407.

El-Jardali, F., Lavis, J. N., Ataya, N., Jamal, D., Ammar, W., and Raouf, S. 2012. "Use of Health Systems Evidence by Policymakers in Eastern Mediterranean Countries: Views, Practices, and Contextual Influences." *BMC Health Services Research* 12(1): 200.

Ellis, L. E., and Kass, N. E. 2016. "How are PCORI-Funded Researchers Engaging Patients in Research and What Are the Ethical Implications?" *AJOB Empirical Bioethics* 8(1): 1–10. doi:10.1080/23294515.2016.1206045.

Faden, R. R., Kass, N. E., Goodman, S. N., Pronovost, P., Tunis, S. and Beauchamp, T. L. 2013. "An Ethics Framework for a Learning Health Care System: A Departure from Traditional Research Ethics and Clinical Ethics." *Hastings Center Report* 43: S16–S27.

Fleurence, R., Selby, J. V., Odom-Walker, K., Hunt, G., Meltzer, D., Slutsky, J. R., et al. 2013. "How the Patient-Centered Outcomes Research Institute Is Engaging Patients and Others in Shaping Its Research Agenda." *Health Affairs* 32(2): 393–400.

Fox, E., and Tulsky, J. 2005. "Recommendations for the Ethical Conduct of Quality Improvement." *Journal of Clinical Ethics* 16(1): 61–71.

Gallo, A., Weijer, C., White, A., Grimshaw, J. M., Boruch, R., Brehaut, J. C., et al. 2012. "What Is the Role and Authority of Gatekeepers in Cluster Randomized Trials in Health Research?" *Trials* 13: 116.

Gilson, L. 2012. *Health Policy and Systems Research: A Methodology Reader* (Geneva: Alliance for Health Policy and Systems Research).

Hoffman, S. J., Røttingen, J.-A., Bennett, S., Lavis, J. N., Edge, J. S., and Frenk, J. 2012. *Background Paper on Conceptual Issues Related to Health Systems Research to Inform a WHO Global Strategy on Health Systems Research* (Geneva: World Health Organization). http://www.who.int/alliance-hpsr/alliancehpsr_backgroundpaperhsrstrat1.pdf.

Hundley, V., Cheyne, H., Bland, J. M., Styles, M., and Barnett, C. A. 2010. "So You Want to Conduct a Cluster Randomized Controlled Trial? Lessons from a National Cluster Trial of Early Labour." *Journal of Evaluation in Clinical Practice* 16: 632–638.

Hunt, M. R., Gogognon, P., and Ridde, V. 2014. "Ethical Considerations Related to Participation and Partnership: An Investigation of Stakeholders' Perceptions of an Action-Research Project on User Fee Removal for the Poorest in Burkina Faso." *BMC Medical Ethics* 15: 13.

Hutton, J. L. 2001. "Are Distinctive Ethical Principles Required for Cluster Randomized Controlled Trials?" *Statistics in Medicine* 20: 473–488.

Hyder, A. A., Bloom, G., Leach, M., Syed, S. B., Peters, D. H., and Future Health Systems: Innovations for Equity. 2007. "Exploring Health Systems Research and Its Influence on Policy Processes in Low Income Countries." *BMC Public Health* 7(1): 309.

Hyder, A. A., Pratt B., Ali, J., Kass, N. E., and Sewankambo, N. 2014. "The Ethics of Health Systems Research in Low- and Middle-Income Countries: A Call to Action." *Global Public Health* 9: 1008–1022. doi:10.1080/17441692.2014.931998.

Hyder, A. A., Rattani, A., Krubiner, C., Bachani, A. M., and Tran, N. T. 2014. "Ethical Review of Health Systems Research in Low- and Middle-Income Countries: A Conceptual Exploration." *American Journal of Bioethics* 14(2): 28–37.

Krubiner, C., and Hyder, A. A. 2014. "A Bioethical Framework for Health Systems Activity: A Conceptual Exploration Applying 'Systems Thinking.'" *Health Systems* 3(2): 124–135.

Krubiner, C., and Hyder, A. A. 2016. "Ethical Challenges in Designing and Implementing Health Systems Research: Experiences from the Field." *AJOB Empirical Ethics* 7(3): 209–221.

Kuruvilla, S., Mays, N., and Walt, G. 2007. "Describing the Impact of Health Services and Policy Research." *Journal of Health Services Research and Policy* 12: 23.

Meyers A. R. and Andresen E. M. 2000. "Enabling our instruments: accommodation, universal design, and access to participation in research." *Archives of Physical Medicine and Rehabilitation* 81: S5–S9.

McRae, A. D., Weijer, C., Binik, A., Grimshaw, J. M., Boruch, R., Brehaut, J. C., et al. 2011. "When Is Informed Consent Required in Cluster Randomized Trials in Health Research?" *Trials* 12: 202.

Mills, A. 2012. "Health Policy and Systems Research: Defining the Terrain; Identifying the Methods." *Health Policy and Planning* 27(1): 1–7.

Ministerial Summit on Health Research. 2004. *The Mexico Statement on Health Research, Mexico City*. http://www.who.int/rpc/summit/agenda/en/mexico_statement_on_health_research.pdf.

National Commission (National Commission for the Protection of Human Subjects of Biomedical and Behavioral Research). 1978. *The Belmont Report: Ethical Principles and Guidelines for the Protection of Human Subjects of Research* (Bethesda, Md.: US Department of Health and Humans Services). https://www.hhs.gov/ohrp/regulations-and-policy/belmont-report/read-the-belmont-report/index.html.

Osrin, D., Azad, K., Fernandez, A., Manandhar, D. S., Mwansambo, C. W., Tripathy, P., et al. 2009. "Ethical Challenges in Cluster Randomized Controlled Trials: Experiences from Public Health Interventions in Africa and Asia." *Bulletin of the World Health Organization* 87: 772–779.

Pratt, B., and Hyder, A. A. 2015a. "Applying a Global Justice Lens to Health Systems Research Ethics: An Initial Exploration." *Kennedy Institute of Ethics Journal* 25(1): 35–66.

Pratt, B., and Hyder, A. A. 2015b. "Global Justice and Health Systems Research in Low and Middle-Income Countries." *Journal of Law, Medicine & Ethics* 43(1): 143–161.

Pratt, B., and Hyder, A. A. 2015c. "Reinterpreting Responsiveness for Health Systems Research in Low and Middle-Income Countries." *Bioethics* 29(6): 379–388.

Pratt, B., Merritt, M., and Hyder, A. A. 2016. "Towards Deep Inclusion for Equity-Oriented Health Research Priority-Setting: A Working Model." *Social Science and Medicine* 151: 215–224.

Pratt, B., Paul, A., Hyder, A. A., and Ali, J. 2017. "Ethics of Health Policy and Systems Research: A Scoping Review of the Literature." *Health Policy and Planning* 32(6): 890–910.

Ruger, J. P. 2011. "Shared Health Governance." *American Journal of Bioethics* 11(7): 32–45.

Ruger, J. P. 2012. "Global Health Justice and Governance." *American Journal of Bioethics* 12(12): 35–54.

Sabin, J. E., Mazor, K., Meterko, V., Goff, S. L., and Platt, R. 2008. "Comparing Drug Effectiveness at Health Plans: The Ethics of Cluster Randomized Trials." *Hastings Center Report* 38(5): 39–48.

SACHRP (US Secretary's Advisory Committee on Human Research Protections). 2014. *Attachment C: Recommendations on Regulatory Issues in Cluster Studies* (Washington, D.C.: US Department of Health & Human Services, Office for Human Research Protections).

Sheikh, K., Gilson, L., Agyepong, I. A., Hanson, K., Ssengooba, F., and Bennett, S. 2011. "Building the Field of Health Policy and Systems Research: Framing the Questions." *PLoS Medicine* 8: e1001073. https://journals.plos.org/plosmedicine/article?id=10.1371/journal.pmed.1001073.

Taljaard, M., Weijer, C., Grimshaw, J. M., and Eccles, M. P. 2013. "The Ottawa Statement on the Ethical Design and Conduct of Cluster Randomised Trials: Precis for Researchers and Research Ethics Committees." *British Medical Journal* 346: f2838.

UK Medical Research Council. 2016. Joint Health Systems Research Initiative. http://www.mrc.ac.uk/funding/science-areas/global-health/joint-health-systems-research-initiative.

UNAIDS (Joint United Nations Programme on HIV/AIDS) and AVAC (AIDS Vaccine Advocacy Coalition). 2011. *Good Participatory Practice: Guidelines for Biomedical HIV Prevention Trials*. 2nd ed. (Geneva: UNAIDS). https://www.avac.org/resource/good-participatory-practice-guidelines-biomedical-hiv-prevention-trials-second-edition.

van Bekkum, J. E., and Hilton, S. 2014. "UK Research Funding Bodies' Views towards Public Participation in Health-Related Research Decisions: An Exploratory Study." *BMC Health Services Research* 14: 318.

Wallwork, E. 2008. "Ethical Analysis of Research Partnerships with Communities." *Kennedy Institute of Ethics Journal* 18(1): 57–85.

Weijer, C., and Anderson, J. A. 2002. "A Critical Appraisal of Protections for Aboriginal Communities in Biomedical Research." *Jurimetrics* 42(2): 187–198.

Weijer, C., Grimshaw, J. M., Eccles, M. P., McRae, A. D., White, A., Brehaut, J. C., et al. 2012. "The Ottawa Statement on the Ethical Design and Conduct of Cluster Randomized Trials." *PLoS medicine* 9(11): e1001346. https://journals.plos.org/plosmedicine/article?id=10.1371/journal.pmed.1001346.

Whicher, D. E., Miller, J. E., Dunham, K. M., and Joffe, S. 2015. "Gatekeepers for Pragmatic Clinical Trials." *Clinical Trials* 12(5): 442–448.

WHO (World Health Organization). 2005. *The Millennium Development Goals Will Not Be Attained without New Research Addressing Health System Constraints to Delivering Effective Interventions* (Geneva: WHO Task Force on Health Systems Research).

WHO (World Health Organization). 2010. *Health Systems Financing: The Path to Universal Coverage* (Geneva: WHO).

WHO (World Health Organization). 2013. *World Health Report 2013: Research for Universal Health Coverage* (Geneva: WHO).

WMA (World Medical Association). 2013. *Declaration of Helsinki* (Seoul: WMA). https://www.wma.net/policies-post/wma-declaration-of-helsinki-ethical-principles-for-medical-research-involving-human-subjects/.

Further Reading

Daniels, N. 2008. *Just Health: Meeting Health Needs Fairly* (Cambridge: Cambridge University Press).

Pogge, T. 2008. *World Poverty and Human Rights: Cosmopolitan Responsibilities and Reforms* (Cambridge: Polity Press).

Powers, M., and Faden, R. 2006. *Social Justice: The Moral Foundations of Public Health and Health Policy* (Oxford: Oxford University Press).

Ruger, J. P. 2009. "Global Health Justice." *Public Health Ethics* 2(3): 261–275.

Ruger, J. P. 2010. *Health and Social Justice* (Oxford: Oxford University Press).

Venkatapuram, S. 2011. *Health Justice: An Argument from the Capabilities Approach* (Cambridge: Polity Press).

CHAPTER 14

THE LEARNING HEALTH CARE SYSTEM AND ETHICS: CHALLENGES AND OPPORTUNITIES

STEPHANIE MORAIN, NANCY E. KASS, AND RUTH R. FADEN

INTRODUCTION

THE idea of a learning health care system (LHCS) is motivated by growing concerns about deficiencies in the current health care system. Developments in medicine and technology have enabled remarkable advances in biomedical research, improving our understanding of disease and identifying better interventions for prevention, diagnosis, and treatment. The rapid expansion of technological capabilities to collect, use, and share electronic data offers further promise to expand the research system's capacity to advance knowledge to improve health. However, concerns persist that health care systems in many countries are falling short in generating and using new knowledge to improve health. In the United States, for example, it is estimated that at least one-third of the $3 trillion spent annually is unnecessary, ineffective, preventable, or harmful (IOM, 2013), with medical errors alone killing tens of thousands of people each year (IOM, 2000; Klevens et al., 2007; HHS, 2008; Winters et al., 2012; Reed and May, 2011).

At the same time, patients are estimated to receive only 55 percent of recommended care (McGlynn et al., 2003). Despite a proliferation of research, there remains insufficient evidence to guide most clinical decisions. The US Institute of Medicine (IOM, now the National Academy of Medicine, or NAM) frames this problem by saying that "too much care that is important is often not delivered, and too much care that is delivered is often not important" (IOM, 2007, xi).

Consequently, there is increasing interest in improving the use of clinical data and the tools of health services research to enhance the efficiency of generating clinically relevant knowledge. There is also increasing interest in finding efficient and reliable ways to transform new knowledge into effective changes that improve health care quality (Califf and Sugarman, 2015).

Defining Characteristics of a Learning Health Care System

The learning health care system (LHCS) model has received considerable attention since at least 2007 as a strategy to drive improvement in the quality and efficiency of medical care. An LHCS is defined as a system in which knowledge generation is built into the ongoing practice of clinical care, and findings based on this knowledge are continuously fed back to improve care delivery. It is a system "in which science, informatics, incentives, and culture are aligned for continuous improvement and innovation, with best practices seamlessly embedded in the delivery process and new knowledge captured as an integral by-product of the delivery experience" (IOM, 2013, 136). Responding to contemporary critiques that research and clinical care are too often "siloed" from one another, the LHCS aims to integrate research into everyday clinical practice, helping to ensure that research is relevant for care, and that care can facilitate the acquisition of new knowledge to drive improvement.

Perhaps the most influential description of an LHCS comes from an IOM report, *Best Care at Lower Cost: The Path to Continuously Learning Health Care in America* (2013), which calls for a substantive transformation in the US health care system. In the report, the IOM presents a vision for addressing shortcomings in the current health care system. Among the opportunities identified are technological advances in the collection, storage, sharing, and analysis of electronic health data; progress in organizational capabilities and management science to improve the reliability and efficiency of care; and increasing patient empowerment.

While the concept of the LHCS has focused mostly on the context of private systems of hospitals, clinics, and health care providers in the United States that are not government-run, the rationales for and importance of creating an LHCS apply as much, if not more, to systems of public health and personal health care services that are financed, managed, or delivered by government institutions. The goals behind the integration of delivery and learning apply to all health systems, including those directly administered by local, regional, and national governments.

Examples of Activities Consistent with a Transition to a Learning Health Care System

In the United States, numerous institutions and other entities have made a public commitment to moving toward the LHCS model. Several European countries and the

United Kingdom (UK) offer promising settings for an LHCS, and recent activities suggest growing interest in the LHCS approach. There is also emerging attention to the implication of the LHCS model for low- and middle-income countries (LMICs).

Public and private actors across the United States have taken steps to move their systems toward an LHCS model. Nonprofit integrated delivery systems like Geisinger Health System in Pennsylvania, Group Health Cooperative (now Kaiser Permanente) in Washington, Kaiser Permanente Colorado, and Intermountain Healthcare in Utah have each implemented comprehensive structural reorganizations of their respective systems consistent with an LHCS. Central to these efforts has been the creation of data systems to collect data from routine clinical care that can be used for research and operations activities to improve health care in their respective systems while improving knowledge across the broader scientific community. Government actors are undertaking similar efforts. For example, the Veterans Health Administration (VHA), the largest integrated health care system in the United States, is increasingly studying the ongoing care that patients receive through both observational designs and randomized and embedded "pragmatic" trials (Rosenthal, 2014). The goal of this work is to accelerate the collection and incorporation of evidence into care, both to improve care more quickly and to reduce the cost associated with traditional clinical trials (D'Avolio et al., 2012).

The LHCS model is also gaining attention outside of the United States. In the United Kingdom, a pilot study was conducted to explore the feasibility of point-of-care trials within the general practitioner (GP) setting (Van Staa et al., 2014). An additional study is underway to explore the "meaning, feasibility, and implications of the LHCS model" within the UK system (Learning Healthcare Project, 2015). Ireland has created Health Atlas Ireland, which enables near real-time use of hospital data, and could serve as the basis for broader learning activities (Friedman and Rigby, 2013). Both the Netherlands and the United Kingdom have relatively high use of primary care electronic record systems, with protocols to enable access to anonymized data for learning activities (Friedman and Rigby, 2013).

LMICs face major challenges to achieve broad coverage of health interventions, optimize health outcomes, address evidence gaps, and translate new evidence into policy and practice. The LHCS is gaining attention as a potential model to respond to these challenges (English et al., 2016; Smith, 2015). In Kenya, for example, a collaborative partnership of researchers, policymakers, professional associations, and providers has formed to establish a pediatric clinical information network across fourteen hospital sites. The goal of such partnerships is to build capacity for research, improve quality of care, and advance evidence-informed policymaking (English et al., 2016). In South Africa, advocates of the LHCS model have identified the potential to expand upon an existing national system that currently advances evidence-based care by providing regularly updated guidelines for tens of thousands of primary care clinicians across the country, creating a basic electronic data platform that could also be used to conduct research (BOLDER Research Group, 2016; Fairall et al., 2015)

Moral Justification for Learning Health Care Systems

Health care institutions arguably have a moral obligation to improve quality, safety, and justice in health care. This obligation is consistent with the goals of an LHCS.[1]

Faden et al. (2013) have put forward three foundational moral reasons for a rapid transformation to an LHCS by invoking three societal goals that ought to be promoted: just health care, high-quality health care, and economic well-being. There are many complex obstacles to securing a just health care system, but among them is the absence of a constantly updated body of evidence about the effectiveness, value, and distribution of (a) health care interventions and (b) alternative ways to deliver and finance health care. The absence of this evidence is also a critical obstacle to securing the hallmarks of high-quality health care, eliminating unnecessary and harmful care, and providing appropriate interventions with the highest achievable patient safety.

The role of the LHCS model in advancing high-quality care is reinforced by Largent Joffe, and Miller (2011), who note in their moral argument for an LHCS that this model can systematically advance the acquisition of evidence-based medicine and promote socially valuable research. Finally, regarding economic well-being, even though the rate of health care cost growth has slowed in recent years (Cuckler et al., 2013), health care spending continues to threaten the economic prospects of families and nations and cannot be effectively reined in without efficient learning. The LHCS model supports economic well-being by addressing the imperative of obtaining greater value in health care.

While these three justifications support the transition towards an LHCS model in all settings, the rationale is arguably even more acute where resources are limited. Given this, LMICs may have a particularly strong justification for adopting an LHCS model.

Ethical Challenges for Learning Health Care Systems

Even with a principled moral justification or mandate in place for transitioning to the LHCS model, the transition process and the ongoing operation of any LHCS raise major ethical issues. Many of these ethical challenges are created by the increased capability of LHCSs to collect, use, and analyze data, and by structural attributes of the institutions that must be involved together in LHCSs. Moreover, a central underlying issue is the poor fit between the needs of an LHCS and existing ethical and regulatory frameworks that have grown out of the traditional "research-practice" distinction. Several ethical challenges identified in the US context are described below. While similar challenges are likely to be encountered in other countries, this list is not intended to be exhaustive; additional ethical challenges may arise, depending on the specifics of the health system in question.

Continuous Data Generation

One set of ethical challenges flows from the increased capability of the LHCS to collect and analyze data about provider performance, which inevitably will identify poorer performing providers. How should health institutions respond to such information? Do they have an ethical obligation to disclose information about specific provider performance to patients?

The enhanced collection and analysis of data also presents challenges related to maintaining the privacy and confidentiality of patient data. The need to maintain standards of privacy and confidentiality is perhaps especially important for data activities involving potentially stigmatizing conditions. Special concern may also exist for rare conditions, given the higher risk of identification due to relatively small patient populations (Ali, Califf, and Sugarman, 2015).

Another set of ethical challenges relates to determining what LHCSs should do with the information they generate pertaining to cost and quality. Much research conducted within an LHCS, including comparative effectiveness research, could and arguably should be constructed to provide information not only about effectiveness, but also about value for money. In some cases, the response to such information will be ethically uncomplicated: an LHCS's decision to switch to a less-expensive treatment based on a finding that it is equally effective, safe, and well-tolerated as a more expensive one is ethically unproblematic. However, when comparisons of treatments reveal that a more expensive treatment provides only a slight improvement in effectiveness or has only slightly fewer side effects, it is not ethically straightforward how an LHCS should respond.

The financial structure of an LHCS may also complicate its ability to respond in an ethically responsible way to continuous learning about health care value. Health care systems that rely on revenue streams from expensive interventions may find information about cost and quality threatening to their financial bottom line when, for example, evidence emerges that these interventions produce relatively little benefit for the costs they incur.

None of these challenges are new. There is a substantial literature on patients' claims to information about provider competence and track record (Gallagher, Studdert, and Levinson, 2007; Jacobs, Cerfolio, and Sade, 2009), and an even more substantial literature on the ethics of cost-quality tradeoffs in health coverage decisions (Povar et al., 2004; Feldman, Novack, and Gracely, 1998; Randel et al., 2001). What is new, however, is that such issues will occur with greater frequency, intensity, and predictability as a result of the design of the LHCS itself. Health care systems must now proactively consider management of these issues. For example, in an LHCS, data about provider performance will be collected continuously, and alternative interventions will be continuously compared. LHCSs will need to establish criteria for determining when they are obligated to act on such information, and in what ways.

Transparency

The question of whether and how health systems should share information on underperforming providers relates to a broader issue of transparency. Specifically, LHCSs will need to determine how and the degree to which they will be transparent with their patients and other stakeholders about specifically which types of data are being analyzed, which decisions are taken based on those data, and whether and how stakeholders should be engaged in these decisions.

Data Interoperability

There are ethical challenges related to obstacles to data interoperability in the US health care system—a challenge also faced by other countries that lack a robust, comprehensive national health care service or national-level data system. While individual institutions can further the integration of research and care to advance quality of care for their own patients, full realization of an LHCS model will require widespread sharing of data and insights from learning activities across providers and systems. Ideally, there would be one, national-level LHCS, in which all providers and institutions, regardless of organization and financing, would participate and freely share information. Such a national system would provide a larger sample size, more care experiences, and a more diverse population from which to learn than is available within any individual institution or system.

The opportunities to learn from a wider sample are relevant both for common conditions, by helping to ensure that recommendations are relevant for a diversity of settings, and for rare conditions, given the importance of aggregation to enable sufficient sample sizes for research. Today's market reality, however, introduces financial incentives for institutions to withhold data. Reports suggest that some technology companies, hospitals, and laboratories in the United States are intentionally obstructing the electronic sharing of health information as part of a business strategy to enhance their "market dominance" (Pear, 2015). A central question is whether it is ethically acceptable for health care organizations to conduct business in this way, or whether policy changes or, at the very least, incentives should be put in place, including by federal funders such as Medicare, to standardize data collection approaches and data platforms to enable sharing across systems.

The Research-Practice Distinction and Ethics Oversight in the Learning Health Care System

A core ethical concern surrounds the continued appropriateness of the research-practice distinction and implications for ethics oversight. Traditional framings of research ethics and regulatory oversight rest upon a sharp delineation between research and practice. Historically, medical care was understood as having a primary moral commitment to the medical best interests of each individual patient, with a model of patient-level data held in individual patient charts for the sole purpose of managing care for that patient. Advancing medical knowledge more broadly, through the aggregation of multiple patients' data, was seen as the primary commitment of clinical research with commitments broadly to "future" patients rather than the patients at hand. In an LHCS, however, this distinction is often difficult to sustain as data systems, treatment recommendations, and strategies to improve care are integrated into the same systems that, by design and simultaneously, serve multiple purposes. Indeed, many activities in an LHCS are not easily classified as either care or research.

As health care institutions begin to move toward the LHCS model, with large data systems created for multiple purposes, the same activity may be designed both to treat a patient and to gather data on outcomes. In such contexts, the continued reliance on the research-practice distinction becomes increasingly problematic, creating a regulatory environment plagued by "delays, confusions, and frustrations" (Kass et al., 2013; Selker et al., 2011; Casarett, Karlawish, and Sugarman, 2000; Baily, 2008; Fiscella et al., 2015). Institutional review boards (IRBs), charged with the oversight of research involving human subjects, struggle to ascertain when an activity should properly be classified as research, and LHCSs struggle with how to develop ethical oversight for activities that are intentionally both practice and research (Kass et al., 2013; Lee et al., 2016).

Ethical Guidance for Learning Health Care Systems

General Ethical Guidance

Several commentators—all supportive of the mission of learning health care—have offered suggestions on how to protect the rights and interest of patients and populations in a system where data collection and learning are built into the system's core structure.

Faden et al. (2013) have proposed an ethical framework for LHCSs. This framework consists of seven obligations: (1) to respect the rights and dignity of patients, (2) to respect the clinical judgment of clinicians, (3) to provide optimal clinical care to each patient, (4) to avoid imposing nonclinical risks and burdens on patients, (5) to reduce health inequalities among populations, (6) to conduct responsible activities that foster learning from clinical care and clinical information, and (7) to contribute to the common purpose of improving the quality and value of clinical care and health care systems (see Table 14.1).

Each of these seven obligations constitutes a necessary condition of adequate ethics within an LHCS. Some obligations within the framework are specific to the LHCS context;

Table 14.1 Seven Ethical Obligations for a Learning Health Care System

Obligation	Implications for health care systems
Respect the rights and dignity of patients	• Assess the impact of learning activities on the rights, respect, and dignity of patients • Assess whether learning activities limit patient choice, including the value to patients of any choices so affected
Respect clinician judgments	• Assess the impact of learning activities on the exercise of physician judgment • Assess the importance of any restriction on clinical judgment for the health and autonomy interests of patients
Provide optimal clinical care to each patient	• Assess the expected net clinical benefit for patients of any learning activity, as compared to the net clinical benefit experienced absent the learning activity
Avoid imposing nonclinical risks and burdens on patients	• Assess the nonclinical risks and burdens to patients affected by a learning activity, as compared to those experienced absent the learning activity
Reduce health inequalities among populations	• Assess whether a learning activity's risks and burdens will fall disproportionately on those already disadvantaged, or, conversely, will disproportionately benefit those who are already socially or economically advantaged • Assess whether a learning activity will help advance the goal of reducing unjust inequalities in health and health care, or whether it can be designed to do so
Conduct responsible activities that foster learning from clinical care and clinical information	• Assess the extent to which a learning activity is likely to contribute to health care quality, fairness, or value • Conduct and contribute to learning activities as a matter of role-specific, professional responsibility
Contribute to the common purpose of improving the quality and value of clinical care and health care systems	• Participate in learning activities that are consonant with other obligations in the framework intended to respect the rights and interest of patients; participate in those deemed acceptable to proceed without patients' express informed consent • Consider participation in learning activities that, because of their impact on the framework's other obligations, cannot ethically proceed without express informed consent

Source: Table modified from Faden et al. (2013).

others are not. Obligations to reduce health inequalities, to foster learning from clinical care, and to contribute to the common purpose of improvement involve substantial revisions to traditional conceptions of the moral foundation of research and clinical ethics. By contrast, obligations to respect patient rights and dignity, respect clinical judgment, avoid imposing nonclinical risks, and provide patients with optimal care are consistent with contemporary discussions of research and professional ethics, but are given a new interpretation within the context of an LHCS.

Ethical Oversight for Activities Designed as Both Practice and Research

Largent, Joffe, and Miller (2011) presented a hypothetical model of an LHCS in which clinical trials would be routinely and systematically integrated into routine care. As part of this model, they recommended a multifaceted system of research review and oversight, including IRBs as well as three additional oversight strategies: (1) a research advisory committee to oversee a system's clinical research portfolio to ensure the research addresses questions of importance to members, is responsive to their medical needs, uses resources wisely, and equitably distributes the benefits and burdens of research activities across the enrolled population; (2) a science review committee, to ensure the clinical and scientific merit of intervention studies before they are sent for IRB review; and (3) a clinical oversight committee, to review trial results to determine which are clinically significant and how results should be incorporated into clinical care.

The US National Academy of Medicine's Leadership Consortium for Value & Science-Driven Health Care advocates for adopting a risk-based oversight framework, whereby oversight and consent requirements would not depend on whether an activity classifies as research, but rather on the level of risk the activity poses to patients (Kupersmith, 2013; Platt, Grossman, and Selker, 2013; Fiscella et al., 2015). The aim is to strike the proper balance between ethical obligations to prevent harm to patients and ethical obligations to rapidly learn and improve care. Others have advanced similar proposals for risk-based frameworks (Fiscella et al., 2015; Casarett, Karlawish, and Sugarman, 2000).

A related view also maintains that oversight and type of consent requirement should not turn on whether an activity is classified as research. Instead, this view holds that risk, particularly risk over and above what patients would encounter in clinical care, is a critical feature. Other relevant features potentially important to determining level of oversight and consent include whether an activity imposes additional burdens on patients, the likelihood that some patients might find the aims or design of the activity problematic in terms of their own values and preferences, and whether there is adequate transparency to the patient community about the activity.

Not all commentators support eliminating the research-practice distinction as a criterion for which activities require oversight, however (Brody and Miller, 2013; Menikoff, 2013). For example, although Largent, Joffe, and Miller (2011) agree that the sharp distinction between research and care is becoming increasingly blurred, they argue that the research-practice distinction continues to be meaningful to patients (Largent, Miller, and Joffe, 2013). Drawing upon empirical research that indicates patients value the research-care distinction (Kelley et al., 2015). Largent (2015) has argued that preserving this distinction as the basis for consent requirements and oversight is important to patient trust, which will be integral to a successful LHCS. Nevertheless, Largent, Miller, and Joffe (2013) share the view that oversight of LHCS activities could be "narrower in scope, more flexible, and better adapted" to the LHCS environment than the current system of IRB review.

A specific question related to regulatory oversight is whether written informed consent should be required for randomized clinical trials that compare widely used, standard therapies—a type of research that LHCSs can be expected to conduct with some frequency. The suggestion that such trials may permissibly be conducted without traditional written informed consent was introduced to the literature nearly two decades ago (Truog et al., 1999). Recently, support for this view has reemerged, although disagreements abound about the precise conditions under which informed consent could ethically be waived and whether or when other forms of patient authorization, such as a streamlined consent process, should be employed (Grady, 2015; Truog et al., 1999; Faden, Beauchamp, and Kass, 2014; Menikoff, 2013; Largent, Joffe, and Miller, 2011). Others disagree that it is ever ethically acceptable to conduct randomized comparative effectiveness studies without written informed consent (Kim and Miller, 2015).

These challenges will grow only more acute as institutions create large data repositories, including with those links to increasingly available biosamples left over from both clinical practice and previous research studies. At Vanderbilt University Medical Center, for example, all data gathered from routine inpatient and outpatient visits are captured through a uniform reporting format that becomes part not only of individual patients' electronic record, but also of a systematic database (Danciu et al., 2014; Roden et al., 2008). These data can be extracted into a research data warehouse where investigators can use de-identified data; the warehouse also includes leftover biosamples if patients have been informed about inclusion of samples and chosen not to opt out (Langanke et al., 2011; Pulley et al., 2000). Such data warehouses offer the potential to improve clinical knowledge and support clinical research. Prior analyses of similar warehouses have been demonstrated to improve disease management support, enable model development to predict health risk assessments, and enhance knowledge about survival rates (Andreu-Perez et al., 2015).

Aggregating data across institutions can be especially important for rare diseases, for which individual institutions are unlikely to encounter sufficient cases for rigorous analysis. For example, thoracic aortic dissection (TAD) is a relatively rare condition that affects fewer than four in 100,000 people each year. Those with one form of TAD generally require surgical intervention, while those with another form instead require long-term careful blood pressure control. While any one institution is unlikely to see sufficient numbers of cases to develop accurate risk stratification models, aggregating diverse data sources across institutions, including imaging results, lifestyle data, and computational fluid dynamics, can enable more accurate risk stratification, supporting appropriate clinical decision-making (Andreu-Perez et al., 2015).

The broad collection and aggregation of data clearly is seen as increasingly important for institutions on a number of grounds related to administrative, economic, clinical, and research efficiencies, and more and more institutions are moving in this direction, often with the inclusion of biological data. Moreover, nongovernmental efforts by entities such as PatientsLikeMe, the Personal Genome Project, and Sage Bionetworks have been creating large databases of biological, clinical, and self-reported data as part of "citizen science," whereby groups either have transparent policies to which users must agree, or give users options for how their data may be used by others (Swan, 2012; Rothstein, Wilbanks, and Brothers, 2015).

All of these efforts are emblematic of the recognition that aggregating data creates enormous potential for learning and improving medical care, while also carrying responsibilities regarding disclosure, privacy, and confidentiality. However, learning health care is organized, and whether efforts reflect smaller, targeted efforts or larger system-wide collaborations, policies will need to be created with regard to protecting individuals' interests while also sharing with individuals what is learned from the analyses of large bodies of data.

Conclusion

The LHCS is gaining interest for its potential to improve the quality and efficiency of health care. Transitioning to an LHCS is supported by several moral justifications, including promotion of societal goals of just health care, high-quality health care, and economic well-being. These justifications notwithstanding, LHCSs also present ethical challenges, including those related to enhanced capacity for continuous data generation, transparency, data interoperability, and the continued relevance of the research-practice distinction as a criterion for assessing the need for ethical oversight. Several commentators have offered general ethical guidance for LHCSs. However, the increasing capability to collect, store, and analyze data will continue to present questions as to the appropriate ethical framework that should govern efforts aimed at continuous improvement in health care.

Note

1. This section draws heavily from Faden et al. (2013) and Kass et al. (2013).

References

Ali, J., Califf, R., and Sugarman, J. 2015. "Anticipated Ethics and Regulatory Challenges in PCORnet: The National Patient-Centered Clinical Research Network." *Accountability in Research* 23(2): 79–96.

Andreu-Perez, J., Poon, C. C. Y., Merrifield, R. D., Wong, S. T. C., and Yang, G. Z. 2015. "Big Data for Health." *IEE Journal of Biomedical and Health Informatics* 19(4): 1193–1208.

Baily, M. A. 2008. "Harming through Protection?" *New England Journal of Medicine* 358(8): 768–769.

BOLDER Research Group. 2016. "Better Outcomes through Learning, Data, Engagement, and Research (BOLDER)—A System for Improving Evidence and Clinical Practice in Low and Middle Income Countries." *F1000Research* 5: 693. https://www.ncbi.nlm.nih.gov/pmc/articles/PMC5089159/.

Brody, H., and Miller, F. 2013. "The Research-Clinical Practice Distinction, Learning Health Systems, and Relationships." *Hastings Center Report* 43(5): 41–47.

Califf, R. M., and Sugarman, J. 2015. "Exploring the Ethical and Regulatory Issues in Pragmatic Clinical Trials." *Clinical Trials* 12(5): 436–441.

Casarett, D., Karlawish, J. H. T., and Sugarman, J. 2000. "Determining When Quality Improvement Initiatives Should Be Considered Research." *JAMA* 283(17): 2275–2280.

Cuckler, G. A., Sisko, A. M., Keehan, S. P., Smith, S. D., Madison, A. J., Poisal, J. A., et al. 2013. "National Health Expenditure Projections, 2012–22: Slow Growth Until Coverage Expands and Economy Improves." *Health Affairs* 32 (10): 1820–1831.

Danciu, I., Cowan, J. D., Basford, M., Wang, X., Saip, A., Osgood, S., et al. 2014. "Secondary Use of Clinical Data: the Vanderbilt Approach." *Journal of Biomedical Informatics* 52: 28–35.

D'Avolio, L., Ferguson, R., Goryachev, S., Woods, P., Sabin, T., O'Neil, J., et al. 2012. "Implementation of the Department of Veteran Affairs' First Point-of-Care Clinical Trial." *JAMA* 19(e1): e170–e176.

English, M., Irimu, G., Agweyu, A., Gathara, D., Oliwa, J., Ayieko, P., et al. 2016. "Building Learning Health Systems to Accelerate Research and Improve Outcomes of Clinical Care in Low- and Middle- Income Countries." *PLoS Medicine* 13 (4): e1001991. https://journals.plos.org/plosmedicine/article?id=10.1371/journal.pmed.1001991.

Faden, R. R., Beauchamp, T. L., and Kass, N. E. 2014. "Informed Consent, Comparative Effectiveness, and Learning Health Care." *New England Journal of Medicine* 370(8): 766–768.

Faden, R. R., Kass, N. E., Goodman, S. N., Pronovost, P., Tunis, S., and Beauchamp, T. L. 2013. "An Ethics Framework for a Learning Health Care System: A Departure from Traditional Research Ethics and Clinical Ethics." *Hastings Center Report* 43(1): S16–S27.

Fairall, L., Bateman, E., Cornick, R., Faris, G., Timmerman, V., Folb, N., et al. 2015. "Innovating to Improve Primary Care in Less Developed Countries: Towards a Global Model." *BMJ Innovations* 1(4): 196–203.

Feldman, D. S., Novack, D. H., and Gracely, E. 1998. "Effects of Managed Care on Physician-Patient Relationships, Quality of Care, and the Ethical Practice of Medicine: A Physician Survey." *JAMA* 158(15): 1626–1632.

Fiscella, K., Tobin, J. A., Carroll, J. K., He, H., and Obgedegbe, G. 2015. "Ethical Oversight in Quality Improvement and Quality Improvement Research: New Approaches to Promote a Learning Health Care System." *BMC Medical Ethics* 16: 63.

Friedman, C., and Rigby, M. 2013. "Conceptualising and Creating a Global Learning Health System." *International Journal of Medical Informatics* 82: e63–e71.

Gallagher, T. H., Studdert, D., and Levinson, W. 2007. "Disclosing Harmful Medical Errors to Patients." *New England Journal of Medicine* 356(26): 2713–2719.

Grady, C. 2015. "Enduring and Emerging Challenges of Informed Consent." *New England Journal of Medicine* 372(22): 855–862.

HHS (US Department of Health and Human Services). 2008. *The Surgeon General's Call to Action to Prevent Deep Vein Thrombosis and Pulmonary Embolism* (Washington, D.C.: HHS).

IOM (Institute of Medicine). 2000. *To Err Is Human: Building a Safer Health System*. Edited by Committee on Quality of Health Care in America, L. T. Kohn, J. M. Corrigan, and M. S. Donaldson (Washington, D.C.: National Academies Press).

IOM (Institute of Medicine). 2007. "Roundtable on Evidence-Based Medicine." In *The Learning Healthcare System: Workshop Summary*, edited by L. A. Olsen, D. Aisner, and J. M. McGinnis (Washington, D.C.: National Academies Press). http://www.ncbi.nlm.nih.gov/books/NBK53484/.

IOM (Institute of Medicine). 2013. *Best Care at Lower Cost: The Path to Continuously Learning Health Care in America*. Edited by M. Smith, R. Saunders, L. Stuckhardt, and J. M. McGinnis (Washington, D.C.: National Academy Press).

Jacobs, J. P., Cerfolio, R. J., and Sade, R. M. 2009. "The Ethics of Transparency: Publication of Cardiothoracic Surgical Outcomes in the Lay Press." *The Annals of Thoracic Surgery* 87: 679–686.

Kass, N. E., Faden, R. R., Goodman, S. N., Pronovost, P., Tunis, S., and Beauchamp, T. L. 2013. "The Research-Treatment Distinction: A Problematic Approach for Determining Which Activities Should Have Ethical Oversight." *Hastings Center Report* 43(Suppl. 1).

Kelley, M., James, C., Kraft, S. A., Korngiebel, D., Wijangco, I., Rosenthal, E., et al. 2015. "Patient Perspectives on the Learning Health System: The Importance of Trust and Shared Decision Making." *American Journal of Bioethics* 15(9): 4–17.

Kim, S. Y., and Miller, F. G. 2015. "Ethical Complexities in Standard of Care Randomized Trials: A Case Study of Morning versus Nighttime Dosing of Blood Pressure Drugs." *Clinical Trials* 12(6): 557–563.

Klevens, R. M., Edwards, J. R., Richards Jr., C. L., Horan, T. C., Gaynes, R. P., Pollock, D. A., et al. 2007. "Estimating Health Care-Associated Infections and Deaths in U.S. Hospitals, 2002." *Public Health Reports* 122(2): 160–66.

Kupersmith, J. 2013. "Advances in the Research Enterprise." *Hastings Center Report* 43(1): S43–S44.

Langanke, M., Brothers, K. B., Erdmann, P., Weinert, J., Krafczyk-Korth, J., Dörr, M., et al. 2011. "Comparing Different Scientific Approaches to Personalized Medicine: Research Ethics and Privacy Protection." *Personalized Medicine* 8(4): 437–444.

Largent, E. A. 2015. "What's Trust Got to Do With It? Trust and the Importance of the Research-Care Distinction." *American Journal of Bioethics* 15(9): 22–24.

Largent, E. A., Joffe, S., and Miller, F. G. 2011. "Can Research and Care Be Ethically Integrated?" *Hastings Center Report* 41(4): 37–46.

Largent, E. A., Miller, F. G., and Joffe, S. 2013. "A Prescription for Ethical Learning." *Hastings Center Report* 43(1): S28–29.

Learning Healthcare Project. 2015. "Project Background." http://www.learninghealthcareproject.org/section/background/methodology.

Lee, S. S. J., Kelley, M., Cho, M. K., Kraft, S. A., James, C., Constantine, M., et al. 2016. "Adrift in the Gray Zone: IRB Perspectives on Research in the Learning Health System." *AJOB Empirical Bioethics* 7(2): 125–134.

McGlynn, E. A., Asch, S. M., Adams, J., Keesey, J., Hicks, J., DeCristofaro, A., et al. 2003. "The Quality of Health Care Delivered to Adults in the United States." *New England Journal of Medicine* 348(26): 2635–2645.

Menikoff, J. 2013. "The Unbelievable Rightness of Being in Clinical Trials." *Hastings Center Report* 43(S1): S30–S31.

Pear, R. 2015. "Tech Rivalries Impede Digital Medical Record Sharing." *New York Times*, May 26. https://www.nytimes.com/2015/05/27/us/electronic-medical-record-sharing-is-hurt-by-business-rivalries.html.

Platt, R., Grossman, C., and Selker, H. P. 2013. "Evaluation as Part of Operations: Reconciling the Common Rule and Continuous Improvement." *Hastings Center Report* 43(1): S37–S39.

Povar, G. J., Blumen, H., Daniel, J., Daub, S., Evans, L., Holm, R. P., et al. 2004. "Ethics in Practice: Managed Care and the Changing Health Care Environment: Medicine as a Profession Managed Care Ethics Working Group Statement." *Annals of Internal Medicine* 141(2): 131–136.

Pulley, J., Clayton, E., Bernard, G. R., Roden, D. M., and Masys, D. R. 2000. "Principles of Human Subjects Protections Applied in an Opt-Out, De-Identified Biobank." *Clinical and Translational Science* 3(1): 42–48.

Randel, L., Pearson, S. D., Sabin, J. E., Hyams, T., and Emanuel, E. 2001. "How Managed Care Can Be Ethical." *Health Affairs* 20(4): 43–56.

Reed, K., and May, R. 2011. *HealthGrades Patient Safety in American Hospitals Study* (Denver, Colo.: Health Grades). https://patientsafetymovement.org/wp-content/uploads/2016/02/Resources_Reports_Patient_Safety_in_American_Hospitals_Study.pdf.

Roden, D. M., Pulley, J. M., Basford, M. A., Bernard, G. R., Clayton, E. W., Balser, J. R., et al. 2008. "Development of a Large-Scale De-identified DNA Biobank to Enable Personalized Medicine." *Clinical Pharmacology and Therapeutics* 84(3): 363–369.

Rosenthal, G. E. 2014. "The Role of Pragmatic Clinical Trials in the Evolution of Learning Health Systems." *Transactions of the American Clinical and Climatological Association* 125: 204–218.

Rothstein, M. A., Wilbanks, J. T., and Brothers, K. B. 2015. "Citizen Science on Your Smartphone: An ELSI Research Agenda." *Journal of Law, Medicine, and Ethics* 43(4): 897–903.

Selker, H., Grossmann, C., Adams, A., Goldmann, D., Dezii, C., Meyer, G., et al. 2011. *The Common Rule and Continuous Improvement in Health Care: A Learning Health System Perspective*. Institute of Medicine Discussion Paper. http://www.imagefirst.com/hs-fs/hub/276565/file-410053658-pdf/docs/1112696053.pdf.

Smith, R. 2015. "How to Fill the Void of Evidence for Everyday Practice?" *BMJ Blog*, August 11. http://blogs.bmj.com/bmj/2015/08/11/richard-smith-how-to-fill-the-void-of-evidence-for-everyday-practice/.

Swan, M. 2012. "Crowdsourced Health Research Studies: An Important Emerging Complement to Clinical Trials in the Public Health Research Ecosystem." *Journal of Medical Internet Research* 14(2): e46.

Truog, R. D., Robinson, W., Randolph, A., and Morris, A. 1999. "Is Informed Consent Always Necessary for Randomized, Controlled Trials?" *New England Journal of Medicine* 340(10): 804–807.

Van Staa, T. P., Dyson, L., McCann, G., Padmanabhan, S., Belatri, R., Goldacre, B., et al. 2014. "The Opportunities and Challenges of Pragmatic Point-of-Care Randomised Trials Using Routinely Collected Electronic Records: Evaluations of Two Exemplar Trials." *Health Technology Assessment* 18(43).

Winters, B., Custer, J., Galvagno, S. M., Colantuoni, E., Kapoor, S.G., Lee, H., et al. 2012. "Diagnostic Errors in the Intensive Care Unit: A Systematic Review of Autopsy Studies." *BMJ Quality and Safety* 12: 894–902.

SECTION FOUR

NEEDS AND ISSUES RELATED TO PARTICULAR POPULATIONS

CHAPTER 15

AN OVERVIEW OF ETHICS ISSUES FOR PUBLIC HEALTH IN PARTICULAR POPULATIONS

RUTH GAARE BERNHEIM
AND ELIZABETH FENTON

Introduction

Populations are a central focus in the fields of public health and public health ethics: public health strategies generally aim to improve, and measure success by, population-wide health outcomes, while public health ethics addresses ethical considerations that arise with these population-focused activities. Public health immunization strategies, for example, illustrate one type of ethical tension in public health that requires weighing the moral imperative to produce population benefit alongside other moral claims, such as the liberty interests of individuals.

Similarly, public health analyses—of infant mortality, for example—can uncover disparities in health among particular individuals and groups within the larger population, raising significant ethical issues related to health equity. Not only are individuals affected by the determinants of health in the broader population within which they live, but they are also impacted by and situated within multiple groups or subpopulations, whether defined by neighborhood, age, or political status, often with a unique cluster of complex and overlapping social, political, and economic characteristics.

Thus, while a population-wide public health strategy may lead to the greatest gains in total population health, such an approach can obscure disparities that continue to exist among particular groups and subpopulations, such as the elderly, immigrants and refugees, and persons with disabilities, that often require unique public health strategies. A population focus that takes into account the interests and characteristics of particular populations as well as those of the entire population is critical for the fields of public health and public health ethics. On the domestic level, for example, a population health perspective highlights those subgroups within a single geopolitical region, such as a nation, who are doing better or worse in terms of health. On a global level, the vast and growing disparities in health between developing and developed countries are especially prominent from the "bird's-eye view" of population health (Wikler and Brock, 2009). Investigation into the reasons for these disparities can help to clarify when they are the result of "upstream" injustices in the distribution of other goods, such as wealth or education, or other forms of social injustice, such as discrimination. The ethical dimensions of a range of challenges in health policy, such as priority-setting for limited health resources, risk distribution, and global aging, also become more vivid, both to ethicists and policymakers, when the focus is on populations and particular subpopulations rather than individuals (Wikler and Brock, 2009).

Defining populations for analyses is complex. The term "population health" is widely used in public health and health policy, and a broadly accepted definition is that given by Kindig and Stoddart (2003, 381), who state that population health is "the health outcomes of a group of individuals, including the distribution of such outcomes within the group." Complexities arise in determining which groups of individuals are considered populations, who defines a population, and for what purpose. An additional complexity is the distinction, if in fact there is one, between population health and public health. To the extent that both are focused on the health of whole populations rather than individuals, and that both recognize the multiple determinants of health as relevant to improving the health of populations, there is little difference between these two fields; that is, both are primarily concerned with "the health of the public." The definition given by the US Institute of Medicine (now the National Academy of Medicine of the National Academies of Sciences, Engineering, and Medicine) underscores that public health is firmly oriented toward improving health on the population level: "Public health is what we, as a society, do collectively to assure the conditions in which people can be healthy" (IOM, 1988, 1). This definition suggests "a far-reaching agenda for public health that focuses attention not only on the medical needs of individuals, but on fundamental social conditions that affect population levels of morbidity and mortality" (Childress et al., 2002, 170).

Chapter Overviews

This section of *The Oxford Handbook of Public Health Ethics* focuses on the public health needs and related ethical issues of particular subpopulations that experience or are exposed to significant health stressors. Stressors generally stem from fundamental social conditions and factors that are pathways for poor health outcomes, including historic injustices, discrimination, and stigmatization, or particular social or physical needs, limitations, or vulnerabilities. In some cases, these stressors contribute to health disparities among these groups and with the larger population. These disparities underscore the importance of the second part of Kindig and Stoddart's definition, which states that population health includes not only overall health outcomes, but also their *distribution* within the population. As Kindig (2015) notes, it is often assumed that improvements in overall population health also reduce disparities for subgroups, but this is not always the case, and in some situations health disparities might even increase. If a positive change in health behavior is more quickly adopted by more educated members of the population, for example, health disparities might increase even as overall population health improves. The chapters in this section illustrate that ethical issues in public health arise not only from tensions with individual moral claims, but also with distributional and equity considerations, which require an examination of the health needs and outcomes of particular populations.

In "Aging Populations and Public Health Ethics," Lois Shepherd examines healthy aging, the reduction of health inequities, and extension of the life span as three primary public health goals related to the needs of the elderly. From a population perspective, each of these goals is important, and there are many public health programs and policies, such as "aging in place" and advance directives, that are designed to promote them. Ethical tensions can emerge, however, with respect to our responsibilities toward older individuals as individuals: to protect them from harm, respect their autonomy, and treat them fairly.

For example, while aging in place has many advantages from a public health perspective, such as health benefits derived from social relationships and community support, for some older adults it might create additional burdens of unmet daily needs, poverty, or social isolation. Similarly, advance directives are important for promoting autonomous decision-making, but they also create ethical challenges as population-wide strategies, such as when choices are circumscribed by the options presented on a standardized form. Public health goals for aging populations can also raise important ethical questions of justice, both within and between population groups. Older individuals on lower incomes can be disadvantaged by limits on government-sponsored insurance programs such as Medicare in the United States, and health resource constraints demand that society decide how to allocate resources between the young and the old, or the old and the poor.

At the other end of the life spectrum, children and adolescents, as a particular population, vary considerably in terms of physical, cognitive, and experiential characteristics, and these variations increase when societal and cultural differences are taken into account. As Margaret Moon argues in "Children, Adolescents, and Public Health: Ethical Considerations," however, three commonalities distinguish this group from others in the general population: disenfranchisement and lack of social and economic power, being subject to stewardship by adults, and a presumed lack of capacity for decision-making. Ethical challenges emerge when these features come into conflict with established public health goals and policies. For example, developmentally appropriate health education and promotion programs are an essential part of public health practice, but in some areas, such as sexual and reproductive health, the values of parents and families, as stewards of children's moral development, must be carefully balanced against the public health goals of comprehensive sex education. Some public health goals, such as reducing sexually transmitted diseases, are more effective when adolescent patients are offered confidentiality, yet this can conflict with the responsibility of health care providers to inform parents or guardians about the care being provided to their children. Parental and governmental failures of stewardship, such as vaccine refusals or lax gun control policies, can also have significant public health impacts for this population.

Whereas everyone in the population can expect, in the course of their life, to become a member of the subgroups that are determined by age, not everyone will be a member of groups that are based on characteristics other than age, such as mental illness, disability, sexual or gender identity, or refugee status. Each of these particular populations faces distinct public health challenges, and ethical considerations are critical to the way in which these challenges are met, in both public health policy and practice. In their chapter "Ethics in Mental Health Care: A Public Health Perspective," Richard J. Bonnie and Heather Zelle begin by examining the implications of the shift in mental health care from institutions to the community. The legal and ethical discourse dominant throughout this shift has been one of individual autonomy and rights to refuse treatment in tension with the perceived individual and social benefits of treatment, leading to ongoing debates over the ethical and legal justifications for coerced or involuntary treatment.

Bonnie and Zelle advance this discourse by taking a population-level perspective, identifying the ethical values that are paramount in a functioning and effective mental health care system. These include the inclusion and integration of people with mental illness into their communities and the health care system, and empowering people with mental illness to gain control over their lives, so they can begin to take responsibility, with the care and support of others, for maintaining that control and managing their illness as they might another form of chronic illness. Recognizing these values is critical to formulating public mental health policy that can address the persistent ethical challenges of inadequate funding for mental health services and community supports; lack of access to services due both to underinsurance and the social stigma attached to mental health care; how to determine the population-level benefits of coerced treatment, such as reductions in violent behavior; and tensions between privacy and the potential benefits of family involvement in mental health care.

Lack of access to and inclusion in public health programs and policies is also an unfortunate hallmark of the history of disability in the United States. In "Persons with Disabilities and Public Health Ethics," Monika Mitra, Linda Long-Bellil, and Robyn Powell highlight the ethical significance of the emergence of the social model of disability, which understands the health and well-being of persons with disabilities as a function of their social environment, and the extent to which they enjoy full rights and inclusion in society. Like people with mental illnesses, persons with disabilities often experience worse health outcomes than the general population because of a lack of investment in the infrastructure needed to provide adequate services, such as accessible equipment, discrimination, and structural and implicit biases held by health care professionals. Reducing these health disparities at the population level requires a renewed focus within public health practice on integrating the needs of persons with disabilities and ensuring their participation in the design and implementation of the policies and programs that affect them.

Sexual and gender minorities also experience a range of health disparities. Despite gains in the recognition of rights, decriminalization of same-sex relationships, and marriage equality, lesbian, gay, bisexual, and transgender (LGBT) populations continue to experience disproportionate burdens of human immunodeficiency virus (HIV) and mental illness, as well as the stigma and discrimination that impede health surveillance efforts and the development of health interventions specifically tailored to their needs. Tonya Littlejohn, Tonia Poteat, and Chris Beyrer argue in "Sexual and Gender Minorities, Public Health, and Ethics," that these inequities form the core social justice challenge for public health in relation to sexual and gender minorities. Advancing social justice, however, requires meeting two further practical challenges: first, collecting robust data on the health status and needs of this population, and second, overcoming criminalization, stigma, discrimination, and violence.

These challenges can be interrelated. For example, attempts to conduct public health research in social or cultural contexts that are hostile toward sexual and gender minorities can be dangerous for participants, or they can be blocked by governments that do not want to legitimize the existence of these groups. HIV/AIDS provides a useful case study of the way in which public health gains in slowing the trajectory of the epidemic must be understood against its persistence among sexual and gender minorities living in hostile environments with high levels of stigma and discrimination. Ensuring that sexual and gender minorities experience the same health gains as others in the population requires that public health efforts be responsive to the cultural, geographic, and structural contexts in which these groups live.

In "Public Health in the Context of Migration: Ethics Issues Related to Immigrants and Refugees," Rachel E. Fabi provides a timely analysis of the ethical and practical challenges of public health for immigrant and refugee populations. The chapter explores three public health challenges experienced by migrants at different points in their journey: (1) immigrant detention, where migrants experience overcrowding, lack of access to medical care, and physical and sexual violence; (2) health screening for immigrants, a process often characterized by entrenched patterns of discrimination; and (3) access to publicly funded health care in the new country, which is typically determined by immigration status and often extremely limited. Public health policies and practices for immigrant and refugee populations are shaped by immigration policies at the national level, which struggle to resolve a fundamental tension between the internationally recognized human right to freedom of movement and the right of sovereign nations to control immigration. In turn, national and international immigration policies are informed by different normative theories about the moral obligations of states with respect to meeting the needs of immigrants.

Conclusion

Taken together, these chapters in *The Oxford Handbook of Public Health Ethics* underscore the ethical significance of particular populations in developing or assessing public health policies. Understanding the needs and interests of different groups within a larger population, as well as historical and contemporary patterns of injustice that create health inequities within a population, is critical to advancing the overarching mission of public health to "assure the conditions in which people can be healthy" (IOM, 1988, 1).

References

Childress, J., Faden, R., Gaare, R. D., Gostin, L. O., Kahn, J., Bonnie, R. J., et al. 2002. "Public Health Ethics: Mapping the Terrain." *Journal of Law, Medicine & Ethics* 30(2): 170–178.

IOM (Institute of Medicine). 1988. *The Future of Public Health* (Washington, D.C.: National Academies Press).

Kindig, D. 2015. "What Are We Talking about When We Talk about Population Health?" *Health Affairs Blog*, April 6. http://healthaffairs.org/blog/2015/04/06/what-are-we-talking-about-when-we-talk-about-population-health/.

Kindig, D., and Stoddart, G. 2003. "What Is Population Health?" *American Journal of Public Health* 93(3): 380–383.

Wikler, D., and Brock, D. W. 2009. "Population-Level Bioethics: Mapping a New Agenda." In *Ethics, Prevention, and Public Health*, edited by A. Dawson and M. Verweij, 78–94 (Oxford, UK: Oxford University Press).

CHAPTER 16

AGING POPULATIONS AND PUBLIC HEALTH ETHICS

LOIS SHEPHERD

INTRODUCTION

THE world's population is aging, and it is aging rapidly. Across the globe, in more- and less-developed countries, populations are experiencing lower fertility rates and longer life spans. Between 2010 and 2050, the number of older adults (generally defined as sixty-five years old and older) is expected to triple, and their portion of the population is predicted to grow from 8 percent to 16 percent. Around the time of the publication of this book, for the first time in history, the number of older adults will exceed that of children aged five and younger, and by 2050 older adults should outnumber young children two to one (He, Goodkind, and Kowal, 2015). In many countries, the oldest old are the fastest growing part of the population (WHO and USNIA, 2011); in some, the share of the population aged eighty and older will quadruple by 2050 (He, Goodkind, and Kowal, 2015).

This chapter will explore three primary ethical questions relating to the health of elderly populations in coming decades. First, what are appropriate *public health goals* for this population? Second, how can programs or policies to advance population-wide goals satisfy *ethical responsibilities to older individuals* in terms of protection from harm, respect for autonomy and dignity, and treating them fairly or justly? Third, how should *public health and public health ethics* be understood in relation to the *particular concerns* of clinical care and clinical ethics, on the one hand, and to *broader social justice efforts*, such as alleviating poverty or protecting the environment, on the other?

Defining the Elderly Population: Realities and Perceptions

Today, the "older person" is commonly described as someone sixty-five years of age or older, but in the early nineteenth century, people over forty were considered to have entered old age. With current extensions of life expectancy, we can expect a steady rise in the age at which people are considered to have reached old age. Perceptions of "old" or "elderly" can also vary by country or culture. Of course, younger people tend to perceive old age as occurring at a much earlier age than older people. Gender may also play a role—some studies reveal that men think the onset of old age occurs earlier than women do (NCPOP, 2009).

Increasingly older populations pose new public health challenges. Safety net programs to provide for financial security and health care for elderly populations are under strain as more people live longer past their productive work years, even as retirement ages rise. Chronic and degenerative diseases, such as heart disease, cancer, and diabetes, rather than communicable diseases, pose increasingly greater burdens to public health (WHO and USNIA, 2011). Even low-income countries, which may still experience high death rates from infectious disease, are seeing a substantial rise in chronic and degenerative diseases.

It is unclear whether elderly populations will experience more or less disability as life spans increase. Some researchers predict an "expansion of morbidity," or "an increase in the prevalence of disability as life expectancy increases," while others posit a decrease in disability prevalence, or a "compression of morbidity" to correspond with healthy aging practices and medical advances (WHO and USNIA, 2011, 12). Alternatively, we may see a decrease in the *severity* of disability even as chronic illness increases if medical advances are able to mitigate the impacts of chronic conditions. There is some historical evidence for this, although rising obesity rates among the aging may counterbalance these improvements (WHO and USNIA, 2011).

Perceptions of older persons can affect employability, receipt of health care services, social inclusion, and overall well-being. Studies of societal and individual perceptions of older persons do reveal positive perceptions, but negative perceptions predominate. Positive stereotypes include perceptions of warmth, sociability, and dependability. But more commonly, older people as a group are perceived as being unhealthy, asexual, set in their ways, isolated, and in a state of mental decline (NCPOP, 2009). Some symptoms are too readily ascribed to age—for example, people may describe a seventy-five-year-old as "senile" but a thirty-five-year-old as "forgetful" for forgetting to buy an item on a shopping list (Friedan, 1993).

Societal and cultural influences can affect perceptions of the elderly; these perceptions also vary among households, communities, and subcultures (NCPOP, 2009). In general, North American and Western cultures, which emphasize individuality and independence, have tended to support less positive perceptions of older persons than Eastern and Middle Eastern cultures, which are associated with more collectivist attitudes that expect and value interdependence. Traditional cultures tend to view older persons as repositories of experience and wisdom. These are broad generalizations, however, and where the world becomes modernized, with an increasing emphasis on individualism, attitudes about older persons can be expected to evolve. These attitudes may also be influenced, positively and negatively, by changes in the proportion of the population made up by older persons, the demands on resources from this subset of the population, the contributions older persons may make to society as a result of healthier aging and technological adaptions, and educational or media portrayals of older people.

Stereotypes can lead to both positive and negative "ageist" behaviors. Positive behaviors include taking care to determine that a very old person can adequately hear what is being said, or holding doors open for older persons. But negative, prejudicial attitudes can result in offensive behavior toward older people, such as unfair discrimination, isolation, neglect, and even abuse. Elderly people may be precluded from full access to health care because of assumptions about their physical and mental abilities, such as when older adults are not adequately screened or provided with health services because a reported ailment is dismissed as a natural part of aging (NCPOP, 2009). Elderly patients may be treated in a patronizing manner by health care providers, through the use of infantilizing language or by being excluded entirely from treatment conversations.

The perception that elderly populations are posing unreasonable burdens on society's resources has been termed "conflictual ageism," which can lead to resentment of older adults. This contrasts with "compassionate ageism," which stereotypes older adults as frail, isolated, and vulnerable (Binstock and Post, 1991). Both forms of ageism can be present at the same time.

Identifying Public Health Goals and Benefits for Elderly Populations

Identifying public health goals for elderly populations is itself an ethical challenge. In determining where to spend their efforts and resources, to what degree should societies focus on improving the well-being of older adults, reducing health inequities, or expanding life spans? Even within these broad, sometimes competing goals lie challenges of definition and translation into policy objectives.

Healthy Aging

"Healthy aging" is frequently cited as an important modern public health goal, but there is much debate about what that term means or whether other terms—suggesting other aims—should predominate, such as "active" or "successful" or "harmonious" aging, each with its own emphasis, such as productivity, independence, or an old age with meaning

(Martinson and Berridge, 2015). While we should expect to see continued debate, a few things seem clear. First, there is increasing emphasis on "adding health to years" (WHO, 2015) rather than adding years to life. Second, healthy aging cannot be defined primarily by simply distinguishing between "healthy" and "unhealthy" individuals, as this perspective fails to appreciate that many people can live well with one or more health conditions as long as they are well-controlled (WHO, 2015). Third, there is increasing recognition that objective measurements of well-being in later life are not sufficient; self-reported, subjective meanings are also essential (Fuchs et al., 2013). And fourth, more typically "Western" perspectives that emphasize independence in old age and individual responsibility for achieving and maintaining independence are increasingly viewed as narrow and incomplete.

The World Health Organization defines "healthy aging" as "the process of developing and maintaining the functional ability that enables well-being in older age" (WHO, 2015). Importantly, the definition offered for "functional ability" includes not just intrinsic physical and mental capacities, but also the individual's interactions with the environment in which he or she lives. The implication is that healthy aging is vitally dependent on an environment—physical, social, relational—that allows people to do the things that are important to them. In emphasizing "well-being," the WHO definition encourages consideration of how life in old age is actually experienced.

"Aging in place" might contribute to healthy aging or be considered as a separate policy goal (WHO, 2015). Even as older adults experience declines in physical and mental capacity, they may prefer to stay in the homes and communities in which they have lived, where they find comfort in familiar surroundings, have social relationships, and feel connected in terms of personal identity. Aging in place may also hold financial benefits for individuals, families, and societies, but this is only possible given the appropriateness of built environments, social arrangements, and access to adequate care. Advances in technology may help, such as devices to track when prescription medicines have been taken, or robots to provide in-home care, an innovation enthusiastically pursued in Japan, whose aging population faces a shortage of caregivers. Critics of current movements toward aging in place point out that while the goal may be reasonable for some older adults, others are likely to suffer from unmet needs in daily living, social isolation, and deteriorating housing conditions; particularly vulnerable are lower-income and frail elderly homeowners (Golant, 2008).

Health Equity in Aging

Advancing health equity in aging is also recognized as an important public health goal. Many of the health differences observed among older people are the result of "social determinants," such as socioeconomic conditions, living and working conditions, education, and the like. The conditions into which one is conceived, born, reared, and educated, and where one eats, sleeps, lives, works, and receives health and social care, have a lifetime cumulative effect on the well-being of a person entering old age. The best way to reduce health inequities—"differences in health that are judged 'unnecessary, avoidable, unfair, and unjust'" (Sadana et al., 2016, S179)—within an elderly population may be to adopt measures or support social changes that affect people at a younger age. But what does this say about how priorities should be established between public health measures to benefit current versus future populations of older people? Directing public health initiatives to benefit existing younger populations may be a final indignity to those who have reached old age despite experiencing health inequities throughout their lives.

Life Extension

Although the focus of recent public health efforts for older populations has moved to healthy aging, aging in place, and reducing health inequities, the goal of longer life expectancy cannot be forgotten. Indeed, public health statistics commonly focus on achievements in extending life expectancy, and part of the more recent focus on well-being in later life is the result of such achievements. But should we continue efforts to expand what we have taken to be a natural life span? If medical care is funded by public monies—and in much of the world, much of medical care is—then the question appears appropriate for public policy analysis. For some, like the philosopher Daniel Callahan, the answer is clear: resources are better, and more fairly, spent on allowing younger people to live out a natural life span. Callahan (2008) writes that "a good society ought to help young people become old people, but is under no obligation to help the old become indefinitely older. The latter is a fiscal black hole, abetted by endless new and costly technologies." But the question of whether to devote resources toward extending the natural life span is not generally posed as a *policy* question to society at large. Instead, medical advances are offered to individual patients in clinical settings, leading incrementally to population-wide life extension. A public policy that denies medical interventions to individuals on account of age suggests age-based discrimination, a controversial proposition.

Ethical Challenges in Pursuing Public Health Goals

Protection from Harm and Promotion of Well-Being

The moral norm of avoiding or preventing harm is seen in efforts to protect older people from falls, isolation, neglect, or abuse. But avoiding and preventing harm through protective measures may come at a cost of reducing autonomy and well-being. The balance is not easy to find. Consider the case of mandatory reporting laws for elder abuse and neglect.

All states in the United States have laws mandating reporting of elder abuse by certain professionals, such as physicians, nurses, attorneys, and clergy. Like mandatory reporting laws for child abuse, these laws appear based on the central assumption that those being "protected" are vulnerable and cannot care for themselves. This assumption is often inappropriate. Laws that include a requirement to report older adults' "self-neglect"—i.e., not just neglect by caregivers—suggest a significant limitation on other important moral norms, such as respecting older people's privacy and their choices and actions in matters such as food, clothing, medication, and health care (Dolgin and Shepherd, 2013). Young and middle-aged adults are—for better or worse—allowed to make all kinds of daily living choices without governmental oversight or intrusion.

Respecting Autonomous Choices

A policy more singularly focused on promoting autonomy might appear to be an easier case, but not always. Take the case of efforts in the United States to promote advance directives for elderly populations. An advance directive is a written statement of a person's wishes regarding medical treatment, should the person later be unable to make decisions for him or herself. A health care agent may be appointed to make decisions and/or provide instructions about what treatments the patient would or would not want in certain conditions, such as terminal illness or permanent unconsciousness (Shepherd, 2014).

Increasing the use of advance directives is clearly an explicitly recognized public health effort in the United States. Most states provide an approved advance directive form, although other forms may also be used. The federal government requires health care facilities to ask all patients upon admission whether they have advance directives and to document their existence. Medicare, the national social insurance program covering older Americans, has recently begun to reimburse health care providers for engaging in advance care planning with patients, including explanation and discussion of advance directives. A few states require physicians to inform patients with a terminal condition of their end-of-life options, including advance directives. The Centers for Disease Control and Prevention (CDC) provides online resources that encourage advance care planning.

Promoting the autonomy of patients to make end-of-life decisions seems like a relatively simple idea, free from the complications of competing ethical considerations—such as balancing this autonomy interest against the individual's welfare interests or the interests of others—but efforts to promote autonomy are ethically complex. This is especially so when those efforts are not individualized but are targeted toward broad swaths of the population. The available instruments are blunt. A standardized form, completed well in advance of an actual treatment decision, may not offer the options desired or later provide the guidance intended by the person who has signed it. When forms do provide more adequate options for individualized choice, they become increasingly legalistic, lengthy, and difficult to understand. Sometimes, advance directives misalign with the current best interests of patients, and it is not clear which should prevail (Dresser, 2003).

Even with the best of forms, advance directives may or may not promote patient autonomy. Because only three in ten Americans have an advance directive, advocates often point to the need for better education, access, and counseling. But skeptics reply that people may avoid them for good reasons: they may not anticipate the medical condition they will later have, or they may not know what they would want done in that situation (Fagerlin and Schneider, 2004). They may prefer to trust family members to make decisions for them when the time arrives. Respecting patients, critics argue, includes respecting the choice *not* to specify medical treatment preferences in advance.

These population-wide efforts may also be biased to encourage individuals to make a socially preferred choice. Early versions of advance directives ("living wills") provided patients only with the option to forgo life-sustaining measures, not to accept them; these forms are still in use in some places. This restricted choice was not necessarily ideologically driven; the assumption at the time was that a living will was not needed if someone *wanted* treatment. On the other hand, some restrictions reflect government-chosen values. In some states, artificial nutrition and hydration will be provided unless specifically refused in an advance directive. Choices have thus been restricted rather than enhanced; only patients with an advance directive have the full panoply of medical choices available to them. The bias most feared, however, is that at some time older people or others with chronic disease or disability will be encouraged to forgo life-prolonging measures (or even hasten their deaths with physician aid, where permitted) in order to reduce governmental health care spending.

Justice

Distributive justice—the fair distribution of benefits and burdens—is a core moral principle of public health ethics (Childress, 2013). But what is fair? Is it just or fair to support *more* or *less* access to health care resources on the basis of old age?

At the *societal level* we make decisions about the allocation of public monies (Dey and Fraser, 2000). In the United States, older adults might be considered to be advantageously positioned vis-à-vis other age groups because of their eligibility for Medicare. Medicare was adopted in 1966 to aid a population that at the time had disproportionately low incomes and was vulnerable to exclusion from private insurance plans. It covers many of the health care needs of older adults, but not all. It does not cover long-term nursing care, for example. Working Americans make income-based contributions to the program through payroll taxes. But some of those receiving Medicare benefits, while they have paid into the program, are not financially needy, and concerns have existed for many years about the financial sustainability of the program through decades of rising medical costs.

We can expect that questions about the extent of health coverage for older adults—e.g., what preventive measures, forms of treatment, and so on, should be paid for with public monies—will be asked with increasing intensity as nations respond to aging populations. How should resources be allocated between the young and the old? Between the poor and the old? Or, within the elderly population, between those who are financially needy and those who are financially secure? Between those with chronic illness or disabilities and those who are aging "well"? In both the United Kingdom and the United States, aging populations are sometimes viewed as posing a heavy burden on public coffers, although some would argue these budgets are unnecessarily and artificially restricted (Dey and Fraser, 2000). Other countries are more accepting of large public expenditures toward health.

Much is made of the frequently cited statistic that a quarter to a third of US government spending on Medicare goes toward medical care in the last year of life. Since the patient dies regardless, these expenditures are often seen as ineffective or wasteful. But many of the most expensive treatments are not known to be ineffective in advance—in other words, "[s]ince there are no reliable ways to identify the patients who will die, it is not possible to say accurately months, weeks, or even days before death which patients will benefit from intensive interventions and which ones will receive 'wasted' care" (Emanuel and Emanuel, 1994, 543). With respect to savings to be achieved by limiting care to the elderly, it is important to note that the oldest old (eighty-five years old and older) already receive less intensive, less hospital-based care when they are near the end of life. Their medical treatment expenses in the last year of life are actually half that of individuals who die between the ages of sixty-five and seventy-five.

Questions also arise about the proper allocation of *programmatic* efforts across ages, such as whether it is appropriate to target prevention, screening, and treatment efforts more intensively toward younger populations. When risk declines with age, then such differential treatment may be justified in terms of limited resources. But such questions become more difficult when risk is not associated with age. Cancer screening programs that have upper age limits even when risks *increase* with age may be justified if treatment will not be effective; otherwise, such age limits seem based on the notion that the extra years of life for an older person are of less value (Daniels, 2008).

Limiting health resources for older adults has been justified by two primary approaches: cost-effectiveness (often discussed in terms of quality-adjusted life years [QALYs]), and the "fair innings" argument. The concern of cost-effectiveness is utilitarian—to maximize the greatest health outcomes (measured in terms of QALYs) relative to cost. QALYs, explicitly adopted in the United Kingdom as a tool in making strategic decisions in public health investments, "are based on life years saved adjusted to take account of impairment of quality, measured in terms of dimensions like ability to function and degree of distress" (Dey and Fraser, 2000, 522). As such, the use of QALYs may mean that public health choices are made that discriminate against older people because "they have fewer life-years ahead of them to be saved" (Childress, 2013, 24). Depending upon how one defines "quality-adjusted," persons with disabilities are also susceptible to discrimination by QALY analysis. Older people who are disabled due to frailty or chronic disease—for which increasing age is a risk factor—can suffer doubly (Brock, 2004).

The "fair innings" argument for limiting resources is based on equity rather than utility or cost-effectiveness, and its effect on older adults is more explicit and unapologetic. Most simply, it posits that if choices about resources have to be made, younger people should have the same opportunity to live a full life that older people have already enjoyed. This will promote equality in "lifetime experiences of health" (Williams, 1997, 822).

Future Directions for Public Health Efforts: The Clinical and the Social

Policy debates about ethics and public health sometimes appear abstract, or removed from the lives of actual persons. Conversely, clinical ethics cases often appear particularized, or removed from public health policies. Any ethically troubling situation relating to health is likely to have both a clinical and a public health component, and to have been borne of hundreds of decisions, made over time by many different actors and made for the intended benefit of various individuals or groups.

Consider the case of a frail man in his late seventies, a lifelong smoker, who has suffered a fall at his rural home, where he lives alone on a small government old-age pension. Hospitalized, he is now ready to be discharged. The hospital social worker and his daughter believe he cannot safely return to his home, but he does not want to move to an assisted-living or nursing facility. He does not want to leave his home, yet his government-provided health insurance will cover only limited home health care assistance.

Situations like this confront hospitals, social workers, families, and older adults every day. This man's story presents a classic example of a conflict in *clinical ethics* between respecting his autonomy (by discharging him to home as he prefers) and protecting him and perhaps others from harm or burden (by persuading or coercing him to move into an assisted-living facility). But this is also a *public health ethics* story. Even with this "thin" presentation of facts, we can identify areas of concern that have population-based application: What transportation, social, health care, and other resources are available that make aging in place more or less possible? What public policies might influence whether an assisted-living or nursing facility is more or less of an attractive option? What effect have past and present public health policies had on this man's current condition? What are societal expectations about family members' involvement?

Looking at particular cases, with particular individuals, can reveal much about the ethics of public policies that affect older populations. Have those policies been, or can those policies in the future, be just? Can they be health-promoting? Can they be respectful of individual dignity and autonomy? An important strategy for advancing public health for older populations is to recognize *patterns of ethical conflict in clinical settings*—such as at the point of discharge—that may have been influenced by past public policy decisions and which population-based strategies may now help reduce or resolve.

But this case example also raises questions about the *social determinants of health*, in terms of both their past and future influence on this man's health. Factors far removed from health systems and traditional health sectors—factors like education and transportation—are increasingly understood to play prominent roles in population health. What does this understanding signal for the future role of public health as a field of inquiry and action, especially as it relates to elderly populations? Growing appreciation of the social determinants of health might suggest that greater efforts should be focused on people's needs early in life, in order to achieve the largest reductions in health inequities across populations and time. But it might also lead to a greater sense of responsibility to those current older adults whose health and other needs are linked to a lifetime of social inequities.

References

Binstock, R. H., and Post, S. 1991. "Old Age and the Rationing of Health Care." In *Too Old for Health Care? Controversies in Medicine, Law, Economics, and Ethics*, edited by R. H. Binstock and S. Post, 1–12 (Baltimore, Md.: Johns Hopkins University Press).

Brock, D. 2004. "Ethical Issues in the Use of Cost-Effectiveness Analysis for the Prioritization of Health Care Resources." In *Handbook of Bioethics*, edited by G. Khushf, 353–380 (Dordrecht, the Netherlands: Springer).

Callahan, D. 2008. "The Economic Woes of Medicare." *New York Times*, November 13.

Childress, J. F. 2013. "Moral Considerations: Bases and Limits for Public Health Interventions." In *Essentials of Public Health Ethics*, edited by R. G. Bernheim, J. F. Childress, R. J. Bonnie, and A. Melnick, 21–41 (Burlington, Md.: Jones and Bartlett Learning).

Daniels, N. 2008. *Just Health: Meeting Health Needs Fairly* (New York: Cambridge University Press).

Dey, I., and Fraser, N. 2000. "Age-Based Rationing in the Allocation of Health Care." *Journal of Aging and Health* 12: 511–537.

Dolgin, J. L., and Shepherd, L. 2013. *Bioethics and the Law*. 3rd ed. (New York: Wolters Kluwer).

Dresser, R. 2003. "Precommitment: A Misguided Strategy for Securing Death with Dignity." *Texas Law Review* 81: 1823.

Emanuel, E. J., and Emanuel, L. L. 1994. "The Economics of Dying—The Illusion of Cost Savings at the End of Life." *New England Journal of Medicine* 330: 540–544.

Fagerlin, A., and Schneider, C. E. 2004. "Enough: The Failure of the Living Will." *Hastings Center Report* 34 (2): 30–42.

Friedan, B. 1993. *The Fountain of Age* (New York: Simon & Schuster).

Fuchs, J., Scheidt-Nave, C., Hinrichs, T., Mergenthaler, A., Stein, J., Riedel-Heller, S. G., et al. 2013. "Indicators for Healthy Ageing—A Debate." *International Journal of Environmental Research and Public Health* 10: 6630–6644.

Golant, S. M. 2008. "Commentary: Irrational Exuberance for the Aging in Place of Vulnerable Low-Income Older Homeowners." *Journal of Aging and Social Policy* 20: 379–397.

He, W., Goodkind, D., and Kowal, P. 2015. *An Aging World: 2015*. International Population Reports (Washington, D.C.: US Census Bureau). https://www.census.gov/content/dam/Census/library/publications/2016/demo/p95-16-1.pdf.

Martinson, M., and Berridge, C. 2015. "Successful Aging and Its Discontents: A Systematic Review of the Social Gerontology Literature." *Gerontologist* 55(1): 58–69.

NCPOP (National Centre for the Protection of Older People). 2009. *Public Perceptions of Older People and Ageing: A Literature Review* (Dublin: NCPOP).

Sadana, R., Blas, E., Budhwani, S., Koller, T., and Paraje, G. 2016. "Healthy Ageing: Raising Awareness of Inequalities, Determinants, and What Could Be Done to Improve Health Equity." *Gerontologist* 56: S178–S193.

Shepherd, L. 2014. "The End of End-of-Life Law." *North Carolina Law Review* 92: 1693.

Williams, A. 1997. "Rationing Health Care by Age: The Case For." *British Medical Journal* 314: 820–822.

WHO (World Health Organization). 2015. *World Report on Ageing and Health* (Geneva: WHO). http://www.who.int/ageing/events/world-report-2015-launch/en/.

WHO (World Health Organization) and USNIA (US National Institute of Aging). 2011. *Global Health and Aging* (Geneva: WHO). http://www.who.int/ageing/publications/global_health/en/.

CHAPTER 17

CHILDREN, ADOLESCENTS, AND PUBLIC HEALTH: ETHICAL CONSIDERATIONS

MARGARET MOON

INTRODUCTION

IDENTIFYING and addressing ethical issues specific to the population comprising children and adolescents is complicated at the outset by definitional and data issues. Children and adolescents account for approximately a third of the extant population, and the age range encompasses such a broad set of physical, cognitive, and experiential characteristics that particularities seem hard to identify. This chapter proposes that there are three fundamental aspects of the experience of children and adolescents that should frame public health approaches: (1) lack of a social and economic power, (2) being subject to stewardship by adults, and (3) a presumed lack of capacity for decision-making.

Interestingly, there is no universal definition of a child or an adolescent. As noted in 1981 by the United Nations Advisory Committee for the first "International Youth Year," "a chronological definition of who is young, as opposed to who is a child or who is an adult, varies with each nation and culture" (Angel, 1995, 133; UN, 1981). For statistical purposes, the United Nations identifies people aged fourteen to twenty-five as "youth," while younger persons are "children." Recent developments in psychology and neuroscience reflect the logic of including young adulthood as part of the developmental range from infant to adult (IOM and NRC, 2014). However, for purposes of policy and law, age eighteen is identified as the beginning of adulthood and the age of majority in most countries (CIA, 2013).

Adolescence, in most cultures, is a term related to puberty, which begins between ages eight and thirteen for girls and between ages nine and fourteen for boys. Adolescence is typically considered to be the period between the beginning of puberty and the onset of adulthood, but the onset of adulthood is socially, not physiologically, determined (United Nations Department of Economic and Social Affairs Population Division, 2012). While formal markers of adulthood, such as age of majority or ability to vote, vary only minimally between countries, the age at which typical experiential markers of adulthood, such as marriage, financial independence, and parenthood, are achieved varies widely between societies and cultures. The variations are not trivial: the experience of young people and the expectations placed on them follow, in large part, from social and cultural age norms. A teenage girl comfortably ensconced in a middle-class family in the United States has expectations of postsecondary education, a protective home environment, and delayed marriage and family. In the poorest areas of sub-Saharan Africa, however, only half the girls of primary school age attend school, and half of all births occur during adolescence (UNESCO, 2003; WHO, 2017a). A focus on the public health issues and the predominant ethical considerations of these complicated age and experience groups requires interpretation beyond the artificial categories of chronologic age, but such a focus can highlight shared experiential characteristics that have profound implications for public health.

Definitional complexities aside, UNICEF estimates that by 2050 there will be nearly 10 billion people in the world, and more than 2.6 billion of them will be younger than eighteen years of age. This is a slight trend downward in the proportion of the world's population under eighteen. Children and adolescents are currently a majority in only the least-developed forty-eight nations. This trend will continue, with children and youth increasingly concentrated in areas where poverty is most entrenched. Interestingly, the actual number of very young children in the world is not well identified. This adds to the difficulty in identifying specific public health issues for this subset of the population, but it also highlights an important ethical concern: fully one-third of children under age five have no birth registration, meaning no state identity at all. These children, estimated at 230 million, are not part of any public health database, and they do not have a birth certificate to register for school, gain legal protection, or, in some areas, access health care. Severe disparities in this very basic benefit of being recognized exist, with almost half of the world's poorest children under age five having no registered identity (UNICEF, 2013).

More positively, the best global estimates of mortality rates for children under age five imply that, for those children who are counted, mortality has been declining steadily for decades, going down by 50 percent between 1990 and 2015 (You et al., 2015). Disparities, however, are remarkable and persistent—the mortality rate for young children in low-income countries (76 per 1,000) is eleven times that in the richest countries (World Bank, 2015). The leading causes of death in children under five are preterm birth complications, pneumonia, birth asphyxia, diarrhea, and malaria. Globally, nearly half of under-five deaths are attributable to undernutrition (World Bank, 2015).

Older children and adolescents are the healthiest sector of the world's population. Mortality rates are low, around 1 per 1,000, and there has been a slight decline in the mortality rate in the past decade. Adolescents tend to be at low risk for diseases that kill young children—such as diarrhea and respiratory disease (UNICEF, 2012)—but they suffer much higher mortality and morbidity from causes that reflect the stereotypical experience of adolescence, including violence, injury, and depression.

Globally, the leading causes of death among adolescents are motor vehicle crashes and road injury, HIV, suicide, lower respiratory infections, and interpersonal violence (Patton et al., 2009). Note that HIV deaths were not on the list of the top ten causes of death in adolescents in 2000, but they tripled between 2008 and 2018.

According to the WHO (2014), the major causes of morbidity in the late childhood and adolescent period include the following:

- depressive disorders
- iron deficiency anemia
- asthma
- back and neck pain
- anxiety disorders
- alcohol use disorders

Unlike the mortality rates for early childhood, the data for the adolescent sector of the population does not vary significantly between poor and wealthy countries or among geographic regions.

Life-course health development models, developed to emphasize the multiple, nested determinants of health, emphasize the trajectory of health or disease from the preconception period to childhood, to adolescence, and through to adulthood (Halfon and Hochstein, 2002). The World Health Organization estimates that 35 percent of the global burden of disease is related to the long-term outcomes of adolescent health and behavior (WHO, 2017b). Life-course models of health raise the stakes for a public health focus on the health of children and adolescents, as the benefits of early good health will support the well-being of a whole population, and the risks of early poor health persist throughout the life span (Sawyer et al., 2012).

Children and Adolescents

Given the differences in health concerns between children and adolescents, as well as the remarkable changes in physical, cognitive, and emotional attributes over this age span, it can seem simplistic to discuss this group as a particular population from the point of view of public health ethics. Children and adolescents are not a disease group. They are not identifiable by a specific incapacity, by any common dependency, or even by an intrinsic vulnerability.

Humans under the age of eighteen make up a "particular population" based on three distinct but interrelated characteristics—each having profound ethical implications for public health: (1) disenfranchisement and lack of social and economic power, (2) status as subject to stewardship, and (3) presumed lack of capacity for decision-making. This chapter will examine several public health challenges affecting children and adolescents with a view to these three defining characteristics and the practical and ethical tensions they create.

Disenfranchisement and Lack of Social and Economic Power

As minors, children and adolescents have no voting rights and no established political voice. As noted earlier, in some of the world's poorest countries, more than half of young children have no birth registration, and hence no political or legal identity at all. The importance of a political identity was recognized in the Convention on the Rights of the Child, an international treaty adopted by the United Nations in 1989 that lays out the human rights of children. These include the right of every child to a name and legal and national identity—just after the right to life (UN, 1989). But even children and adolescents with established legal identities still have a very limited political voice. In their relatively powerless state, minors rely on the wisdom and foresight of those with power to enact and enforce policies that support their well-being. Essential conflicts arise when the interests of children are weighed against the interests of parents, families, or the state.

Article 3(1) of the Convention on the Rights of the Child states, "In all actions concerning children,... the *best interests of the child* shall be a primary consideration" (UN, 1989; emphasis added). Despite the powerful language of the Convention and its widespread acceptance, nations struggle to make the "best interests of the child" standard anything more than aspirational. In any political arena, there are many interests competing for limited resources, and the voice of the powerless is easily lost. Examples abound: while global morbidity and mortality statistics imply that the best interests of children require a focus on mental health for children and adolescents, resources fall far short of the need, competition for financial resources affects mental health disproportionately, and social stigma remains a significant barrier to care (WHO, 2003). Similarly, gun-related deaths and injuries remain a leading cause of morbidity and mortality in the adolescent and young adult age groups, but progress on gun control meets obstacles from increasing numbers of pro-gun lobby groups, and, particularly in the United States even research on the prevention of gun deaths, routinely falls prey to political interests (Wellford, Pepper, and Petrie, 2005). Despite evidence that simple programs to enhance maternal preconception health lead to healthier mothers and children, key components of these programs, such as maternal education and birth planning, fail to gain and maintain traction in the development of health and social policy (Moos, 2010; Africa Progress Panel, 2010).

Comparing Articles 3 and 5 of the Convention on the Rights of the Child offers insight into one of the potential conflicts of interest that weaken Article 3's strongly worded "best interest" standard. Article 5 asserts, "States Parties shall respect the *responsibilities, rights and duties of parents*... to provide, in a manner consistent with the evolving capacities of the child, appropriate direction and guidance in the exercise by the child of the rights recognized in the present Convention" (UN, 1989; emphasis added). Article 5's conflation of parental responsibilities with parental rights introduces the idea of stewardship and its limits on the best interest standard.

Stewardship and Ownership: The Rights and Duties of Parents

Within the family or community, the best interests of an individual child is a very high standard for acceptable decisions. In societies that promote and protect the importance of family, parents are presumed to have the right to raise a child according to parental cultural, religious, and philosophical values, along with the duty to provide an environment compatible with healthy development. Therein lies the challenge of "stewardship."

Most societies have moved away from considering children as parental property or chattel, and children are now widely viewed as having moral status equal to their parents and, in some cases, an opportunity to be recognized as having decision-making authority. While the law in most countries asserts that parents must not violate the rights of their children, must not allow others to violate the rights of their children and should promote the interests of the child, it also gives parents substantial leeway in determining best interests and sets a high threshold for state infringement of parental rights. Instead of ownership, parents can be understood as having *stewardship* rights over their children, and as stewards they are charged with overseeing and protecting something of value that they do not "own" (Brennan and Noggle, 1997). Environmental stewardship, in a similar vein, does not imply that we cannot make use of the environment, but only that we are charged with protecting environmental resources and making any use sustainable. Stewardship is a limited duty; stewards are free to pursue their own interests as long as the stewardship obligations are fulfilled. Parents, correspondingly, are not asked to support the best interests of a child to the exclusion of their own interests. Parents, as stewards, evaluate their own interests alongside the interests of their children, seeking an appropriate balance (Austin, 2007).

Legal authorities do not generally hold parents to a best interests standard when evaluating the decisions made on behalf of a child. Instead, they apply the more practical "good enough interest" standard, offering parents broad leeway in parenting without state interference, and recognizing that within families there is a constant evolution in the balance of interests between children, parents, and family. The limit to parental authority over children is not a failure to promote best interests, but a material risk of avoidable harm to the child (Diekema, 2011). Within the stewardship model of parental obligations, some limited harms are acceptable when balanced against the well-being of the family.

Children thrive when parents, the community, and the state function as good stewards, making choices that promote the best possible interests of the child. Tremendous disparities exist, however, between families, between communities, and between nations in the extent to which children are protected and nurtured.

Presumption of Incapacity

The third unique characteristic that is common to children and adolescents is that of presumed incapacity. Essential to the logic of stewardship is the idea that children and adolescents are incapable of managing their own interests effectively and lack capacity for informed decision-making. The role of the steward is to protect the child while promoting and encouraging the development of independence. While the presumption of incapacity and the need for stewardship is clear and reasonable for much of early childhood, the ethical tensions rise as children develop independent skills and begin to approximate adult capacity for decision-making sometime in early or middle adolescence (Lipstein, Brinkman, and Fiks, 2015; Ruhe et al., 2015).

Public Health Challenges

Health Information and Health Promotion for Children and Adolescents

A mainstay of public health practice is the development and implementation of health promotion and health education programs. Challenges around health promotion activities arise from the competing duties to give children and adolescents access to developmentally appropriate information necessary to promote their own healthy development while avoiding harmful messaging, and to respect family and community values regarding the content and presentation of information.

Effective programs are targeted to specific populations and make use of salient characteristics of the target population. During childhood and adolescence, however, the only constant characteristic is change. The age range from childhood to adolescence involves remarkable transitions in cognitive capacity and emotional maturity. Successful health information and health promotion programs must be designed to incorporate capacity-specific messaging. For example, a smoking cessation program targeted toward the fourteen- to sixteen-year-old demographic must be mindful of the specific cognitive capacities of middle adolescence. Middle adolescence is marked by a heightened sense of anxiety about attractiveness, a newly emerging capacity for abstract thought, and a limited ability to consider the future. Concerns about long-term health complications of smoking are likely to miss the mark, while presentation of the negative effect of smoking on physical attractiveness will get attention. The same campaign directed toward early adolescents (ages ten to thirteen) should employ concrete logic and make use of early adolescents' anxiety about being different from their peers, emphasizing that smoking makes a teen an outlier. The late adolescent to young adult group (ages seventeen to twenty-five) has a richer capacity for abstract thought and is more future-focused, so that discussion of smoking as a long-term health risk might be effective.

Complicating the situation, cognitive and emotional capacities may develop at a different pace than physical capacities. Families may be attuned to a child's emotional or cognitive age, but in social environments, physical appearance becomes the most common guide to frame interactions with a child. Children who mature physically before maturing cognitively and emotionally are at risk of being exposed to information beyond their capacity to comprehend. Community-based public health programs may have a limited ability to attend to the nuance between physical and cognitive/emotional development.

School-based education about sexual and reproductive health has been a flashpoint for a challenge between family values and public health goals. Some of the reported benefits of comprehensive sex education include pregnancy avoidance, increased condom use, delay in initiation of sex, and increased monogamy (Advocates for Youth, 2009). However, some families and communities have rejected these health promotion efforts as contrary to religious or other closely held views about sexuality and reproduction. Families argue, from the stewardship perspective, that their duties and rights as stewards of their children's moral development limit the schools' right to present a curriculum around sexuality, challenging the ethical justifiability of sex education programs.

With any public health activity, the ethical justification depends on several considerations, including the importance of the public health problem, the likelihood that this activity will meet the goal of reducing the problem, the burden the program places on the community or the individual, and whether less burdensome alternatives are available (Kass, 2001; Upshur, 2002; Childress et al., 2002). School-based sex education in the United States illustrates the challenges presented by public health programming for the school-aged child and adolescent. Specifically, it illustrates how the ethical justifiability of a public health program can be challenged. There has been little debate about the importance of the problem of high-risk sexual behavior and unwanted pregnancy. However, debates about the use of school-based sex education as part of a public health program to promote safer sex have been vigorous. In the United States, the debates have focused predominantly on two considerations related to ethical justification: the effectiveness of sex education programs, and whether sex education encourages early initiation of sexual behavior or high-risk sexual behavior. Although federal funding was, for many years, limited to abstinence-only education, detractors cited scant evidence of effectiveness (Kirby, 2008). Without evidence of effectiveness, abstinence-only programs are hard to justify.

Even without evidence of harm from abstinence-only programs, their ineffectiveness implies a lost opportunity to meet the public health goal and misdirection of limited public health resources. Comprehensive sex education, on the other hand, has been shown to increase knowledge and change behavior, but detractors have continued to raise concerns that comprehensive sex education promotes early sexual activity. If evidence of that harm ever materialized, it would create a strong argument that comprehensive school-based sex education creates an undue risk or burden to the community and was unjustifiable as a public health program.

In addition to beliefs about sexual morality, a key component of the concern about promotion of sexual behavior has been the appropriate target age for sex education. While sex education is most effective when introduced in early adolescence, the variability in cognitive and emotional capacities of early adolescents has generated concerns that sex education might have the unintended consequence of encouraging sexual behavior in cognitively or emotionally young teens.

Although there has not been any evidence that school-based sex education encourages sexual activity among young adolescents, the concern that health promotion activities might have harmful unanticipated consequences for children and adolescents is very real. Obesity has become a serious threat to public health, and obesity prevention is on the agenda of many governments. Health promotion messages about obesity must be carefully gauged to avoid creating a second burden of anxiety, shame, or even disordered eating for children who are overweight or obese (Toftemo, Glavin, and Lagerlov, 2013; Salas, 2015). Similarly, sexual assault prevention messages have been criticized as blaming the victims for failing to be in control, and sexually transmitted disease prevention messages have raised concerns about increasing stigma to the extent that adolescents will not seek care. In each of these cases, ethical justification for the program rests in large part on ensuring that any risks of the messaging, particularly those related to the cognitive and emotional vulnerabilities of children and adolescents, are carefully considered and addressed.

Access to Confidential Health Services for Adolescents

Children and adolescents typically rely on parents or other caretaking adults for access to health care when access requires financial payment or insurance. When access to care or specific treatment requires informed consent, children and adolescents are, with few exceptions, legally prevented from authorizing care and are usually presumed to be incapable of fully informed consent. An important practical tension arises when adolescents limit their use of necessary or beneficial care due to a concern for confidentiality. Public health programs that provide confidential reproductive health care to adolescents, for example, are designed to reduce disease transmission and unwanted pregnancy by removing obstacles that might dissuade an adolescent from seeking reproductive health care. Decades of evidence confirm that adolescents are more likely to seek care for reproductive health when confidentiality is offered (Carroll et al., 2012; Cheng et al., 1993). Confidentiality has been seen as instrumental in achieving the public health goal of optimizing access to reproductive health care for adolescents.

An ethical tension in access to health care arises from conflicting duties to ensure that adolescents have access to necessary care while respecting the family's interest in being informed about health risks to which the adolescent is exposed and treatments an adolescent might undergo. In this arena, confidentiality for adolescent patients has both intrinsic and instrumental value. One of the central principles of biomedical ethics is the duty to respect autonomy (Beauchamp and Childress, 2013). For pediatric and adolescent patients, the duty to respect autonomy is complicated by the fact that autonomy, as capacity for self-rule, is a developmental construct. As children develop cognitive and emotional capacities, the autonomy-related duty moves from protecting and promoting the developing autonomy of young children toward respecting the decisions made by adolescents who have decision-making capacity similar to that of adults. As an intrinsic value, protection of confidentiality for adolescent patients is a commitment to respect the autonomy and the dignity of people who are in need of care. The duty is limited by the actual capacity for decision-making, but the presumption that adolescents and older children lack capacity is unrealistic.

As an instrumental value, the promise of confidential care increases the likelihood that adolescent patients will seek care and offer frank disclosures of health concerns. Both values, intrinsic and instrumental, are important in the care of adolescents, who, from a developmental perspective, are seeking to achieve autonomy from their parents and are learning to make appropriate decisions about a variety of issues, including healthy behaviors and seeking health care.

The challenge in adolescent reproductive health care is to balance these intrinsic and instrumental values of confidentiality with the duties to promote adolescents' well-being and avoid harms. While adolescents are developmentally programmed to seek independence, families remain, in most situations, their primary source of moral and financial support and protection. Programs offering confidential care should seek to enrich family connections while encouraging healthy independence. Communities and families can be engaged in program planning and implementation so that the rationale for confidential care is clear and the limits of confidentiality—specifically related to disclosure of high-risk behavior—are established and accepted.

Failures of Stewardship

Children and adolescents suffer avoidable harms when parents or legislative groups, as stewards of children, obstruct access, fail to protect access, or fail to promote access to highly valuable care. Vaccination against common infectious diseases is a current example. Childhood immunization has been one of the most significant public health successes of the modern era. Immunization programs meet all criteria for an ethically justifiable public health program. In recent decades, however, vaccine refusal has rendered large populations of children (and others in the community, such as the immunocompromised) vulnerable to highly preventable disease. The best available scientific evidence does not support vaccine refusal. Stewardship requires the capacity and willingness to protect the child against irrevocable and avoidable harms. In the vaccination case, government policies can exacerbate failures of parental stewardship (Omer et al., 2006). Vaccine refusal is most common in states or jurisdictions where public health policies routinely grant nonmedical exemptions, such as religious or philosophical exemptions, to immunization requirements for school admission. Similarly, policies that allow religious exemptions from medical neglect statutes allow parents to reject effective medical care for their children without legal repercussions. This can result in limited access to necessary care for vulnerable children and adolescents (Antommaria and AAP Committee on Bioethics, 2013).

Global morbidity and mortality data highlight specific failures in the stewardship duties of political systems. Mental health concerns, for example, particularly depression, are a major cause of morbidity and mortality for children and adolescents. However, access to mental health services is inadequate, hampered by government policies and inadequate funding (Kieling et al., 2011). Interpersonal violence has held a spot in the most prominent causes of death in adolescents for decades, but gun control and even research into firearm injuries fails to clear political obstacles in the United States. These and other public health concerns of particular relevance to children and adolescents should be comprehensively addressed to reduce the burden on disease on this population. In addition, epidemiological data now identify the population-level risk factors for childhood health disparities that could be addressed early to promote lifelong health and well-being, both in this population and in society more broadly. Stewardship, informed by principles of health equity and the rights of the child, requires policies and practices that not only ensure access to health care, but also address the socioeconomic, environmental, and behavioral determinants of children's health (AAP, 2010).

Conclusion

Ethical issues in public health approaches to the fascinatingly complex and diverse population of children and adolescents arise from three themes that connect this population: lack of political and economic power, stewardship of parents and the state, and presumption of incapacity. While the Convention on the Rights of the Child seeks to establish the "best interests of the child" as the threshold for ethically justifiable public policy, this standard remains mostly aspirational. Children do not vote and do not hold much, if any, financial or political power, so their interests require the protection of other, self-interested, parties. A "good enough interests" standard, as a pragmatic compromise of aspirations, liberal theory, and political reality, comports with a stewardship model of parenting and state action in the lives of children.

Stewardship is as beneficial as the steward is capable, willing, and free to steward. But disparities within and between societies are profound. The legal presumption of incapacity flies in the face of the logic of child and adolescent cognitive and emotional development. Public health policies and practices can support children and adolescents at these critical periods along the health trajectory by anticipating the risks related to disenfranchisement, advocate for enlightened stewardship within both families and political leadership, and promote respect for developing capacity and autonomy.

References

AAP (American Academy of Pediatrics, Council on Community Pediatrics and Committee on Native American Child Health). 2010."Policy Statement: Health Equity and Children's Rights." *Pediatrics* 125(4): 838–849.

Advocates for Youth. 2009. *Comprehensive Sex Education: Research and Results*. http://www.advocatesforyouth.org/publications/1487#ref.

Africa Progress Panel. 2010. *Policy Brief: Maternal Health: Investing in the Lifeline of Healthy Societies and Economies*. http://www.africaprogresspanel.org/policy-papers/maternal-health-investing-in-the-lifeline-of-healthy-societies-economies/.

Angel, W. D., ed. 1995. "Resolutions on Youth Rights and Responsibilities Adopted by the General Assembly and Economic and Social Council of the United Nations 1965–1993." In *The International Law of Youth Rights: Source Documents and Commentary*, 129–256 (Boston: Martinus Nijhoff).

Antommaria A., and AAP Committee on Bioethics. 2013. "Conflicts between Religious or Spiritual Beliefs and Pediatric Care: Informed Refusal, Exemptions, and Public Funding." *Pediatrics* 132(5): 962–965.

Austin, M. W. 2007. *Conceptions of Parenthood: Ethics and the Family*. Aldershot, UK: Ashgate.

Beauchamp, T., and Childress J. 2013. *Principles of Biomedical Ethics*. 7th ed. (New York, NY: Oxford University Press).

Brennan, S. and Noggle, R. 1997. "The Moral Status of Children: Children's Rights, Parents' Rights and Family." *Social Theory and Practice* 23(1): 1–27.

Carroll, C., Lloyd-Jones, M., Cooke, J., and Owen, J. 2012. "Reasons for the Use and Non-use of School Sexual Health Services: A Systematic Review of Young People's Views." *Journal of Public Health* 34(3): 403–410.

Cheng, T., Savageau, J., Sattler, A., and DeWitt, T. 1993. "Confidentiality in Health Care: A Survey of Knowledge, Perceptions and Attitudes among High School Students." *JAMA* 269(11): 1404–1407.

Childress, J., Faden, R., Gaare, R., Gostin, L., Kahn, J., Bonnie, R., et al. 2002, "Public Health Ethics: Mapping the Terrain." *Journal of Law, Medicine & Ethics* 30(2): 170–178.

CIA (Central Intelligence Agency). 2013. *The World Factbook*. https://www.cia.gov/library/publications/the-world-factbook/fields/2123.html.

Diekema, D. 2011. "Revisiting the Best Interest Standard: Uses and Misuses." *Journal of Clinical Ethics* 22(2): 128–133.

Halfon, N., and Hochstein, M. 2002. "Life Course Health Development: An Integrated Framework for Developing Health, Policy, and Research." *Milbank Quarterly* 80(3): 433–479.

IOM (Institute of Medicine) and NRC (National Research Council). 2014. *Investing in the Health and Well-Being of Young Adults*. Washington, DC: National Academies Press. https://www.nap.edu/catalog/18869/investing-in-the-health-and-well-being-of-young-adults.

Kass, N. 2001. "An Ethics Framework for Public Health." *American Journal of Public Health* 91(11): 1776–1782.

Kieling, C., Baker-Hennington, H., Belfer, M., Conti, G., Ertem, I., Omigbodun, O., et al. 2011. "Child and Adolescent Mental Health Worldwide: Evidence for Action." *Lancet* 378(9801): 1515–1525.

Kirby, D. 2008. "The Impact of Abstinence and Comprehensive Sex and STD/HIV Education Programs on Adolescent Sexual Behavior." *Sexuality Research and Social Policy* 5: 18.

Lipstein, E., Brinkman, W., and Fiks, A. 2015. "An Emerging Field of Research: Challenges in Pediatric Decision Making." *Medical Decision Making* 35(3): 403–408.

Moos, M. 2010. "From Concept to Practice: Reflections on the Preconception Health Agenda." *Journal of Women's Health* 19(3): 561–567.

Omer, S., Pan, W., Halsey, N., Stokley, S., Moulton, L., Navar, A., et al. 2006. "Nonmedical Exemptions to School Immunization Requirements: Secular Trends and Association of State Policies with Pertussis Incidence." *JAMA* 296(14): 1757–1763.

Patton, G., Coffey, C., Sawyer, S., Viner, R., Haller, D., Bose, K., et al. 2009. "Global Patterns of Mortality in Young People: A Systematic Analysis of Population Health Data." *Lancet* 374(9693): 881–892.

Ruhe, K., Wangmo, T., Badrau, D., Elger, B., and Niggli, F. 2015. "Decision-Making Capacity of Children and Adolescents—Suggestions for Advancing the Concept's Implementation in Pediatric Healthcare." *European Journal of Pediatrics* 174(6): 775–782.

Salas, X. 2015. "The Ineffectiveness and Unintended Consequences of the Public Health War on Obesity." *Canadian Journal of Public Health*. 106(2): e79–e81.

Sawyer, S., Afifi R., Bearinger, L., Blakemore, S., Dick, B., Ezeh, A., et al. 2012. "Adolescence: A Foundation for Future Health." *Lancet* 379(9826): 1630–1640.

Toftemo, I., Glavin, K., and Lagerlov, P. 2013. "Parents' Views and Experiences When Their Preschool Child Is Identified as Overweight: A Qualitative Study in Primary Care." *Family Practice* 30(6): 719–723.

UN (United Nations). 1981. *Report of the Advisory Committee for the International Youth Year*. http://www.un.org/esa/socdev/unyin/documents/A_res_37_48.pdf.

UN (United Nations).1989. Convention on the Rights of the Child. http://www.ohchr.org/EN/ProfessionalInterest/Pages/CRC.aspx.

UNESCO (United Nations Educational, Scientific and Cultural Organization). 2003. *Education for All (EFA) Global Monitoring Report 2003/4*. http://unesdoc.unesco.org/images/0013/001325/132550e.pdf.

UNICEF (United Nations Children's Fund). 2012. *Progress for Children: A Report Card on Adolescents*. https://www.unicef.org/publications/files/Progress_for_Children_-_No._10_EN_04232012.pdf

UNICEF (United Nations Children's Fund). 2013. *Every Child's Birthright: Inequities and Trends in Birth Registration* (UNICEF Data and Analytics Section, Division of Policy and Strategy). https://www.un.org/ruleoflaw/files/Embargoed_11_Dec_Birth_Registration_report_low_res.pdf

United Nations Department of Economic and Social Affairs Population Division. 2012. *World Population Monitoring: Adolescents and Youth—A Concise Report*. http://www.un.org/en/development/desa/population/publications/pdf/fertility/12_66976_adolescents_and_youth.pdf.

Upshur, R. 2002. "Principles for the Justification of Public Health Intervention." *Canadian Journal of Public Health* 93(2): 101–103.

Wellford, C., Pepper, J. and Petrie, C., eds. 2005. *Firearms and Violence: A Critical Review*. Committee to Improve Research Information and Data on Firearms, and Committee on

Law and Justice, Division of Behavioral and Social Sciences and Education (Washington, DC: National Academies Press.)

WHO (World Health Organization). 2003. *Caring for Children and Adolescents with Mental Disorders: Setting WHO Directions*. http://www.who.int/mental_health/media/en/785.pdf.

WHO (World Health Organization). 2014. *Health for the World's Adolescents: A Second Chance in the Second Decade*. http://apps.who.int/iris/bitstream/10665/112750/1/WHO_FWC_MCA_14.05_eng.pdf.

WHO (World Health Organization). 2017a. "Adolescent Pregnancy." Fact Sheet. http://www.who.int/mediacentre/factsheets/fs364/en/.

WHO (World Health Organization). 2017b. "Maternal, Newborn, Child and Adolescent Health: Adolescent Health Epidemiology." http://www.who.int/maternal_child_adolescent/epidemiology/adolescence/en/.

World Bank. 2015. *Levels and Trends in Child Mortality: Estimates Developed by the UN Inter-agency Group for Child Mortality Estimation (IGME)*. http://documents.worldbank.org/curated/en/306381468000931160/Levels-and-trends-in-child-mortality-estimates-developed-by-the-UN-Inter-agency-Group-for-Child-Mortality-Estimation-IGME-report-2015.

You, D., Hug, L., Ejdemry, S., Idele, P., Hogan, D., Mathers, C., et al. 2015. "Global, Regional, and National Levels and Trends in Under-5 Mortality between 1990 and 2015, with Scenario-Based Projections to 2030: A Systematic Analysis by the UN Inter-agency Group for Child Mortality Estimation." *Lancet* 386(10010): 2275–2286.

CHAPTER 18

ETHICS IN MENTAL HEALTH CARE: A PUBLIC HEALTH PERSPECTIVE

RICHARD J. BONNIE AND HEATHER ZELLE

Introduction

Mental illness is a broad term encompassing a wide range of problems, and it requires an open-ended definition. [1] Mental illness is "generally characterized by some combination of abnormal thoughts, emotions, behavior and relationships with others" (WHO, 2013, 38). More specifically,

> A mental disorder is a syndrome characterized by clinically significant disturbance in an individual's cognition, emotion regulation, or behavior that reflects a dysfunction in the psychological, biological, or developmental processes underlying mental functioning. Mental disorders are usually associated with significant distress or disability in social, occupational, or other important activities. (APA, 2013, 20)

In contrast, mental *health* is "a state of well-being in which an individual realizes his or her own abilities, can cope with the normal stresses of life, can work productively and is able to make a contribution to his or her community" (WHO, 2013, 38). Mental health is "an essential element" of overall health, "a state of complete physical, mental and social well-being" (WHO, 2013, 43). Importantly, mental illness (and health) implicate a person's functioning, not merely the presence or absence of symptoms.

Epidemiology of Mental Illness

Incidence and burden estimates for mental illness depend upon definitional, demographic, and geographic factors. Nonetheless, it is widely accepted that mental illness is a pervasive health condition around the globe. For example, 18 percent of US adults experienced a diagnosable mental disorder in 2014, with a little over 4 percent experiencing a serious mental illness (i.e., an illness that results "in serious functional impairment, which substantially interferes with or limits one or more major life activities"; NIMH, 2017). Similar estimates have been made elsewhere in the world (Kessler et al., 2009). Around the world, mental and substance use disorders were the leading cause of years lived with disability in 2010 (Whiteford et al., 2013), and an estimated $16 trillion will be lost between 2011 and 2030 due to the direct costs of care and lost income as a result of disability or mortality attributable to mental disorder (Bloom et al., 2011). Complicating the matter, mental illnesses tend to accrue high rates of comorbidity with other diseases, including cardiovascular disease, diabetes, and substance use disorders. As a result, mental illness is associated with increased mortality: a recent meta-analysis found the median reduction in life expectancy was 10.1 years, with a range from 1.4 to 32 years (Walker, McGee, and Druss, 2015).

The costs of mental illness are further amplified by lack of access to treatment. The WHO reports that 76 to 85 percent of people with serious mental illness in low-income and middle-income countries receive no treatment, and between 35 and 50 percent of people in high-income countries do not receive care (WHO, 2013). In the United States, the public mental health system, which may be a resource for the uninsured, is strained because it provides approximately two-thirds of all mental health care. Despite a significant decline in the number of uninsured persons in recent years attributable to federal legislation, mental health care is typically underinsured, leading to insufficient and/or low-quality care (Barry, Goldman, and Huskamp, 2016; Bartlett and Manderscheid, 2016; Goplerud, 2013).

Compounded Disparities

Review of the determinants of mental health reveals a Gordian knot, as mental illness tends to perpetuate many of the social determinants that can give rise to or exacerbate mental illness. Disparities in housing, employment, and criminal justice involvement, for example, are closely linked with mental illness because of the ways that mental illness can impact functioning (WHO, 2014). Disruption in mood, thinking, and/or relationships can destabilize employment and/or housing, yet without stable housing and income, mental illness is exacerbated. Disturbing behavior related to mental illness may attract the attention of law enforcement and begin a process of cycling in and out of the criminal justice system, which is highly disruptive to continuity of care and often worsens symptoms. Even seemingly less-related determinants can have large impacts: elements of the built environment (e.g., public transportation) can be critical barriers to obtaining consistent care, for example.

One social determinant that must be singled out is stigma. Cultural and social norms around the world have long marginalized people with mental illness, eroded their rights, and stymied development of supportive health care practices and policies. Despite the gains of the last few decades, stigma remains a prevalent problem.

In short, many social disparities are risk factors for mental illness, and mental illness often widens social disparities. It is important to recognize these relationships because they underscore the complex nature of mental illness and mental health care and make clear that public health efforts are needed across multiple levels and sectors—not just at the individual level in the health care sector (WHO, 2014).

A Brief History of Mental Health Policy in the United States

During the American colonial era, people with mental illness[2] in America were generally considered the responsibility of their family and friends (Slobogin et al., 2013). During the Enlightenment period in the 1700s, an era of therapeutic optimism emerged, characterized by a belief that scientific study would reveal the causes of mental illness and would yield a cure. The United States established its first state hospital dedicated to the provision of mental health care in 1773, and the number of psychiatric hospitals in Europe and America increased dramatically during the 1800s (Eghigian, 2010).

Emergence of the Psychiatric Hospital as the Model of Care

Reliance on institutional care grew during the nineteenth century in the United States and elsewhere in the Western world, undergirded by civil commitment laws authorizing involuntary confinement of mentally ill persons. Legal authority in the United States was firmly grounded in the state's "police power" to protect public health and safety and in its obligation (as "*parens patriae*") to protect citizens unable to protect themselves. Although late nineteenth-century reformers complained about poor conditions in the institutions and questioned the effectiveness of institutional treatment, the medically grounded institutional model survived and was broadened by a new generation of paternalistic commitment statutes in the mid-twentieth century, which sought to make commitment easier due to optimism in new advances in treatment (Slobogin et al., 2013; Boldt, 2014).

Deinstitutionalization

During the 1960s, the modern era of mental health policy began to emerge, marked by the downsizing and closing of state psychiatric hospitals. Deinstitutionalization was driven by several factors, including the high costs of institutional care, critiques of institutional care as oppressive and dehumanizing, nascent sensitivity to the civil rights of persons with mental illness, allegations that psychiatry was used as a form of social control, and a renewed optimism about the ameliorative effects of new pharmacotherapies and community-based mental health services.

Broadly speaking, the civil rights movement of the 1960s and expansion of federal funding for community mental health services propelled the public mental health system in the United States toward a community-based model (Petrila, 2001). Litigation led to landmark decisions vindicating rights of persons with mental illness, including due process in civil commitment proceedings, freedom from coerced treatment in the absence of danger to self or others (e.g., *O'Connor v. Donaldson*, 422 U.S. 563 [1975]), and a right to treatment upon commitment. Federal policies, including Medicaid and Social Security expansion, aimed to increase availability of services in the community as alternatives to institutionalization (Petrila, 2001). As a result, the census of public mental health facilities decreased dramatically: in 1956 the average daily census was 551,390 out of 169 million Americans, but by 2004 the average daily census was 55,000 out of 275 million Americans (Slobogin et al., 2013).

Individuals' Rights versus Treatment Needs

Legal and ethical discourse in mental health policy during the period of deinstitutionalization largely focused on the tension between benevolence and respect for patient autonomy, and on the meaning and normative significance of decisional capacity (Appelbaum, 1994). Physicians traditionally acted to benefit their patients based on their own judgments about patients' needs (both for information and for treatment), but respect for patient autonomy demands protection of patients' rights to receive full information and to make their own judgments about what treatment they receive. In the legal context, this theme translated into debates, which continue into the present day, about the justifications for coercive confinement/treatment and the scope of the individual's right to refuse psychiatric treatment.

On one side, courts have insisted on narrow and specific criteria to justify involuntary hospitalization or forcible medication of involuntarily hospitalized patients. For example, courts may require that there be a substantial likelihood of harm to self or others as a result of the mental illness, the likelihood of which must be demonstrated by "clear and convincing" evidence in most jurisdictions. On the other side, critics of the "right to refuse" treatment have argued that the commitment laws should focus on the "needs" (i.e., treatment) of persons with mental illness and have bemoaned the tragic consequences of allowing suicidal or helpless persons with mental illness to "die with their rights on" (i.e., respecting autonomy to the point of allowing harm to occur; Treffert, 1973).

A current iteration of this ongoing tension in mental health policy focuses on the legitimacy of "mandated outpatient treatment" (MOT).[3] MOT is the provision of treatment in an outpatient setting, but under the constraint of a court order. A person who fails to meet requirements of an MOT plan may be taken into custody for evaluation or treatment. MOT is an appealing option to many because it serves benevolent aims of providing treatment to those in need of it through a less intrusive method than institutional confinement. Opponents, however, highlight the increased paternalism of extending involuntary treatment into community settings and widening the net of social control.

Ethical Principles for Contemporary Mental Health Policy

Deinstitutionalization has been the distinguishing feature of twentieth-century mental health policy in the United States. However, shifting the locus of mental health services from institutions to communities amounts simply to ending an old policy rather than creating a new one. First, there has been a collective failure to establish the community-based services and supports that are needed to enable persons with mental illness to function safely and successfully in the community. Second, reducing unwarranted coercion, by itself, provides a thin and inadequate ethical foundation for the transformative mental health policies needed to vindicate both the rights and needs of persons with mental illness and to assure the mental health and well-being of the population. We next highlight several ethically salient strands of contemporary mental health policy in the United States (which are echoed in international human rights documents and may inform global policy as well [see UN, 2006]).

One policy strand emphasizes inclusion and integration. The Americans with Disabilities Act (42 US Code §§ 12101–12213 [1990]), a US civil rights law prohibiting disability discrimination, has become a charter for freedom for persons with mental illness. Its passage signaled the overarching importance of facilitating inclusion and integration of persons with disabilities, including mental disabilities, into the community, and pressed state and local governments to establish services and supports in the community to enable persons with mental disabilities to achieve equal citizenship.

Another policy strand reflects empowerment and recovery. As used in the behavioral health field, "recovery" describes an ongoing process of gaining greater control over one's own life, partly through gaining control over symptoms, but also through attending to needs in other domains, such as work and relationships. The recovery model emerged from the psychiatric rehabilitation movement, which expanded the view of mental health treatment to encompass consumers'[4] psychosocial needs, and the mental health consumer movement, which emphasized the importance of basic human rights and decried social discrimination and stigma (Pouncey and Lukens, 2010). Although it is difficult to define recovery concretely, several key concepts include autonomy, empowerment, respect, responsibility, and human rights (Davidson et al., 2005; Jacobson and Greenley, 2001).

Yet another salient policy strand concerns the emergence of personal responsibility for managing chronic health conditions. A corollary of empowerment is responsibility. Advances in treatment and the emergence of recovery-oriented frameworks have highlighted the nature of mental illness as a chronic health condition because they have increased the ability to attain and *maintain* wellness. Thus, like persons with other chronic conditions, such as diabetes, persons with a mental illness have the opportunity to view their treatment with a preventive and maintenance orientation and to interact with their families and clinicians accordingly. This counteracts the tendency to see a person with mental illness as a crisis waiting to happen that must be controlled by coercive means.

In this context, it is important to assist persons with mental illness to take control of their treatment; for example, an *advance directive* can be a tool of empowerment in mental health treatment (Elbogen et al., 2007; Scheyett et al. 2007), and facilitating the use of advance directives as part of routine care of persons with serious mental illness should be an explicit goal of contemporary mental health policy (Kemp, Zelle, and Bonnie, 2015; Zelle, Kemp, and Bonnie, 2015). The emphasis on taking responsibility for managing one's own condition also has the potential effect of eroding stigma, because it highlights the similarities (rather than the differences) between mental illness and other chronic health conditions. Mental illnesses (and neurological conditions, such as epilepsy) differ from diabetes because they affect the brain, but they are similar because they are rooted etiologically in the genetic predispositions, environmental exposures, and gene-environment interactions that account for all health conditions. Indeed, advances in understanding of the neurobiological underpinnings of mental illnesses help to normalize them as health problems.

Three Ethical Challenges

This final part of the chapter focuses the population-level ethical discourse on three ethical issues related to persons with mental illness: enhancing access to and utilization of services, preventing harm, and respecting the interests of families.

Justice, Access, and Utilization of Services and Supports

In the United States, as well as many other countries, many people with mental illness have no meaningful access to mental health care at all or are severely underserved. For example, in 2015, 34.7 percent of adults with serious mental illness did not receive any treatment (CBHSQ, 2016). The unfinished business of deinstitutionalization is the creation of the mental health services and supports that are needed to enable persons with mental illness to function successfully in the communities where they live. The creation of services and supports implicates the general ethical discussions of justice in health care and the ongoing debate regarding the best path to universal access to health care in the United States. This section focuses on two distinctive features of that debate regarding mental health care: lack of access (or parity in access) to health insurance (or free services), and the role of stigma in deterring utilization of available services.

Historically, mental health services in the United States were not covered by health insurance or were severely underinsured. Medicaid, which is government-funded, covered some services for the poor, but most medically indigent people were not eligible for Medicaid. The result was that states and localities provided a safety net of emergency services for persons experiencing mental health crises. As recently as 2011, mental health care was financially inaccessible for 51 percent of the population (SAMHSA, 2013). The Patient Protection and Affordable Care Act (Pub. L. No. 111-148, 124 Stat. 119 [2010]) and the Mental Health Parity and Addiction Equity Act (26 U.S.C. § 9812, 29 U.S.C. § 1185a, 42 U.S.C. § 300gg-5 [2012]) significantly increased access to covered mental health services for many people: one estimate suggested that Medicaid expansion would increase mental health and substance use coverage to approximately 16 million people by 2019 (Kessler, 2014; Sipe et al., 2015). However, as of 2014, 1.9 million uninsured people with a mental illness or substance use disorder lived in states that had not adopted Medicaid expansion under the ACA (HHS, 2016) and were entirely dependent on care from a severely underfinanced public mental health services system.

What is more, the gaps in mental health services are accompanied by gaps in subsidized and supportive housing and other community supports. These gaps in services and community supports are widely believed to be at least partially responsible for the increasing number of arrests and detentions of persons with mental illness in local jails, as well as the steady stream of police shootings of persons with mental illness (Kennedy-Hendricks et al., 2016; Steadman et al., 2009; Wilper et al., 2009). Whatever one's position on the demands of justice in access to health care or the underlying causes of "criminalization" of people with mental illness, the substantial number of people with mental illness who are incarcerated presents a significant public health challenge for many communities. Only public action can ameliorate this problem (see, e.g., Harki, 2016; Kennedy-Hendricks et al., 2016; Kindy and Elliott, 2015; Morse, 2016; Swanson, 2016).

The insufficiency of public mental health services is not due solely to lack of insurance and lack of public funding for direct care. Even when services are accessible, persons with mental illness are often deterred from accessing them (or continuing to engage with them) due to social stigma, which has a pervasive history across cultures and dating back to ancient times (Hill et al., 2016; Nadeem et al., 2007; SAMHSA, 2013; VanSickle et al., 2016). Most studies have found positive signs in destigmatizing mental illness and in raising public understanding, including worldwide adoption of Mental Health First Aid training (see also, e.g., Crisanti et al., 2016; Kenny and Bizumic, 2016). The growing movement toward the integration of behavioral health care into primary (medical) health care in the United States also should help counter stigma and help people understand that mental health is a component of overall health. A cross-systems approach that connects and coordinates mental health services across health, justice, education, and social service agencies is needed.

Another avenue to reducing the current ethical tension around access to mental health care is for public mental health to ensure that people with mental illness have a voice in policymaking. The widespread adoption of the recovery model is laudable in part because it does just that. For example, peer support specialists (individuals who identify as having a mental illness and commit themselves as volunteers or employees of mental health care providers) effectuate procedural justice by bringing the affected people directly into the process of shaping public mental health services. Here, *procedural justice* refers to the public health moral consideration of ensuring public participation in practice and policy decisions such that they feel an ownership of policies, rather than the conceptualization of procedural justice as people's assessment of the fairness of a legal decision-making process, as described by Tom R. Tyler (2003). The recovery model's adoption has also led to a definition of quality of life by people with mental illness, rather than by a paternalistic society—people do not seek to be "cured" and made "normal," but rather to achieve a level of wellness that allows them to take meaningful control over their lives. Continued movement in these directions may contribute a great deal to empowering people with mental illness to utilize health care services.

Preventing Harm

As noted earlier, the ethics of coercion has been a preoccupying concern in mental health law. The question to be addressed here is how the lens of public health ethics sheds new light on the ethics of coercion in mental health care. Traditionally, each instance of involuntary treatment is considered to affect only that case: Did the intervention prevent suffering by, or injury to, the person (e.g., suicide) or someone else (e.g., assault), or did the failure to intervene result in an otherwise avoidable suffering or injury? To evaluate the justification for coercion in the individual case, the balance is struck at the clinical level, taking the patient's decisional capacity, the risk of harm, and the availability and effects of alternative interventions into account. But how does one evaluate involuntary treatment *from a population perspective*?

Ethical analysis of civil commitment (and other preventive or coercive interventions, such as warning a potential victim or taking other precautionary action) can be analogized to traditional public health crisis management. Treatment of persons with dangerous contagious diseases, such as tuberculosis, includes restraint of a person for treatment, whether through isolation (i.e., separation from people without the disease), directly observed therapy (i.e., provision of treatment by a health professional who observes the patient take the medication), or aggressive community treatment (e.g., intensive preventive treatment of those without the disease). Interventions like these implicate justificatory conditions,[5] such as necessity (i.e., the strategy is necessary to achieve the public health goal) and least infringement (i.e., the strategy is the least restrictive and least intrusive possible), at the level of the *individual*, but the benefits of the interventions are assessed by measuring the incidence of disease in the *population* (e.g., the number of new infections prevented by the intervention). In comparison, restricting the liberty of a person with mental illness is justified because of the need to reduce a specific threat of harm to the patient or someone else at the time of the intervention. The population benefits are obtained by aggregating the benefits of each individual intervention.

The legal changes in the 1970s that were noted earlier included case law that narrowed the parameters for civil commitment. Courts and subsequent legislation made clear that a person's liberty cannot be infringed merely because treatment may be beneficial; people have a right to refuse treatment, no matter how "unwise" that decision may be, unless a person poses a serious danger to themselves or others. The justification for coercion is measured one case at a time, and the courts generally insist on proof of a serious and immediate threat.

From a population perspective, what were the effects of narrowing these criteria? Were commitments reduced? With what effect on individuals and on the population? Not surprisingly, there have been no controlled trials on the application of civil commitment criteria, and the few before/after studies on this question tend to show that narrowing or broadening the criteria has had relatively little effect compared to other influences on hospitalization and commitment practices, such as reducing the number of beds or the level of insurance reimbursement. Recent controlled trials of mandatory outpatient treatment, however, have suggested that being under an MOT order for at least six months increased treatment engagement and reduced violent behavior, as compared with receiving outpatient services without the order (e.g., Phelan et al., 2010; Swartz et al., 2010). Results of other studies have been mixed, though, so it is not yet clear whether a strong balance of benefits is accrued and whether infringement of autonomy is offset by claims of effectiveness. Another interesting question is whether disqualifying persons who have been involuntarily committed from purchasing or carrying a firearm reduces suicides or firearm-related injuries and deaths to other victims. Systematic research on these long overlooked questions is just emerging (e.g., Swanson et al., 2015), posing the ethical challenge of weighing the population benefits of categorical restrictions against the principle of individualized decision-making that has generally characterized mental health law and ethics.

Privacy and Relational Autonomy

Advances in treatment may allow for activities at the secondary prevention level, but they also implicate autonomy interests. For example, psychotic symptoms (e.g., hallucinations and delusions) often first present in late adolescence or early adulthood, and recent clinical research has underscored the importance of intervening as early as possible with emergent psychotic disorders. Although proactive family involvement in such programs may be viewed by consumers as overly paternalistic and intrusive, the programs may be supported by the theory of relational autonomy, which posits that an individual's autonomy is informed by and even promoted through the person's relationships with others because her sense of self and what is moral and ethical is informed by these relationships. Thus, a program that increases family involvement may ultimately increase a person's autonomy rather than infringe it.

Unrelated to such programs, proposals to increase access by families to otherwise private health information have been advanced, with proponents arguing that allowing the person's support system to be engaged in treatment can avoid a worsening of symptoms and result in benefits to the community as well as the individual (Castro, 2015; Johnston, 2008). Critics, however, argue that such policies weight population (including family) interests over the individual's rights and may further stigmatize mental illness (e.g., Mathis, 2016).

Considering earlier sections of this chapter, it is worth asking whether improved access and decreased stigma would encourage a young person in the early stages of mental illness to engage in treatment and share information, and thus abate the tension between privacy and well-being.

Conclusion

A rich discourse on the ethics of mental health policy and law has emerged since the beginning of deinstitutionalization. That discourse has focused almost entirely on balancing the benefits to the individual and society achieved by involuntary treatment and unwanted disclosure of information against the affront to individual liberty and privacy that they entail. In this chapter, we have shifted the focus of ethical discourse to the population level and to the values that ought to be sought in a system for delivering mental health services. The key values are enhancing access, promoting recovery and empowerment, nurturing community integration and equality of citizenship, and encouraging personal responsibility for managing one's own chronic health condition. Systems and policies that promote these values can be expected to reduce mortality and morbidity in and the accompanying social burden of mental illness.

Notes

1. In the absence of a specific reference, such as the US National Survey on Drug Use and Health (NSDUH), or unless a specific technical meaning is intended, this chapter uses the terms mental disorder and mental illness interchangeably.
2. Throughout this chapter we utilize "person-first language" in which the individual is recognized as a person before specifying that he or she happens to have a mental illness. This language-sensitive approach is widely applied in the behavioral health field and is not just "politically correct" but is actually reflective of an enhanced emphasis on autonomy and empowerment, because it does not reduce a person to a mere diagnostic label.
3. Many statutes refer to "assisted outpatient treatment," but we use the term "mandatory outpatient treatment" because it directly expresses the coercive element of such policies. Another common term is "outpatient commitment."
4. Indeed, the preference for terms other than "patient" to identify those receiving treatment is one product of increased respect for autonomy and empowerment of those receiving treatment: many view the term "patient" to embody the traditional "doctor knows best" power differential, and prefer terms that instead reflect the sense of a person's engagement with treatment (e.g., a mental health treatment "consumer").
5. Justificatory conditions are considerations that rebut the presumption in favor of individual rights concerns such as liberty, privacy, and confidentiality. When considering the ethics of public health situations, individual rights are typically given priority over government considerations; however, a public health action that infringes on those rights could be justified if certain considerations are deemed to outweigh the importance of individual rights (Childress and Gaare Bernheim, 2015).

References

APA (American Psychiatric Association). 2013. *Diagnostic and Statistical Manual of Mental Disorders*. 5th ed. (Washington, D.C.: American Psychiatric Publishing).

Appelbaum, P. S. 1994. *Almost a Revolution: Mental Health Law and the Limits of Change* (New York: Oxford University Press).

Barry, C. L., Goldman H. H., and Huskamp, H. A. 2016. "Federal Parity in the Evolving Mental Health and Addiction Care Landscape." *Health Affairs* 35: 1009–1016.

Bartlett, J., and Manderscheid, R. 2016. "What Does Mental Health Parity Really Mean for the Care of People with Serious Mental Illness." *Psychiatric Clinics of North America* 39: 331–342.

Bloom, D. E., Cafiero, E. T., Jané-Llopis, E., Abrahams-Gessel, S., Reddy Bloom, L., Fathima, S., et al. 2011. *The Global Economic Burden of Noncommunicable Diseases*. Report presented at the World Economic Forum, Geneva, September 2011.

Boldt, R. C. 2014. "Perspectives on Outpatient Commitment." *New England Law Review* 49: 39.

Castro, J. 2015. "Piercing the Privacy Veil: Toward a Saner Balancing of Privacy and Health in Cases of Severe Mental Illness." *Hastings Law Journal* 69: 1769.

CBHSQ (Center for Behavioral Health Statistics and Quality). 2016. *2015 National Survey on Drug Use and Health: Detailed Tables*. https://www.samhsa.gov/data/sites/default/files/NSDUH-DetTabs-2015/NSDUH-DetTabs-2015/NSDUH-DetTabs-2015.pdf.

Childress, J. F., and Gaare Bernheim, R. 2015. "Introduction: A Framework for Public Health Ethics." In *Essentials of Public Health Ethics*, edited by R. G. Bernheim, J. F. Childress, R. J. Bonnie, and A. L. Melnick, 3–19 (Burlington, Mass.: Jones and Bartlett Learning).

Crisanti, A. S., Luo, L., McFaul, M., Silverblatt, H., and Pyeatt, C. 2016. "Impact of Mental Health First Aid on Confidence Related to Mental Health Literacy: A National Study with a Focus on Race-Ethnicity." *Psychiatric Services* 67: 350–353.

Davidson, L., O'Connell, M. J., Tondora, J., Lawless, M., and Evans, A. C. 2005. "Recovery in Serious Mental Illness: A New Wine or Just a New Bottle?" *Professional Psychology: Research and Practice* 36: 480–487.

Eghigian, G., ed. 2010. *From Madness to Mental Health: Psychiatric Disorder and Its Treatment in Western Civilization* (New Brunswick, N.J.: Rutgers University Press).

Elbogen, E. B., Swanson, J. W., Swartz, M. S., Van Dorn, R., Ferron, J., Wagner, H. R., et al. 2007. "Effectively Implementing Psychiatric Advance Directives to Promote Self-Determination of Treatment among People with Mental Illness." *Psychology, Public Policy, and Law* 13: 273–288.

Goplerud, E. 2013. *Consistency of Large Employer and Group Health Plan Benefits with Requirements of the Paul Wellstone and Pete Domenici Mental Health Parity and Addiction Equity Act of 2008* (Washington, D.C.: US Department of Health and Human Services). https://aspe.hhs.gov/report/consistency-large-employer-and-group-health-plan-benefits-requirements-paul-wellstone-and-pete-domenici-mental-health-parity-and-addiction-equity-act-2008.

Harki, G. A. 2016. "Virginia Is Outpacing the Nation in Police Shootings of the Mentally Ill." *Virginian-Pilot*, June 4. http://pilotonline.com/news/government/virginia/virginia-is-outpacing-the-nation-in-police-shootings-of-the/article_de1e5f1d-d893-51fb-9d9d-4c47f034ba66.html.

HHS (US Department of Health and Human Services). 2016. "New Report Shows Medicaid Expansion Can Improve Behavioral Health Care Access." http://www.hhs.gov/about/news/2016/03/28/new-report-shows-medicaid-expansion-can-improve-behavioral-health-care-access.html.

Hill, S. K., Cantrell, P., Edwards, J., and Dalton, W. 2016. "Factors Influencing Mental Health Screening and Treatment among Women in a Rural South Central Appalachian Primary Care Clinic." *Journal of Rural Health* 32: 82–91.

Jacobson, N. and Greenley, D. 2001. "What Is Recovery? A Conceptual Model and Explication." *Psychiatric Services* 52: 482–485.

Johnston, S. G. 2008. "The Mental Health Security for America's Families in Education Act: Helping Colleges and Universities Balance Students' Privacy and Personal Safety." *Duquesne Law Review* 46: 211.

Kemp, K., Zelle, H., and Bonnie, R. J. 2015. "Embedding Advance Directives in Routine Care for Persons with Serious Mental Illness: Implementation Challenges." *Psychiatric Services* 66: 10–14.

Kennedy-Hendricks, A., Huskamp, H. A., Rutkow, L., and Barry, C. L. 2016. "Improving Access to Care and Reducing Involvement in the Criminal Justice System for People with Mental Illness." *Health Affairs* 35: 1076–1083.

Kenny, A., and Bizumic, B. 2016. "Learn and ACT: Changing Prejudice Towards People with Mental Illness Using Stigma Reduction Interventions." *Journal of Contextual Behavioral Science* 5: 178–185.

Kessler, R. C., Aguilar-Gaxiola, S., Alonso, J., Chatterji, S., Lee, S., Ormel, J., et al. 2009. "The Global Burden of Mental Disorders: An Update from the WHO World Mental Health (WMH) Surveys." *Epidemiologia e Psichiatria Sociale* 18: 23–33.

Kessler, S. 2014. "Mental Health Parity: The Patient Protection and Affordable Care Act and the Parity Definition Implications." *Hastings Science and Technology Law Journal* 6: 145, 158–160.

Kindy, K., and Elliott, K. 2015. "2015 Police Shootings Investigation." *Washington Post*, December 26. https://www.washingtonpost.com/graphics/national/police-shootings-year-end/.

Mathis, J. 2016. "Mental Health Privacy: Do Inquiring Minds Really Need to Know?" *Human Rights* 41: 10.

Morse, D. 2016. "Mental-Health Crisis Ensnares Inmates, Judges, Jailers and Hospitals." *Washington Post*, June 7. https://www.washingtonpost.com/local/public-safety/mental-health-crisis-ensnares-inmates-judges-jailers-and-hospitals/2016/06/07/b5379c7c-2aa1-11e6-a3c4-0724e8e24f3f_story.html.

Nadeem, E., Lange, J. M., Edge, D., Fongwa, M., Belin, T., and Miranda, J. 2007. "Does Stigma Keep Poor Young Immigrant and U.S.-Born Black and Latina Women from Seeking Mental Health Care?" *Psychiatric Services* 58: 1547–1554.

NIMH (National Institute of Mental Health). 2017. "Serious Mental Illness (SMI) among U.S. Adults." https://www.nimh.nih.gov/health/statistics/mental-illness.shtml.

Petrila, J. 2001. "From Constitution to Contracts: Mental Disability Law at the Turn of the Century." In *The Evolution of Mental Health Law*, edited by L. E. Frost and R. J. Bonnie, 75–100 (Washington, D.C.: American Psychological Association).

Phelan, J. C., Sinkewicz, M., Castille, D. M., Huz, S., and Link, B. G. 2010. "Effectiveness and Outcomes of Assisted Outpatient Treatment in New York State." *Psychiatric Services* 61: 137–143.

Pouncey, C. L., and Lukens, J. M. 2010. "Madness versus Badness: The Ethical Tension between the Recovery Movement and Forensic Psychiatry." *Theoretical Medicine and Bioethics* 31: 93–105.

SAMHSA (Substance Abuse and Mental Health Services Administration). 2013. "Affordability Most Frequent Reason for Not Receiving Mental Health Services." *NSDUH Report*,

September 24. http://www.samhsa.gov/data/sites/default/files/spot075-services-affordability-2013/spot075-services-affordability-2013.pdf.

Scheyett, A. M., Kim, M. M., Swanson, J. W., and Swartz, M. S. 2007. "Psychiatric Advance Directives: A Tool for Consumer Empowerment and Recovery." *Psychiatric Rehabilitation Journal* 31: 70–75.

Sipe, T. A., Finnie, R. K. C., Knopf, J. A., Qu, S., Reynolds, J. A., Thota, A. B., et al. 2015. "Effects of Mental Health Benefits Legislation: A Community Guide Systematic Review." *American Journal of Preventive Medicine* 48: 755–766.

Slobogin, C., Hafemeister, T. L., Mossman, D., and Reisner, R. 2013. *Law and the Mental Health System: Civil and Criminal Aspects*. 6th ed. (St. Paul, Minn.: West Academic Publishing).

Steadman, H. J., Osher, F. C., Robbins, P. C., Case, B., and Samuels, S. 2009. "Prevalence of Serious Mental Illness among Jail Inmates." *Psychiatric Services* 60: 761–765.

Swartz, M. S., Wilder, C. M., Swanson, J. W., Van Dorn, R. A., Robbins, P. C., Steadman, H. J., et al. 2010. "Assessing Outcomes for Consumers in New York's Assisted Outpatient Treatment Program." *Psychiatric Services* 61: 976–981.

Swanson, J., 2016. "Mental Illness, Release from Prison, and Social Context." *JAMA* 316: 1771–1772.

Swanson, J. W., McGinty, E., Fazel, S., and Mays, V. 2015. "Mental Illness and Reduction of Gun Violence and Suicide: Bringing Epidemiologic Research to Policy." *Annals of* Epidemiology 25: 366–376.

Treffert, D. A. 1973. "Dying with One's Rights On." *JAMA* 12: 1649.

Tyler, T. R. 2003. "Procedural Justice, Legitimacy, and the Effective Rule of Law." *Crime and Justice* 30: 283–357.

UN (United Nations). 2006. Convention on the Rights of Persons with Disabilities. https://www.un.org/development/desa/disabilities/convention-on-the-rights-of-persons-with-disabilities.html.

VanSickle, M., Werbel, A., Perera, K., Pak, K., DeYoung, K., and Ghahramanlou-Holloway, M. 2016. "Perceived Barriers to Seeking Mental Health Care among United States Marine Corps Noncommissioned Officers Serving as Gatekeepers for Suicide Prevention." *Psychological Assessment* 28: 1020–1025.

Walker, E. R., McGee, R. E., and Druss, B. G. 2015. "Mortality in Mental Disorders and Global Disease Burden Implications: A Systematic Review and Meta-Analysis." *JAMA Psychiatry* 72: 334–341.

Whiteford, H. A., Degenhardt, L., Rehm, J., Baxter, A. J., Ferrari, A. J., Erksine, H. E., et al. 2013. "Global Burden of Disease Attributable to Mental and Substance Use Disorders: Findings from the Global Burden of Disease Study 2010." *Lancet* 382: 1575–1586.

Wilper, A. P., Woolhandler, S., Boyd, W., Lasser, K. E., McCormick, D., Bor, D. H., et al. 2009. "The Health and Health Care of US Prisoners: Results of a Nationwide Survey." *American Journal of Public Health* 99: 666–672.

WHO (World Health Organization). 2013. *Mental Health Action Plan: 2013–2020* (Geneva, Switzerland: WHO Document Production Services). http://www.who.int/mental_health/action_plan_2013/en/.

WHO (World Health Organization). 2014. *Social Determinants of Mental Health* (Geneva, Switzerland: WHO Document Production Services). http://www.who.int/mental_health/publications/gulbenkian_paper_social_determinants_of_mental_health/en/.

Zelle, H., Kemp, K., and Bonnie, R. J. 2015. "Advance Directives for Mental Health Care: Innovation in Law, Policy, and Practice." *Psychiatric Services* 66: 7–9.

Further Reading

CBHSQ (Center for Behavioral Health Statistics and Quality). 2015. *Behavioral Health Trends in the United States: Results from the 2014 National Survey on Drug Use and Health.* HHS Publication No. SMA 15–4927, NSDUH Series H-50. http://www.samhsa.gov/data/sites/default/files/NSDUH-FRR1-2014/NSDUH-FRR1-2014.pdf.

Kaiser Family Foundation. 2016. *Key Facts about the Uninsured Population.* http://kff.org/uninsured/fact-sheet/key-facts-about-the-uninsured-population/.

CHAPTER 19

PERSONS WITH DISABILITIES AND PUBLIC HEALTH ETHICS

MONIKA MITRA, LINDA LONG-BELLIL, AND ROBYN POWELL

Introduction

Disability is a complex term that can be defined and conceptualized in numerous ways. While the medical model conceptualizes disability as a problem or impairment localized in the individual body or mind, a social perspective suggests disability is a phenomenon created by social oppression and prejudices on society's construction of what is "normal" versus "abnormal." Disability can also be examined within a legal framework. Laws and public policies have changed and adapted over time as the conception of disability has evolved in the medical, social, and political contexts. Disability is now explicitly defined under US law, and individuals with disabilities are granted certain rights and protections.

The chapter will begin with a brief historical perspective of disability in the United States as a context for examining key ethical issues related to public health policy and practice. The chapter will then examine the ethical dimensions of practice and policy flowing from medical, social, and legal perspectives on disability in public health.

Disability and Public Health: Historical Perspectives

Federal programs and data and surveillance systems have differing definitions of disability, so there is no single definition that has been adopted for use in all laws and policies. Nonetheless, six questions used in the American Community Survey are reflected in

US federal law as the data standard for survey questions on disability (HHS, 2011). These include questions relating to whether an individual has serious difficulty hearing, seeing, walking or climbing stairs, dressing or bathing, doing errands or concentrating, and remembering or making decisions because of a physical, mental, or emotional condition. Based on a definition suggested by these questions, there are approximately 61 million adults living with disabilities in the United States (Okoro et al., 2018). Disability rates vary by age, with the prevalence of disability increasing with age. Non-Hispanic black and Hispanic adults are more likely to have a disability than are white non-Hispanic adults. Those with lower education levels, lower incomes, and who are unemployed are also more likely to report a disability.

The United States has a long history of excluding and mistreating persons with disabilities. Changing social and political perspectives on poverty during the seventeenth and eighteenth centuries in Europe and the United States, together with the increasing medicalization of disability during the nineteenth and twentieth centuries, resulted in increasing segregation and stigmatization of persons with disabilities (Braddock and Parish, 2001). Indeed, beginning in the 1800s, persons with disabilities were institutionalized and segregated from society (Braddock and Parish, 2001). Institutionalization hit its peak during the 1950s. Also during the twentieth century, women with disabilities were often involuntarily sterilized (Braddock and Parish, 2001). The 1970s marked the beginning of the deinstitutionalization movement, resulting in persons with disabilities being increasingly integrated into their communities.

Progress has been made in reducing discrimination against and segregation of individuals with disabilities since the passage of the Americans with Disabilities Act of 1990 (ADA), a civil rights law prohibiting discrimination. Nonetheless, studies show that persons with disabilities have poorer health than persons without disabilities, and many health issues related to their health status are preventable. Moreover, compared to persons without disabilities, persons with disabilities are more likely to be unemployed, live in poverty, and participate in social safety-net programs (Brucker and Houtenville, 2015).

Implications for Public Health

Historically, the needs of persons with disabilities have often been unrecognized in public health, and efforts to address these needs since the 1990s have been sporadic and fragmented (Krahn, Walker, and Correa-De-Araujo, 2015). Public health professionals and researchers increasingly recognize that the needs of persons with disabilities must be integrated into all facets of public health, and that disability-related disparities are inequities. Yet few state public health departments have taken specific steps to address these inequities. In the United States, federal agencies with responsibility for public health often fail to include disabled people in public health programs, policies, and research. One notable exception is the Disability and Health Program within the National Center on

Birth Defects and Developmental Disabilities at the US Centers for Disease Control and Prevention (CDC), which since 1997 has funded state capacity-building to improve the health and well-being of persons with disabilities in some states. Nonetheless, a 2016 public health survey, conducted by the National Association of County and City Health Officials (NACCHO), found only 11 percent of local health department administrators recognized persons with disabilities as a population that experiences health inequities (Leser et al., 2016). Although a large number of public health professionals reported including persons with disabilities in emergency preparedness efforts, only between 16 and 47 percent reported including persons with disabilities in health promotion programs such as tobacco cessation, obesity prevention, or screenings (Leser et al., 2016).

In 2002, the Public Health Leadership Society (PHLS) issued "Principles of the Ethical Practice of Public Health" (PHLS, 2002). This code of ethics was designed for reference and use by US public and other institutions with explicit public health missions, and it was subsequently adopted by the American Public Health Association. Underlying the code's twelve principles is the belief that human beings are interdependent and that people and their environments are interdependent as well (PHLS, 2002). This perspective is consistent with more contemporary conceptualizations of disability. For example, the World Health Organization's International Classification of Functioning, Disability and Health (ICF), discussed below, goes beyond the individualistic orientation of the medical model and emphasizes the interaction of individuals with their physical and social environments. The PHLS principles go further to state that "public health should advocate and work for the empowerment of disenfranchised community members... [and] be implemented in a manner that most enhances the physical and social environments" (4). Given the historical disenfranchisement of individuals with disabilities, the code demands an emphasis on comprehensive public health efforts to benefit persons with disabilities at the national, state, and local levels, and places an important and necessary focus on the interaction between the person and the environment.

Conceptual Frameworks and Approaches to Disability

To better identify some key ethical issues pertaining to disability in the United States, three distinct conceptual frameworks might be considered. A purely medical model represents a traditional approach to disability, although it has less influence currently because of its limited considerations of the environment. The social model, which emphasizes society's role in influencing group identity and oppression, is considered the "new paradigm," although it also has not gone without criticism (Beaudry, 2016). Finally, the legal framework provides historical context on how US policy has changed as the understanding of what it means to be disabled has evolved.

Medical Model

Historically, public health research and policies related to improving the well-being of persons with disabilities were based on a traditional "medical model," which considers disabilities to be defects that harm a person's functioning (Shakespeare, 2006). Under this view, persons with disabilities are assumed to have worse health than nondisabled people, which makes disparities inevitable, uninteresting, and even unimportant. This perspective leads practitioners, researchers, and policymakers to consider how persons with disabilities are different and inferior, and it perceives persons with disabilities as inherently limited in their ability to be included fully in society (Evans, 2004). This medical model offers insufficient answers to key questions about the health of persons with disabilities, as examining individual impairments fails to explain the wide gaps in health, function, and access to care between persons with and without disabilities (Meade, Mahmoudi, and Lee, 2015).

Social Model

The social model of disability, developed in reaction to the medical model, argues that the health of persons with disabilities depends on external and contextual factors—namely, the interaction between individuals and their physical and social environment (Shakespeare, 2006). Health is therefore affected by the degree to which persons with disabilities enjoy full rights and inclusion in society. The social model yields novel questions about the social determinants of health and health care disparities for persons with disabilities. Consistent with other disparity populations (e.g., racial and ethnic minorities), public health research and policies focused on the physical and social environment are crucial in terms of understanding and reducing disability-based disparities (Drum et al., 2005).

In 2001, the WHO published the ICF, a framework that integrates the medical and social models of disability. The ICF framework defines disability as an umbrella term that includes bodily impairments, activity limitations, or participation restrictions that relate to a health condition. Hence, these limitations, which interact with personal and contextual factors of the environment, result in disability. The ICF framework is viewed as the most widely accepted model of disability in public health, although the United States has been slow to adopt it (Iezzoni and Freedman, 2008; Krahn et al., 2015).

Legal Framework

Nondiscrimination, the Americans with Disabilities Act, and Related Laws

Two laws, the landmark Americans with Disabilities Act (ADA) and its predecessor, the Rehabilitation Act of 1973, established national mandates prohibiting discrimination based on disability. Collectively, these vital laws prohibit public and private health care providers from discriminating on the basis of disabilities and ensure persons with disabilities have an equal opportunity to participate in and benefit from health care services.

The Rehabilitation Act of 1973 was the first federal civil rights law to protect persons with disabilities. The most well-known provision of the Act is Section 504, which prohibits discrimination against persons with disabilities under any program or activity that receives federal financial assistance.[1] Hence, health care entities and providers that receive federal monies through Medicaid or Medicare must comply with the Act.

On July 26, 1990, President George H. W. Bush signed the ADA into law, extending the protections and prohibitions of the Rehabilitation Act to private entities. Titles II and III of the ADA prohibit disability discrimination and require health care providers to be physically and programmatically accessible to persons with disabilities. Health care providers have legal obligations to comply with the ADA unless they can prove that doing so would cause an undue burden or fundamentally alter the service.

Despite these requirements, health care facilities and services are often not fully accessible. Although national data are unavailable, a recent survey of nearly 2,400 primary care facilities serving Medicaid patients in California revealed that fewer than half of the facilities were fully architecturally accessible, only 8.4 percent had accessible examination tables, and less than 4 percent had accessible weight scales (Mudrick et al., 2012). Moreover, according to Krahn et al. (2015), persons with disabilities often receive incomplete medical examinations because equipment such as weight scales, exam tables, and mammography equipment do not accommodate their disability. Notably, in 2013 the United States Architectural and Transportation Barriers Compliance Board (US Access Board, 2013) released standards to define accessibility of medical equipment. However, the standards are voluntary, and no research yet exists on their effectiveness.

Laws Relating to Health Care for Persons with Disabilities

Although the ADA was a significant step forward in advancing the rights of individuals with disabilities, it failed to improve access to private health insurance due to its inclusion of a "safe harbor" provision for health insurers, which permitted them to continue discriminatory practices, such as denying coverage for persons with preexisting medical conditions, as long as those practices were "based on or not inconsistent with state law" and not "used as a subterfuge to evade the purposes of" the ADA.[2] This provision has been construed to permit insurers to exclude individuals from or limit their health coverage if such exclusions or limitations are "based on sound actuarial principles or related to actual or reasonably anticipated experience"[3] (EEOC, 1993). The Patient Protection and Affordable Care Act of 2010 addressed this interpretation of the ADA by prohibiting the use of preexisting condition exclusions in individual health insurance policies.[4] This change in insurance practices increases access to individual private health insurance coverage among individuals with disabilities.

Public Health Law and Policy Relating to Persons with Disabilities

Public health was historically the province of the states as one of the powers reserved to them by the Tenth Amendment of the US Constitution. Within the last century, however, the federal government has increasingly relied upon its spending power and its authority under the Constitution's Supremacy Clause. That clause establishes the primacy of federal law over state law to implement various public health policies and practices nationwide through the CDC and other federal agencies. The federal government's efforts to exercise its authority in the field of public health have generally been guided by traditional public health principles emphasizing a population focus and prevention orientation coupled with considerations of social justice (Gostin, 2016).

With respect to disability, the principles requiring a focus on population health and prevention have historically been interpreted as requiring a focus on primary prevention, with disability viewed primarily as an outcome that public health initiatives should endeavor to minimize in the general population. Only recently has an understanding of the principle of social justice begun to change the perception of persons with disabilities as a distinct social group who have the same rights to health and well-being as others, and who deserve access to the resources necessary to make that possible.

Ethical Dimensions of Public Health Approaches

Expanding Access to Public Health Programs

Despite the increased awareness of the health needs of persons with disabilities in the United States, persons with disabilities still fare significantly worse than those without disabilities on most health indicators. Persons with disabilities report higher rates of smoking, lack of daily moderate and vigorous physical activity, and higher rates of overweight and obesity. They also report higher rates of chronic diseases, such as asthma, diabetes, hypertension, and cardiovascular disease. Other challenges include negative clinician attitudes, inaccessible medical equipment, and lack of information and knowledge from health care providers (Mitra et al., 2015).

Social justice has been described as "captur[ing] the twin moral impulses that animate public health," which are "to advance human well-being by improving health and to do so particularly by focusing on the needs of the disadvantaged" (Gostin, 2016, 18). Health equity, then, is essential to the ethical practice of public health. The emphasis on social justice in public health has resulted in efforts to reduce health disparities through a variety of measures. For racial and ethnic groups, these efforts included the creation of the federal government's Office of Minority Health, which the Affordable Care Act subsequently imbued with greater importance by placing it high up in the administrative hierarchy in the Office of the Secretary of the Department of Health and Human Services. Health disparities experienced specifically by persons with disabilities, however, have not received the same level of recognition and resources, and they have not been included in these equity initiatives (Krahn et al., 2015).

Public health research and policies concerning multiple identities of persons with disabilities and how disabilities intersect with other identities and affect access to health care has slowly emerged. This emergence is noteworthy, as intersectionality—defined as the recognition that multiple social categories such as race, ethnicity, gender, and disability status intersect at the micro level to reflect macro-level systems of oppression—provides an important framework for public health (Bowleg, 2012). Notably, the limited existing research on intersectionality indicates that people of color with disabilities, as well as lesbian, gay, bisexual, and transgender (LGBT) individuals with disabilities, experience additional significant disparities and difficulties accessing care as a result of their multiple identities and the many layers of discrimination they face (ACMH, 2011; Tarasoff, 2016).

Research indicates that disability is more prevalent among non-Hispanic blacks, which has been attributed to low socioeconomic status, as well as environmental and social factors and poorer health status (Courtney-Long et al., 2015; Goyat, Vyas, and Sambamoorthi, 2016; Kubzansky et al., 2001). The increased rates of disability among racial minorities are notable because studies have revealed that persons of color with disabilities are more likely to experience substantial health care disparities. For example, the life expectancy for whites/Caucasians with Down syndrome is about fifty-five years compared to twenty-five years for blacks/African Americans with Down syndrome (ACMH, 2011). Jones and Sinclair (2008) found persons with both mobility limitations and minority status experienced greater health disparities than adults with either minority status or mobility limitations alone. Moreover, a recent study revealed that Latino and black adults with intellectual and developmental disabilities (IDDs) had worse health outcomes compared to white adults with IDDs, as well as worse health outcomes than nondisabled adults from the same racial and ethnic group (Magaña et al., 2016). These findings indicate that significant gaps in health persist, and that further research is needed to understand the impact of social determinants on the health of persons with disabilities, particularly those from racial and ethnic minority groups.

Likewise, the prevalence of disability is higher among LGBT adults compared with heterosexual adults, which has been attributed to health-related behaviors, decreased access to health care, and socioeconomic factors (Fredriksen-Goldsen, Kim, and Barkan, 2012; Landers and Gilsanz, 2009). Public health research concerning LGBT persons with disabilities is scarce, but it indicates that this population, particularly youth, experience multiple stigmatized identities, which impacts access to appropriate health care (Duke, 2011). Moreover, LGBT persons with disabilities may have an increased need for mental health services, and may face many challenges to accessing appropriate care and services (Olkin, 1999).

Addressing Implicit and Structural Biases

Implicit and structural biases have a negative impact on trust and health care outcomes for persons with disabilities and other historically marginalized communities. Emerging evidence indicates that health care providers, similar to the general population, hold implicit biases (Green et al., 2007; Sabin et al., 2009). In its 2003 report titled *Unequal Treatment*, the US Institute of Medicine (IOM, now the National Academy of Medicine) concluded that implicit bias against members of a social group may negatively affect communication or the care offered to those individuals (IOM, 2003). Structural bias, which is defined by Schulz and Mullings (2006) as the "privileging [of] some groups and denying others access to the resources of society," can also result in significant health disparities (quoted in Yearby, 2011, 87).

Remarkably, research has found that the attitudes of physicians and other health care providers toward persons with disabilities are as negative as those of the general public, if not more so (National Council on Disability, 2009; Pendo, 2008). Indeed, the difference between health care providers and persons with disabilities in evaluating life with disability is striking. For example, in a survey of attitudes of emergency care providers, only 18 percent of physicians, nurses, and technicians believed they would be glad to be alive with a severe spinal cord injury, as compared to 92 percent of persons with a high spinal cord injury who reported they were glad to be alive (Gerhart et al., 1994). More recently, Hausmann et al. (2015) found that health care providers harbored implicit bias toward persons with spinal cord injuries, which can lead to worse outcomes for patients.

Structural biases also impact the ability of persons with disabilities to access appropriate health care. Persons with disabilities are disproportionately poor and are more likely to receive publicly funded health insurance (i.e., Medicaid or Medicare), limiting access to certain health care providers (National Council on Disability, 2009). Limited transportation options also create significant barriers to accessible and appropriate health care providers (National Council on Disability, 2015). Other structural biases experienced by persons with disabilities include professional training and competency of providers, inadequate or no health insurance coverage for visits to specialists, and poor physical access to usable and adapted or specialized examination and diagnostic equipment (National Council on Disability, 2009; Pendo, 2008).

Public health professionals must address the implicit and structural biases experienced by persons with disabilities to ensure that public health practice upholds the principles of social justice. One strategy is to provide training that addresses implicit bias and discrimination. The results of the 2014 NACCHO survey (Leser et al., 2016) demonstrate the need for additional training of local health department staff to ensure that they understand the health needs of persons with disabilities, and to ensure their inclusion in local public health programs. This has led to a response by public health officials. Healthy People 2020 is a federal framework issued by the US Department of Health and Human Services that provides ten-year national goals to improve American health. Significantly, one objective is to "increase the number of Tribes, States, and the District of Columbia that have public health surveillance and health promotion programs for people with disabilities and caregivers" (ODPHP, 2016). In addition, NACCHO has a Health and Disability Project, which provides local health departments with "practical strategies and recommendations to promote the inclusion and engagement of people with disabilities in the planning, implementation, and evaluation of public health programs, products, and services" (NACCHO, 2016).

Similarly, medical providers require additional training in caring for persons with disabilities. Krahn et al. (2015, S203) note that "[e]very major report addressing the poor health of persons with disabilities has called for improvements in the training of health care providers." These include reports issued in 2002 and 2005 by the Office of the

Surgeon General and a 2009 report by the National Council on Disability (HHS, 2002, 2005; National Council on Disability, 2009). The IOM has similarly acknowledged that "today's physicians may be poorly prepared to meet the complex medical and psychosocial needs of people with disabilities" (Field and Jette, 2007, 130).

Empowerment and Procedural Justice

The ethical practice of public health demands greater attention to policies and programs that integrate and address the needs of persons with disabilities and that require representation of persons with disabilities in the decision-making process to define and clarify what their needs are in the social and political contexts in which they live. Increased systematic collection and analysis of data regarding this population are critical, particularly to inform programs that focus on health, wellness, and the prevention of secondary conditions for persons with disabilities. These efforts will require the allocation of resources to reduce the physical and social barriers to participation. A significant increase in resources for both data collection about and participation of persons with disabilities is ethically justifiable to ensure parity in public health and the integration of considerations about disability in all programs.

Reducing these barriers also requires training the public health and health care workforce to enhance their willingness and capacity to engage individuals with disabilities in decision-making. Training should be supported by providing health professionals with appropriate infrastructure and by holding them accountable both for legally required accessibility standards and for developing administrative processes, grounded in procedural justice, that include community stakeholders, such as persons with disabilities, in decision-making.

It is also critical to include persons with disabilities in health research. According to Krahn et al. (2015, S203), "routinely including people with disabilities in general health research will help close the knowledge gap on effective interventions." Some notable efforts to this end at the federal level include the establishment of the Interagency Committee on Disability Research (ICDR) in 1978 and implementation of requirements to include persons with disabilities in public health research and programs by agencies such as the National Institute on Disability, Independent Living, and Rehabilitation Research (NIDILLR); the Agency for Healthcare Research and Quality (AHRQ); and the CDC (CDC, 2006; US Department of Education, 2012; AHRQ, 2016). Notwithstanding some efforts to include persons with disabilities in public health decision-making, the inclusion of persons with disabilities should be required on decision-making panels in public health and health policy agencies.

Conclusion

This chapter has drawn on medical, social, and legal perspectives to identify and highlight key ethical issues pertaining to the treatment, representation, and inclusion of disabled persons in public health policy and practice. A public health approach, grounded in social justice, supports local, state, and federal policies and programs that aim to reduce discrimination and stigmatization of persons with disability, as well as their higher risk factors for chronic disease or chronic disease catalyzers, such as physical exercise and smoking. Public health professionals, animated by PHLS principles to "ensure that the basic resources and conditions necessary for health are accessible to all," should advocate for programs and resources that address health disparities arising from biological impairment and the social and political context.

Notes

1. Rehabilitation Act of 1973, as amended, 29 U.S.C. §§ 794 et seq.
2. Americans with Disabilities Act of 1990. Public Law 101–336. 108th Congress, 2nd session §§ 12131 et seq. (July 26, 1990).
3. 749 H.R. Rep. No. 45, 101st Cong., 2d Sess., pt. 3, at 70 (1990).
4. Patient Protection and Affordable Care Act. 42 USC. §§ 4302, 5307, and 4203; 2010.

References

ACMH (Advisory Committee on Minority Health). 2011. *Assuring Health Equity for Minority Persons with Disabilities*. https://minorityhealth.hhs.gov/Assets/pdf/Checked/1/ACMHHealthDisparitiesReport.pdf.

AHRQ (Agency for Healthcare Research and Quality). 2016. *Priority Populations*. http://www.ahrq.gov/health-care-information/priority-populations.

Beaudry, J. S. 2016. "Beyond (Models of) Disability?" *Journal of Medical Philosophy* 41(2): 210–228.

Bowleg, L. 2012. "The Problem with the Phrase *Women and Minorities*: Intersectionality—An Important Theoretical Framework for Public Health." *American Journal of Public Health* 102(7): 1267–1273.

Braddock, D., and Parish, S. 2001. "Disability History from Antiquity to the Americans with Disabilities Act." In *Handbook of Disability Studies*, edited by G. L. Albrecht, K. D. Seelman, and M. Bury, 11–68 (Thousand Oaks, Calif.: SAGE).

Brucker, D. L., and Houtenville, A. 2015. "People with Disabilities in the United States." *Archives of Physical Medicine and Rehabilitation* 96: 771–774.

CDC (Centers for Disease Control and Prevention). 2006. "Environmental Barriers to Health Care among Persons with Disabilities: Los Angeles County, California, 2002–2003." *Morbidity and Mortality Weekly Report* 55(48): 1300–1303.

Courtney-Long, E. A., Carroll, D. D., Zhang, Q. C., Stevens, A. C., Griffin-Blake, S., Armour, B. S., et al. 2015. "Prevalence of Disability and Disability Type among Adults—United States, 2013." *Morbidity and Mortality Weekly Report* 64(29): 777–783.

Drum, C. E., Krahn, G., Culley, C., and Hammond, L. 2005. "Recognizing and Responding to the Health Disparities of People with Disabilities." *Californian Journal of Health Promotion* 3(3): 29–42.

Duke, T. S. 2011. "Lesbian, Gay, Bisexual, and Transgender Youth with Disabilities: A Meta-Synthesis." *Journal of LGBT Youth* 8: 1–52.

EEOC (Equal Employment Opportunity Commission). 1993. "Interim Enforcement Guidance on the Application of the Americans with Disabilities Act of 1990 to Disability-Based

Distinctions in Employer Provided Health Insurance." EEOC Notice Number 915.002. https://www.eeoc.gov/policy/docs/health.html.

Evans, J. E. 2004. "Why the Medical Model Needs Disability Studies (and Vice-Versa): A Perspective from Rehabilitation Psychology." *Disability Studies Quarterly* 24(4): 93–98.

Field M., and Jette A. 2007. *The Future of Disability in America* (Washington, D.C.: Institute of Medicine of the National Academies).

Fredriksen-Goldsen, K. I., Kim, H.-J., and Barkan, S. E. 2012. "Disability among Lesbian, Gay, and Bisexual Adults: Disparities in Prevalence and Risk." *American Journal of Public Health* 102(1): e16–e21.

Gerhart, K. A., Koziol-McLain, J., Lowenstein, S. R., and Whiteneck, G. G. 1994. "Quality of Life Following Spinal Cord Injury: Knowledge and Attitudes of Emergency Care Providers." *Annals of Emergency Medicine* 23: 807–812.

Gostin, L. 2016. *Public Health Law: Power, Duty, Restraint* (Oakland: University of California Press).

Goyat, R., Vyas, A., and Sambamoorthi, U. 2016. "Racial/Ethnic Disparities in Disability Prevalence." *Journal of Racial and Ethnic Health Disparities* 3: 635–645.

Green, A. R., Carney, D. R., Pallin, D. J., Ngo, L. H., Raymond, K. L., Iezzoni, L. I., et al. 2007. "Implicit Bias among Physicians and its Prediction of Thrombolysis Decisions for Black and White Patients." *Journal of General Internal Medicine* 22(9): 1231–1238.

Hausmann, L. R. M., Myaskovsky, L., Niyonkuru, C., Oyster, M. L., Switzer, G. E., Burkitt, K. H., et al. 2015. "Examining Implicit Bias of Physicians Who Care for Individuals with Spinal Cord Injury: A Pilot Study and Future Directions." *Journal of Spinal Cord Medicine* 38(1): 102–110.

HHS (US Department of Health and Human Services). 2002. *Closing the Gap: A National Blueprint to Improve the Health of Persons with Mental Retardation: Report of the Surgeon General's Conference on Health Disparities and Mental Retardation* (Rockville, Md.: Office of the Surgeon General).

HHS (US Department of Health and Human Services). 2005. *The Surgeon General's Call to Action to Improve the Health and Wellness of Persons with Disabilities* (Rockville, Md.: Office of the Surgeon General).

HHS (US Department of Health and Human Services). 2011. *Implementation Guidance on Data Collection Standards for Race, Ethnicity, Sex, Primary Language, and Disability Status.* http://aspe.hhs.gov/datacncl/standards/ACA/4302/index.pdf.

Iezzoni, L. I., and Freedman, V. A. 2008. "Turning the Tide: The Importance of Definitions." *JAMA* 299(3): 332–334.

IOM (Institute of Medicine). 2003. *Unequal Treatment: Confronting Racial and Ethnic Disparities in Health Care* (Washington, D.C.: National Academies Press). https://www.nap.edu/read/12875/.

Jones, G. C., and Sinclair, L. B. 2008. "Multiple Health Disparities among Minority Adults with Mobility Limitations: An Application of the ICF Framework and Codes." *Disability and Rehabilitation* 30(12–13): 901–915.

Krahn, G. L., Walker, D. K., and Correa-De-Araujo, R. 2015. "Persons with Disabilities as an Unrecognized Health Disparity Population." *American Journal of Public Health* 105(S2): S198–S206.

Kubzansky, L. D., Krieger, N., Kawachi, I., Rockhill, B., Steel, G. K., and Berkman, L. F. 2001. "United States: Social Inequality and the Burden of Poor Health." In *Challenging Inequities in Health: From Ethics to Action*, edited by T. Evans, M. Whitehead, F. Diderichsen, A. Bhuiya, and M. Wirth, 104–121 (New York: Oxford University Press).

Landers, S. J., and Gilsanz, P. 2009. *The Health of Lesbian, Gay, Bisexual and Transgender (LGBT) Persons in Massachusetts: A Survey of Health Issues Comparing LGBT Persons with their Heterosexual and Non-Transgender Counterparts* (Boston, Mass.: Department of Public Health).

Leser, K. A., Jetty, A., Yates, S. C., and Li, J. 2016. "NACCHO's Baseline Assessment of Disability Inclusion within Local Health Departments." *Journal of Public Health Management and Practice* 22(5): 496–497.

Magaña, S., Parish, S. L., Morales, M. A., Li, H., and Fujiura, G. 2016. "Racial and Ethnic Health Disparities among People with Intellectual and Developmental Disabilities." *Intellectual and Developmental Disabilities* 54(3): 161–172.

Meade, M. A., Mahmoudi, E., and Lee, S. Y. 2015. "The Intersection of Disability and Healthcare Disparities: A Conceptual Framework." *Disability and Rehabilitation* 37(7): 632–641.

Mitra, M., Parish, S. L., Clements, K. M., Cui, X., and Diop, H. 2015. "Pregnancy Outcomes among Women with Intellectual and Developmental Disabilities." *American Journal of Public Health* 48(3): 300–308.

Mudrick, N. R., Breslin, M. L., Liang, M., and Yee, S. 2012. "Physical Accessibility in Primary Health Care Settings: Results from California On-Site Reviews." *Disability Health Journal* 5(3): 159–167.

NACCHO (National Association of County and City Health Officials). 2016. "Health and Disability." http://archived.naccho.org/topics/HPDP/healthdisa/.

National Council on Disability. 2009. *The Current State of Health Care for People with Disabilities*. http://www.ncd.gov/publications/2009/Sept302009.

National Council on Disability. 2015. *Transportation Update: Where We've Gone and What We've Learned*. http://www.ncd.gov/publications/2015/05042015.

ODPHP (Office of Disease Prevention and Health Promotion). 2016. *Healthy People 2020*. https://www.healthypeople.gov/2020/topics-objectives/topic/disability-and-health/objectives.

Okoro, C. A., Hollis, N. D., Cyrus, A. C., Griffin-Blake, S. 2018. "Prevalence of Disabilities and Health Care Access by Disability Status and Type among Adults — United States, 2016." *Morbidity and Mortality Weekly Report* 67(32): 882–887.

Olkin, R. 1999. *What Psychotherapists Should Know about Disability* (New York: Guilford Press).

Pendo, E. 2008. "Disability, Equipment Barriers, and Women's Health: Using the ADA to Provide Meaningful Access." *Saint Louis University Journal of Health Law and Policy* 2: 15–56.

PHLS (Public Health Leadership Society). 2002. *Principles of the Ethical Practice of Public Health*. https://www.apha.org/-/media/files/pdf/membergroups/ethics/ethics_brochure.ashx.

Sabin, J. A., Nosek, B. A., Greenwald, A. G., and Rivara, F. P. 2009. "Physicians' Implicit and Explicit Attitudes about Race by MD Race, Ethnicity, and Gender." *Journal of Health Care for the Poor and Underserved* 20(3): 896–913.

Schulz, A., and Mullings, L. 2006. "Intersectionality and Health: An Introduction." In *Gender, Race, Class and Health: Intersectional Approaches*, edited by A. J. Schulz and L. Mullings, 3–20 (Hoboken, N.J.: Wiley).

Shakespeare, T. 2006. "The Social Model of Disability." *Disability Studies Reader* 2: 197–204.

Tarasoff, L. 2016. "'We Exist': The Health and Well-Being of Sexual Minority Women and Trans People with Disabilities." In *Eliminating Inequities for Women with Disabilities*, edited by S. E. Miles-Cohen and C. Signore, 179–207 (Washington, D.C.: American Psychological Association).

US Access Board. 2013. *Advancing Equal Access to Diagnostic Services: Recommendations on Standards for the Design of Medical Diagnostic Equipment for Adults with Disabilities.* https://www.access-board.gov/guidelines-and-standards/health-care/about-this-rulemaking/advisory-committee-final-report.

US Department of Education. 2012. "National Institute on Disability and Rehabilitation Research: Notice of Proposed Long-Range-Plan for Fiscal Years 2013–2017." *Federal Register* 77(75): 23231–23237.

Yearby, R. 2011. "Breaking the Cycle of Unequal Treatment with Health Care Reform: Acknowledging and Addressing the Continuation of Racial Bias." *Connecticut Law Review* 44(4): 1281–1324.

Further Reading

Gill, C. J. 2001. "Divided Understandings: The Social Experience of Disability." In *Handbook of Disability Studies*, edited by G. Albrecht, K. D. Seelman, and M. Bury, 351–372 (Thousand Oaks, Calif.: SAGE).

Grob, G. N. 1994. *The Mad among Us: A History of the Care of America's Mentally Ill* (New York: Free Press).

Koelen, M. A., Lenneke, V., and Colomér, C. 2001. "Health Promotion Research: Dilemmas and Challenges." *Journal of Epidemiology and Community Health* 55(4): 257–262.

O'Toole, C. J., and Brown, A. A. 2002. "No Reflection in the Mirror." *Journal of Lesbian Studies* 7(1): 35–49.

Roberts, J. L. 2013. "Health Law as Disability Rights Law." *Minnesota Law Review*. http://dx.doi.org/10.2139/ssrn.2027534.

Robey, K. L., Minihan, P. M., Long-Bellil, L. M., Hahn, J. E., Reiss, J. G., Eddey, G. E., et al. 2013. "Teaching Health Care Students about Disability within a Cultural Competency Context." *Disability and Health Journal* 6(4): 271–279.

Stone, D. A. 1984. *The Disabled State* (Philadelphia: Temple University Press).

WHO (World Health Organization). 2001. *International Classification of Functioning, Disability and Health* (Geneva, Switzerland: World Health Organization).

CHAPTER 20

SEXUAL AND GENDER MINORITIES, PUBLIC HEALTH, AND ETHICS

TONYA LITTLEJOHN, TONIA POTEAT, AND CHRIS BEYRER

INTRODUCTION

SEXUAL and gender minorities—lesbian, gay, bisexual, and transgender (LGBT) persons—are a diverse and multifaceted population. Although the communities that make up this particular population are increasingly visible, engaged, and mobilized, there have been uneven gains in advancing their health status and a range of health disparities remains prevalent. The inequities are exacerbated by a relative paucity of data that could otherwise inform public health surveillance, interventions, and policies unique to the needs of these communities, as well as by structural factors that reinforce health inequities.

Present-day health inequities experienced by sexual and gender minorities have a social and historical precedent that has profoundly shaped their collective story (Mayer et al., 2008; IOM, 2011). For most of the twentieth century in the United States, homosexuality—understood as same-sex desire, attraction, or sexual activity—was seen as pathological (Drescher, 2015) and same-sex behavior illegal (IOM, 2011). The pathologization of homosexuality was challenged by the work of Alfred Kinsey, Clellan Ford and Frank Beach, and Evelyn Hooker, who debunked the psychiatric belief that homosexuality was a sign of psychological disturbance (Drescher, 2015; IOM, 2011). Confronted with mounting empirical evidence at a time of shifting cultural and social norms, fueled in part by events such as the Stonewall Riots in 1969, the American Psychiatric Association removed homosexuality from its *Diagnostic and Statistical Manual* (*DSM*) in 1973 (Daniel and Butkus, 2015). The diagnostic revision of homosexuality marked an important shift of the role of medicine in the "social stigmatization of homosexuality" to the moral and political domains (Drescher, 2015; see also Reed et al., 2016; Drescher, 2010).

The history of gender variance and transgender both echoes and provides a contrast to that of homosexuality and sexual orientation. The inclusion of gender identity disorder (GID) in *DSM-III* in 1980 drew criticism from those in the transgender community who felt that labeling the expression of gender as a symptom of a mental disorder would lead to further stigmatization and harm. Others felt the omission of a formal diagnosis would limit access to critical medical and surgical care (Drescher, 2010). The most recent version of the manual, *DSM-5*, revised GID to gender dysphoria, intending to depathologize gender variance while improving access to clinical care. *DSM-5* continues to classify transgender as a mental disorder. Significantly, in the updated World Health Organization's International Classification of Diseases (ICD-11) gender incongruence is considered to be a sexual health condition rather than a mental disorder.

The stigma, discrimination, and criminalization experienced by sexual and gender minorities have a deleterious effect on health and are a fundamental cause of health disparities (IOM, 2011; Link and Phelan, 2005). Institutions, attitudes, and perceptions that have evolved in societies that stigmatize sexual and gender minorities have important implications for the ability of public health to address their needs (IOM, 2011). As a result, sexual and gender minorities may be harder for public health to reach, posing a challenge for health surveillance and the development of tailored, culturally contextualized public health interventions.

To understand the health disparities that sexual and gender minorities face, it is essential to acknowledge the homophobia and transphobia of health care systems, and to recognize that health care systems and worldviews of providers arose from, and were developed within, heteronormative cultures and structures. This chapter identifies the key ethical issues and debates their impacts on the advancement of health for sexual and gender minorities. The chapter begins by identifying perspectives on public health discourse—that is, language, meaning, and constructs—pertaining to sexual and gender minorities. It suggests that how identity and behavior are described has important implications for public health inquiry. The second section, drawing on principles of equity and distributive justice, considers health disparities and the social determinants of health affecting sexual and gender minorities.

Next, we consider the moral dilemmas that emerge in public health surveillance, including methodological issues and the challenge of context, and how social and political impediments, such as stigma and criminalization, can prevent protection of the most vulnerable. We explore ethical issues that have emerged in relation to the human immunodeficiency virus/acquired immunodeficiency syndrome (HIV/AIDS) epidemic as it affects sexual and gender minorities. The chapter concludes with a discussion of how frontline research in partnership with these populations can lead to best practices in public health. It offers options that enable an inclusive, culturally competent, affirming public health for all.

The Sexual and Gender Minority Framework: Defining the Landscape

The language and discourse of sexuality, gender identity, and gender expression are dynamic, evolving, and reflect shifting paradigms of cultural and social meaning. In the Global North lexicon, sexuality and gender-identity diversity is often referred to under the umbrella term of LGBT, encompassing lesbian, gay, bisexual, and transgender—with variants of LGBTI (adding intersex), LGBTQ (adding queer or questioning) , or LGBT+ (adding indeterminate or intersex)—to further distinguish binary from nonbinary, or to describe non-heteronormative and cisnormative (i.e., the alignment of gender identity with assigned sex at birth) notions of gender identity and sexual orientation (Logie et al., 2012). The diversity of characterization and categories across other cultural contexts is vast and has been addressed elsewhere, so the LGBT frame will be used here (Carroll, 2016; Parker, Aggleton, and Perez-Brumer, 2016; Reisner et al., 2016). LGBT represents a diverse population of individuals and groups with a multiplicity of races, ethnicities, and ages, as well as cultural and social constructs of sexuality, gender identity, and gender expression.

Sexuality and *sexual orientation* are terms used to describe sexual behavior, identity, and attraction to the same sex, another sex, or more than one sex (Richards et al., 2016; Bailey et al., 2016; IOM, 2011). *Gender* refers to the norms, roles, and behaviors that typically characterize individuals as male or female, genderqueer, or gender nonbinary (Richards et al., 2016). Sexual orientation and gender identity are universal aspects of the self, but they vary greatly in their interpretation and their specificity to different cultural contexts (Bailey et al., 2016). The term *transgender* describes individuals whose gender identity or expression differs from the sex assigned to them at birth. It may include those who have had gender-affirming chest, breast, or genital surgery; hormonal treatment to masculinize or feminize their body; both; or neither. Transgender people may be sexually oriented toward any gender.

A variety of conditions that lead to atypical development of physical sex characteristics are collectively referred to as intersex conditions or differences of sexual development (DSD) (Malouf and Wisniewski, 2016). These conditions can involve differences of the external genitals, internal reproductive organs, sex chromosomes, or sex-related hormones. These individuals may have undergone genital reconstructive surgery and/or hormone therapy early in life, and they may express a gender identity that is different from that which was assigned at birth.

The use of categorization and the meanings ascribed to sexual and gender minorities, and their variants, must undergo continual evaluation and reflection to ensure ongoing relevance. The allocation of sexual and gender minorities into standardized, replicable, continuous categories, and the omission of context, may fail to capture the diversities that exist within categories as well as the intersections between them (Perez-Brumer et al., 2016). Similarly, categorization with a reliance on behavior as a risk determinant can erase social and cultural contexts (Young and Meyer, 2005).

Intersectionality, a term first coined by civil rights advocate and the legal scholar Kimberlé Williams Crenshaw, makes a useful contribution to the discourse on sexual and gender minorities by offering a way to understand and reflect on the complicated lived reality of individuals (Bauer, 2014; Larson et al., 2016). It suggests that categories of social identity (such as gender, sexual orientation, age, and race) are inextricably linked to social structures and systems of power and representations of dominance, privilege, and oppression in ways that are dynamic and contextually grounded. Inclusion, exclusion, marginalization, and disadvantage are therefore not static, inevitable, or silo concepts, but may be experienced simultaneously at any given point. Intersectionality guides a more nuanced system of inquiry that is not reliant on dichotomous categories or a layering of multiple categories in an additive manner (e.g., black race plus female plus impoverished equals disempowered), but instead sees social inequity as mutually constitutive (Larson et al., 2016). Intersectionality acknowledges complex configurations of social determinants of health, as well as how these social constructs produce health inequities and directly impact sexual and gender minority health. The emphasis is on the embeddedness of identity within social constructs that are contextual and dynamic, rather than universal.

Health Disparities and Inequities of Sexual and Gender Minorities

Justice is a core value and guiding principle of public health, as it seeks to enable the collective advancement of health for all while minimizing systematic inequities and disparities. Lawrence Gostin and Madison Powers (2006, 1054) describe these as the "twin moral impulses" motivating public health. Dan Beauchamp, one of the earliest scholars of justice and public health, observed that the critical barrier to achieving improvements in public health is not a lack of technology but rather an unwillingness by the advantaged to give up any of their advantages to benefit those worse off. He describes this unwillingness as "a social ethic that unfairly protects the most numerous or most powerful from the burdens of prevention" (Beauchamp, 1976, 101). Justice, understood as a fair and equitable distribution of the benefits and burdens of society, or "the fair disbursement of common advantages and the sharing of common burdens" (Gostin and Powers, 2006, 1054), is an antidote to this social ethic. When public health is guided by or pursues justice, it can help to overcome or eliminate powerful social, political, and environmental forces that create, shape, and sustain patterns of systematic disadvantage (Beauchamp, 1976; Gostin and Powers, 2006).

A central issue of justice for sexual and gender minorities is the disproportionate burden of disease and ill health they often experience as a result of issues such as access to and the quality of health care. These challenges, and the resultant health deficits, can be experienced differently by individuals within the group, or according to cultural context and geographical location. Some groups of individuals within sexual and gender minority populations have increased risks and needs, which have been expressed in health prevalence data and disease burdens (Daniel and Butkus, 2015; Cochran and Mays, 2017). For example, gay men and other men who have sex with men, and transgender women who have sex with men, have increased rates of sexually transmitted infections (STIs) and bear a disproportionate burden of HIV (Beyrer et al., 2012; Baral et al., 2013). Disparities in modifiable cardiovascular disease risk factors such as smoking, obesity, and stress have been identified among lesbian and bisexual women based in the United States (Simoni et al., 2017; Caceres et al., 2017). Mounting data support an increased burden of depression and suicidality among transgender populations globally (Grant et al., 2011) compared to their cisgender counterparts. Although health equity in sexual and gender minorities is still a relatively recent area of investigation, such findings highlight the significance of differences attributable to social harms of discrimination and stigma. Data on other disease systems and disparities are more sparse and urgently needed.

Public Health Research and the Challenge of Context

Understanding the nature of the health burden and inequities that sexual and gender minorities face is critical to framing public policy discussions accurately and targeting public health interventions appropriately. There are several significant challenges to collecting robust data to inform health knowledge of this population.

First, as highlighted in the 2011 Institute of Medicine (IOM, now known as the National Academy of Medicine, or NAM) report on the health of LGBT people, there is a challenge to develop and standardize valid and reliable measures of sexual orientation and gender identity (Temple-O'Connor and Wehr, 2013). In part, this may be due to the allocation of sexual and gender minorities to discrete categories, or not adjusting for socially significant variables, that obscure the unique vulnerabilities within the group (Fiereck, 2015). For example, transgender women have historically been categorized according to assigned sex at birth and have been conflated with men who have sex with men. This conflation is troublesome, as it limits insight into attributable differences due to sex or gender, the contribution of specific social and structural determinants of health, and the responsiveness and effectiveness of the public health intervention (Poteat, German, and Flynn, 2016; Perez-Brumer et al., 2016; Reisner et al., 2016; Fiereck, 2015).

There are related issues affecting the integrity and robustness of epidemiological inquiry that must be resolved. As Fiereck (2015, 32) notes, "the effacement or elision of differences between sex and gender" influences how the disease of interest is mapped in the population. It is clear that contextualization of language and meaning in sexuality and gender frame public health surveillance efforts, and a lack of consistency in standardized methods and survey instruments across studies limits the generalizability and relevance of findings (Reisner et al., 2016).

Second, the way in which sexual and gender minorities are conceptualized, and the terminology and categories used to describe the individuals within the population, is dynamic, and this presents both a challenge and an opportunity for the use of epidemiological methodologies for health surveillance. The challenge is how comprehensively to ascertain variations and differences that exist between groups at a global level, and how these differences shape the public health response and effort.

This final point engages with the notion that those who bear the burden of the research (or intervention), particularly when targeted toward the most vulnerable, must also be the ones with the greatest likelihood to benefit from it (Cohen, Kass, and Beyrer, 2007). While sexual and gender minorities are situated in culturally specific contexts, they are concurrently connected to greater political and structural inequalities that occur at a global scale (Padilla et al., 2007). It is therefore incumbent on epidemiologists, public health researchers, and practitioners continually to reflect on and critically engage with cultural meanings, geographical variations, and social constructs of sexuality, identity, and behavior, and with how these impact health burdens and inequities (Perez-Brumer et al., 2016; Conron et al., 2014). This pursuit ensures that both quantitative and qualitative dimensions are captured, and it levers public health researchers and advocates into uncharted areas of inquiry or advocacy.

Stigma, Criminalization, and the Risk-Benefit Ratio

Systematic and persistent violence and discrimination leveled at individuals on the basis of their sexual and gender identity remains one of the great challenges for the human rights agenda. Despite efforts to advance the health of sexual and gender minorities in some countries, they have been stymied by repugnant laws and policies that criminalize same-sex behavior as well as gender nonconformity. In 2016, seventy-two countries recognized by the United Nations (UN) had laws criminalizing homosexuality between consenting adults (Carroll, 2016). The vast majority of these countries are in Africa, Asia, and the Middle East (Schwartz et al., 2015). A further number of nations and political entities, including Russia and Gaza/Palestine, prohibit same-sex relations or have laws against "homosexual propaganda." Thirteen countries have a death penalty that may be applied as a sanction for same-sex sexual acts (Carroll, 2016). In the United States, the US Supreme Court ruled antisodomy laws unconstitutional in 2003; as of 2016 the thirteen states with such laws had not formally repealed them (Carroll, 2016), so they remain visible yet unenforceable in practice. Criminalization strengthens stigmatization, which in turn fortifies discrimination and vulnerability.

Criminalization by nation-states on the basis of sexual identity and behavior contravenes basic human rights instruments that safeguard the rights of sexual and gender minorities, with a profound effect on access to public health goods and interventions. States, as signatories to international treaties and covenants, assume obligations and duties to protect and promote the full realization of rights, including the right of everyone to the enjoyment of the highest attainable standard of physical and mental health articulated in the International Covenant on Economic, Social and Cultural Rights, Article 12(1) (UN, 1967). The legal obligations of states, under international law, prohibit discrimination on the basis of sexual orientation or gender identity and outline obligations to protect individuals from homophobic and transphobic violence; prevent inhuman, cruel, or degrading treatments; repeal laws that criminalize homosexuality, including arbitrary arrest and detainment; and safeguard freedom of expression, association, and peaceful assembly for all sexual and gender minorities (OHCHR, 2012).

However, the legal obligations of states neither guarantee nor provide moral guidance on how states should behave and act to secure health and well-being for all. Zahn et al. (2016) note that even in settings such as South Africa, where protective legal frameworks are in place, including protection of confidentiality and disclosure, these protections alone are insufficient to address violence, discrimination, and attitudes affecting sexual minorities. In a study in Russia on men who have sex with men, the risk of violence and discrimination perpetrated toward study participants was so great that the risks of proceeding did not justify the potential benefits of the findings, and the study was subsequently withdrawn (Hylton et al., 2017).

There are important ethical considerations concerning how to engage and operate in public health practice and research in settings where the population of interest is not recognized or is repressed within the target community. There are examples in which a government has actively opposed public health research and interventions directed toward sexual and gender minorities, based on the belief that it would legitimize the existence of these populations in their country (Amon et al., 2012). If the protective function of public health is abandoned, and the position of the state is given primacy over the health of marginalized groups, who, or what institutions, will protect the well-being of sexual and gender minorities? Responding to changing contexts and awareness of when the safety of individuals is compromised by public health research or intervention has been a devastating reality of operating in contexts that favor stigma and criminalization.

Studies have consistently demonstrated that sexual and gender minorities who encounter high levels of experienced, anticipated, or internalized stigma and discrimination are more vulnerable to negative health outcomes (Poteat et al., 2015; Winskell and Sabben, 2016; Zahn et al., 2016). In one study on HIV risk among men who have sex with men in Senegal, it was noted that even when preventive services were available, fear of violence and arbitrary arrest and related loss of trust in institutions led to decreased uptake of health care and interruptions to service provision (Poteat et al., 2011). The 2013 Same-Sex Marriage Prohibition Act in Nigeria extended existing criminalization of same-sex sexual practices by prohibiting participation in organizations and other forms of association that are supportive of same-sex relationships and sexual practices. Gay men and men who have sex with men experienced greater stigma and discrimination, reported an increased fear associated with seeking health care, and experienced an absence of safe spaces to socialize with others (Schwartz et al., 2015).

By contrast, in Sweden, one of the most progressive countries with regard to sexual and gender minorities, a supportive policy environment has contributed to a reduction of health vulnerabilities experienced by sexual and gender minorities. The removal of the requirement for a sterilization order to change the gender marker on legal documents is a policy that represents the conditions necessary for broader health equity for sexual and gender minorities, and for the fulfillment of basic human rights for all (EU FRA, 2015).

Case Study: HIV/AIDS

The HIV/AIDS epidemic has been at the epicenter of multiple ethical issues concerning the health of sexual and gender minorities. The ongoing global epidemic of HIV reinforces the centrality of justice in the public health mission. Debates related to public health surveillance and intervention testing, consent, disclosure, disproportionate burdens, access to treatment, and stigma have profoundly shaped the global response to HIV among sexual and gender minorities (Cohen et al., 2007; Bayer and Fairchild, 2004).

The earliest cases of AIDS were identified in otherwise healthy young gay men in New York and California in 1981. What followed, with devastating impact, was a tsunami of loss and collective trauma as the epidemic took hold. Gay men, bisexual men, and other men who have sex with men were the most affected. In the public domain, homosexuality became synonymous with AIDS, and this indelibly marked the global response to the epidemic, which stigmatized those living with the virus, limited effective public health responses in some cases, and drove coercive and punitive ones in others (Beyrer et al., 2012). The gay rights movement undoubtedly had an impact on the epidemic from early on, with politically mobilized groups driving advocacy, access, and treatment and prevention strategies (Bayer and Fairchild, 2004). However, at the same time, the gay community was confronted with the paradox that increased social organization, empowerment, and visibility also translated to increased stigma and discrimination, and to fewer protections at a local level. This legacy continues in the present day.

At the global level, the trajectory of HIV has been slowed by advances in understanding of biomedicine and modes of transmission, and by public health–based interventions to mitigate impact, such as the use of condoms, routine testing, and access to treatment (Cohen et al., 2007). The emergence of primary prevention and treatment as prevention, including access to and use of lifesaving antiretroviral drugs (ARVs) to decrease susceptibility to the virus in the uninfected or infectiousness in those living with HIV, has been similarly transformative (Caceres et al., 2015). The efficacy of pre-exposure prophylaxis (PrEP), a combination of two HIV medicines made available to individuals at very high risk for HIV, has been demonstrated, but as a preventive public health strategy PrEP has not been universally adopted, and the uptake at the country level is slow (Beyrer et al., 2016).

Despite gains in arresting transmission at the global level, the epidemic continues unabated among sexual and gender minorities in places where stigma and discrimination prevail, and in key populations of gay men, other men who have sex with men, and transgender people who have sex with men (Beyrer et al., 2016). In 2014, more than 90 percent of new HIV infections in Central Asia, Europe, North America, the Middle East, and North Africa were among key populations, which also included sex workers, people who use drugs, and incarcerated persons (UNAIDS, 2016).

Remaining ethical challenges for the HIV response include advancing access to HIV prevention and treatment options to ensure sexual and gender minorities are not left behind. The cornerstone achievement will be to situate the public health agenda—discourse, surveillance, and intervention—in the cultural, geographical, and structural contexts that define the lived reality of sexual and gender minorities. Such a response will need to be supported by community partnerships to inform research methods and data points required to develop service models that maximize benefit for all.

Best Practices for Gender and Sexual Minority Health

Safe environments and spaces to access health care initiatives that engage sexual and gender minorities are fundamental to advancing the health of sexual and gender minorities. The disproportionate burden among this group of HIV and mental health challenges, including depression, anxiety, and suicide risk, have been well documented. There are limited data on specific health conditions and risk determinants in underrepresented population groups, including those pertaining to lesbians, bisexual females, and transgender populations, and to adolescent sexual and gender minorities. Understanding intersecting themes of identity, culture, geography, and structural disadvantage is critical to guide a more nuanced approach aimed at resolving key ethical issues in public health surveillance, policy, and programming.

For researchers, ethics review board members, and those seeking to improve the health and well-being of sexual and gender minority communities, there are a number of important best practice approaches that have emerged in the past decades of sexual and gender minority health research.

First and foremost is the importance of context. A relatively low-risk epidemiologic study that includes capture of personal identifiers and assessment of sexual identity or practices may be of little concern in settings where same-sex behavior is legal and sexual and gender minority persons are protected by the state. The same study, however, may be life-threatening for participants in states like Iran, Saudi Arabia, or the Sharia states of northern Nigeria. In contrast, transgender identity and persons may be acceptable in Iran, but face intense medical, social, and community opprobrium in Jamaica, where "cross-dressing" has led to mob violence and extrajudicial execution (US Department of State, 2015).

The centrality of context leads to a second tenet: the need for public health professionals to work closely and consistently with sexual and gender minority communities, leaders, and activists in assessing the risks and benefits of health research or interventions. Community members typically know a great deal more than professional voices about the realities on the ground, what is safe and not safe, and who is best placed to implement needed work. Arguably, more than for any other population, the centrality of genuine community participation is essential to ensuring minimization of risks and maximization of benefits, both in public health research and practice.

Both contextual awareness and community engagement must also be sustained over time, as context is dynamic, can change rapidly, and requires vigilance on the part of investigators and human subjects committees. In Russia, the passage of new national antigay legislation by the Putin administration, and the widespread tolerance for antigay vigilante violence, including the physical intimidation of gay men and staff members at sexual and gender minority–friendly clinics, has led to a rapidly deteriorating safety environment. Such secular trends can develop quickly and significantly alter risk-benefit ratios.

Addressing the needs of sexual and gender minority minors and adolescents is also an area fraught with numerous special challenges and concerns. One particularly contentious issue is the current debate over "conversion therapy" or "reparative therapy." These purported therapies have the goal of attempting to change sexual orientation to heterosexual, and gender-variant gender identity to sex assigned at birth. There is a clear scientific consensus that there is no evidence for efficacy of such therapies, and abundant evidence for harm (IOM, 2011). Indeed, they have been made illegal in a number of US states and in other countries, based on the evidence of an array of harms. Yet they remain common, widely practiced in many settings, and the subject of intense political debate. Because minors may be subject to these abuses when consent is obtained from parents, youth are particularly vulnerable to these violations of the right to personhood.

In conclusion, sexual and gender minority health is an emerging area of public health that urgently needs expansion, investigation, and engagement. There is an ethical imperative to address the health disparities faced by these individuals, families, and communities, through research, policies, and interventions that are responsive to particular needs, attentive to the social and political context, and guided by the principles of social justice, health equity, and the protection of basic human rights.

References

Amon, J. J., Baral, S. D., Beyrer, C., and Kass, N. 2012. "Human Rights Research and Ethics Review: Protecting Individuals or Protecting the State?" *PLoS Medicine* 9(10): e1001325. https://journals.plos.org/plosmedicine/article?id=10.1371/journal.pmed.1001325.

Bailey, J. M., Vasey, P. L., Diamond, L. M., Breedlove, S. M., Vilain, E., and Epprecht, M. 2016. "Sexual Orientation, Controversy, and Science." *Psychological Science in the Public Interest* 17(2): 45–101.

Baral, S., Poteat, T., Stromdahl, S., Wirtz, A., Guadamuz, T. E., and Beyrer, C. 2013. "Worldwide Burden of HIV in Transgender Women: A Systematic Review and Meta-analysis." *Lancet* 13(3): 214–222.

Bauer, G. R. 2014. "Incorporating Intersectionality Theory into Population Health Research Methodology: Challenges and the Potential to Advance Health Equity." *Social Science and Medicine* 111: 10–17.

Bayer, R., and Fairchild, A. L., 2004. "The Genesis of Public Health Ethics." *Bioethics* 18(6): 473–492.

Beauchamp, D. 1976. "Public Health as Social Justice." *Inquiry* 13: 1–14.

Beyrer, C., Baral, S. D., Collins, C., Richardson, E. T., Sullivan, P., Sanchez, J., et al. 2016. "The Global Response to HIV in Men Who Have Sex with Men." *Lancet* 388(10040): 198–206.

Beyrer, C., Baral, S.D., van Griensven, F., Gooreau S., Chariyalertsak S., Wirtz A., et al. 2012. "Global Epidemiology of HIV Infection in Men Who Have Sex with Men." *Lancet* 380 (9839) 367–377.

Caceres, B. A., Brody, A., Luscombe, R. E., Primiano, J. E., Marusca, P., Sitts, E. M., et al. 2017. "A Systematic Review of Cardiovascular Disease in Sexual Minorities." *American Journal of Public Health* 107(4): e13–e21.

Caceres, C. F., Koechlin, F., Goicochea, P., Sow, P-S., O'Reilly, K. R., Mayer, K., et al. 2015. "The Promises and Challenges of Pre-exposure Prophylaxis as Part of the Emerging Paradigm of Combination HIV Prevention." *Journal of the International AIDS Society*. 18(Suppl. 3): 1–9.

Cochran, S. D., and Mays, M. 2017. "Advancing the LGBT Health Research Agenda: Differential Health Trends within the Lesbian, Gay, and Transsexual Populations." *American Journal of Public Health* 107(4): 497–498.

Cohen, J., Kass, N., and Beyrer, C. 2007. "Human Rights and Public Health Ethics: Responding to the Global HIV/AIDS Pandemic." In *Public Health and Human Rights: Evidence-Based Approaches*, edited by C. Beyrer and H. F. Pizer (Baltimore, Md: Johns Hopkins University Press).

Conron, K., Landers, S., Reisner, S., and Sell, R. 2014. "Sex and Gender in the U.S. Health Surveillance System: A Call to Action." *American Journal of Public Health*. 104(6): 970–976.

Carroll, A. 2016. *State Sponsored Homophobia 2016: A World Survey of Sexual Orientation Laws: Criminalisation, Protection and Recognition* (Geneva: International Lesbian, Gay, Bisexual, Trans and Intersex Association).

Daniel, H., and Butkus, R. 2015. "LGBT Health Disparities." *Annals of Internal Medicine* 163(2): 135–137.

Drescher, J. 2010. "Queer Diagnoses: Parallels and Contrasts in the History of Homosexuality, Gender Variance, and the *Diagnostic and Statistical Manual*." *Archives of Sexual Behaviour* 39: 427–460.

Drescher, J. 2015. "Out of *DSM*: Depathologizing Homosexuality." *Behavioral Sciences* 5: 565–575.

EU FRA (European Union Agency for Fundamental Rights). 2015. *The Fundamental Rights Situation of Intersex People* (Vienna: EU FRA).

Fiereck, K. 2015. "Cultural Conundrums: The Ethics of Epidemiology and the Problems of Population in Implementing Pre-exposure Prophylaxis." *Developing World Bioethics* 15(1): 27–39.

Gostin, L. O., and Powers, M. 2006. "What Does Social Justice Require for the Public's Health?" *Health Affairs* 25(4): 1053–1060.

Grant, J. M., Mottet, L. A., Tanis, J., Harrison, J., Herman, J. L., and Keisling M. 2011. *Injustice at Every Turn: A Report of the National Transgender Discrimination Survey* (Washington, DC: National Center for Transgender Equality and National Gay and Lesbian Task Force).

Hylton, E., Wirtz, A. L., Zelaya, C. E., Latkin, C., Peryshkina, A., Mogilnyi, V., et al. 2017. "Sexual Identity, Stigma, and Depression: The Role of the 'Anti-gay Propaganda Law' in Mental Health among Men Who Have Sex with Men in Moscow, Russia." *Journal of Urban Health* 94(3): 319–329.

IOM (Institute of Medicine). 2011. *The Health of Lesbian, Gay, Bisexual, and Transgender People: Building a Foundation for Better Understanding* (Washington, DC: National Academies Press).

Larson, E., George, A., Morgan, R., and Poteat, T. 2016. "10 Best Resources on . . . Intersectionality with an Emphasis on Low- and Middle-Income Countries." *Health Policy and Planning* (Online First, April 27). doi:10.1093/heapol/czw020.

Link, B., and Phelan, J. 2005. "Fundamental Sources of Health Inequalities." In *Policy Challenges in Modern Health Care*, edited by L. Rogut, J. R. Knickman, D. Mechanic, and D. Colby (New Brunswick, NJ: Rutgers University Press).

Logie, C. H., James, L., Tharao, W., and Loutfy, M. R. 2012. "'We Don't Exist': A Qualitative Study of Marginalization Experienced by HIV-Positive Lesbian, Bisexual, Queer and Transgender Women in Toronto, Canada." *Journal of International AIDS Society* 15(2). https://onlinelibrary.wiley.com/doi/full/10.7448/IAS.15.2.17392.

Malouf, M. A., and Wisniewski, A. B. 2016. "Differences of Sex Development/Intersex Populations." In *Lesbian, Gay, Bisexual, and Transgender Healthcare: A Clinical Guide to Preventive, Primary, and Specialist Care*, edited by K. L. Eckstrand, and J. M. Ehrenfeld (Cham, Switzerland: Springer International).

Mayer, K., Bradford J. B., Makadon H., Stall R., and Goldhammer H., 2008. "Sexual and Gender Minority Health: What We Know and What Needs to Be Done." *American Journal of Public Health* 98(6): 989–995.

OHCHR (Office of the High Commissioner of Human Rights). 2012. *Born Free and Equal: Sexual Orientation and Gender Identity in Human Rights Law* (New York: United Nations).

Padilla, M., Vásquez del Aguila, E., and Parker, R. 2007. "Globalization, Structural Violence, and LGBT Health: A Cross-Cultural Perspective." In *The Health of Sexual Minorities: Public Health Perspectives on Lesbian, Gay, Bisexual and Transgender Populations*, edited by I. Meyer and M. Northridge (New York: Springer).

Parker, R., Aggleton, P., and Perez-Brumer A. G. 2016. "The Trouble with 'Categories': Rethinking Men Who Have Sex with Men, Transgender and Their Equivalents in HIV Prevention and Health Promotion." *Global Public Health* 11(7–8): 819–823.

Perez-Brumer, A. G., Oldenburg, C. E., Reisner, S. L., Clark, J. L., and Parker, R. 2016. "Towards 'Reflexive Epidemiology': Conflation of Cisgender Male and Transgender Women Sex Workers and Implications for Global Understandings of HIV Prevalence." *Global Public Health* 11(7–8): 849–865.

Poteat, T., Diouf, D., Drame, F. M., Ndaw, M., Traore, C., Dhaliwal, M., et al. 2011. "HIV Risk among MSM in Senegal: a Qualitative Rapid Assessment of the Impact of Enforcing Laws that Criminalize Same Sex Practices." *PLoS One* 6(12). https://journals.plos.org/plosone/article?id=10.1371/journal.pone.0028760.

Poteat, T., German, D., and Flynn, C. 2016. "The Conflation of Gender and Sex: Gaps and Opportunities in HIV Data among Transgender Women and MSM." *Global Public Health*. 11(7–8): 835–48.

Poteat, T. C., Logie, C. H., Adams, D., Mothopeng, T., Lebona, J., Letsie, P., et al. 2015. "Stigma, Sexual Health and Human Rights among Women Who Have Sex with Women in Lesotho." *Reproductive Health Matters* 23(46): 107–116.

Poteat, T., Scheim, A., Xavier, J., Reisner, S., and Baral, S. 2016. "Global Epidemiology of HIV Infection and Related Syndemics Affecting Transgender People." *Journal of Acquired Immune Deficiency Syndromes* 72(Suppl. 3): S210–S219.

Reed, G. M., Drescher, J., Krueger, R. B., Atalla, E., Cochran, S., First, M. B., et al. 2016. "Disorders Related to Sexuality and Gender Identity in the ICD-11: Revising the ICD-10 Classification Based on Current Scientific Evidence, Best Clinical Practices, and Human Rights Considerations." *World Psychiatry* 15: 205–221.

Reisner, S. L., Poteat, T., Keatley, J., Cabral, M., Mothopeng, T., Dunham, E., et al. 2016. "Global Health Burden and Needs of Transgender Populations: A Review." *Lancet* 388 (10042): 412–436.

Richards, C., Bouman, W. P., Seal, L., Barker, M. J., Nieder, T. O., and T'Sjoen, G. 2016. "Non-binary or Genderqueer Genders." *International Review of Psychiatry*. 28(1): 95–102.

Schwartz, S. R., Nowak, R. G., Orazulike, I., Keshinro, B., Ake, J., Kennedy, S., et al. 2015. "The Immediate Effect of the Same-Sex Marriage Prohibition Act on Stigma, Discrimination, and Engagement on HIV Prevention and Treatment Services in Men Who Have Sex with Men in Nigeria: Analysis of Prospective Data from the TRUST Cohort." *Lancet HIV* 2(7): e299–e306.

Simoni, J. M., Smith, L., Oost, K. M., Lehavot, K., and Fredriksen-Goldsen, K. 2017. "Disparities in Physical Health Conditions among Lesbian and Bisexual Women: A Systematic Review of Population-Based Studies." *Journal of Homosexuality* 64(1): 32–44.

Temple-O'Connor, and M., Wehr E. 2013. *Consideration of the Institute of Medicine (IOM) Report on the Health of Lesbian, Gay, Bisexual, and Transgender (LGBT) Individuals* (Washington, DC: NIH LGBT Research Coordinating Committee).

UN (United Nations). 1967. International Covenant on Economic, Social and Cultural Rights. https://www.ohchr.org/en/professionalinterest/pages/cescr.aspx.

UNAIDS (Joint United Nations Programme on HIV/AIDS). 2016. *Prevention Gap Report* (New York: United Nations).

US Department of State. 2015. *Jamaica 2015 Human Rights Report*. Washington, DC: United States Department of State, Bureau of Democracy, Human Rights and Labor.

Winskell, K., and Sabben, G. 2016. "Sexual Stigma and Symbolic Violence Experienced, Enacted and Counteracted in Young Africans' Writing about Same-Sex Attraction." *Social Science and Medicine* 161: 143–150.

Young, R., and Meyer, I. 2005. "The Trouble with "MSM" and "WSW": Erasure of the Sexual-Minority Person in Public Health Discourse." *American Journal of Public Health* 95(7): 1144–1149.

Zahn, R., Grosso, A., Scheibe, A., Bekker, L-G., Ketende, S., Dausab, F., et al. 2016. "Human Rights Violations among Men Who Have Sex with Men in Southern Africa: Comparisons between Legal Contexts." *PLoS One* 11(1): 1–12. https://journals.plos.org/plosone/article?id=10.1371/journal.pone.0147156.

CHAPTER 21

PUBLIC HEALTH IN THE CONTEXT OF MIGRATION: ETHICS ISSUES RELATED TO IMMIGRANTS AND REFUGEES

RACHEL E. FABI

INTRODUCTION

THIS chapter explores the ethics and public health issues associated with immigrant and refugee populations, both in the United States and globally. It is organized by the phases of the journey of migrants from their home country to the community they join in their new country. We explore these issues for multiple categories of immigrants, including refugees, documented immigrants, and undocumented or irregular immigrants. This first section provides an overview of the types of immigrants and the motivating reasons people migrate internationally. The second section reviews three areas of political or moral theory related to immigration, and the third section provides an ethics analysis of three public health issues that occur at different phases of immigration.

It should be noted that the public health needs and threats facing this population vary widely across various immigrant groups, as well as by stage of migration. Migrants fleeing violence in their home country or living in a refugee camp are subject to very different challenges than immigrants who have settled into a new country where they do not speak the language. Because of this heterogeneity, this chapter reviews three distinct health challenges facing immigrants at different stages of migration: immigration detention, immigrant health screening, and access to health coverage for undocumented immigrants. These examples are not meant to be exhaustive, but rather illustrative of the sorts of public health issues that can arise in the immigration process and their ethical implications.

Types of Immigrants

There are many terms used to describe the movement of individuals between countries, many of which are tied to their motivation for movement. *Immigration* refers to the "movement of persons across national borders for purposes other than travel or short-term residence," while *emigration* refers to "the exodus of people from their country of origin for settlement, usually permanently, in a new country" (Messina and Lahav, 2006, 9). For the sake of simplicity, we will refer to all people who cross international borders for a significant period of time as immigrants. Immigrants can be divided into two categories: *voluntary* and *involuntary*.

Voluntary immigrants include *economic migrants*, who leave their host country for economic reasons and may be *documented* or *undocumented*, depending on whether their presence in the host country is legally sanctioned. Other voluntary immigrants migrate not for economic reasons, but for *family reunification*, or to join relatives living in other countries (Messina and Lahav, 2006). Involuntary immigrants are those who are forced to flee their home country to escape violence or persecution; these include *refugees* and *asylees*, who migrate for similar reasons but through different avenues. Article 1 of the UN Convention Relating to the Status of Refugees defines a refugee as

> any person who, owing to a well-founded fear of being persecuted for reasons of race, religion, nationality, membership in a particular social group or political opinion, is outside the country of his nationality and is unable or, owing to such fear, is unwilling to avail himself of the protection of that country.
>
> (UNGA, 1951, Article 1)

An asylee must meet this definition and submit a request for asylum while inside the destination country or at a port of entry, whereas refugees are generally granted refugee status while located outside the destination country (USCIS, 2015).

Normative Positions

Whether these various immigration statuses or motivations for immigration are morally relevant in determining the justice obligations of receiving countries is the subject of much debate. This section will outline several of the normative positions and political theories that address this question, including cosmopolitanism, nationalism, and communitarianism.

Cosmopolitanism is based on a belief in the moral equality of all human beings and the idea that "all human beings' needs and interests deserve equal consideration," regardless of where they are located on the globe, all else being equal (Brock, 2015, 113). It also shares with the human rights paradigm a commitment to a right to freedom of movement within and between countries. The logical conclusion of these two ideas is a position that dictates that justice obligations do not distinguish between compatriots and noncompatriots, so immigrants and refugees have equal claims to a nation's resources as its citizens. Indeed, strict versions of cosmopolitanism argue that our duties of justice are not geographically restricted (Singer, 1972). Cosmopolitanism does not necessarily provide guidance for the just distribution of resources, but rather insists that we treat nationality and immigration status as morally irrelevant, or at least not of paramount moral importance, in devising distribution schemes. Broader justice questions of whether these schemes demand only that we rescue those in dire emergency positions regardless of immigration status or location on the globe, or whether they demand that we provide full and equal access to the complete spectrum of human rights, are left for the cosmopolitan reader to consider.

On the other end of the spectrum from cosmopolitanism is *nationalism*, or the position that legitimate states have the right to political self-determination, including the freedom to associate (or not associate) with others (Wellman and Cole, 2011). Implicit in this understanding of political legitimacy is the idea that states do not have any obligations to noncitizens, including immigrants, and that they cannot be morally compelled to provide assistance to outsiders. Thomas Nagel (2005, 121) refers to this as the "political conception of justice," and argues that "justice is something we owe through our shared institutions only to those with whom we stand in a strong political relation. It is . . . an *associative* obligation." Nationalism thus conflicts with the cosmopolitan approach to justice in that it regards as incoherent questions of justice obligations to noncompatriots. The nationalist might concede that foreigners both beyond and within our borders may be owed humanitarian assistance in times of emergency, but these obligations are generated by concerns distinct from justice, such as duties of beneficence.

The final category of normative positions that we will consider are *communitarian* positions, which hold that the strength of an individual's claim on public resources is based on the strength of the individual's relationship to the community in which he or she is situated. These positions differ from cosmopolitanism in that many hinge on different levels of "deservedness," which a cosmopolitan would reject on the grounds that all humans are equally deserving simply by virtue of being human. Different societies may endorse different characteristics that determine entitlement to social benefits, although membership in the society is typically considered relevant. Another distinction between this position and nationalism is that the boundaries of communities are not necessarily those of nation-states—the key moral issue is community rather than nationality.

Ethical Issues in the Migrant's Journey

Ethics in Migration: Freedom of Movement and Human Rights

Debates about the ethics of immigration can often be boiled down to a conflict between two rights: the right of sovereign nations to freedom of association (that is, the right to decide who will be permitted to enter their countries), and the right of individuals to freedom of movement across borders. Arguments for freedom of movement across borders typically fall into one of two camps: either immigration is a "remedial right" that allows the disadvantaged to recover resources and opportunities denied to them in their home countries, or it is a "primary right" that cannot be restricted without justification (Bauböck, 2009, 2). If it is a remedial right, then it should only exist as long as global injustices persist, and should cease to be necessary once all nation-states are able to provide similar levels of quality of life (Carens, 1987). Others construe this freedom as a primary human right that is not only instrumentally valuable but also "an essential component of human agency, such that it is a crucial part of the ability of people to be free and equal choosers, doers, and participators in their local, national, and global communities" (Wellman and Cole, 2011, 297).

A formalization of the right to freedom of movement can be found in Article 13 of the UN Declaration of Human Rights (1948), which states, "(1) Everyone has the right to freedom of movement and residence within the borders of each state," and "(2) Everyone has the right to leave any country, including his own, and to return to his country." The Declaration of Human Rights is not legally binding, and most political theorists recognize that the right to freedom of movement is not absolute and must be balanced against other considerations (Miller, 2016). Nonetheless, the right to leave one's home country (and to return to it) is also enshrined in several other international covenants, including the International Covenant on Civil and Political Rights (UNGA, 1966a).

The right to freedom of movement is complicated, however, by the fact that a right to leave one's home country does not equate to the right to enter another. The fundamental tension between a sovereign nation's right of association to control immigration and the right of an individual to emigrate raises significant challenges to the exercise of freedom of movement, especially to the global poor and disenfranchised, who often find themselves unwelcome in wealthier nations and therefore unable to emigrate legally (Wellman and Cole, 2011; Zolberg, 1981; Jordan and Düvell, 2003). Whether a right to freedom of movement entails the complementary right to enter another country hinges on whether and to what extent borders should be open to free immigration.

Ethics at the Border: Open and Closed Borders

The question of whether there is a human right to freedom of movement across borders, or a human right to immigration, is a subject of much debate among political theorists. David Miller (2016) argues that there is no human right to immigration, and that states can be justified in limiting inward movement across their borders to control overall numbers, prevent major cultural shifts, and maintain the composition of the citizen body. Typically, theorists who argue that the right to freedom of association trumps the right to freedom of movement support closed borders as well. Christopher Wellman, for example, argues that legitimate states are entitled to political self-determination, of which freedom of association is an integral component that entails the right not to associate with others (Wellman and Cole, 2011). Miller, Wellman, and many other nationalist theorists do support a humanitarian obligation to assist people in dire need, but they do not believe that this obligation requires political communities to admit migrants and refugees (though Miller concedes that there are "human rights questions to be asked about the criteria used to select immigrants who do not qualify as asylum seekers" [Miller, 2016, 30]).

Joseph Carens (2013) takes a cosmopolitan position in his defense of open borders. He argues that freedom of movement is necessary to preserve equality of opportunity, and that immigration control policies therefore require justification. Carens suggests that "a commitment to equal moral worth entails some commitment to economic, social, and political equality, partly as a means of realizing equal freedom and equal opportunity and partly as a desirable end in itself," and that freedom of movement would contribute to a reduction of these inequalities (228). Thus, Carens's argument for open borders is two-pronged: freedom of movement both supports equality of opportunity and reduces global inequalities, so restrictions of it must be justified rather than accepted as the status quo.

Ethics in the Destination Country: Communitarian Obligations to Noncitizens

Once an immigrant has reached her destination country, the question of what obligations her new home has toward her as a noncitizen must be considered. A communitarian might argue that she is not different in a morally relevant way from the citizens with whom she shares her community, and thus she is entitled to the same benefits of community membership, including claiming public resources. This position is shared by Michael Walzer, who argues that once an immigrant has been admitted and resides among citizens, he must receive equal rights and a plausible path to citizenship. Walzer writes that "the principle of political justice is this: that the processes of self-determination through which a democratic state shapes its internal life, must be open, and equally open, to all those men and women who live within its territory, work in the local economy, and are subject to local law" (Walzer, 1983, 60). This is an ideal theory position, but it is related to a variety of practical arguments.

One practical communitarian argument in favor of an obligation to provide at least some level of public assistance to immigrants is that they "contribute to social welfare in the same ways that other productive members of society do, including paying at least some taxes" (Hall and Perrin, 2015, 134). A recent report by the nonpartisan Institute on Taxation and Economic Policy in the United States found that undocumented immigrants paid $11.84 billion in US state and local taxes in 2012, at an effective tax rate of 8 percent (Gardner, Johnson, and Wiehe, 2015), but the claim that undocumented immigrants pay sufficient taxes to merit access to public services is disputed (Edwards, 2010; Camarota, 2009; Martin, 2012). Either way, it could be argued that basing entitlement on who pays taxes is ethically problematic, and may not be the most morally appropriate approach (Dwyer, 2004).

Another communitarian position is the *social embeddedness* argument that "even when immigrants' social contributions cannot be quantified, they are nevertheless tangible in more diffused or qualitative senses of communitarianism" (Hall and Perrin, 2015, 135). Many immigrants live in neighborhoods and work in businesses, and through the formation of social relationships they become deeply embedded in the society in which they live. Carens argues that the amount of time an immigrant has resided in a community is morally relevant, and that social embeddedness increases with time, as does the strength of a noncitizen's claim to public resources.

Public Health Issues in the Migrant's Journey

Public Health in Migration: Immigrant Detention

Closely related to the right to freedom of movement is the issue of immigrant or immigration detention, which is a policy of detaining immigrants who are suspected of entering or remaining in a country without legal permission. Immigrant detainees include undocumented men, women, and children awaiting deportation proceedings and refugees petitioning for asylum, as well as those who have been arrested for committing a crime. Immigration detention policies differ from country to country. The United States and Australia have policies of mandatory detention, under which all illegal immigrants and asylum seekers are compulsorily detained, although in the United States they may be released if they do not have a criminal history and are not deemed a threat to national security by the Immigration and Customs Enforcement Agency (ICE).

Conditions in many immigrant detention facilities in the United States are notoriously poor. Reports by the ACLU (American Civil Liberties Union), Amnesty International, the US Commission on Civil Rights, and several other independent bodies have documented overcrowded conditions, inappropriate use of isolation, inadequate access to necessary medical care, restricted access to federally mandated legal services and books, and physical and sexual abuse of detainees, among other rights violations (Amnesty International, 2009; IACHR, 2010; ACLU, 2014; USCCR, 2015; Migration and Refugee Services, 2015). Many of these claims are corroborated by a 2009 report by ICE itself (Schriro, 2009). These issues are compounded by the dramatic increase in the number of immigrants in US detention facilities, rising from around 85,000 in 1995 to a peak of 477,523 in FY 2012 (Global Detention Project, 2016).

Particularly troubling is the recent surge in juvenile detention in the United States; between October 2013 and September 2014, authorities apprehended 68,541 unaccompanied children at the US–Mexico border, nearly 80 percent of whom were from Central American countries (Phippen, 2015). The detention of children, many of whom risked incredibly dangerous conditions and physical and sexual abuse while fleeing violence in their home countries, has been met with strong criticism from immigrant rights groups. Juvenile detainees are at particular risk for psychological distress and the development of mental health conditions due to a variety of factors. These include the trauma they experienced in their home countries and along the journey to the country in which they seek asylum, as well as the effects of separation from family, malnutrition, disease, and neglect (Newman and Steel, 2008; Silove, Austin, and Steel, 2007).

Of course, the United States is not detaining immigrants out of malice; a massive influx of migrants with no resources and significant physical and mental health needs can mean major costs to the local communities in which they settle. Receiving localities may not be equipped to accept thousands of migrant children with minimal English proficiency, and while federal law guarantees all children a free public education, the costs of educating undocumented children are largely borne by local school districts (Pierce, 2015). These costs create incentives for communities to reject unaccompanied minors and urge stronger enforcement of federal immigration law.

Public Health at the Border: Immigrant Health Screening

Immigrant health screening is a controversial topic in public health ethics, as it pits the health of the citizen population against that of the individual immigrant, severely restricting her autonomy and freedom of movement in order to protect the public good. In a world of semi-porous closed borders, states must set specific criteria for the admission of new immigrants, and one common criterion is the immigrant's health status.

In the United States, immigrant health screening has been a key component of the refugee and immigrant admission process since the Immigration Act of 1882, which called for the exclusion of "any person unable to take care of him or herself without becoming a public charge," including the mentally ill, the sick, and the disabled (Immigration Act of 1882, 22 Stat. 214, Sec 2). This exclusion was further specified in the Immigration and Nationality Act of 1952 (INA), which established that immigrants "who are afflicted with tuberculosis . . . leprosy, or any dangerous contagious disease" are "ineligible to receive visas and shall be excluded from admission into the United States" (Immigration and Nationality Act of 1952, Pub.L. 414, Sec. 212).

Health screening is mandatory for all immigrants applying for permanent residence in the United States, including asylum seekers and refugees. The public health purpose of these policies was ostensibly to protect citizens from contracting potentially deadly and highly contagious diseases, although they were often applied in a discriminatory fashion to keep out immigrants seen as undesirable, including homosexual immigrants, who were explicitly barred from entry until the Immigration Act of 1990 removed "sexual deviance" as an excludable category (Forrester, 1987; Shoop, 1993).

In 1987, in response to the growing human immunodeficiency virus/acquired immunodeficiency syndrome (HIV/AIDS) epidemic, the Centers for Disease Control and Prevention's (CDC's) list of dangerous contagious diseases (now called "communicable diseases of public health significance") was expanded to include HIV, mandating that all immigrants seeking permanent residence undergo blood testing. Although proponents of this measure argued that it would protect the public's health, many ultimately supported a ban because of the perceived financial burden of providing care for patients with HIV/ AIDS. One US legislator declared that "it is simply not in the interests of this nation to allow into this country as permanent immigrants people who have a noncurable disease. Our health care system is already inundated trying to keep up with the health needs of... citizens" (Gladwell, 1991; Shoop, 1993, 533). Opponents to the HIV exclusion, including representatives of the international community and several international health agencies, argued that it would not be an effective way of preventing the spread of disease, given that tourists and other visitors were not subjected to the same ban, and that it could not be spread through casual contact (UNAIDS and IOM, 2004).

The ban was kept in place for over twenty years, and the measure prevented HIV-infected would-be immigrants from entering the United States in search of medical care for their condition at the peak of the epidemic. HIV remained on the list of excludable conditions until November 2009, when the CDC removed it and all references to mandatory serologic testing of new immigrants (CDC, 2009).[1] Although the United States has eliminated its ban, many other nations continue to impose harsh restrictions on the movement of HIV-positive immigrants. In 2016, fifty-six countries still had special entry regulations related to HIV (Wiessner and Lemmen, 2016). While this represents an improvement since 1999, when 104 countries were found to have HIV-specific travel restrictions, there is still much work to be done on the global scale to improve freedom of movement for people living with HIV/AIDS.

Public Health in the Destination Country: Undocumented Immigrants and Publicly Funded Health Care in the United States

Although many international covenants recognize access to medical services as a human right, including the International Covenant on Economic, Social and Cultural Rights (which the United States has not ratified), immigrants are frequently barred from accessing publicly funded health care (UNGA, 1966b). Policies regarding immigrant eligibility for public health care in the United States have evolved significantly since the late 1990s, and many reflect the various normative positions outlined above.

Eligibility for social services in the United States varies greatly by immigration status. The Personal Responsibility and Work Opportunity Reconciliation Act of 1996 (PRWORA, or "welfare reform") divides immigrants into eligibility categories that have implications for which public benefits they may access, creating an eligibility spectrum that privileges certain types of immigrants over others. Immigrants who qualify for some public insurance coverage include legal permanent residents who have resided in the United States for five or more years (known as the five-year bar), refugees, asylees, and several other humanitarian immigrant groups. The five-year bar reflects the communitarian notion of social embeddedness (i.e., that one's claim to public resources depends on how long one has resided in the community), although five years may seem like an arbitrary cut-off point for eligibility. States wishing to provide nonexempt qualified immigrants with access to public benefits during the five-year bar, or to unqualified immigrants, must do so with state-only funds, since the use of federal funds for these populations is illegal. Waiving the five-year bar for refugees and asylees demonstrates a commitment to a humanitarian ethic: immigrants who have entered the United States for their own safety (through accepted legal mechanisms) deserve protection.

The United States treats unqualified immigrants quite differently. Asylum applicants, students, tourists, and undocumented immigrants are ineligible for almost all forms of public medical insurance, although they can access some services on a sliding fee scale at Federally Qualified Health Centers (FQHCs) (Gusmano, 2012). Many undocumented and otherwise unqualified immigrants access health care through emergency rooms under the Emergency Medical Treatment and Active Labor Act (EMTALA), which requires hospitals to accept patients in life-threatening condition or active labor without ascertaining immigration or insurance status (Siskin, 2004). In specific circumstances, treatment provided under EMTALA will be covered by Emergency Medicaid, which is an encounter-based payment by a government insurance program (Medicaid) to the institution providing care that covers the emergency medical costs of some unqualified patients, including low-income pregnant women, children under nineteen, and disabled persons (Siskin, 2004; GAO, 2004). Providing unqualified immigrants with coverage only for emergency care indicates a minimalist humanitarian position under which we owe no more than what is required to save a life.

Limiting the time-dependent public benefits to just legal permanent residents does not comport with Carens's social embeddedness theory, because many undocumented immigrants are deeply embedded in their communities. It does, however, reflect "deservedness" objections that "illegality disqualifies [undocumented immigrants] for at least some social services they would otherwise merit" (Hall and Perrin, 2015, 135). There is an aspect of punishment or retributive justice in the view that, having broken the law to enter the country, undocumented immigrants are undeserving of public benefits, yet many citizens violate the law every day without being disqualified from health care coverage (although in practice the care that prisoners receive is often far below accepted health care guidelines standards) (Dwyer, 2015; Hall and Perrin, 2015; Wilper et al., 2009). Even if the punishment argument were convincing, however, it could be argued that denying care to undocumented children unjustly punishes them for a crime they did not commit. Several states, including New York, California, and Illinois, provide coverage for undocumented children, reflecting this objection.

Guaranteeing the right to health care for immigrants will likely require progressive realization. As this section shows, most countries' patchwork and minimalist protections for undocumented immigrants fall far short of meeting minimal humanitarian, let alone substantive communitarian or cosmopolitan, obligations toward noncitizen residents and community members. Correcting this injustice will require states to reevaluate their health policies toward immigrants, a process unlikely to occur overnight.

Conclusion

Immigration across borders raises a number of ethical questions and creates significant public health concerns. What we believe we owe to our fellow humans who leave their home country in search of a better life hinges on the normative position we take, be it cosmopolitan, nationalist, or something in between. In an increasingly globalized society in which humanity grows more interconnected through modern communication and economic interaction, it is necessary that we reevaluate our ethical obligations to noncitizens both within and beyond our borders.

Note

1. Diseases that remain excludable include "active tuberculosis, infectious syphilis, gonorrhea, infectious leprosy," among others, as well as "any quarantinable, communicable disease specified by Executive Orders," which currently include pandemic flu, severe acute respiratory syndrome (SARS), viral hemorrhagic fevers (such as Ebola virus disease), and plague (USCIS, 2016).

References

ACLU (American Civil Liberties Union). 2014. *Warehoused and Forgotten: Immigrants Trapped in Our Shadow Private Prison System*. New York: American Civil Liberties Union. https://www.aclu.org/other/warehoused-and-forgotten-immigrants-trapped-our-shadow-private-prison-system.

Amnesty International. 2009. *Jailed without Justice: Immigrant Detention in the USA* (London: Amnesty International). https://www.amnestyusa.org/pdfs/JailedWithoutJustice.pdf.

Bauböck, R. 2009. "Global Justice, Freedom of Movement and Democratic Citizenship." *European Journal of Sociology* 50(1): 1–31.

Brock, G. 2015. "Global Justice, Cosmopolitan Duties and Duties to Compatriots: The Case of Healthcare." *Public Health Ethics* 8(2): 110–120. doi:10.1093/phe/phu039.

Camarota, S. A. 2009. *Illegal Immigrants and HR 3200* (Washington, DC: Center for Immigration Studies). https://cis.org/Illegal-Immigrants-and-HR-3200.

Carens, J. 1987. "Aliens and Citizens: The Case for Open Borders." *Review of Politics* 49(2): 251–273.

Carens, J. 2013. *The Ethics of Immigration* (New York: Oxford University Press).

CDC (Centers for Disease Control and Prevention). 2009. "Medical Examination of Aliens—Removal of Human Immunodeficiency Virus (HIV) Infection from Definition of Communicable Disease of Public Health Significance." *Federal Register* 74(210): 56547–56562.

Dwyer, J. 2004. "Illegal Immigrants, Health Care, and Social Responsibility." *Hastings Center Report* 34(1): 34–41.

Dwyer, J. 2015. "On Taking Responsibility for Undocumented Migrants." *Public Health Ethics* 8(2): 139–147.

Edwards, J. R. 2010. "The Medicaid Costs of Legalizing Illegal Aliens" (Washington, DC: Center for Immigration Studies).

Forrester, W. R. 1987. "Medical Examination of Aliens." *In Defense of the Alien* 10: 258–263.

GAO (Government Accountability Office). 2004. *Undocumented Aliens: Questions Persist about Their Impact on Hospitals' Uncompensated Care Costs* (Washington, DC: GAO).

Gardner, M., Johnson, S., and Wiehe, M. 2015. *Undocumented Immigrants' State & Local Tax Contributions* (Washington, D.C.: Institute on Taxation and Economic Policy).

Gladwell, M. 1991. "Reversal of AIDS Exclusion Is Said to Be Shelved: 4-Year Bar to Immigration Criticized as Discriminatory and Medically Unjustified." *Washington Post*, May 25, A6.

Global Detention Project. 2016. *United States Immigration Detention* (Geneva: Global Detention Project). https://www.globaldetentionproject.org/immigration-detention-in-the-united-states.

Gusmano, M. K. 2012. *Undocumented Immigrants in the United States: U.S. Health Policy and Access to Care* (Garrison, NY: Hastings Center).

Hall, M. A., and Perrin, J. 2015. "Irregular Migrant Access to Care: Mapping Public Policy Rationales." *Public Health Ethics* 8(2):130–138. doi:10.1093/phe/phv016.

IACHR (Inter-American Commission on Human Rights). 2010. *Report on Immigration in the United States: Detention and Due Process* (Washington, D.C.: Organization of American States). https://www.oas.org/en/iachr/migrants/docs/pdf/migrants2011.pdf.

Jordan, B., and Düvell, F. 2003. *Migration: The Boundaries of Equality and Justice* (Cambridge: Polity Press).

Martin, J. 2012. *Deterring Illegal Immigrant Settlement: A Guide to State and Local Action* (Washington, DC: Federation for American Immigration Reform).

Messina, A. M., and Lahav, G. 2006. *The Migration Reader: Exploring Politics and Policies* (Boulder, CO: Lynne Rienner).

Migration and Refugee Services. 2015. *Unlocking Human Dignity: A Plan to Transform the U.S. Immigrant Detention System* (Migration and Refugee Services, U.S. Conference of Catholic Bishops, and the Center for Migration Studies). https://doi.org/10.14240/jmhs.v3i2.48.

Miller, D. 2016. "Is There a Human Right to Immigrate?" In *Migration in Political Theory: The Ethics of Movement and Membership*, edited by S. Fine and L. Ypi (New York: Oxford University Press).

Nagel, T. 2005. "The Problem of Global Justice." *Philosophy & Public Affairs* 33(2): 113–147.

Newman, L. K., and Steel, Z. 2008. "The Child Asylum Seeker: Psychological and Developmental Impact of Immigration Detention." *Child and Adolescent Psychiatric Clinics of North America* 17(3): 665–683.

Phippen, J. W. 2015. "Young, Illegal, and Alone." *The Atlantic*, October 15.

Pierce, S. 2015. *Unaccompanied Child Migrants in U.S. Communities, Immigration Court, and Schools* (Brussels: Migration Policy Institute). https://www.migrationpolicy.org/research/unaccompanied-child-migrants-us-communities-immigration-court-and-schools.

Schriro, D. 2009. *Immigration Detention: Overview and Recommendations* (Washington, DC: US Immigration and Customs Enforcement). https://www.ice.gov/doclib/about/offices/odpp/pdf/ice-detention-rpt.pdf.

Shoop, L. G. 1993. "Health Based Exclusion Grounds in United States Immigration Policy: Homosexuals, HIV Infection and the Medical Examination of Aliens." *Journal of Contemporary Health Law and Policy* 9: 521–544.

Silove, D., Austin, P., and Steel, Z. 2007. "No Refuge from Terror: The Impact of Detention on the Mental Health of Trauma-Affected Refugees Seeking Asylum in Australia." *Transcultural Psychiatry* 44(3): 359–393. doi:10.1177/1363461507081637.

Singer, P., 1972. "Famine, Affluence, and Morality." *Philosophy and Public Affairs* 1(3): 229–243, http://personal.lse.ac.uk/robert49/teaching/mm/articles/Singer_1972Famine.pdf.

Siskin, A. 2004. *Federal Funding for Unauthorized Aliens' Emergency Medical Expenses*. CRS Report for Congress (Washington, D.C.: Congressional Research Service).

UN (United Nations). 1948. Universal Declaration of Human Rights (New York: United Nations General Assembly).

UNAIDS (Joint United Nations Programme on HIV/AIDS) and IOM (Institute of Medicine). 2004. *UNAIDS/IOM Statement on HIV/AIDS-Related Travel Restrictions* (UNAIDS International Organization for Migration).

UNGA (United Nations General Assembly). 1951. Convention relating to the Status of Refugees. https://treaties.un.org/pages/ViewDetailsII.aspx?src=TREATY&mtdsg_no=V-2&chapter=5&Temp=mtdsg2&clang=_en.

UNGA (United Nations General Assembly). 1966a. International Covenant on Civil and Political Rights. https://www.ohchr.org/en/professionalinterest/pages/ccpr.aspx.

UNGA (United Nations General Assembly). 1966b. International Covenant on Economic, Social and Cultural Rights. https://www.ohchr.org/en/professionalinterest/pages/cescr.aspx.

USCCR (United States Commission on Civil Rights). 2015. *With Liberty and Justice for All: The State of Civil Right at Immigration Detention Facilities* (Washington, D.C.: USCCR). https://reliefweb.int/sites/reliefweb.int/files/resources/Statutory_Enforcement_Report2015.pdf.

USCIS (United States Citizenship and Immigration Services). 2015. *Refugees & Asylum*. Washington, DC: USCIS. https://www.uscis.gov/humanitarian/refugees-asylum.

USCIS (US Citizenship and Immigration Service). 2016. "Communicable Diseases of Public Health Significance." In *USCIS Policy Manual* (Washington, D.C.: USCIS).https://www.uscis.gov/policymanual/HTML/PolicyManual-Volume8-PartB-Chapter6.html.

Walzer, M. 1983. *Spheres of Justice: A Defense of Pluralism and Equality*. New York: Basic Books.

Wellman, C. H., and Cole, P. 2011. *Debating the Ethics of Immigration: Is There a Right to Exclude?* (New York: Oxford University Press).

Wiessner, P., and Lemmen, K. 2016. *Quick Reference: Entry and Residence Regulations for People Living with HIV* (Berlin: Deutsche AIDS-Hilife).

Wilper, A. P., Woolhandler, S., Boyd, J. W., Lasser, K. E., McCormick, D., Bor, D. H., et al. 2009. "The Health and Health Care of US Prisoners: Results of a Nationwide Survey." *American Journal of Public Health* 99(4): 666–672. doi:10.2105/AJPH.2008.144279.

Zolberg, A. R. 1981. "International Migrations in Political Perspective." In *Global Trends in Migration: Theory and Research on International Population Movements*, edited by M. Kritz, C. Keely, and S. Tomasi, 3–27 (New York: Center for Migration Studies).

SECTION FIVE

HEALTH DISPARITIES

CHAPTER 22

AN OVERVIEW OF HEALTH DISPARITIES IN THE CONTEXT OF PUBLIC HEALTH ETHICS

ANDREW W. SIEGEL

INTRODUCTION

PUBLIC health researchers have long understood that differences in socioeconomic status (SES, or status as defined by income, education, and occupation) are associated with disparities in health among individuals. In early studies looking at the health effects of SES, researchers compared persons at the low end of the socioeconomic ladder with those above the poverty line. These studies demonstrated substantial disparities between the health of impoverished and well-off (or at least better-off) persons (Antonovsky, 1967). Those data appeared to reveal that adverse effects of poverty can explain the impact of SES on health. Inadequate medical care, crowded and unsanitary living conditions, poor nutrition, and the like were thought to account for the health disparities between the poor and the well-off. Based on this understanding, eliminating serious health disparities requires eliminating poverty.

Poverty does indeed play a quite substantial role in accounting for some health disparities, particularly those that exist between low-income and high-income countries. Males in low-income countries have an average life expectancy of about sixty years, in contrast to a life expectancy of seventy-six years for males in high-income countries. Likewise, females in low-income countries have an average life expectancy of about sixty-three years, in contrast to a life expectancy of eighty-two years for females in high-income countries (WHO, 2014). The disparities are even more dramatic when considering life expectancies at the far ends of the spectrum, with a thirty-eight-year difference between the average life expectancies in Sierra Leone (forty-six years) and Japan (eighty-four years) (WHO, 2014). More than half of the deaths in low-income countries are caused by communicable diseases, malnutrition, maternal causes, and complications that emerge in pregnancy and childbirth. In high-income countries, these causes account for less than 7 percent of deaths (WHO, 2017).

Raising the standard of living in poor countries would go a long way toward addressing some of the major causes of death in those countries, and in narrowing the existing gaps in life expectancy between low-income and high-income countries. Much of the literature on global justice and health focuses on the obligation to promote measures that would improve life expectancy in low-income countries (Lenard and Straehle, 2012; Millum and Emanuel, 2012).

However, while eliminating poverty would do much to reduce global health disparities, health disparities also exist in high-income countries between different socioeconomic groups that are above the poverty line, and even where all the groups have the same access to health care. Numerous studies over the last few decades have established that SES and health are in fact associated at every point in the socioeconomic hierarchy. The seminal study supporting this proposition is the Whitehall study, which was a screening study of 17,000 men employed by the British Civil Service. The workers in each category were fully employed and had full access to the health care provided by the National Health Service, the publicly funded single-payer system in England. The British Civil Service operates with ranked grades of employment, which, from the lowest to highest grade, include unskilled workers, clerical workers, professionals and executives, and top administrators. The study revealed a social gradient in which the relative risk of mortality over ten years increased at each point at which the employment grade decreased (Marmot, Shipley, and Rose, 1984).

Other studies have similarly found a graded relationship between income and mortality, and also between years of education and mortality (McDonough et al. 1997; Montez and Zajacova, 2013). Some have further interpreted the data on income and mortality as showing that an individual's health is affected by the level of inequality in society as a whole, and not just by her or his own level of income (Wilkinson, 1996).

Being in a position of social disadvantage relative to others unquestionably has a negative impact on health. But what are the causal pathways that connect one's position on the socioeconomic hierarchy to health? Differences in individual behaviors (e.g., the greater incidence of smoking, poor diet, and alcohol and drug abuse among low-status persons) and the physical environments in which persons live (e.g., greater exposure to environmental pollutants among low-status persons) partly explain the health disparities between lower- and higher-status individuals. But there is support for accounts that identify more complex psychosocial causes. In the occupational context, evidence indicates that the differing levels of control experienced by workers at different points in the hierarchy influence health outcomes (Marmot, 2015). Outside of work, lower-status individuals are more likely to live in neighborhoods with a lack of social cohesion and more hostility and violence, which are associated with poor health outcomes (Kawachi, 1999; Diez Roux et al., 2001). Generally, lower-status persons may feel less respected by virtue of their place on the social hierarchy. As Richard Wilkinson writes,

> Wider income differences mean that more people are excluded from the jobs and incomes that are the usual sources of status.... [W]hat matters most about relative deprivation is not so much the lower living standards in themselves, but the affront to dignity and respect, and the imputation of inferiority that accompanies relative poverty. (Wilkinson, 2000, 27)

All of these factors—lower levels of control at work, less cohesive and more hostile neighborhoods, and experiencing a lack of respect—put low-status persons at heightened risk of chronic stress, which in turn increases the risk of heart disease, cancer, and other illnesses (Marmot and Theorell, 1988; McEwen and Seeman, 1999; McEwen, 2012).

Chapter Overviews

The four chapters in this section of *The Oxford Handbook of Public Health Ethics* are dedicated to examining ethical considerations related to health disparities. They are introduced below.

Ethics, Social Justice, and the Reduction of Health Disparities

Once we recognize the nature and scope of the social determinants of health, it becomes critical to consider the ethical obligation to address them as a means of reducing health disparities. In "Health Disparities and the Social Determinants of Health: Ethical and Social Justice Issues," Sridhar Venkatapuram discusses this issue. Venkatapuram highlights the fact that addressing the social determinants of health requires transforming a wide range of societal conditions. In this vein, Sol Levine (1994, 10) has suggested that we must revise our conception of health policy in light of the impact socioeconomic factors have on health: "Health policy should not be separated from social and economic policy. Indeed, health leaders might find themselves becoming involved in issues ordinarily viewed as distant from health concerns—such as tax policy, ways to fight inflation, and the kind of remedies we use for unemployment."

However, as Venkatapuram argues, we cannot simply assume that it is appropriate to intervene in other social spheres to improve public health. In some cases, social interventions to improve health may generate improvements in other spheres. For example, creating greater equality of opportunity may advance both health and employment. But in other instances, interventions may raise concerns. For example, radical redistributions of wealth might reduce health disparities, but they might also reduce incentives to produce wealth to such a degree that, overall, everyone ends up worse off.

Identifying what social interventions are appropriate requires a theory of social justice. Venkatapuram notes that theories of justice specify both a good that is sought and a principle for the distribution of the good. The standard goods appealed to are welfare, resources, and capabilities, while the competing principles of distribution include equality, sufficiency, and priority. As Venkatapuram points out, most social justice theorists hold that inequalities are permissible under certain conditions. For example, prioritarians allow inequalities where they benefit those who are worst off (Rawls, 1971; Daniels, 2008), and sufficientarians hold that what matters for justice is that everyone has enough of the goods essential to leading a decent life, not that all persons have an equal amount of goods (Frankfurt, 1987; Powers and Faden, 2006). These theories of justice thus allow some health disparities, though giving priority to the least well off or ensuring sufficient health for everyone would substantially reduce current disparities.

Racial and Ethnic Health Disparities

The discussion above about SES and health focused on the social gradients related to income, occupation, and education. But there is more to the connection between social status and health than is revealed by these standard measures of SES. There are racial health disparities that the standard measures do not fully capture. Not only do black Americans have a substantially higher death rate than white Americans, but a differential persists even where blacks and whites have the same level of education and income (Isaacs and Schroeder, 2004; Wong et al., 2002). This suggests that racial disparities require both their own analysis and additional modes of intervention.

In "Racial and Ethnic Health Disparities as a Public Health Ethics Issue," Stephen B. Thomas discusses the empirical data on racial and ethnic disparities, the social determinants of these disparities, and the moral imperative to reduce the disparities. Thomas identifies racism and systematic discrimination as the fundamental causes of the disadvantages that racial and ethnic groups suffer. He locates the moral foundation for a public health focus on the discriminatory underpinnings of racial health disparities in both the ethical obligation to address the primary causes of disease and the obligation to pay special attention to systematically disadvantaged groups.

Thomas notes that while progress has been made in reducing racial disparities, much remains to be done. The legacy of slavery and racism persists and continues to have a detrimental impact on the health of minorities. Researchers, he suggests, should seek to learn from historical injustices. Thomas argues that we need to move beyond the public health science of health disparities and develop a new generation of health disparities research that identifies strategies for reducing racial and ethnic health disparities.

Conflicts between Reducing Health Disparities and Advancing Population Health

While the chapters in this section on socioeconomic disparities and racial and ethnic disparities identify moral arguments for reducing health disparities, in the chapter "Reconciling Two Ethics Goals of Public Health: Reducing Health Disparities and Improving Population Health," Norman Daniels examines some conflicts that arise between reducing unjust health disparities and advancing population health. Sometimes the public health interventions that maximize aggregate health produce or heighten health disparities. For example, directing resources in low-income countries to subgroups that are better off and more readily accessible may yield the best overall health outcomes, but it also results in intracountry inequality. Similarly, smoking cessation and vaccine campaigns in the United States improve aggregate health but disproportionately benefit persons with higher incomes and education.

Daniels argues that these kinds of conflicts give rise to a set of rationing problems concerning what priority we should give the worst off, when we should permit modest aggregate gains to large numbers of persons to outweigh significant gains to a smaller number, and when we should privilege giving persons fair chances at a health benefit over seeking the best aggregate health outcome. The issues become more complex where the relevant background inequalities are unjust. For example, when the inequalities between the best off and worst off are unjust, the problem about what priority to give the worst off also involves the question of what weight to attach to the background injustice.

Daniels submits that reasonable people will disagree about how to solve these rationing problems. He proposes that they be addressed through a procedure that is fair to everyone. Such a fair procedure would require that (a) the rationales for decisions be made public, (b) decisions be based on reasons that everyone considers relevant, (c) decisions be revised where warranted on the basis of new arguments and evidence, and (d) there is a mechanism in place to enforce that these conditions are met. While a fair procedure will not yield outcomes that everyone can agree to, it should yield outcomes that everyone can accept.

Measuring Health Inequities

The health inequalities that are of greatest concern are those involving inequities. In such instances, public health policy decisions about how much priority to give the worst off must place weight on existing health inequities. But public health policy can determine how much weight to give these inequities in setting priorities only where it has a measurement of them. In "Measuring Health Inequity: A Public Health Ethics Inquiry," Yukiko Asada discusses the central tasks involved in measuring health inequities and describes how ethical considerations play a critical role at each stage of the measurement process.

Asada identifies three tasks involved in measuring health inequities: definition, operationalization, and quantification. First, to measure health inequities, one needs a definition of health inequity. Asada discusses accounts of health inequity from the public health, economics, and philosophy literatures. Second, measurement requires the operationalization of the chosen definition of health inequity. For example, if we adopt a theory of health justice that is concerned with capabilities or functionings, then it would be most appropriate to use a measure of capacity or functional status rather than one that just tracks the presence of certain medical conditions. Third, measuring health inequity requires quantification of the magnitude of health inequity. One's approach to quantification involves adopting various indices, which, in turn, must be informed by value judgments. For example, if we hold that ten years in a short life matter more than ten years in a long life, then we should quantify the magnitude of health inequity with a relative index rather than an absolute one.

Asada's examination reveals that the measurement of health inequity is not simply a technical exercise. Instead, the measurement of health inequity must take considerations of ethics and social justice into account. This is true as well with the analyses of health disparities in the contexts of SES, racial and ethnic disparities, and population health: ethics must inform assessments and interventions related to health disparities.

Conclusion

Collectively, the chapters in this section of *The Oxford Handbook of Public Health Ethics* offer a public health ethics foundation for addressing health disparities. Ongoing work in these areas will continue to expand our understanding of its complexity and the importance of attending to ethical considerations in the public health sphere.

References

Antonovsky, A. 1967. "Social Class, Life Expectancy and Overall Mortality." *Milbank Memorial Quarterly* 45(2): 31–73.

Daniels, N. 2008. *Just Health: Meeting Needs Fairly* (New York: Cambridge University Press).

Diez Roux, A. V., Merkin, S. S., Arnett, D., Chambless, L., Massing, M., Nieto, F. J., et al. 2001. "Neighborhood of Residence and Incidence of Coronary Heart Disease." *New England Journal of Medicine* 345(2): 99–106.

Frankfurt, H. 1987. "Equality as a Moral Ideal." *Ethics* 98(1): 21–42.

Isaacs, S. L., and Schroeder, S. A. 2004. "Class: The Ignored Determinant of the Nation's Health." *New England Journal of Medicine* 351(11): 1137–1142.

Kawachi, I. 1999. "Social Capital and Community Effects on Population and Individual Death." *Annals of the New York Academy of Sciences* 896(1): 120–130.

Lenard, P. T., and Straehle, C., eds. 2012. *Health Inequalities and Global Justice* (Edinburgh: Edinburgh University Press).

Levine, S. 1994. "If Our Government Really Cared About Health." *Social Policy* 24(3): 6–12.

Marmot, M. 2015. *The Health Gap: The Challenge of an Unequal World* (London: Bloomsbury).
Marmot, M., Shipley, M. J., and Rose, G. 1984. "Inequalities in Death: Specific Explanations of a General Pattern?" *Lancet* 323(8384): 1003–1006.
Marmot, M., and Theorell, T. 1988. "Social Class and Cardiovascular Disease: The Contribution of Work." *International Journal of Health Services* 18(4): 659–674.
McDonough, P., Duncan, G. J., Williams, D., and House, J. 1997. "Income Dynamics and Adult Mortality in the United States, 1972 through 1989." *American Journal of Public Health* 87(9): 1476–1483.
McEwen, B. S. 2012. "Brain on Stress: How the Social Environment Gets under the Skin." *Proceedings of the National Academy of Sciences* 109(S2): 17180–17185.
McEwen, B. S., and Seeman, T. 1999. "Protective and Damaging Effects of Mediators of Stress." *Annals of the New York Academy of Sciences* 896(1): 30–47.
Millum, J., and Emanuel, E., eds. 2012. *Global Justice and Bioethics* (New York: Oxford University Press).
Montez, J. K., and Zajacova, A. 2013. "Trends in Mortality Risk by Education Level and Cause of Death among US White Women from 1986 to 2006." *American Journal of Public Health* 103(3): 473–479.
Powers, M., and Faden, R. 2006. *Social Justice: The Moral Foundations of Public Health and Health Policy* (New York: Oxford University Press).
Rawls, J. 1971. *A Theory of Justice* (Cambridge, Mass.: Harvard University Press).
WHO (World Health Organization). 2014. *World Health Statistics 2014* (Geneva: WHO). http://www.who.int/gho/publications/world_health_statistics/2014/en/.
WHO (World Health Organization). 2017. "The Top 10 Causes of Death." http://www.who.int/mediacentre/factsheets/fs310/en/index1.html.
Wilkinson, R. G. 1996. *Unhealthy Societies: The Afflictions of Inequality* (New York: Routledge).
Wilkinson, R. G. 2000. *Mind the Gap: Hierarchies, Health and Human Evolution* (London: Weidenfeld and Nicolson).
Wong, M. D., Shapiro, M. F., Boscardin, W. J., and Ettner, S. L. 2002. "Contribution of Major Diseases to Disparities in Mortality." *New England Journal of Medicine*. 347(20): 1585–1592.

CHAPTER 23

HEALTH DISPARITIES AND THE SOCIAL DETERMINANTS OF HEALTH: ETHICAL AND SOCIAL JUSTICE ISSUES

SRIDHAR VENKATAPURAM

Introduction

HEALTH *disparities* is a term most commonly used in the United States to refer to the differences in health states or outcomes across individuals and social groups. Elsewhere, such as in European countries and international institutions such as the World Health Organization (WHO), the term *health inequalities* is more commonly used to refer to the same phenomena. One explanation for the use of different terms is that *disparities* is seen to be less value-laden, and to more objectively describe natural facts. *Inequality*, in contrast, is seen to describe and implicitly evaluate a difference as a problematic deviation from equality (NIH, 2008). That is, inequalities are usually perceived to be bad, while disparities describe phenomena and leave open the valuation of goodness or badness. Furthermore, the phrase *social determinants of health* (SDOH) is also not as straightforward as it may seem. Most people who research, make policies about, or implement interventions to address SDOH are more than likely working on the social determinants of disease, illness, impairments, mortality, and related concepts. In a paradigm where health is understood as the absence of disease, addressing the determinants of disease is seen as realizing health.

The link between the terminology and underlying phenomena is that while disparities/inequalities describe the distribution patterns of health across individuals and social groups, SDOH describes certain types of causes of ill health in individuals. Importantly, SDOH are also identified to be the causes of the distribution patterns of health across social groups. Consequently, reducing disparities across social groups would require addressing SDOH that operate at the group level, not just at the individual level (Rose, 1985). While the scientific research on health disparities and SDOH is relatively new, ethical reasoning about them is even newer. Nevertheless, both areas of research are evolving quickly, mutually informing each other, and are raising many questions even as they provide new insights. This chapter presents some of the revolutionary scientific findings regarding SDOH, and examines how health disparities and SDOH raise profound questions in public and global health ethics and social justice philosophy.

It should be noted at the outset that this chapter does not present a comprehensive survey of the scientific literature or of the relevant philosophical literature. It presents some of the central scientific concepts, and situates them in ethics and social justice philosophy. In fact, health disparities and SDOH have relevance for many branches of philosophy, such as epistemology and philosophy of science. Nevertheless, the discussion emphasizes the ethics and social justice philosophy aspects.

Epidemiology and the Social Determinants of Health

Epidemiology is the study of the distribution and determinants of health-related states or events, and as such it is the informational engine of medicine, public health, and health policy. The knowledge epidemiology produces is then deployed toward addressing disease and other health problems. Though not easily apparent to outsiders, there is ongoing turmoil within the field of epidemiology concerning its central paradigm, as well as fundamental disagreements about what kind of science it is and what kind of values it may have. At the center of this turmoil is the question of whether it is appropriate to study social phenomena as causes of disease.

This question may seem surprising to some, as there is a long history of identifying the role of the social environment in the causal pathways to disease and mortality. It was central to the epidemiological work of Louis-René Villermé and Rudolph Virchow in the nineteenth century, for example (see Julia and Valleron, 2011; Virchow and Rather, 1985). And social conditions were very much a visible part of community and social medicine that began to flourish in the mid-twentieth century (Trostle, 2005). However, as epidemiology developed into a distinct and sophisticated scientific discipline in the twentieth century in the United States, its research paradigm or scope was increasingly narrowed down to individual-level factors (Krieger, 1994). That is, the primary focus became individuals, and disease came to be understood to be caused by the independent or interactive result of individual-level natural factors such as individual biology, behaviors, and harmful proximate exposures to the body.

Social Gradient in Health

However, in the 1970s, epidemiologists began to produce compelling evidence that health outcomes (e.g., life expectancy, mortality rates, obesity, cognitive development) are distributed along a social gradient, showing that each socioeconomic class—defined by income, occupational grade, or educational attainment—has worse health outcomes than the one above it (Kawachi, Subramanian, and Almeida-Filho, 2002; Macintyre, 1997; Marmot et al., 1997). In other words, there is a health-illness gradient from the top to the bottom of the social hierarchy within societies.

To press the point further, health and disease are not simply divided between the haves and have-nots, as often thought; instead, there is a health-illness gradient that parallels the social hierarchy within all societies. Such a step-wise gradient in health outcomes suggests a "dose-response" pathway between determinants related to social hierarchy/inequality and health outcomes. Research also shows that the steeper the socioeconomic gradient (i.e., the more social inequality), the lower the overall health and well-being of the entire population. Everyone in that society is worse off in the domain of health, and in many other domains, than they could be otherwise (Daniels, Kennedy, and Kawachi, 1999; Deaton, 2003; Wilkinson and Pickett, 2009).

Social Determinants of Health and the Health Gradient

The remarkable findings about the particular social distribution patterns of ill health have motivated numerous research studies on the underlying causal determinants. This is often the usual or normal practice in epidemiology. First, it is recognized that some individuals have a disease and others do not. Then, the aim is to find out what caused the disease in some individuals but not in the others. The important thing about social epidemiology is that unlike studies which try to identify what causes a disease in one individual rather than another, these studies aim to identify what causes disease in certain individuals, as well as in differing amounts in different social groups. The main hypothesis is that the causal factors are found in the social conditions (i.e., the factors affecting social groups differently in different places on the social hierarchy). Where one stands on the social gradient determines the types and levels of harmful exposures and protective factors in pathways to ill health and mortality.

The research has so far identified a whole range of social determinants (discrete exposures as well as pathways) of ill health over the entire life cycle, starting from the social conditions surrounding one's mother while one is still in utero to the amount and quality of one's social relationships in old age. To be clear, while availability of health care is crucial for health, other more influential causal determinants include such things as early infant care and stimulation, safe and secure employment, housing conditions, discrimination, self-respect, personal relationships, community cohesion, and income inequality (Berkman, Kawachi, and Glymour, 2014; Marmot and Wilkinson, 1999). Furthermore, these determinants operate at levels ranging from the micro, such as material deprivations and individual-level psychosocial mechanisms, to the macro, such as community cultures, national political regimes, and global processes affecting trade and respect for human rights. The possibility that extra-national, global determinants may have a significant impact on the health and longevity of some individuals and social groups within a society means that the causal analysis, as well as the ethical analysis, has to include a global perspective.

Keeping in mind that most of social epidemiological research so far has been done in high-income countries and may not be generalizable everywhere, Mackenbach (2012) presents a good review of the extant theories that could explain the persistence of health inequalities in developed countries. The WHO's Commission on the Social Determinants of Health (CSDH, 2008) presented a causal or explanatory model for all societies and human beings. The commission identified factors from the individual level all the way to national level, such as political leadership, governance, and cultural and social norms. More recently, a *Lancet*-University of Oslo Commission on Global Governance for Health pushed forward the commission's analysis and considered the transnational social and political factors that affect health and health inequalities, such as economic crises, foreign investment treaties, irregular migration, and transnational corporate activity (Ottersen, Frenk, and Horton, 2011).

These types of social epidemiological research and analyses challenge both the dominant individual-level explanatory paradigm in epidemiology, which largely focuses on genetics and personal "lifestyle choices," and the lack of domestic and global action regarding harmful social or "structural" conditions. While the level of expenditures and quality of health care, individual behaviors, and genetic risk factors clearly have a causal role, social conditions are more closely correlated with prevalence of preventable ill health and mortality in a society. That is, social conditions explain the causes and distribution patterns of ill health better than individual-level phenomena do. Such findings compel the recognition that mitigating preventable ill health and premature mortality in individuals, as well as health inequalities across groups, requires substantial changes to basic social institutions, processes, policies, and values (CSDH, 2008; Krieger and Birn, 1998; Marmot, 2006).

The empirical or scientific research in social epidemiology thus implies that existing social concern for health and health inequalities in a society warrants a scope of moral concern that goes beyond health care or even public health, reaching deep into the basic structures of domestic and, indeed, global society. However, many extant philosophical approaches to social equity and justice are simply ill-equipped to evaluate the ethics of such a broad relationship between social and global arrangements and ill health or health inequalities. On the one hand, the traditional reliance on moral philosophy in bioethics that focuses on the actions of individuals does not capture the social aspects of SDOH or health disparities across groups. On the other hand, modern debates in political philosophy have largely side-stepped the topic of health, which was long considered the domain of bioethics, and very few are aware of the profound findings in social epidemiology. However, a confluence of events such as globalization, the global spread of HIV/AIDS, and the WHO SDOH Commission, as well as philosophical interest in global justice and development, has instigated a flurry of activity at the intersection of social epidemiology and philosophy.

Obligations to Address Health Disparities and SDOH

Equality is one the most important social values of liberal democracies in the modern world. And equality—in particular, the equal status of all human beings—is a central tenet of the Universal Declaration of Human Rights as well as national and regional constitutions throughout the world. Moreover, for any theory of social justice or conception of a good society to persevere in the modern world, it would have to treat human beings equally in some meaningful way. However, the profound importance of equality as a social value throughout the world and across diverse societies still leaves open a further question: In which domains of human life is equality important? Does a shared starting point of equal moral status of individuals—that no human being is morally worth more or less than another—mean that we must ensure that everything about them is equal? It seems unlikely that we could adequately justify the position that the moral equality of persons means that we must ensure that all persons have equal hair length, have equal access to pottery classes, are equally able to run a marathon, and so forth. Clearly, equality matters in some domains and not in others. And perhaps equality matters more in some domains and less in others.

Equality, or, more accurately, inequality, in the domain of income and resources has been a central and motivating concern in various political philosophies and ideologies, as have political, social, and violent revolutions throughout the world over the past few centuries. Income and wealth are valued and valuable because of their instrumental nature (i.e., what they enable people to do). Inequalities in resources are seen to be morally bad or socially unjust for a number of reasons. A lack of resources constrains people's well-being, resource inequalities can corrode social relationships, extreme inequalities can allow the haves to dominate the have-nots, and so forth. But if these are some of the reasons why resource inequalities are ethically troubling and have motivated revolutions, health inequalities should be as, or even more, troubling.

Like income and wealth, health is instrumentally valuable. The state of one's health determines what one is practically able to be and do on a daily basis, as well as one's ability to make and realize long-term life plans. However, unlike income and wealth, health is also valuable because of its intrinsic aspects, because it partly constitutes a person's well-being. Resources, such as a pile of minerals or a stack of parchment paper, have no intrinsic value. Their value derives wholly from what human beings are able to be and do through their possession and conversion. Human well-being, in contrast, with health as a constituent component, is valuable in itself. The instrumental and intrinsic nature of health, then, should elevate the concern about inequalities in health to the same level as that of the worry about inequalities in resources, if not higher. But health has some other unique ethical aspects that would be missed if it is primarily understood as analogous to income and wealth, or something that can be purchased through income and wealth.

Any practical policy deliberations striving to identify the right social response to ill health in individuals or groups unavoidably confront ethical questions. Health policies are profoundly political because they distribute significant and diverse benefits and burdens across individuals and groups. In contemporary health policy debates, ethical ideas are often used to justify how limited resources are distributed across individuals and groups, or to constrain individual rights. But just beyond these familiar and immediate policy questions about the distribution of resources or individual liberties, there exist more fundamental questions and complex problems regarding how and why there should be any social interventions to address ill health in the first place. What is it about health or ill health that compels a social response or makes it a concern for social justice? Is it the types of causes of ill health, the absolute levels of health achievements, their relative inequalities, or the consequences of ill health that must be addressed as a matter of social justice? There are good reasons to believe that all of these multiple dimensions of health should matter in realizing social equity and justice (Sen, 2002). Even so, how do we then morally evaluate the different dimensions of the types of causes, levels of ill health, and consequences of ill health in relation to each other? Which dimension should social action address first, second, and so on? Furthermore, how does the understanding of what matters about these different dimensions change when the moral concern for individuals is supplemented by a concern for groups?

SDOH research complicates these numerous and difficult ethical questions even further by showing how narrowing absolute and/or relative health inequalities requires making changes to a range of basic social practices and institutions. In light of SDOH research, the scope of social interventions to address health concerns has now become much larger than just providing health care or addressing individual-level material causal factors. In fact, SDOH research expands the scope of social intervention to encompass all social environments, as it strives to identify and address any and all possible social determinants of impairment and mortality. While some social determinants are the social bases of autonomy, freedom, dignity, or respect, interventions to transform such determinants could mean redistributing economic resources and opportunities, material goods, and choices and duties of individuals and institutions. This means that addressing inequalities in the realm of individual or group health achievements may have to manipulate or, indeed, create inequalities in other realms of individual life and societal functioning.

Health and Distributive Justice

In the language of distributive justice debates, mitigating or manipulating social determinants of ill health and mortality means that there must be a redistribution of some valued goods or "things" in different social spheres. While SDOH research has provided information on some social bases of causal pathways to impairments and mortality, the literature has given little attention to the possible consequences in other nonhealth social spheres that would follow from transforming such causal pathways. It is often implicit in the SDOH literature that the logical social response to the identification of social determinants of ill health is to transform them. Ideally, transforming or redistributing a particular social determinant will improve health achievements, which in turn will create even more positive social determinants. For example, improving the social bases of dignity by creating opportunities for income and wealth could improve health achievements. Individuals who take advantage of those opportunities could in turn create more opportunities for income and wealth, and thus also create more social bases of dignity for themselves and others. Where such a virtuous circle does not exist, however, what sort of criteria should be used to decide how to balance the goals of improving absolute levels and relative inequalities in health functioning against goals regarding how things function or are distributed in other social realms?

Within the health sector, it seems self-evident that the primary goals of health interventions are to transform the causes, levels, and consequences of health. All things being equal, it may be a good thing to lessen health inequalities. Yet, as SDOH research has made clear, health policies are also cross-sector social policies. Thus, determining the right social response will require determining how the moral concern for the multiple dimensions of health of individuals and groups relates to the right and just functioning of a variety of social spheres. Ideally, a general theory of social justice would provide a clear framework that would help guide social action by identifying the justification for addressing health concerns in relation to pursuing other social goals, as well as determining how to address these concerns. However, there is no general theory of social justice that is commonly accepted within a particular society or across the societies in the world.

Social Justice Theory

Throughout the nineteenth century, and most of the twentieth, the dominant conception of social justice in philosophical discussions was utilitarianism. Simplifying greatly, an action or society was considered to be just if it produced the greatest happiness or welfare for the greatest number of individuals. However, since the 1970s, due to the profound critiques of utilitarianism and a meaningful alternative proposed by the philosopher John Rawls, debates on alternative conceptions of social and, indeed, global justice are flourishing again (Kymlicka, 2002). Nevertheless, utilitarian thought continues to profoundly shape public policymaking around the world—particularly public health policy.

All liberal theories of social justice begin from the premise that the individual is the primary unit of analysis or moral agent, and that every individual has equal moral worth. The equal moral worth of individuals is seen to arise from the capacity of human beings to reason, and thereby conceive and pursue a life plan. Equal moral worth and the freedom to conceive and pursue one's life plans are seen as interrelated concepts. From this common starting point, different theories go on to articulate what that means for how society must treat the individual. This central question of how individuals should be treated by society has been transformed into the question of what should be distributed to individuals. The reason treatment has turned into distribution is because social contract theories have had a profound influence on liberal conceptions of social justice, of which John Rawls's theory is the most recent (Rawls, 1971, 2001). Such influence has meant that liberal social justice, or how society should justly treat its members, is predominantly understood as being a conception of how to distribute the benefits and burdens of social cooperation fairly across individuals (Brighouse and Robeyns, 2010).

In reviewing the range of alternative theories, Amartya Sen has argued that the various modern conceptions of liberal social justice can be understood to differ most fundamentally according to the "thing" that is valued, and to how the theory distributes that thing across individuals (Sen, 1992). Among the range of different theories of social justice, the "things" to be distributed include welfare (preferences, objective welfare), resources (income, primary goods, personal and impersonal resources, negative liberties), and capabilities (basic capabilities, ten central human capabilities). Underlying both the identification of the things and the distribution schemes for them is the profound concern for inequality. Each of the different theories provides reasoning as to how the equal moral worth of individuals allows or disallows inequalities in different aspects of the lives of individuals thought to be relevant to social justice. Importantly, what has come to be accepted is that equal respect and concern for every individual does not necessarily mean that things are distributed equally to all individuals (Clayton and Williams, 2002; Daniels, 1996; Sen, 1992).

Despite the resurgence of philosophizing about social justice since the 1970s, only since the late 1990s have concerns about health, health inequalities, and SDOH been given significant attention by social justice philosophers. One explanation for this may be that philosophers, like most others, also thought ill health was caused by the natural lottery of biology, personal behaviors, and proximate exposures. The important thing to note is that knowledge about SDOH shifts both the causal story and the moral responsibility for ill health from the individual and nature squarely onto social institutions and choices. Because social conditions, choices, and, indeed, neglect are directly linked to ill health in individuals and social group inequalities in health, the fairness and justness of social institutions is at stake. Various philosophers have sought to rise to the challenge of developing a theory of social justice or health justice that takes account of SDOH as well as other health-related issues (Daniels, 2008; Powers and Faden, 2008; Sen, 1999; Venkatapuram, 2011; Weinstock, 2015). The comparative evaluation of these theories is just beginning, but it is clear they are being developed in conversation with each other and with an eye toward the frontiers of research in social epidemiology.

Global Health Disparities and Global Social Determinants of Health

Regarding global health inequalities, a number of political philosophers have begun to provide some insight. The moral concern for the "global poor" underlying global justice discussions of the early 2000s most often starts with concerns regarding the scale of their premature deaths and high levels of impairments. Low life expectancies of populations and inequalities in life expectancies across countries are often the first facts presented, and they are said to raise moral dilemmas to do with (global) justice. Yet these facts are not presented as raising moral problems regarding health and justice or SDOH. Instead, by focusing largely on premature mortality or life expectancy, the subject of health is circumvented. Often implicitly, life expectancy is treated as the "absolutist core" of human well-being. And like the equal moral worth of every human being, premature mortality as a moral bad is treated as something not needing explanation or justification; it is something that is assumed to resonate with the moral intuitions of most individuals, though they will hold a wide variety of philosophical views about justice. From there, reasoning is presented for the ethical claims all human beings can make about their well-being, or for the scope of obligations to the well-being of foreigners (Brock, 2005; Nussbaum, 2006; Singer, 2004). Some have identified the causal role of nondomestic actors in premature deaths and impairments of the "global poor" and the relevant moral obligations this entails (Pogge, 2002). That is, in contrast to positive duties to help ensure the wellbeing of foreigners, negative duties not to harm foreigners or to correct the harms caused to them would be stronger and more urgent. In real world examples, this would mean that a person's duty to correct for harms to people they have caused on a foreign holiday would be stronger and more urgent than for providing money directly or indirectly for healthcare for foreigners whom they did not harm. And when it can be shown that international institutions, regulations and processes are harming people such as certain trade regimes, the people benefitting have a strong duty to correct the harms.

Meanwhile, other philosophers have also made arguments that while stark health inequalities across societies may be a moral worry, such inequalities do not necessarily involve injustice (Daniels, 2008; Nagel, 2005). In comparison to the rapid growth of academic global health centers and interventions, the ethical reasoning about global health seems to be lagging behind. It may be that just as bioethics became productive when moral philosophy and medical sciences truly became integrated, for ethical reasoning on global health disparities to progress requires theories or approaches that reflect the closer integration of public/global health sciences and social/global justice philosophy.

Conclusion

There is much more that can be said about the science of health disparities and SDOH, as well as what may be the required social responses. Nevertheless, the present chapter has aimed to present a clear explanation of health disparities and their links to SDOH. While individual-level factors may explain the causes of disease in individuals, SDOH explain both diseases in individuals and the distribution patterns of disease across social groups within and across countries. In fact, SDOH are said to explain the social gradient in health that has been found to exist in all societies. The profound findings regarding

SDOH have also directly impacted how modern philosophers are conceptualizing theories or approaches to social and global justice. Fundamentally, the shift in thinking about the causes of disease from personal choices and tragic genetic luck to social determinants requires a reconsideration and reconceptualization of a good society or social justice. As SDOH also function across countries, they also require reconsidering approaches to global justice and, more specifically, global health justice. The potential for understanding preventable suffering in the world, as well as the possibility of changing it, has never seemed greater.

References

Berkman, L. F., Kawachi, I., and Glymour, M. M., eds. 2014. *Social Epidemiology*. 2nd ed. (New York: Oxford University Press).

Brighouse, H., and Robeyns, I., eds. 2010. *Measuring Justice: Primary Goods and Capabilities* (Cambridge: Cambridge University Press).

Brock, G. 2005. "Needs and Global Justice." In *The Philosophy of Need*, edited by S. Reader, 51–72 (Cambridge: Cambridge University Press).

Clayton, M., and Williams, A. 2002. *The Ideal of Equality* (Basingstoke, UK: Palgrave).

CSDH (Commission on Social Determinants of Health). 2008. *Closing the Gap in a Generation: Health Equity through Action on the Social Determinants of Health. Final Report of the Commission on Social Determinants of Health* (Geneva: World Health Organization).

Daniels, N. 1996. *Justice and Justification: Reflective Equilibrium in Theory and Practice*. Cambridge Studies in Philosophy and Public Policy (New York: Cambridge University Press).

Daniels, N. 2008. *Just Health: Meeting Health Needs Fairly* (New York: Cambridge University Press).

Daniels, N., Kennedy, B. P., and Kawachi, I. 1999. "Why Justice Is Good for Our Health: The Social Determinants of Health Inequalities." *Daedalus* 128(4): 215–251.

Deaton, A. 2003. "Health, Inequality, and Economic Development." *Journal of Economic Literature* 41(1): 113–158.

Julia, C., and Valleron, A. J. 2011. "Louis-René Villermé (1782–1863), a Pioneer in Social Epidemiology: Re-analysis of His Data on Comparative Mortality in Paris in the Early 19th Century." *Journal of Epidemiology and Community Health* 65(8): 666–670. doi:10.1136/jech.2009.087957.

Kawachi, I., Subramanian, S. V., and Almeida-Filho, N. 2002. "A Glossary for Health Inequalities." *Journal of Epidemiology and Community Health* 56(9): 647–652.

Krieger, N. 1994. "Epidemiology and the Web of Causation: Has Anyone Seen the Spider?" *Social Science & Medicine* 39(7): 887–903.

Krieger, N., and Birn, A. E. 1998. "A Vision of Social Justice as the Foundation of Public Health: Commemorating 150 Years of the Spirit of 1848." *American Journal of Public Health* 88(11): 1603–1606.

Kymlicka, W. 2002. *Contemporary Political Philosophy: An Introduction*. 2nd ed. (New York: Oxford University Press).

Macintyre, S. 1997. "The Black Report and Beyond: What Are the Issues?" *Social Science & Medicine* 44(6): 723–745.

Mackenbach, J. P. 2012. "The Persistence of Health Inequalities in Modern Welfare States: The Explanation of a Paradox." *Social Science & Medicine* 75(4): 761–769.

Marmot, M. 2006. "Health in an Unequal World." *Lancet* 368(9552): 2081–2094.

Marmot, M., Bosma, H., Hemingway, H., Brunner, E., and Stansfeld, S. 1997. "Contribution of Job Control to Social Gradient in Coronary Heart Disease." *Lancet* 350(9088): 1404–1405.

Marmot, M., and Wilkinson, R. G. 1999. *Social Determinants of Health* (New York: Oxford University Press).

Nagel, T. 2005. "The Problem of Global Justice." *Philosophy and Public Affairs* 33(2) 113–147.

NIH (National Institutes of Health). 2008. "Social Determinants of Health: From Research to Action." Recorded on December 11. NIH Videocast. http://videocast.nih.gov/launch.asp?14827.

Nussbaum, M. C. 2006. *Frontiers of Justice: Disability, Nationality, Species Membership* (Cambridge, Mass.: Harvard University Press).

Ottersen, O. P., Frenk, J., and Horton, R. 2011. "*The Lancet*-University of Oslo Commission on Global Governance for Health, in Collaboration with the Harvard Global Health Institute." *Lancet* 378(9803): 1612–1613. doi:10.1016/S0140-6736(11)61617-6.

Pogge, T. 2002. *World Poverty and Human Rights: Cosmopolitan Responsibilities and Reforms* (Cambridge: Polity Press).

Powers, M., and Faden, R. R. 2008. *Social Justice: The Moral Foundations of Public Health and Health Policy* (New York: Oxford University Press).

Rawls, J. 1971. *A Theory of Justice* (Cambridge, Mass.: Harvard University Press).

Rawls, J. 2001. *Justice as Fairness: A Restatement*. Edited by E. Kelly (Cambridge, Mass.: Harvard University Press).

Rose, G. 1985. "Sick Individuals and Sick Populations." *International Journal of Epidemiology* 14(1): 32–38.

Sen, A. 1992. *Inequality Reexamined* (Cambridge, Mass.: Harvard University Press).

Sen, A. 1999. *Development as Freedom* (New York: Knopf).

Sen, A. 2002. "Why Health Equity?" *Health Economics* 11(8): 659–666. doi:10.1002/hec.762.

Singer, P. 2004. *One World: The Ethics of Globalization*. 2nd ed. (New Haven, Conn.: Yale University Press).

Trostle, J. A. 2005. *Epidemiology and Culture*. Cambridge Studies in Medical Anthropology 13 (New York: Cambridge University Press).

Venkatapuram, S. 2011. *Health Justice: An Argument from the Capabilities Approach* (Cambridge: Polity Press).

Virchow, R. L. K., and Rather, L. J. 1985. *Collected Essays on Public Health and Epidemiology*. 2 vols. Resources in Medical History (Canton, Mass.: Science History Publications).

Weinstock, D. M. 2015. "Health Justice after the Social Determinants of Health Revolution." *Social Theory & Health* 13(3–4): 437–453. doi:10.1057/sth.2015.11.

Wilkinson, R. G., and Pickett, K. 2009. *The Spirit Level: Why More Equal Societies Almost Always Do Better* (London: Allen Lane).

CHAPTER 24

RACIAL AND ETHNIC DISPARITIES AS A PUBLIC HEALTH ETHICS ISSUE

STEPHEN B. THOMAS

INTRODUCTION

IMAGINE two men of the same age in the United States standing together on a Metro platform in Washington, D.C., heading to their respective homes. One boards a train that takes him to Montgomery County, Maryland. The other rides a train to his home in Prince George's County, Maryland. The men live just ten miles from each other. Can you predict how long each will live based on where the subway stops? The answer is yes, as illustrated in Figure 24.1.

The graphical presentation of data in Figure 24.1 has been repeated for cities across the United States, and the same pattern emerges each time (RWJF, 2015). And while the these differences in life expectancy based on "place" may seem startling, differences in life expectancy based on race are even more staggering. For example, a black man living in Washington, D.C. can expect to live 68.8 years, while a white man who lives in Washington can anticipate living 83.2 years—more than 14 years longer (Department of Health Systems Administration, Georgetown University School of Nursing & Health Studies, 2016). Both place *and* race contribute to health in the United States.

Differences in life expectancy between black and white men provide just one of many examples of how the color of one's skin is reflected in one's health. Racial and ethnic minorities in the United States suffer more from numerous health conditions than their white counterparts. Racial differences in illness and death from many of the leading causes of death (e.g., cardiovascular disease, diabetes, cancer) would be easy to ignore were they not so well documented. Cancer incidence rates for all cancers combined are highest for black men compared to all other racial and ethnic groups, and mortality

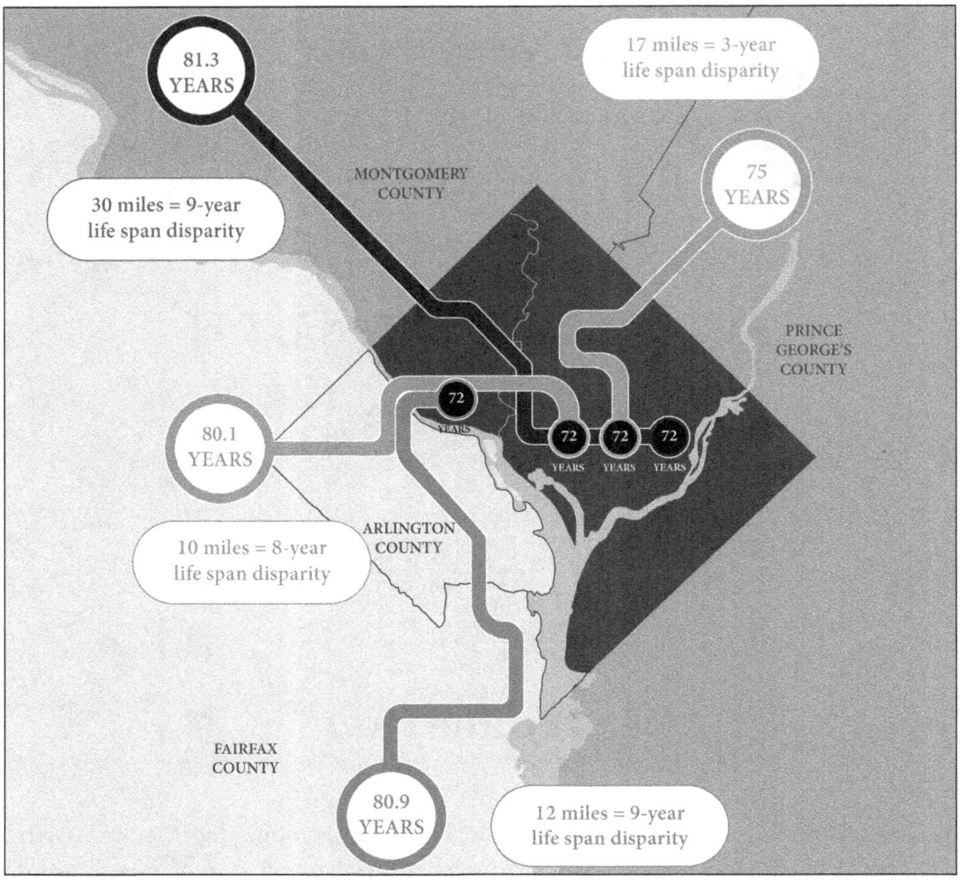

FIGURE 24.1 A Short Distance to Large Disparities in Health

Source: RWJF, 2013. *Copyright 2013. Robert Wood Johnson Foundation. Used with permission from the Robert Wood Johnson Foundation.*

from most major cancers is highest among African Americans. An African American woman with a college degree is more likely to have her baby die in the first year of life than a white woman without a high school diploma (Reeves and Matthew, 2016). American Indians and Alaska Natives continue to have the poorest five-year survival rates among all racial and ethnic groups for all cancers combined (HHS, 2012). Notably, cervical cancer statistics differ significantly for Hispanic women when compared to non-Hispanic white women: they are nearly two times as likely to have the disease and 1.4 times more likely to die from it (CDC, 2016). According to the American Diabetes Association (2018), Latinos are 70 percent more likely to have diagnosed diabetes compared to non-Latino Caucasians, and racial and ethnic minority populations have a higher risk of complications of diabetes compared to non-Hispanic whites. Excess death and disease among racial and ethnic minority groups compared to the majority white population constitute health disparities, defined by the US Department of Health and Human Services as "a particular type of health difference that is closely linked with social, economic, and/or environmental disadvantage. Health disparities adversely affect groups of people who have systematically experienced greater obstacles to health based on their racial or ethnic group" (NCHS, 2016).

Racial and ethnic minority health disparities are closely linked with socioeconomic status (SES), which is an individual's or group's position or standing in society, as determined by a combination of factors, including occupation, education, income, wealth, and place of residence (Williams and Jackson, 2005). Yet research shows that even at "equivalent" levels of SES, racial and ethnic minorities still suffer more from many health conditions than whites, indicating that factors additional to SES are responsible for determining one's health. After controlling for SES (as defined by income and education), researchers found that "few of the already described racial/ethnic health differentials disappear" (Crimmins, Hayward, and Seeman, 2004, 334).

Based on the work of the Robert Wood Johnson Foundation's Commission to Build a Healthier America, Figure 24.1 is a graphic description of how life-span disparities reflect differences in wealth, education, and environment across all community residents (RWJF, 2013). SES also determines what social determinants of health people face. Social determinants of health (SDOH) are defined by the US Centers for Disease Control and Prevention (CDC) as "conditions in the places where people live, learn, work, and play [that can] affect a wide range of health risks and outcomes" (CDC, 2018). In addition to SDOH, other determinants of health include biology and genetics, health care access, and personal lifestyle behaviors, among others. However, though the numbers have yet to be conclusively determined, researchers suggest that SDOH are major contributors to health. Early estimates suggested that SDOH accounted for around 15 percent of overall health, while more recent research increases the significance of social, economic, and environmental determinants to 50 percent, with individual biology, behaviors, and health care accounting for the other 50 percent (McGinnis, Williams-Russo, and Knickman, 2002; Department of Health Systems Administration, Georgetown University School of Nursing & Health Studies, 2016). Some might argue that individual behaviors are largely influenced by the social and economic conditions in which one lives. Likewise, genetics and biology can be influenced by physical environment and other social determinants. Thus, the conclusion is clear: SDOH, factors beyond medical care, are significant contributors to health.

In what follows, this chapter (a) describes public health policy initiatives that address racial and ethnic health disparities, (b) situates racial disparities in the current social and political milieu, (c) examines what progress has been made in reducing racial and ethnic disparities, (d) offers an account of the moral foundations for further efforts to reduce disparities, and (e) suggests a way forward for eliminating racial and ethnic health disparities.

Health Disparities and Public Health Policy

The emergence of health disparities as a US public health priority was first codified in 1980 with the publication of a seminal report by the Secretary of the US Department of

Health, Education and Welfare (DHEW, a predecessor agency to the Department of Health and Human Services). The *Report of the Secretary's Task Force on Black and Minority Health* (also known as the Heckler Report) documented the evidence of excess death among black and other minority groups compared to the white population (Heckler, 1985). In 2002 the Institute of Medicine (now the National Academy of Medicine) released *Unequal Treatment: Confronting Racial and Ethnic Disparities in Health Care*, which further delineated a significant body of research documenting the existence of disparities in actual delivery of health care services (Smedley, Stith, and Nelson, 2002). According to the report, minorities are less likely to be given appropriate cardiac medications or to undergo bypass surgery, and are less likely to receive kidney dialysis or transplants, compared to their white counterparts.

In 1979, prior to the release of the Heckler Report, the Healthy People Initiative began with the Surgeon General's Report *Healthy People: Health Promotion and Disease Prevention* (US Public Health Service, 1979). Since that inaugural report, the Healthy People Initiative has continued to set science-based national health goals to improve the health of Americans in ten-year increments. In its initial iteration, the Healthy People goals called for the reduction of preventable illness and death, but it stopped short of specifically identifying health disparities as a focus. The Healthy People 2000 goals included, for the first time, the reduction of health disparities (ODPHP, 2018). That same year, Congress passed legislation creating the National Center on Minority Health and Health Disparities (Minority Health and Health Disparities Research and Education Act of 2000, Public Law 106-525), just after new guidelines were issued on the collection of race and ethnicity data in biomedical and public health research (HHS, 1999). In 2003 the Agency on Health Research & Quality (AHRQ) released its inaugural annual report on health care disparities, representing the first comprehensive national effort to measure differences in quality of and access to health care services overall and by various populations (Kelley et al., 2005). Beginning with *Healthy People 2010*, and continuing with *Healthy People 2020*, the elimination of health disparities became a central goal of the initiative. Additionally, for the first time, the 2020 plan included addressing the social determinants of health (Breen, 2017).

The reinvigorated mission to eliminate health disparities was furthered by the passage of the Affordable Care Act (ACA) in 2010, which ushered in a new era of federal provisions designed to close the health disparities gap. These provisions included the establishment of individual Offices of Minority Health within a number of federal agencies and departments. Additionally, it called for the establishment of the National Institute on Minority Health and Health Disparities. Passage of the ACA also helped millions of Americans without health insurance to finally obtain coverage, decreasing disparities in access to care. The ACA also supports new prevention initiatives that address health disparities, including, but not limited to, the National Prevention Council, which involves twenty federal departments, agencies, and offices and is chaired by the Surgeon General (HHS, 2016). However, various efforts to repeal and actively undermine the ACA have created some uncertainty about whether these initiatives will remain in place.

Public Health Ethics in the Era of Black Lives Matter

In 2002 the Public Health Leadership Society (PHLS), a highly regarded group of senior public health officials and others, published the often cited *Principles of the Ethical Practice of Public Health* (PHLS, 2002). This code delineates twelve principles to guide the ethical practice of public health. Two principles stand out as useful for addressing health disparities:

> **Principle 1**: Public health should address principally the fundamental causes of disease and requirements for health, aiming to prevent adverse health outcomes.
>
> **Principle 4**: Public health should advocate and work for the empowerment of disenfranchised community members, aiming to ensure that the basic resources and conditions necessary for health are accessible to all.

Principle 1 is important because there is growing scientific consensus that racism is a *fundamental cause* of premature illness and death among racial and ethnic minority groups in the United States (Phelan and Link, 2015). Principle 4 is also significant because black men in general, and young black men in particular, are *the most disenfranchised demographic* in the nation. It is ironic that since the 2008 election of Barack Obama, the first self-identified African American/black person to become president of the United States, the plight of black men has garnered national and international attention largely due to staggering high school dropout rates, high unemployment, and high rates of incarceration. Sociologists coined the metaphor of the "school-to-prison pipeline" to describe disturbing vestiges of historic subjugation manifest in the pattern of black men involved with the juvenile and adult criminal justice system. President Obama's election did not immediately eliminate the legacy of slavery that undergirds the persistent racism and discrimination shaping the social determinants of health that disproportionately impact people of color in general, or African American men in particular.

Violence is also a public health issue, and young black males are more at risk of death by homicide than other racial and ethnic groups. On the night of February 26, 2012, Trayvon Martin, an unarmed seventeen-year-old black high school student encountered George Zimmerman, a twenty-eight-year-old mixed-race Hispanic man who served as the Neighborhood Watch coordinator for a gated community in Sanford, Florida, where Martin was living with his father. Before the night was over, Martin was shot and killed by Zimmerman. Zimmerman was charged with murder, his case went to trial, and a jury acquitted him in July 2013.

Just over a year after Zimmerman's acquittal, on August 9, 2014, the police shooting of another young black man made national news. Michael Brown, an unarmed black eighteen-year-old, was shot and killed by a white police officer while walking down his neighborhood street in Ferguson, Missouri. His dead body lay in the street, sweltering uncovered in the summer heat, for hours, fueling outrage that sparked riots in Ferguson and protests outside the region, as far away as Baltimore. This marked the beginning of an unrest that continued and reignited when a November 2014 grand jury declined to indict the police officer who shot Brown. While each case is made more complicated by details of the criminal justice proceedings, the pattern fit what far too many African Americans believe to be true—black lives are perceived as having no value.

These two events ignited what has become a national movement, "#BlackLivesMatter," which is more than a Twitter hashtag. Black Lives Matter is "a call to action and a response to the virulent anti-black racism that permeates our society" (Black Lives Matter, n.d.). While the hashtag was originally coined just after the acquittal of Zimmerman, it did not catch on until the following months brought national and international attention to the plight of far too many unarmed black men killed at the hands of law enforcement and the resulting riotous tumult in Ferguson and Baltimore.

These events, and others like them, made clear that the United States has yet to achieve the hoped-for postracial society many believed had been ushered in by President Obama and echoed by the president himself in his "A More Perfect Union: The Race Speech," delivered March 18, 2008, in Philadelphia:

> We do not need to recite here the history of racial injustice in this country. But we do need to remind ourselves that so many of the disparities that exist in the African-American community today can be directly traced to inequalities passed on from an earlier generation that suffered under the brutal legacy of slavery and Jim Crow
>
> (Obama, 2008)

While homicide may not be included among the ten leading causes of death in the United States, African Americans experience disparate rates of incidence and death for many of the ten, which include heart disease, cancer, and diabetes (Kochanek, Anderson, and Arias, 2015; Logan et al., 2013). The United States has made progress in extending the length and quality of life for everyone, but even with that progress there is clear evidence that certain racial and ethnic groups—black, Latino, American Indian, Asian and Pacific Islander— suffer a disproportionate burden of premature illness and preventable death compared to whites (Kochanek, Anderson, and Arias, 2015; Mozaffarian et al., 2016). As racial and ethnic populations continue to grow toward becoming the numerical majority, their health and well-being will become the health baseline status for the nation.

Have We Made Progress?

Since national attention was brought to the existence of health disparities, first with the Heckler Report, and then with the extensive research and documentation of the problems that followed, the question is, has the United States made progress? In short, the answer is obviously yes. But any enthusiasm for the progress that has been made must be tempered by the work still to come. First, the progress: The gap in life expectancy between African Americans and whites is narrowing. In 1990 there was an 8.2-year disparity in life expectancy at birth between a white male and African American male. In 2000 the gap had decreased to 6.5 years, and in 2013 it had further narrowed to 4.4 years. The narrowing in the gap is largely attributed to larger decreases in death rates for African Americans due to heart disease, cancer, and HIV/AIDS. While life expectancy increased for both white and African American males from 1990 to 2013, it increased more for African Americans (+4.0 years vs. +7.8 years). A similar trend is seen with women. In 1990 there was a 5.8-year disparity in life expectancy, which shrank to 4.8 years in 2000, and to 3.0 years in 2013. Again, this trend is due to larger decreases in death rates for African American women from heart disease, HIV, and cancer, resulting in greater gains in life expectancy (Kochanek, Anderson, and Arias, 2015).

Second, the reality of how far we have to go: African Americans still live shorter lives than whites do. In 2013 life expectancy for African American males was equivalent to that of white males in 1990. Even more striking, the life expectancy of African American females is equivalent to that of white women all the way back to 1980 (Kochanek, Anderson, and Arias, 2015).

In addition to improvements in the disparities between blacks and whites in terms of life expectancy, the racial gap for different diseases is narrowing as well. Rates of many diseases, including heart disease, cancer, infant mortality, and HIV/AIDS, among others, are decreasing more for African Americans than for other racial and ethnic groups. These accomplishments do demonstrate progress and movement in the right direction, but the disparities, while narrowing, still persist. For example, while African American women saw a nearly 20 percent decrease in the infant mortality rate between 2005 and 2013, the 2013 rate of 11.11 (infant deaths per 100,000) is still over two times the rate for non-Hispanic white women (5.06), and almost three times more than that for Cuban Americans (who experience the lowest rate, at 3.09) (Mathews and Macdorman, 2013). The sobering reality is that promising signs of progress to date are not enough to claim victory in the national goal to achieve health equity, which "requires valuing everyone equally with focused and ongoing societal efforts to address avoidable inequalities, historical and contemporary injustices, and the elimination of health and health care disparities" (ODPHP, 2018). Such an understanding of health equity requires a commitment to a set of core principles to guide action.

Social Movements and a Moral Foundation: Pillars of Public Health

Since the mid-1980s, minority heath has been elevated from the margins of academe to the mainstream of government-funded health disparities research, along with federal, state, and local public policy initiatives addressing the social determinants of health—all designed to achieve health equity (ODPHP, 2018). The emergence of health disparities as a science (Dankwa-Mullan et al., 2010) and health equity as a public policy goal begs the question of whether this is a public health social movement rooted in a moral foundation, similar to the environmental justice movement (leading to the Clean Air Act of 1963) or the national campaign to provide quality medical care for people with AIDS (leading to the Ryan White Act of 1990). Is there a moral foundation of public health that provides a philosophical framework for health disparity research designed to achieve health equity? Some theorists answer in the affirmative.

Madison Powers and Ruth Faden (2006) argue that social justice is the moral foundation of public health. At its core, public health is concerned with the well-being of people in social communities—populations of people where they live, learn, work, play, and worship. According to Powers and Faden,

> Public health is the social institution charged with promoting human welfare by bringing about a certain kind of human good, the good of health. The moral foundation for public health thus rests on the general obligations in beneficence to promote good or welfare.... [T]he moral imperative in public health to produce health must be tempered with concern for who experiences these health benefits as well as who is exposed to hazards that harm health. (81)

Powers and Faden rightly call for public health research and programs to be grounded in social justice. This call has even greater salience for health disparity research, because inequalities between groups are the most urgent ones to address. Social justice is not only about how individuals live, but also about how groups live. Systematic discrimination linked to gender, ethnicity, race, religion, social class, sexual orientation, and disability makes groups and entire communities even more disadvantaged and vulnerable to health disparities.

Health disparities remain the unfinished business of public health. Over the years, efforts to reduce and ultimately eliminate health disparities and achieve health equity have focused primarily on access to medical care designed to cure and/or treat disease at the individual level. Far less attention has been focused on the social and economic conditions in society that fuel persistent disparities in health care access and individual and community health status. Health is more than freedom from disease or infirmity. To eliminate health disparities, we must address cultural and environmental conditions that shape the lived experience of people and communities suffering from health disparities.

It is also critical that we look to the past to guide our future plans. We need to understand why these disparities exist in order to understand where and how to focus our efforts to eliminate them. Research is needed, and the historical injustices and mistreatments of racial and ethnic minorities is a legacy that cannot be ignored by researchers today. There are well-known examples of this legacy, including the US Public Health Service Syphilis Study done in Tuskegee (1932–1972), where approximately four hundred black men from rural Alabama were recruited into a natural history study to determine what would happen if syphilis went untreated. Unfortunately, the men were not told the truth about the study, and the government doctors went to great lengths to ensure that even when penicillin became available in the 1950s, the men in the Tuskegee Study did not receive treatment (Jones, 1993).

The Tuskegee Study is just one of many examples of research abuse that cast a shadow of mistrust on biomedical and public health researchers today. Trust, and mistrust, play an important role in the decisions of individuals to participate in the very research studies that help investigators understand health and health disparities. Minorities remain underrepresented in many clinical research studies, including those investigating the very diseases in which the greatest disparities are seen (Murthy, Krumholz, and Gross, 2004; Oh et al., 2015; Sardar et al., 2014). We also know, from a limited number of research reports, that different racial and ethnic groups have different risk factors for different disease conditions, and that they respond differently to specific treatments (Cubeddu et al., 1986; Exner et al., 2001).

Toward a New Generation of Health Disparities Research

In their publication "Toward a Fourth Generation of Disparities Research to Achieve Health Equity," Thomas et al. (2011) delineate generations of health disparities research. First-generation disparities research is focused on surveillance (incidence and prevalence trends); second-generation research is focused on associated risk factors (e.g., heart disease and diet high in saturated fat); and third-generation research is focused on randomized controlled trials (what works). According to Thomas et al., now is the time to launch a fourth generation of health disparities research, focused on taking action. This approach translates the science of medical and public health research into culturally tailored community-based interventions designed to reduce exposure to risk factors for chronic disease and ultimately eliminate health disparities to achieve health equity.

This call to take action must address racism within the context of the social determinants of health, and it reflects moving beyond documenting and understanding the existence of health disparities to actively implementing solutions. Additionally, expanding access to health care is critical to moving the nation closer to health equity; it represents a moral and ethical obligation that "public health should advocate and work for the empowerment of disenfranchised community members, aiming to ensure that the basic resources and conditions necessary for health are accessible to all" (PHLS, 2002, 4).

There is no one right way to conduct fourth-generation research. However, there are ethical characteristics that should be embodied in these efforts, especially Principle 6 from the *Principles of the Ethical Practice of Public Health*: "Public health institutions should provide communities with the information they have that is needed for decisions on policies or programs and should obtain the community's consent for their implementation" (Thomas et al., 2002, 1058). Fourth-generation disparities research efforts include strategic partnerships with community groups, sustained outreach efforts, and the involvement of local media to help spread awareness. Researchers are called on to critically examine themselves, their team, and their unconscious biases through self-reflection. They must also become comfortable with feeling uncomfortable (Thomas et al., 2011).

Conclusion

Race and racism continue to be the color line that, as first described by W. E. B. Du Bois defines the great challenge of our democracy:

> Herein lie buried many things which if read with patience may show the strange meaning of being black here at the dawning of the Twentieth Century. This meaning is not without interest to you, . . . for the problem of the Twentieth Century is the problem of the color line. . . . [T]he relation of the darker to the lighter races of men in Asia and Africa, in America and the islands of the sea.
>
> (Du Bois, 1903, Forethought)

In the twenty-first century, that color line runs through population health. It is sometimes easier to gloss over race and racism, rather than face them head on and acknowledge how pervasive they are in today's society. But the mounting scientific evidence that structural racism can get under your skin and make you sick must not be dismissed, because the demographic transformation from majority white to majority minority is here to stay: as people of color become the numerical majority in the nation, the health of these populations will constitute and represent the health of the United States. We must be filled with the urgency of how to ensure that the color of your skin, or where you live, or how much money you make, does not define your life expectancy. The political climate following the 2016 US election is full of uncertainty about how the Trump administration will impact US health policy. Thus, public health researchers must stand on principle and not depend on shifting political idiosyncrasies. We must be ever vigilant about the ethics of public health and how race and ethnicity still define one's health status, and we must focus on educating and inspiring the public to demand ethical treatment and end social injustice.

Acknowledgment

I would like to thank Erica Casper, who was very helpful to me on this project.

References

American Diabetes Association. 2018. "Health Disparities." http://www.diabetes.org/advocacy/advocacy-priorities/health-disparities.html?referrer=https://www.google.com/.

Black Lives Matter. http://blacklivesmatter.com/about/.

Breen, N. 2017. *For the First Time, Healthy People Initiative Focuses on Social Determinants of Health* (Washington, D.C.: National Institute on Minority Health and Health Disparities). https://nimhd.blogs.govdelivery.com/2017/04/20/for-the-first-time-healthy-people-initiative-focuses-on-social-determinants-of-health/.

CDC (Centers for Disease Control and Prevention). 2016. "Cervical Cancer Rates by Race and Ethnicity." https://www.cdc.gov/cancer/cervical/statistics/race.htm.

CDC (Centers for Disease Control and Prevention). 2018. "Social Determinants of Health: Know What Affects Health." https://www.cdc.gov/socialdeterminants/.

Crimmins, E. M., Hayward, M. D., and Seeman, T. E. 2004. "Race/Ethnicity, Socioeconomic Status, and Health." In *Critical Perspectives on Racial and Ethnic Differences in Health in Late Life*, edited by B. Cohen, R. A. Bulateo, and N. B. Anderson, 310–352 (Washington, D.C.: National Academies Press).

Cubeddu, L. X., Aranda, J., Singh, B., Klein, M., Brachfeld, J., Freis, E., et al. 1986. "A Comparison of Verapamil and Propranolol for the Initial Treatment of Hypertension: Racial Differences in Response." *JAMA* 256(16): 2214–2221.

Dankwa-Mullan, I., Rhee, K. B., Williams, K., Sanchez, I., Sy, F. S., Stinson N., Jr., et al. 2010. "The Science of Eliminating Health Disparities: Summary and Analysis of the NIH Summit Recommendations." *American Journal of Public Health* 100(S1): S12–S18.

Department of Health Systems Administration, Georgetown University School of Nursing & Health Studies. 2016. *The Health of the African American Community in the District of Columbia: Disparities and Recommendations* (Washington, D.C.: Georgetown University School of Nursing & Health Studies). https://www.georgetown.edu/sites/www/files/The%20Health%20of%20the%20African%20American%20Community%20in%20the%20District%20of%20Columbia.pdf.

Du Bois, W. E. B. 1903. *The Souls of Black Folk*. Edited with an Introduction and Notes by B. H. Edwards (New York: Oxford University Press, 2008).

Exner, D. V., Dries, D. L., Domanski, M. J., and Cohn, J. N. 2001. "Lesser Response to Angiotensin-Converting–Enzyme Inhibitor Therapy in Black as Compared with White Patients with Left Ventricular Dysfunction." *New England Journal of Medicine* 344(18): 1351–1357.

Heckler, M. 1985. *Report of the Secretary's Task Force on Black and Minority Health* (Washington, D.C.: US Department of Health, Education and Welfare).

HHS (US Department of Health and Human Services). 1999. *Improving the Collection and Use of Racial and Ethnic Data in HHS* (Rockville, Md.: HHS).

HHS (US Department of Health and Human Services). 2012. *The National Cancer Program: Managing the Nation's Research Portfolio, an Annual Plan and Budget for Fiscal Year 2013* (Rockville, Md.: HHS).

HHS (US Department of Health and Human Services). 2016. *2015 National Healthcare Quality and Disparities Report and 5th Anniversary Update on the National Quality Strategy* (Rockville, Md.: HHS).

Jones, J. H. 1993. *Bad Blood* (New York: Simon & Schuster).

Kelley, E., Moy, E., Stryer, D., Burstin, H., and Clancy, C. 2005. "The National Healthcare Quality and Disparities Reports: An Overview." *Medical Care* 43(3): I-3–I-8.

Kochanek, K. D., Anderson, R., and Arias, E. 2015. "Leading Causes of Death Contributing to Decrease in Life Expectancy Gap between Black and White Populations: United States, 1999–2013." *NCHS Data Brief* 218(November): 1.

Logan, J. E., Hall, J., McDaniel, D., and Stevens, M. R. 2013. "Homicides—United States, 2007 and 2009." *CDC Health Disparities and Inequalities Report—United States, 2013* 62(3): 164.

Mathews, T., and MacDorman, M. F. 2013. "Infant Mortality Statistics from the 2009 Period Linked Birth/Infant Death Data Set." *National Vital Statistics Reports* 61(8): 1–28.

McGinnis, J. M., Williams-Russo, P., and Knickman, J. R. 2002. "The Case for More Active Policy Attention to Health Promotion." *Health Affairs* 21(2): 78–93. doi:10.1377/hlthaff.21.2.78.

Mozaffarian, D., Benjamin, E. J., Go, A. S., Arnett, D. K., Blaha, M. J., Cushman, M., et al. 2016. "Executive Summary: Heart Disease and Stroke Statistics—2016 Update: A Report from the American Heart Association." *Circulation* 133(4): 447–454.

Murthy, V. H., Krumholz, H. M., and Gross, C. P. 2004. "Participation in Cancer Clinical Trials: Race-, Sex-, and Age-Based Disparities." *JAMA* 291(22): 2720–2726.

NCHS (National Center for Health Statistics). 2016. *Health, United States, 2015: With Special Feature on Racial and Ethnic Health Disparities* (Washington, D.C.: US Government Printing Office). https://www.cdc.gov/nchs/data/hus/hus15.pdf.

Obama, B. 2008. "A More Perfect Union: 'The Race Speech.'" http://obamaspeeches.com/E05-Barack-Obama-A-More-Perfect-Union-the-Race-Speech-Philadelphia-PA-March-18-2008.htm.

ODPHP (Office of Disease Prevention and Health Promotion). 2018. "*Healthy People 2020*: Disparities." https://www.healthypeople.gov/2020/about/foundation-health-measures/Disparities.

Oh, S. S., Galanter, J., Thakur, N., Pino-Yanes, M., Barcelo, N. E., White, M. J., et al. 2015. "Diversity in Clinical and Biomedical Research: A Promise Yet to Be Fulfilled." *PLoS Medicine* 12(12): e1001918.

Phelan, J. C., and Link, B. G. 2015. "Is Racism a Fundamental Cause of Inequalities in Health?" *Annual Review of Sociology* 41(1): 311–330. doi:10.1146/annurev-soc-073014-112305.

PHLS (Public Health Leadership Society). 2002. *Principles of the Ethical Practice of Public Health.* https://www.apha.org/-/media/files/pdf/membergroups/ethics/ethics_brochure.ashx.

Powers, M., and Faden, R. 2006. *Social Justice: The Moral Foundations of Public Health and Health Policy* (Oxford: Oxford University Press).

Reeves, R. V., and Matthew, D. B. 2016. "6 Charts Showing Race Gaps within American Middle Class." Brookings Social Mobility Memos (Washington, D.C.: Brookings Institution). https://www.brookings.edu/blog/social-mobility-memos/2016/10/21/6-charts-showing-race-gaps-within-the-american-middle-class/.

RWJF (Robert Wood Johnson Foundation). 2013. "Metro Map: Washington, D.C." RWJF Commission to Build a Healthier America. https://www.rwjf.org/en/library/infographics/washington-dc-map.html.

RWJF (Robert Wood Johnson Foundation). 2015, "City Maps: Short Distances to Large Gaps in Health." http://www.rwjf.org/en/library/articles-and-news/2015/09/city-maps.html.

Sardar, M. R., Badri, M., Prince, C. T., Seltzer, J., and Kowey, P. R. 2014. "Underrepresentation of Women, Elderly Patients, and Racial Minorities in the Randomized Trials Used for Cardiovascular Guidelines." *JAMA Internal Medicine* 174(11): 1868–1870.

Smedley, B. D., Stith, A. Y., and Nelson, A. R. 2002. *Unequal Treatment: Confronting Racial and Ethnic Disparities in Health Care* (Washington, D.C.: National Academies Press).

Thomas, J. C., Sage, M., Dillenberg, J., and Guillory, V. J. 2002. "A Code of Ethics for Public Health." *American Journal of Public Health* 92(7): 1057–1059.

Thomas, S. B., Quinn, S. C., Butler, J., Fryer, C. S., and Garza, M. A. 2011. "Toward a Fourth Generation of Disparities Research to Achieve Health Equity." *Annual Review of Public Health* 32: 399–416.

US Public Health Service. 1979. *Healthy People: The Surgeon General's Report on Health Promotion and Disease Prevention* (Washington, D.C.: Government Printing Office).

Williams, D. R., and Jackson, P. B. 2005. "Social Sources of Racial Disparities in Health." *Health Affairs* 24(2): 325–334.

CHAPTER 25

RECONCILING TWO ETHICS GOALS OF PUBLIC HEALTH: REDUCING HEALTH DISPARITIES AND IMPROVING POPULATION HEALTH

NORMAN DANIELS

INTRODUCTION

REDUCING health inequalities is an important objective of social justice in the United States, where race "disparities" (a euphemism for "inequities") are significant and generally thought to be unjust (IOM, 2003). It is a more developed feature of public policy in Europe, where a Health for All strategy has evolved (WHO, 1999, 2002). Globally, the World Health Organization (WHO) has made equity in health central to its agenda, including in its recent emphasis on universal coverage (Norheim et al., 2014).

It is argued that health inequality between social groups is unjust when it results from an unjust distribution of the socially controllable factors affecting population health (Daniels, Kennedy, and Kawachi, 1999; Daniels, 2007). Norman Daniels (2007) illustrates the idea using Rawls's account of justice as fairness, since Rawls's principles of justice capture key socially controllable determinants of health and, thus, concerns about race or gender inequalities in health, as well as about socioeconomic status (SES) inequalities. If social policy has produced health inequality, there may be additional reasons for wanting to reduce it; in any case, people have a social obligation to meet these health needs however they arise.

But life is not so simple, even where injustice is involved. This chapter argues that many policies that would reduce inequities between groups encounter the same foci of disagreement about distributive justice that elsewhere have been called "unsolved rationing problems" (Daniels, 1993); namely, the priorities problem (How much priority should we give to those who are worst off?), the aggregation problem (When should we allow a modest benefit to a larger number of people outweigh a significant benefit to a smaller number?), and the best outcomes/fair chances problem (When should we give people fair chances at a benefit rather than favor getting a best outcome?). These problems, so common in medical resource allocation contexts, describe the baseline distributions of health neutrally. In the priority problem, for example, no moral judgment is made about whether the inequality between the health of better- and worse-off people is itself unfair or unjust. This moral neutrality regarding the baseline may carry over from the neutrality that seems appropriate in medical contexts, where the focus is properly on the medical need and not on a moral account of how it arose.

The morally problematic features of the baseline are what make health inequalities into inequities. Inequalities in the prevalence of some diseases between blacks and whites are the result of the unjust distribution of many socially controllable factors, including income, job opportunity, education, housing quality and location, and racial discrimination itself. Some inequalities in health outcomes may well be the result of racially distinct utilization decisions by clinicians—perhaps the result of conscious or unconscious stereotyping. Similarly, the higher prevalence of human immunodeficiency virus/acquired immune deficiency syndrome (HIV/AIDS) among young females than among males in southern Africa is the result of an unjust distribution of property and marriage rights, extreme poverty leading to transactional sex, and the lack of empowerment of women to control their sexual and reproductive choices. Justice opposes health inequality in such cases.

Suppose a high degree of priority can be given to reducing an unjust racial inequality in health only by foregoing a more effective use of resources that improves the health of a larger number of other people. What price in aggregate health should be paid in order to reduce unjust health disparities? A smoking cessation campaign may be more effective for better-off groups, such as professionals and groups with higher income and higher education levels, than for manual workers or lower SES groups (Barbeau, Krieger, and Soobader, 2004), so that if it is implemented, the existing gap in smoking rates may increase. What should be done when efforts to improve population health increase health disparities? It is important to examine this troubling conflict between reducing unjust health disparities and promoting population health fairly.

Race and Gender Inequities Illustrated

Consider the following examples of health inequalities that most people would consider unjust.

Inequity in Access by Race

Controlling for type of payer, treatment site, and clinical condition, physicians underutilize important treatments, such as cardiac catheterization (Schulman et al., 1999) and renal transplantation (Epstein et al., 2000), in blacks (and women) compared to whites. The Schulman study videotaped interactions between physicians and black and white actors, both male and female, who were dressed similarly and had matching educational and occupational profiles and identical clinical descriptions. Black women received the lowest referral rate for catheterization. In the Epstein study, meanwhile, there was overutilization of transplantation among whites and underutilization for blacks. Whether there is overt racism among providers or subconscious stereotyping that is not malicious, the effect is an inequality of access to crucial interventions. Understanding the source of the discrimination is important to devising effective interventions.

Health Inequity from the Experience of Racism

A review by Williams, Neighbors, and Jackson (2003) showed a strong association between the experience of discrimination and (i) psychological distress, (ii) major depression, and (iii) physiological measures of stress, such as blood pressure (see also Harrell, Hall, and Taliaferro, 2003). Some evidence suggests that people who "internalize" rather than "resist" discrimination have higher blood pressure (Krieger and Sidney, 1996; Noh and Kaspar, 2003). Since the racism people experience is diverse, remedying the health inequity that results from it is probably more difficult than altering the discriminatory behavior of providers, but this is an empirical question.

Health Inequity from Institutional Racism

In 1990 black men at age twenty could expect to live 7.6 fewer years, but with more disability, than white men at the same age (Hayward and Heron, 1999). Black males aged fifty-one to sixty-one had a higher prevalence of hypertension, stroke, diabetes, kidney and bladder problems, and stomach ulcers than white males of the same age. Whites, meanwhile, had a higher prevalence of cardiac and chronic obstructive pulmonary disease, high cholesterol, and back and eye problems. Altogether, blacks had higher mortality and disability rates in middle age.

While SES explains most of the aggregate black-white differences in health, this fact understates the role of unfair social and economic disadvantage suffered by blacks (Kawachi, Daniels, and Robinson, 2005). The broad legacy of overt and institutional racism in American society disproportionately confines blacks to lower SES groups. At the same time, within each SES level, the health of blacks is worse than that of whites (House and Williams, 2000). In addition, segregation—including hyper-segregation and other severe forms of segregation—is associated with multiple risk factors for blacks as compared to whites (Acevedo-Garcia et al., 2003).

All the major risky health behaviors (smoking, immoderate drinking and eating, lack of exercise) explain but 10 to 20 percent of SES inequalities in health. Since the health inequalities produced by SES and race vastly exceed in scope those produced by inequalities in access to health care, reducing them will require broad intersectoral efforts.

Gender Inequity in the HIV/AIDS Epidemic

Girls and young women (ages fifteen to twenty-four) have a significantly higher incidence of HIV/AIDS than comparable males in sub-Saharan Africa (UNAIDS, UNFPA, and UNIFEM, 2004). Despite the biological vulnerability of young girls to HIV, the key determinants of the health inequality are extensive poverty, leading to early transactional sex to pay for school fees; and gender inequalities in property, marriage, and divorce rights, which give women little room to protect themselves from unsafe sex and early marriage.

These examples are all relatively uncontroversial instances of health inequities. There are clear reasons of justice to intervene to reduce these health inequalities. But reducing them requires investing resources, and such investments have distributive implications that must be attended to.

Encounters with Unsolved Rationing Problems

The Millennium Development Goals (MDGs) of inequality reduction, developed by the UN in 2000, did not explicitly state that inequality is unjust, although they assumed that inequalities should be reduced. Five of the eight internationally negotiated MDGs were aimed directly at reducing inequality, since their targets aimed at poverty reduction or providing primary education to those who lack it. The three health targets were stated in terms of reducing health outcome measures that apply to the whole population, such as the under-five child mortality rate.

David Gwatkin (2002) models two extreme approaches to these aggregate health goals. A maximizing approach seeks rapid achievement of the target by directing resources to better-off (easier to reach and improve) subgroups in the population. A maximizing approach increases intracountry inequality but is likely to be attractive to international donors aiming to show rapid progress from their investment. An egalitarian approach first helps those who are worst off (within each country), then the next worst off, and so on. It sacrifices some aggregate health benefit to the goal of giving priority to those who are worst off. But how much sacrifice of aggregate mortality of children under age five should be accepted? The problem is a conflict between best outcomes and fair chances. Best aggregate outcomes get the numbers up quickly, but the approach does not give the worst-off groups a fair chance at benefits.

Gwatkin's example more closely resembles the cases of inequity discussed in the previous section if the worst-off group with regard to child mortality is an ethnic group long excluded and discriminated against. Does making the injustice of the baseline more explicit affect thinking about what trade-offs between equity and maximization are considered acceptable? Will reasonable people disagree about the trade-offs involved?

How Much Priority Should Be Given to Reducing Existing Health Inequities?

If the determinants of the gender inequality in HIV/AIDS prevalence among people aged fifteen to twenty-four in the southern African region are as described above, then the health inequality is an inequity. Many will then believe that one indicator of fair access to treatments would be to match prevalence to treatment rates—we should treat more women than men, in other words, though this goal is difficult to achieve because of the social stigma facing infected women. Accordingly, efforts to enroll proportionally more women for treatment mean treating fewer people overall, because it is easier and quicker to enroll men. (To redress the inequality in prevalence itself would require non-health-sector efforts, as well as public health measures that reduce sexually transmitted diseases and provide effective education about safe sexual practices.) An international agency understanding this situation might conclude that it should follow a best outcomes strategy that would maximize the numbers treated, and not invest heavily in trying to break down the gender barriers to treatment. Others would accept lower treatment rates in order to invest in a more equitable policy. Reasonable people may disagree about how to make these trade-offs, even if they all agree that the health inequality that results from the gender bias against women violates concerns of justice.

What can be said about the priority problem? There are social obligations to avoid racist or sexist treatment of people, and also a social obligation to try to preserve normal functioning in the whole population. The latter would apply even if the source of the inequality was morally neutral, but remedy is now owed to the worse off for two weighty reasons of justice, not one. This fact of extra reasons might translate into giving them more priority than they would otherwise have.

In addition, suppose the better-off groups in both cases were partly responsible for the discriminatory practices, and that some also derived benefit from them. (Some argue that whites benefit from racism in the United States, but, although whites are better off than blacks and have often obtained privileges that blacks lack, racism also prevents blacks and most whites from uniting to seek better conditions for all [Kawachi, Daniels, and Robinson, 2005].) One might then think that people who compromise the health of others and sustain advantages should thereby lose some of their claims on health care.

But how much more priority should be given to those made worse off by racism or gender bias? Many argue they should not be given complete priority, for it seems wrong to give priority to meeting the health needs of blacks or women whose health status is not as bad as that of more seriously ill members of other groups. The concern to rectify intergroup inequities, reflected in giving some additional priority to meeting their needs and closing the gap, should not lead us to ignore other considerations of equity across individuals, and it should not lead us to ignore completely the aggregate impact on population health. Additionally, knowing that some groups that are largely responsible for racist or sexist health policies are also the ones that also enjoy relative health advantage as a result does not imply that their health needs may be ignored altogether. In general, it is not held that the proper punishment for criminal misdeeds that harm others is the denial of medical care.

This brings the discussion back to the main features of the unsolved rationing problems: implausible extreme views, such as giving no priority to those worst off, or, on the other hand, giving complete priority to them. Reasonable people will continue to disagree about how much additional priority to grant. Some of this disagreement may be the result of the original disagreement about how to make the trade-offs in the morally neutral distributive problems. But some of it may be specifically a result of disagreements about how much weight to give to the underlying fact of injustice, be it race- or gender-based.

The following points emerge from this discussion. Knowing that the health inequality between two groups is unjust may justify giving some extra weight to the priority assigned to the worst off, or it may add to concerns that the worst off be given fair chances at some benefit. There are, however, limits to the sacrifices in population health that would be acceptable as a result of attempting to reduce health inequity. Other people also have claims of justice on measures that protect their health. In addition, the fact that racism and gender bias are reprehensible forms of injustice does not mean that those who may be complicit in them, or derive some benefit from them, lose all claim on health protection themselves. In short, reasonable people will disagree about how to make the trade-offs involved.

Improving Health at the Expense of Exacerbating Inequities

Consider now cases where the aim is to improve population health, but the methods used either create or exacerbate health inequalities, some of which may be admittedly unjust. What is fair treatment in these cases? David Mechanic (2002) notes that some interventions that improve population health avoid generating inequalities, while others do not. The kind of intervention that improves population health while not increasing health inequalities is relatively unusual and has distinctive properties. Fluoridation of water, for example, improves the health of all who must use the water supply, independently of their demographic and behavioral features. In contrast, smoking cessation and vaccination campaigns improve population health while disproportionately helping groups who are better off in terms of income and education (lower-status groups actually try to stop smoking as frequently as better-off groups, but they succeed less often [Barbeau, Krieger, and Soobader, 2004]).

Black infant mortality rates (IMRs) in the United States were 64 percent higher than whites in 1954, but they were 130 percent higher in 1998, even though white rates dropped by 20.8 per 1,000 and black IMRs dropped by 30.1 per 1,000 (Mechanic, 2002). Mechanic concludes about this, and other cases, that it is reasonable to accept increasing health inequalities (as measured by the ratios) that result from policies that improve population health, as long as the health of all groups is being improved. Accordingly, there should be no real complaint about the ongoing (and increasing, from the perspective of ratios) inequality, given the fact of improving black IMRs.

Suppose, however, that there are two interventions (in any sector, and involving any novel technology), both of which raise the health of all groups. If intervention A does less for those who are worse off than intervention B, but does much more for those much better off, then both satisfy Mechanic's criterion. His criterion then fails to tell us how to choose between these options. If the initial inequality is one that society is responsible for causing through unfair policies, there may be a special obligation to give more weight to equity than to maximization of aggregate population health. But just how much sacrifice of benefits to others should be made is something reasonable people will disagree about.

There are also issues about speed as well as magnitude. Historical injustices that underlie many health inequalities, as in the racism and gender bias examples discussed above, are long-standing. Surely we owe some reasonable rate of progress toward eliminating them—let alone not increasing them (Held, 1973). But how fast is fast enough? Here, too, people are likely to disagree.

Mechanic's criterion, in short, runs afoul of the same distributive problems we have been considering. Reasonable people will disagree about which policy, A or B, to pursue. The scope of the problem raised by these unsolved rationing problems is very great, as they go well beyond medical resource allocation for individuals and pose dilemmas for population health. They pose these dilemmas regardless of whether the baseline distribution is described in morally neutral terms or is a clear case of injustice. They pose these dilemmas whether we are trying to reduce health inequities or simply avoid making them greater.

The Complexity of Inequality Itself

A further source of complexity to the problem of reducing health disparities derives from what Larry Temkin (1993, 76) has identified as the "complexity of inequality."

Temkin gives a schematic description of situations in which two or more groups of individuals differ in their levels of well-being. He then asks a question: Which situation has the worse inequality? The question is normative, not descriptive, for he is not asking which has more inequality. Specifically, someone who is worse off has a legitimate complaint, he argues, about the unfairness of the inequality. The strength of that complaint, however, depends on whether we compare those who are worst off (a) with those who are best off, (b) with all those better off than they are, or (c) with the average to determine the magnitude of their complaint. To determine when one inequality is worse than another, one must not only assess the strength of each complaint, but also aggregate those complaints within each situation. Here, too, there are different approaches to aggregation: we can adopt a maximum egalitarian view that aggregates the complaints of those who are worst off, an additive view that simply adds them up, or a weighted additive view that weights complaints by seriousness before adding them. The nine combinations of these bases for judging inequalities as better or worse yield somewhat divergent judgments about cases, including ones with multiple groups and ones involving welfare transfers among groups. Though all nine approaches, for example, might make the worst-off individual or group better before adding comparable benefits to any of the other individuals or (equal-sized) groups, judgments may differ about many other cases.

Temkin argues that none of these nine combinations can be dismissed outright as inconsistent or otherwise completely implausible. Thus, reasonable people—even egalitarian people—will often disagree about which situation is worse with regard to inequality than another. Disagreement about when one inequality is worse than another may be part of what underlies disagreements about how much priority to give worst-off individuals or groups. The reasoning behind the disagreements is something that needs to be addressed in a fair deliberative process.

Reasonable Disagreements and Accountability for Reasonableness

The central argument put forth here is that reducing unjust inequalities faces a complexity one might not have expected in the pursuit of justice. Even where health inequalities between groups are avowedly unjust and there are good reasons of justice for reducing them, we still encounter unsolved distributive problems. Three sources of reasonable disagreement are identified: (1) preexisting disagreements about how to address the priorities, aggregation, and best outcomes/fair chances problems that arise in all resource allocations, including these decisions aimed at reducing health inequalities; (2) disagreement about how much to weigh the injustice of the baseline against other issues of fair distribution posed by these distributive problems; and (3) Temkin-type disagreements about when one inequality is worse than another, which may interact with the second disagreement about weighing injustice. These three sources of disagreement also arise in the more common case where we are not setting out to remove injustice but only to improve population health, and we discover that our interventions tend to sustain or increase health inequalities, many of which are unjust. In short, the problem is both complex and pervasive.

What should be done about making decisions in the face of these controversies? These resource allocation decisions need to be made in real time and in a way that is perceived to be fair by all affected by them, despite the underlying moral disagreements. As in the simpler case of the distributive problems taken alone, one must resort to a form of procedural justice. In the absence of prior agreement on principles that can resolve such disputes, decisions must be made in a process that is fair to all (assuming all can agree on what that means). The outcome of the fair process can then be accepted as fair.

One proposal for such a process is that institutions be established at different decision-making levels in health systems, and that the procedures for decision-making meet the following conditions (Daniels and Sabin, 2002):

- Publicity: rationales for decisions are made public.
- Relevance: decision-makers, ideally including a broad range of relevant stakeholders, make decisions on the basis of reasons all consider relevant.
- Revisability: decisions are revised in the light of new evidence and arguments.
- Enforcement: the above conditions are met.

Meeting these conditions makes decisions accountable for their reasonableness. Why think adhering to this process yields greater fairness, even if we concede there is enhanced legitimacy?

There are two main forms of procedural justice (Rawls, 1971). In pure procedural justice, prior agreement on a relevant principle for determining just outcomes is lacking. Rawls offers gambling as an example: the outcome of a fair spin of the roulette wheel is considered to be fair. Criminal trials constitute an example of impure procedural justice, since there is prior agreement on a relevant principle: convict all and only the guilty. Who the guilty are is determined through trials that pit adversaries against each other but are judged by neutral parties. If conclusive evidence is later found that someone found guilty in a trial is in fact innocent (say through DNA evidence), then the trial result should be overturned.

The proposed process is like pure procedural justice in that there is a lack of prior agreement on distributive principles specific enough to yield outcomes to decisions about allocating health care resources. But the situation differs in two important ways from Rawls's example of gambling. Unlike gambling, outcomes that violate requirements of justice, say about nondiscrimination, should be rejected. Further, one can imagine arriving at a philosophically persuasive view about how to solve the priorities problem, or any of the other unsolved rationing problems. Such a view might "defeat" decisions about fairness arrived at through the process. The most that can be claimed for the outcome of fair process is that it is "defeasibly" fair.

I conclude by emphasizing that work must still be done if a fair process is to be implemented. First, there must be a body of research on how the four conditions can best be achieved at the different institutional levels at which decisions are made. Second, we must learn more about the actual magnitudes of the trade-offs that are involved in one type of intervention rather than another. Deliberations about options should be informed by the best evidence and arguments. Integrating these two bodies of research with clear normative thinking is a major challenge facing the bioethics of population health.

Acknowledgments

This chapter has been modified from "Reducing Health Disparities: No Simple Matter" (Daniels, 2013), with permission of Oxford University Press.

References

Acevedo-Garcia, D., Lochner, K. A., Osypuk, T. L., and Subramanian, S. V. 2003. "Future Directions in Residential Segregation and Health Research: A Multilevel Approach." *American Journal of Public Health* 93(2): 215–221.

Barbeau, E. M., Krieger, N., and Soobader, M. J. 2004. "Working Class Matters: Socioeconomic Disadvantage, Race/Ethnicity, Gender, and Smoking in NHIS 2000." *American Journal of Public Health* 94(2): 269–278.

Daniels, N. 1993. "Rationing Fairly: Programmatic Considerations." *Bioethics* 7(2–3): 224–233.

Daniels, N. 2007. *Just Health: Meeting Health Needs Fairly*. New York: Cambridge University Press.

Daniels, N. 2013. "Reducing Health Disparities: No Simple Matter." In *Inequalities in Health: Concepts, Measures, and Ethics*, edited by N. Eyal, S. A. Hurst, O. F. Norheim, and D. Wikler (New York: Oxford University Press).

Daniels, N., Kennedy, B., and Kawachi, I. 1999. "Why Justice Is Good for Our Health: The Social Determinants of Health Inequalities." *Daedalus* 128(4): 215–251.

Daniels, N., and Sabin, J. 2002. *Setting Limits Fairly: Can We Learn To Share Medical Resources?* (New York: Oxford University Press).

Epstein, A. M., Ayanian, J. Z., Keogh, J. H., Noonan, S. J., Armistead, N., Cleary, P. D., et al. 2000. "Racial Disparities in Access to Renal Transplantation—Clinically Appropriate or Due to Underuse or Overuse?" *New England Journal of Medicine* 343(21): 1537–1544.

Gwatkin, D. R. 2002. *Who Would Gain Most from Efforts to Reach the Millennium Development Goals for Health* (Washington, D.C.: World Bank).

Harrell, J. P., Hall, S., and Taliaferro, J. 2003. "Physiological Responses to Racism and Discrimination: An Assessment of the Evidence. *American Journal of Public Health* 93(2): 243–248.

Hayward, M. D., and Heron, M. 1999. "Racial Inequality in Active Life among Adult Americans." *Demography* 36(1): 77–91.

Held, V. 1973. "Reasonable Progress and Self-Respect." *The Monist* 57(1): 12–27.

House, J., and Williams, D. R. 2000. "Understanding and Reducing Socioeconomic and Racial/Ethnic Disparities in Health." In *Promoting Health: Intervention Strategies from Social and Behavioral Research*, edited by B. D. Smedley and S. L. Syme, 81–124 (Washington, D.C.: National Academy Press).

IOM (Institute of Medicine). 2003. "*Unequal Treatment: Confronting Racial and Ethnic Disparities in Health Care* (Washington, D.C.: The National Academies Press).

Kawachi, I., Daniels, N., and Robinson, D. E. 2005. Health Disparities By Race and Class: Why Both Matter." *Health Affairs* 24(2): 343–352.

Krieger, N., and Sidney, S. 1996. "Racial Discrimination and Blood Pressure: The CARDIA Study of Young Black and White Adults." *American Journal of Public Health* 86(10): 1370–1378.

Mechanic, D. 2002. "Disadvantage, Inequality, and Social Policy." *Health Affairs* 21(2): 48–59.

Noh, S., and Kaspar, V. 2003. "Perceived Discrimination and Depression: Moderating Effects of Coping, Acculturation, and Ethnic Support." *American Journal of Public Health* 93(2): 232–238.

Norheim, O., Ottersen, T., Berhane, F., Chitah, B., Cookson, R., Daniels, N., et al. 2014. *Making Fair Choices on the Path to Universal Health Coverage: Final Report of the WHO Consultative Group on Equity and Universal Health Coverage* (Geneva: World Health Organization).

Rawls, J. 1971. *A Theory of Justice* (Cambridge, Mass.: Harvard University Press).

Schulman, K. A., Berlin, J. A., Harless, W., Kerner, J. F., Sistrunk, S., Gersh, B. J., et al. 1999. "The Effect of Race and Sex on Physicians' Recommendations for Cardiac Catheterization." *New England Journal of Medicine* 340(8): 618–626.

Temkin, L. S. 1993. *Inequality* (New York: Oxford University Press).

UNAIDS (Joint United Nations Programme on HIV/AIDS), UNFPA (United Nations Population Fund), and UNIFEM (United Nations Development Fund for Women). 2004. *Women and HIV/AIDS: Confronting the Crisis* (New York: United Nations Population Fund) http://www.unfpa.org/publications/women-and-hivaids.

WHO (World Health Organization). 1999. *Health 21: The Health for All Policy Framework for the WHO European Region* (Copenhagen: WHO Regional Office for Europe). http://www.euro.who.int/en/publications/abstracts/health21-the-health-for-all-policy-framework-for-the-who-european-region.

WHO (World Health Organization). 2002. *The World Health Report 2002: Reducing Risks, Promoting Healthy Life* (Geneva: World Health Organization). http://www.who.int/whr/2002/en/.

Williams, D. R., Neighbors, H. W., and Jackson, J. S. 2003. "Racial/Ethnic Discrimination and Health: Findings from Community Studies." *American Journal of Public Health* 93(2): 200–208.

CHAPTER 26

MEASURING HEALTH INEQUITY: A PUBLIC HEALTH ETHICS INQUIRY

YUKIKO ASADA

INTRODUCTION

A healthy population is an ultimate goal of public health. Regardless of the specific focus of a public health intervention—be it smoking cessation, water fluoridation, chronic disease management, or health insurance coverage—all public health interventions ultimately aim to improve population health. Overall health outcomes, such as life expectancy or the prevalence rate of a disease in the population, have traditionally been used as indicators of the health of a population. Such overall health outcomes, however, could mask potentially diverse health and illness experiences of persons in the population. Many jurisdictions now acknowledge the importance of paying attention to differences in health outcomes across individuals or population groups in addition to overall health outcomes in the assessment of population health (Graham, 2004; Hines et al., 2011; CSDH, 2008)

The consideration of differences in health has a long history in public health. Differences in health are often referred to as health *inequalities* (Farr, 1856). Some health inequalities are judged as ethically or morally problematic and referred to as health *inequities* (Kawachi, Subramanian, and Almeida-Filho, 2002). Measurement of health inequities is essential to support public health policy (Truman et al., 2011; CSDH, 2008). It offers information regarding the magnitude of health inequities that currently exist, the impact of interventions to address health inequities identified as priorities, and changes and comparisons of health inequities observed across time and populations. Measuring health inequities, however, is complex, because it requires attention to ethical considerations (Asada, 2007).

This chapter discusses ethical considerations that arise in three essential tasks for the measurement exercise: *definition*, *operationalization*, and *quantification*. The first section introduces some of the definitions of health inequity proposed in relevant literatures. The second section discusses some of the important strategies used to incorporate, explicitly and transparently, these various perspectives of health inequity into its measurement. The third section outlines some of the key ethical considerations that arise in choosing indices to quantify the magnitude of health inequity. To conclude, the chapter underscores the importance of interdisciplinary integration of ethics, methods, and policy considerations in the measurement of health inequity.

Definition

The first task required for measuring health inequity is defining health inequity. There is no agreed-upon definition, however, and efforts to articulate critical elements of health equity persist in various disciplines (Braveman, 2006; Daniels, 2007; Fleurbaey and Schokkaert, 2012; Hausman, 2007, 2009; Powers and Faden, 2008; Ruger, 2010; Segall, 2010; Venkatapuram, 2011; Whitehead, 1991). Lack of consensus is sometimes frustrating for public health practitioners and policymakers who are deeply worried about inequalities in health outcomes observed in a population but are unable to find clear guidance regarding what exactly "health inequity" means. A challenge for them is how best to take advantage of multidisciplinary contributions to these conceptual debates. Relevant writings are often scattered in diverse disciplines, with variations in language and style depending on the particular disciplinary audience. This section introduces some of the widely used definitions of health inequity in the public health, economics, and philosophy literatures.

Arguably, the most accepted definition of health inequity in the public health literature is that of Margaret Whitehead (1991, 431), who states that health inequities are "differences [in health] which are unnecessary and avoidable but, in addition, are considered unfair and unjust." In much of the public health literature, social inequalities in health are considered unfair and unjust. For example, Michael Marmot, who chaired the highly influential World Health Organization Commission on Social Determinants of Health (CSDH, 2008), regards as unfair social inequalities in health that "could be avoidable by reasonable means" (Marmot, 2013, 284). "Social inequalities" in health here refers to graded levels of health corresponding to social status. Thus, for Marmot, higher breast cancer incidence rates among women with higher socioeconomic status, for example, are not unfair.

The interpretation of what constitutes social inequalities in health is increasingly expansive in the public health literature. For example, *Healthy People 2020*, a decennial national health plan in the United States, defines a health disparity—a more common term used in the United States than health inequity—as

> a particular type of health difference that is closely linked with social, economic, and/ or environmental disadvantage...adversely affect[ing] groups of people who have

> systematically experienced greater obstacles to health based on their racial or ethnic group; religion; socioeconomic status; gender; age; mental health; cognitive, sensory, or physical disability; sexual orientation or gender identity; geographic location; or other characteristics historically linked to discrimination or exclusion."
>
> (HHS, 2008, 28)

The list of group characteristics included in the definition has been getting longer over the years, with little consideration for intersectionality of these group characteristics (e.g., a person can be described by sex, racial or ethnic, *and* socioeconomic characteristics). Accordingly, it is unclear how to make sense of health inequalities across a multitude of social groups, especially when a person belongs to disadvantaged groups in some characteristics and, at the same time, advantaged groups in other characteristics (e.g., a person is male, professional, and disabled).

While social identification plays a key role when considering inequity in public health, it does not always do so in other disciplines. In economics, for example, the study of income inequality is almost always about the distribution of income across individuals. Bringing in this tradition, in 1999, Christopher Murray and colleagues focused on the distribution of health across individuals regardless of group associations and argued that this distribution is ethically important (Murray, Gakidou, and Frenk, 1999). This proposal was met with fierce criticism in the public health literature and has since had little influence on the definitions of health inequity used in public health (Almeida et al., 2001; Braveman, Krieger, and Lynch, 2000; Braveman, Starfield, and Geiger, 2001; Braveman, 2001; Szwarcwald, 2002; Ugá et al., 2001).

Recent developments in economics, however, can be seen as an extension of the Murray definition. Fleurbaey and Schokkaert (2009; 2012), for example, hold that it is too broad to view all health inequalities across individuals as inequitable, but too narrow to focus on health inequalities only in terms of socioeconomic status. To seek an answer somewhere in-between, they argue that one needs to think about causes of health inequalities. One must distinguish between "legitimate" and "illegitimate" causes of health inequalities, with the former being ethically acceptable and the latter being ethically unacceptable. Health inequalities caused by illegitimate—ethically unacceptable—causes are, thus, considered as unfair. With this framework, the core tension among different definitions of health inequity can be understood as a disagreement regarding the legitimate-illegitimate distinction. The particular application of this framework to define health inequity chosen by Fleurbaey and Schokkaert is a view of equal opportunity for health. This view posits that differences in health resulting from persons' efforts (or lack thereof) are ethically permissible, while those from persons' circumstances are inequitable.

It is not just economists, but also philosophers, who now vigorously debate what constitutes health inequity. Traditionally, philosophers did not emphasize health when discussing justice and fairness, because health was viewed largely as determined by luck. But, informed by evidence on social determinants of health, they began to expand existing theories of justice and proposed a variety of views on health inequity. The aforementioned view of equal opportunity for health, for example, is a particular application of a general theory known as *luck egalitarianism* to health. Luck egalitarianism is concerned with unfairness understood as inequalities for which persons cannot be held responsible (Roemer, 1995).

Another—and arguably the most developed—application of an existing philosophical theory to derive a definition of health inequity is Norman Daniels's expansion of John Rawls's theory of justice as fairness (Daniels, 2007; Rawls, 1971). Rawls argues that free and equal persons would agree with three principles of justice: (1) ensuring equal basic liberty; (2) providing fair equality of opportunity for power and offices; and (3) limiting inequalities in all-purpose means, such as income and wealth, to those that benefit the worst off. In Rawls's theory, all persons are assumed to be healthy, and he thus does not consider inequalities in health as relevant to justice. To argue for health as relevant in the pursuit of social justice, Daniels first broadens the interpretation of fair equality of opportunity to include the ability to form and carry out life plans. Viewing health as a function, Daniels then argues that ensuring a certain range of human functioning through prevention and treatment of disease or disability—referred to as species-typical normal functioning—is critical in the pursuit of fair equality of opportunity. Health inequalities are unjust, Daniels continues, when access to health care is inequitable and social determinants are distributed in a manner that does not benefit the worst off.

In these and many other expansions of general theories of justice to health, the extended views typically discuss health inequality in isolation from other inequalities. Dan Hausman questions this practice (Hausman, 2007, 2009; Hausman and Waldren, 2011). He argues that what we are ultimately concerned about is general inequality—inequality in opportunity or welfare, for example—and inequality in health can tell us about general inequality only when it is *remediable* (i.e., possible to eliminate inequality in health) and *incompensable* (i.e., not possible to make up for health inequality through some means other than eliminating health inequality).

The brief introduction above shows a diversity of views proposed in multidisciplinary literatures. Some views are competing; for example, there is a question of whether the distribution of health in itself is of ethical concern, or whether it is only those inequalities associated with socially important group characteristics that are of ethical concern. Other views can be complementary; for example, Daniels's view might provide a further articulation of the popular view in the public health literature that avoidable social inequalities in health are unfair, and it might be able to provide an insight as to which social inequalities are more important than others in light of Rawls's theory. Whichever view one might adopt, articulating a chosen definition of health inequity and the reason for the choice is critical in the measurement exercise because, as we will see in the next section, such articulation informs many choices involved in the measurement of health inequity.

Operationalization

The second task for measuring health inequity is empirically operationalizing the chosen definition of health inequity. Doing so requires examination of typical decisions in empirical quantitative analyses through an ethical lens. Such decisions include, but are not limited to, the choice of the health outcome measure (e.g., life years or self-reported health), the unit of analysis (e.g., groups or individuals), and the time period (e.g., longitudinal or cross-sectional) with which to measure health inequity. To illustrate that these typical empirical decisions are not merely technical, but also ethical, this section focuses on the choice of the unit of analysis (Asada, 2013).

The majority of public health studies use groups as the focal point of the measurement of health inequity. They examine a relationship between health and another ethically and policy-relevant group characteristic (e.g., income). These studies then compare the average health between groups (e.g., high-, middle-, and low-income groups). Numerous descriptions of health inequalities between groups collectively embody the widely shared definition of health inequity: social inequalities in health are unfair and unjust. However, this group approach has two shortcomings.

First, based on these numerous group-based descriptions of health inequalities, it is very difficult to answer the deceptively simple question of whether, on the whole, society is making progress in terms of health equity. Suppose differences in low birthweight between education groups become smaller but differences in low birthweight between racial/ethnic groups become larger. Has health equity, on the whole, improved? The answer depends on which of these group characteristics may be prioritized and why. The challenge of gaining a comprehensive understanding of inequalities across a multitude of groups is increasing as the list of group characteristics used in health inequality studies is growing (see the example of *Healthy People 2020* discussed in the previous section).

In addition, the exclusive group focus poses serious concerns. The examination of one group characteristic at a time (e.g., income) hinders a broader appreciation of intersectionality across group characteristics (e.g., income, race, and sexual orientation). In addition, the group approach compares inequalities between groups by focusing on group averages. One would expect that health outcomes of individuals within each group (e.g., low-, middle-, or high-income group) differ, just as some individuals in a socially disadvantaged group may do well. At the same time, one would assume that a group average reasonably represents the overall health of each group. Studies examining inequalities both within and between groups cast doubt on this assumption (Ferrer and Palmer, 2004; Muir, 2016; Pradhan, Sahn, and Younger, 2003; Smits and Monden, 2009; Wagstaff and Doorslaer, 2004). They show that in each group there are always healthy individuals. What makes some groups, on average, less healthy than others is a difference in the proportion of less healthy individuals. Moreover, inequalities within groups are usually much larger than inequalities between groups. We might then ask: How should we identify the socially disadvantaged—those with low socioeconomic status or those with sickness? And among whom should we wish to distribute health equitably—across individuals or groups? (Asada, 2013; Lippert-Rasmussen, 2013; Temkin, 1993)

Most issues related to the exclusive group focus can be overcome by considering multiple group characteristics at the same time. For example, rather than examining health inequity by income (e.g., poor and rich) and by race (e.g., white and nonwhite) separately, we could examine health inequity by income and race simultaneously (e.g., poor-white, rich-white, poor-nonwhite, rich-nonwhite). As the number of group characteristics increases, however, this strategy becomes cumbersome. Alternatively, we can start with individual-level data and incorporate as many group characteristics as we wish in the measurement. A promising method doing just that is called the *fairness-standardization method* (Asada et al., 2014, 2015; Fleurbaey and Schokkaert, 2012). This method estimates ethically problematic health more tightly connected to a chosen definition of health inequity. It has been primarily developed by economists through empirical implementation of the view of equal opportunity for health (Fleurbaey and Schokkaert, 2009; García-Gómez et al., 2015; Jusot, Tubeuf, and Trannoy, 2013; Rosa Dias, 2009).

Using individual-level data, the fairness-standardization method starts by modeling health. "Modeling health" means quantifying the association between health and its determinants. This is a descriptive task, and the goal is to statistically explain variation in health as much as possible with the data at hand. After identifying the best-fit model, the next step, which is a normative task, classifies each variable used in the health model as an ethically acceptable or unacceptable cause of ill health according to the chosen definition of health inequity. On the account of health inequity that appeals to equal opportunity for health, for example, health inequalities due to factors beyond individual control are inequitable. One might classify age and health behavior variables (e.g., smoking, body mass index, physical activity, etc.) as ethically acceptable and other variables indicating social background (e.g., income, education, marital status, visible minority, etc.) and care and support (e.g., self-reported unmet need, having regular medical doctor, drug insurance, etc.) as ethically unacceptable causes of ill health. Age is not under individual control but can be considered as ethically acceptable, because aging is a universally shared biological process among all persons. Health behaviors are not solely under individual control but are also influenced by an individual's circumstances. This fact can be accommodated by estimating the effects of health behavior on the health outcomes that are conditional on social background and treating the interaction between health behavior and social background as ethically unacceptable.

Having classified each variable as ethically acceptable or unacceptable, we then remove the influence of the ethically acceptable or fair component (i.e., legitimate variables according to a chosen definition of health inequity) on the observed health through fairness standardization. This standardization leaves us with inequality due to unfair sources. Fairness standardization is similar to age standardization in epidemiological studies, which removes the influence of age when estimating mortality rates. In this context, standardization removes the influence of all legitimate, or fair, sources of inequality. Consequently, the standardization generates the inequitable distribution of health in the population.

There are two challenges in this approach. Often, empirical data have much less granularity, and statistical methods much less sophistication, to convey important nuances of the concepts. Also, those who agree on the definition of health inequity could disagree on particular empirical implementation, such as the classification of ethically acceptable and unacceptable variables. Still, this method makes all decisions and the rationales underpinning them explicit, and thereby allows for further debate.

The discussion above shows how ethical considerations are woven into the seemingly technical choice of the unit of analysis. Ethical considerations should also apply to other aspects of measurement strategies. For example, when measuring health inequity, the choice of the measure of health outcome should reflect what it is about health we wish to distribute fairly. Some theories are silent about this question, but others do provide guidance. For example, in Daniels's view, health is understood in terms of species-typical functioning. Thus, if applying his view to empirical analysis, it would be more fitting to use a measure of functional status rather than, for example, the presence of certain medical conditions. As this section illustrates, to produce clear health inequity information, the articulation of a chosen definition of health inequity is merely a first step, and the explicit and transparent incorporation of the chosen definition of health inequity must follow as a second step.

Quantification

The third task for measuring health inequity is quantifying the magnitude of health inequity using an index. Various indices are available for the quantification. As with the operationalization discussed in the previous section, the choice of an index involves both technical and ethical considerations. This section discusses some of the key ethical issues, particularly those that arise in the choice between absolute and relative indices.

Why is the quantification of the magnitude of health inequity important? It facilitates communication and comparison. Consider, for example, a difference in life expectancy between American women in the top 1 percent of income distribution and American women in the bottom 1 percent. The life expectancy of the former is eighty-nine years, while that of the latter is seventy-nine years, pooling data from 2001 to 2014 (Chetty et al., 2016). Suppose, based on a view that social inequalities in health are unfair and unjust, we regard this inequality as inequitable and wish to quantify the magnitude of this inequity. To do so, we might decide to use an absolute range measure, thereby expressing the degree of health inequity as ten life years (by taking the difference between eighty-nine and seventy-nine), or we might use a relative range measure, thereby expressing the degree of health inequity as 1.12 (the quotient when eighty-nine is the dividend and seventy-nine is the divisor). Using these calculated numbers, we can communicate how much inequity exists, and by obtaining comparable numbers from the past or from different populations, we can assess trends or rank populations in terms of health inequity.

There are many indices to choose from for the quantification (Coulter, 1989; Harper and Lynch, 2005; Keppel et al., 2005; Regidor, 2004a, 2004b; Sen, 1973). While some of these indices were developed particularly for health distributions, others involve the application of indices developed and used primarily in other topic areas, such as income inequality and social segregation. The same mathematical index, in principle, can summarize both unequal distributions of health (i.e., index of health inequality) and inequitable distributions of health (i.e., index of health inequity).

The choice of an index is often considered as a technical exercise. Yet when the purpose of the quantification is to express the magnitude of health inequity in numbers, the process of selecting an index involves value judgments (Asada, 2007; Harper et al., 2010; Kjellsson, Gerdtham, and Petrie, 2015). There are established literatures that examine the value judgments underlying inequality and inequity indices. The income inequality literature is one of them, and the common approach it takes is often referred to as the axiomatic approach. It identifies axioms—rules or principles—that are backbones of indices and also examines value judgments involved in supporting or rejecting these axioms (Sen, 1973; Temkin, 1993).

There are several questions relevant to the choice of a health inequity index that involve value judgments: (1) Who is compared against whom in the population? (2) How are differences that arise from the comparison aggregated at the population level? (3) Should the judgment of inequity be sensitive to the total population size? (4) How should the judgment of inequity be sensitive to subgroup characteristics, such as subgroup population size? (5) Should the judgment of inequity be sensitive to the mean level of the population? (Asada, 2007).

The last question in this list has been of particular interest in the public health literature, which understands the question as the choice between absolute and relative indices (Keppel et al., 2005; King, Harper, and Young, 2012; Low and Low, 2006). In the life expectancy example above, the question typically asked in the public health literature is whether we should use the absolute range measure and express the degree of health inequity as ten life years, or instead use the relative range measure and express the degree of health inequity as 1.12. To answer this question, discussion in the public health literature is mostly technical in nature. Yet a critical question regarding the choice between absolute and relative indices relates to value judgment: Does the same absolute difference matter more in a sicker population (Asada, 2007; Temkin, 1993)?

In the life expectancy example above, with a life expectancy of eighty-nine years among American women in the top 1 percent of income distribution and that of seventy-nine years among American women in the bottom 1 percent, we can say American women are, on average, healthy. Imagine women in a hypothetical country with a life expectancy of forty years for rich women and thirty years for poor women. The absolute difference in life expectancy between the rich and the poor is the same ten years in both countries. But we might think that the ten-year difference matters more in the sicker country, given that women in that country have much lower life expectancy. Do ten years in a short life matter more than ten years in a long life? We are answering "yes" to this question when using the relative indices and "no" when using the absolute indices.

As the above discussion related to the question of the sensitivity to the mean, or, as framed in the public health literature, the choice between absolute and relative indices, illustrates, questions and related value judgments that arise in the process of quantification are unique. That is, the first two steps of measuring health inequity—defining health inequity and operationalizing the chosen definition—do not automatically yield the value judgments or particular indices involved in quantifying the magnitude of health inequity. Hence, the third step calls for distinct ethical considerations in measuring health inequity.

Conclusion

This chapter highlights some of the key ethical issues that arise in each of the three essential tasks for measuring health inequities: definition, operationalization, and quantification. This overview underscores a wide range of ethical issues that are important in a seemingly technical exercise of measuring health inequity. It also demonstrates the multidisciplinary nature of the topic. Cross-fertilization across the relevant disciplines and interdisciplinary integration of considerations of ethics, methods, and policy are vital for further advancement of the measurement of health inequity, which in turn offers a strong foundation for public health research and policy.

References

Almeida, C., Braveman, P., Gold, M. R., Szwarcwald, C. L., Ribeiro, J. M., Miglionico, A., et al. 2001. "Methodological Concerns and Recommendations on Policy Consequences of the World Health Report 2000." *Lancet* 357(9269): 1692–1697.

Asada, Y. 2007. *Health Inequality: Morality and Measurement* (Toronto: University of Toronto Press).

Asada, Y. 2013. "A Summary Measure of Health Inequalities: Incorporating Group and Individual Inequalities." In *Inequalities in Health: Concepts, Measures, and Ethics*, edited by N. Eyal, S. A. Hurst, O. F. Norheim, and D. Wikler, 37–51 (New York: Oxford University Press).

Asada, Y., Hurley, J., Norheim, O. F., and Johri, M. 2014. "A Three-Stage Approach to Measuring Health Inequalities and Inequities." *International Journal for Equity in Health* 13: 98. https://equityhealthj.biomedcentral.com/articles/10.1186/s12939-014-0098-y.

Asada, Y., Hurley, J., Norheim, O. F., and Johri, M. 2015. "Unexplained Health Inequality—Is It Unfair?" *International Journal for Equity in Health* 14: 11. https://equityhealthj.biomedcentral.com/articles/10.1186/s12939-015-0138-2.

Braveman, P. 2001. "Epidemiology and (Neo-)Colonialism." *Journal of Epidemiology & Community Health* 55(3): 160–161.

Braveman, P. 2006. "Health Disparities and Health Equity: Concepts and Measurement." *Annual Review of Public Health* 27(1): 167–194.

Braveman, P., Krieger, N., and Lynch, J. 2000. "Health Inequalities and Social Inequalities in Health." *Bulletin of the World Health Organization* 78(2): 232–235.

Braveman, P., Starfield, B., and Geiger, H. J. 2001. "World Health Report 2000: How It Removes Equity from the Agenda for Public Health Monitoring and Policy." *British Medical Journal* 323(7314): 678–681.

Chetty, R., Stepner, M., Abraham, S., Lin, S., Scuderi, B., Turner, N., Bergeron, A., et al. 2016. "The Association between Income and Life Expectancy in the United States, 2001–2014." *JAMA* 315(16): 1750–1766.

Coulter, P. B. 1989. *Measuring Inequality: A Methodological Handbook* (Boulder, Colo.: Westview Press).

CSDH (Commission on Social Determinants of Health). 2008. *Closing the Gap in a Generation: Health Equity through Action on the Social Determinants of Health: Commission on Social Determinants of Health Final Report* (Geneva: World Health Organization).

Daniels, N. 2007. *Just Health: Meeting Health Needs Fairly* (New York: Cambridge University Press).

Farr, W. 1856. *Report on the Nomenclature and Statistical Classification of Diseases*. In *Annual Report of the Registrar-General of Births, Deaths, and Marriages in England* (London: Great Britain General Registrar Office).

Ferrer, R., and Palmer, R. 2004. "Variations in Health Status within and between Socioeconomic Strata." *Journal of Epidemiology* & *Community Health* 58(5): 381–387.

Fleurbaey, M., and Schokkaert, E. 2009. "Unfair Inequalities in Health and Health Care." *Journal of Health Economics* 28(1): 73–90.

Fleurbaey, M., and Schokkaert, E. 2012. "Equity in Health and Health Care." In *Handbook of Health Economics*, edited by M. V. Pauly, T. G. Mcguire, and P. P. Barros (Oxford: North Holland).

García-Gómez, P., Schokkaert, E., Van Ourti, T., and Bago d'Uva, T. 2015. "Inequity in the Face of Death." *Health Economics* 24(10): 1348–1367.

Graham, H. 2004. "Social Determinants and Their Unequal Distribution: Clarifying Policy Understandings." *Milbank Quarterly* 82(1): 101–124.

Harper, S., King, N. B., Meersman, S. C., Reichman, M. E., Breen, N., and Lynch, J. 2010. "Implicit Value Judgments in the Measurement of Health Inequalities." *Milbank Quarterly* 88(1): 4–29.

Harper, S., and Lynch, J. 2005. *Methods for Measuring Cancer Disparities: Using Data Relevant to "Healthy People 2010" Cancer-Related Objectives*. NCI Cancer Surveillance Monograph Series (Bethesda, Md.: National Cancer Institute). https://seer.cancer.gov/archive/publications/disparities/measuring_disparities.pdf.

Hausman, D. M. 2007. "What's Wrong with Health Inequalities?" *Journal of Political Philosophy* 15(1): 46–66.

Hausman, D. M. 2009. "Benevolence, Justice, Well-Being and the Health Gradient." *Public Health Ethics* 2(3): 235–243.

Hausman, D. M., and Waldren, M. S. 2011. "Egalitarianism Reconsidered." *Journal of Moral Philosophy* 8(4): 567–586.

HHS (US Department of Health and Human Services). 2008. *The Secretary's Advisory Committee on National Health Promotion and Disease Prevention Objectives for 2020. Phase I Report: Recommendations for the Framework and Format of Healthy People 2020. Section IV: Advisory Committee Findings and Recommendations* (Washington, D.C.: HHS). https://www.healthypeople.gov/sites/default/files/PhaseI_0.pdf.

Hines, R., Dobrzynski, L., Huang, D., Pearcy, J., Rose, C., Rosendorf, K., et al. 2011. *Healthy People 2010 Final Review* (Hyattsville, Md.: National Center for Health Statistics). https://www.cdc.gov/nchs/healthy_people/hp2010/hp2010_final_review.htm.

Jusot, F., Tubeuf, S., and Trannoy, A. 2013. "Circumstances and Efforts: How Important Is Their Correlation for the Measurement of Inequality of Opportunity in Health?" *Health Economics* 22(12): 1470–1495.

Kawachi, I., Subramanian, S., and Almeida-Filho, N. 2002. "A Glossary for Health Inequalities." *Journal of Epidemiology & Community Health* 56(9): 647–652.

Keppel, K., Pamuk, E., Lynch, J., Carter-Pokras, O., Kim, I., Mays, V., et al. 2005. "Methodological Issues in Measuring Health Disparities." *Vital and Health Statistics, Series 2: Data Evaluation and Methods Research* 2(141): 1–16.

King, N. B., Harper, S., and Young, M. E. 2012. "Use of Relative and Absolute Effect Measures in Reporting Health Inequalities: Structured Review." *British Medical Journal* 345: e5774.

Kjellsson, G., Gerdtham, U.-G., and Petrie, D. 2015. "Lies, Damned Lies, and Health Inequality Measurements: Understanding the Value Judgments." *Epidemiology* 26(5): 673–680.

Lippert-Rasmussen, K. 2013. "When Group Measures of Health Should Matter." In *Inequalities in Health: Concepts, Measures, and Ethics*, edited by N. Eyal, S. A. Hurst, O. F. Norheim, and D. Wikler, 52–65 (New York: Oxford University Press).

Low, A., and Low, A. 2006. "Health Economics: Importance of Relative Measures in Policy on Health Inequalities." *British Medical Journal* 332(7547): 967–969.

Marmot, M. 2013. "Fair Society, Healthy Lives." In *Inequalities in Health: Concepts, Measures, and Ethics*, edited by N. Eyal, S. A. Hurst, O. F. Norheim, and D. Wikler, 282–298 (New York: Oxford University Press).

Muir, A. 2016. "Describing Health Inequalities within and between Groups." MS diss., Dalhousie University.

Murray, C. J., Gakidou, E. E., and Frenk, J. 1999. "Health Inequalities and Social Group Differences: What Should We Measure?" *Bulletin of the World Health Organization* 77(7): 537–543.

Powers, M., and Faden, R. 2008. *Social Justice: The Moral Foundations of Public Health and Health Policy* (New York: Oxford University Press).

Pradhan, M., Sahn, D. E., and Younger, S. D. 2003. "Decomposing World Health Inequality." *Journal of Health Economics* 22(2): 271–293.

Rawls, J. 1971. *A Theory of Justice* (Cambridge, Mass.: Belknap Press).

Regidor, E. 2004a. "Measures of Health Inequalities: Part 1." *Journal of Epidemiology & Community Health* 58(10): 858–861.

Regidor, E. 2004b. "Measures of Health Inequalities: Part 2." *Journal of Epidemiology & Community Health* 58(11): 900–903.

Roemer, J. 1995. "Equality and Responsibility." *Boston Review* 20(2): 3–7.

Rosa Dias, P. 2009. "Inequality of Opportunity in Health: Evidence from a UK Cohort Study." *Health Economics* 18(9): 1057–1074.

Ruger, J. P. 2010. *Health and Social Justice* (New York: Oxford University Press).

Segall, S. 2010. *Health, Luck, and Justice* (Princeton, N.J.: Princeton University Press).

Sen, A. 1973. *On Economic Inequality* (Oxford: Clarendon Press).

Smits, J., and Monden, C. 2009. "Length of Life Inequality around the Globe." *Social Science & Medicine* 68(6): 1114–1123.

Szwarcwald, C. L. 2002. "On the World Health Organisation's Measurement of Health Inequalities." *Journal of Epidemiology & Community Health* 56(3): 177–182.

Temkin, L. S. 1993. *Inequality* (New York: Oxford University Press).

Truman, B. I., Smith, K., Roy, K., Chen, Z., Moonesinghe, R., Zhu, J., et al. 2011. "Rationale for Regular Reporting on Health Disparities and Inequalities—United States." *MMWR Surveillance Summaries* 60(Suppl. 01): 3–10.

Ugá, A. D., Almeida, C. M., Szwarcwald, C. L., Travassos, C., Viacava, F., Ribeiro, J. M., et al. 2001. "Considerations on Methodology Used in the World Health Organization 2000 Report." *Cadernos de Saúde Pública* 17(3): 705–712.

Venkatapuram, S. 2011. *Health Justice* (Cambridge, Mass.: Polity Press).

Wagstaff, A., and Doorslaer, E. V. 2004. "Overall versus Socioeconomic Health Inequality: A Measurement Framework and Two Empirical Illustrations." *Health Economics* 13(3): 297–301.

Whitehead, M. 1991. "The Concepts and Principles of Equity and Health." *Health Promotion International* 6(3): 217–228.

Further Reading

Braveman, P. A., Kumanyika, S., Fielding, J., LaVeist, T., Borrell, L. N., Manderscheid, R., et al. 2011. "Health Disparities and Health Equity: The Issue Is Justice." *American Journal of Public Health* 101(S1): S149–S155.

Eyal, N., Hurst, S. A., Norheim, O. F., and Wikler, D. 2013. *Inequalities in Health: Concepts, Measures, and Ethics* (New York: Oxford University Press).

SECTION SIX

DATA COLLECTION

CHAPTER 27

AN OVERVIEW OF ETHICS AND PUBLIC HEALTH DATA COLLECTION

HOLLY A. TAYLOR

Introduction

The recorded history of public health surveillance in Europe begins with the Venetian Republic counting the victims of the pneumonic plague in the 1300s and the republic's implementation of a quarantine of travelers from plague-endemic regions (Declich and Carter, 1994). The measurement of morbidity and mortality has remained the core of everyday practice of public health. Before the 1950s, surveillance efforts in the United States focused on the observation of *individuals* exposed to a communicable disease (Declich and Carter, 1994). Alexander Langmuir, who directed the US Epidemic Intelligence Service for almost twenty years, is credited with promoting the principles of surveillance for observation of disease in *populations* (Brachman, 1996). With this shift in focus, the practice of surveillance allowed for the detection of patterns and potential control of disease.

A key ethical challenge with the collection of public health data has been, and will remain, how best to balance the health of the community with the respect owed to individual citizens. The early use of public surveillance techniques led to the quarantine of travelers who had been exposed, or were assumed to be exposed, to a communicable disease. As we know from more modern examples, labeling an individual or population at risk of disease can have consequences beyond quarantine, such as stigma (Mahajan et al., 2008). Stigma can result in discrimination that unfairly restricts access to basic social goods such as employment and housing.

As the methods of public health data collection, analysis, interpretation, and dissemination have advanced, so has the need to consider and adopt robust ethical principles to guide the handling and use of such data. For example, as the ability to store and process large data sets compiled from multiple data sources advances, the more information those who have access to and are responsible for stewarding this data will know about the health and welfare of individuals and communities. In addition, aggregated data from individuals that are maintained electronically, such as electronic health record data, may be valuable for public health research. Entities and researchers who collect, hold, aggregate, and use those data have stewardship obligations, including the need to inform individuals how their data may be used for research purposes, including whether and how it will be linked with data from other sources, such as social media (Vayena et al., 2015).

Those who hold, aggregate, or use data also must commit to transparency, a responsibility that may not have been as relevant in the past. Similarly, an aggregator of data from across multiple sources must now think carefully about the use and release of findings and their implications for individuals and communities, including avoiding harms such as those that may result from unintentional breaches in confidentiality (Allen et al., 2013).

Chapter Overviews

This section of *The Oxford Handbook of Public Health Ethics* is dedicated to the examination of ethics and public health data collection. Public health data is generally collected in two ways: through the public health surveillance system, and through a variety of public health research methods. The four chapters in the section each address the collection of a particular type of public health data and examine related ethical challenges.

In "Public Health Surveillance: Ethical Considerations," Lisa M. Lee explains that the public health surveillance system relies on health care providers and public health laboratories to report test results for particular diseases and health conditions to local or state health departments. Some of these data are also shared with national authorities. This collection of data is relatively routine and constant, and as such it can be used to monitor community health. The goal is to identify and track potential risks to the health and well-being of the community. Fueling the surveillance system must therefore be balanced with a commitment to protect data confidentiality. A public health surveillance system must be built in a way that protects the privacy of those whose data is captured in the system to serve the goal of the community accruing the benefits of the system.

In some instances, the routine reporting of information has implications for individuals other than those who were tested (e.g., contact tracing). The handling and disclosure of this information require a commitment to limit the potential for a breach of confidentiality to maximize the likelihood that such efforts can achieve various public health goals, such as working to stem the tide of disease. Lee notes that as our understanding of disease, risk of disease, and biomedical markers has advanced, so too have public health surveillance systems. She explains how the core values and tensions in public health ethics are in play in the ethics of public health surveillance.

The bulk of the chapter is devoted to a description of the core components of a robust public health surveillance system—from creating the infrastructure to manage the data collected to the use and dissemination of data—presenting both key ethical considerations and best practices along the way. Lee lastly identifies and considers the ethical implications of recent advances in information systems that have allowed for the aggregation of public health surveillance data along with other data sources to advance knowledge beyond the traditional limits of public health.

The work of public health relies on more than the collection of surveillance data, including carrying out research whose data are used in service of public health. Public health research, conducted by government agencies, nongovernmental agencies, academics, and other stakeholders can take a variety of shapes and forms. As is the case with human subject research more generally, the goal of public health research is to produce generalizable knowledge to promote health and prevent disease. As the promotion of health and prevention of disease are also key goals of public health practice, the boundary between public health research and public health practice can be blurred. This blurring can lead to confusion about how best to balance the benefit of the production of new knowledge with whether and how the individuals from whom the data collected ought to be informed about their participation in the production of that knowledge.

In "Framing Public Health Research Ethics," Holly A. Taylor examines the distinctions and boundaries between public health practice and research, focusing on two criteria that public health investigators and practitioners ought to consider: intent and experimentation. She then compares public health research with biomedical research, identifying a critical distinction that deserves ethical attention: communities, rather than individuals, are often the population of interest. Because communities are made up of individuals, the traditional concerns of respect for persons, minimizing risk to subjects, and the equitable distribution of risks and benefits apply, but other considerations are relevant as well. These include respect for the community, minimizing risks to the community, and considerations as to whether the planned research further disadvantages an already disadvantaged group.

One approach to public health research fully embraces the principle of respect for community. Community-based participatory research (CPBR) is a relatively recent addition to the research methods used by public health researchers. As its name implies, CPBR is a method that expects and relies on the community to have an essential role in the research process as a beneficiary of the research and a partner in its conduct. In general, *community* refers to members of the population who are a part of the community to be studied—individuals who have a unique perspective as members of the community who partner with a study team. The community members and study team collaborate from beginning to end, from identifying the research question(s) to disseminating results. Engagement in CBPR requires commitment from the study team and community members. This relationship between the research subjects and study team is unique to CPBR and has resulted in a number of ethical challenges.

The ethical "promise" of CBPR is that its inclusive and deliberative approach has the potential to minimize community harm and avoid exploitation, and in so doing better serve the interests of the community and its members. In "Community-Based Participatory Research: Ethical Considerations," David R. Buchanan explores the nature of community harm and how adopting a CBPR approach can lead researchers to act in ways that respect communities through researching in partnership with them. Buchanan identifies several unresolved ethical questions related to CBPR: Who is the "community" with which researchers ought to engage? What are the hallmarks of a successful partnership? What is the scope of responsibility a "community" has when engaged in CBPR? How do researchers make clear to communities that their participation in research may not lead to direct benefit to the community? The collaboration between Arizona State University (ASU) and the Havasupai Indian tribe is a cautionary tale. It began as a promising example of the use of CBPR to address health concerns prioritized by the tribe. Later, however, data were used to answer research questions without input from, or even knowledge of, the tribe, leading to what the tribe considered community harms and a breach of trust (Mello and Wolf, 2010).

An even more recent addition to public health research methods is the use of "big data" to answer questions about the promotion of health and prevention of disease. While the term has been defined in a number of ways, here "big data" refers to the aggregation and analysis of data from large data sources, including data from sources as diverse as routine public health surveillance activities and social media activity. Advances in computational capacity have made big data approaches possible. As with the other examples of public health research mentioned above, big data research puts the potential benefit to the health and well-being on the community in tension with the privacy rights of the individual.

In "Navigating the Ethics of Big Data in Public Health," Effy Vayena and Lawrence Madoff scrutinize ethical issues arising out of the increasing use of big data as a novel tool in public health research and practice. Big data's two core components are the variety of sources of data that can be brought together in a big data set, and the variety of techniques available to find meaning in the data once aggregated. The techniques developed to bring multiple data sources together allow for the blending of data collected for research purposes along with diverse sources of data, such as that collected for clinical or commercial purposes, social media postings, and behavior and activity trackers. This boundary-crossing raises ethical issues related to what is owed to those individuals who have, knowingly or unknowingly, become a data point (or many data points) in one or many data sets, introducing potentially novel risks to privacy and confidentiality.

Vayena and Madoff review the current technical challenges that limit the current potential of big data initiatives and highlight the importance of considering privacy concerns and protections as these technical challenges are overcome. The main sources of data currently being brought together under the banner of big data in an effort to improve public health include electronic health record systems, social media data, and electronic self-reporting, such as those designed for real-time tracking of infectious disease outbreaks like the flu. The authors posit that the ethical challenges in the establishment of big data resources that can benefit public health revolve around the blurring of once clear lines along three axes: "personal health data and nonhealth data; . . . private and the public sphere in the online world; and, . . . the powers and responsibilities of state and nonstate actors" (Vayena and Madoff, this volume).

Conclusion

Data collection is a core function of public health. So too are the obligations of the collectors, aggregators, and users of that data to ensure that individual interests are respected in the pursuit of knowledge benefiting the health and well-being of populations. The value and promise of public health data must be balanced against the potential harm it can bring to individuals and communities through its collection, handling, and dissemination.

References

Allen, J., Hulman, D., Meslin, E. M., and Stanley, F. 2013. "Privacy Protectionism and Harms to Health: Is There Any Redress?" *Journal of Law and Medicine* 21: 473–485.

Brachman, P. S. 1996. "Epilogue: Alexander Duncan Langmuir." *American Journal of Epidemiology* 144 (Suppl. 8): S74–S75.

Declich, S., and Carter, A. O. 1994. "Public Health Surveillance: Historical Origins, Methods and Evaluation." *Bulletin of the World Health Organization* 72(2): 285–304.

Mahajan, A. P., Sayles, J. N., Patel, V. A., Remien, R. H., Ortiz, D., Szekeres, G., et al. 2008. "Stigma in the HIV/AIDS Epidemic: A Review of the Literature and Recommendations for the Way Forward." *AIDS* 22(Suppl. 2): S67–S79.

Mello, M. M., and Wolf, L. E. 2010. "The Havasupai Indian Tribe Case—Lessons for Research Involving Stored Biologic Samples." *New England Journal of Medicine* 363(3): 204–207. https://www.nejm.org/doi/full/10.1056/NEJMp1005203.

Vayena, E., Salathé, M., Madoff, L. C., and Brownstein, J. S. 2015. "Ethical Challenges of Big Data in Public Health." *PLoS Computational Biology* 11(2): e1003904. doi:10.1371/journal.pcbi.1003904.

CHAPTER 28

PUBLIC HEALTH SURVEILLANCE: ETHICAL CONSIDERATIONS

LISA M. LEE

Introduction

Public health surveillance is the "ongoing, systematic collection, analysis, and interpretation of health-related data with the a priori purpose of preventing or controlling disease or injury, or of identifying unusual events of public health importance, followed by the dissemination and use of information for public health action" (Lee and Thacker, 2011, Figure 1). Public health professionals gather evidence for action in response to their governmental duty to promote and protect the health of the community. Public health surveillance is one of a growing number of ways public health professionals collect data to inform public health policy. It is most often implemented by trusted state actors, but it increasingly includes nongovernmental professionals. In some cases, participation in public health surveillance is legally mandated and requires health care providers—regardless of patient knowledge or consent—to report specific health outcomes (e.g., cases of syphilis, influenza, or cancer) to health officials, who must then discharge their duty to citizens and take action to protect the public's health.

The ethical dimensions of public health surveillance evolve as populations progress through the epidemiologic transition. This transition occurs when the primary causes of morbidity and mortality in a population change from communicable diseases to chronic conditions and injuries. In the presence of threats from infectious diseases, governments have an ethical (and often legal) duty to protect citizens from the infectious harm. The harm principle, along with public beneficence, supports the development of infectious disease surveillance activities. The harm principle articulates not only the liberty that a state owes its citizens, but also what individuals owe their community. According to John Stuart Mill ([1859] 2008), a state's imposition on individual liberty is acceptable only when it is necessary to prevent harm to others. Mill also recognized that the state can limit absolute autonomy by compelling positive acts that benefit others in particular circumstances (Mill, [1859] 2008; Lee, 2014). Public beneficence is the duty of a government to maximize public benefits and minimize public harm, and to promote activities that have great potential to improve the well-being of the population (PCSBI, 2010). In the case of some infectious diseases, the duty of public health professionals to minimize potential harm to the community can be in conflict with the potential economic or social harm that might result if private information about individuals is disclosed.

As the proportion of ill-health effects from infectious diseases declines and the impact of noncommunicable conditions increases, a population begins the epidemiologic transition. Public health professionals' responsibilities begin to expand to encompass the prevention of chronic conditions, including injuries, and the role of social determinants as predictors of health outcomes. A shift in public health surveillance efforts toward the identification and tracking of social determinants of health—such as income inequity, poverty, and lack of access to quality education and affordable health care—prompts a shift in emphasis from secondary prevention to primary prevention. Primary prevention (preventing the onset of disease and disability, rather than diagnosis and treatment of disease) reduces costs, both fiscal and social, and improves the health and well-being of both individuals and communities (Maciosek et al., 2010).

A further epidemiologic shift occurs with advances in genetics, epigenetics, and the ability to identify predispositions to particular diseases or conditions. The public health response to this shift includes new approaches to prevention, with an emphasis on what has been described as "primordial prevention"—the use of policy and intersectional action to identify and address the far upstream factors that create biologic, social, economic, and environmental conditions that result in morbidity and mortality (Porta, 2008). The types of data that public health professionals need to collect in order to support primordial prevention are often associated with behaviors or genetic predispositions that some individuals and communities view as sensitive, since their collection might stigmatize groups or communities, revealing predispositions or behaviors leading to increased disease risks. From an ethics perspective, arguments for prevention are a matter of both utility and public beneficence.

The Values of Public Health

The values that motivate the collection, storage, and use of personal information for public health surveillance are based on values that motivate the field of public health more generally. While there is not a universally agreed upon list of values that make up our common professional morality in public health, several themes have emerged over the past quarter of a century of thought by leaders in public health ethics. These themes include justice, equity, respect for communities and individuals, evidence-based action, professionalism, transparency, public trust, interdependence, and collective action (Lee and Zarowsky, 2015; Lee, 2012), which has been explicated as solidarity (Dawson and Jennings, 2012) and communitarianism (Jennings, 2007). At times these public health values conflict. For example, respect for individual privacy (as a form of respect for persons) might conflict with advancing public health science (as a form of public beneficence) when public health professionals need to collect sensitive data to inform and support public health action. This value conflict arose at the beginning of the HIV/AIDS epidemic when public health officials needed to collect information about infected individuals' sexual and drug use behaviors to better understand modes of transmission in order to prevent the spread of the virus.

Value conflicts also occur in noncommunicable disease surveillance. In 2005 the New York City Department of Health and Mental Hygiene proposed the establishment of a novel public health surveillance system—mandatory name-based laboratory reporting of A1C results (Chamany et al., 2009). (The A1C blood test provides information about a person's glucose levels and can be used in diabetes management.) The goal of the system was to identify and link to care those suffering with uncontrolled diabetes, reflected by an A1C test result of more than 9 percent. The overarching goal of the effort was to address geographic disparities among city residents with inadequate access to health care, and to address an unjust distribution of poor outcomes. Under the proposal, the health department would follow up with both the ordering clinician and the patient when results indicated uncontrolled disease. Some opposed the proposal, however, noting that mandatory reporting was an infringement on individual liberty. Through a process of deliberate engagement via public comment, a pilot program that included public feedback, and critical discourse in the peer-reviewed literature, the city and the community ultimately agreed on a system that would balance the tension between these two conflicting values (Chamany et al., 2009).

Ethical Drivers for the Development and Implementation of Public Health Surveillance Systems

As a practical matter, integrating ethical considerations throughout the development and implementation of a public health surveillance system can help public health professionals anticipate and, in some cases, avoid ethical conflicts. Conflicts might still arise, but public health surveillance professionals who have articulated and attended to potential ethical considerations will be better prepared to address them. Ethical considerations ought to drive the development and implementation of each step of a public health surveillance system, from designing a system through the use and dissemination of information to improve the public's health.

Public Health Surveillance System Design

Numerous factors can motivate the decision to develop and design a public health surveillance system for a particular condition of interest, including severity of disease or condition, years of productive life lost due to morbidity or mortality caused by a condition, communicability of a pathogen, cost of treating a condition, public interest, and even political motivations and availability of funding. But the ethical drivers of the surveillance system design rest on the governmental obligation to promote and protect the health of the population. Public health professionals should ensure that public health surveillance systems are developed—and their data used—for legitimate public health purposes only, and that, on balance, the benefits of adopting a system outweigh the risks (WHO, 2017). Benefits might include longer life, reduction in morbidity, improved productivity, and other socially valued outcomes. Risks might include potential harms to individuals or groups about whom private information is disclosed, or to groups about whom aggregated information might be shared. Privacy and confidentiality are critical ethical considerations for any public health data collection effort (Lee and Gostin, 2009), but they take on heightened significance for public health surveillance.

Public health surveillance systems often collect private information without individual consent, which is necessary for public health surveillance systems to provide complete coverage and equitable and just results. Given the necessary impingement on autonomy, public health professionals have learned the value of actively and intentionally engaging communities affected by a proposed public health surveillance system. Transparent engagement builds trust and includes articulation of the goals and benefits of the system, data to be collected and stored, potential risks and plans to mitigate these risks, and planned uses of individual-level and aggregated data. Public trust requires that public health professionals respectfully handle and use private, confidential public health surveillance data. Public health professionals use a variety of approaches to build trust and address potential value conflicts, including engaging affected communities in deliberations throughout all stages of a surveillance system and promoting professional ethics among the public health workforce to ensure professionals honor their contract with communities. Public engagement and deliberation were essential, for example, in the development of the national HIV infection reporting system in the United States. Throughout the 1990s, federal and state public health surveillance experts worked with affected communities—men who have sex with men, injection drug users, heterosexuals with partners at high risk—to outline the goals of the system and permitted uses of the data (Glynn, Lee, and McKenna, 2007).

Collection and Collation of Data

Collection and collation of high-quality, valid data is required to provide the best evidence, arrive at accurate conclusions, and meet the goals of any public health surveillance system. Data collected and collated for such systems are often sensitive and sometimes even incriminating. Given that obtaining informed consent is not always possible or desirable in population-based public health surveillance, public health professionals must be thoughtful about—and provide a publicly accessible justification for—collecting such data. Alternative ways to respect individual autonomy in the context of a public health surveillance system include collecting the minimum information necessary to achieve the public health goal and establishing privacy and security standards to ensure data are protected from intrusion during all phases of the system—starting with collection and collation.

Whether data are collected manually, electronically, or through both means, public health professionals must have access to and be required to use the tools necessary to access, record, transport, and store data safely and securely. Coded data collection forms, locking briefcases, encryption software, secure data transport protocols, secure networks, and physically and digitally secured storage servers are some of the ways that public health professionals maintain data security. It is incumbent on every public health professional to ensure that data collected without individual consent are not accessed by unauthorized persons or used for unauthorized purposes; unlike participants in research or in-person health surveys, individuals whose identifiable information is reported to public health surveillance systems have not been advised of the benefits, nor have they consented to the potential risks.

Patient privacy is becoming more difficult to maintain in the digital era. Confidentiality is at greater risk due to our increased connectedness through ubiquitous digital systems. The widespread erosion of the ability to keep personal information private affects all aspects of life and can be especially challenging when stigma and discrimination accompany a health condition. If confidential information from a public health surveillance system were to be disclosed, it could have devastating social and even financial consequences for individuals. Such disclosures would also dramatically diminish the public's trust, reducing the ability of public health professionals to disrupt the transmission of communicable diseases or reduce morbidity and mortality of chronic conditions. In the United States, there have been very few documented disclosures of public health surveillance information, though the disclosure of patient identity by others is often misattributed to public health professionals (Enserink, 2015). Swift and severe consequences for inappropriate disclosure of private information are needed in all spheres, and are especially important for maintaining trust in public health.

In addition to respecting autonomy, a commitment to justice is foundational to the collection and collation of public health surveillance data. The principle of justice and a commitment to health equity require that surveillance systems be *population*-based, so that the public health actions proposed based on surveillance data available address the needs of all affected persons and communities. For example, collecting data from one group at risk of a particular disease and not from others at similar risk reduces both the utility of data collected and the success of any intervention directed at the disease in question. Often, special efforts are required to ensure that hidden or hard-to-reach populations are included in data collection efforts.

Analysis and Interpretation of Data

Embedded in the analysis and interpretation of public health surveillance data are two ethical considerations: professional integrity and public beneficence. Public health scientists are accountable to the public. They are professionally obligated to intellectual honesty and accuracy, including conducting valid analyses and interpreting results considering—and stating—limitations. The local, state, and national public health infrastructure, including public health agencies and associated organizations, is obligated to provide an environment in which integrity is fostered and best evidence is produced (IOM, 2002). Public health professionals also have a professional duty to produce public benefits. Their analysis and interpretation of public health surveillance data should promote community well-being and reveal health inequities to support effective interventions.

Use and Dissemination of Data

Once public health surveillance data are analyzed, public health officials ought to use the information in planning and implementing public health programs, as well as disseminate the information to relevant stakeholders through appropriate venues. Putting the public health surveillance data to use in promoting public health justifies the risks posed to individuals in the collection and storage of the data. Sharing resulting information with affected communities, policymakers, and public health interventionists honors transparency and increases the chance that positive change will be implemented. In some circumstances, however, dissemination of negative public health surveillance findings can introduce additional burden or bring potential harm to members of at-risk communities. To reduce such harms, stewards of public health surveillance data should consult with community members and advisors to plan the most beneficial use of surveillance data. For example, a discussion of findings with community leaders might lead to more beneficial action than releasing information in a news release or public report.

In some instances, sharing public health surveillance data across jurisdictional borders is required to protect communities and ensure equitable distribution of burden and benefits. As demonstrated by several international outbreaks of infectious diseases in the early twenty-first century, there are legitimate prudential and ethical justifications for sharing public health surveillance data within and across jurisdictions (PCSBI, 2015). The revised International Health Regulations (IHR), in effect since 2007, require that the 196 country signatories report data to the World Health Organization when authorities suspect a public health event of international concern (WHO, 2018). Sharing these public health surveillance data helps governments—whether local or national—fulfill their duty to promote and protect health. To ensure that jurisdictions also respect individuals and communities, data-sharing agreements should be in place and should include elements that require that data be shared and subsequently used for public health purposes only; that data disposition be clarified; and that the minimum information necessary be shared, preferably in aggregate. If it is necessary to share individual-level data, personally identifying information should be excluded if possible. In addition to respecting individuals when sharing data, concerns arise about the just distribution of benefits that result from data sharing. Officials in low- and middle-income countries fear that countries with more advanced laboratory and scientific capacity will use their data, including specimens, to develop technologies or public health approaches that only higher-income countries can afford. Justice requires an equitable distribution of burdens and benefits, and therefore data contributors are entitled to equitable benefits that result from data sharing. In the case of pandemic influenza, the World Health Organization's *Pandemic Influenza Preparedness Framework* outlines this expectation (WHO, 2011).

Ethics and Advances in Public Health Surveillance

Several recent advances in technology and data science, as well as changing expectations of how public health surveillance can serve the public good, have implications for how public health professionals design and conduct ethical surveillance systems. Advances in digital technology, the role of public health in preparedness and response, and the inclusion of nonstate actors in the development of public health programs are changing the public health surveillance landscape.

Technological Advances

New digital data collection and storage technologies are changing the way public health professionals collect, collate, disseminate, and share public health surveillance data. Increasingly, "big data"—stores of electronic information left behind from digital activity such as web searches, social media, electronic commerce and banking, and use of mobile applications—are serving as a source for public health surveillance (see "Navigating the Ethics of Big Data in Public Health," this volume). While public health officials increasingly use these data stores to identify potential events of public health importance, the aggregation of multiple data sources itself is not a public health *surveillance system*: Big data initiatives generally do not meet the definition, noted above, of an "ongoing, systematic collection, analysis, and interpretation of health-related data with the a priori purpose of preventing or controlling disease or injury." However, as a source for data collection and collation, big data can powerfully augment public health surveillance systems. Risks to privacy and confidentiality can increase as additional data sets are merged with surveillance records. Re-identification of individuals becomes easier as additional characteristics or personal data are added, even in the absence of names. It is critical for public health surveillance professionals to identify and address these risks and weigh whether the additional data are worth the increased risks to the security of the information.

In addition to taking advantage of big data as a data source for surveillance, public health professionals increasingly store data electronically and use web-connected computers for analysis and dissemination. The ethical concerns—individual privacy, data security, and misuse of data—are similar whether data are on paper or in digital format, but the tools to manage these risks are different. In place of coded paper forms and locked briefcases, tools such as state-of-the-art encryption software and password-restricted access protect data in many public health surveillance systems that use digital data collection. When public health surveillance professionals are planning a system, they must consider these digital risks and incorporate ways to minimize them.

Public Health Preparedness and Biosurveillance

Public health professionals have long been involved in preparedness for and response to natural and human-made disasters. After the September 11, 2001, terrorist attacks in the United States, however, investment in public health surveillance to enhance early warning of bioterrorism events surged. As a result, biosurveillance—the science and practice of managing health-related data for early warning of threats and detection of events, and the rapid characterization of an event so that action can be taken to mitigate adverse health effects (CDC, 2010)—became a priority. Biosurveillance incorporates components of public health surveillance, national security, and big data to create situation awareness. Public health surveillance is a key input to situation awareness, and the ethical components of data sharing apply. A common tension in sharing public health surveillance data with biosurveillance systems is that the latter's focus on security often requires release of information from the system to other governmental agencies for non–public health purposes, which is counter to the ethical use of public health surveillance data and might impact public trust.

Nonstate Actors

Public health surveillance is typically considered a public sector task and is conducted by public health professionals employed by local, state, or national governments (Rein, 2010). Although only governments can compel public health reporting, nongovernmental actors—including universities, charitable foundations, and private sector contractors—are often involved in the execution of one or more steps in a surveillance system. For example, a state or provincial government might mandate reporting of malignant tumors, but the resulting cancer surveillance registry might be run by and housed at a large academic medical center where many cancer cases are referred for treatment. In cases of private-public collaboration, ownership of and access to data are areas for potential ethical concern and should be fully addressed during the planning and contracting phases. Because nonstate actors act on behalf of the governmental public health surveillance system, all should be knowledgeable about and required to honor the ethical responsibilities that come with the creation and maintenance of a public health surveillance system. Professional ethics expectations (and consequences for noncompliance) apply to all persons who have contact with public health surveillance data.

Ethical Review of Public Health Surveillance Systems

As data sources for and potential uses of public health surveillance become more complex, some scholars have questioned whether formal ethical review and independent oversight of public health surveillance ought to be implemented (Fairchild and Bayer, 2004). However, other scholars and public health professionals have argued that public health surveillance is a standard activity of public health practice, and that designing and conducting it ethically falls under professional ethics of public health practitioners (Middaugh et al., 2004). Books and guidance on designing and conducting public health surveillance often address the profession's expectations for the ethical conduct of public health surveillance (Lee et al., 2010). In January 2017, US regulations covering research with human participants (known as the Common Rule) were updated (with a 2019 effective date). The revised rules state that public health surveillance is excluded from oversight by institutional review boards (IRBs, elsewhere referred to as research ethics committees, or RECs), which are committees that review research activities to ensure the protection of human participants. The stated rationale for this exclusion in the revised rules is that

> when a public health authority conducts public health surveillance activities to fulfill its legal mandate to protect and maintain the health and welfare of the populations it oversees, the regulatory protections of the Common Rule should not impede its ability to accomplish its mandated mission of promoting this recognized public good, in keeping with the principle of beneficence. Other protections independent of the Common Rule exist that serve to protect the rights and welfare of individuals participating in such activities, including privacy, confidentiality and security safeguards for the information collected. (HHS, 2015, 53949)

The issue of whether public health surveillance systems ought to undergo review by an ethics board—similar to the way research protocols undergo IRB/REC review—or if ethical conduct of such systems ought to be included in the professional ethics standards for all of public health practice, remains unresolved. It is clear that public health surveillance systems must be ethically sound to be effective—to collect, store, and use the information necessary to promote health and prevent morbidity. It is also clear that these systems must be agile and responsive, qualities uncharacteristic of many overburdened ethics review processes. The unanswered question is whether professional ethics expectations and best practices of public health professionals are adequate to ensure the development and implementation of an ethically sound public health surveillance system, or if it is necessary to engage a responsive independent surveillance review board to provide approval and oversight.

Conclusion

For three centuries, public health surveillance has anchored and informed public health action. Population-based public health surveillance ensures that public health professionals can execute their duties to prevent morbidity and mortality, protect the health of communities, and reduce health inequities. These duties are motivated by a combination of liberal and collective ethical principles, such as justice, equity, respect for communities and individuals, evidence-based action, professionalism, transparency, public trust, interdependence, and collective action, including solidarity and communitarianism.

As public health professionals design and implement public health surveillance systems, ethical principles can come into conflict. These professionals must make decisions about how to move forward to meet their duties and respectfully honor commitments to the public. Decisions about the path forward depend on both the empirical information—including the severity of the health condition, the emergent nature of the threat, and the consequences of inaction—as well as moral duties to the public. Attention to and integration of ethical considerations throughout the development and implementation of public health surveillance systems will better prepare professionals to identify and address the inevitable ethical conflicts that arise.

The digital era has presented us with many new tools and technologies to improve both the quality and efficiency of public health surveillance. Regardless of the ways we obtain, store, and disseminate surveillance data, we do so to create the conditions that lead to healthy lives for all people. Engaging communities, developing and maintaining trust with the public, and deliberating together about how best to create these conditions will remain essential inputs into the development and conduct of successful and ethically acceptable public health surveillance systems for centuries to come.

References

CDC (Centers for Disease Control and Prevention). 2010. *National Biosurveillance Strategy for Human Health, Version 2.0* (Atlanta: CDC).

Chamany, S., Silver, L. D., Bassett, M. T., Driver, C. R., Berger, D. K., Neuhaus, C. E., et al. 2009. "Tracking Diabetes: New York City's A1C Registry." *Milbank Quarterly* 87(3): 547–570. https://www.ncbi.nlm.nih.gov/pmc/articles/PMC2881457/.

Dawson, A., and Jennings, B. 2012. "The Place of Solidarity in Public Health Ethics." *Public Health Reviews* 34: 65–79.

Enserink, M. 2015. "Risk of Exposure: When New or Dangerous Infectious Diseases Strike, Public Health Often Trumps Personal Privacy." *Science* 347(6221): 498–500.

Fairchild, A. L., and Bayer, R. 2004. "Ethics and the Conduct of Public Health Surveillance." *Science* 303(5658): 631–632.

Glynn, M. K., Lee, L. M., and McKenna, M. T. 2007. "The Status of National HIV Case Surveillance, United States 2006." *Public Health Reports* 122(Suppl. 1): 63–71.

HHS (US Department of Health and Human Services). 2015. Notice of Proposed Rulemaking. *Federal Register* 80(173): 53931–54061. https://www.gpo.gov/fdsys/pkg/FR-2015-09-08/pdf/2015-21756.pdf.

IOM (Institute of Medicine). 2002. *Integrity in Scientific Research: Creating an Environment That Promotes Responsible Conduct* (Washington, D.C.: National Academies Press).

Jennings, B. 2007. "Public Health and Civic Republicanism: Toward an Alternative Framework for Public Health Ethics." In *Ethics, Prevention, and Public Health*, edited by A. Dawson and M. Verweij, 30–58 (New York: Oxford University Press).

Lee, L. M. 2012. "Public Health Ethical Theory: Review and Path to Convergence." *Journal of Law, Medicine & Ethics* 40(1): 85–98.

Lee, L. M. 2014. "Health Information in the Background: Justifying Public Health Surveillance without Patient Consent." In *Emerging Pervasive Information and Communication Technologies (PICT): Ethical Challenges, Opportunities and Safeguards*, edited by K. D. Pimple, 39–53 (Dordrecht, the Netherlands: Springer).

Lee, L. M., and Gostin, L. O. 2009. "Ethical Collection, Storage, and Use of Public Health Data: A Proposal for National Privacy Protection." *JAMA* 302(1): 82–84.

Lee, L. M., Teutsch, S. M., Thacker, S. B., and St. Louis, M. E. 2010. *Principles and Practice of Public Health Surveillance* (New York: Oxford University Press).

Lee, L. M., and Thacker S. B. 2011. "Public Health Surveillance and Knowing about Health in the Context of Growing Sources of Health Data." *American Journal of Preventive Medicine* 41(6): 636–640.

Lee, L. M., and Zarowsky, C. 2015. "Foundational Values for Public Health." *Public Health Reviews* 36(2): 5.

Maciosek, M. V., Coffield, A. B., Flottemesch, T. J., Edwards, N. M., and Solberg, L. I. 2010. "Greater Use of Preventive Services in U.S. Health Care Could Save Lives at Little or No Cost." *Health Affairs* 29(9): 1656–1660.

Middaugh, J. P., Hodge, J. G., Cartter, M. L., Fairchild, A. L., and Bayer, R. 2004. "The Ethics of Public Health Surveillance." Author Reply. *Science* 304(5671): 681–682.

Mill, J. S. (1859) 2008. "On Liberty." Reprint. In *John Stuart Mill: On Liberty and Other Essays*, edited by J. Gray, 5–130 (New York: Oxford University Press).

Porta, M. 2008. *A Dictionary of Epidemiology*. 5th ed. (New York: Oxford University Press).

PCSBI (Presidential Commission for the Study of Bioethical Issues). 2010. *New Directions: The Ethics of Synthetic Biology and Emerging Technologies* (Washington D.C.: PCSBI).

PCSBI (Presidential Commission for the Study of Bioethical Issues). 2015. *Ethics and Ebola: Public Health Planning and Response* (Washington, D.C.: PCSBI).

Rein, D. B. 2010. "Economic and Policy Justification for Public Health Surveillance." In *Principles and Practice of Public Health Surveillance*, edited by L. M. Lee, S. M. Teutsch, S. B. Thacker, and M. E. St. Louis, 32–43 (New York: Oxford University Press).

WHO (World Health Organization). 2011. *Pandemic Influenza Preparedness Framework* (Geneva: WHO).

WHO (World Health Organization). 2018. "International Health Regulations (IHR)." http://www.who.int/topics/international_health_regulations/en/.

WHO (World Health Organization). 2017. *WHO Guidelines on Ethical Issues in Public Health Surveillance* (Geneva: WHO).

CHAPTER 29

FRAMING PUBLIC HEALTH RESEARCH ETHICS

HOLLY A. TAYLOR

INTRODUCTION

THE mission of public health is "assuring conditions in which people can be healthy," through its core functions of "assessment, policy development, and assurance" (IOM, 1988, 7). The systematic collection and analysis of public health data is central to this assessment function and spans a number of activities, including "surveillance, identifying needs, analyzing the causes of problems, collecting and interpreting data, case-finding, monitoring and forecasting trends, research, and evaluation of outcomes" (IOM, 1988, 44). Thus, data are collected and analyzed in the context of public health practice, such as ongoing infectious disease surveillance to detect epidemics, or in the context of frank research, such as studies designed to better understand the causes and preventability of infectious disease. The goal of this chapter is to offer a framing of the ethics of the latter, *public health research.*

Some public health activities are easily classified as either research or nonresearch, while the distinction for other activities is more nuanced and classification becomes more challenging. How an activity gets classified has ethical implications—additional oversight, requirements for consent of participants, and potentially whether the activity can be undertaken at all. One way to frame the ethics of public health research is to distinguish it from public health practice. While public health professionals engaged in systematic data collection in support of public health practice activities are subject to professional codes of ethical conduct, the conduct of public health research is subject to an additional set of ethical principles as well as regulations (National Commission, 1979; Public Health Leadership Society, 2002; Soskolne, 1991, 1997; Coughlin, Beauchamp, and Weed, 2009; Coughlin, 2009). The research-practice distinction is ethically important, because in the conduct of public health practice the needs of the public can override the rights of the individual, which is much more difficult to defend in the context of research. For example, public health mandates to collect, report, and share identifiable information potentially infringe individual autonomy but are justified by the expected benefit to the public's health. In contrast, the conduct of public health research must respect the rights of individual participants (e.g., through practices such as informed consent), despite the potential benefit to the public. Public health research is also subject to the ethical principles of human subject research and is likely to be subject to regulatory review and oversight. The three principles informing the ethics of human subject research—respect for persons, beneficence, and justice (specifically distributive justice, rather than other types of justice)—guide researchers in carrying out their research (e.g., seeking informed consent from participants, minimizing risk of harms and maximizing the likelihood of potential benefits, and engaging in fair recruitment practices) (National Commission, 1979). This chapter begins by examining various attempts to distinguish public health research from practice, and it highlights the ethical implications of both.

Practitioners often work for local and state agencies responsible for the protection and promotion of the health of their communities. In the context of public health practice, *community* refers to the citizens of the local jurisdiction for which the local public health agency is responsible. How, though, should researchers account for community in the context of the ethics of public health research? The standard formulation of human subject research fails to account for community: the stakeholders are the researcher, the participant, and society; or, rather, the researcher recruits participants to generate knowledge to benefit society broadly. A conventional application of research ethics principles to public health research may fail to account for risks and benefits to the community in which the research is being conducted, resulting in avoidable harm to the community. The second part of this chapter contends that the ethics of public health research must be framed to include the community perspective (i.e., traditional ethics principles must be extended to include the community as a key stakeholder in the conduct of public health). The community, in this framing, deserves respect and ought to be protected from harm and exploitation, and benefits to the community should be maximized.

Distinguishing Public Health Research from Practice

Public health practice involves the systematic collection of data to protect and promote the health of the public. Public health practitioners must strike a balance between the private nature of the data they collect and the benefit to the population whose health the data is meant to protect and promote. Codes of ethics are directed at helping public health practitioners navigate this balance. In the United States, two relevant principles from the Public Health Leadership Society's *Principles of the Ethical Practice of Public*

Health, adopted as the standard for public health practitioners by the American Public Health Association, serve as examples:

> "Public health should achieve community health in a way that respects the rights of individuals in the community.... Public health institutions should protect the confidentiality of information that can bring harm to an individual or community if made public. Exceptions must be justified on the basis of the high likelihood of significant harm to the individual or others."
>
> (Public Health Leadership Society, 2002, 4)

Public health surveillance is a prototypical example of the systematic collection of public health data. A close examination reveals what is at stake in striking the right balance between individual rights to privacy and what is best for the health of the community.

The goal of public health surveillance is to identify and track trends to guide and target public health interventions. It can include the collection of identifiable information to pinpoint the source of disease (see "Public Health Surveillance: Ethical Considerations," this volume). In the United States, for example, health care providers and laboratories are required by state law to report cases of sexually transmitted infection (STI) to public health authorities. An individual seeking STI testing will be informed that positive results will be reported to public health authorities. So while the individual's testing decision is voluntary, the health care provider's reporting of the individual's results is mandatory, and may also result in additional individual follow-up and contact of sexual contacts. In this example, the public health mandate of reporting is justified by the benefit to the community, even though the practice conflicts with both the self-determination of and the protection of private information about the tested individual.

Identifiable information is collected to make sure that the individual diagnosed with the STI is connected to appropriate care, and that those who may have been exposed to infection are notified (Faden, Kass, and Powers, 1991). The burden of inclusion in public health surveillance efforts (i.e., the risk of a potential breach of confidentiality) falls on a particular group of individuals—in this case, those diagnosed with an STI. An individual experiencing the symptoms of an STI could choose to avoid testing to avoid the reporting of the diagnosis, but the individual would then be forgoing referral for treatment. In some instances, states have conditionally mandatory testing programs for STIs to facilitate testing and diagnosis (Faden, Kass, and Powers, 1991). While many, if not all, of those diagnosed with an STI will directly benefit as a result of being tested, the goal of this public health surveillance activity is to benefit the broader community by preventing the further spread of the STI (Fairchild and Bayer, 2004; Taylor and Johnson, 2007; Public Health Ontario, 2012). This balance in favor of the health of the population is common to much of public health practice. For example, school-age children in the United States are subject to state vaccination mandates, and individuals presumed to have a highly contagious disease can be isolated or quarantined (Bensimon and Upshur, 2007; Omer et al., 2009).

Public health practice is most often carried out by public health practitioners affiliated with local public health agencies. Public health research, on the other hand, can be conducted by public health practitioners as well as by independent public health investigators (e.g., those affiliated with an academic institution or nongovernmental organization). In the same way that public health practitioners are subject to codes of ethical conduct, public health researchers are held to professional codes regarding the responsible conduct of (all) research (National Academy of Sciences, 2009). When practitioners or researchers are engaged in public health research involving human subjects, they are also subject to policy oversight informed by the principles relating to the ethics of research on human subjects as articulated in the *Belmont Report* (National Commission 1979; HHS, 2017). Regulations include requirements for independent review of the proposed research and informed consent from those asked to supply data. Clear distinctions between public health research and practice are necessary to avoid misclassifications that could hamper or limit the collection of critical public health information, on the one hand, or fail to require oversight and consent of participants, on the other. Clear definitions are essential for guiding public health activities and for helping public health practitioners and researchers appropriately balance the interests of the individuals, groups, and communities the activities are intended to serve or benefit.

Given the implications of whether systematic data collection is defined as public health practice or public health research, numerous authors have proposed criteria to distinguish the two (NBAC, 2001; Amoroso and Middaugh, 2002; Hodge and Gostin, 2004; Hodge, 2005; Taylor and Johnson, 2007; CDC, 2010; Otto, Holodniy, and DeFraites, 2014; Barrett et al., 2016). The two most common and promising criteria among those proposed are the intent of the public health activity and whether the activity involves experimentation. Each of these criteria is discussed further below.

Intent

Numerous authors and the US Centers for Disease Control and Prevention (CDC) conclude that the *intent* of systematic public health data collection is the core consideration for determining whether the activity is public health practice or public health research (CDC, 1999, 2010; Hodge and Gostin, 2004; Otto, Holodniy, and DeFraites, 2014). The argument is that the intent of systematic public health data collection is to "assure conditions in which people can be healthy," while the intent of human subject research is to contribute to generalizable knowledge (IOM, 1988; NBAC, 2001; CDC, 2010; Otto, Holodniy, and DeFraites, 2014).

Another way to consider the intent of systematic public health data collection is through recognition of the actor collecting the data: public health data is most often collected by local authorities. Local public health authorities serve local jurisdictions and are ethically obligated to protect the health and safety of their local communities. Thus, the intent of local public health data collection is to promote the health of those who reside in the local jurisdiction, (i.e., everyone in the local community). The intent of public health research, on the other hand, is to contribute to generalizable knowledge (i.e., the ethical obligation of the public health researcher is to the health and safety of the research participants). Research participants may be members of a local community, but the researcher is ethically obligated to protect the health and safety only of those enrolled in their research. The knowledge generated by public health research *could be* applied to and benefit those living in the local community from which the subjects were recruited, but the intent of the effort is to contribute generalizable knowledge that may be useful beyond the local community. When the intent of the systematic public health data collection is to benefit those beyond the borders of the local jurisdiction, it is then classified as public health research. Indeed, the risk-benefit assessment required when conducting human subject research allows for the potential risks to individual participants to be offset by benefits to society (National Commission, 1979). For example, if a public health research project was conducted in the City of Baltimore, the potential risks to those enrolled may be offset by the potential benefit that may accrue to those who reside in similar cities.

Experimentation

Whether experimentation is a component of systematic public health data collection is another criterion that authors have proposed as a way to distinguish public health practice from public health research (Hodge and Gostin 2004; Taylor and Johnson, 2007; Otto, Holodniy, and DeFraites, 2014). Experimentation can be defined to include the exposure of an individual or community to an activity not yet proven effective (i.e., not yet standard practice). In general, public health practice does not include experimentation. Public health practice utilizes standard interventions previously proven effective to prevent disease and promote health. While there may be some risk to the individuals or communities exposed to a standard public health intervention, the intended, known benefits of the intervention outweigh the potential risk. Testing a novel public health intervention where individuals or groups of individuals may be exposed to risk ought to be tested against the standard intervention (or placebo if no standard exists) before it is adopted more broadly. It is in the testing of a novel intervention that the ethics of human subject research become relevant. It would be unethical to expose an individual or group of individuals to a public health intervention with known risks and unknown potential benefit without their informed consent.

Knowing the intent of systematic data collection activity and whether experimentation is involved are key to distinguishing public health practice from research. While these two criteria on their own may not be adequate to accurately classify every proposed systematic data collection activity as practice or research, they narrow the number of projects about which practitioners, researchers, and oversight bodies are uncertain.

Community as Stakeholder

The Belmont principles of respect for persons, beneficence, and justice are most easily applied by those conducting conventional biomedical and behavioral research (National Commission, 1979). The term *conventional* is meant to refer to research conducted to determine whether a novel intervention is as good as or better than the standard intervention (or placebo if no standard exists). An investigator formulates a research question, recruits individual participants to participate, and collects data with the intent of generating findings to benefit future patients. The Belmont principles help the investigator to navigate how to obtain informed consent from potential participants, how to strike an appropriate balance between the benefits and risks to the participants enrolled and to future patients, and to assure that the benefits and risks of participation are fairly distributed among those who participate. A number of authors endorse holding public health research to these principles but find the principles wanting in their failure to consider the community as a key stakeholder in research (Taylor and Johnson, 2007; Verweij and Dawson, 2009; Barrett et al., 2016; Taylor et al., 2016). Failing to consider the community as a key stakeholder in the conduct of public health research may result in ethical harms that could otherwise be avoided. What follows is a proposal that the Belmont principles of respect for persons and beneficence can be extended to accommodate the community as a stakeholder.

Respect for Persons/Respect for Community

One way to ensure that the interests of the community are considered in the ethical evaluation of a public health research project is to extend the principle of respect for persons to encompass the community as a stakeholder (National Commission, 1979; Public Health Ontario, 2012; Taylor et al., 2016). Such an extension places an affirmative obligation on the public health researcher(s) to acknowledge the community as a key stakeholder in the proposed research and respect the community when considering how best to seek permission to include the community as a participant in research. The community in this formulation is an identifiable group that has a stake in the conduct of the proposed research. The community is the group from which the participants will be drawn (i.e., eligible by virtue of their membership in the community) and may be affected by the outcome of the research. While a community can be defined by a variety of borders, whether geographic, cultural, racial, or another classification, it does have recognizable borders. Nonetheless, engagement with "the community" is not without challenges, including determining those boundaries and identifying who is authorized to represent the values and beliefs of the community. Taylor et al. (2016) conclude that, at a minimum, public health researchers must inform the community of their presence and intent and disseminate the findings of the research conducted. That is, disclosure, rather than informed consent, is required, and findings are disseminated out of respect for the community's contribution to the research effort. Community-based participatory research (CBPR) engages the community as an active partner from the development of the research question through to how the results ought to be disseminated (Israel et al., 2005; see also "Community-Based Participatory Research: Ethical Considerations," this volume). Public health researchers who engage in CBPR are held to a higher ethical standard regarding their obligation to engage with the community as a stakeholder. In practical terms, this disclosure may take a variety of forms. In some cases, a community has a recognizable leader or set of leaders who must be approached first to gain access to the larger community. While the permission of the leader is important, respect for community does not mean the investigator should not also obtain informed consent from the individuals approached to participate. An ethically acceptable exception to this rule may be when a researcher is engaged in a cluster randomized trial (CRT).

A CRT is designed to study an intervention's effects on identified groups or populations rather than individuals. Randomization is accomplished at the level of communities. CRTs are commonly used to test the effect of an intervention to increase awareness about a particular health risk (Barrett et al., 2016). For example, one community may be targeted for a media campaign, while no such campaign is used in a different but comparable community. The research is designed to compare differences in subsequent awareness of the health risk. Investigators identify eligible communities, meant to be geographically distant in order to minimize "contamination" across communities, and randomly assign them to receive or not receive the novel intervention. Data are collected on awareness in all communities, and the outcomes are compared.

Seeking individual consent in this example would likely be resource-intensive, as well as likely to undermine the ability of the investigators to answer their research question when and if people choose not to participate. Under such circumstances, the investigator might seek the option to waive individual consent and propose engaging in a community consultation in advance of the study, the goal of which would be to disclose their presence and intent as well as seek permission to engage the community. As noted above, at the very least the study team would need to seek permission from the relevant authorities to collect data in the study communities, and be prepared to justify their presence in each community during the data collection phases of the project. Whether or not such an approach would be considered ethically acceptable would likely hinge on the risk of the intervention, the type and magnitude of the data collected from community members, and the dissemination plans of the investigators (Taylor and Johnson, 2007; Taylor et al., 2016).

Risks and Potential Benefits to Communities

The ethical principle of beneficence can also be extended to consider the community as a stakeholder in research. The principle of beneficence requires that researchers "do no harm and maximize possible benefits and minimize possible harms" (National Commission, 1979). Because some research must expose participants to risk in order to answer an important research question, investigators must carefully consider the balance of potential benefits and harms. The principle of beneficence can and should be extended to the community as a stakeholder. The practical application of the principle of beneficence is to identify the potential risks to which research participants may be exposed, the potential benefits that may accrue to participants, and the benefits that may accrue to future patients or society. Once identified, the investigator must consider whether potential benefits to the individual and society outweigh the potential risks to the individual participants. Verweij and Dawson (2009) note that the utility of beneficence is limited in the conduct of public health research if it is not extended to the potential risks that may accrue to the community from which the research participants are drawn. Extending the risk assessment beyond the individual participants may result in the identification of community-wide harms such as stigma or economic loss. Failure to acknowledge that the community may be at risk can foster mistrust of investigators and compromise the research enterprise beyond the particular project being conducted (Public Health Ontario, 2012; Pacheco et al., 2013; Taylor et al., 2016).

For example, researchers involved in public health research projects that use media campaigns must consider the risk of harm such campaigns may bring to the community. A media campaign meant to encourage good dental hygiene is different from a media campaign to prevent human immunodeficiency virus (HIV) infection or interpersonal violence. An HIV or violence prevention media campaign, for example, should consider the potential for harm to communities, including the potential association of the research or its findings with public assumptions that the participating communities are at high risk for HIV or have a high prevalence of interpersonal violence. The potential for such assumptions should not mean the research ought not to go forward, but rather that researchers consider the potential harm to communities in balancing research risks and benefits, and consider approaches to appropriately managing it, for example by disclosure to the community prior to implementing the research. Indeed, the community may endorse research on the understanding that the potential benefits it offers to the community, as well as to broader society, sufficiently outweigh the potential risks of community-level harm.

Justice/Social Justice

The principle of justice as articulated in the *Belmont Report* is a principle of distributive justice (National Commission, 1979), which demands that an investigator and the oversight process assure that the burdens and benefits of participation in research are allocated fairly, through equitable selection and participation of participants and the groups they are deemed to represent. Since the publication of the *Belmont Report*, the understanding of the principle of justice has been expanded to include the consideration that groups ought not to be excluded from the potential benefits of participation in research (Mastroianni and Kahn, 2001).

Attention to distributive justice in the conduct of public health research is essential. Public health researchers must make sure that particular groups are not excluded arbitrarily from participation, and at the same time ensure that particular groups do not take on more than their fair share of the burden of research participation (National Commission, 1979; Mastroianni and Kahn, 2001). An extension of distributive justice to the community as stakeholder could bring attention to whether a particular community (or communities) is bearing more than its share of the burdens of research. This question is relevant to at least two kinds of public health research. The term *parachute research* refers to research where the investigator may drop into a community to collect biological samples and leave as soon as the data collection is complete, never to return to the community (Flicker et al., 2007). Longitudinal epidemiologic cohort studies may also place burdens on the communities in which they are conducted. Such studies are ethically acceptable if the community bears some benefit from the presence of the study. For example, a community may benefit if its clinical infrastructure is enhanced by raising the level of health care received.

In addition to reflecting on how the principle of justice can be extended to acknowledge the community as a stakeholder, Verweij and Dawson (2009) and Taylor et al. (2016) argue that the ethical conduct of public health research should attend to social justice. Powers and Faden (2006) argue that attention to the least advantaged is a "hallmark of public health" and among the fundamental aims of public health research. By extension, public health researchers ought to also attend to health inequities while focusing on health promotion and the prevention of disease (i.e., those differences in health status that result from unfair institutional arrangements rather than biology) (Taylor et al., 2016). Two ways to make this attention to social justice real would be to engage in public health research designed to identify barriers and facilitators to health equity or to prioritize the public health needs of the most disadvantaged (Public Health Ontario, 2012).

Conclusion

Whether an activity is considered public health practice or public health research has important ethical implications, including additional oversight such as prospective approval, and requirements for consent, of participants. The criteria of intent of the activity and whether it is experimentation are useful factors for helping to distinguish public health practice from public health research, though it is difficult to prevent some public health practice activities from being misclassified as research and some research activities misclassified as practice.

The principles relevant in the conduct of research on human subjects—respect for persons, beneficence, and justice—are applicable but not sufficient in consideration of the ethics of public health research. The additional principle of community is a critical and necessary addition. The so-called Belmont principles were drafted in response to a series of ethical violations that resulted in direct harm to and exploitation of research subjects (National Commission, 1979). In retrospect, it makes sense that the community was not acknowledged as a stakeholder in the conduct of human research, given the attention the principles bring to the need to protect vulnerable populations. The focus of the Belmont principles was on the recruitment of competent adults able to make informed decisions about enrollment in research that may put them at risk of harm but meant to benefit them or future patients. Extending the principles to accommodate the community as a stakeholder will bring attention to the interests of the community and require that public health researchers consider the implications of their work beyond the individuals they approach to enroll. Such an extension may also encourage researchers to engage more directly with the communities whose health they want to protect and promote.

References

Amoroso P. J., and Middaugh J. P. 2002. "Research vs. Public Health Practice: When Does a Study Require IRB Review?" *Preventive Medicine* 36: 250–253.

Barrett, D. H., Brown, N., DeCausey, B. R., Saenz, C., and Dawson, A. 2016. "Public Health Research." In *Public Health Ethics: Cases Spanning the Globe*, edited by D. H. Barrett, L. H. Ortmann, A. Dawson, C. Saenz, A. Reis, and G. Bolan (Cham, Switzerland: Springer International). http://www.springer.com/us/book/9783319238463.

Bensimon, C. M, and Upshur, R. E. G. 2007. "Evidence and Effectiveness in Decision-Making for Quarantine." *American Journal of Public Health* 97(Suppl. 1): S44–S48.

CDC (Centers for Disease Control and Prevention). 1999. *Guidelines for Defining Public Health Research and Public Health Non-Research* (Atlanta: CDC). https://www.cdc.gov/od/science/integrity/docs/defining-public-health-research-non-research-1999.pdf.

CDC (Centers for Disease Control and Prevention). 2010. *Distinguishing Public Health Research and Public Health Non-research* (Atlanta: CDC). https://www.cdc.gov/od/science/integrity/docs/cdc-policy-distinguishing-public-health-research-nonresearch.pdf.

Coughlin, S. S., ed. 2009. *Ethics in Epidemiology and Public Health Practice*. 2nd ed. (Washington D.C.: American Public Health Association).

Coughlin, S. S., Beauchamp, T. L., and Weed D. L., eds. 2009. *Ethics and Epidemiology*. 2nd ed. (New York: Oxford University Press).

Faden, R. R., Kass, N. E., and Powers, M. 1991. "Warrants for Screening Programs: Public Health, Legal and Ethical Frameworks. "In *AIDS, Women and the Next Generation: Towards a Morally Acceptable Public Policy for HIV Testing of Pregnant Women and Newborns*, edited by R. R. Faden, G. Geller, and M. Powers, 3–26 (New York: Oxford University Press).

Fairchild, A., and Bayer R. 2004. "Ethics and the Conduct of Public Health Surveillance." *Science* 303(5658): 631–632.

Flicker, S., Travers, R., Guta, A., McDonald, S., and Meagher, A. 2007. "Ethical Dilemmas in Community-Based Participatory Research: Recommendations for Institutional Review Boards." *Journal of Urban Health* 84(4):478–493.

HHS (US Department of Health and Human Services). 2017. "45 CFR 46: Protection of Human Subjects." https://www.hhs.gov/ohrp/regulations-and-policy/regulations/45-cfr-46/.

Hodge, J. G. 2005. "An Enhanced Approach to Distinguishing Public Health Practice and Human Subjects Research." *Journal of Law, Medicine & Ethics* 33(1): 125–141.

Hodge, J. G., and Gostin L. O. 2004. *Public Health Practice vs. Research: A Report for Public Health Practitioners Including Cases and Guidance for Making Distinctions* (Atlanta: Council of State and Territorial Epidemiologists). http://www.cste2.org/webpdfs/CSTEPHResRptHodgeFinal.5.24.04.pdf.

IOM (Institute of Medicine). 1988. *The Future of Public Health* (Washington, D.C: National Academies Press).

Israel, B., Eng, E., Schulz, A. J., and Parker, E. A., eds. 2005. *Methods in Community-Based Participatory Research for Health* (San Francisco: Jossey-Bass).

Mastroianni, A., and Kahn J. 2001. "Swinging on the Pendulum: Shifting Views of Justice in Human Subjects Research." *Hastings Center Report* 31(3): 21–28.

National Academy of Sciences. 2009. *On Being a Scientist: A Guide to Responsible Conduct in Research*. 3rd ed. (Washington, D.C.: National Academies Press) https://www.nap.edu/catalog/12192/on-being-a-scientist-a-guide-to-responsible-conduct-in.

National Commission (National Commission for the Protection of Human Subjects of Biomedical and Behavioral Research). 1979. *The Belmont Report: Ethical Principles and Guidelines for the Protection of Human Subjects of Research* (Washington, D.C.: US Department of Health, Education, and Welfare). https://www.hhs.gov/ohrp/regulations-and-policy/belmont-report/index.html.

NBAC (National Bioethics Advisory Commission). 2001. *Ethical and Policy Issues in Research Involving Human Participants* (Bethesda, Md.: NBAC) https://bioethicsarchive.georgetown.edu/nbac/human/overvol1.pdf.

Omer, S. B., Salmon, D. A., Orenstein, W.A., DeHart, P., and Halsey, N. 2009. "Vaccine Refusal, Mandatory Immunization, and the Risks of Vaccine-Preventable Diseases." *New England Journal of Medicine* 360(19): 1981–1988.

Otto, J. L., Holodniy, M., and DeFraites, R. F. 2014. "Public Health Practice Is Not Research." *American Journal of Public Health* 104(4): 596–602.

Pacheco, C. M, Daley, S. M., Brown, T., Filippi, M., Greiner, K. A., and Daley, C. M. 2013. "Moving Forward: Breaking the Cycle of Mistrust between American Indians and Researchers." *American Journal of Public Health* 103(12): 2152–2159.

Powers, M., and Faden, R. 2006. *Social Justice: The Moral Foundations of Public Health and Health Policy* (New York: Oxford University Press).

Public Health Leadership Society. 2002. *Principles of the Ethical Practice of Public Health, Version 2.2*. https://www.apha.org/-/media/files/pdf/membergroups/ethics/ethics_brochure.ashx?la=en&hash=1E9425A9C96347E42AC0D6B0D2000AA6A8717C3C.

Public Health Ontario. 2012. *A Framework for the Ethical Conduct of Public Health Initiatives* (Ontario: Public Health Ontario). https://www.publichealthontario.ca/en/eRepository/PHO%20%20Framework%20for%20Ethical%20Conduct%20of%20Public%20Health%20Initiatives%20April%202012.pdf.

Soskolne, C. 1991. "Ethical Decision Making in Epidemiology: A Case Study Approach." *Journal of Clinical Epidemiology* 44(Suppl. 1): 125S–130S.

Soskolne, C. 1997. "Ethical, Social, and Legal Issues Surrounding Studies of Susceptible Populations and Individuals." *Environmental Health Perspectives* 106(Suppl. 4): 837–841.

Taylor, H. A., McGee, S. J., Faden, R. R., and Kass, N. 2016. "Ethics of Public Health Research: Moral Obligations to Communities." In *International Encyclopedia of Public Health*, edited by K. Heggenhougen and S. Quah, 423–427 (Amsterdam and Boston: Elsevier).

Taylor, H. A., and Johnson, S. 2007. "Ethics of Population-Based Research." *Journal of Law Medicine and Ethics* 35(2): 295–299.

Verweij, M., and Dawson, A. 2009. "Public Health Research Ethics: A Research Agenda." *Public Health Ethics* 2(1): 1–6.

CHAPTER 30

COMMUNITY-BASED PARTICIPATORY RESEARCH: ETHICAL CONSIDERATIONS

DAVID R. BUCHANAN

INTRODUCTION

INTEREST and investment in community-based participatory research (CBPR) began in earnest in the United States in the 1990s. After more than twenty-five years of experience with CBPR projects, the ethical significance of this prominent public health activity merits careful examination. Meredith Minkler and Nina Wallerstein (2003) define CBPR in their dedicated textbook as follows: "Although often and erroneously referred to as a research method, CBPR and other participatory approaches are not methods at all but *orientations to research*" (4, emphasis in original). They specify the fundamental characteristics of CBPR: it is cooperative, engaging community members and researchers in a joint process in which both contribute equally; it achieves a balance between research and action; it involves systems development and local community capacity building; and it is an empowering process through which participants can increase control over their lives.

Buchanan and colleagues (2007) further identified three purposes that CBPR aims to fulfill: (1) to elicit ideas from community members for novel public health interventions; (2) to strengthen participant skills in research, communication, leadership, advocacy, and other areas; and (3) to demonstrate respect for community autonomy. CBPR is thus a method for developing innovative interventions, an intervention itself intended to change the respective partners positively as a result of their participation, and a means to fulfill an ethical obligation. Although these distinct purposes are emphasized to differing degrees in evaluations of CPBR projects, in practice they operate simultaneously in a mutually reinforcing process. Proponents assert that, by fulfilling these purposes, CBPR advances the cause of social justice in the public health domain (Israel et al., 2005; Wallerstein and Duran, 2006, 2010). The fundamental tenet of CBPR is to achieve maximum feasible participation of the affected population in all phases of the research, by sharing equal power to review and shape research projects that directly impact their lives.

Evolution and Practical Challenges of CBPR

The origins of CBPR can be traced to several influences. One major stream dates to the philosophy of "participatory action research," associated with the work of Kurt Lewin starting in the 1930s, when social scientists thought that active community engagement was critical to bring about social change (Minkler and Wallerstein, 2003). Growing out of a different tradition in education, the work of Paolo Freire (1970) and his focus on critical consciousness (*conscientização*) for social change was highly influential on researchers in the Americas. Another significant influence was concern with healing the breach of trust that resulted from the Tuskegee Syphilis Experiment, the notorious US Public Health Service study that came to light in newspaper reports in the mid-1970s. Public outcry led to the creation of the first national commission on the ethical conduct of health research and the publication of its landmark *Belmont Report* in 1978. Advocates see CBPR as essential for engaging African American and other minority communities in a respectful, equal power-sharing, and fully transparent relationship regarding the goals and methods of public health research. In light of this history, the US Institute of Medicine (now the National Academy of Medicine) published *The Future of Public Health* in 1988, which lamented the state of "disarray" of the US public health care system (IOM, 1988, 1). In follow-up, the W. K. Kellogg Foundation (2001) launched its groundbreaking Community-Based Public Health (CBPH) initiative in the early 1990s. The CBPH initiative was premised on concern about the lack of progress in reducing health disparities. It aimed to strengthen programs by calling for fully equal partnerships among three key parties: academic researchers, public health practitioners, and community members.

Practical Challenges

CBPR collaborations start with forming partnerships and identifying priority health problems. Community priorities may differ from priorities set by government officials. Typically, government funding priorities are determined by a utilitarian calculus aimed at achieving the greatest good for the greatest number, which results in the allocation of resources proportional to the leading causes of morbidity and mortality (IOM, 1998).

As a result, significant resources are now allocated to reduce smoking and obesity rates. Impoverished communities, however, may not perceive smoking and obesity to be the most urgent health threats that they face (Wolff et al., 2003). As differences between the priorities of government public health officials and community members have come up often in CBPR projects, the federal government and private foundations have created new funding mechanisms that support a two- to three-year start-up period. During that time, the researchers and community participants can work out agreements about the problem(s) to be addressed and the methods for addressing them. Reports on CBPR projects indicate that such partnerships have been most successful in tackling the first steps involved in designing and conducting health research, and less successful in the latter stages (Viswanathan et al., 2004; Wallerstein et al., 2008).

One significant challenge in conducting CBPR has been in gaining extensive community participation in data analysis (Flicker and Nixon, 2014). This shortcoming is attributed to a number of factors, including the lack of necessary technical skills, the uneven distribution of financial resources to support community member versus researcher time, and the respective levels of interest (Wallerstein and Duran, 2006). As a result, the hope that CBPR would bring to light new constructs and significant yet previously overlooked social and social structural factors remains largely unfulfilled (Minkler and Wallerstein, 2003; Israel et al., 2005).

CBPR projects have shown greater success in disseminating the results of the research, both by publishing in the academic literature and in using various more accessible channels to distribute findings to the populations in need. Although gaining community review and approval of articles for publication in scientific journals can take longer than other types of research, and faculty face mounting "publish-or-perish" pressures, CBPR projects have found considerable community support for publishing in scholarly journals (Chen et al., 2010). Because journal articles are generally considered a poor means to reach community members, community partners have developed many strategies for updating the community, including using social media such as Facebook and Twitter, in addition to the more traditional means of newsletters and community forums (Minkler et al., 2012). Also, the Community-Campus Partnerships for Health (2018) has set up an online repository, called CES4Health, which provides access to products of CBPR projects that might not be suitable for a journal article, but are still valuable to the field.

The Ethical Promise and Challenges of CBPR

The ethical significance of CBPR lies in its potential to provide safeguards against community harm and exploitation and in demonstrating respect for community autonomy. Because harms can occur at both the individual and the community level, the conduct of CBPR is one of the few processes currently available that attends to the need to gain the informed consent of the community as a whole, and thus demonstrates respect for *community* autonomy.

Harms

One major impetus for developing CBPR has been to provide protections against potential harms to and exploitation of the community. From a public health perspective, the conceptualization of ethically relevant risks and benefits must be broadened to take into account not only the risks and benefits to individuals, but also the risks and benefits to the population as a whole. Potential harms to the community include (1) stigmatization; (2) lost opportunity costs; (3) the spread of fear, through unfounded rumors; (4) the loss of the potential benefits of research participation, due to distrust and withdrawal from health research; and (5) the potential for the misappropriation of limited community resources (Buchanan et al., 2008).

Health research has significant potential for generating stigma that falls on socially identifiable groups. Long after human immunodeficiency virus/acquired immune deficiency syndrome (HIV/AIDS) was labeled "gay-related immune deficiency," female Ashkenazi Jews were found to be at elevated risk for breast cancer; in each case, entire groups of people were stigmatized based on their membership in a group regardless of their individual behavior or actual genetic risk (National Institute of General Medical Sciences, 2000). Similarly, in an unprecedented legal settlement, Arizona State University paid $700,000 to the Havasupai Indian tribe in 2010 to "remedy the wrong that was done" by using their blood samples for unauthorized genetic research (as cited in Gilbert, 2010). Tribe members believed that they had donated blood for research on diabetes, but investigators subsequently used the samples for unrelated purposes, including studies of the genetic basis of schizophrenia. The tribe sued the university, claiming that they had not consented to these uses and that the potential threat of being labeled as prone to schizophrenia could cause harm to the tribe's identity and self-understanding. Current research-review processes do not take into account the potential for such harms to the broader community, but CBPR enables community representatives to review the implications of the research for the community as a whole.

Communities should also have the collective right to decide about the use of limited fiscal or social resources (e.g., health clinic personnel and facilities) and whether potentially important opportunities are being lost as a result (Brody et al., 2005). This right raises the issue of protection against exploitation, where exploitation is defined as one party taking unfair advantage of another. As Wertheimer (1996) explains, for exploitation to occur, it is not necessary for one party to harm another—only that the benefit to one side be disproportionate compared to the benefit to the other. Given the power and prestige of health research institutions, it is imperative to set up a representative body with sufficient standing to serve as an effective counterweight to the research institution's terms and conditions and set fair terms of participation.

The community bears other types of risks that cannot be reduced to the individual level. Rumors start easily, and fears can spread rapidly, particularly with respect to the goals or results of a particular research project. Seroconversion due to participation in HIV/AIDS vaccine trials has a high potential for family, workforce, and community disruption if there is not widespread understanding of its significance (London et al., 2012). Community members may be skeptical of researcher claims and need a more trusted source of information to address their fears. Moreover, the success of many health interventions depends on their adoption by the population. To the extent that the conduct of the research reinforces negative attitudes (e.g., human beings used as "guinea pigs"), it undermines trust in health research, which impedes the adoption of effective interventions. Finally, the use of public resources also calls for public accountability, a standard that transcends individual consent and is not part of standard human subjects research review. If researchers claim that making referrals to a research project will not sap clinic resources, there needs to be a body to monitor whether the research project is not, in fact, interfering with the timely care of patients or otherwise impeding the delivery of services.

The community should also have the capacity to determine due compensation in return for their participation. The "ancillary duties" of researchers have received increasing attention in recent years, taking up questions about the extent of researcher obligations, for instance, to provide supplemental medical care for study participants, or to offer other related health services (e.g., HIV testing and counseling) (Belsky and Richardson, 2004; Macklin, 2004; Wendler, Emanuel, and Lie, 2004). The scope of fair, non-exploitative recompense cannot be established by individual participants nor research-institution-based IRBs, but only by the community itself.

Respect for Community Autonomy

Respect for community autonomy acknowledges the fundamental right of the community itself to have a meaningful role in determining the conduct of research that affects the lives of community members, especially about deciding whether the potential benefits of participation outweigh the risks for the community as a whole. Communities should have the right to decide whether participation is consistent with their collective goals and interests. Researchers may hypothesize that needle-exchange programs will reduce transmission of HIV/AIDS, but the community must have a role in deciding whether they want to participate in such experiments or not.

In the wake of debates about the HIV perinatal transmission trials in Africa, Emanuel et al. (2004) proposed an ethical requirement for community collaboration in international health research. They identify seven indicators to assess the degree to which this ethical requirement has been met: (1) developing partnerships between researchers, policymakers, and the community; (2) involving community partners in identifying health problems; (3) involving community partners in assessing the value of the research; (4) involving community partners in planning, conducting, and overseeing research; (5) involving community partners in integrating the results into the health care system; (6) respecting the community's values, culture, and social practices; and (7) ensuring that community members benefit from the research. CBPR is one crucial and viable means of meeting this proposed ethical standard.

Unresolved Ethical Issues in the Conduct of CBPR

Although CBPR aims to satisfy important ethical purposes, several unresolved issues remain (Dickert and Sugarman, 2005). The most important normative question concerns who has legitimated authority to represent the interests of the larger community (Friedman, 1990; Raz, 1990; Richardson, 2003). The issue of representation, in turn, raises the question of how *community* is defined. Broadly, *community* is most commonly defined either geographically or sociologically (Clark, 1973), and CBPR projects generally fall along one of these lines, either working in a particular geographic location or with a socially identifiable group. In either case, identifying legitimated, authorized representatives remains a thorny issue, including who sits at the table, how they are selected, how many are selected, the scope of their powers, and related concerns. Any group charged with responsibility for assuring community input and oversight must be vested with authority duly recognized by the community affected by the research.

Legitimated Representation

In practice, the most common model for identifying CBPR community partners is purposeful selection, based on mutual interest in addressing a particular public health problem (Duran et al., 2012). In years past, these relationships were typically initiated by academic researchers who had identified a funding opportunity, and so would reach out through their professional networks to identify a community organization or community coalition invested in alleviating the problem. However, as the parties to such ad hoc relationships were often motivated by the pursuit of their respective self-interests (i.e., research publications for academics, program resources for communities), such partnerships often foundered in squabbling over resources and the primary objectives to be achieved (Israel et al., 1998; Lantz et al., 2001). Although the issue of building trust between the respective partners has received greater attention and been addressed more successfully (e.g., funding two- to three-year start-up periods), the critical ethical question remains the basis for claiming authority to speak on behalf of the broader community. For example, can an organization whose membership is primarily African American fairly represent the interests of the Latino or gay communities on the issue of HIV/AIDS prevention?

In the United States, although various proposals have been put forward in the literature (Woodsong and Karim, 2005), there are no standards that stipulate that geographically or sociologically defined communities should elect or appoint a board to represent their interests in approving proposed research projects, with the significant exception of Native American territories.

Native American nations are the only communities whose collective authority to regulate the conduct of research on their territories is recognized by the US government. Positively, these regulations provide a model that could be emulated elsewhere. However, the regulations of the Navaho Nation and other tribal organizations confer absolute veto power over publishing study results to the appointed board (American Indian Law Center, 1999). The authority to withhold permission to publish appears to threaten the principle of academic freedom. This tension, in turn, raises complicated issues about notions of "objective truth," the right not to be slandered or defamed, and the desire to control the image of a people projected to the world (Taylor, 1992). Although by no means unique to this sphere of activities, it is common to encounter these issues in CBPR.

Scope of Responsibilities

Outside of Native American communities, the scope of responsibilities of any such ad hoc community research bodies is unspecified, with wide variation in practice. Should they have legal authority, like institutional review boards (IRBs, also known as research ethics committees, or RECs), to stop or prohibit a research project from proceeding? If exploitation involves taking unfair advantage, what standards should be used to determine whether the community is gaining equitable benefit? Determining the right level of compensation for community projects is complex, with open questions about the appropriate balance between offering few or no benefits to the community, which may discourage participation, versus offering substantial benefits, which raises concerns about undue inducement. In response to calls for setting up representative boards with regulatory powers, it is also important to note that researchers have objected that mandating another layer of review would make an already protracted process even more burdensome, and thereby discourage research aimed at addressing health problems among those most in need (Berkley, 2003; Dawson and Kass, 2005). As these issues remain unresolved, beyond the relatively benign process of community consultation in the design and execution of CBPR projects, there is now no political drive toward further recognition of community rights to regulate public health research.

Issues in Research Design

It is well established that many individuals assume that by participating in clinical research investigations, they are availing themselves of the most advanced therapies devised by medical scientists—an idea known as the "therapeutic misconception" (Miller and Brody, 2003; Miller and Rosenstein, 2003). Analogously, many people assume that participation in community-based research projects also provides access to the most effective interventions developed to date (a perception compounded by community involvement in their design). As a result, there is growing interest in and recourse to crossover research designs (where the control/comparison group "crosses over" to gain access to the experimental intervention). Community-wide interventions, however, generally require significant resources to have a measurable impact, so that extending an experimental intervention to the comparison group may nearly double the costs of the study, while its potential benefits remain unknown. The potential waste of limited resources in CBPR projects with cross-over research designs deserves more careful ethical consideration (Rosen et al., 2006).

With greater numbers of people involved in conducting the research and collecting and analyzing data, comes a greater risk of failure to protect the confidentiality or anonymity of participants. Federally qualified health centers are important sites for CBPR projects, for example, but they are often used by the community research team as well as the intended research participants. Research on novel approaches to increase rates of HIV screening, for example, may lead to unintentional encounters in waiting rooms (Buchanan et al., 2002). Similarly, the recent interest in digital storytelling and other social media poses higher risks of inadvertent disclosures than the one-on-one interactions involved in clinical trials (Gubrium, Hill, and Flicker, 2014).

Fair compensation for community research team members is also unresolved. The division of research grant funds often looks lopsided in favor of the academic researchers, which may foster perceptions of inequities and exploitation. There are no established norms regarding a fair wage for community representatives in CBPR, and attempts to narrow the differences often generate pushback from university or agency human resource divisions, questioning the rationale for paying someone at a rate that appears inconsistent with established measures of qualifications. Relatedly, concerns are frequently raised about the respective levels of power and influence that attach to the different social positions of the researchers vis-à-vis community members, especially in the deliberations and decision-making of the executive committee charged with directing the project (Wallerstein, 1999). However, as the level of interactions has increased over time and community members have grown more accustomed to these types of collaborations, the weight of this concern appears to be diminishing.

Conclusion

Community-based participatory research has emerged as a widespread and ethically significant public health activity. It would be fair to say that, after more than twenty-five years of experience with the approach, a palpable degree of skepticism about the value of CBPR has settled in among independent third parties with respect to developing effective community interventions to address significant public health problems. There is limited evidence that one principal aim of CBPR—to develop novel culturally attuned programs that would be readily taken up by disenfranchised communities, and thus more effectively reduce health disparities—has been realized to the degree once hoped. Less attention has focused on the capacity-building aim of CBPR and the degree to which community members have learned new skills; the few studies to date have found mixed results (Wallerstein et al., 2008). Even less research has been conducted on the effects of CBPR participation on academic researchers (e.g., whether they become more culturally sensitive, less racist, etc.), outcomes that are difficult to tease out due to the significant self-selection bias involved in evaluating the effects of participation on researchers who choose to conduct CBPR. Based on these observations, it may be fair to say that the leading contribution of CBPR lies in its ethical significance.

From a public health perspective, it is essential to recognize that there are categorically distinct threats of harm to the community that cannot be reduced to the individual level, and that individual consent procedures are inadequate to assure protection against such macro-level harms. CBPR is one of the few options available to gain community-level assent regarding the value of the goals and methods of the proposed research. Moreover, just as individual research participants can never be treated merely as a means to an end, communities should also have the collective right to decide if they want to participate in any proposed research. In clinical trials, one meaningful demonstration of respect for autonomy is through the procedural requirement of written informed consent. There is now no equivalent ethical standard that recognizes the right to community autonomy. CBPR is a signficant if imperfect (in its current form) solution to this critical ethical challenge.

A general principle to guide the development of policies aimed at securing community consent is that the higher the potential for harm, the greater the level of community participation should be (Buchanan, Miller, and Wallerstein, 2007). IRBs are currently mandated by US law to have one community representative seated on the board. One possibility would be to increase the number of community representatives and expand the scope of IRB responsibilities to encompass the potential community impacts enumerated above. This action may suffice in many instances, but local communities should still have the right to decide whether they want to participate in a particular project. Thus, another possibility would be to set up a community review board composed of duly appointed local community representatives, where the procedures for electing or appointing local boards of health offer one model for securing legitimated authority (granted, it would also require changes in federal legislation to recognize their authority). Finally, to have a measurable impact at the community level, public health interventions often have multiple components. Hence, depending on their complexity, local boards may need to supplement their deliberations through various means common to CBPR, such as interviews with stakeholders and key informants, focus groups, community surveys, community forums, partnerships with community associations, and other efforts to maximize community participation and understanding of the research (Duran et al., 2012).

To test more powerful community interventions, review committee approval alone cannot suffice. With an appropriately revised mandate and expanded scope of responsibilities and membership, a community ethical review process should require researchers to use a progressively more inclusive process proportionately geared to the potential risks and threat of exploitation. To protect against community exploitation, to ensure fair terms of cooperation, to ratify that the interventions to be tested are regarded as appropriate by community members, and to minimize potential misunderstandings about the purpose of the research, there needs be a process whereby a collective decision representing the interests of the body politic can be made. CBPR is currently the most significant and most viable attempt to demonstrate respect for community autonomy in public health research.

References

American Indian Law Center. 1999. *Model Tribal Research Code: With Materials for Tribal Regulation for Research and Checklist for Indian Health Boards*. 3rd ed. (Albuquerque, N.M.: American Indian Law Center). https://ccph.memberclicks.net/assets/Documents/CBPR Curriculum/AppendixF/mdl-code.pdf.

Belsky, L., and Richardson, H. S. 2004. "Medical Researchers' Ancillary Clinical Care Responsibilities." *BMJ* 19(328): 1494–1496.

Berkley, S. 2003. "Thorny Issues in the Ethics of AIDS Vaccine Research." *Lancet* 362(9388): 992.

Brody, B. A., McCullough, L. B., and Sharp, R. R. 2005. "Consensus and Controversy in Clinical Research Ethics." *JAMA* 294(11): 1411–1414.

Buchanan, D., Khoshnood, K., Stopka, T., Shaw, S., Santelices, C., and Singer, M. 2002. "Ethical Dilemmas Created by the Criminalization of Status Behaviors: Case Examples from Ethnographic Research with Injection Drug Users." *Health Education and Behavior* 29(1): 30–42.

Buchanan, D., Miller, F. G., and Wallerstein, N. 2007. "Ethical Issues in Community-Based Participatory Research: Balancing Rigorous Research with Community Participation in Community Intervention Studies." *Progress in Community Health Partnerships: Research, Education, and Action* 1(2): 153–160.

Buchanan, D., Reddy, P., Sifunda, S., and James, S. 2008. "Assuring Adequate Protections in International Health Research: A Principled Justification and Practical Recommendations for the Role of Community Oversight." *Public Health Ethics* 1(3): 246–257.

Chen, P., Diaz, N., Lucas, G., and Rosenthal, M. 2010. "Dissemination of Results in Community-Based Participatory Research." *American Journal of Preventive Medicine* 39(4): 372–378.

Clark, D. B. 1973. "The Concept of Community: A Re-examination." *Sociological Review* 21: 397–416.

Community-Campus Partnerships for Health. 2018. "CES4Health." https://www.ccphealth.org/ces4health/.

Dawson, L., and Kass, N. E. 2005. "Views of US Researchers about Informed Consent in International Collaborative Research." *Social Science and Medicine* 61: 1211–1222.

Dickert, N., and Sugarman, J. 2005. "Ethical Goals of Community Consultation in Research." *American Journal of Public Health* 95: 1123–1127.

Duran, B., Wallerstein, N., Avila, M., Belone, L., Minkler, M., and Foley, K. 2012. "Developing and Maintaining Partnerships with Communities." In *Methods for Community-Based Participatory Research for Health, Second Edition*, edited by B. A. Israel, E. Eng, A. J. Schulz, and E. A. Parker, 43–68 (San Francisco: Jossey-Bass).

Emanuel, E. J., Wendler, D., Killen, J., and Grady, C. 2004. "What Makes Clinical Research in Developing Countries Ethical? The Benchmarks of Ethical Research." *Journal of Infectious Diseases* 189(5): 930–937.

Flicker, S., and Nixon, S. A. 2014. "The DEPICT Model for Participatory Qualitative Health Promotion Research Analysis Piloted in Canada, Zambia and South Africa." *Health Promotion International* 30(3): 616–624.

Freire, P. 1970. *Pedagogy of the Oppressed* (New York: Bloomsbury).

Friedman, R. B. 1990. "On the Concept of Authority in Political Philosophy." In *Authority*, edited by J. Raz, 56–91 (New York: New York University Press).

Gilbert, S. 2010. "Behind the Curtain of Personalized Medicine: The Havasupai Tribe Settlement." *Bioethics Forum*, June 14. https://www.thehastingscenter.org/behind-the-curtain-of-personalized-medicine-the-havasupai-tribe-settlement/.

Gubrium, A., Hill, A., and Flicker, S. 2014. "A Situated Practice of Ethics for Participatory Visual and Digital Methods in Public Health Research and Practice: A Focus on Digital Storytelling." *American Journal of Public Health* 104(9): 1606–1614.

IOM (Institute of Medicine). 1988. *The Future of Public Health* (Washington, D.C.: National Academies Press).

IOM (Institute of Medicine). 1998. *Scientific Opportunities and Public Needs: Improving Priority Setting and Public Input at the National Institute of Health* (Washington, D.C.: National Academy Press).

Israel, B., Eng, E., Schulz, A. J., and Parker, E. A., eds. 2005. *Methods in Community-Based Participatory Research for Health* (San Francisco: Jossey-Bass).

Israel, B., Schulz, A. J., Parker, E., and Becker, A. 1998. "Review of Community-Based Research: Assessing Partnership Approaches to Improve Public Health." *Annual Review of Public Health* 19: 173–202.

Lantz, P. M., Viruell-Fuentes, E., Israel, B. A., Softley, D., and Guzman, R. 2001. "Can Communities and Academia Work Together on Public Health Research? Evaluation Results from a Community-Based Participatory Research Partnership in Detroit." *Journal of Urban Health* 78(3): 495–507.

London, L., Kagee, A., Moodley, K., and Swartz, L. 2012. "Ethics, Human Rights and HIV Vaccine Trials in Low-Income Settings." *Journal of Medical Ethics* 38: 286–293.

Macklin, R. 2004. *Double Standards in Medical Research in Developing Countries* (New York: Cambridge University Press).

Miller, F. G., and Brody, H. 2003. "A Critique of Clinical Equipoise: Therapeutic Misconception in the Ethics of Clinical Trials." *Hastings Center Report* 33(3): 19–28.

Miller, F. G., and Rosenstein D. L. 2003. "The Therapeutic Orientation to Clinical Trials." *New England Journal of Medicine* 348(14): 1383–1385.

Minkler, M., Garcia, A., Rubin, V., and Wallerstein, N. 2012. *Community-Based Participatory Research: A Strategy for Building Healthy Communities and Promoting Health through Policy Change* (Berkeley: University of California, Berkeley School of Public Health). http://community-wealth.org/content/community-based-participatory-research-strategy-building-healthy-communities-and-promoting.

Minkler, M., and Wallerstein, N., eds. 2003. *Community-Based Participatory Research for Health* (San Francisco: Jossey-Bass).

National Institute of General Medical Sciences. 2000. "First Community Consultation on the Responsible Collection and Use of Samples for Genetic Research." https://www.nigms.nih.gov/News/meetings/Pages/FirstCommunityConsultationResponsibleCollectionUseSamplesGeneticResearch.aspx.

Raz, J. 1990. "Authority and Justification." In *Authority*, edited by J. Raz, 115–141 (New York: New York University Press).

Richardson, H. S. 2003. *Democratic Autonomy: Public Reasoning about the Ends of Policy* (New York: Oxford University Press).

Rosen, L., Manor, O., Engelhard, D., and Zucker, D. 2006. "In Defense of the Randomized Controlled Trial for Health Promotion Research." *American Journal of Public Health* 96: 1181–1186.

Taylor, C. 1992. *The Ethics of Authenticity* (Cambridge, Mass.: Harvard University Press).

Viswanathan, M., Ammerman, A., Eng, E., Gartlehner, G., Lohr, K., Griffith, D., et al. 2004. *Community-Based Participatory Research: Assessing the Evidence*. Summary, Evidence Report/ Technology Assessment No. 99, AHRQ Publication 04-E022-1 (Rockville, Md.: Agency for Healthcare Research and Quality).

Wallerstein, N. 1999. "Power Dynamics between Researcher and Community: A Case Study of New Mexico's Healthier Communities." *Social Science and Medicine* 49(1): 39–53.

Wallerstein, N., and Duran, B. 2006. "Using Community-Based Participatory Research to Address Health Disparities." *Health Promotion Practice* 7(3): 312–323.

Wallerstein, N. and Duran, B. 2010. "Community-Based Participatory Research Contributions to Intervention Research: The Intersection of Science and Practice to Improve Health Equity." *American Journal of Public Health* 100(Suppl. 1): S40–S46.

Wallerstein, N., Oetzel, J., Duran, B., Tafoya, G., Belone, L., and Rae, R. 2008. "What Predicts Outcomes in CBPR?" In *Community-Based Participatory Research for Health: Process to Outcomes*, 2nd ed., edited by M. Minkler and N. Wallerstein, 371–392 (San Francisco: Jossey-Bass).

Wendler, D., Emanuel, E., and Lie, R. 2004. "The Standard of Care Debate: Can Research in Developing Countries be Both Ethical and Responsive to Those Countries Health Needs?" *American Journal of Public Health* 94(6): 923–928.

Wertheimer, A. 1996. *Exploitation* (Princeton, N.J.: Princeton University Press).

W. K. Kellogg Foundation. 2001. *An Overview of the Community-Based Public Health Initiative* (Battle Creek, Mich.: W. K. Kellogg Foundation). http://www.wkkf.org/resource-directory/resource/2001/12/overview-of-the-community-based-public-health-initiative.

Wolff, M., Bates, T., Beck, B., Young, S., Ahmed, S., and Maurana, C. 2003. "Cancer Prevention in Underserved African-American Communities: Barriers and Effective Strategies—A Review of the literature." *Wisconsin Medical Journal* 102(5): 36–40.

Woodsong, C., and Karim, Q. A. 2005. "A Model Designed to Enhance Informed Consent: Experiences From the HIV Prevention Trials Network." *American Journal of Public Health* 95(3): 412–419.

CHAPTER 31

NAVIGATING THE ETHICS OF BIG DATA IN PUBLIC HEALTH

EFFY VAYENA AND LAWRENCE MADOFF

Introduction

Digitalization and advanced methods of storing, curating, mining, and analyzing data have ushered in in the era of big data. "Big data" is a broadly defined phenomenon that seems to touch upon nearly all aspects of human activity, and to have the potential of revolutionizing modern life (Mayer-Schönberger and Cukier, 2013). There are two fundamental aspects to big data: The first is the plurality of sources from which data are generated. They span a broad spectrum from Internet clicks, to social media activity, geolocation, and the use of apps, to genomic data and health and credit records. The second aspect is the data analytics and data mining techniques deployed to distill meaning from the data themselves. Such tools enable important inferences and identification of non-obvious patterns in human behavior as well as other structures in organizations and networks. This understanding allows the development of predictive models, and it is precisely this predictive power that makes big data valuable (Vayena and Gasser, 2016b; Pentland et al., 2013).

Big data is widely thought to offer an unprecedented opportunity to improve both public health research and practice (Shaw, 2014). The digital transformation we are witnessing is unprecedented in several ways, including the amount and diversity of data that are generated and stored; the possibilities of linking diverse data for analysis, even if some of these sets do not appear to have any bearing on health (e.g., cell phone metadata, Internet clicks); the speed with which data can be analyzed; and the predictive power that such analyses can yield. Furthermore, big data makes available information that may previously have been public in a technical sense but is now made available widely and, in many cases, at no cost to the user (Google Street View is an example, as is access to tax and real estate records).

Despite the excitement about big data in public health, attention has been drawn to various challenges such applications pose (Vayena, Mastroianni, and Kahn, 2012; Goodman and Meslin, 2014; Vayena et al., 2015; Mittelstadt and Floridi, 2015). Some of these challenges are technical in nature, such as interoperability and analysis of unstructured data, filtering "noise" from data, among others (Khoury and Ioannidis, 2014; Palfrey and Gasser, 2012). As a result, much of the promise of big data in public health still remains in the domain of imagined possibility. Nonetheless, this chapter will describe and anticipate ethical challenges for big data in the public health domain, with a special focus on the following non-exhaustive list of concerns: privacy, control and sharing of data, roles of state and nonstate actors, fair distribution of benefits and burdens, civic empowerment, and accountability.

It is worth noting the complex interplay between the technical and ethical concerns. For example, it could be argued that, given the current limited uptake of big data in public health, addressing trade-offs between privacy and public benefit are not yet called for. On the other hand, it might be argued that there is a moral responsibility to take measures that will enable big data approaches to fulfill their as yet unrealized potential. We can readily see that a dilemma may arise—big data cannot fulfill its public health potential because of ethical constraints (e.g., privacy concerns), which are in turn justified by a claim that technical approaches to address those ethical constraints (e.g., privacy protections) are not yet sufficiently reliable.

The Big Data Phenomenon and its Potential for Public Health

Big Data from the Health Care System

Early hopes about big data were initially fueled by the advent and increasing adoption of electronic health records (EHRs) (Ross, Wei, and Ohno-Machado, 2014; Birkhead, Klompas, and Shah, 2015; Hoffman and Podgurski, 2013). EHRs are rich sources of data, including not just the patients' health data, but basic demographic data as well. EHR systems may have additional functionalities and even allow for some practice-level statistics. Therefore, analysis of EHR data can be used to carry out quality improvement, "real-world" research, and public health surveillance for communicable and noncommunicable diseases (Ross et al., 2014). In some countries, institutions that have established EHR systems are obliged to submit data to the health authorities, including lab results, syndromic surveillance, and immunization data. Several studies have also demonstrated the potential of EHR data mining for pharmacovigilance. More recent studies have shown that analysis of open notes on health records can pick up adverse events earlier than standard pharmacovigilance, leading to faster examination of suspected adverse events (LePendu et al., 2013).

Routine electronic reporting from health system EHRs results in calculation of population-level immunization rates. A system dubbed ESP (Electronic Support for Public Health) that sits alongside and communicates with EHRs has been used to monitor events of potential public health significance such as vaccine adverse events (Baker et al., 2015). However, it is fair to say that the full potential of EHRs in public health has not yet been adequately realized due to a variety of factors, including lack of interoperability across EHR systems, lack of data analytics specific to public health, lack of standard implementation practices, and unanticipated challenges in the disruption of work flow in the clinical context (Cresswell and Sheikh, 2012).

Big Data beyond the Health Care System

Another promising use of big data in public health is the use of data sources from outside the health care system. Internet searches, social media, cell phone metadata, and other sources can be mined for a variety of public health purposes. For example, predictive analytics (data analytics tools that make predictions about future events) can be used to identify communities, neighborhoods, and eventually individuals that are in need of health services. Early examples of this have been reported by the Chicago Department of Public Health, which used predictive analytics to develop microtargeting campaigns for mammography screening. (Bhatt and Mansour, 2015). Furthermore, computational analyses of opinions expressed in social media (sentiment analysis) can point to the specific types of health information that would be most relevant for these communities. On the basis of such information, health promotion programs can be better targeted and result in better outcomes (Ayers et al., 2016). Examples of applications in the public health sphere are increasing and include complex issues such as vaccination coverage and utilization of mental health services, including interventions for suicide prevention (Costa-Roberts, 2015).

Perhaps most notably, big data sources outside the health care system can be used as a source of early and reliable information for public health surveillance. This activity is better known as "digital disease detection" (DDD) (Brownstein et al., 2009). (Other terms that have been used for this category of surveillance include "informal" or "unstructured" surveillance, "epidemic intelligence," and "event-based" surveillance, or EBS.) Many examples of DDD systems have developed over approximately twenty-five years. ProMED-mail (the International Society for Infectious Diseases's Program for Monitoring Emerging Diseases, [http://promedmail.org]), for example, is an expert-moderated system that is widely used in the global public health community (Yu and Madoff, 2004), and HealthMap is an automated system that retrieves data on disease outbreaks via the Internet (Harvard Medical School and Boston Children's Hospital, 2018).

Other innovations have used alternative data sources. A notable and well-documented example was Google Flu Trends (and later Google Dengue Trends), which used geolocalized search query data to detect or predict disease outbreaks. The ever-expanding sources of data that have been studied for disease-detection purposes now include cell phone usage patterns, *Wikipedia* access, online access to medical textbooks, and Amazon.com queries (Wesolowski et al., 2014; Santillana et al., 2014; McIver and Brownstein, 2014).

Syndromic surveillance, based on reports of symptoms of illness that are collected (e.g., fever, headache, vomiting), is often categorized as part of traditional or official public health systems. One innovative syndromic approach, outside of the formal health system, aggregates self-reports of symptoms to monitor potential disease events. Sometimes called "participatory surveillance," and including systems such as Flu Near You in the United States and Salud Boricua in Puerto Rico, their results closely parallel more established public health surveillance.

Finally, another concept that can potentially impact public health is that of the digital phenotype. It is based on the idea of the extended phenotype, first introduced by Richard Dawkins, who argued that our phenotype cannot be limited strictly to our biological processes (Dawkins, 1982). Instead, our interactions with the environment and the ways in which we modify it are part of our wider phenotype. Capturing and understanding these interactions allows for greater understanding of how we function, and therefore of our health status. Jain et al. (2015) take this idea further, opening the notion of the phenotype to our daily digital interactions. We interact with personal digital technologies, we modify them and they affect us, and they constitute a major part of our environment; as such, they are natural extensions of our phenotypes. In this understanding, the digital phenotype serves as a normative guide that aims to offer (a) an alternative, but not exclusive, approach to the standard biomedical paradigm that typically starts with a fixed hypothesis about biological processes and aims to collect evidence to refute or confirm it; and (b) a more unified take on big data, whereby all data that can be captured about, or from, a person can contribute to understanding biology, health, and disease. The "digital phenotype" gives an answer to several calls over recent years to exploit all kinds of data in relation to the individual (Murdoch and Detsky, 2013; Ayers et al., 2014). Several epistemic arguments have been offered in support of such efforts, including the identification of new hypotheses, real time insight, and assumption-free insight (Weber et al., 2014).

Key Ethical Challenges

Ethical challenges to adopting the methods described above revolve around the blurring of three previously clearer boundaries: between personal health data and nonhealth data; between the private and the public sphere in the online world; and, finally, between the powers and responsibilities of state and nonstate actors in relation to big data. In this section, we explore some key ethical questions that arise in the new context in which these familiar divisions can no longer be assumed to be fixed. Towards that end,

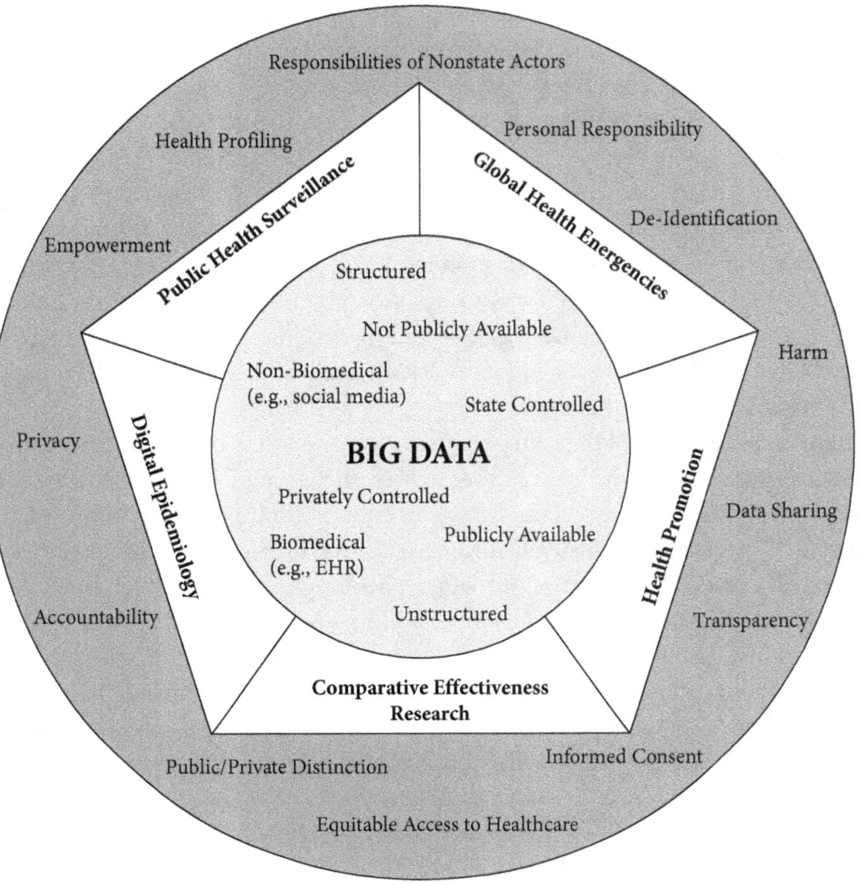

FIGURE 31.1 Key Ethical Issues in Big Data and Public Health. The inner circle contains different features of big data, the middle sections refer to possible applications of big data in the field of public health, and the broadest circle lists key ethical issues arising from the use of big data in the public health sector.

Figure 31.1 articulates features of big data and specifies their potential public health applications, identifying key ethical issues that may arise from big data's use in the public health sector.

Privacy

Privacy is often cited as the most difficult ethical challenge in uses of big data (Gasser, 2015). Several reasons account for this difficulty. First, to increase utilization of data, access should be granted to several users (researchers or public health practitioners) for uses that were not necessarily intended or anticipated when the data were collected. Widening access to data in this way can aggravate the risk of breaches of confidential information. Second, routine measures adopted in the past to ensure privacy protection, such as de-identification or even anonymization, may no longer be adequate to protect the confidentiality of data (Rothstein, 2010; de Montjoye et al., 2015). As a result of advanced analytical and computational methods, linking different data sets increases the risk of re-identification (Sweeney, 2000). Third, a primary mechanism for assuring the protection of privacy has been respect for individual consent (Vayena and Gasser, 2016a). However, the consent model is stretched to the breaking point when what is in prospect is consenting to unknown uses and linkages of data by various unknown users (Vayena, Mastroianni, and Kahn, 2013; Koenig, 2014; Cate and Mayer-Schönberger, 2013). A powerful feature of big data is that data from diverse data sources are linked and analyzed for an infinite variety of purposes that cannot be foreseen at the time that consent is obtained from an individual. It is therefore impossible for an individual to make an informed decision about the risks and benefits of data use when both the purpose of use and future users are unknown. Finally, underlying all these challenges is the deeper challenge of articulating a method to protect the confidentiality of private information that does not unduly inhibit the use of information for the common good.

Complicating all these challenges is the way in which the distinction between the public and private spheres has been called into question in recent years (Gleibs, 2014; Zimmer, 2010). Studies of social media users have shown that being online and sharing information about oneself is not necessarily the same as having decided to "go public" with the same information (O'Brien et al., 2015). Users may have expectations of privacy despite being active online, and this includes the expectation that they are not being tracked or having personal data (beyond actual postings on a social medium) used and shared by the owners of the interface they are using (e.g., Facebook sharing with Google).

An example that illustrates these tensions is the use of Twitter data for public health surveillance. It is unlikely that those who tweet are aware of all the ways their tweets may be put to use (e.g., as public health surveillance or pharmacovigilance). Although Twitter data are in the public domain, questions have been raised about the ethics of their use (Rivers and Lewis, 2014). Two different arguments have been constructed: one relates to the earlier point about people who tweet being unaware of the uses of their data, including potential risks that such uses may carry; the second, which represents a more European perspective on the value of privacy, relates to the point that even if people made their personal data publicly available, that does not automatically translate into unconditional permission for use by anyone for any purpose. The latter point is of particular interest in the following sense: What an individual makes publicly available, such as a symptom she experiences, like a "headache," will be combined with similar data from others; algorithms will then be applied to the data; and novel information will be derived that reveals more about her—for example, that she may be suffering from a specific health condition. It is not the data point "headache" that this person considers private (she made this publicly accessible), but rather the end result of the analysis of this and other data points—in this example, that she may be suffering from a specific health condition. Given the stigma associated with many diseases and conditions, real harm can occur to individuals and groups, if either can be identified in the reporting on results.

Despite such concerns, the ease with which such data sets can be analyzed and the increasing evidence about their potential value make it tempting for various organizations to utilize them. Consider the example of suicide prevention (O'Dea et al., 2015). Big social media platforms (e.g., Facebook, Reddit's SuicideWatch) have developed suicide prevention programs. In 2014 Twitter partnered with Samaritans, a suicide prevention charity, on an app (Samaritans Radar) that screened tweets for suicide-relevant content and alerted followers of the person considered to be at risk. The project was enthusiastically launched, only to be suspended a week after the launch due to concerns about privacy and stigmatization. This example highlights the tension between achieving some public health goals while respecting the right to privacy (Lee, 2014; Samaritans, 2014).

Control of Data and Data Sharing

A number of ethical issues arise from the question of who controls data sets, including the mechanisms that determine how data may be shared. Sharing of data for public health purposes, even within the same nation, is challenging, but it is even more so across international borders. Public health emergencies often bring the difficulties in data sharing to the forefront. The barriers to sharing data include logistical, political, economic, legal, and ethical factors. Notably, there is no global framework for data sharing in public health, or even specifically for surveillance.

Moreover, many data sources that constitute big data, and that have potentially valuable public health uses, typically belong to private companies, such as those that operate social media platforms or search engines. One question that requires deeper exploration is what obligations, if any, such private companies have to make their data (or metadata) accessible to public health researchers or authorities for purposes such as public health surveillance. Many such companies treat personal data that they have in their possession as a key business asset. This in turn raises further questions about the conditions that need to be met in order for access to be granted, and about the means by which possible uses of data may be communicated to the public. In the post-Snowden era of concern about state surveillance, public concerns about the legitimacy of state surveillance for security purposes may negatively affect public acceptance of public health surveillance. Therefore, it is crucial to distinguish the role (and/or intent) of public health surveillance from other forms of surveillance, whether conducted by state or nonstate actors.

Nonstate Actors in Public Health

No adequate account of the ethics of big data in public health is possible without an extended analysis of the nature and capabilities of the agents involved. The state, of course, is a key player in public health. Others include powerful nonstate actors (e.g., corporations), some with a global reach in their activities and with the capacity to draw on levels of resources that surpass those possessed by many states. In a space with a plurality of highly diverse actors, it is all the more important to explore the question of the public health role that can be properly assigned to each. Consider, for example, that a private company running analytics on large data is able to discover—perhaps without even seeking to do so—a pattern of disease related to a behavior, a region threatened by an outbreak, or even a particular individual as a source of an infectious disease outbreak. Is this company obliged to report its findings to health authorities? Or is it obliged to communicate its findings to the broader public, or to individuals who are specially affected? What are the duties of nonstate actors to anticipate such concerns through incorporating a public health dimension into their due diligence procedures (Kahn et al., 2014)? As argued in the United Nations' *Guiding Principles on Business and Human Rights*, nonstate actors, such as corporations, have responsibilities toward global justice and human rights quite independent of their legal duties (UN OHCHR, 2011). Therefore, some nonstate actors may bear specific responsibilities to contribute to public health activities (e.g., corporations collecting data that can be used for surveillance in a country that is lacking a state surveillance system), while they simultaneously have the duty to respect individual rights.

Finally, beyond the role of nonstate actors as *subjects* of norms, it is also important to consider the role they play in the process of norm *creation* in the sphere of big data. This role partly arises out of the fact that powerful nonstate actors are often in possession of the data sets, have special control and expertise regarding their handling (e.g., encryption), and operate globally and hence are able to influence standard-setting across a variety of jurisdictions. Naturally, the assumption of unaccountable nonstate actors, motivated by profit maximization, having a quasi-legislative role clearly gives rise to a serious concern about the legitimacy of the ensuing norms. Serious questions arise as to whether nonstate actors should have any such role and, if they do, under what conditions, relating to such factors as accountability and transparency.

Harm Mitigation

Various kinds of harms potentially arise when individuals or communities are identified within the context of some public health activity. Such harms may include the infringement of individual rights, discrimination, and stigmatization, which may result in economic and social sanctions, social exclusion, damaged family and social relationships, among other harms. The risk of these harms is in various ways exacerbated because big data approaches to public health are in an early stage of technical development (e.g., misidentification, false predictions). Some of the most commonly discussed methodological challenges for big data in public health involve difficulties in filtering out "noise" from data and validating and adjusting algorithms, including the entire spectrum of relevant data versus data that may give a skewed result. An example often cited with respect to the methodological issues is Google Flu Trends, which initially appeared to be very successful in identifying influenza trends in the United States, doing so as accurately, but much faster, than the US Centers for Disease Control and Prevention (CDC). Eventually, however, the Google flu algorithms failed to deliver similarly accurate results, becoming a landmark case of the potential hype and risks associated with big data analytics in the public health sphere (Cook et al., 2011; Butler, 2013; Lazer et al., 2014).

The question of redressing harms in public health has also been raised in the opposite way: If people are harmed by inaction or, in the case of big data, failure to use available technologies and means to improve public health, what means are available to individuals of groups for redress? Allen et al. (2013) have argued that there is no redress mechanism for such harms. This argument can be extended to the big data context, particularly as novel methods are developed that enhance the value of big data analytics in advancing the public's health.

Fair Distribution of Benefits

Big data uses for public health can generate both benefits (e.g., improvements in health) and burdens (e.g., risk of privacy breaches) for individuals and communities. This leads to a series of questions about whether the burdens and benefits of big data approaches to public health are fairly distributed. In 2013 the National Health Service (NHS) in England introduced the care.data initiative, aiming to collect patients' records from general practitioners to a centralized database. The data would be used for research as well as for quality improvement in service provision. However, many critics felt that the burden that may accrue to individual users of the NHS if their confidential data was disclosed was not balanced with the benefit that would likely accrue to profit-making companies that were provided access to their health data. These concerns were consolidated into a strong public opposition to the initiative, which led to its discontinuation in 2016 (UK Department of Health, 2016). Such imbalances will likely arise in the future when big data collected in resource-poor settings is used to benefit those in high-resource settings.

Civic Empowerment

Big data offers the prospect of an actively engaged citizenry, one that voluntarily takes up opportunities to make valuable contributions to public health that serve the common good. Participatory models may counteract the negative image that, in the perspective of big data analysis, individuals are reduced to merely the source of valuable data to be used for the benefit of someone other than themselves. We should be wary of a potential dark side, however, to the rhetoric of empowerment. This is the risk that under the banner of giving people enhanced options one is in fact burdening them with responsibilities that they are not equipped to discharge. For example, in a future scenario in which the delivery of health care depends on a widespread use of participatory methods, those ill-equipped to make use of those methods (e.g., elderly people who are not adept at using smart phones or other technologies) may enjoy only an illusory form of empowerment (Robinson et al., 2015).

Accountability

The foregoing is a non-exhaustive list of the kinds of considerations that are central to the regulation of the use of big data in public health. In addition to these "first-order" concerns, it is necessary also to bring into play "second-order" institutional mechanisms of accountability (Vayena et al., 2018). These mechanisms monitor the extent to which the first-order concerns are being addressed and provide methods for improving performance and avenues for seeking appropriate remedies in the case of failure. These accountability mechanisms should apply to both state and nonstate actors, although their nature may differ in line with differences in the kinds of actors, their goals in using big data, the degree of power they enjoy, and so on.

Conclusion

New streams of data, from both inside and outside the health care system, along with techniques to analyze them, will only increase. Our interconnected devices that automatically communicate and exchange data within networks are already offering a glimpse of the future of ubiquitous and continuous data generation and capture. These technologies can offer benefits to public health. However, for them to serve the purpose of public health successfully, they need to be carefully balanced against potential harms, including the loss of privacy and the diminishment of autonomy and equity (Vayena and Gasser, 2016b). Public health must respect individual human rights (Childress et al., 2002), but it must also draw its moral legitimacy from considering the common good (Tasioulas and Vayena, 2016). Both respect of individual rights and promotion of the common good of health are not just a matter of state responsibility. Nonstate actors are increasingly playing important roles in data control and data uses, which can impact the conduct of public health research and activity. Therefore, their responsibilities in relation to their interaction with state actors need to be clearly spelled out. Ultimately, public health success will rely on the public's trust and cooperation, and for that, transparency and accountability are crucial. Big data in public health cannot afford the shadow of opacity about potential harms relating to privacy, discrimination, and fair distribution of benefits. It needs to identify, balance, and mitigate them in order to legitimate its application and harness its immense potential.

References

Allen, J., Hulman, D., Meslin, E. M., and Stanley, F. 2013. "Privacy Protectionism and Harms to Health: Is There Any Redress for Harms to Health?" *Journal of Law and Medicine* 21: 473–485.

Ayers, J. W., Althouse, B. M., and Dredze, M. 2014. "Could Behavioral Medicine Lead the Web Data Revolution?" *JAMA* 311(14): 1399–1400. doi:10.1001/jama.2014.1505.

Ayers, J. W., Westmaas, J. L., Leas, E. C., Benton, A., Chen, Y., Dredze, M. et al. 2016. "Leveraging Big Data to Improve Health Awareness Campaigns: A Novel Evaluation of the Great American Smokeout." *JMIR Public Health and Surveillance* 2(1): e16. doi:10.2196/publichealth.5304.

Baker, M. A., Kaelber, D. C., Bar-Shain, D. S., Moro, P. L., Zambarano, B., Mazza, M., et al. 2015. "Advanced Clinical Decision Support for Vaccine Adverse Event Detection and Reporting." *Clinical Infectious Diseases* 61(6): 864–870. doi:10.1093/cid/civ430.

Bhatt, J., and Mansour, R. 2015. "How Chicago Is Using Predictive Analytics to Improve Public Health." Paper presented at the Annual Meeting of the American Public Health Association, November 3. https://apha.confex.com/apha/143am/webprogram/Paper335084.html

Birkhead, G. S., Klompas, M., and Shah, N. R. 2015. "Uses of Electronic Health Records for Public Health Surveillance to Advance Public Health." *Annual Review of Public Health* 36: 345–359.

Brownstein, J. S., Freifeld, C. C., and Madoff, L. C. 2009. "Digital Disease Detection—Harnessing the Web for Public Health Surveillance." *New England Journal of Medicine* 360(21): 2153–2157. doi:10.1056/NEJMp0900702.

Butler D. 2013. "When Google Got Flu Wrong." *Nature* 494(7436): 155–156.

Cate, F. H., and Mayer-Schönberger, V. 2013. "Notice and Consent in a World of Big Data." *International Data Privacy Law* 3(2): 67–73. doi:10.1093/idpl/ipt005.

Childress, J. F., Faden, R. R., Gaare, R. D., Gostin, L. O., Kahn, J., Bonnie, R. J., et al. 2002. "Public Health Ethics: Mapping the Terrain." *Journal of Law, Medicine & Ethics* 30(2): 170–178.

Cook, S., Conrad, C., Fowlkes, A. L., and Mohebbi, M. H. 2011. "Assessing Google Flu Trends Performance in the United States during the 2009 Influenza Virus A (H1N1) Pandemic." *PLoS ONE* 6(8): e23610. doi:10.1371/journal.pone.0023610.

Costa-Roberts, D. 2015. "South Korea Announces App to Combat Student Suicide." *PBS NewsHour*, March 15. http://www.pbs.org/newshour/rundown/south-korea-announces-app-prevent-student-suicides/.

Cresswell, K., and Sheikh, A. 2012. "Effective Integration of Technology into Health Care Needs Adequate Attention to Sociotechnical Processes, Time and a Dose of Reality." Letter to the Editor. *JAMA* 307(21): 2255. doi:10.1001/jama.2012.3520.

Dawkins, R. 1982. *The Extended Phenotype: The Gene as the Unit of Selection* (San Francisco: W.H. Freeman).

de Montjoye, Y. A., Radaelli, L. Singh, V. K., and A. Pentland. 2015. "Unique in the Shopping Mall: On the Reidentifiability of Credit Card Metadata." *Science* 347 (6221): 536–539. doi:10.1126/science.1256297.

Gasser, U. 2015. "Perspectives on the Future of Digital Privacy." *ZSR* II(134): 426–427.

Gleibs, I. H. 2014. "Turning Virtual Public Spaces into Laboratories: Thoughts on Conducting Online Field Studies Using Social Network Sites." *Analyses of Social Issues and Public Policy* 14: 352–370.

Goodman, K. W., and Meslin, E. M. 2014. "Ethics, Information Technology, and Public Health: Duties and Challenges in Computational Epidemiology." In *Public Health Informatics and Information Systems*, 2nd ed., edited by J. A. Magnuson and P. Fu, 191–209 (New York: Springer).

Harvard Medical School and Boston Children's Hospital. 2018. http://www.healthmap.org.

Hoffman, S., and Podgurski, A. 2013. "Big Bad Data: Law, Public Health, and Biomedical Databases." *Journal of Law, Medicine & Ethics* 41 (Suppl. 1): 56–60.

Jain, S. H., Powers, B. W., Hawkins, J. B., and Brownstein, J. S. 2015. "The Digital Phenotype." *Nature Biotechnology* 33(5): 462–463.

Kahn, J. P., Vayena, E., and Mastroianni, A. C. 2014. "Opinion: Learning as We Go: Lessons from the Publication of Facebook's Social-Computing Research." *Proceedings of the National Academy of Sciences* 111(38): 13677–13679. doi:10.1073/pnas.1416405111.

Khoury, M. J., and Ioannidis, J. P. A. 2014. "Big Data Meets Public Health: Human Well-Being Could Benefit from Large-Scale Data if Large-Scale Noise Is Minimized." *Science* 346(6213): 1054–1055.

Koenig, B. A. 2014. "Have We Asked Too Much of Consent?" *Hastings Center Report* 44(4): 33–34.

Lazer, D., Kennedy, R., King, G., and Vespignani, A. 2014. "The Parable of Google Flu: Traps in Big Data Analysis." *Science* 343(6176): 1203–1205.

Lee, N. 2014. "Trouble on the Radar." *Lancet* 384(9958): 1917.

LePendu, P., Iyer, S. V., Bauer-Mehren, A., Harpaz, R., Mortensen, J. M., Podchiyska, T., et al. 2013. "Pharmacovigilance Using Clinical Notes." *Clinical Pharmacology and Therapeutics* 93(6): 547–555. doi:10.1038/clpt.2013.47.

Mayer-Schönberger, V., and Cukier, K. 2013. *Big Data: A Revolution That Will Transform How We Live, Work, and Think* (London: John Murray).

McIver, D. J., and Brownstein, J. S. 2014. "*Wikipedia* Usage Estimates Prevalence of Influenza-Like Illness in the United States in Near Real-Time." *PLoS Computational Biology* 10(4): e1003581. doi:10.1371/journal.pcbi.1003581.

Mittelstadt, B. D., and Floridi, L. 2015. "The Ethics of Big Data: Current and Foreseeable Issues in Biomedical Contexts." *Science and Engineering Ethics* 22(2): 303–341. doi:10.1007/s11948-015-9652-2.

Murdoch, T. B., and Detsky, A. S. 2013. "The Inevitable Application of Big Data in Health Care." *JAMA* 309(13): 1351–1352. doi:10.1001/jama.2013.393.

O'Brien, D., Ullman, J., Altman, M., Gasser, U., Bar-Sinai, M., Nissim, K., et al. 2015. *Integrating Approaches to Privacy Across the Research Lifecycle: When Is Information Purely Public?* Berkman Center Research Publication No. 2015–2017 (Cambridge, Mass.: Berkman Center for Internet & Society). doi:10.2139/ssrn.2586158.

O'Dea, B., Wan, S., Batterham, P. J., Calear, A. L., Paris, C., and Christensen, H. 2015. "Detecting Suicidality on Twitter." *Internet Interventions* 2(2): 183–188.

Palfrey, J., and Gasser, U. 2012. *Interop: The Promise and Perils of Highly Interconnected Systems* (New York: Basic Books).

Pentland, A., Reid, T. G., and Heibeck, T. 2013. *Big Data and Health: Revolutionizing Medicine and Public Health*. Report of the WISH Big Data and Health Working Group. https://kit.mit.edu/sites/default/files/documents/WISH_BigData_Report.pdf.

Rivers, C. M., and Lewis, B. L. 2014. "Ethical Research Standards in a World of Big Data." *F1000Research* 3. https://f1000research.com/articles/3-38/v2.

Robinson, L., Cotten, S. R., Ono, H., Quan-Haase, A., Mesch, G., Chen, W., et al. 2015. "Digital Inequalities and Why They Matter." *Information, Communication and Society* 18(5): 569–582. doi:10.1080/1369118X.2015.1012532.

Ross, M. K., Wei, W., and Ohno-Machado, L. 2014. "'Big Data' and the Electronic Health Record." *Yearbook of Medical Informatics* 9(1): 97. doi:10.15265/IY-2014-0003.

Rothstein, M. A. 2010. Is Deidentification Sufficient to Protect Health Privacy in Research?" *American Journal of Bioethics* 10(9): 3–11. doi:10.1080/15265161.2010.494215.

Samaritans. 2014. "Samaritans Launches Twitter App to Help Identify Vulnerable People." Press Release, October 29. https://www.samaritans.org/news/samaritans-launches-twitter-app-help-identify-vulnerable-people.

Santillana, M., Nsoesie, E. O., Mekaru, S. R., Scales, D., and Brownstein, J. S. 2014. "Using Clinicians' Search Query Data to Monitor Influenza Epidemics." *Clinical Infectious Diseases* 59 (10): 1446. doi:10.1093/cid/ciu647.

Shaw, J. 2014. "Why 'Big Data' Is a Big Deal." *Harvard Magazine*, March-April. http://harvard-magazine.com/2014/03/why-big-data-is-a-big-deal.

Sweeney, L. 2000. "Simple Demographics Often Identify People Uniquely." Data Privacy Working Paper 3 (Pittsburgh: Carnegie Mellon University). https://dataprivacylab.org/projects/identifiability/paper1.pdf.

Tasioulas J, and Vayena E. 2016. "Public Health and Human Rights." *JAMA* 316(1): 103–104. doi:10.1001/jama.2016.5244.

UK Department of Health. 2016. "Review of Health and Case Data Security and Consent." Written statement to Parliament, July 6. https://www.gov.uk/government/speeches/review-of-health-and-care-data-security-and-consent.

UN OHCHR (United Nations Office of the High Commissioner for Human Rights). 2011. *Guiding Principles on Business and Human Rights* (Geneva: United Nations). http://www.ohchr.org/Documents/Publications/GuidingPrinciplesBusinessHR_EN.pdf.

Vayena, E., and Gasser, U. 2016a. "Between Openness and Privacy in Genomics." *PLoS Medicine* 13(1): e1001937.

Vayena, E., and Gasser, U. 2016b. "Strictly Biomedical? Sketching the Ethics of the Big Data Ecosystem in Biomedicine." In *Ethics of Biomedical Big Data*, edited by B. Mittelstadt and L. Floridi, 17–40 (Cham, Switzerland: Springer).

Vayena, E., Mastroianni, A., and Kahn, J. 2012. "Ethical Issues in Health Research with Novel Online Sources." *American Journal of Public Health* 102(12): 2225–2230. doi:10.2105/AJPH.2012.300813.

Vayena, E., Mastroianni, A., and Kahn, J. 2013. "Caught in the Web: Informed Consent for Online Health Research." *Science Translational Medicine* 5(173): 173fs6. doi:10.1126/scitranslmed.3004798.

Vayena, E., Salathé, M., Madoff, L. C., and Brownstein, J. S. 2015. "Ethical Challenges of Big Data in Public Health." *PLoS Computational Biology* 11(2): e1003904. doi:10.1371/journal.pcbi.1003904.

Vayena, E., Dzenowagis, J., Brownstein, J. S., and Sheikh, A., 2018 "Big Data Implications for Public Health." *Bulletin of the World Health Organization* 96: 66–68.

Weber, G. M., Mandl, K. D., and Kohane, I. S. 2014. "Finding the Missing Link for Big Biomedical Data." *JAMA* 311(24): 2479–2480. doi:10.1001/jama.2014.4228.

Wesolowski, A., Buckee, C. O., Bengtsson, L., Wetter, E., Lu, X., and Tatem, A. J. 2014. "Commentary: Containing the Ebola Outbreak—the Potential and Challenge of Mobile Network Data." *PLoS Currents Outbreaks*, September 29. http://currents.plos.org/outbreaks/index.html%3Fp=42561.html.

Yu, V. L., and Madoff, L. C. 2004. "ProMED-mail: An Early Warning System for Emerging Diseases." *Clinical Infectious Diseases* 39(2): 227–232.

Zimmer, M. 2010. "'But the Data Is Already Public': On the Ethics of Research in Facebook." *Ethics Information Technology* 12: 313–325. doi:10.1007/s10676-010-9227-5.

Further Reading

Crawford, K., and Schultz, J. 2014. "Big Data and Due Process: Toward a Framework to Redress Predictive Privacy Harms." *BCL Review* 55: 93. http://lawdigitalcommons.bc.edu/bclr/vol55/iss1/4.

The Economist. 2014. "Ebola and Big Data: Waiting on Hold." *The Economist*, October 25. https://www.economist.com/news/science-and-technology/21627557-mobile-phone-records-would-help-combat-ebola-epidemic-getting-look.

European Commission. 2014. *The Use of Big Data in Public Health Policy and Research*. Background information document. A report from the Directorate-General for Health and Consumers Unit D3 eHealth and Health Technology Assessment (Brussels: European Commission). https://ec.europa.eu/health/sites/health/files/ehealth/docs/ev_20141118_co07b_en.pdf.

Freifeld, C. C., Brownstein, J. S., Menone, C. M., Bao, W., Filice, R., Kass-Hout, T., et al. 2014. "Digital Drug Safety Surveillance: Monitoring Pharmaceutical Products in Twitter." *Drug Safety* 37(5): 343–350. doi:10.1007/s40264-014-0155-x.

Nahass, T. A., and Nahass, R. G. 2012. "Electronic Health Record Technology." *JAMA* 307(21): 2255. doi:10.1001/jama.2012.3520.

O'Neill, O. 2013. "Can Data Protection Secure Personal Privacy?" In *Genetic Privacy: An Evaluation of the Ethical and Legal Landscape*, edited by T. S. H. Kaan and C. W. L. Ho, 25–40 (London: Imperial College Press).

Vayena, E., Dzenowagis, J., Brownstein, J. S., and Sheikh, A. 2018. "Policy Implications of Big Data in the Health Sector." *Bulletin of the World Health Organization* 96(1): 66. doi:10.2471/BLT.17.197426.

White, R. W., Tatonetti, N. P., Shah, N. H., Altman, R. B., and Horvitz, E. 2013. "Web-Scale Pharmacovigilance: Listening to Signals from the Crowd." *Journal of the American Medical Informatics Association* 20: 404–408. doi:10.1136/amiajnl-2012-001482.

SECTION SEVEN

SEXUAL AND REPRODUCTIVE HEALTH

CHAPTER 32

AN OVERVIEW OF SEXUAL AND REPRODUCTIVE HEALTH IN THE CONTEXT OF PUBLIC HEALTH ETHICS

LESLIE MELTZER HENRY

Introduction

SINCE the mid-1990s, the concept of sexual and reproductive health has evolved from a limited focus on discrete health issues, such as maternal and child health, to a broad understanding of the many factors, such as gender inequality, that can affect people's sexual and reproductive lives. The move toward a more expansive vision of sexual and reproductive health is frequently traced to the landmark 1994 United Nations International Conference on Population and Development (ICPD). In a paradigm shift, the ICPD replaced traditional fertility control programs, which emphasized demographic goals, with a "Programme of Action" (PoA) that not only placed the sexual and reproductive health of *individuals*—and particularly women and girls—at its core, but also affirmed sexual and reproductive health, reproductive rights, and gender equality as human rights and cornerstones of sustainable development (UN, 1994).

The PoA committed ICPD member states to providing universal access to a core set of health services: education related to sexuality and reproduction, prevention of sexually transmitted infections (STIs), family planning, safe abortion, and maternal and newborn care. Despite occasional setbacks, efforts to build on that vision continue. The United Nations 2030 Agenda for Sustainable Development includes universal access to sexual and reproductive health as a target (UN, 2015), and the 2018 report of the Guttmacher-*Lancet*

Commission on Sexual and Reproductive Health and Rights calls for universal access to sexual and reproductive health, comprehensively defined as a state of "physical, emotional, mental, and social well-being in relation to all aspects of sexuality and reproduction, not merely the absence of disease, dysfunction, or infirmity" (Starrs et al., 2018, 11).

Sexual and reproductive health is an important aspect of individual health and well-being, but it also functions as a significant determinant of public health. The intersection between the deeply personal consequences of sexual and reproductive ill health, and its profound affect on public health outcomes, is reflected in the chapters of this section of *The Oxford Handbook of Public Health Ethics*, which examines public health ethics in the context of STI control measures, contraception, abortion, and pregnancy-related services. Some of the ethical complexities arising across the spectrum of sexual and reproductive health more generally are highlighted below.

Ethical Complexities

Individual and public health outcomes associated with sexual and reproductive health have generally improved worldwide as a consequence of greater support for gender equality, wider access to educational opportunities, higher rates of contraceptive use, and lower incidences of maternal morbidity and mortality (Snow, Laski, and Mutumba, 2015). When examined through the lens of public health ethics, however, a number of moral considerations come into greater focus (Childress et al., 2002). Three of the many areas of moral complexity are highlighted as examples: social justice, contested views of harms and benefits, and self-determination. Although there is interplay between these moral considerations, they are presented individually for ease of understanding.

Social Justice

While improvements in aggregate sexual and reproductive health outcomes are noteworthy, they can conceal considerable global inequalities. Often, these disparities stem from economic, social, cultural, and structural determinants of health, several of which are briefly highlighted in the discussion that follows.

Wealth inequality is a significant determinant of sexual and reproductive health, both between and within countries. Women in low-income countries are more likely than those in high-income countries to have unmet contraceptive needs, unintended pregnancies, unsafe abortions, and inadequate maternity care (Singh, Darroch, and Ashford, 2014). Within countries, women living in poverty are similarly disadvantaged as compared to their wealthier counterparts (Singh, Darroch, and Ashford, 2014).

Globally, the most significant risk factor for poverty is female gender (Rogers, 2006). Gender norms continue to limit women's access to education, information, employment, and health services. As a result, women remain disproportionately represented among the global poor. The "feminization of poverty" can prevent women from gaining influence and authority to challenge societal gender-power imbalances, which only reinforces the gender norms at the crux of their poverty (Pearce, 1978, 28).

Women who are socially and economically dependent on men generally have less power to negotiate condom use and access contraception. Although they are at heightened risk for contracting STIs and having unintended pregnancies (Glasier et al., 2006), their social and financial dependency diminishes their ability to access sexual and reproductive health care services (Cottingham and Ravindran, 2011). They consequently face higher than average rates of morbidity and mortality associated with STI-related complications, unsafe abortions, and unattended births (Starrs et al., 2018). Women who carry unintended pregnancies to birth are also more likely to lose economic, educational, and social opportunities (Cook and Dickens, 2009)—the very same factors that contribute to poverty, gender inequality, and dependency. Inequality begets further inequality, and women can become trapped in a socially unjust cycle from which it is increasingly difficult to escape.

Some populations are more likely than others to confront barriers to sexual and reproductive health information and services, and in turn to experience adverse health outcomes. Individuals whose communities view their sexual activities and identities as unacceptable (e.g., sex workers, men who have sex with men) are among those at highest risk because social stigma, discrimination, violence, and fear of criminal penalties can deter them from seeking health services (Starrs et al., 2018). Survivors of gender-based violence also report forgoing medical and legal services because of community perceptions of gender-based violence as a private matter, justified, or even a reason to shun or punish the survivor (Glasier et al., 2006).

Contested Views of Harms and Benefits

Sexual and reproductive health practices, programs, and policies raise some of the most contested issues in public discourse. Is it ethically permissible to provide HIV-prevention drugs to at-risk adolescents without parental consent? To require employers to provide employees with insurance that covers contraception? To use reproductive technology to enhance offspring? These and similar questions prompt disputes in health clinics and courts, religious venues and voting booths, and private conversations and public protests. Often at the crux of such debates are differing views about what constitutes harm, and what types of benefits, if any, can outweigh that harm.

Although moral considerations of harms and benefits are well-marked features on the "terrain of public health ethics" (Childress et al., 2002, 170), addressing them in the context of sexual and reproductive health can prove especially challenging in several respects. The first is that sexuality and reproduction frequently implicate personal preferences, sociocultural attitudes, and religious beliefs in ways that can provoke visceral responses and reveal deep—and sometimes irreconcilable—divides about what constitutes harm. Public policies and laws involving sex education, same-sex marriage, and abortion are notoriously contentious in this regard, because they collide with contested values related to sexual activity, marriage, and human life itself.

A second, related difficulty involves how to assess competing harms and benefits, particularly when they are incommensurate. Sex education in public schools is proven to reduce adolescent pregnancy and STI transmission, but opponents argue that it violates their religious liberty by normalizing premarital sex. How should decision-makers resolve conflicts between the harms set forth by each side? Are some harms, such as intrusion on religious liberty, absolute constraints on government action? Or can public health benefits justify such an intrusion in some circumstances? Without concrete ethical guidance (Childress et al., 2002), it is unclear how to resolve such conflicts.

These challenges are compounded when population benefits are offered as a justification for government interventions in sexuality and reproduction. Throughout history, governments have appealed to the common good to justify policies that employ coercion, incentives, and disincentives to alter fertility rates. Some policies have deprived individuals of their ability to reproduce, based on factors such as race, class, or perceived mental health (e.g., US state sterilization laws), while other policies have forced women to continue pregnancies (e.g., Romania's ban on contraception and abortion) or terminate pregnancies (e.g., China's one-child policy) against their will. Collectively, they are a reminder that governments, and those subject to their policies, may have conflicting views about what constitutes population benefit.

Self-determination

Self-determination is a significant determinant of sexual and reproductive health. Often used interchangeably with "autonomy," self-determination is the individual freedom to live in accordance with one's own values and decisions. Much of the literature about self-determination focuses on whether a specific individual has the rational capacity to make a certain decision, from a set of options, in an informed and reasonable manner and without external coercion. That model, however, can overlook the range of ways in which background social conditions—such as poverty and gender inequality—can limit, or even eliminate, an individual's ability to exercise self-determination with regard to a particular choice (Sherwin, 1998).

In the context of sexual and reproductive health, a number of factors can affect self-determination, three of which are mentioned here. To make informed decisions, individuals must have *access to comprehensive and scientifically accurate information*. Evidence-based sex education for adolescents is critical in this respect, as it dispels myths, confronts biases, and fosters informed decision-making (Starrs et al., 2018). Conversely, policies that prevent the dissemination of information about abortion availability, as well as laws that require the distribution of scientifically inaccurate information (e.g., a claim that abortion increases the risk of breast cancer), undermine informed decision-making and self-determination.

To exercise self-determination, individuals must be respected as persons with *authority to make choices* about their sexual and reproductive life, *without discrimination, coercion, or violence*. Laws and customs that require spousal consent before married women can access contraception, abortion, and sterilization services deny women authority to determine if and when they will have children, and also fail to respect them as persons. Stigmatization, discrimination, and the threat of violence—as well as laws that criminalize same-sex sexual activity, ban same-sex marriage, and require sterilization before transgender and intersex people can obtain birth certificates that match their preferred gender—constrain the choices of people with nonconforming sexual orientations and identities. Cultural practices such as child marriage and female genital cutting can also negatively impact self-determination by precluding girls, and the women they will become, from decisions that profoundly affect their sexual and reproductive health.

Self-determination not only requires access to information and the authority to make choices, but also the *socioeconomic means to access those choices*. A woman who continues her pregnancy because she cannot afford an abortion, the cost of which may include travel to a distant clinic (sometimes more than once) and child care expenses, has not made a fully autonomous choice. Her socioeconomic circumstances limit her to one option: pregnancy.

Chapter Overviews

The chapters in this section of *The Oxford Handbook of Public Health Ethics* provide a public health ethics perspective in each of four areas of sexual and reproductive health: STI control measures, contraception, abortion, and pregnancy-related services.

In "Sexually Transmitted Infections and Public Health Ethics," Mary A. Ott and John Santelli examine STI control, which the authors define as public health programs, policies, and practices that aim to prevent, treat, and limit the transmissibility of STIs. Mandatory reporting, contact tracing, and outreach education are examples of STI control activities. In striving to maximize population sexual health, however, STI control activities can pose significant ethical challenges. Ott and Santelli offer thoughtful approaches that strive to balance the sexual health and well-being of populations with the liberty and equality interests of individuals.

In "Contraception and Public Health Ethics," Saumya RamaRao and John Townsend focus on contraception, not only as a core component of public health, but also as a locus for ethical conflict between population goals and individual rights. Relying on the ethical principles of respect for persons, beneficence, and justice, they explore how tensions between public health goals and individual rights unfold in two contexts: routine contraceptive services and contraceptive research. The authors highlight the consequences of these tensions for health systems, providers, and contraceptive users, optimistically concluding that the relevant stakeholders can manage these conflicts in ways that are beneficial to all.

In "Abortion and Public Health Ethics," Mahmoud F. Fathalla offers a global public health ethics perspective on abortion. Given the magnitude of public health harms resulting from unsafe abortion, and the health inequities and social injustices stemming from insufficient access to safe abortion, Fathalla argues that the global community has an obligation to address, and ultimately eliminate, unsafe abortion. That responsibility is heightened, he contends, by women calling on governments to address unsafe abortion, an international consensus that eliminating unsafe abortion is central to the global reproductive agenda, and economic data demonstrating that greater access to safe abortion produces cost savings. Fathalla concludes that the global community must stand with women as they assert their right to health.

In "Access to Pregnancy-Related Services: Public Health Ethics Issues," Anne Drapkin Lyerly, Elana Jaffe, and Margaret Olivia Little address ethical challenges that arise when the value or utility of pregnancy-related services are contested. They first identify features of pregnancy-related care that contribute to such conflicts. For example, some pregnancy-related services, such as pregnancy termination due to fetal abnormality, involve a complex interplay between public health programs (e.g., prenatal screening) and individual women's values, which are known to differ. Using prenatal testing and modes of childbirth to ground their discussion, the authors explore how societal and cultural values affect access to pregnancy-related care.

Conclusion

Since the mid-1990s, the international community has made progress toward the goals set forth at the ICPD, but the promise of universal access to sexual and reproductive health services remains elusive in much of the world. Public health ethics sheds light on the moral complexities involved in achieving that goal. It recognizes that factors such as poverty and gender inequality can lead to a cycle of systematic disadvantage, in which sexual and reproductive ill health is the result, and the cause, of other deprivations. Public health ethics also highlights tensions that arise when sexual and reproductive health issues collide with contested values, and it draws attention to the far-reaching political, economic, and individual health implications of those conflicts. Despite, and because of, these challenges to achieving universal sexual and reproductive health, a renewed and bold commitment to the ICPD's vision is essential.

References

Childress, J. F., Faden, R. R., Gaare, R. D., Gostin, L. O., Kahn, J., Bonnie, R. J., et al. 2002. "Public Health Ethics: Mapping the Terrain." *Journal of Law, Medicine and Ethics* 30: 170–178.

Cook, R. J., and Dickens, B. M. 2009. "From Reproductive Choice to Reproductive Justice." *International Journal of Gynecology and Obstetrics* 106: 106–109.

Cottingham, J. C., and Ravindran, T. K. S. 2011. "Gender Aspects of Sexual and Reproductive Health." In *Sexual and Reproductive Health: A Public Health Perspective*, edited by P. F. A. Van Look, H. K. Heggenhougen, and S. R, Quah, 302–308 (San Diego, Calif.: Elsevier).

Glasier, A., Gülmezoglu, A. M., Schmid, G. P., Moreno, C. G., and Van Look, P. F. A. 2006. "Sexual and Reproductive Health: A Matter of Life and Death." *Lancet* 368: 1595–607.

Pearce, D. 1978. "The Feminization of Poverty: Women, Work and Welfare." *Urban and Social Change Review* 11: 28–36.

Rogers, W. A. 2006. "Feminism and Public Health Ethics." *Journal of Medical Ethics* 32(6): 351–354.

Sherwin, S. 1998. *The Politics of Women's Health: Exploring Agency and Autonomy* (Philadelphia: Temple University Press).

Singh, S., Darroch, J. E., and Ashford, L. S. 2014. *Adding It Up: Investing in Contraception and Maternal and Newborn Health* (New York: Guttmacher Institute).

Snow, R.C., Laski, L., and Mutumba, M. 2015. "Sexual and Reproductive Health: Progress and Outstanding Needs." *Global Public Health* 10(2): 149–173.

Starrs, A. M., Ezeh, A. C., Barker, G., Basu, A., Bertrand, J. T., Blum, R., et al. 2018. "Accelerate Progress—Sexual and Reproductive Health and Rights for All: Report of the Guttmacher–*Lancet* Commission." *Lancet* 391(10140): 2642–2692. doi:10.1016/S0140-6736(18)30293-9.

UN (United Nations). 1994. "Programme of Action." *Report of the International Conference on Population and Development, Cairo.* A/CONF.171/13/Rev.1 (New York: United Nations Secretariat).

UN (United Nations). 2015. *Transforming Our World: The 2030 Agenda for Sustainable Development.* A/RES/70/1 (New York: United Nations). https://sustainabledevelopment.un.org/post2015/transformingourworld/publication.

CHAPTER 33

SEXUALLY TRANSMITTED INFECTIONS, PUBLIC HEALTH, AND ETHICS

MARY A. OTT AND JOHN SANTELLI

INTRODUCTION

A core function of public health systems is to prevent and treat sexually transmitted infections (STIs). STIs are infectious diseases transmitted through vaginal, anal, or oral sexual contact. These include bacterial infections such as gonorrhea, syphilis, and chlamydia; viral infections such as hepatitis B, human immunodeficiency virus (HIV), herpes simplex virus, and human papillomavirus (HPV); protozoal infections such as trichomoniasis; and parasites such as pubic lice.[1] Globally, more than one million STIs are acquired each day, and in the United States the number of new STI infections has reached an all-time high (WHO, 2016b; CDC, 2017b). In addition to any symptoms of the infections themselves, STIs are associated with higher than average morbidity and mortality, poor reproductive outcomes, increased health care expenditures, and negative economic growth (HHS, 2017). While STIs differ from each other in type and severity of sequelae, treatment, potential for cure, and transmission through other routes (e.g., blood, mother to child), public health activities focused on their prevention and treatment raise similar ethics issues stemming from their sexual transmissibility.[2]

STI control activities are public health programs, policies, and practices focused on preventing and treating STIs. These practices may concentrate on the virus (e.g., through universal HIV screening as a part of routine health care [Murphy et al., 2015]), or on human "hosts" (e.g., by providing increased access to condoms, or brief counseling interventions focused on behavior change [Kamb, 1998]). STI control may involve interventions at multiple points along the STI-care continuum, including prevention, early identification, linkage to treatment, engagement in care, and the interruption of subsequent transmission. Control activities also may involve multiple actors, including individuals (e.g., contact tracing for HIV), health systems (e.g., confidentiality policies), communities (e.g., outreach and education), and governments (e.g., disease surveillance, outbreak investigation, and mandated reporting laws).

STI control is part of a broader initiative by the World Health Organization (WHO, 2017) and the US Centers for Disease Control and Prevention (CDC, 2015) to improve sexual health and well-being. The WHO (2006) describes sexual health broadly as

> a state of physical, emotional, mental and social well-being in relation to sexuality; it is not merely the absence of disease, dysfunction or infirmity. Sexual health requires a positive and respectful approach to sexuality and sexual relationships, as well as the possibility of having pleasurable and safe sexual experiences, free of coercion, discrimination, and violence. For sexual health to be attained and maintained, the sexual rights of all persons must be respected, protected and fulfilled.

As applied to STI control, the twin goals of public health are to maximize population sexual health and individual sexual well-being, and to ensure social justice by reducing disparities in STI outcomes (Munthe, 2008).

In STI control, there are two broad areas of ethical concerns. First are the concerns raised by public health practices to control STIs. These practices include surveillance, contact tracing, and public health laws requiring disclosure, consent, and confidentiality. The second are the ethical concerns raised by STI-related health disparities in access to information, prevention, screening and treatment, and STI outcomes. This chapter first focuses on the balance between individual liberties and population health in STI control practices, drawing upon the harm principle. It then turns to issues of social justice related to inequities in STI services and sexual health outcomes, drawing on a human rights framework to highlight current system failures.

Differences between high- and low-income countries—in terms of STI prevalence, sequelae, and social impact—often raise distinct ethical issues. To illustrate ethically relevant differences, we use examples from both the United States and lower-income countries. We consider ethical issues that arise with both adults and adolescents, because some ethics concerns span the age range, such as mandated reporting of STIs to health departments, while other issues are particularly salient with adolescents, such as confidentiality and consent for one's own services.

STI Control Practices: Balancing Individual Liberty and Population Health

STI control practices span the STI care continuum, and include prevention, early identification, linkage to treatment, engagement in care, and the interruption of subsequent transmission (Murphy et al., 2015). Operating on multiple levels, these practices have the potential to improve the sexual health and well-being of the individual (e.g., through early identification and linkage to care), their current and former sexual partner(s) (e.g., through disruption of HIV transmission with interventions such as pre-exposure prophylaxis, or treatment-as-prevention for HIV); and communities (e.g., through disruption of transmission and a lower community burden of disease). STI control practices also have risks to the individual, however, including the potential loss of confidentiality associated with mandated reporting, the absence of a requirement for individual consent prior to contact tracing, and a provider's duty to warn partners at risk.

The Harm Principle

The ethics of STI control practices involve a balance between respecting individuals' liberty to make their own sexual health decisions and protecting communities from the harms of STIs. The political and legal authority for STI control programs is vested in governments. The moral justification for STI control laws and policies can be understood through John Stuart Mill's work on the harm principle (Diekema, 2008). Mill ([1859] 2011) writes that in a civil society, the only purpose for which power can be rightfully exercised over individuals against their will is to prevent harm to others. The harm principle recognizes not only the moral importance of individual liberties in a just society, but also that individual liberties can be limited to ensure the health and well-being of others. A corollary is that if liberties must be limited, then the least restrictive approach should be sought (Diekema, 2008). The harm principle incorporates both considerations of effectiveness of public health measures and the importance of always choosing the least intrusive means to achieve the desired effect.

Operationalizing the harm principle requires public health data and careful consideration of contexts. Public health agencies should assess the effectiveness of the intervention, the magnitude and probability of harm to individuals, and the degree of restriction on individual liberties.

Mandatory Reporting and Contact Tracing

To satisfy the harm principle, there must be reasonably strong evidence that STI surveillance activities that limit individual liberty will improve the health and well-being of both the individual and the community. Mandatory reporting laws are an example of an STI surveillance activity that satisfies the harm principle. Mandatory reporting laws require health care providers, hospitals, and/or laboratories to report cases of STIs, as well as identifiable information about the patients (e.g., full name, date of birth), to health departments when those STIs are identified. This information allows health departments to identify cases where immediate disease control and prevention activities are needed (CDC, 2017a). The consent of infected individuals is not required before personal information is provided to health departments. Although there is a risk of violating individual confidentiality, mandatory reporting is justified under the harm principle because the surveillance data can directly benefit individuals and communities.

Contact tracing is the notification of those who may be at risk of contracting an infection from an index case. In the case of STIs, the individuals at risk are sexual partners or injection drug and needle-sharing partners. Health departments notify these contacts to let them know that they may have been exposed to a STI and should be tested and/or treated, but they are not told who referred them (National Coalition of STD Directors, 2016). They are then asked about their contacts so that networks can be created. The index patient's consent is not required for public health officials to contact his or her present and former partners.

Mandatory reporting and contact tracing can benefit individuals, allowing for early detection and facilitating treatment of STIs for both the index case and contacts. For example, during an HIV outbreak in a small US community in southern Indiana, HIV and hepatitis C testing, followed by contact tracing, identified 181 new HIV infections (Peters et al., 2016). HIV-infected individuals' health outcomes are markedly improved with early diagnosis and access to antiretroviral medications, shifting HIV from a progressive, deadly disease to a manageable chronic illness in which one can live a long and productive life (WHO, 2016a). Mandated reporting and contact tracing can also benefit communities, as data can be used to better target prevention programs and directly disrupt STI transmission. In the southern Indiana HIV epidemic, contact tracing enabled CDC investigators to demonstrate that HIV infections were transmitted through sharing needles in injection drug networks, rather than sexual networks, permitting scarce public health resources from that rural community to be directed to interventions, such as needle exchanges, that were most likely to interrupt transmission (Conrad et al., 2015).

While powerful tools in STI control, particularly in epidemics, mandatory reporting and contact tracing carry the potential to violate the confidentiality of both the index patient and her or his partners, with resulting stigma and social harms. Although contacts are not provided with the name of the index patient, when a person has a limited number of sexual partners or resides in a small community, the index patient's name may be easy to deduce. All STIs carry the risk of stigma and social harm. Those harms will vary by infection (e.g., HIV carries a high risk of stigma) and the contexts of transmission (e.g., via anal sex or via mother-to-child transmission). Applying the harm principle, the use of mandatory reporting and contact tracing should be limited to those infections with strong evidence for improved individual and community health outcomes, and they must be done in the least restrictive manner and with the highest levels of protections for individual confidentiality.

HPV and School Vaccination Mandates

From the harm principle, it can also be argued that if there is sufficient evidence of effectiveness, and if the limitations on personal liberties can be minimized, then an STI control initiative should be undertaken. An example is the use of school mandates to improve HPV vaccination rates for eleven- to twelve-year-olds. School mandates, or policies requiring immunization for entry into schools, are a highly effective method of increasing vaccination rates (Brandt et al., 2016). The rates of serious side effects from the HPV vaccine are low, and there is clear evidence that the vaccine reduces the incidence of HPV-related disease, including cervical, penile, oral, and anal cancers (Kahn et al., 2016). However, in most US states, HPV has not been added to school vaccine mandates, and HPV vaccination rates remain low. Other childhood vaccines, such as measles, mumps, and rubella (MMR), which are mandated for public school attendance, boast high rates of vaccination.

Opponents of HPV vaccination mandates have argued that the mandates violate their right to individual liberty, including religious liberty, to make decisions regarding their children's health care (Ferrer et al., 2014). Some argue that because HPV is sexually transmitted, mandating the vaccine gives adolescents permission to have sex. That argument, which is unique to STI vaccines, is not supported by data linking HPV vaccination to increased risk behaviors (Coles et al., 2015).

Stronger arguments against school mandates for the HPV vaccine have been based upon the harm principle. Because HPV is sexually transmitted, nonvaccination does not present a direct risk to other school children in the same way that nonvaccination against diseases spread by respiratory illness, such as measles, does (Ferrer et al., 2014). Thus, HPV mandates limit parents' liberty to choose not to vaccinate their children, without sufficient benefit to other children in the school. However, this harm/benefit analysis shifts if one considers the health of the community as a whole. School vaccine mandates present a unique opportunity to markedly increase community-wide vaccine rates, and to improve public health through the prevention of cervical, penile, oral, and anal cancers, along with the pain and suffering and costs associated with these vaccine-preventable cancers. Additionally, high levels of vaccination provide "herd immunity" (also known as "community immunity"), preventing transmission even if a disease enters a community, resulting in protection of those who cannot be vaccinated for medical reasons (Diekema, 2014).

In ethics, an error of omission may be considered as ethically problematic as an error of commission (e.g., not enacting a policy that can effectively reduce pain and suffering may be considered as ethically problematic as enacting a policy that causes pain and suffering). This applies to STI control interventions that can improve public health outcomes with an acceptably low impact on individual liberties. Given the low rate of serious side effects from HPV vaccination, the effectiveness of the vaccine for both individuals and communities in preventing cancer and other HPV-related illness, and the effectiveness of school mandates in increasing community vaccination rates, an ethical argument can be made for school HPV vaccine mandates using the harm principle.

Criminalizing HIV Transmission

Conversely, if public health policies lack evidence of effectiveness or have evidence to suggest harm, the harm principle may also be violated. The harm principle requires that there be some potential for effectiveness if STI control interventions threaten individual liberties. An example is criminalizing HIV transmission. On the surface, laws that permit a state to prosecute an HIV-infected individual who knowingly infects another person may appear to make sense. HIV is a potentially life-threatening illness that is frequently asymptomatic. The presumptive purposes of these laws are to encourage disclosure and to punish HIV-infected individuals who knowingly expose others to harm by choosing not to disclose their HIV status. Disclosure of HIV status between sexual partners allows disruption of transmission through safer sex behaviors, such as condom use.

Data, however, do not support criminalization of HIV transmission as an effective way to encourage disclosure or to decrease transmission. Awareness of criminalization laws has not been associated with increased disclosure or behavior change (Harsono et al., 2017). A review of published research in Canada suggests that, particularly for women, criminalization laws may actually act as a barrier to access at all points in the HIV care cascade, discouraging testing, linkage to treatment, and engagement in care (Patterson et al., 2015). Because empiric data do not support the presumptive purpose (increased disclosure and interrupted transmission), almost all STI control professionals oppose this type of legislative intervention (Harsono et al., 2017; Lazzarini et al., 2013).

The second purpose of criminalization laws is to punish an HIV-infected individual who knowingly exposes another person to harm without providing a warning through disclosure. Disclosure would provide the at-risk individual an opportunity to take preventive action (e.g., avoid intercourse, use condoms, or engage in other safer sex behaviors). The argument in favor of punishing individuals for knowingly transmitting HIV is predicated on the co-occurrence of three factors—transmissibility, (in)curability, and severity. Some STIs, like syphilis, have the potential for equally severe sequelae but are curable. Other STIs, like herpes, are not curable, but their clinical course is usually more indolent. In HIV, there is both lack of a cure and the potential for severe medical and social sequelae.

The ethical reasoning for universal criminal punishment for nondisclosure of HIV is less compelling, given our current understanding of HIV transmission and treatment. The effectiveness of HIV treatment has led to a "treatment as prevention" approach. Individuals living with HIV who maintain undetectable viral loads have almost no chance of transmission. While there is still no HIV cure, with modern antiretroviral treatment and good adherence, HIV is no longer a certain death sentence and is now considered a chronic disease. Per the harm principle, in an HIV-infected individual with good adherence and an undetectable viral load, one could argue that broad criminalization of HIV transmission is an unacceptable restriction on personal liberties. In contrast, nondisclosure from a person living with HIV who knows his or her diagnosis, has a high viral load, and has sexual practices that put the encounter at highest risk for transmitting HIV presents a different harm scenario. These contrasting cases support the necessity of flexibility and individualization.

The duty to warn is related to criminalization of HIV, but instead of obliging individuals living with HIV to disclose their HIV status to prospective partners, it obliges health care providers to warn potential partners of their risk of contracting HIV. The legal duty to warn is most often associated with psychiatry, and in the United States it is grounded in a court case, *Tarasoff v. Regents of the University of California*, in which a patient disclosed to a therapist his intention to commit homicide, which he later proceeded to commit (Huprich, Fuller, and Schneider, 2003). The court found the therapist at fault because he did not warn the victim of the threat to her life. The duty to warn is codified in the American Medical Association (AMA) Code of Medical Ethics, which allows providers to break confidentiality when they judge that there is a "reasonable probability" that a patient will "inflict serious physical harm on an identifiable individual"

(AMA, Opinion 3.2.1). The provider's duty to warn has been applied to HIV in cases where individuals living with HIV neither disclose their HIV status to a partner nor practice safer sex, putting their partner(s) at risk for HIV infection (Odunsi, 2007).

The duty of providers to warn at-risk partners, like criminalization of HIV, is based upon an belief that HIV is always highly transmissible and uniformly fatal. As described above, current antiretroviral therapy has reduced HIV transmissibility in individuals with very low viral loads, shifting the course toward that of a chronic illness. The harm principle would argue against a universal policy of warning all partners who can be identified and have not been disclosed to. An individual living with HIV, who has an undetectable viral load but has not disclosed, may not present a "reasonable probability" of harm to others through HIV transmission to justify the loss of confidentiality and individual liberty posed by a universal duty to warn policy (Huprich, Fuller, and Schneider, 2003). Because of the importance of case specifics in the probability and severity of harm, the duty to warn should be flexible and individualized to account for individual circumstances, risks to partner, and provider judgment.

Social Justice and Human Rights

STI-Related Health Disparities

Inequalities in sexual and reproductive health intersect with several cross-cutting health disparities of high importance to public health ethics, including poverty, ethnic minority status, gender, sexual violence, sexual minority status, and youth (OHCHR, 2016b). STIs track with poverty and inequities in wealth. The global burden of HIV and STIs is concentrated in the countries with the lowest per capita incomes (OHCHR, 2016b). Within high-income countries, STIs cluster in high-poverty communities (UNAIDS, 2014). In many cases, the poor not only experience higher rates of STIs and lower access to services, but also higher levels of stigma and fear (Harling et al., 2013; Holtgrave and Crosby, 2003). Similarly, racial and ethnic minorities bear a disproportionate burden of STIs, including HIV (Wabiri and Taffa, 2013). In the United States, for example, rates of gonorrhea for African American individuals are almost ten times those of white individuals, and rates of syphilis are five times higher (CDC, 2016b).

Of global importance, large disparities in STIs can be attributed to gender and sexual violence. Women, particularly young women, have some of the highest rates of STIs, most notably HIV (UNAIDS, 2014). In the United States, young women have the highest rates of chlamydia and gonorrhea, with attendant sexual health sequelae, including infertility (CDC, 2016b). Globally, even when STI prevention and treatment are available, women are less likely to utilize those services because of disproportionately high levels of discrimination and stigma associated with STIs coupled with inequalities in economic power that limit women's ability to access and utilize services independently (OHCHR, 2016b). For example, in rural South Africa, for every 1 percent increase in community-level stigma, women's rates of HIV testing dropped 3 percent (Treves-Kagan et al., 2017). Sexual violence exacerbates the situation, such that the population most in need of sexual health services is the least able to access it (Dunkle et al., 2004).

Sexual and gender minorities also experience inadequate access to sexual health information and STI-related services. In the United States, most new HIV infections occur in African American and Latino men who have sex with men (MSM) (CDC, 2016a). Broad structural disparities directly contribute to these disparities in both STI information and services. Among MSM, HIV and unprotected anal intercourse happen in the contexts of structural factors such as mental health disorders, substance abuse, violence, sexual stigma, and homelessness (Santos et al., 2014).

Globally, lesbian, gay, bisexual, and transgender (LGBT) individuals are frequently denied basic civil rights, including denial of the right to marry and criminalization of same-sex relationships (OHCHR, 2015). LGBT individuals experience discrimination in accessing economic and social rights and are often targets for hate crimes and violence (Hatzenbuehler and Pachankis, 2016). LGBT individuals also report high rates of STI risk factors, including sexual violence (Whitton et al., 2016). Human rights approaches to STIs support broad access to sexual health care and freedom from discrimination. This is of particular importance for LGBT individuals and obliges states to take action to address these disparities in access and outcomes, and to change the above discriminatory practices and policies (O'Flaherty and Fisher, 2008).

Adolescents also experience disparities in access to sexual health information, STI care, and STI outcomes. While access to medically accurate sexual health information to maximize sexual health and well-being is a basic human right (Coliver, 1995), many sex education programs in the United States and globally focus on abstinence and heterosexual youth, and do not provide essential information on STI prevention, risk reduction, gender, discrimination, or sexual orientation (Santelli et al., 2006). Although human rights documents support confidential STI care (OHCHR, 2016a), and adolescents report that a lack of confidentiality will decrease the likelihood that they will access care (Jones and Boonstra, 2004), many adolescents still find themselves unable to access confidential sexual health care. As a consequence, they may delay STI prevention, diagnosis, and care (Sam-Agudu, Folayan, and Ezeanolue, 2016), any one of which may put the adolescents and their communities at heightened risk.

Failure to respect the human rights of marginalized populations, such as the poor, women, racial and ethnic minorities, sexual minorities, and adolescents, impedes effective STI control. Discrimination and stigma cause these at-risk, marginalized populations to remain hidden, which in turn reduces their access to screening, treatment, referral, and prevention programs, and ultimately limits the effectiveness of STI control. To counter that outcome, STI control must include efforts to address the social injustices underpinning existing health disparities.

A Human Rights Framework for STIs

A human rights approach best addresses issues of social injustice in the context of access to STI information and care. Persons are at increased vulnerability to STIs in part because they are unable to realize their civil, political, economic, social and cultural rights (OCHR, 2016b). Social justice in STI control involves securing a sufficient level of sexual health for all, as well as narrowing inequalities in access to sexual health information, access to STI prevention and treatment, and STI outcomes. Notions of social justice can be derived from human rights principles, including the right to the best attainable sexual health, as well as the right to access STI services, including education, prevention, testing, and treatment.

Poor or marginalized communities experience a higher prevalence of treatable STIs, likely due, in part, to their lack of access to STI treatment. A recent global analysis of trends in STIs found that syphilis was most prevalent in the African World Bank region and was associated with low national income and more limited access to antenatal syphilis testing in those areas (Newman et al., 2015). The discrimination and stigma accompanying STI (particularly HIV) diagnoses can lead to human rights violations, which frequently hamper effective public health responses (OHCHR, 2016b). For example, women living with HIV in low- and middle-income countries experience higher levels of interpersonal violence and economic marginalization, which in turn impedes linkage, access to, and retention in treatment (Ippoliti, Nanda, and Wilcher, 2017). The WHO's (2017) consolidated guideline on sexual and reproductive health and rights of women living with HIV recognizes the associations among discrimination, stigma, and HIV, and incorporates recommendations such as universal screening for violence, empowerment interventions focused on the individual woman, and economic interventions focused on the broader community.

Multiple human rights documents make specific recommendations that STI policies and programs include the human rights to sexual health information, sexual health services (both prevention and treatment), and freedom from discrimination—including the Convention on the Elimination of All Forms of Discrimination against Women (OHCHR, 2016b), the Convention on the Rights of the Child (OHCHR, 1990), and the International Covenant on Economic, Social and Cultural Rights (United Nations, 2000; UNAIDS, 2016). These documents support an individual's right to the best attainable sexual health and emphasize the importance of upholding human rights as a mechanism to address the disparities in STI and HIV prevalence. Because governments are often the source of stigma and discrimination, these documents clearly address the role of the state in supporting human rights and eliminating stigma and discrimination—steps that are critical for STI control (OHCHR, 1990).

Summary and Recommendations

Enormous disparities in STI rates exist among groups, both between and within countries. These disparities in disease outcomes track with disparities in access to sexual health information, STI prevention modalities, and STI treatment services. Marginalized groups, such as women, ethnic minorities, sexual minorities, adolescents, and individuals in poverty, are disproportionately affected, meaning that those with the greatest need have the least access to the knowledge and resources necessary to improve health outcomes.

Ethical approaches to STI control are supported by the harm principle and the protection of human rights. The harm principle protects individual liberties up to the point at which those liberties have a high potential to harm the community. Even then, individual liberties should be infringed upon in the least restrictive manner. Policies that threaten individual liberties, such as contact tracing, should be conducted in a manner that is respectful of individual rights while protecting the health of others within the community.

Human rights approaches are essential to achieving social justice in STI control. This ethical position is supported by the WHO, which recommends that STI control programs be delivered with respect for human rights and the dignity of persons with STIs (OHCHR, 2016b). By maintaining a human rights focus, STI control policies can potentially reduce, rather than reinforce, disparities in information, prevention, and treatment modalities, while at the same time interrupting STI transmission and preventing future infection.

Notes

1. STI and HIV control activities are often separated because of differences in funding streams; however, HIV is sexually transmitted, and there is substantial overlap between STI and HIV control activities and the ethical issues those activities raise. For the purposes of this chapter, we consider the ethics of STI and HIV control together, except where we specifically indicate HIV.
2. Detailed information on transmissibility, clinical syndromes, diagnosis, and treatment of each STI is available through the World Health Organization's website (WHO 2016b).

References

AMA (American Medical Association). Opinion 3.2.1 Confidentiality. *Code of Medical Ethics*. https://www.ama-assn.org/delivering-care/confidentiality.

Brandt, H. M., Pierce, J. Y., and Crary, A. 2016. "Increasing HPV Vaccination through Policy for Public Health Benefit." *Human Vaccine Immunotherapy* 12(6): 1623–1625.

CDC (US Centers for Disease Control and Prevention). 2015. *National Center for HIV/AIDS, Viral Hepatitis, STD, and TB Prevention Strategic Plan through 2020* (Atlanta, Ga.: CDC). https://www.cdc.gov/nchhstp/strategicpriorities/default.htm.

CDC (US Centers for Disease Control and Prevention). 2016a. *HIV Surveillance Report, 2015*; vol. 27 (Atlanta, Ga.: CDC). https://www.cdc.gov/hiv/pdf/library/reports/surveillance/cdc-hiv-surveillance-report-2015-vol-27.pdf.

CDC (US Centers for Disease Control and Prevention). 2016b. *STD Surveillance Report, 2015* (Atlanta, Ga.: CDC). https://www.cdc.gov/std/stats15/toc.htm.

CDC (US Centers for Disease Control and Prevention). 2017a. "National Notifiable Diseases Surveillance System (NNDSS)—Data Collection and Reporting." https://wwwn.cdc.gov/nndss/data-collection.html.

CDC (US Centers for Disease Control and Prevention). 2017b. *Sexually Transmitted Disease Surveillance 2016* (Atlanta, Ga.: CDC). https://www.cdc.gov/std/stats16/CDC_2016_STDS_Report-for508WebSep21_2017_1644.pdf.

Coles, V. A., Patel, A. S., Allen, F. L., Keeping, S. T., and Carroll, S. M. 2015. "The Association of Human Papillomavirus Vaccination with Sexual Behaviours and Human Papillomavirus Knowledge: A Systematic Review." *International Journal of STD and AIDS* 26(11): 777–788.

Coliver, S. 1995. "The Right to Information Necessary for Reproductive Health and Choice under International Law." In *The Right to Know: Human Rights and Access to Reproductive Health Information*, edited by S. Coliver, 38–82 (Philadelphia: University of Pennsylvania Press).

Conrad, C., Bradley, H. M., Broz, D., Buddha, S., Chapman, E. L., Galang, R. R., et al. 2015. "Community Outbreak of HIV Infection Linked to Injection Drug Use of Oxymorphone—Indiana, 2015." *Morbidity and Mortality Weekly Report* 64(16): 443–444.

Diekema, D. S. 2008. "Public Health, Ethics, and State Compulsion." *Journal of Public Health Management Practice* 14(4): 332–334.

Diekema, D. S. 2014. "Personal Belief Exemptions from School Vaccination Requirements." *Annual Review of Public Health* 35: 275–292.

Dunkle, K. L., Jewkes, R. K., Brown, H. C., Gray, G. E., McIntyre, J. A., and Harlow, S. D. 2004. "Gender-Based Violence, Relationship Power, and Risk of HIV Infection in Women Attending Antenatal Clinics in South Africa." *Lancet* 363(9419): 1415–1421.

Ferrer, H. B., Trotter, C., Hickman, M., and Audrey, S. 2014. "Barriers and Facilitators to HPV Vaccination of Young Women in High-Income Countries: A Qualitative Systematic Review and Evidence Synthesis." *BMC Public Health* 14: 700. https://bmcpublichealth.biomedcentral.com/articles/10.1186/1471-2458-14-700.

Harling, G., Subramanian, S., Barnighausen, T., and Kawachi, I. 2013. "Socioeconomic Disparities in Sexually Transmitted Infections among Young Adults in the United States: Examining the Interaction between Income and Race/Ethnicity." *Sexually Transmitted Diseases* 40(7): 575–581.

Harsono, D., Galletly, C. L., O'Keefe, E., and Lazzarini, Z. 2017. "Criminalization of HIV Exposure: A Review of Empirical Studies in the United States." *AIDS and Behavior* 21(1): 27–50.

Hatzenbuehler, M. L., and Pachankis, J. E. 2016. "Stigma and Minority Stress as Social Determinants of Health among Lesbian, Gay, Bisexual, and Transgender Youth: Research Evidence and Clinical Implications." *Pediatric Clinics of North America* 63(6): 985–997.

HHS (US Department of Health and Human Services). 2017. "Global Statistics: The Global HIV/AIDS Epidemic." https://www.hiv.gov/hiv-basics/overview/data-and-trends/global-statistics.

Holtgrave, D. R., and Crosby, R. A. 2003. "Social Capital, Poverty, and Income Inequality as Predictors of Gonorrhoea, Syphilis, Chlamydia and AIDS Case Rates in the United States." *Sexually Transmitted Infections* 79(1): 62–64.

Huprich, S. K., Fuller, K. M., and Schneider, R. B. 2003. "Divergent Ethical Perspectives on the Duty-to-Warn Principle with HIV Patients." *Ethics and Behavior* 13(3): 263–278.

Ippoliti N. B., Nanda G., and Wilcher, R. 2017. "Meeting the Reproductive Health Needs of Female Key Populations Affected by HIV in Low- and Middle-Income Countries: A Review of the Evidence." *Studies in Family Planning* 48(2): 121–151.

Jones, R. K., and Boonstra, H. 2004. "Confidential Reproductive Health Services for Minors: The Potential Impact of Mandated Parental Involvement for Contraception." *Perspectives on Sexual Reproductive Health* 36(5): 182–191.

Kahn, J. A., Widdice, L. E., Ding, L., Huang, B., Brown, D. R., Franco, E. L., et al. 2016. "Substantial Decline in Vaccine-Type Human Papillomavirus (HPV) among Vaccinated Young Women during the First 8 Years after HPV Vaccine Introduction in a Community." *Clinics in Infectious Diseases* 63(10): 1281–1287.

Kamb, M. L., Fishbein, M., Douglas, J. M., Jr., Rhodes, F., Rogers, J., Bolan, G., et al. 1998. "Efficacy of Risk-Reduction Counseling to Prevent Human Immunodeficiency Virus and Sexually Transmitted Diseases: A Randomized Controlled Trial. Project RESPECT Study Group." *JAMA* 280(13): 1161–1167.

Lazzarini, Z., Galletly, C. L., Mykhalovskiy, E., Harsono, D., O'Keefe, E., Singer, M., et al. 2013. "Criminalization of HIV Transmission and Exposure: Research and Policy Agenda." *American Journal of Public Health* 103(8): 1350–1353.

Mill, J. S. (1859) 2011. *On Liberty* (Luton: Andrews UK).

Munthe, C. 2008. "The Goals of Public Health: An Integrated, Multidimensional Model." *Public Health Ethics* 1(1): 39–52.

Murphy, R. D., Wohl, A. R., Ma, Y., Kobeissi, L., Oduyemi, O., and Perez, M. J. 2015. "Adaptation of the HIV Care Continuum as a Method for Evaluating Syphilis and Gonorrhea Disease Control Activities in Los Angeles County." *Sexually Transmitted Diseases* 42(12): 686–690.

National Coalition of STD Directors. 2016. "Sexually Transmitted Disease (STD) Contact Tracing."http://www.ncsddc.org/resource/sexually-transmitted-disease-std-contact-tracing-infographic-2/.

Newman L., Rowley J., Vander Hoorn S., Wijesooriya, N. S., Unemo, M., Low, N., et al. 2015. "Global Estimates of the Prevalence and Incidence of Four Curable Sexually Transmitted Infections in 2012 Based on Systematic Review and Global Reporting." *PLoS ONE* 10(12): e0143304. https://journals.plos.org/plosone/article?id=10.1371/journal.pone.0143304.

Odunsi, B. 2007. "Should Caregivers Be Compelled to Disclose Patients' HIV Infection to the Patients' Sex Partners without Consent?" *Studies in Family Planning* 38(4): 297–306.

O'Flaherty M., and Fisher, J. 2008. "Sexual Orientation, Gender Identity and International Human Rights Law: Contextualising the Yogyakarta Principles." *Human Rights Law Review* 8(2): 207–248.

OHCHR (Office of the United Nations High Commissioner on Human Rights). 1990. Convention on the Rights of the Child, General Assembly Resolution 44/25. UN Doc. A/44/49 (1989), Article 13. http://www.un.org/documents/ga/res/44/a44r025.htm

OHCHR (Office of the United Nations High Commissioner for Human Rights). 2015. *Discrimination and Violence against Individuals Based on their Sexual Orientation and Gender Identity*. http://repository.un.org/handle/11176/312186.

OHCHR (Office of the United Nations High Commissioner for Human Rights). 2016a. "Committee on the Rights of the Child: General Comment on the Implementation of the Rights of the Child during Adolescence, CRC/GC/2003/4." http://www.youthpolicy.org/library/documents/general-comment-on-adolescence/.

OHCHR (Office of the United Nations High Commissioner for Human Rights). 2016b. "HIV/AIDS and Human Rights." http://www.ohchr.org/EN/Issues/HIV/Pages/HIVIndex.aspx.

Patterson, S. E., Milloy, M., Ogilvie, G., Greene, S., Nicholson, V., Vonn, M., et al. 2015. "The Impact of Criminalization of HIV Non-disclosure on the Healthcare Engagement of Women Living with HIV in Canada: A Comprehensive Review of the Evidence." *Journal of the International AIDS Society* 18(1): 20572. https://www.ncbi.nlm.nih.gov/pmc/articles/PMC4689876/.

Peters, P. J., Pontones, P., Hoover, K. W., Patel, M. R., Galang, R. R., Shields, J., et al. 2016. "HIV Infection Linked to Injection Use of Oxymorphone in Indiana, 2014–2015." *New England Journal of Medicine* 375(3): 229–239.

Sam-Agudu, N. A., Folayan, M. O. and Ezeanolue, E. E. 2016. "Seeking Wider Access to HIV Testing for Adolescents in Sub-Saharan Africa." *Pediatric Research* 79(6): 838–845.

Santelli, J. S., Ott, M. A., Lyon, M., Rogers, J., Summers, D., and Schleifer, R. 2006. "Abstinence and Abstinence-Only Education: A Review of US Policies and Programs." *Journal of Adolescent Health* 38(1): 72–81.

Santos, G. M., Do, T., Beck, J., Makofane, K., Arreola, S., Pyun T., et al. 2014. "Syndemic Conditions Associated with Increased HIV Risk in a Global Sample of Men Who Have Sex with Men." *Sexually Transmitted Infections* 90(3): 250–253.

Treves-Kagan, S., El Ayadi, A. M., Pettifor, A., MacPhail, C., Twine, R., Maman, S., et al. 2017. "Gender, HIV Testing and Stigma: The Association of HIV Testing Behaviors and Community-Level and Individual-Level Stigma in Rural South Africa Differ for Men and Women." *AIDS and Behavior* 21(9): 2579–2588.

UNAIDS (Joint United Nations Programme on HIV/AIDS). 2014. *The Gap Report* (Geneva: UNAIDS). http://files.unaids.org/en/media/unaids/contentassets/documents/unaidspublication/2014/UNAIDS_Gap_report_en.pdf.

UNAIDS (Joint United Nations Programme on HIV/AIDS). 2016. "Sexually Transmitted Diseases: Policies and Principles for Prevention and Care." http://data.unaids.org/publications/irc-pub04/una97-6_en.pdf.

United Nations. 2000. "General Comment 14: The Right to the Highest Attainable Standard of Health." Committee on Economic, Social and Cultural Rights, UN Doc. E/C.12/2000/4.

Wabiri, N., and Taffa, N. 2013. "Socio-economic Inequality and HIV in South Africa." *BMC Public Health* 13: 1037.

Whitton, S. W., Newcomb, M. E., Messinger, A. M., Byck, G., and Mustanski, B. 2016. "A Longitudinal Study of IPV Victimization among Sexual Minority Youth." *Journal of Interpersonal Violence*. doi:10.1177/0886260516646093

WHO (World Health Organization). 2006. "Defining Sexual Health." http://www.who.int/reproductivehealth/topics/sexual_health/sh_definitions/en/.

WHO (World Health Organization). 2016a. "HIV/AIDS." http://www.who.int/mediacentre/factsheets/fs360/en/.

WHO (World Health Organization). 2016b. "Sexually Transmitted Infections (STIs)." http://www.who.int/mediacentre/factsheets/fs110/en/.

WHO (World Health Organization). 2017. *Consolidated Guideline on Sexual and Reproductive Health and Rights of Women Living with HIV* (Geneva, Switzerland: WHO). http://www.who.int/reproductivehealth/publications/gender_rights/Ex-Summ-srhr-women-hiv/en/

CHAPTER 34

CONTRACEPTION AND PUBLIC HEALTH ETHICS

SAUMYA RAMARAO AND JOHN TOWNSEND

INTRODUCTION

CONTRACEPTION is a core public health issue. It has the potential to reduce family size and improve birth spacing, which in turn lead to better health outcomes for infants, children, and women. In addition, contraception provides women with choices to pursue their education, participate in the labor force, and contribute in economic and other ways to the lives of their families and communities. Furthermore, some contraceptives, such as male and female condoms, provide protection not only against unintended pregnancy, but also against sexually transmitted infections (STIs), including human immunodeficiency virus (HIV) (WHO, 2018). For all these reasons, ensuring access to contraception and family planning services is recognized as a policy decision that will facilitate economic development.

The decision to use contraception, however, is one that women and men make in private as they decide if and when they want to have children. Many factors affect that decision—the nature of the relationship between the sexual partners, including power dynamics; availability of and access to contraceptive services; the broader family context; and wider socioeconomic and cultural factors. Family planning programs have sought to increase access to contraceptives, based on the 1968 International Conference on Human Rights in Tehran, which affirmed the basic human right of men and women to decide freely and responsibly the number and spacing of their children (UN, 1968). Since the Tehran conference, three decennial World Population Conferences (Bucharest, 1974; Mexico City, 1984; and Cairo, 1994) have reaffirmed the central role that individual rights and family planning programs have in advancing individual and national development interests (UNFPA, 1974, 1984, 1994).

In response, government-sponsored family planning programs in many developing countries began to actively promote and provide contraceptive services to their citizens.

By the time of the 1984 Mexico City conference, many governments of developing countries expressed firm support for family planning and population programs, as did some donor countries, although their implementation strategies varied. In contrast to programs that promoted helping individuals plan their families, some countries promoted population policies that emphasized the demographic imperative of reducing national birth rates (e.g., China, India), prompting unease about potential state regulation of individual reproductive decisions and behaviors (Jain, 1998). However, the 1994 Cairo conference reaffirmed the importance of respecting and protecting individual reproductive health and rights over the achievement of demographic targets. Other global policy frameworks—originating from the 1995 Fourth World Conference on Women in Beijing, the Sustainable Development Goals (SDGs), and Family Planning 2020 (often referenced as FP2020)—have continued the trend of framing reproductive health and family planning within the context of human rights, including the right to health. Despite that acknowledgment, there continues to be a tension in balancing individual rights and well-being with demographic and public health goals.

This chapter discusses how the potential conflict between individual rights and public health goals can be managed in the delivery of routine contraceptive services and in the conduct of research on contraceptive product development and innovative service models. The following discussion illustrates how the tension plays out in the application of three ethical principles—respect for persons, beneficence, and justice—and highlights the consequences of those tensions for health systems, family planning providers, and users of health systems.

The Three Ethical Principles

Numerous ethical guidelines, including the Nuremberg Code, the Declaration of Helsinki, the Belmont Report, relevant US federal regulations, and the International Conference on Harmonisation's Guideline for Good Clinical Practice (GCP), emphasize three guiding ethical principles: respect for persons; beneficence; and justice. Each of these principles plays out in different ways in service delivery and research as illustrated in the following discussion (Fischer, 2006; RamaRao, Friedland, and Townsend, 2007).

Respect for Persons

Most ethical guidelines highlight that respect for persons, sometimes referred to as autonomy, is critical to the ethical conduct of health care delivery and clinical research (Fischer, 2006). For example, the 1979 Belmont Report, issued by the US National Commission for the Protection of Human Subjects of Biomedical and Behavioral Research (National Commission, 1979), explains that the principle of respect for persons means that individuals with decision-making capacity should be treated as autonomous agents, and that those with diminished capacity should be entitled to protections.

Respect for persons embodies the notion that individuals are given the opportunity to decide for themselves if, and to what extent, they wish to participate in therapy or research. The operationalization of that principle occurs through the informed consent process, which involves providing relevant information to patients, clients, or research subjects in a format they can understand, and ensuring that decisions about therapy or research participation are made voluntarily (i.e., without undue influence or coercion).

Application in Service Delivery

In contraceptive service delivery, public health systems and family planning providers bear primary responsibility for ensuring respect for persons. Health advocates can facilitate respectful care through third-party monitoring and accountability of services, and by educating service users about their rights and what to expect from services in a range of settings. The intended outcome is a satisfied service user who has made an informed decision about his or her contraceptive use and provider after receiving relevant, accurate, comprehensive, and comprehensible information.

Informed *choice* is an essential component of contraceptive decision-making. Users and potential users need to be informed about how available contraceptive methods work, their potential side effects, the location and skills of providers, and the time frames required for health checkups and ongoing contraceptive supply. With that information, individuals can determine which method best meets their needs, preferences, stage of reproductive life cycle, and life circumstances. From both ethical and programmatic points of view, there is clear evidence suggesting that users who receive the contraceptive of their choice and are well-informed tend to be satisfied users who adhere to the requirements of their chosen contraceptive method (Jain et al., 2012; Pariani, Heer, and Van Arsdol, 1991; RamaRao and Mohanam, 2003). Satisfied contraceptive users contribute to the success of public health programming and health impact while meeting their own personal needs.

Informed consent, however, is only one aspect of respect for persons. In many developing countries, for example, sexually active adolescents face barriers to the sexual and reproductive health care that are critical to their well-being (Bankole and Malarcher, 2010). Family planning providers may refuse to provide information or care to adolescents for a variety of reasons. The cultural milieu may stigmatize sexual activity among unmarried adolescents, promote pro-natalist attitudes among married adolescents, or offer contraceptives and service outlets that do not match adolescent preferences or lifestyles. Furthermore, existing laws and policies may restrict the provision of contraception to unmarried adolescents or those below a certain age (Chandra-Mouli et al., 2014). The failure to respect adolescents as persons too often leaves them with unmet contraceptive needs that place them at substantially greater risk of unintended pregnancy and unwanted infection (WHO, 2018).

Even in family planning programs that intend to improve access to good quality contraceptives and services, tensions can arise between individual decision-making, provider preferences, and public health. For example, long-acting reversible contraceptives (LARCs) are increasingly seen as a panacea by family planning program managers and other decision-makers for addressing plateauing unintended pregnancy rates and for providing long-term contraceptive protection for women who may not be able to access services easily (Gomez, Fuentes, and Allina, 2014; Jacobstein, 2018). While LARCs certainly add to women's contraceptive options, how women receive information about LARCs can shape their decisions, and even nudge them to make choices that may not be in line with their preferences or needs (Gomez, Fuentes, and Allina, 2014). In a highly influential project that demonstrated the feasibility of promoting LARC uptake, providers presented women with information from the most to least effective contraceptive. As Gomez, Fuentes, and Allina, (2014, 173) argue, the counseling model adopted by the project prioritized the effectiveness of the method over the "range of concerns, preferences and priorities that individual women bring to their contraceptive decision making." Such a counseling model has the potential to override the preferences of individual women, thereby reducing their autonomy, but it can be successful in achieving the public health goal of more effective contraceptive protection.

Application in Research

In research, informed consent is a critical first step in respecting persons. The onus of ensuring informed consent lies with researchers, their institutions, and the sponsors supporting the scientific inquiry. In the research context, the intended outcome should be a fully informed individual who understands the nature of the research as well as its potential risks and benefits, and who has voluntarily agreed to participate in the research and comply with its requirements. Examples of clinical research include safety and efficacy trials of a new contraceptive, feasibility studies to determine the costs and benefits of deploying new cadres of providers to deliver family planning services, and studies examining new ways of counseling family planning clients. In all research studies, investigators should use accessible language to inform participants about the nature and scope of the research.

Issues and Consequences

Ensuring informed consent and respect for individual choice is a resource-consuming process, but the effort is necessary. Supportive policies and programmatic frameworks, such as performance incentives, can help facilitate these goals if they are in harmony with the principle of respect for persons. Individual contraceptive choice and public health goals need not be in tension, as treating contraceptive users and research participants with respect and providing them with information and choice will result in win-win situations for all stakeholders. The public health program will achieve impacts in terms of improved health and well-being of women, men, and their offspring. High contraceptive uptake and continuation will avert unintended pregnancy, birth, and unsafe abortion while promoting better planned and spaced pregnancies. Health system users will be satisfied with services and empowered to use contraception in ways that help them achieve their reproductive intentions. Providers, too, will be gratified that they contributed to their clients' health and well-being by addressing their needs.

Beneficence

Beneficence requires that service providers and researchers maximize possible benefits and minimize possible harms to users and research participants. Beneficence is assessed by comparing the potential risks and benefits that a service user or research participant may experience as a result of the contraceptive service/method or proposed research. The ethical rationale for conducting the activity is met if the potential benefits outweigh the potential risks. Such an assessment is complex, because contraceptives offer benefits, such as avoiding unintended pregnancy, along with risks, such as side effects and potential contraceptive failure, even when used correctly.

Furthermore, while risks are borne solely by the service user or research participant, the benefits might accrue both to them and to the broader society. For example, contraceptive research can generate knowledge useful to all in society, and the benefits of individuals using contraception can result in better public health outcomes due to reductions in rates of unintended pregnancy, unsafe abortion, and maternal mortality. The risk need not be confined to health risks but may include risks to clients' interests (e.g., how they would like to deal with associated bleeding or amenorrhea, which add a more nuanced social dimension to the assessment).

Application in Service Delivery

The ethical conundrum that arises when individual risk is balanced against societal benefit is well illustrated by the use of Depo-Provera (DMPA) in countries with high HIV prevalence. DMPA is a progestin-only injectable contraceptive that has received significant attention since 2010 (Polis et al., 2014) because observational studies indicate that women using DMPA might be at higher risk of acquiring HIV (Heffron et al., 2012; Polis et al., 2016). A risk-benefit assessment of DMPA involves weighing its benefits to women (e.g., avoiding unintended pregnancy) and society (e.g., improved maternal health outcomes) against its potential risks to women (e.g., heightened susceptibility to HIV). In settings where HIV infection rates are high and contraceptive use is low, risk-benefit assessments are especially challenging (Covshoff, Sauer, and Pittrof, 2015; Haddad, Philpott-Jones, and Schonfield, 2015a, 2015b; Han et al., 2017).

In many sub-Saharan African countries, where DMPA is the most commonly used contraceptive, the challenge is providing appropriate guidance to women and family planning providers about a popular method that may also increase the risk of HIV acquisition for some women. For example, what type of counseling on HIV-risk reduction, or restrictions on DMPA use, should be put in place?

One view is that restrictions on the use of DMPA, while intended to protect women from a heightened risk of HIV acquisition, would limit access to an effective contraceptive for many women, thereby exposing them to unwanted harm (Haddad, Philpott-Jones, and Schonfield, 2015a, 2015b) and increasing maternal mortality (Rodriguez, Reeves, and Caughey, 2012). Others have argued that such restrictions limit women's opportunity to make informed decisions about whether they wish to use DMPA (Covshoff, Sauer, and Pittrof, 2015).

Recognizing the alternate viewpoints on public health benefits versus individual risks, the state of existing scientific evidence, and the need for clear policy guidance, the World Health Organization (WHO) issued an update to the Medical Eligibility Criteria for progestin-only injectables in women at high individual risk of HIV (WHO, 2017). The updated guidance changes the provision of those contraceptives from Category 1 (no restriction) to Category 2 (benefits outweigh risks), and reflects the WHO's attempt to balance public health concerns with individual rights.

Application in Research

Many countries of sub-Saharan Africa and Asia are challenged by health worker shortage and retention, which limit access to and availability of essential family planning services. Task shifting and task sharing have been proposed as mechanisms for improving access and cost-effectiveness within health systems in these regions (WHO, 2012). Under these strategies, lower cadres (occupational groups) of health staff, including "lay health workers," would be trained and enabled to deliver the same family planning services currently offered by higher-level or specialized staff. From an ethical perspective, task shifting and sharing may improve equity of access to family planning services, especially for remote and underserved communities, without compromising quality of care, providing the associated training is appropriate.

Since the early years of the twenty-first century, research evidence has been slowly accumulating on the types of health workers and the types of contraceptives they can safely deliver. For example, studies from Kenya, Madagascar, Nigeria, and Uganda have documented the feasibility, effectiveness, and acceptability of community-based distribution of injectable contraceptives through non-medically trained workers (Hoke, Brunie, et al., 2012; Hoke, Wheeler, et al., 2012).

Conducting a risk-benefit assessment of research on task shifting and task sharing involves balancing potential risks to research participants against potential benefits that they or society may gain, including knowledge emanating from the research. Early participants, for example, may bear harms, such as those arising from poor contraceptive services, stemming from the limited training of lower cadres of health workers and community-based health workers. Research participants who wish to keep their contraceptive use secret also face risks related to their privacy and confidentiality, particularly in small communities. Research participants should be provided information on the various types of risks during the informed consent process to enable their decision-making about participation. If those risks are outweighed, however, by benefits that will accrue to individuals and underserved communities, such as increased or early access to novel contraceptives, then the proposed research may satisfy the principle of beneficence.

Issues and Consequences

The two examples discussed above—of restrictions on injectable use and task shifting and task sharing—highlight the weighing of risks and benefits and the balancing of public health goals and individual benefits. In both cases, the consequences are borne by health systems (including providers), contraceptive users, and society at large. In the case of DMPA, the extent to which all three stakeholders may bear the impact of reduced access will depend on the extent to which contraceptive users are provided with a choice of alternate methods and are able to make an educated and informed decision that enhances their reproductive health.

Research on task sharing and shifting benefits health systems in two ways—first, through the identification of cost-efficiencies associated with the decreased cost of deploying lower cadres of health workers, and second, by increasing family planning coverage. Higher cadres of family planning providers benefit by reduced pressure to serve large volumes of clients, and lower cadres of workers gain opportunities for training, employment, and social prestige. Overall, contraceptive users benefit from easier and more convenient access to family planning services.

Distributive Justice

Distributive justice refers to the equitable distribution of benefits and burdens across members of society. There are numerous theories of distributive justice, each of which offers a moral principle to guide decisions about how society ought to distribute goods fairly. One frequently invoked principle requires that societies distribute benefits and burdens in a manner that provides the greatest benefit to the least advantaged groups (Rawls, 1971). In the context of family planning, political and institutional decision-makers who adhere to that principle might conclude, for example, that they have an obligation to ensure that vulnerable groups—as defined by factors such as age, gender, poverty level, and ethnicity—not only benefit from the full range of contraceptive delivery services, but also are protected from burdens associated with overrepresentation in research.

Application in Service Delivery

Historically, contraceptive services targeted women of reproductive age because doing so was viewed as a cost-effective way to achieve a substantial public health impact. That approach, however, led to a dearth of services for significant subpopulations, including men and young people (both girls and boys). Other factors, most notably medical and social norms, have further exacerbated the lack of services for those subpopulations. Once contraceptive services were medicalized for women (e.g., oral contraceptives, IUDs, implants, injectables, and female sterilization), they were provided in settings largely devoted to women's health. As a consequence, products and services for men—beyond condoms—were largely ignored, even for contraceptive methods that require men's cooperation in the timing of intercourse and nature of sexual activity. Local norms that suggest unmarried people should not be sexually active, and therefore should not have access to information and services for "family planning," have similarly led to the exclusion from family planning services of young unmarried people below the age of eighteen. As a matter of social justice, however, men and sexually active youth need contraception and protection from sexually transmitted infection as much as any other sexually active group.

Increasing access to vasectomy and investments in emerging male technologies would allow men to share the responsibility and risks of contraception (health, social, and financial) fairly and in a just manner. This may be easier to achieve before a range of safe and effective male contraceptive products become available with the backup of safe abortion services. Nevertheless, distributive justice requires that underserved groups receive additional protections, particularly when the burden of side effects, costs, and complications currently fall on women. In the current context of private-sector services and a reliance on short-term methods, a case may be made that older women seeking to terminate childbearing are also underserved by the current constellation of services, particularly in resource-poor countries.

Universal health coverage (UHC), policy initiatives such as conditional cash transfers, and provider incentives for performance aim to increase access to underserved groups and bypass barriers such as geography and gender. However, such policies often do not include explicit investments in contraceptive supplies, information, and services that are consistent with the long-term policy goals of helping families at the community level have the children they want, and of slowing unwanted population growth at the country level. The emphasis is on achieving a public health impact by increasing the coverage and quality of basic health care, but individuals or vulnerable groups may still not benefit from contraceptive or other maternal health services as intended if these services are ignored or inadequately covered in the policy's essential care packages.

New contraceptives are often introduced in urban markets aimed at paying consumers. This is a strategy for ensuring quick and easy returns on investments made by market players. Consequently, less privileged or less wealthy consumers may not have the opportunity to benefit from the new product, even though they may potentially benefit more from it, and may indeed have participated in greater numbers in the clinical trials, thus shouldering many of the early risks. With decreasing engagement of the public sector in family planning service delivery, contraception is viewed as more of a routine commodity in the family budget. At the same time, the extent to which the private sector serves poor and underserved populations is evolving and highly variable by context. Given the flow of benefits both to users and health systems in terms of unwanted pregnancies and births avoided, the state has an obligation to serve those populations with unmet need, so as to facilitate their access to beneficial services and products.

Application in Research

Justice demands that all subpopulations relevant to a research inquiry be represented in the study population. For example, product development and implementation research should ensure that adequate samples of young people are represented in early-phase clinical studies, as well as in planning and piloting interventions designed for testing strategies to scale up services. At the end of the study, justice demands that the public, including the segment represented by research participants, and policymakers have access to the results of the research in a way that might address their interests and facilitate their use of the data. If the results of the research are positive for segments of the participant pool, efforts must be made by duty bearers—that is, public-sector decision-makers in health and finance leadership roles—to utilize the results, as appropriate, in the development and implementation of policies, guidelines, and services. For early research on product development, this may mean making reasonable efforts to support translational research to facilitate the movement of the product along the development pipeline from small phase I proof-of-concept studies to large phase III studies on efficacy, safety, and acceptability.

Issues and Consequences

Paying attention to distributive justice in contraceptive services will lead to greater coverage and cost efficiencies. Individuals will benefit from contraceptive protection when they need it, and states and health systems will benefit by reducing the costs associated with unintended pregnancies and, in turn, poor maternal and child health outcomes. When the local standard of care differs from international research standards on implementation, international consensus suggests that care is ethical if it is based on a valid scientific purpose for using a lesser standard, provides social benefits for the local host community, and shows a favorable risk-benefit ratio for the individual research participants (Wendler, Emmanuel, and Lie, 2004).

Conclusions

Ethical analysis of family planning services and research remains as critical now as it was a half-century ago, when human rights were first recognized by world governments. In part, this is due to the unique role contraception plays in the context of health systems. It is a service for healthy individuals, and, at the same time, it is one of the most cost-effective, "smart investments" for international development (Copenhagen Consensus, 2015). As a result, issues of population growth—and more often, issues of contraceptive access and use—become a locus of conflict between individual decisions on reproduction, the preferences and biases of researchers and health providers, and the objectives of the state to preserve health and simultaneously influence overall population size and social welfare.

Can these apparent tensions be managed in such a way that governments, health systems, societies, and individuals all benefit from investments in family planning services and research? We believe that renewed commitment to the rights of individuals, coupled with efforts to develop approaches to the application and oversight of these principles, hold promise for duty bearers (i.e., policymakers and health providers) and potential beneficiaries alike. While the principles have remained the same (i.e., respect for persons, beneficence, and justice), their applications have become much more diversified, including, for example, the use of social media to recruit research participants and the delivery of contraceptive services in a wide variety of settings (e.g., community health workers, pharmacies, health centers, and even Internet-based distribution of information and supplies). Moreover, new mechanisms are being employed to oversee the provision of consent, the analysis of risks and benefits, and, above all, the accountability of health systems in the distribution of the benefits of contraceptive services and research. Contraception for men, outside of condom use, remains one of the few areas where both research on methods for men and services for men remain marginal to most health system investments.

Persistent issues remain that require continuous reflection on our assumptions and ethical standards. We must be cognizant of the evolving context in which contraceptive services and research take place, as well as the regulatory environments that govern them. Development programs now have a more diverse range of stakeholders beyond government, including the community, private-sector entities, and religious groups. When implementing protections in challenging environments, we must seek the right balance between compliance with prevailing policy practice and adherence to sound ethical principles.

Acknowledgments

The authors would like to acknowledge the generous support of USAID, NICHD, the Packard Foundation, and the Hewlett Foundation in the development of the ideas and organization of the paper. The opinions expressed in this paper are solely those of the authors and do not necessarily reflect the views of the funding agencies.

References

Bankole, A., and Malarcher, S. 2010. "Removing Barriers to Adolescents' Access to Contraceptive Information and Services." *Studies in Family Planning* 41(2): 117–124.

Chandra-Mouli, V., McCarraher, D. R., Phillips, S. J., Williamson, N. E., and Hainsworth, G. 2014. "Contraception for Adolescents in Low and Middle Income Countries: Needs, Barriers, and Access." *Reproductive Health* 11: 1. https://reproductive-health-journal.biomedcentral.com/articles/10.1186/1742-4755-11-1.

Copenhagen Consensus. 2015. "Population and Demography." www.copenhagenconsensus.com/post-2015-consensus/populationanddemography.

Covshoff, E., Sauer, U., and Pittrof, R. 2015. "Human Rights and Clinical Ethics Are the Right Framework to Address the Probable DMPA-HIV Interaction." *BMJ Sexual and Reproductive Health Care* 41(2): 156. https://srh.bmj.com/content/41/2/156.1.

Fischer, B. A., IV. 2006. "A Summary of Important Documents in the Field of Research Ethics." *Schizophrenia Bulletin* 32(1): 69–80.

Gomez, A. M., Fuentes, L., and Allina, A. 2014. "Women or LARC First? Reproductive Autonomy and the Promotion of Long-Acting Reversible Contraceptive Methods." *Perspectives in Sexual and Reproductive Health* 46(3): 171–175.

Haddad, L. B., Philpott-Jones, S., and Schonfield, T. 2015a. "Contraception and Prevention of HIV Transmission: A Potential Conflict of Public Health Principles." *Journal of Family Planning and Reproductive Health Care* 41(1): 20–23.

Haddad, L. B, Philpott-Jones, S., and Schonfield, T. 2015b. "Human Rights and Clinical Ethics are the Right Framework to Address the Probable DMPA-HIV Interaction: Authors' Response." *BMJ Sexual and Reproductive Health* 41(2). http://dx.doi.org/10.1136/jfprhc-2015-101204.

Han, L., Patil, E., Kidula, N., Gaffield, M. L., and Steyn, P. S. 2017. "Guidelines on the Potential Risks of HIV Acquisition and Progestogen-Only Contraception Use." *Global Health Science and Practice* 5(4): 540–546.

Heffron, R., Donnell, D., Rees, H., Celum, C., Nelly Mugo, E. W., de Bruyn, G., et al. 2012. "Hormonal Contraceptive Use and Risk of HIV-1 Transmission: A Prospective Cohort Analysis." *Lancet Infectious Diseases* 12(1): 19–26.

Hoke, T. H., Brunie, A., Krueger, K., Dreisbach, C., Akol, A., Rabenja, N L., et al. 2012. "Community-Based Distribution of Injectable Contraceptives: Introduction Strategies in Four Sub-Saharan African Countries." *International Perspectives on Sexual and Reproductive Health* 38(4): 214–219.

Hoke, T. H., Wheeler, S. B., Land, K., Green, M. S., Razafindravony, B. H., Rasamihajamanana, E., et al. 2012. "Community-Based Provision of Injectable Contraceptives in Madagascar: 'Task Shifting' to Expand Access to Injectable Contraceptives." *Health Policy and Planning* 27(1): 52–59.

Jacobstein, R. 2018. "Liftoff: The Blossoming of Contraceptive Implant Use in Africa." Global *Health Science and Practice* 6(1): 17–39.

Jain, A. 1998. *Do Population Policies Matter? Fertility and Politics in Egypt, India, Kenya, and Mexico* (New York: Population Council).

Jain, A. K., RamaRao, S., Kim, J., and Costello, M. 2012. "Evaluation of an Intervention to Improve Quality of Care in a Family Planning Program in the Philippines." *Journal of Biosocial Science* 44(1): 27–41.

National Commission (National Commission for the Protection of Human Subjects of Biomedical and Behavioral Research). 1979. *The Belmont Report: Ethical Principles and Guidelines for the Protection of Human Subjects of Research*. DHEW Publication No. (OS) 78-0012 (Washington, D.C.: Government Printing Office). https://www.hhs.gov/ohrp/sites/default/files/the-belmont-report-508c_FINAL.pdf.

Pariani, S., Heer, D. M., and Van Arsdol, M. D., Jr. 1991. "Does Choice Make a Difference to Contraceptive Use? Evidence from East Java." *Studies in Family Planning* 22(6): 384–390.

Polis, C. B., Curtis, K. M., Hannaford, P. C., Phillips, S. J., Chipato, T., Kiarie, J. N., et al. 2016. "An Updated Systematic Review of Epidemiological Evidence on Hormonal Contraceptive Methods and Risk of HIV Acquisition in Women." *AIDS* 30(17): 2665–2683.

Polis, C. B., Phillips, S. J., Curtis, K. M., Westreich, D. J., Steyn, P. S., Raymond, E., et al. 2014. "Hormonal Contraceptive Methods and Risk of HIV Acquisition in Women: A Systematic Review of Epidemiological Evidence." *Contraception* 90(4): 360–390.

RamaRao, S., Friedland, B., and Townsend, J. W. 2007. "A Question of Ethics: Research and Practice in Reproductive Health." *Studies in Family Planning* 38(4): 229–241.

RamaRao, S., and Mohanam, R. 2003. "Quality of Family Planning Programs: Concepts, Measurements, Interventions, and Effects." *Studies in Family Planning* 34(4): 227–248.

Rawls, J. 1971. *A Theory of Justice* (Cambridge, Mass.: Belknap Press of Harvard University Press).

Rodriguez, M., Reeves, M., and Caughey, A. 2012. "Evaluating the Competing Risks of HIV Acquisition and Maternal Mortality in Africa: A Decision Analysis." *British Journal of Obstetrics and Gynecology* 119(9): 1067–1073.

UN (United Nations). 1968. *Resolution XVIII: Human Rights Aspects of Family Planning, Final Act of the International Conference on Human Rights.* International Conference on Human Rights Tehran, Republic of Iran, 22 April to 13 May 1968. U.N. Doc. A/CONF. 32/41, p.15.

UNFPA (United Nations Population Fund). 1974. *World Population Plan of Action.* Adopted by the World Population Conference, Bucharest, 19–30 August 1974 (New York: UNFPA). https://www.unfpa.org/sites/default/files/event-pdf/World%20Population%20Plan%20of%20Action_1.pdf.

UNFPA (United Nations Population Fund). 1984. *Report of the International Conference on Population, 1984,* Mexico City, 6–14 August 1984 (New York: UNFPA). https://www.unfpa.org/sites/default/files/event-pdf/ICP_mexico84_report.pdf.

UNFPA (United Nations Population Fund). 1994. *Programme of Action: Adopted at the International Conference on Population and Development,* Cairo, 5–13 September 1994 (New York: UNFPA). https://www.unfpa.org/sites/default/files/event-pdf/PoA_en.pdf.

Wendler D., Emmanuel, E. J., and Lie, R. K. 2004. "The Standard of Care Debate: Can Research in Developing Countries Be Both Ethical and Responsive to Those Countries' Health Needs?" *American Journal of Public Health* 94(6): 923–928.

WHO (World Health Organization). 2012. *WHO Recommendations: Optimizing Health Worker Roles to Improve Access to Key Maternal and Newborn Health Interventions through Task Shifting* (Geneva: WHO).

WHO (World Health Organization). 2017. *Hormonal Contraceptive Eligibility for Women at High Risk of HIV: Guidance Statement* (Geneva: WHO). http://apps.who.int/iris/bitstream/handle/10665/254662/WHO-RHR-17.04-eng.pdf;jsessionid=0B123FC93F926142C8C219514C590F9A?sequence=1. Accessed June 17, 2018.

WHO (World Health Organization). 2018. "Family Planning/Contraception." Fact Sheet, February 8. http://www.who.int/news-room/fact-sheets/detail/family-planning-contraception.

CHAPTER 35

ABORTION AND PUBLIC HEALTH ETHICS

MAHMOUD F. FATHALLA

UNSAFE ABORTION: A GLOBAL PUBLIC HEALTH CHALLENGE

UNSAFE abortion has been described as a preventable pandemic (Grimes et al., 2006). Each year, approximately 25 million abortions worldwide meet the World Health Organization (WHO) definition of "unsafe abortion": they are performed either by individuals without the necessary skills or in an environment that does not conform to minimum medical standards, or both (WHO, 2017). Importantly, *unsafe abortion* and *illegal abortion* are not synonyms. Illegal abortion involves terminating, or attempting to terminate, a pregnancy when doing so is against the law. Illegal abortion is often, but not always, unsafe. In many countries where abortion is illegal, for example, private physicians may perform safe abortions for wealthy patients who can afford their high medical fees (Warriner, 2006). Also, not all legal abortions are safe. Some developing countries have liberalized their abortion laws, but because their health care systems are inadequate to meet the demand for abortion, women in those countries may go to medically unqualified abortionists for the procedure (Warriner, 2006).

The public health rationale for addressing unsafe abortion was first highlighted in 1967 by the World Health Assembly, which declared that "abortions and... high maternal and child mortality constitute a serious public health problem in many countries," warranting international action (WHO, 1967, 25). In addition to the public health justification for addressing unsafe abortion, there is an ethical imperative to do so as well. The moral obligation is dictated by the magnitude of the health problems caused by unsafe abortion (in terms of prevalence, mortality, and morbidity), the health inequities and social injustices that poor women experience when they cannot access safe abortion, the many women who have called for action, and an international consensus—including statements and guidelines from the WHO—that recognizes unsafe abortion as a global public health problem. The availability of affordable and appropriate public health interventions, coupled with the cost savings from fewer abortion complications, reinforce the ethical imperative to prevent unsafe abortions.

Magnitude of the Problem

The global prevalence of unsafe abortion is staggering. A 2017 study supported by the WHO and the World Bank, among others, reported that each year between 2010 and 2014, approximately 25 percent of all pregnancies globally ended in an induced abortion, which accounts for an estimated 56 million induced (safe and unsafe) abortions each year worldwide during that time period (WHO, 2017; Ganatra et al., 2017). Of those induced abortions, more than 25 million met the WHO definition of unsafe abortion, and almost all of these (97 percent) occurred in developing countries (WHO, 2017).

When performed safely, induced abortion can be markedly safer than childbirth. Even in a developed country like the United States, the risk of death associated with childbirth is reported to be approximately fourteen times higher than that with safe induced abortion; similarly, the overall morbidity associated with childbirth exceeds that associated with safe abortion (Raymond and Grimes, 2012).

Unsafe abortion, however, is a significant factor in maternal morbidity and mortality. The major life-threatening complications resulting from unsafe abortion are hemorrhage, infection, and injury to the genital tract and internal organs. In developing countries, about 7 million women are admitted to the hospital each year for complications related to unsafe abortion (WHO, 2017; Singh and Maddow-Zimet, 2016). Complications of unsafe abortion are also responsible for approximately 47,000 pregnancy-related deaths each year, accounting for 4.7–13.2 percent of all maternal deaths (Say et al., 2014). Because stigma and fear of punishment may deter reliable reporting, particularly following illegal abortion procedures, deaths and disabilities resulting from unsafe abortion are probably underestimated. In addition, unsafe abortion can have major emotional, social, and financial costs for women and their families.

Inequity, Injustice, and Women's Voices

Public health ethics has always concerned itself with equity and social justice in population health. At the global level, unsafe abortion is a glaring inequity. In developed regions, it is estimated that 30 women die as a consequence of unsafe abortion for every 100,000 abortions performed; that number rises to 220 deaths per 100,000 unsafe abortions in developing regions, and 520 deaths per 100,000 unsafe abortions in sub-Saharan Africa (WHO, 2017). Mortality from unsafe abortion disproportionately affects women in Africa. While the continent accounts for 29 percent of all unsafe abortions, it sees 62 percent of unsafe-abortion-related deaths (WHO, 2011b).

Within countries in which abortion is legal but highly restricted, unequal access to safe abortion can result in socially unjust outcomes. While "[u]nsafe abortions threaten the lives of a large number of women" and represent "a grave public health problem," the Fourth World Conference on Women in Beijing in 1995 noted that "it is primarily the poorest and youngest [women] who take the highest risk" (UN, 1996, para. 97). Abortions that meet safety requirements can become the privilege of the rich, while poor women have little choice but to resort to unsafe abortions. Young adolescent girls are especially vulnerable to unsafe abortions, because they may delay the procedure to later in their pregnancies, when there often are more legal restrictions on the procedure and fewer skilled providers offering safe abortion (Woog et al., 2015).

Recognizing the inequity and injustice associated with unsafe abortion, women at the Beijing Conference called upon "[a]ll governments and relevant intergovernmental and non-governmental organizations . . . to strengthen their commitment to women's health, to deal with the health impact of unsafe abortion as a major public health concern" (UN, 1996, para.106, k).

International Consensus

In 1994 the world government community at the United Nations International Conference on Population and Development recognized unsafe abortion as a major public health concern (UNFPA, 1994, para. 8.25). A decade later, the World Health Assembly adopted a global reproductive health strategy in which eliminating unsafe abortion is a key component (WHO, 2004). The strategy is stated to be "grounded in international human rights treaties and global consensus declarations that call for the respect, protection, and fulfilment of human rights" to health, including "the right of women to have control over, and decide freely and responsibly on matters related to their sexuality, including sexual and reproductive health, . . . the right of access to relevant health information, and the right of every person to enjoy the benefits of scientific progress and its applications" (WHO, 2012, sec. 1.2). To realize these rights, and to save women's lives, the WHO strategy calls on the international community to address the programmatic, legal, and policy aspects of providing safe abortion worldwide.

Preventing Unsafe Abortion: The Practical and Economic Rationale

The ethical imperative to address unsafe abortion is further bolstered by practical and economic considerations. A variety of public health actions, including effective contraception services, provision of safe and legal induced abortion, timely management of complications, and provision of post-abortion care are feasible steps toward preventing almost every death and disability caused by unsafe abortion (WHO, 2017).

One of the ethical challenges in public health is the rationing of limited resources for different health and disease conditions. In countries that face competing demands for the limited resources their health systems can afford, safe abortion is rarely, if ever, a top priority, and unsafe abortion is thus more likely to become a public health problem. Treating complications of unsafe abortion is costly and can overwhelm health systems in low-income countries (WHO, 2012). For example, estimates suggest that the total annual cost to the health system in the developing world for management of serious, post-abortion medical complications that require hospitalization lies between $375 and $838 million, with a central estimate of around $500 million (Vlassoff et al., 2008). If the millions of women who currently receive no treatment from a health system for serious, post-abortion complications were to do so, approximately $375 million more would be required each year to cover their care. The cost of long-term morbidities, mainly infertility and chronic reproductive tract infections, may cost many billions of dollars annually. In addition, estimates suggest that women and their families may pay $600 million in out-of-pocket expenses, and developing countries may face economic losses of more than $400 million each year from lower productivity caused by unsafe abortion.

Against this background, it is important to emphasize that safe abortion services are a cost-saving measure. For example, unsafe abortion was estimated to cost the Mexico City health system $2.6 million in 2005, prior to the legalization of abortion (Levin et al., 2009). Although studies to document cost savings are needed, it was estimated that with access to safe abortion, the system could potentially save $1.7 million annually, by shifting abortion management from emergency in-patient procedures to routine outpatient procedures as well as use of medical abortion (Levin et al., 2009). Eliminating unsafe abortion would result in significant savings that health systems could then conserve and redirect to other urgent public health needs.

Abortion at the Intersection of Morality, Religion, Law, and Human Rights

Abortion has been, and continues to be, a controversial topic in reproductive health (Cook, Dickens, and Fathalla, 2003). The ethical obligation of public health to eliminate unsafe abortion must, therefore, consider the ways in which abortion intersects with morality, religion, law, and human rights.

The public debate on the moral status of the human embryo and fetus, as a person requiring protection independent of the mother, remains, and probably will remain, unsettled (Araujo et al., 2015; Catlin, 2015). Some people believe the fetus lacks personhood status until birth, while others believe it warrants protection as a person from the moment of conception. This debate can have a potential impact on public health policy, which led the American Public Health Association (APHA) to issue a statement renouncing the adoption or misapplication of laws to recognize fetuses as independent of pregnant women (APHA, 2013).

Although world religions have not been silent on the question of induced abortion, there is not a unanimous view shared by all religions. Religious perspectives on induced abortion range from very conservative to more permissive, with leniency—where allowed—more likely for early-term abortions (Maguire, 2016). There can also be a variety of views within individual religious traditions. From a public health perspective, institutionalized religions may influence laws and policies limiting access to abortion (Marecek, Macleod, and Hoggart, 2017).

Because abortion laws and policies vary by country, any global public health efforts to stem unsafe abortions must consider the legal context in which unsafe abortions are occurring. At the start of the twentieth century, abortion was illegal in almost every country of the world. During the second half of the twentieth century, as a part of the social movement for women's rights, countries that otherwise prohibited abortion began to enact laws that allow abortion on specified grounds. Currently, the exceptions for which abortion is allowed vary widely by country, and may include risk to the woman's life; risk to her physical and, sometimes, mental health; pregnancy resulting from rape or sexual abuse; serious fetal anomaly; social and economic reasons; and permission by request. The permissibility of abortion on each of those grounds also varies greatly between regions. For example, recent studies report that abortion is permitted upon request in 65 percent of developed countries but only 14 percent of developing countries, and for economic and social reasons in 75 percent of developed countries but only 19 percent of developing countries (Berer, 2017).

Where abortion is not against the law, abortion access may still be restricted by legally introduced procedural barriers, such as mandatory and biased counseling requirements, waiting periods, third-party consent and notification requirements, limitations on the range of permissible abortion methods, and limitations on public funding (Finer and Fine, 2013). In June 2017, to enhance global and country-specific efforts to address unsafe abortion, the WHO Human Reproduction Programme, in collaboration with the Population Division of the United Nations Department of Economic and Social Affairs, launched the open-access Global Abortion Policies Database (Human Reproduction Programme, 2017). The database is a tool that tracks evolving abortion policies by country and is intended to inform policymaking and advocacy to eliminate unsafe abortion.

When prohibitions and restrictions on abortion threaten women's lives and conflict with their individual liberty, human rights violations may occur. Recognizing women as competent and conscientious decision makers in their own lives, one legal view places abortion as one procedure within a spectrum of services to which women should have safe access as a matter of human rights and social justice (Cook and Dickens, 2003). Abortion policies should be geared to respecting, protecting, and fulfilling the human rights of women (WHO, 2012). Offering access to safe abortion also recognizes women as competent and conscientious decision-makers in their own lives. A tension in public health ethics may occur, however, when abortion policies appear to contravene human rights, which can occur in two ways.

The first way in which abortion policy can conflict with human rights is when action for a real or perceived public good conflicts with individual liberty. For example, population growth is a legitimate concern, and the state may make voluntary, safe pregnancy termination an option for women. However, human rights "red lines" are crossed when women are forced to terminate wanted pregnancies, as was reported in China during the implementation of its "one-child policy"—a government mandate in effect from 1979 through 2015 to limit families to one child in order to restrain population growth (Howden and Zhou, 2014). Human rights were similarly abridged under the authoritarian leadership of Nicolae Ceauşescu in Romania where women were forced to do the opposite under his population-promoting policies; that is, they were compelled to keep unwanted pregnancies for the public good, because the fetus was considered the socialist property of the state, and women who resorted to abortion were viewed as deserters and betrayers (Hord et al., 1991).

The second way in which abortion policy can conflict with human rights is when individual liberty conflicts with a perceived public good, as in the case of sex-selective abortion. The availability of ultrasounds and other technologies has enabled parents to detect the sex of a fetus during prenatal screenings. In cultures where son preference prevails, parents may arrange to abort female fetuses. This can result in gender imbalances in the population, which is of increasing concern in some South Asian, East Asian, and Central Asian countries (Fathalla, 1994; WHO, 2011a). The individual liberty to choose sex-selective abortion not only reflects the persistent, low status of women and girls, but it also results in a female deficit that may have damaging effects on societies.

Public Health Actions

Inaction Is Not an Ethical Option

Inaction, by denial or neglect, is not an ethically justifiable response to the global tragedy of unsafe abortion. Denying or neglecting a major health problem does not take it off the ethical radar screen. Whether or not it is wanted by society, abortion is needed by women. They have needed it throughout human history, and they have often risked their health or lives in the process. The oath of Hippocrates, which has at times been taken by those who become physicians, includes an injunction against abortion: "I will not give to a woman a pessary to cause abortion." However, Hippocrates himself, writing in 400 BCE, could not ignore the reality that women nevertheless resort to abortion, often with serious consequences to their health:

> When the woman is afflicted with a large wound as a consequence of abortion, or the womb is damaged by strong suppositories, as many women are always doing, doctoring themselves, or when the fetus is aborted and the woman is not purged of the afterbirth, and the wound inflames, closes and is not purged, if she is treated promptly she will be cured but will remain sterile. (Cited in McLaren, 1990, 28)

In developed countries, the global public health problem of unsafe abortion may be neglected because it is considered to be only a problem of the poor. In developing countries, the problem may be neglected because it is perceived as a woman's issue in societies where women are undervalued. It is an inconvenient truth that many "women are not dying because of untreatable conditions... [t]hey are dying because societies have yet to make the decision that their lives are worth saving" (Fathalla, 2006, 409).

Four Components of an Ethical Public Health Strategy

The growing international consensus, as adopted by the United Nations General Assembly, is that unsafe abortion can, and should, be dealt with through a public health strategy with four components: reducing the need for abortion by provision of family planning services, making safe abortion services available to the full extent of the law, offering quality services for management of post-abortion complications, and providing post-abortion care to help avoid repeat abortions (UNFPA, 1999).

Reducing the Need for Abortion

Making contraceptive information and services available, accessible, and affordable can reduce women's need for abortion (Bongaarts and Westoff, 2000). In the United States, the availability and appropriate use of affordable, effective, and safe contraception has been associated with decreasing numbers of abortions (Chescheir, 2017). Data from countries in Eastern Europe and Central Asia, where induced abortion was once the main method for regulating fertility, show that when the use of modern contraceptive methods increased, the incidence of induced abortion decreased (Westoff, 2005). Rates of induced abortion are the lowest in Western Europe, where modern contraceptive use is high and abortion is generally legally available on request (WHO, 2012).

Although impressive gains have been made in contraceptive use worldwide, an unmet need for family planning continues to persist. Defined broadly, unmet need for family planning is "the number of women who want to avoid or postpone a pregnancy but are not using any method of contraception" (WHO, 2012, 23). The WHO (2017) estimates that 214 million women of reproductive age in developing countries who want to avoid pregnancy are not using a modern contraceptive method. Women will continue to face unintended pregnancies as long as their family planning needs are not met.

Given the reality of gendered power relationships, women are often exposed to unprotected sexual intercourse. This dictates the need for backup methods that women can use in such instances to reduce the need for abortion. Methods for emergency contraception (often referred to as the "morning-after pill") exist and can be used within a few days of unprotected sexual intercourse to prevent pregnancy. This "retroactive contraception" would also be suited to the particular needs of adolescents, where the decision to contracept may not be made before having sex. Emergency contraception is also greatly needed in refugee situations and cases of sexual assault (Fathalla, 2003). It is not enough that services for emergency contraception are made available. Although they cannot be a substitute for regular contraception, information about emergency contraception methods should be widely distributed. A multi-country analysis of the knowledge and use of emergency contraception highlighted the need to broaden the dissemination of information about this service (Palermo, Bleck, and Westley, 2014).

Although contraceptive use reduces the number of unintended pregnancies, it does not eliminate the need for access to safe abortion. Data from 2007 on contraceptive prevalence and the typical failure rates of contraceptive methods estimated that approximately 33 million women worldwide experience an accidental pregnancy while using contraception every year (WHO, 2012). Some of the accidental pregnancies are terminated by induced abortions, and some end up as unplanned births.

Where Abortion Is Not Against the Law, It Should Be Safe

In 1994 the Programme of Action of the United Nations International Conference on Population and Development stated that in "circumstances where abortion is not against the law, such abortion should be safe" (UNFPA, 1994, para. 8.25). At a Special Session of the UN General Assembly in June 1999, governments agreed that "in circumstances where abortion is not against the law, health systems should train and equip health-service providers and should take other measures to ensure that such abortion is safe and accessible" (UNFPA, 1999, para. 63, I, iii).

The legal status of abortion has "no effect on a woman's need for an abortion, but it dramatically affects her access to safe abortion" (WHO, 2012, 17). Although laws vary widely by country, they generally permit abortion to save a woman's life and (in the majority of countries) to preserve the woman's physical and/or mental health, or on other grounds such as rape or incest and fetal impairment. Safe abortion services, including medication abortion, should be available and accessible for all women, to the full extent of the law. Patients and health care providers should be familiar with conditions where abortion is not against the law. Keeping this information hidden is not ethically justifiable.

The WHO provides and updates technical and policy guidance for safe abortion services (WHO, 2012; Fathalla and Cook, 2012). There is an ethical responsibility to provide safe abortion services within the limits of the law. Conscientious objection is allowable but should not be used to hide the fear of the stigma associated with abortion (Faúndes, 2017). It should be remembered that when women are denied access to legal, safe abortion services, they often resort to an unsafe abortion, and in many cases they suffer its consequences. As asserted by the Committee for the Ethical Aspects of Human Reproduction and Women's Health of the International Federation of Gynecology and Obstetrics (FIGO, 2012, 29): "The primary conscientious duty of obstetrician–gynecologists is at all times to treat, or provide benefit and prevent harm, to the patients for whose care they are responsible. Any conscientious objection to treating a patient is secondary to this primary duty." Pharmacists, too, where abortion is not against the law, cannot ethically justify denying women access to drugs used for medication abortion.

Access to Treatment for Abortion Complications

Health care providers are ethically obliged to provide life-saving medical care to any woman who suffers abortion-related complications, regardless of the legality of abortion in that locality. The WHO (2012) has developed technical and policy guidance for the provision of these services. From a public health perspective, the practice of extracting confessions from women seeking emergency medical care as a result of illegal abortion is not ethically acceptable. Such a practice puts women's lives at risk because it prevents women from seeking care. It is also ethically objectionable for a state to conscript health care providers as police informants to report patients who have undergone abortion to relevant authorities. Not only does this practice create a conflict of interests, it also violates patient confidentiality, a central principle of medical ethics and professionalism (WHO, 2017).

Post-abortion Care

Following an abortion, women should, at a minimum, receive information and be offered counseling that addresses post-abortion health care, including how to avoid a future abortion. All women should receive contraceptive information and be offered counseling for and methods of post-abortion contraception, including emergency contraception, before leaving the health care facility (WHO, 2015).

An Ethical and Social Duty for the Public Health Community

Abortion laws and policies impact women's lives and health. The public health community has an ethical and social duty to educate legislators, policymakers, health administrators, and the public at large about any adverse health impact of such laws and policies. Examples of such collective public health action include the APHA's statement "urging federal and state legislatures, law enforcement and judiciary bodies, election commissions, and health care providers to renounce any and all personhood claims or misapplications of child welfare laws that recognize fetuses as persons and infringe on women's reproductive, constitutional, and human rights" (APHA, 2013), as well as the association's position that "restricted access to abortion violates human rights, precludes reproductive justice, and demands public health intervention" (APHA, 2015).

There will always be ideological views opposed to any attempt to interrupt the establishment of pregnancy after an ovum has been fertilized, or even to any form of artificial contraception. Those views are entitled to full respect. They should not, however, be imposed on those who do not share them, nor should they be enforced to adversely impact women's lives, rights, and health.

Unsafe abortion is a global public health problem requiring worldwide attention and the necessity of a multi-actor response. Members of the health profession should be among those at the forefront. Women trust their health and life to the health profession. They expect more than technicians and services to fix their diseased body, organs, and systems. They expect a health profession that stands beside them and behind them as they claim the human rights voiced by women when they gathered at the Fourth World Conference on Women in Beijing in 1995: "The human rights of women include their right to have control over and decide freely and responsibly on matters related to their sexuality, including sexual and reproductive health, free of coercion, discrimination and violence" (UN, 1996, para. 96).

References

APHA (American Public Health Association). 2013. "Renouncing the Adoption or Misapplication of Laws to Recognize Fetuses as Independent of Pregnant Women." Policy Number 20139. https://www.apha.org/policies-and-advocacy/public-health-policy-statements/policy-database/2014/07/14/14/03/renouncing-laws-to-recognize-fetuses-as-independent-of-pregnant-women.

APHA (American Public Health Association). 2015. "Restricted Access to Abortion Violates Human Rights, Precludes Reproductive Justice, and Demands Public Health Intervention." Policy Number 20152. https://www.apha.org/policies-and-advocacy/public-health-policy-statements/policy-database/2016/01/04/11/24/restricted-access-to-abortion-violates-human-rights.

Araujo, J., Carvalho, A.S., Silvestre, M., and da Silva, P.M. 2015. "Embryo." In *Encyclopedia of Global Bioethics*, edited by H. ten Have, 1–12 (Cham, Switzerland: Springer Science). https://link.springer.com/referenceworkentry/10.1007/978-3-319-09483-0_169

Berer, M. 2017. "Abortion Law and Policy around the World: In Search of Decriminalization." *Health and Human Rights Journal* 19: 13–27.

Bongaarts, J., and Westoff, C. 2000. "The Potential Role of Contraception in Reducing Abortion." *Studies in Family Planning* 31: 193–202.

Catlin, A. 2015. "Fetus." In *Encyclopedia of Global Bioethics*, edited by H. ten Have, 1–7 (Cham, Switzerland: Springer Science).

Chescheir, N.C. 2017. "Worldwide Abortion Rates and Contraception Access." *Obstetrics & Gynecology* 129: 783–785.

Cook, R. J., and Dickens, B. M. 2003. "Human Rights Dynamics of Abortion Law Reform." *Human Rights Quarterly* 25: 1–59.

Cook, R. J., Dickens, B. M., and Fathalla, M. F. 2003. *Reproductive Health and Human Rights: Integrating Medicine, Ethics, and Law* (New York: Oxford University Press).

Fathalla, M. F. 1994. "The One Hundred Million Missing Women Are Dead: Let It Happen Never Again." *International Journal of Gynecology & Obstetrics* 40: 101–104.

Fathalla, M. F. 2003. "Reducing the Need for Abortion." *Contraception* 68: 397–399.

Fathalla, M. F. 2006. "Human Rights Aspects of Safe Motherhood." *Best Practice & Research: Clinical Obstetrics & Gynaecology* 20: 409–419.

Fathalla, M. F., and Cook, R. J. 2012. "Women, Abortion and the New Technical and Policy Guidance from WHO." *Bulletin of the World Health Organization* 90: 712.

Faúndes, A. 2017. "The Responsibility of Gynecologists and Obstetricians in Providing Safe Abortion Services within the Limits of the Law." *International Journal of Gynecology & Obstetrics* 139: 1–3.

FIGO (International Federation of Gynecology and Obstetrics). 2012. *Ethical Issues in Obstetrics and Gynecology*. A report by the Committee for the Study of Ethical Aspects of Human Reproduction and Women's Health (London: FIGO). https://www.figo.org/sites/default/files/uploads/wg-publications/ethics/English%20Ethical%20Issues%20in%20Obstetrics%20and%20Gynecology.pdf.

Finer, L., and Fine, J. B. 2013. "Abortion Law around the World: Progress and Pushback." *American Journal of Public Health* 103: 585–589.

Ganatra, B., Gerdts, C., Rossier, C., Johnson, R. R., Jr., Tunçalp, Ö., Assifi, A., et al. 2017. "Global, Regional and Subregional Classification of Abortions by Safety, 2010–2014: Estimates from a Bayesian Hierarchical Model." *Lancet* 390(10110): 2372–2381. doi:10.1016/S0140-6736(17)31794-4.

Grimes, D. A., Benson, J., Singh, S., Romero, M., Ganatra. H., Okonofua, F. E., et al. 2006. "Unsafe Abortion: The Preventable Pandemic." *Lancet* 368: 1908–1919.

Hord, C., David, H. P., Donnay, F., and Wolf, M. 1991. "Reproductive Health in Romania: Reversing the Ceausescu Legacy." *Studies in Family Planning* 22: 231–240.

Howden, D., and Zhou, Y. 2014. "China's One-Child Policy: Some Unintended Consequences." *Economic Affairs* 34: 353–369.

Human Reproduction Programme. 2017. Global Abortion Policies Database. http://srhr.org/abortion-policies/.

Levin, C., Grossman. D., Berdichevsky, K., Diaz, C., Aracena, B., Garcia, S. G., et al. 2009. "Exploring the Costs and Economic Consequences of Unsafe Abortion in Mexico City before Legalisation." *Reproductive Health Matters* 17: 120–132.

Maguire, D. C. 2016. "Abortion and Religion." In *The Wiley Blackwell Encyclopedia of Gender and Sexuality Studies*, edited by N. A. Naples, 1–5 (Malden, Mass: Wiley-Blackwell). doi:10.1002/9781118663219.wbegss267.

Marecek, J., Macleod, C., and Hoggart, L. 2017. "Abortion in Legal, Social, and Healthcare Contexts." *Feminism & Psychology* 27: 4–14.

McLaren, A. 1990. *A History of Contraception: From Antiquity to the Present Day* (Cambridge, Mass.: Basil Blackwell).

Palermo, T., Bleck, J., and Westley, E. 2014. "Knowledge and Use of Emergency Contraception: A Multicountry Analysis." *International Perspectives on Sexual and Reproductive Health* 40: 79–86.

Raymond, E. G., and Grimes, D. A. 2012. "The Comparative Safety of Legal Induced Abortion and Childbirth in the United States." *Obstetrics & Gynecology* 119: 215–219.

Say, L., Chou, D., Gemmill, A., Tunçalp, Ö., Moller, A.B., Daniels, J., et al. 2014. "Global Causes of Maternal Death: A WHO Systematic Analysis." *Lancet Global Health* 2: e323–333.

Singh, S., and Maddow-Zimet, I. 2016. "Facility-Based Treatment for Medical Complications Resulting from Unsafe Pregnancy Termination in the Developing World, 2012: A Review of Evidence from 26 Countries." *BJOG: An International Journal of Obstetrics & Gynaecology* 123: 1489–1498.

UN (United Nations). 1996. *Report of the Fourth World Conference on Women: Beijing, 4–15 September 1995*. http://www.un.org/womenwatch/daw/beijing/pdf/Beijing%20full%20 report%20E.pdf.

UNFPA (United Nations Population Fund). 1994. Programme of Action. Adopted at the International Conference on Population and Development, Cairo, 5–13 September 1994. https://www.unfpa.org/sites/default/files/pub-pdf/programme_of_action_Web%20 ENGLISH.pdf.

UNFPA (United Nations Population Fund). 1999. "Key Actions for the Further Implementation of the Programme of Action of the International Conference on Population and Development." Adopted at the Twenty-first Special Session of the UN General Assembly, New York, 8 November 1999. http://www.unfpa.org/sites/default/files/resource-pdf/key_actions.pdf.

Vlassoff, M., Shearer, J., Walker, D., and Lucas, H. 2008. *Economic Impact of Unsafe Abortion-Related Morbidity and Mortality: Evidence and Estimation Challenges*. IDS Research Reports 59 (Brighton, UK: Institute of Development Studies). http://www.abortionresearchconsortium.org/reports/Rr59.pdf.

Warriner, I. K. 2006. "Unsafe Abortion: An Overview of Priorities and Needs." In *Preventing Unsafe Abortion and its Consequences: Priorities for Research and Action*, edited by I. K. Warriner and I. H. Shah, 1–15 (New York: Guttmacher Institute).

Westoff, C. F. 2005. *Recent Trends in Abortion and Contraception in 12 Countries*. DHS Analytical Studies 8 (Calverton, Md.: ORC Macro).

WHO (World Health Organization). 1967. Resolution WHA20.41: "Health Aspects of Population Dynamics." In *Twentieth World Health Assembly, Geneva, 23 May 1967 (WHA20/1967/Rec/1)* (Geneva: WHO).

WHO (World Health Organization). 2004. World Health Assembly Resolution WHA57.12: "Reproductive Health: Strategy to Accelerate Progress Towards the Attainment of International Development Goals and Targets" (Geneva: WHO). http://apps.who.int/gb/ebwha/pdf_files/WHA57/A57_R12.en.pdf.

WHO (World Health Organization). 2011a. *Preventing Gender-Biased Sex Selection: An OHCHR, UNFPA, UNICEF, UN Women and WHO Interagency Statement* (Geneva: WHO). http://www.who.int/reproductivehealth/publications/gender_rights/9789241501460/en/.

WHO (World Health Organization). 2011b. *Unsafe Abortion: Global and Regional Estimates of the Incidence of Unsafe Abortion and Associated Mortality in 2008*. 6th ed. (Geneva: Department of Reproductive Health and Research). http://www.who.int/reproductivehealth/publications/unsafe_abortion/9789241501118/en/.

WHO (World Health Organization). 2012. *Safe Abortion: Technical and Policy Guidance for Health Systems*. 2nd ed. (Geneva: WHO). http://who.int/reproductivehealth/publications/unsafe_abortion/9789241548434/en/.

WHO (World Health Organization). 2015. *Health Worker Roles in Providing Safe Abortion Care and Post-abortion Contraception* (Geneva: WHO). http://www.who.int/reproductivehealth/publications/unsafe_abortion/abortion-task-shifting/en/.

WHO (World Health Organization). 2017. "Preventing Unsafe Abortion." WHO Fact Sheet. http://www.who.int/mediacentre/factsheets/fs388/en/.

Woog, V., Singh, S., Browne, A., and Philbin, J. 2015. *Adolescent Women's Need for and Use of Sexual and Reproductive Health Services in Developing Countries* (New York: Guttmacher Institute). www.guttmacher.org/pubs/Adolescent-SRHS-Need-Developing-Countries.pdf.

CHAPTER 36

ACCESS TO PREGNANCY-RELATED SERVICES: PUBLIC HEALTH ETHICS ISSUES

ANNE DRAPKIN LYERLY, ELANA JAFFE, AND MARGARET OLIVIA LITTLE

Introduction

Access to pregnancy-related services raises several important issues for public health ethics. Most obvious are inequalities in access to services that are critical to important health outcomes for the pregnant woman and her child.[1] Access to focused antenatal care saves lives, as newborns are 40–50 percent more likely to die in the first month of life if mothers have not received antenatal care (Vintzileos et al., 2002). Access to skilled birth attendants and other evidence-based interventions, such as magnesium sulfate for eclampsia prevention, are associated with reduced rates of maternal mortality (Nour, 2008). Yet there are enormous disparities between and within countries in access to such interventions, raising issues of justice. For instance, Millennium Development Goal 5 for 2015 was universal access to antenatal care, yet the global average of women accessing the World Health Organization's (WHO's) recommended minimum of four antenatal care visits is only around 60 percent (UNICEF, 2018; WHO, 2016). Even within high-income countries, disparities in outcomes, including maternal mortality, are significant and problematic (APHA, 2011). A critical issue for public health ethics is addressing the often complex sources of these inequalities, and working toward universal access to the key health care services that reduce maternal and neonatal mortality and morbidity.

But there is another layer to public health ethics and pregnancy-related services that is less well explored. Much of pregnancy-related care is about provision of services and care whose value or utility is not primarily or exhaustively about direct medical benefit. These include access to termination for women who do not want to become mothers; access to assistance in achieving a biologically related child; and access to meaningful choice and control in how a woman will give birth, care for her newborn, and integrate parenting, work, and future reproductive planning. These are services that merit highly personal decisions, and that intersect with individual and societal values in ways that can be hidden, contested, and varied.

For instance, when describing barriers to access to pregnancy-related services, implicit value judgments about *whose* reproduction is valued can inform and tacitly shape analyses regarding fertility, and whether to assist or control it. Social scientists have coined the term "stratified reproduction" to characterize differences in how fertility, reproduction, and maternity in some groups are valued and ascribed meaning compared to other groups (Harris and Wolfe, 2014). Stratified reproduction is emblematized by the shameful history in the United States of eugenic sterilization programs that targeted immigrants as well as individuals who were working class, poor, mentally disabled, or racial minorities. But stratified reproduction continues to operate today, albeit in more nuanced ways. It manifests as implicit biases about whose reproduction is valued (and how), which in turn shape access to a range of reproductive and pregnancy-related services.

More familiar are ways in which certain pregnancy-related services run into profoundly contested values. Access to abortion is the obvious example. Much discussion has addressed whether and under what conditions abortion services should be made available, as well as what individuals or institutions should pay for or provide them (Stulberg, Jackson, and Freedman, 2016). More subtle, though, if only because they shadow public health discussions even for those generally supportive of abortion access, are discussions of selective abortion for disability or sex, and how public health decisions about access should frame the values at stake.

Further, even when values are not publicly contested in the way they are for abortion, many important pregnancy-related services involve value-based decisions, where women's individual values are known to differ, raising complex questions about how public health programs should intersect with individuals' important personal priorities. Many decisions around pregnancy are less like decisions about setting broken bones (i.e., clear directives based on medical utility calculations), and more like decisions around end of life care (i.e., deeply laden with personal values, bodily integrity, and issues of existential meaning), with a wide range of reasonable decisions that ideally are not only tolerated but supported with information, contextualized counseling, sympathetic alliance, and access to required care consistent with individuals' value- and evidence-informed choices. Yet this ideal masks the challenges and ethical trade-offs that are inherent in such contexts. Accommodating choice itself comes with costs, including social resources. And biases about the "correct" or "most reasonable" choice can affect institutional structures in often hidden ways.

In this chapter we highlight issues in this deeper layer of public health ethics around pregnancy-related services by exploring illustrative examples from two areas of maternity care: access to prenatal testing, and access to preferred modes of birth. In each case we highlight the ways in which issues of access are complicated by social and cultural ideas about what is valued; discuss contested questions about what is ethically responsible or required of patients, providers, and public health systems in these reproductive health contexts; and address areas of needed research and further ethical analysis.

Pregnancy: Access to Prenatal Testing

Antenatal care is a prime example of a service whose remit has been expanding in ways that magnify several underlying ethical complexities inherent to health care. Prenatal genetic testing[2] is a paradigm case. Driven by a range of factors—including a focus on genetics and health, advancing technologies that predict illness with less expense and less intervention, and financial incentives—prenatal testing has become an expected part of many antenatal care programs. Certainly this is true in high-income countries (HICs). For example, the American College of Obstetricians and Gynecologists (ACOG, 2016) now recommends that all pregnant women, regardless of age, "be offered the option of aneuploidy screening or diagnostic testing for fetal genetic disorders." Prenatal genetic testing has also been increasingly deployed in low- and middle-income countries (LMICs), notably reflected in the 2010 resolution on the prevention and care of birth defects by the World Health Assembly and the 2011 WHO publication of the first global report on community genetic services in LMICs (WHO, 2012). With the advent of new tests for cell-free fetal DNA in maternal serum, the use of prenatal genetic testing is widely expected to increase, given that these screening tests can be done starting as early as nine weeks of gestation, do not require particular technical skill or instrumentation, do not present immediate risk for the woman or fetus, and can indicate certain genetic abnormalities with high sensitivity and specificity at low cost.

Yet the public health community and relevant governing bodies have struggled with how to think about the role of prenatal genetic testing in health agendas. Certainly, in LMICs, challenging questions persist about how these services compare with foundational antenatal care as ethical priorities for scarce resources. More broadly, though, there are ethical challenges that exist across economic contexts.

For instance, there are deep value-based tensions about how to appropriately frame the social value of prenatal genetic testing. When prenatal genetic testing is offered, it is often done under the rubric of a "preventive" service. Yet, as the disability rights community has made vivid, this characterization is problematic (Parens and Asch, 2003). While most preventive services are aimed at preventing a disease (e.g., blood pressure screening to prevent a woman from developing pre-eclampsia), prenatal testing is aimed—primarily at least—at preventing a birth of an affected child. Down syndrome, for example, can only be prevented by preventing birth, though some of its attendant morbidities, such as heart defects, can be treated and their effects mitigated. Indeed, some have offered that there may be health-related benefits to prenatal diagnosis, such as planning for risk-appropriate delivery location and, in rare contexts, therapeutic intervention before birth. Treatment prospects notwithstanding, for the most part, prevention in the context of prenatal genetic testing is achieved through abortion of the entity that would experience disease, rather than preventing a disease harm to an extant person; abortion rates after Down syndrome diagnosis range from approximately 67 percent in the United States to nearly 100 percent in Iceland (Natoli et al., 2012). Such testing cannot be justified by the usual case for advancing the health status of the person who would have disease.

Further, prenatal genetic testing raises vexing ethical questions about the proper role of public health in selective abortion. Clearly, there are general disagreements about the morality of abortion. But terminations based on characteristics of the fetus, including sex and congenital abnormalities, can raise distinct concerns even among those who view abortion in other contexts as morally permissible. If used for sex selection, there are concerns that prenatal testing may reinforce the gendered norms it might be expected to redress. Also, the disability community has raised serious concerns about abortion based on congenital abnormality. What is perceived as a disability stems from a lack of experience with or understanding of a condition; notions of disability are often determined by social institutions and structures that privilege the interests of those with certain intellectual or physical abilities over others; and difference is often turned into disadvantage rather than appreciated as intrinsic to the condition itself. Furthermore, the value of the information gained from prenatal testing varies by context. For example, it is only when women have access to care at high-quality medical centers that prenatal testing may have a role in diagnosing a fetal condition that is possible to repair; conversely, the value of prenatal testing (particularly when it uses limited public health resources) is less certain in contexts where neither medically advanced services nor termination are accessible. These are not just debates over how to set priorities; they interrogate how to understand what values and whose interests are at issue in ensuring access to selective abortion. And the nature and role of these values and interests is contested.

There is yet another layer here. Many believe that, as important as the cultural criticism of selective abortion is, at the end of the day women should have the ability to make choices about their reproductive life, including such private and personal matters as whether to test for or give birth to a child with a disability, and whether or not they are financially or emotionally able to care for a child with disabilities. Reproductive choice as such emerges as a second-order and critical goal for all women, not just those with financial and other resources. Even here, though, there is a distinct group of ethical challenges to ensuring meaningful access to prenatal testing that has nothing to do with either access or dollars, but rather with the ways in which a test is made available.

First are the challenges that arise out of the important but often blurred distinction between *offering* and *recommending* a test or intervention in the context of elective and value-laden care—and that manifest in how the day-to-day exchanges between health care providers and patients relate to public health guidelines (Little et al., 2008). For instance, in the state of California, all medical care providers since 1986 have been required to inform patients in their second trimester of pregnancy about the Prenatal Screening Program, a statewide service that provides optional prenatal screening and follow-up diagnostic testing to all women in the state (California Department of Health, 2018). Notice that the requirement is that patients be *informed* of the *optional* program—not that they actually undergo screening or testing.

But as several studies have demonstrated, with the routinization of testing, the message has shifted, and access to informed decision-making has been constrained (Press and Browner, 1994). First, routinization can lead patients to believe that a test *offered* in the context of pregnancy—particularly one with no immediate medical risks and which can provide information about the health of the fetus—is *recommended* (Little et al., 2008). Second, it can obscure the merits and even the possibility of *not* undergoing testing: patients may not be informed about or appreciate the emotional stress and morally complicated choices that testing can engender (Suter, 2002). Indeed, as testing of the fetal genome has expanded to include such technologies as genomic microarray, genomic variations of uncertain significance can be experienced as "toxic"—creating anxiety both among women who carry their pregnancy to term and those who end it (Bernhardt et al., 2013). And third, women who decline testing—particularly those at elevated risk because of age or other factors—may face repeated pressure to undergo testing despite their informed choice (Rapp, 1994; Press and Browner, 1997).

No doubt, practitioners and institutions in some clinical settings have held fast to the importance of patient-centered decision-making and have worked to ensure meaningful informed consent for their patients, including clearing space for decisions to decline screening or forego invasive testing in the context of elevated risk, or referrals to genetic counselors. Even here, there is a further set of challenges, ensconced in guidelines and manifested in the way that results are reported and options are framed—indeed in the very notion of "elevated risk." For instance, the threshold of risk at which a test is deemed "abnormal" is based on presumptions that do not reflect the range of values that women bring to the prenatal testing context (Kuppermann et al., 2004). As Kuppermann and others have argued, in the United States this threshold has been linked to the risk of having an affected fetus for a healthy thirty-five-year-old woman (Kuppermann et al., 2000). It turns out that this risk is roughly equal to the risk that was associated with procedure-related miscarriage among women undergoing invasive testing. But, of course, individual women vastly differ in their views of the two outcomes. There is no recoverable generalized trade-off between the outcomes—reflecting again challenges to ensuring informed decisions about, and meaningful access to, this important if contested pregnancy-related service.

Birth: Access to Maternity Care Options

As the prenatal testing context makes clear, how public health interventions should ensure access in the context of pregnancy is a value-laden issue. Maternity care also reflects this extra layer of complexity. Should the focus be put on improving delivery care in medical institutions or improving resources for deliveries occurring in the range of settings, including freestanding birth centers and homes? Safety remains a top priority of public health interventions around birth, but disagreement around quality measures complicates how delivery of care is evaluated by standards of established public health ethics frameworks. Further, once a threshold of safety can be established, other aspects of giving birth that matter deeply to women come to the fore, raising questions about how they should inform public health approaches to maternity care.

The process of shaping interventions to ensure safety often gets entangled in disputes about what is a "normal" or a "good" birth. It is pertinent here to consider varying definitions of a "normal" or "good" birth, and to question who has access to them. Conceptions of what comprises a "good birth" vary, both on a cultural level and on an individual level. Central to reproductive justice is the ability of individuals to make their own choices about reproduction, including decisions about whether, when, and under what conditions they would like to give birth. A focus on patient preference and access to services is crucial and goes hand in hand with examining differing standards to measure the quality of maternity care.

From the standpoint of medical obstetrics, the "success" of a birth is usually measured in terms of discrete health outcomes (e.g., rates of prematurity, Apgar scores, hemorrhage, NICU [neonatal intensive care unit] transfer, maternal or neonatal mortality). In contrast, within the midwifery literature, the "success" of a birth is often measured by its physiologic "normalcy" which usually tracks with avoidance of medical intervention (e.g., birth without anesthesia or instrumentation). Yet neither of these approaches fully captures the priorities of those giving birth (Lyerly, 2013). Those who may need medical intervention—say a person for whom labor is unsafe because of previous uterine surgery—will not have access to a "good" birth according to the midwifery model standards, due to a medical indication for a cesarean section. On the flip side, a woman who experiences a difficult or traumatic birth (especially in a hospital setting), but from which she and her baby emerge physically healthy, may find her story of difficulty to be discounted due to the view in obstetrics that good medical outcomes should be "enough." Described as the "birth wars," these polarizing frameworks often leave women stuck between opposing narratives of what comprises a "good" birth—and without a narrative that captures what it is that they themselves value in the birthing process (Lyerly, 2013).

This conflict is further reflected in the ways that biomedical and global health policy interventions are working toward shaping the developing maternity care systems of

LMIC countries. Take, for example, conditional cash transfer programs that incentivize women to give birth in medical institutions. Many countries have implemented such programs, which conceptually equate "safer delivery" with "institutional delivery" (Lim et al., 2010; Barrett et al., 2016). However, a major critique of these initiatives is that parallel efforts have not been made to ensure that the respective health care systems have the facilities or capacities to accommodate or ensure quality care for increased institutional births. Nepal's Safe Delivery Inventive Program and India's Janani Suraksha Yojana initiatives failed to significantly decrease neonatal mortality and maternal mortality (respectively) among women who received incentives and gave birth in institutions or with a skilled attendant present (Lim et al., 2010; Gaarder, Glassman, and Todd, 2010).

Evaluations of a program in Cambodia made vivid the reasons that many women did not deliver in hospitals even with a voucher incentive, including transportation constraints, an inability to leave home given child-care responsibilities, and poor staff attitudes at health centers (Ir et al., 2010). All participants pointed to a strong preference for home delivery. Indeed, the authors note that many who did participate in the program already had access to skilled birth attendants at home, raising the question of whether the program served those most in need. Improving safety of delivery is therefore likely to depend not simply on clearing a path to birth in medical centers, but also on ensuring home births are attended by skilled health care providers. Not only does the preference for facility-based birth fail to attend to the priorities and desires of childbearing women, but it also often fails to achieve optimal health outcomes for those most at risk for harm.

There is also a way in which increased accessibility of interventions can set back maternal and infant health interests. For example, increasing rates of cesareans demonstrate how overuse of technology can occur as an unintended consequence of a confluence of policy, technology, and shifting cultural norms. The WHO estimates that approximately 15 percent of cesarean sections are medically necessary (WHO, 2015). When countries have rates significantly lower than that, there is cause to worry that women are not receiving medically necessary care. Yet the opposite concern has also emerged, particularly in HIC countries like the United States, where the cesarean rate rose 60 percent between 1996 and 2009, and now is around 32 percent (Martin et al. 2018). Cesareans, like any operation, carry risks, such as infection, hemorrhage, and complications of anesthesia. Additionally, a prior cesarean creates increased risks for future deliveries, whether vaginal or cesarean (WHO, 2015). Higher than medically necessary rates of cesareans mean childbearing women will face higher levels of risk, and for non-medical reasons. Elevated rates of cesarean in the United States reflect several such non-medical factors, among them liability concerns, constraints on patient choice, hospital policy, and cultural valuation of a medicalized birth. Efforts to remedy inequalities in access to medical care do not always address such complex questions around when and under what circumstances a procedure is beneficial. When a medical center–based birth or a cesarean is explicitly or structurally incentivized in an implementation program or public health system, the question of how to ensure appropriate access to maternity care is ethically complex.

These examples illustrate that when prenatal care focuses on a narrow or unexamined set of services, and when resources are focused on improving access to those specific services, many women are either left behind entirely or experience care shaped by values they do not share, resulting in inequalities endemic to and often perpetuated by the current public health infrastructure. Institutional structures, including procedural and administrative issues such as staffing patterns, can put pressure on women's meaningful access to certain types of services, especially for those whose idea of valued care, while reasonable, does not match those of an aggregated mean or majority (Obstetrics and Gynecology Risk Research Group et al., 2009).

The rate of cesarean sections in the United States also serves as an example of stratified access to delivery services. Women on Medicaid—a public health insurance program in the United States—were more likely to report an inability to plan a vaginal birth after cesarean than women with private insurance, and also more likely to report provider unwillingness to accommodate vaginal birth after cesarean (VBAC) requests (Childbirth Connection, 2013). Thus, how a birth occurs is all too often related not to patient "choice" but to identity and correlative social determinants of health. Between 2008 and 2010, Medicaid funded 48 percent of births in the United States, as well as the greatest number of births in the American South, where there are higher numbers of black and Hispanic people enrolled in Medicaid (Kaiser Family Foundation, 2015; Markus et al., 2013). Among births supported by Medicaid, people of color were more likely to feel as though they did not have a choice in their birthing attendant/obstetrics provider, and were more likely to "report poor treatment" in hospitals (Childbirth Connection, 2013). Doula services—preferred by many and associated with shorter labors and lower rates of cesarean and instrumental births—are not covered by Medicaid.

Thus, access to appropriate maternity care is stratified in a way that is reinforced by the current system. While the global maternal mortality rate is declining, the rate in the United States is rising and is significantly higher than in other HICs. Despite significant investment in the US health care system and the fact that the public cost of maternal and newborn care is much higher than in other developed countries, the majority of maternal deaths in the United States are preventable (Agrawal, 2015). In addition, maternal mortality is correlated to race, ethnicity, and socioeconomic status in the United States—in 2005 the rate of maternal mortality for black women was almost four times the rates for Hispanic and white women (Kung et al., 2008; APHA, 2011).

For some, meaningful access to delivery care includes hospital care and medical intervention, while for others it is the ability to choose a delivery option that minimizes medical intervention and is more cost-effective, such as a delivery at a birthing center or a home birth. For some, it means access to anesthesia during labor (e.g., an epidural), while for others it is having their decision to refuse an epidural respected. Meaningful and equal access on an individual level means that all people who are giving birth be advised and informed respectfully and neutrally about the risks and benefits of all options, and be given a choice in the setting, manner, and companionship for delivery. "Respectful maternity care" advocates work both nationally and globally to improve access to and quality of maternity care. But there is complexity even here. Some advocate for a strong shift toward evidence-based practice, while others give attention to nuance, noting that what counts as evidence can be shaped by priorities of the research community and cultural understandings, as well as by challenges to understanding, interpreting, and applying clinically the assessments of risk in the context of pregnancy (De Vries and Lemmens, 2006; Lyerly et al., 2009).

Conclusion

Issues of access in pregnancy-related care must attend to broad issues of justice and access, as well as to the often very particular ways that pregnancy services are valued, debated, and made available to women who might—or might not—benefit from them. Maternity care is in many ways an issue at the crux of public health and ethics, as it is the literal first step in improving health outcomes for individuals in the global community. It is also an arena that intersects with deeply personal, varied, and sometimes contested values. Those charged with developing, evaluating, and deploying pregnancy-related services for the public health sphere need to be mindful of several critical issues: values vary among women—and can change over the course of a given woman's life; vigilance is required to limit the harms from biases of stratified reproduction, in which some women's reproduction is valued but that of others is not; and pregnancy-related care must be mindfully shaped around the lives of the women who need it in order to remain ethically relevant.

Notes

1. Although we use the term *women* throughout this chapter, we recognize that not all individuals with female reproductive systems identify as women. The ethical complexities we discuss are meant to be inclusive of the intersectionality of individuals who do not identify as women but can become pregnant and give birth.
2. Used here, the term *prenatal genetic testing* includes screening tests that use serologic tests, maternal age and history, and sometimes ultrasound to offer a likelihood of fetal aneuploidy; and also invasive diagnostic testing that can definitively diagnose a genetic disorder by testing amniotic fluid or chorionic villous tissue.

References

Agrawal, P. 2015. "Maternal Mortality and Morbidity in the United States of America." *Bulletin of the World Health Organization* 93: 135.

American College of Obstetrics and Gynecology. 2016. "Practice Bulletin No. 162: Prenatal Diagnostic Testing for Genetic Disorders." *Obstetrics and Gynecology* 127(5): e108–e122.

APHA (American Public Health Association). 2011. "Reducing US Maternal Mortality as a Human Right." Policy Number 201114. https://www.apha.org/policies-and-advocacy/public-health-policy-statements/policy-database/2014/07/11/15/59/reducing-us-maternal-mortality-as-a-human-right/.

Barrett, D. H., Ortmann, L. H., Dawson, A., Saenz, C., Reis, A., and Bolan, G., eds. 2016. *Public Health Ethics: Cases Spanning the Globe*. Vol. 3 (Cham, Switzerland: Springer International).

Bernhardt, B. A., Soucier, D., Hanson, K., Savage, M. S., Jackson, L., and Wapner, R. J. 2013. "Women's Experiences Receiving Abnormal Prenatal Chromosomal Microarray Testing Results." *Genetics in Medicine* 15 (2): 139–145.

California Department of Health. 2018. "California Prenatal Screening Program." https://www.cdph.ca.gov/Programs/CFH/DGDS/Pages/pns/default.aspx.

Childbirth Connection. 2013. "Listen to Mothers: Surveying the Experience of Birth." Medscape. https://www.medscape.com/viewarticle/809905_1.

De Vries, R., and Lemmens, T. 2006. "The Social and Cultural Shaping of Medical Evidence: Case Studies from Pharmaceutical Research and Obstetric Science." *Social Science & Medicine* 62 (11): 2694–2706.

Gaarder, M. M., Glassman, A., and Todd, J. E. 2010. "Conditional Cash Transfers and Health: Unpacking the Causal Chain." *Journal of Development Effectiveness* 2(1): 6–50.

Harris, L. H., and Wolfe, T. 2014. "Stratified Reproduction, Family Planning Care and the Double Edge of History." *Current Opinion in Obstetrics and Gynecology* 26(6): 539–544.

Ir, P., Horemans, D., Souk, N., and Damme W. V. 2010. "Using Targeted Vouchers and Health Equity Funds to Improve Access to Skilled Birth Attendants for Poor Women: A Case Study in Three Rural Health Districts in Cambodia." *BMC Pregnancy and Childbirth* 10(1): 1. https://bmcpregnancychildbirth.biomedcentral.com/articles/10.1186/1471-2393-10-1.

Kaiser Family Foundation. 2015. "Births Financed by Medicaid." https://www.kff.org/medicaid/state-indicator/births-financed-by-medicaid/.

Kung, H. C., Hoyert, D. L., Xu, J. Q., and Murphy, S. L. 2008. "Deaths: Final Data for 2005." *National Vital Statistics Reports* 56(10): 1–120. https://www.cdc.gov/nchs/data/nvsr/nvsr56/nvsr56_10.pdf.

Kuppermann, M., Nease, R. F., Jr., Gates, E., Learman, L. A., Blumberg, B., Gildengorin, V., et al. 2004. "How Do Women of Diverse Backgrounds Value Prenatal Testing Outcomes?" *Prenatal Diagnosis* 24 (6): 424–429.

Kuppermann, M., Nease, R. F., Jr., Learman, L. A., Gates, E., Blumberg, B., and Washington, A.E. 2000. "Procedure-Related Miscarriages and Down Syndrome–Affected Births: Implications for Prenatal Testing Based on Women's Preferences." *Obstetrics and Gynecology* 96(4): 511–516.

Lim, S. S., Dandona, L., Hoisington, J. A., James, S. L., Hogan, M. C., and Gakidou, E. 2010. "India's Janani Suraksha Yojana, a Conditional Cash Transfer Programme to Increase Births in Health Facilities: An Impact Evaluation." *Lancet* 375(9730): 2009–2023.

Little, M. O., Lyerly, A. D., Mitchell, L. M., Armstrong, E. M., Harris, L. H., Kukla, R. et al. 2008. "Mode of Delivery: Toward Responsible Inclusion of Patient Preferences." *Obstetrics and Gynecology* 112(4): 913–918.

Lyerly, A. 2013. *A Good Birth: Finding the Positive and Profound in Your Childbirth Experience* (New York: Penguin Group).

Lyerly, A. D., Mitchell L. M., Armstrong E. M., Harris, L. H., Kukla, R., Kuppermann, M., et al. 2009. "RISK and the Pregnant Body." *Hastings Center Report* 39(6): 34–42.

Markus, A. R., Andres, E., West, K. D., Garro, N., and Pellegrini C. 2013. "Medicaid Covered Births, 2008 through 2010, in the Context of the Implementation of Health Reform." *Women's Health Issues* 23 (5): e273, 280.

Martin J. A., Hamilton B. E., Osterman M. J. K., Driscoll A. K., and Drake P. 2018. "Births: Final Data for 2017." National Vital Statistics Reports 67(8): 1–50. https://www.cdc.gov/nchs/data/nvsr/nvsr67/nvsr67_08-508.pdf.

Natoli, J. L., Ackerman, D. L., McDermott, S., and Edwards, J. G. 2012. "Prenatal Diagnosis of Down Syndrome: A Systematic Review of Termination Rates (1995–2011)." *Prenatal Diagnosis* 32(2): 142–153.

Nour, N. M. 2008. "An Introduction to Maternal Mortality." *Reviews in Obstetrics and Gynecology* 1(2): 77–81.

Obstetrics and Gynecology Risk Research Group, Kukla, R., Kuppermann, M., Little, M., Lyerly, A. D., Mitchell, L. M., et al. 2009. "Finding Autonomy in Birth." *Bioethics* 23(1): 1–8.

Parens, E., and Asch, A. 2003. "Disability Rights Critique of Prenatal Genetic Testing: Reflections and Recommendations." *Mental Retardation and Developmental Disabilities Research Reviews* 9(1): 40–47.

Press, N. A., and Browner, C. H. 1994. "Collective Silences, Collective Fictions: How Prenatal Diagnostic Testing Became Part of Routine Prenatal Care." In *Women and Prenatal Testing: Facing the Challenges of Genetic Technology*, edited by K. Rothenberg and E. J. Thomson, 201–218 (Columbus: Ohio State University Press).

Press, N. A., and Browner, C. H. 1997. "Why Women Say Yes to Prenatal Diagnosis." *Social Science and Medicine* 45 (7): 979–989.

Rapp, R. 1994. "Women's Responses to Prenatal Diagnosis: A Sociocultural Perspective on Diversity." In *Women and Prenatal Testing: Facing the Challenges of Genetic Technology*, edited by K. Rothenberg and E. J. Thomson, 219–233 (Columbus: Ohio State University Press).

Stulberg, D. B., Jackson, R. A., and Freedman, L. R. 2016. "Referrals for Services Prohibited in Catholic Health Care Facilities." *Perspectives on Sexual and Reproductive Health* 48(3): 111–17.

Suter, S. M. 2002. "The Routinization of Prenatal Testing." *American Journal of Law and Medicine* 28: 233–270.

UNICEF (United Nations Children's Fund). 2018. "Only Half of Women Worldwide Receive the Recommended Amount of Care during Pregnancy." https://data.unicef.org/topic/maternal-health/antenatal-care/.

Vintzileos, A. M., Ananth, C. V., Smulian, J. C., Scorza, W. E., and Knuppel R. A. 2002. "The Impact of Prenatal Care on Neonatal Deaths in the Presence and Absence of Antenatal High-Risk Conditions." *American Journal of Obstetrics and Gynecology* 186(5): 1011–16.

WHO (World Health Organization). 2012. "Screening the Genes." *Bulletin of the World Health Organization* 90(8): 557–632.

WHO (World Health Organization). 2015. "WHO Statement on Caesarean Section Rates." https://apps.who.int/iris/bitstream/handle/10665/161442/WHO_RHR_15.02_eng.pdf.

WHO (World Health Organization). 2016. "Pregnant Women Must Be Able to Access the Right Care at the Right Time, Says WHO." News Release, November 7, WHO Media Centre. http://www.who.int/news-room/detail/07-11-2016-pregnant-women-must-be-able-to-access-the-right-care-at-the-right-time-says-who.

SECTION EIGHT

COMMUNICABLE DISEASES

CHAPTER 37

AN OVERVIEW OF ETHICS, PUBLIC HEALTH, AND COMMUNICABLE DISEASES

HOLLY A. TAYLOR

INTRODUCTION

THERE are at least three key factors, alone and in combination, that are relevant to the ethics of the public health response to communicable diseases: ease of transmission, the severity of disease, and the availability of effective prevention and treatment. In general, as both the ease of transmission and the severity of a disease increase, public health authorities need to consider whether infected or exposed individuals should be separated from the general public. Consider tuberculosis (TB) and human immunodeficiency virus (HIV). Both are most likely to be transmitted from person to person when the mycobacterium or virus is not suppressed with treatment. But TB, which is airborne, is much more easily transmitted from person to person than HIV, which requires an exchange of bodily fluids. Anyone near a TB patient with active, untreated TB is at risk of exposure. The ease of transmission and resulting risk to the community can therefore justify the adoption of interventions that limit the free movement of the individual with TB (Coker et al., 2007). In such a situation, the principle of beneficence (i.e., protecting the community from harm) is in tension with the respect owed to the individual.

Severity of disease is also important in terms of how readily public health authorities will and should consider adopting interventions that may restrict movement to prevent transmission of disease. For example, during the 2014–2015 Ebola outbreak in West

Africa, public health authorities were quick to recommend the isolation and quarantine of those diagnosed and exposed (Nyenswah et al., 2015).

Finally, the availability of effective prevention and treatment can dramatically reduce—at both the individual and the public health level—the risks of contracting or dying from an infectious disease. As such, when diseases are severe and easily spread, public health has often mandated preventive interventions when the risk of the intervention is considered far less significant than the risk of the disease. The near eradication of childhood diseases such as measles and mumps in the United States can be attributed to the requirement that children be vaccinated before they start school (Ventola, 2016).

This section of *The Oxford Handbook of Public Health Ethics* is devoted to examining the ethical issues relevant to the prevention and treatment of communicable disease. These issues can vary based on multiple factors, including ease of disease transmission, the severity of disease, and the availability of effective approaches to disease prevention and treatment. A chapter on immunization is followed by chapters in which specific diseases are used to raise a number of ethical considerations; namely, tuberculosis (TB), mosquito-borne illnesses, and HIV/AIDS.

Chapter Overviews

Immunization is arguably *the* most important advance in public health in terms of its ability, through a single technology, to successfully prevent morbidity and mortality. At the same time, it generates a paradigmatic ethical tension often found at the core of public health debates: When does the likely benefit to others result in justifiable infringement of individual liberty? While immunization has a direct benefit to individuals who are vaccinated, the true public health benefit of the intervention comes when enough individuals are vaccinated to interrupt the spread of the infectious agent in an entire community.

While vaccination can result in harm to an individual, immunization only becomes incorporated into public health policy when the risk of harm from vaccination is considerably less, on a population level, than suffering from the illness it is intended to prevent. In "Immunization and Ethics: Beneficence, Coercion, Public Health, and the State," James Colgrove points out that the first debates about the uptake of vaccines came with the development of a smallpox vaccine in the 1700s. The state of biomedical science at the time meant that vaccination indeed came with many more risks than any vaccine produced today, but it was also generally effective at preventing an otherwise deadly disease. Very early in the history of immunization policy, various "states" made vaccination mandatory, placing the benefits to the community above the rights of the individual to abstain. As much as *Jacobson v. Massachusetts* (197 U.S. 11 [1905]) is a landmark in US public health law and ethics, it is also a landmark in immunization policy. The case, decided in 1905, endorsed the state's power to mandate vaccination.

Colgrove notes that the key argument in the case was that an individual who refuses vaccination might bring harm to another person.

Colgrove goes on to provide a critical analysis of additional ethical arguments in favor of compulsory vaccination—the harm principle, the prevention of free riders, and *parens patriae*— while also discussing nonmedical exemption laws across the United States and related legal challenges posed by outbreaks of infectious disease long considered eradicated from the United States. The author evaluates two cases—the compulsory human papillomavirus (HPV) vaccination of middle schoolers, and influenza vaccination of health care workers—to articulate the myriad of ethics factors to consider when deciding whether to adopt a mandatory vaccination policy. Finally, Colgrove considers the ethics of vaccine scarcity in the context of public health emergencies and public policy surrounding compensation for vaccine injury.

The ethical issues relevant to a public health response to an infectious disease pandemic can be illustrated with a case study of TB. According to the World Health Organization, in 2016 more than 10 million individuals were diagnosed with TB (WHO, 2017). TB is also the leading cause of death of those with HIV (WHO, 2017). While TB remains a global disease, the burden of disease has settled on those living in low- and middle-income countries, disadvantaging already disadvantaged populations. As an airborne infectious disease, TB thrives in overcrowded communities that lack access to basic knowledge and means to prevent transmission. Diego Silva and Michael Selgelid begin the next chapter, "Prevention and Treatment of Tuberculosis in Low- and Middle-Income Countries: Ethical Challenges," with an overview of the epidemiology of TB and the emergence of TB strains resistant to some or all of the current treatments available. The authors then take on three ethical challenges faced when responding to TB: isolation, third-party notification, and incorporating new TB medications into an already complex treatment regimen. The use of isolation in the case of an airborne virus is a straightforward example of where the harm principle can be invoked. While nonresistant TB can be made noninfectious rather quickly with strict adherence to treatment, an untreated patient or a patient who struggles with compliance can become a threat to the health of others. While the majority of patients understand their status and comply with social distancing advice, there are some for whom isolation may be required as a last resort. The authors argue that in the instance of voluntary or compulsory isolation, the public health authority ought to provide the isolated patient with adequate resources to address her or his basic needs (e.g., adequate food and water) for the duration of the isolation period.

Another ethics challenge for public health in managing TB is when and how to notify third parties about their possible TB exposure. Most patients comply with requests to name those with whom they have been in close contact when told they may have exposed them to TB. Notification of third parties, according to these authors, becomes problematic when the patient also has HIV or refuses to name possible contacts. In the case of the latter, the right of the individual patient to privacy conflicts with the professional responsibility of the public health authority to prevent the further spread of a serious disease within the community.

The chapter concludes with a description of the ethical challenges encountered in the development and dissemination of novel TB medications. The development of novel TB medications has lagged behind the incidence and prevalence of disease. Effective treatment of nonresistant TB requires the ingestion of multiple drugs for up to six months. The treatment of multidrug-resistant TB requires up to twenty-four months of treatment, including a daily painful injection for the first six months. However, this regimen is an effective cure only 50 percent of the time. Noncompliance with either regimen can result in the development and transmission of even deadlier strains of TB. The authors review the recent addition of two new TB medications, neither of which are free of side effects. According to the clinical trials conducted to date, these novel drugs may ease the burden of TB treatment. But the authors note that their effectiveness can be maximized only if the health system is capable of supporting patient adherence and closely monitoring patients for side effects and adverse events, a challenge in low- and middle-income countries with limited resources.

An extraordinary number of individuals globally are threatened each year by infectious diseases spread by mosquitoes. For many of these diseases, interventions targeted at the community, rather than specifically to individuals, is often how public health responds. These community-based interventions raise their own set of ethics considerations. Laura Greisman, Barbara Koenig, and Michele Barry examine these issues in "Control of Mosquito-Borne Illnesses: A Challenge to Public Health Ethics." The authors review ethical issues in surveillance of mosquito-borne illnesses, and then consider the ethical implications of three different interventions: the provision of insecticide-treated nets (ITNs), the spraying of pesticides, and the introduction of genetically modified mosquitoes. Heightening the ethical tension around each of these strategies is uncertainty about the effectiveness of each of these interventions. These strategies also raise unique challenges. ITNs, while considered a community-focused intervention, require the cooperation of the individuals in the community to use the nets as directed. Moreover, the spraying of pesticides or the introduction of genetically modified mosquitoes, while directed at the mosquito, may affect the humans who live in the communities where the interventions are deployed. Ethically, all of these factors require that public health professionals considering the deployment of these interventions first engage the affected communities.

The chapter concludes with a case study of the Zika outbreak in 2015–2016. The case highlights the value of robust surveillance systems as well as the challenges of navigating the ethical issues that surround the maternal-fetal transmission of a virus and balancing the risks of recommending the use of insect repellent and assuring universal access to reproductive health and contraception. The case of Zika is also a reminder that the burden of communicable disease is almost always carried disproportionately by those living in poverty.

A review of the public health response to HIV/AIDS over the last forty years highlights the range of ethical concerns and tensions that arise when responding to an infectious disease. In "Global HIV/AIDS Prevention and Treatment: Public Health

Ethics Considerations," Mark Barnes and Devin Cohen begin this story in the 1980s, when clusters of previously rare diseases began appearing among otherwise healthy individuals. The authors argue that, because those affected were generally members of already stigmatized populations, the policy debates quickly evolved into efforts needed to protect "us against them."

A test for HIV antibodies was developed in 1986. At that time there were no effective treatments for HIV. While testing might result in individuals changing their behavior to reduce transmission to others, their personal prognosis was bleak. Once effective treatments were available, the ethical argument tipped in favor of advocating testing for the benefit of the individual who could access treatment and for the implementation of partner notification programs. This approach has only gained momentum as the development of effective drugs have been developed and made readily available to those in high-income settings. And while access to treatment has improved in low- and middle-income countries, disparities remain. The examples of Cuba and South Africa are a historic and a more contemporary case of national responses to the epidemic. The authors track the advances in HIV treatment from the first trials of AZT, to the landmark trial "ACTG 076," which proved AZT to be effective in preventing mother-to-infant transmission of HIV, to the current array of medications. They also describe efforts to encourage HIV testing among those at greatest risk of infection.

As the effectiveness of HIV treatment advanced, so too did calls for shifts from voluntary, anonymous testing to universal testing and named reporting. Debates swirled about whether to advocate for "opt-in" or "opt-out" policies, trying to balance the autonomy of the individuals involved with the benefits that both knowledge and treatment of HIV could bring to individuals and their intimate contacts, and to the public's health more generally. Barnes and Cohen conclude their chapter with a discussion of the current challenges faced by low- and middle-income countries. Despite the growing number of options to prevent and treat HIV, these countries may lack the financial and human resources to fully support comprehensive efforts.

Conclusion

Two questions dominate the examination of the ethics of infectious disease. First, under what circumstances is it permissible for a public health authority to restrict the movement or liberty of an individual infected with or exposed to a communicable disease, or to require an individual submit to a preventive measure, in the name of preventing the spread of disease? Second, how do conditions of social inequity contribute to infectious disease spread, and what does ethics require in this social context? This section of *The Oxford Handbook of Public Health Ethics*, focused on the public health ethics of communicable diseases, addresses these questions, providing a window into the ethics of much of public health response more broadly.

References

Coker. R., Thomas. M., Lock, K., and Martin, R. 2007. "Detention and the Evolving Threat of Tuberculosis: Evidence, Ethics, and Law." *Journal of Law, Medicine and Ethics* 35(4): 609–615.

Nyenswah, T., Blackley, D. J., Freeman, T., Lindblade, K. A., Arzoaquoi, S. K., Mott, J. A., et al. 2015. "Community Quarantine to Interrupt Ebola Virus Transmission—Mawah Village, Bong County, Liberia, August–October, 2014" *Morbidity and Mortality Weekly Report* 64(7): 179–182.

Ventola, C. L. 2016. "Immunization in the United States: Recommendations, Barriers, and Measures to Improve Compliance, Part 1: Childhood Vaccination." *Pharmacy and Therapeutics* 41(7): 426–436.

WHO (World Health Organization). 2017. "Tuberculosis Fact Sheet." http://www.who.int/mediacentre/factsheets/fs104/en/.

CHAPTER 38

IMMUNIZATION AND ETHICS: BENEFICENCE, COERCION, PUBLIC HEALTH, AND THE STATE

JAMES COLGROVE

INTRODUCTION

IMMUNIZATION against infectious disease is one of the most beneficial and cost-effective public health activities. For more than 200 years, vaccines have reduced rates of sickness and death, improved well-being, and enhanced human flourishing (Plotkin and Plotkin, 2013). A vaccine provides a dual benefit: a direct benefit to the person receiving it, and an indirect benefit to other members of the community through the creation of herd immunity. Thus, there are both self-interested and altruistic reasons for being vaccinated. Like any medical intervention, immunization also carries a risk of adverse events. Most such events are transient and superficial, such as mildly elevated fever or pain at the injection site, but rare serious harms do occur. For example, the oral polio vaccine carries a risk of vaccine-associated paralytic polio in about 1 in 750,000 first doses (WHO, 2015). But in most circumstances, the risk of suffering severe illness or death if one contracts a vaccine-preventable disease is far greater than the risk of suffering an adverse event from the vaccine.

Individual decisions about immunization involve weighing risks and benefits. When the prevalence of a vaccine-preventable disease is high, the benefit to the individual from undergoing vaccination is greatest. As disease prevalence declines, however, the benefits of undergoing vaccination accrue primarily to society as a whole in the form of reduced disease prevalence. Decisions about whether or not to receive a vaccine are influenced by risk perceptions and psychological biases, such as a preference for errors of omission over errors of commission, and for natural over man-made risks.

The more disease incidence declines, the less firsthand experience people have with the disease, and the more they take their freedom from it for granted. Thus, any successful vaccination program eventually becomes a victim of its success. Finally, because most vaccines today are given to infants and children, decisions about immunization may also involve a determination of the best interests of minors and the state's role in safeguarding that interest.

The collective implications of immunization have led states—both national and subnational governments—to enact policies and laws designed to achieve high rates of vaccine coverage among their populations. These policies have been both persuasive and coercive. For example, governments have sponsored educational and promotional efforts through mass media or in school or clinical settings, allocated public funds to pay for a vaccine, required that private health insurers pay for vaccinations, offered incentives to health care providers who achieve high levels of uptake among their patients, and required vaccination as a condition of school or day-care attendance (Briss et al., 2000).

As medical products given to healthy people (mostly children) at least partly for the benefit of others, vaccines raise a uniquely challenging set of ethical questions and a corollary set of legal and policy issues. Chief among these questions are: What ethical obligations do governments have to minimize the risk of vaccine-preventable diseases, and health risks more generally, among their citizens? What ethical obligations do individuals have to be vaccinated, or to assure that their children are vaccinated? What strategies may governments use to achieve high rates of acceptance? How can vaccines be distributed equitably? How should society deal most ethically with the inevitable rare harms that vaccines cause?

Historical Overview of Vaccination Ethics, Law, and Policy

The first vaccine was developed in the 1790s. The ability of this smallpox vaccine to control the spread of one of the most feared killers of the era quickly led to its wide adoption. Nevertheless, smallpox vaccination was well known for causing both minor side effects, such as swollen arms, rashes, and blisters, as well as the rare but severe chance of one death per million doses. Moreover, the relatively crude and often unsanitary procedures for vaccination sometimes led to the transmission of blood-borne illnesses. As smallpox declined in subsequent decades, many people chose to take their chances with the disease rather than undergo what they saw as an unpleasant and risky procedure. In the 1870s, a New York City health official lamented his fellow citizens' complacency toward smallpox and resistance to vaccination: "It is easy to be bold against an absent danger, to despise the antidote while one has no experience of the bane" (cited in Colgrove, 2006, 9).

One strategy that governments used to overcome such reluctance was legal compulsion. In England, the vaccination of all infants was made mandatory in 1853, and parents who refused faced fines or prison terms. Where health officials saw a rational way to guard against the danger of resurgent smallpox, however, many British citizens saw a violation of their bodies that could be painful and even fatal. Legal compulsion thus gave rise to a large and vocal anti-vaccination movement that resisted the law through protests, demonstrations, and riots. The British anti-vaccinationists won a significant victory in 1898, when the government added a "conscience clause" that excused parents who believed that vaccination would harm their children's health, a provision that was expanded in a 1907 act. The effect of these provisions was dramatic. By 1911 only about 56 percent of newborns were being vaccinated (Durbach, 2005). Vaccination was also made mandatory in some circumstances in several other European nations. Germany passed its compulsory vaccination law in 1873, in part because of its experience in the Franco-Prussian War two years earlier, in which German troops suffered lower smallpox mortality than their French opponents, among whom rates of vaccination were lower (Huerkamp, 1985).

During the nineteenth century, compulsory vaccination laws were enacted in some US cities and states in an uneven patchwork that reflected a more decentralized public health system than in Europe. The laws provoked many court challenges from people who considered them a violation of constitutional liberties. Conflicting decisions in these cases culminated in the landmark Supreme Court case *Jacobson v. Massachusetts* (197 U.S. 11 [1905], hereafter *Jacobson*), which held that compulsory vaccination was a legitimate exercise of state governments' "police powers" to guard the health, welfare, safety, and morals of citizens. The ruling's most famous passage offers a robust defense of the right of governments to impose compulsory vaccination:

> The liberty secured by the Constitution of the United States to every person within its jurisdiction does not import an absolute right in each person to be, at all times and in all circumstances, wholly freed from restraint. There are manifold restraints to which every person is necessarily subject for the common good.... Real liberty for all could not exist under the operation of a principle which recognizes the right of each individual person to use his own, whether in respect of his person or his property, *regardless of the injury that may be done to others.* (*Jacobson*, 26, emphasis added)

Thus, a key argument in the *Jacobson* decision is that legal compulsion is justified because people who refuse vaccination may harm others. The next section will examine this claim more closely.

Over the twentieth century, the armamentarium of vaccines steadily expanded. Vaccines against diphtheria, tetanus, and pertussis were developed before World War II (and combined into a single combination vaccine in 1948), and in the postwar era, a flurry of research and development brought forth vaccines against the childhood scourges of polio, measles, mumps, and rubella. As vaccines grew more numerous, a new set of ethical issues related to equity emerged. Uptake of vaccines was uneven, with wide disparities based on socioeconomic status and much lower rates of protection among poor children (Colgrove, 2006). Policies at the federal level have sought to achieve equity in vaccine coverage. In 1993 the US Congress created the Vaccines for Children Program, which provided funding to distribute vaccines free of charge to parents of children eligible for Medicaid, children who lacked insurance, and Native American children (CDC, 2016b). The Vaccines for Children Program covers all vaccines recommended by the Centers for Disease Control and Prevention (CDC) for routine administration (CDC, 2016b). In part as a response to the problem of "underinsurance"—children missing recommended vaccines because their private insurance plan did not cover them—the 2010 Patient Protection and Affordable Care Act (also known as Obamacare) included a provision mandating that health insurers provide coverage for all CDC-recommended vaccines with no cost-sharing (HHS, 2016). Addressing financial barriers was especially important because some new vaccines, including those against invasive pneumococcal disease, meningococcal disease, and human papillomavirus, are much more expensive than older vaccines. Today, the CDC recommends vaccines against fourteen diseases for children zero to six years of age (CDC, 2016a).

Since the 1970s, transnational organizations have sought to increase vaccine uptake worldwide and, more specifically, to address the global disparities in access to vaccines between high- and low-income countries, and thus reduce the disproportionate burden of disease in the latter. The World Health Organization established the Expanded Program on Immunization in 1974 in an effort to provide children in developing countries with access to vaccines against tuberculosis, polio, and measles (Mitchell et al., 2013). Since 2000, the Global Alliance for Vaccines and Immunization (GAVI, now Gavi, The Vaccine Alliance), a public-private partnership involving the Bill and Melinda Gates Foundation, the World Health Organization, UNICEF, and the World Bank, has pursued a similar goal. As of 2015, almost 580 million children have been immunized with Gavi support, and an estimated eight million deaths from ten targeted diseases have been prevented (Gavi, 2016).

One potential benefit of vaccination programs is to provide freedom from disease for future generations. The global campaign to eradicate smallpox through vaccination, one of the most massive public health efforts ever undertaken, achieved success in 1980 (WHO, 1980). Smallpox remains the only human disease to be eradicated. A global campaign to eradicate polio has been under way since 1988; as of 2016, the worldwide incidence of the disease had decreased by more than 99 percent (WHO, 2016).

The Ethics of Compulsory Vaccination

The most controversial ethics question raised by immunization has been whether, or under what circumstances, states may make it compulsory. The most common justification for these policies has been a utilitarian one. Although some members of the community will be harmed by vaccine adverse events, most harms are relatively minor, serious harms are relatively infrequent, and harms are greatly outweighed by resulting gains in health and well-being and reductions in disease incidence. At least two plausible principled justifications may also be offered: the harm principle and the prevention of free riders.

The harm principle, set forth by John Stuart Mill in *On Liberty*, holds that the only justification for coercive action against an individual is the presence of imminent harm to other members of society (Mill, 1863). A person's own good, Mill wrote, is insufficient reason. According to supporters of mandates, people who refuse to be vaccinated or to have their children vaccinated harm others; this is the justification given in the 1905 *Jacobson* ruling. A harm principle–based argument is not iron-clad, however. While being vaccinated clearly benefits others, it is less obvious that the failure to be vaccinated harms others. Many factors influence the likelihood of disease transmission in any given situation, including the prevalence and contagiousness of the infectious agent, and some ethicists have argued that the potential harm that an unvaccinated person poses to other susceptible people in the community is too distal or uncertain to invoke the harm principle (Dare, 1998).

Another potential challenge to a harm principle–based argument is that each individual has within his or her power the ability of self-protection: anyone who wishes to escape contracting a disease can choose to receive a vaccine, and therefore has no moral claim to force another person to receive it (Veatch, 1987). This reasoning is flawed, however. Some people cannot safely undergo vaccination because of medical contraindications, and some people, notably infants, lack the biological capacity to develop immunity in response to a vaccine. Also, no vaccine is 100 percent effective; a small number of people who receive a vaccine will fail to develop the intended immunity (cases known as "vaccine failures"), and it is not practically possible to identify these individuals. All these people may be placed in danger by infectious diseases that unvaccinated members of the community may spread. Therefore, declining to be vaccinated (or declining to have one's child vaccinated) does have other-regarding consequences.

A second potential rationale for the use of compulsion is to prevent the problem of free riders (Diekema and Marcuse, 1998). In economic and political theory, "free riders" are people who use a public good without assuming their fair share of the cost. The herd immunity created by high levels of immunization can plausibly be considered a public good, according to the classic definition: It is nonexcludable (if it is available to some people in the community, it is necessarily available to everyone), and it is nonrivalrous (the protection that one individual derives from it does not diminish another's protection). The optimal situation for the community occurs when each member assumes the small risk of undergoing vaccination in order to protect both himself and the group as a whole, but an individual's most self-interested strategy would be to allow everyone else to assume the small risk of vaccination but avoid vaccination himself.

Herd immunity is also susceptible to another type of collective action problem—what has been termed the "tragedy of the commons" (Hardin, 1968). In this situation, the availability of a shared resource is undermined by self-interested actions. The decision of any one individual in a community to refuse vaccination will not affect the group's protection, but if many people make that choice, herd immunity will eventually be eroded and the community will be left vulnerable to disease outbreaks. Free riding and the tragedy of the commons represent problems of distributive justice, in that the benefits and burdens of immunization are not fairly distributed among all members of society.

A final justification for coercive policies, specifically relevant to childhood immunization, is the principle of *parens patriae* (Silverman and May, 2001). This is the legal doctrine that the state has both a right and a duty to protect minors and incompetent persons from harm. That it is appropriate for the state to intervene to protect minor children from the harmful acts of their parents is well-accepted in both ethics and law, but the question of when society has a right to override parental choice can be far from straightforward. In general, governments give wide discretion to parents to raise their children as they see fit, and they step in only in cases of clear danger to a child.

This issue has sparked controversy in both medical and nonmedical contexts around issues such as compliance with mandatory education laws, prohibitions on child labor, and, most famously, consent for life-saving blood transfusions. A *parens patriae* argument would be strongest when a serious disease is prevalent in the community and would weaken as the incidence or severity of disease declined. Considerations of justice could also complement a *parens patriae* argument. To the extent that compulsory vaccination can be used in conjunction with policies to reduce barriers of cost and access, they can raise coverage rates among socioeconomically disadvantaged children who are less likely to be vaccinated, and thus serve the cause of justice by narrowing systematic disparities in uptake (Morita, Ramirez, and Trick, 2008).

Nonmedical Exemptions to Compulsory Immunization

The principle of least restriction holds that liberty-infringing policies should be implemented in ways that impose the fewest burdens on individual autonomy while still achieving their goals. Compulsory vaccination laws, for example, have been made less burdensome by including exemptions for people with strongly held objections to them. Almost all US states offer exemptions for people with religiously based objections to vaccination, and almost half allow opting out based on philosophical or "personal belief" objections. The arguments that support compulsory vaccination laws as either ethically acceptable or required would, as a corollary, militate against provisions that weaken the effect of these laws. A large literature demonstrates that higher rates of exemptions to compulsory vaccination laws are associated with higher risk of disease outbreaks (Omer et al., 2006, 2008; Atwell et al., 2013). Some public health officials have argued against elimination of nonmedical exemptions, however, on the grounds that such an action would trigger a political backlash that could undermine public trust and support for the immunization system (Opel and Diekema, 2012). An alternate approach, based on the principle of least restriction, would be a policy making exemptions difficult but not impossible to claim. States have implemented various procedural hurdles to parents seeking to opt out, such as requiring educational counseling from a health care provider or annual renewal of the exemption (Diekema, 2014).

It might be argued that vaccine refusal grounded in religious belief warrants greater deference than general philosophical opposition. It is difficult in practice to distinguish between religious beliefs and other strongly held philosophical or moral values, however (Salmon and Siegel, 2001). Although few religions have explicit doctrinal objections to vaccination, many people have found language in sacred texts (such as commandments to keep the body pure before God) that they have interpreted as proscribing vaccination (Colgrove, 2006). It is not clear, moreover, that an individual's religious belief should trump basic duties of nonmaleficence. In a 1944 case, the US Supreme Court held that the "right to practice religion freely does not include liberty to expose the community or the child to communicable disease or the latter to ill health or death" (Veatch, 1987).

Compulsory HPV Immunization of Middle-School Students

Human papillomavirus (HPV) is a common sexually transmitted infection that is associated with cancer of various sites, including cervix, larynx, anus, mouth, and penis. The licensing of the HPV vaccine in 2006 for the prevention of cervical cancer in women, and the subsequent approval in 2009 for the prevention of anal cancer and genital warts in boys, raised a distinct set of ethical issues related to compulsory vaccination. Some religious conservatives argued that it was inappropriate for the state to mandate protection against a disease that is sexually transmitted (Charo, 2007). This reasoning speciously focused on the route of transmission rather than the consequences of the infection, however. School mandates for immunization against hepatitis B, which also can be sexually transmitted and causes a deadly cancer, had been widely adopted and recognized as beneficial previous to HPV licensure.

Some public health advocates, implicitly drawing upon Mill's harm principle, argued that mandates should be used only to prevent imminent danger to third parties from diseases that are casually transmissible (Gostin and DeAngelis, 2007). An alternate ethical reasoning, however, would conclude that HPV vaccine mandates are justified on grounds of justice and beneficence. There is a disproportionate epidemiological burden of cervical cancer in poor women of color, who are less likely to receive regular Pap smears and follow-up after abnormal results (Smith, 2008). Middle school compulsory vaccination against hepatitis B has been shown to raise coverage rates among young people with racial and ethnic minority backgrounds who are less likely to be vaccinated otherwise (Morita, Ramirez, and Trick, 2008). Such effects highlight the ways that vaccination programs can advance health equity.

Health Care Workers and Mandatory Flu Immunization

Although the severity of seasonal influenza varies each year, in recent years it has been responsible for between approximately 3,000 and 49,000 US deaths annually (CDC, 2010), with victims disproportionately older and sicker. Nevertheless, rates of flu vaccine uptake remain low among many health care providers. These rates are of particular public health concern because of the life-saving role health care providers play, and because of the risk they could pose to their patients should they become infected with a contagious airborne infection. Reasons for these low rates vary, including doubts about the vaccine's efficacy, the erroneous belief that the vaccine can cause the flu, and simple inconvenience. Health care organizations have offered a range of incentives to encourage voluntary uptake, with limited success. Since about 2005, many hospitals have enacted mandatory flu vaccination for their employees and have achieved uptake rates of more than 95 percent (Nowalk et al., 2013). The most severe penalty for noncompliance with the policies has been termination; less restrictive alternatives include requirements to wear a mask, restriction from direct patient care duties, and placement on unpaid leave during flu season (Nowalk et al., 2013).

Arguments in favor of these requirements may be grounded not just in the harm principle, but also in professional duties of beneficence and nonmaleficence. Hospitals and health care facilities are settings where disease transmission is more likely to occur, and the consequences are more likely to be severe because of the high number of sick and immune-compromised individuals in them. Codes of medical ethics, from the Hippocratic Oath to contemporary codes in medicine, nursing, and other allied health professions, all emphasize the unique responsibility of health care providers not to place their patients at undue risk of harm. Health care providers are widely recognized to have special duties to promote the well-being of their patients that laypeople are not considered to have toward each other (Cortes-Penfield, 2014).

Vaccine Scarcity and Rationing

Pandemics or emergency situations, during which vaccine supplies may be scarce, raise ethics questions about who should be vaccinated when not all can be. A variety of frameworks for prioritization have been put forth, based on a mixture of principled and consequentialist justifications. They are discussed in turn.

Many systems give first priority to professionals responsible for guarding health, welfare, and public safety. Typically, doctors, nurses, emergency medical technicians, and people directly involved in the production and distribution of vaccines are included in the first priority tier, but those providing police and fire protection or performing other essential societal functions, such as food transportation and distribution, may also be included (Arras, 2005). The justifications for this approach are twofold: first, society asks these people to fulfill special obligations, and thus has a reciprocal duty to protect them from harm they may encounter in executing their roles; second, protecting these people will maximize the chances of saving the most lives overall.

An alternate or complementary framework would give highest priority to protect the most vulnerable: infants or those who are elderly, infirm, or immune-compromised (and their contacts) who would be most likely to die should they become infected. (The precise profile of who will be most likely to die may vary according to the nature of the pandemic. In many cases, mortality presents a U-shaped curve, with the highest death rates at the beginning or end of life; in the 1918 Spanish flu epidemic, however, the mortality curve was W-shaped, with high death rates found among young adults [Morens et al., 2010].)

In contrast to a "protect the vulnerable" principle, a "save the most lives" principle would give priority to those with the best prognosis for survival (Persad, Wertheimer, and Emanuel, 2009). Another system carries a "life cycle" justification: each person should have the opportunity to experience all stages of life. In some forms, this framework would prioritize any younger person over an older person; a variant on this system would give first priority to people between early adolescence and middle age, on the grounds that they have a greater "investment" in their life and more developed interests and goals than infants or small children (Emanuel and Wertheimer, 2006). Finally, the principle of justice might demand a lottery system, on the grounds that society has an obligation to treat all citizens equally (McLachlan, 2012).

Compensation for Vaccine Injuries

The inherent and unavoidable risks of vaccine adverse events have been recognized since the nineteenth century. Not until the 1960s, however, did governments begin to establish systems to provide compensation to individuals suffering vaccine-induced harms. In addition to providing monetary compensation to individuals who experienced adverse events (or to survivors in the case of individuals who died), such systems typically indemnify vaccine manufacturers from damages for non-negligently caused harm. West Germany instituted the first government-run vaccine injury compensation program in 1961, and over the next two decades, many other countries, including Denmark, France, Japan, New Zealand, Sweden, and the United Kingdom, followed suit (Evans, 1999). In the United States, legislation in 1986 created the National Vaccine Injury Compensation Program, which provides reimbursement for medical and rehabilitative care for people injured by any vaccine designated by the CDC for routine administration to children (Mariner, 1992). The system allows no punitive damages against manufacturers unless there is evidence of gross negligence. Claims are reviewed by a special master in the US Court of Federal Claims, and normal rules of evidence are relaxed. Petitioners may pursue a claim in civil court only if they first go through the special master and either reject that decision or have the claim denied (Mariner, 1992; HRSA, 2017).

Historically, injury compensation plans arose in response not to a perceived ethical problem, but rather to a market failure. People who believed they or their children had suffered a vaccine adverse event were pursuing tort claims, and the fear of having to pay high damage awards in court drove many vaccine manufacturers from the market (Colgrove, 2006). A government no-fault compensation system is ethically preferable to tort litigation, which is a more adversarial and uncertain environment, both for people who believe they have been harmed and for vaccine manufacturers who would often otherwise leave the marketplace. Such a system promotes justice: since people receive vaccines or vaccinate their children at least partially for altruistic reasons, in order to help safeguard community welfare, it is fair that they be compensated for harms that may occur. Such a rationale is even stronger when vaccines are required by law. A compensation system also expresses the principle of solidarity, in which all members of a community share in the risks (Mello, 2007). By assuring a stable supply of vaccines, government compensation systems fulfill society's obligations to all who undergo vaccination.

Conclusion

Immunization policy in the twenty-first century presents a host of complex ethical challenges. In the United States, the coverage targets set in *Healthy People 2020* are currently met for several recommended vaccines, including polio, MMR, hepatitis B, and varicella, but are lagging for several others, including *Haemophilus influenzae* B and diphtheria-tetanus-acellular pertussis (Hill et al., 2015). Although significant progress has been made overcoming socioeconomic disparities in routine childhood immunization, coverage gaps remain between rich and poor children for some vaccines (Zhao and Smith, 2013). Inequities at the global level remain more intractable, although improvements in coverage have been achieved through the strengthening, through public and philanthropic funds, of immunization systems in low- and middle-income countries, and their health care systems more generally, and through economic measures such as tiered pricing (Hinman and McKinlay, 2015).

Even as public health policymakers confront the challenges of assuring access to vaccines, they must also contend with doubts among many people about the safety and efficacy of vaccines. "Vaccine hesitancy" is a complex phenomenon encompassing a spectrum of behaviors ranging from complete rejection of all vaccines to selective or modified immunization inconsistent with standard medical guidelines. It has diverse motivations, including mistrust of the pharmaceutical industry, antigovernment animus, and devotion to "natural" or alternative healing methods. Responding to vaccine hesitancy requires that policymakers balance their duties of beneficence and justice with their respect for individual and parental autonomy. Navigating this difficult environment will demand careful ethical analysis that also takes into account procedural and distributive justice, nonmaleficence, transparency of decision-making, and least restriction. Because of the uniquely important role of vaccines in the public health toolkit—they have done more in both rich and poor nations to prevent sickness and death, and to improve health and overall quality of life, than any other intervention—it is critical to achieve ethical consensus so that the potential benefits of immunization may be realized.

References

Arras, J. 2005. "Rationing Vaccine during an Avian Influenza Pandemic: Why It Won't Be Easy." *Yale Journal of Biology and Medicine* 78: 287–300.

Atwell, J. E., Van Otterloo, J., Zipprich, J., Winter, K., Harriman, K., Salmon, et al. 2013. "Nonmedical Vaccine Exemptions and Pertussis in California, 2010." *Pediatrics* 132 (2013): 624–630.

Briss, P. A., Rodewald, L. E., Hinman, A. R., Shefer, A. M., Strikas, R. A., Bernier, R. R., et al. 2000. "Reviews of Evidence Regarding Interventions to Improve Vaccination Coverage in Children, Adolescents, and Adults." *American Journal of Preventive Medicine* 18: S97–S140.

CDC (US Centers for Disease Control and Prevention). 2010. "Estimates of Deaths Associated with Seasonal Influenza—United States, 1976–2007." *Morbidity and Mortality Weekly Report* 59: 1057–1062.

CDC (US Centers for Disease Control and Prevention). 2016a. "Immunization Schedules." https://www.cdc.gov/vaccines/schedules/index.html.

CDC (US Centers for Disease Control and Prevention). 2016b. "Vaccines for Children Program (VFC)." http://www.cdc.gov/vaccines/programs/vfc/index.html.

Charo, R.A. 2007. "Politics, Parents, and Prophylaxis—Mandating HPV Vaccination in the United States." *New England Journal of Medicine* 356: 1905–1908.

Colgrove, J. 2006. *State of Immunity: The Politics of Vaccination in 20th Century America* (Berkeley: University of California Press).

Cortes-Penfield, Nicolas. 2014. "Mandatory Influenza Vaccination for Health Care Workers as a New Standard of Care: A Matter of Patient Safety and Nonmaleficent Practice." *American Journal of Public Health* 104(2014): 2060–2065.

Dare, T. 1998. "Mass Immunisation Programmes: Some Philosophical Issues." *Bioethics* 12: 125–149.

Diekema, D. S. 2014. "Personal Belief Exemptions from School Vaccination Requirements." *Annual Review of Public Health* 35: 275–292.

Diekema, D. S., and Marcuse, E. K. 1998. "Ethical Issues in the Vaccination of Children." In *Primum Non Nocere Today*, edited by G. R. Burgio and J. D. Lantos (New York: Elsevier).

Durbach, N. 2005. *Bodily Matters: The Anti-Vaccination Movement in England, 1853–1907* (Durham, N.C.: Duke University Press).

Emanuel, E., and Wertheimer, A. 2006. "Who Should Get Influenza Vaccine When Not All Can?" *Science* 312: 854–855.

Evans, G. 1999. "Vaccine Injury Compensation Programs Worldwide." *Vaccine* 17: S25–S35.

Gavi (Gavi, The Vaccine Alliance). 2016. "Facts and Figures." http://www.gavi.org/about/mission/facts-and-figures/.

Gostin, L. O., and DeAngelis, C. D. 2007. "Mandatory HPV Vaccination: Public Health vs Private Wealth." *Journal of the American Medical Association* 297: 1921–1923.

Hardin, G. 1968. "The Tragedy of the Commons." *Science* 162: 1243–1248.

HHS (US Department of Health and Human Services). 2016. "The Affordable Care Act and Immunization." http://www.hhs.gov/healthcare/facts-and-features/fact-sheets/aca-and-immunization/index.html.

Hill, H. A., Elam-Evans, L. D., Yankey, D., Singleton, J. A., and Kolasa, M. 2015. "National, State, and Selected Local Area Vaccination Coverage among Children Aged 19–35 Months—United States, 2014." *Morbidity and Mortality Weekly Report* 64: 889–896.

Hinman, A., and McKinlay, M. A. 2015. "Immunization Equity." *American Journal of Preventive Medicine* 49: S399–S405.

HRSA (US Health Resources & Services Administration). 2017. "National Vaccine Injury Compensation Program." Fact Sheet. https://www.hrsa.gov/sites/default/files/hrsa/vaccine-compensation/faq/vicp-fact-sheet.pdf.

Huerkamp, C. 1985. "The History of Smallpox Vaccination in Germany: A First Step in the Medicalization of the General Public." *Journal of Contemporary History* 20: 617–636.

Mariner, W. 1992. "The National Vaccine Injury Compensation Program." *Health Affairs* 11: 255–265.

McLachlan, H. V. 2012. "A Proposed Non-consequentialist Policy for the Ethical Distribution of Scare Vaccination in the Face of an Influenza Pandemic." *Journal of Medical Ethics* 38: 317–318.

Mello, M. 2007. "Rationalizing Vaccine Injury Compensation." *Bioethics* 22: 32–42.

Mill, J. S. 1863. *On Liberty* (Boston: Ticknor and Fields).

Mitchell, V., Dietz, V. J., Okwo-Bele, J. M., and Cutts, F. T. 2013. "Immunization in Developing Countries." In *Vaccines*, 6th ed., edited by S. A. Plotkin, W. A. Orenstein, and P. A. Offit (New York: Elsevier).

Morens, D. M., Taubenberger, J. K., Harvey, H. A., and Memoli, M. J., 2010. "The 1918 Influenza Pandemic: Lessons for 2009 and the Future." *Critical Care Medicine* 38: e10–e20.

Morita, J. Y., Ramirez, E., and Trick, W. E. 2008. "Effect of a School-Entry Vaccination Requirement on Racial and Ethnic Disparities in Hepatitis B Immunization Coverage Levels among Public School Students." *Pediatrics* 121: e547–e552.

Nowalk, M. P., Lin, C. J., Raymund, M., Bialor, J., and Zimmerman, R. K. 2013. "Impact of Hospital Policies on Health Care Workers' Influenza Vaccination Rates." *American Journal of Infection Control* 41: 697–701.

Omer S. B., Enger K. S., Moulton L. H., Halsey N. A., Stokley, S., and Salmon, D. A. 2008. "Geographic Clustering of Nonmedical Exemptions to School Immunization Requirements and Associations with Geographic Clustering of Pertussis." *American Journal of Epidemiology* 168: 1389–1396.

Omer, S. B., Pan, W. K., Halsey, N. A., Stokley, S., Moulton, L. H., Navar, A. M., Pierce, M., and Salmon, D. A. 2006. "Nonmedical Exemptions to School Immunization Requirements: Secular Trends and Association of State Policies with Pertussis Incidence." *Journal of the American Medical Association* 296: 1757–1763.

Opel, D. J., and Diekema, D. S. 2012. "Finding the Proper Balance between Freedom and Justice: Why We Should Not Eliminate Personal Belief Exemptions to Vaccine Mandates." *Journal of Health Policy, Politics, and Law* 37: 141–147.

Persad, G., Wertheimer, A., and Emanuel, E. J. 2009. "Principles for Allocation of Scarce Medical Resources." *Lancet* 373: 423–431.

Plotkin, S. L., and Plotkin, S. 2013. "A Short History of Vaccination." In *Vaccines*, 6th ed., edited by S. A. Plotkin, W. A. Orenstein, and P. A. Offit (New York: Elsevier).

Salmon, D. A., and Siegel, A. W. 2001. "Religious and Philosophical Exemptions from Vaccination Requirements and Lessons Learned from Conscientious Objectors from Conscription." *Public Health Reports* 116: 289–295.

Silverman, R. D., and May, T. 2001. "Private Choice Versus Public Health: Religion, Morality, and Childhood Vaccination Law." *University of Maryland Law Journal of Race, Religion, Gender, and Class* 1: 505–521.

Smith, J. S. 2008. "Ethnic Disparities in Cervical Cancer Illness Burden and Subsequent Care: A Prospective View." *American Journal of Managed Care* 14: S193–S199.

Veatch, R. 1987. "The Ethics of Promoting Herd Immunity." *Family and Community Health* 10: 44–53.

WHO (World Health Organization). 1980. *The Global Eradication of Smallpox: Final Report of the Global Commission for the Certification of Smallpox Eradication* (Geneva: WHO).

WHO (World Health Organization). 2015. "Poliomyelitis (Polio)." http://www.who.int/ith/vaccines/polio/en/.

WHO (World Health Organization). 2016. *Global Polio Eradication Initiative-Annual Report 2015* (Geneva: World Health Organization).

Zhao, Z., and Smith, P. J. 2013. "Trends in Vaccination Coverage Disparities among Children, United States, 2001–2010." *Vaccine* 31: 2324–2327.

CHAPTER 39

PREVENTION AND TREATMENT OF TUBERCULOSIS IN LOW- AND MIDDLE-INCOME COUNTRIES: ETHICAL CHALLENGES

DIEGO S. SILVA AND MICHAEL J. SELGELID

Introduction

Although tuberculosis (TB) affects persons from all socioeconomic classes worldwide, it overwhelmingly burdens those in low- and middle-income countries (LMICs) and the most economically impoverished within both LMICs and high-income countries (HICs) (WHO, 2016a). While all countries are confronted with ethical challenges related to the treatment and prevention of TB, the greater resource constraints of LMICs can exacerbate the ethical challenges themselves, as will be noted below.

This chapter outlines three key ethical challenges in TB care and control, particularly within the context of LMICs: isolation and involuntary isolation, third-party notification, and the introduction of new antitubercular drugs. It begins with a background on TB to better ground the exploration of the challenges identified herein. There are many ethical challenges faced by those in both HICs and LMICs, and it is impossible to cover all of them here. Therefore, the chapter focuses on some of the most pertinent, difficult, or unresolved issues.

BACKGROUND ON TB

TB is a bacterial pathogen (*Mycobacterium tuberculosis*) transmitted between people through the air. Although it can affect different parts of a person's body, it most often affects the lungs. Approximately one-third of the world's population has latent TB (WHO, 2014c). Those with latent TB have been infected and their bodies harbor live TB bacilli. They do not, however, suffer active illness, nor can they transmit TB to others. Approximately 10 percent of those with latent TB eventually fall ill and require care. However, persons with compromised immunities (e.g., persons living with human immunodeficiency virus [HIV]) and those who suffer from malnutrition are at greater risk of both being infected and becoming ill (WHO, 2015). In general, the economically impoverished are at greater risk of acquiring TB and developing active TB. In addition to commonly suffering from physical ailments that increase the risk of infection (e.g., compromised immunity, malnutrition, etc.), the poor often live or work in crowded conditions that facilitate the spread of TB (Oxlade and Murry, 2012). Furthermore, because they often lack access to proper and timely primary medical care, the poor suffer greater mortality and morbidity when illness does occur.

Symptoms of active TB include cough (potentially with blood and sputum), fever, and weight loss (WHO, 2017b). Though it can be deadly (especially in the absence of adequate treatment), TB is curable in the vast majority of cases. Recommended treatment for ordinary drug-sensitive TB (active illness), which accounts for approximately 95 percent of all active TB cases, involves "a standard 6 month course of 4 antimicrobial drugs that are provided with information, supervision and support to the patient by a health worker or trained volunteer" (WHO, 2017b). The support and supervision provided to patients aim to ensure that medications are taken regularly, clinical complications are addressed as soon as possible, and patients receive any and all social supports that are locally available (e.g., government disability grants in South Africa) (Foster et al., 2015). In order to prevent the further spread of TB, patients may be asked to remain in isolation, either within their homes or, in some circumstances, in hospitals, usually for a short duration of time (approximately two weeks, by which time treatment normally renders patients noncontagious). However, a minority of patients remain infectious for much longer during treatment and are thus isolated for an extended period of time (e.g., several months) (Lange et al., 2014).

In 2015 an estimated 10.4 million people worldwide fell ill with TB, including 1 million children and over a million HIV-positive persons (WHO, 2016a). Newly diagnosed patients have a treatment success rate of 83 percent. The good news is that, globally, the incidence of TB fell by an average of 1.5 percent per year between 2000 and 2015. Unfortunately, there were still an estimated 1.8 million deaths associated with TB in 2015, approximately 400,000 of which involved persons who were HIV positive. The burden of TB is highest in the World Health Organization's (WHO's) Southeast Asia and Western Pacific regions. India, Indonesia, and China have the highest incidence rates of TB (WHO, 2016a).

In addition to drug-sensitive TB, global public health is threatened by the increasing spread of multidrug-resistant tuberculosis (MDR-TB). MDR-TB strains do not respond to at least the two most powerful first-line TB drugs (isoniazid and rifampicin). They account for 3.9 percent of new cases and approximately 5 percent of all cases (Sharma et al., 2017; WHO, 2014b). Treatment for MDR-TB can take up to twenty-four months. In addition to needing to take potentially toxic antitubercular drugs, long periods of isolation are often required for those infected with extensively drug-resistant TB (XDR-TB) (i.e., strains that do not respond to most first-line and second-line drugs; see WHO, 2017b). There were an estimated 480,000 new cases of MDR-TB globally during 2015, with a 52 percent rate of successful treatment; 45,000 of these cases involved XDR-TB, with a 28 percent rate of successful treatment (WHO, 2016a).

Ethical Challenges

Numerous ethical issues are raised by the prevention and treatment of TB in LMICs. Among others, such issues include surveillance (e.g., how to conduct ethical surveillance in the absence of consent); the need for greater monetary investment on the part of HICs toward new drugs and diagnostics; care for special or vulnerable populations, such as children, migrants, or prisoners; diagnosis in the absence of treatment; addressing issues of risk and benefit in the treatment of latent TB infection; and health care rights and responsibilities in caring for persons with TB (Denholm, Matteelli, and Reis, 2015; Frick, 2016; Selgelid, 2008b; WHO, 2016c, 2017a). In what follows, we examine three especially pertinent, difficult, or unresolved issues faced by those who work in TB care and control in LMICs: isolation and involuntary isolation, third-party notification, and the introduction of new antitubercular drugs.

Isolation and Involuntary Isolation

The isolation of persons with easily transmissible airborne infectious diseases, like TB, is commonly justified by an appeal to the harm principle (Coker et al., 2007). The harm principle states that a person should be free to behave as she or he chooses so long as the person's actions do not cause harm to another person (Mill, 2009). In TB care, isolation is a public health measure commonly employed to protect others from contracting TB, particularly those in frequent contact with the TB patient. Patients are usually isolated only as long as they remain infectious, which is usually a few weeks into treatment for routine drug-sensitive cases (Ritchie et al., 2007).

In the vast majority of cases, patients willingly abide by social distancing requests, including isolation orders. Patients generally wish to avoid infecting others—including their loved ones, who, given routine close contact, are often at greatest risk of transmission. In some instances, patients struggle to remain in isolation, not because they fail to understand the risks they pose to others, but for circumstantial reasons. If a TB patient is a sole breadwinner with limited job security, for example, that person may be tempted to return to work before he or she is no longer infectious. In all instances, but particularly where a patient lacks basic resources, it is imperative for the state to provide social supports to those who undergo TB treatment, especially during periods of isolation (WHO, 2015).

The need to provide social supports can be justified by appeal to the principle of reciprocity, which states that one ought to return good for good received and rectify any wrong one has done to another person (Becker, 1990). Given that isolation can result in loss of income, and that the primary benefit of isolation is to the community, the principle of reciprocity demands that TB patients have their essential needs (e.g., food, water, income) met while in isolation in order to minimize the burden to them and maximize the benefit to the community (Silva, Dawson, and Upshur, 2016). It is generally understood that the state is responsible for discharging reciprocal obligations in these cases, since the state is primarily in charge of public health activities. For example, the WHO's End TB Strategy calls for the implementation of "social protection" and "poverty alleviation" to assist TB patients during treatment (WHO, 2015). The disabilities grants offered by the South African Social Security Agency to TB patients, intended to offset personal costs associated with an inability to work, is a concrete example of social supports provided by the state; however, how readily available these supports are in practice has come into question (Foster et al., 2015). Discharging obligations that emerge out of reciprocity does not amount to charity, meaning that the state is not being charitable when it supports a patient with TB to maintain isolation, but is rather providing what patients are owed, since the state is actively preventing them from seeking income or support for themselves.

In some exceptional circumstances, patients may refuse isolation orders even if support measures are provided to help them. In these instances, involuntary isolation might be justified—again, by appeal to the harm principle. If involuntary isolation is invoked, it is commonly agreed that it must be a last resort, and, as such, it is agreed that alternative and less restrictive methods must be attempted first (WHO, 2017a). Moreover, there must be evidence to suggest that isolation is, in fact, indicated, and that the patient is not subject to arbitrary or unreasonable types of detention (e.g., involuntary isolation of a patient who is homeless and suffers from a mental illness—not because the patient is a public health threat, but because he or she may prove to be a difficult patient to assist) (Coker et al., 2007).

Still, a fundamental ethics question remains: How great does the public health threat need to be for isolation of a person to be justified, or, stated differently, how much risk of infection should the public bear to protect the rights and freedoms of a person infected with TB? (Coker et al., 2007; Selgelid, 2008b). Exactly how much risk of harm society should be willing to accept to protect basic freedoms, such as freedom of movement, remains a contentious issue. Likewise, it is unclear when such freedoms should be sacrificed for the sake of the broader public's well-being. This question is of even greater concern in the context of XDR-TB, where the likelihood of cure is low and some patients may need to remain in isolation indefinitely to avoid infecting others (Singh, Upshur, and Padayatchi, 2007). In such circumstances, the reciprocal obligation to support the patient is especially important. As Singh and colleagues note, "[t]he use of legally sanctioned restrictive measures for the control of XDR-TB should not obscure the fact that being infected is not a crime. A strong reciprocal obligation is borne by authorities so wishing to invoke these measures." However, the greater the number of social supports that ought to be given to a TB patient, the greater the costs that society and the state must bear. Given that XDR-TB largely occurs in LMICs, the greatest costs associated with providing social supports fall on those states that are least able to afford them.

Third-Party Notification

Once a person is diagnosed with active TB, public health officials will often (as a legal requirement) be notified, and they will then work with the patient to identify those with whom the patient has close contact to alert them and make sure they are tested for TB. Such routine contact tracing on the part of public health authorities usually occurs without objection from the patient. In the vast majority of cases, as noted above, TB patients wish to cooperate with health workers in order to prevent the spread of TB, especially to their loved ones (Jin et al., 2008). However, there are instances when a patient may resist assisting in the process of identifying and notifying other persons (i.e., "third parties"). The reasons may stem from the stigma and discrimination they may face, which can lead to a host of additional nonclinical harms to the patient, such as being ostracized from their families or communities, loss of income, and so on—all of which can be exacerbated in cases of HIV/AIDS coinfection (Courtwright and Turner, 2010). In such instances, health workers must be attentive to the needs and desires of the TB patient while also fulfilling their duties to notify third parties that they may be at risk for TB.

The most ethically problematic situation arises when a TB patient refuses to cooperate even after all efforts have been made by health workers to protect the patient from potentially harmful consequences associated with the disclosure of the TB infection. In these situations, the right of the patient to confidentiality regarding private health information clashes with the need to protect others from harm (Selgelid, 2008a). Rights to confidentiality and privacy are often grounded in the principle of autonomy (i.e., that persons should be free to direct their lives as they see fit), which includes making choices about what health care to accept, and whether, how, and to whom to disclose personal medical information. In most clinical encounters, maintaining patient confidentiality is of utmost importance, outweighing other morally worthy considerations.

However, in the case of TB, given the risk to third parties of being infected, what is good for the health of others (i.e., protecting their right not to be harmed) may conflict with the right of TB patients to autonomously choose to keep their TB status private. Patients may also face harm in having their confidentiality breached; stigma and discrimination from their families and communities, as well as the loss of trust in the therapeutic relationship with their health workers, are nontrivial harms. The loss of trust could potentially have a chilling effect in other cases, whereby persons who think they might be infected with TB do not seek treatment, or do not seek treatment as early as they otherwise would have, out of fear that their diagnosis will be made known to others against their wishes (Selgelid, 2008a).

In situations where a TB patient's right to confidentiality conflicts with a third party's right not to be harmed, a health worker might consider breaching the patient's right to confidentiality in order to protect others on two separate (nonexclusive) grounds. First, one might maintain that even if the right to confidentiality is important, it should not be thought to have absolute priority over other values in health care. It might be that the right to confidentiality should be balanced against other rights and values, and that, in certain contexts at least, other rights or values will sometimes be deemed more important. In the case of contacting third parties for TB care, it might be argued that the right of others not to be (potentially severely) harmed trumps the right a TB patient may have to keep aspects of their private health information confidential. If so, a TB health worker may be morally permitted (or arguably required) to inform others that they may be at risk of infection and try to protect the patient's identity as well as possible, knowing that the patient may end up being identified by those other persons who have been contacted.

Second, one might alternatively (or additionally) argue that a TB patient who refuses to assist public health authorities with contact tracing is acting in a negligent manner, or in some manner that is morally wrong (i.e., in violation of the duty to avoid harming others) by choosing to put others at risk of TB. In such circumstances, one might conclude that the TB patient thereby forfeits the right to confidentiality, and that therefore the right of others not to be harmed can be protected through contact tracing despite the risk of disclosing the status of the patient (Selgelid, 2008a).

Assuming either of these arguments is sound, a further consideration is whether a health worker is merely *permitted* to contact third parties, knowing it may breach the confidentiality of the TB patient, or *required* to contact third parties. If it is deemed that the health worker is required to do so, and if such a requirement will become part of policy and practice within a public health unit or TB program, then what formal mechanisms should be in place to facilitate the health worker's obligation to contact third parties? What, if any, penalties should be in place if health workers choose not to go ahead with third-party notifications? Such questions would need further consideration and answers prior to requiring health workers to notify third parties in such instances of noncooperation on the part of the patient.

Complicating matters is the reality that many factors may increase or decrease the risk of others contracting TB. How drug sensitive the patient's strain of TB is, how prevalent TB is in a particular geographical area, the type of job a TB patient has (e.g., a teacher interacting with young children), the patient's daily movements (e.g., taking public transportation to work versus walking to work)—these all affect the risk of others being infected. Since these factors affect the nature and magnitude of risk imposed on third parties, they must be taken into consideration when making judgments about whether breach of patient confidentiality (and thus trust) is justified by the reduction of risk to third parties.

Implementing New Antituberculars: Bedaquiline and Delamanid

Given the dearth of new TB drug development in recent decades, bedaquiline (approved by the Food and Drug Administration in the United States in 2012) and delamanid (approved by the European Medicines Agency in 2014) have been heralded as important new antituberculars to be used in combination with other drugs for the treatment of M/XDR-TB when all other treatment options have failed (WHO, 2014a). The accelerated approval of these drugs was given based on Phase IIb data. Both drugs are currently undergoing further Phase III testing, with results likely within the next few years (Stop TB Partnership, 2017). Both bedaquiline and delamanid were demonstrated to be more effective than standard treatment regimens for M/XDR-TB when used in combination with other second-line drugs; however, serious side effects were noted in both, including issues associated with the heart's electrical system that could lead to serious or fatal heart disease, known as QT interval prolongation (WHO, 2014a). In the case of bedaquiline, there were ten deaths among the seventy-nine participants randomized to the experimental arm, compared with two deaths among eighty-one participants in the treatment-as-usual arm of the study. Although a significant cause for concern, five of the ten deaths in the experimental arm were attributed to TB, and another to a motor vehicle accident, leaving four deaths without a (recognized) common cause (Cox, 2014). When drafting recommendations regarding the use of these drugs, the WHO expert groups had a "very low level of confidence" in the evidence presented for the efficacy and safety of both bedaquiline and delamanid (WHO, 2013, 2014d).

The prominent ethical issue regarding the use of bedaquiline and delamanid involves risk-benefit considerations that need to be undertaken prior to their use at a programmatic level or for individual patients. The risk stems from the potential adverse effects related to the drugs, which are poorly understood to date given the limited data. The benefit is a potentially effective treatment for M/XDR-TB, which has historically had a poor prognosis given previously available pharmaceuticals (Cox, 2014). Regulatory officials have placed the balance in favor of approval for bedaquiline and delamanid—despite the drugs' poorly understood risks—given the morbidity and mortality of drug-resistant TB (Cox, 2014). Moreover, the balance of risks and benefits associated with bedaquiline and delamanid is also context-dependent, as noted by Horsburgh and colleagues:

> This balance can be positively altered by a high standard of care at the clinical sites managing the administration of the new drugs and careful monitoring of patient responses. The risk-benefit trade-off may thus vary from country to country and from site to site within a given country. The identification or establishment of clinical

> centers that possess the required expertise, monitoring and laboratory capability will certainly favorably alter the balance. (Horsburgh et al., 2013, 150)

A goal, therefore, as with all clinical medicine, is to further implement mechanisms that reduce the risks associated with bedaquiline and delamanid.

The WHO's recommendations regarding the use of bedaquiline and delamanid for national TB programs center on mechanisms to reduce the risk of harm to patients. For example, the WHO (2013, 10) states that treatment should be "administered under closely monitored conditions, adhering to best practices in treatment delivery, to enable optimal drug effectiveness and safety." A key component of best practices is well-planned pharmacovigilance to monitor the safety of those prescribed bedaquiline and delamanid. Building and maintaining the trust of patients, as well as the broader public, is also pivotal, given the uncertainty surrounding these new drugs. As such, the WHO recommends that "[t]reatment protocols are preferably submitted to, and approved by the relevant national ethics authority in the country, prior to patient enrolment on treatment," and that an "oversight of treatment programmes is provided by an independent group of experts in clinical management and public health" (WHO, 2014d, 8). Part of what it means to build and maintain trust is to have transparent processes administered by groups independent of those administrating the new drugs.

Another safety mechanism that the WHO recommends when introducing bedaquiline and delamanid into the clinical setting is ensuring that the informed consent of patients is sought carefully. The WHO's expert group notes that patients need to be explicitly informed about the "novel nature" of these drugs, be able to understand why one of these new drugs is being offered, and be cognizant of the risks and benefits associated with taking them (WHO, 2014a). Informed consent is traditionally conceived as a means of upholding patients' autonomy vis-à-vis the choices they make regarding what will happen to their bodies, including whether or not to take certain medications. Although all drugs have risk-benefit profiles, the balancing of the risks and benefits associated with bedaquiline and delamanid becomes that much more important in the context of clinically treating M/XDR-TB. Therefore, the balancing of risks and benefits related to these drugs occurs on at least two levels: first, at a programmatic level where policymakers decide whether or not to even offer these new drugs; and second, at an individual/clinical level, where patients must choose whether or not to take them (if offered), knowing that not taking them may very well lead to death, but that they have significant risks that are not well understood.

Given that the burden of M/XDR-TB is most acutely felt in LMICs, the ethical challenges and recommendations on how to best introduce bedaquiline and delamanid, and other future pharmaceuticals, will need to be applicable in the context of resource constraints. For example, pharmacovigilance is often a challenge in LMICs due to the number of patients a health care worker will see during the day (which often leaves little to no time to fill out pharmacovigilance paperwork), the unavailability of reporting structures in local languages, and challenges maintaining and using electronic networks necessary for the reporting itself (Olsson, Pal, and Dodoo, 2015). In light of these challenges, the broader global TB community should consider what resources need to be dedicated to LMICs in order for countries to safely implement bedaquiline and delamanid, as well as the extent to which these drugs should even be administered in the absence of robust pharmacovigilance.

Conclusion

With the advent of new technologies, such as new drugs and diagnostics, coupled with the continuing public health efforts across high-burden countries and the global health community more broadly, there are reasons to believe that the rates of TB will continue to fall. However, ethical challenges will persist as long as TB exists, and the brunt of these challenges will likely be felt most strongly in LMICs faced with acute and chronic resource constraints.

References

Becker, L. 1990. *Reciprocity* (Chicago: University of Chicago Press).

Coker, R., Thomas, M., Lock, K., and Martin, R., 2007. "Detention and the Evolving Threat of Tuberculosis: Evidence, Ethics, and Law." *Journal of Law, Medicine & Ethics* 34(4): 609–615.

Courtwright, A., and Turner, A. 2010. "Tuberculosis and Stigmatization: Pathways and Interventions." *Public Health Reports* 125(Suppl. 4): 34–42.

Cox, E. 2014. "FDA Approval of Bedaquiline: The Benefit-Risk Balance for Drug-Resistant Tuberculosis." *New England Journal of Medicine* 371: 689–691.

Denholm, J. T., Matteelli, A., and Reis, A. 2015 "Latent Tuberculous Infection: Ethical Considerations in Formulating Public Health Policy." *International Journal of Tuberculosis and Lung Disease* 19(2):137–140.

Foster, N., Vassall, A., Cleary, S., Cunnama, L., Churchyard, G., and Sinanovic, E. 2015. "The Economic Burden of TB Diagnosis and Treatment in South Africa." *Social Science and Medicine* 130: 42–50.

Frick, M. 2016. *2016 Report on Tuberculosis Research Funding Trends, 2005–2015: No Time to Lose* (New York: Treatment Action Group).

Horsburgh, C. R., Jr., Haxaire-Theeuwes, M., Lienhardt, C., Wingfield, C., McNeeley, D., Pyne-Mercier, L., et al. 2013. "Compassionate Use of and Expanded Access to New Drugs for Drug-Resistant Tuberculosis." *International Journal of Tuberculosis and Lung Disease* 17(2): 146–152.

Jin, J., Sklar, G. E., Oh, V. M. S., and Li, S. C. 2008. "Factors Affecting Therapeutic Compliance: A Review from the Patient's Perspective." *Therapeutics and Clinical Risk Management* 4(1): 269–286.

Lange, C., Abubakar, I., Alffenaar, J. W. C., Bothamley, G., Caminero, J. A., Carvalho, A. C. C., et al. 2014. "Management of Patients with Multidrug-Resistant/Extensively Drug-Resistant Tuberculosis in Europe: A TBNET Consensus Statement." *European Respiratory Journal* 41(1): 23–63.

Mill, J. S. 2009. *On Liberty and Other Essays* (New York: Kaplan).

Olsson, S., Pal, S. N., and Dodoo, A. 2015. "Pharmacovigilance in Resource-Limited Countries." *Expert Review of Clinical Pharmacology* 8(4): 449–460.

Oxlade, O., and Murry, M. 2012. "Tuberculosis and Poverty: Why Are the Poor at Greater Risk in India?" *PLoS One* 7(11): e47533. doi:10.1371/journal.pone.0047533.

Ritchie, S. R., Harrison, A. C., Vaughan, R. H., Calder, L., and Morris, A. J. 2007. "New Recommendations for Duration of Respiratory Isolation Based on Time to Detect Mycobacterium Tuberculosis in Liquid Culture." *European Respiratory Journal* 30(3): 501–507.

Selgelid, M. J. 2008a. "Ethics, Tuberculosis and Globalization." *Public Health Ethics* 1(1): 10–20.

Selgelid, M. J. 2008b. "Improving Global Health: Counting Reasons Why." *Developing World Bioethics* 8(2): 115–125.

Sharma, A., Hill, A., Kurbatova, E., van der Walt, M., Kvasnovsky, C., Tupasi, T. E., et al. 2017. "Estimating the Future Burden of Multidrug-Resistant and Extensively Drug-Resistant Tuberculosis in India, the Philippines, Russia, and South Africa: A Mathematical Modelling Study." *Lancet Infectious Disease* 17(7): 707–715. doi:10.1016/S1473-3099(17)30247-5.

Silva, D. S., Dawson, A., and Upshur, R. E. G. 2016. "Reciprocity and Ethical Tuberculosis Treatment and Control." *Journal of Bioethical Inquiry* 13(1): 75–86.

Singh, J., Upshur, R. E. G., and Padayatchi, N. 2007. "XDR-TB in South Africa: No Time for Denial or Complacency." *PLoS Medicine* 4(1): e50.

Stop TB Partnership. 2017. "Clinical Pipeline." Working Group on New TB Drugs. http://www.newtbdrugs.org/pipeline/clinical.

WHO (World Health Organization). 2013. *The use of Bedaquiline in the Treatment of Multidrug-Resistant Tuberculosis: Interim Policy Guidance* (Geneva: WHO).

WHO (World Health Organization). 2014a. *Companion Handbook to the WHO Guidelines for the Programmatic Management of Drug Resistant TB* (Geneva: WHO).

WHO (World Health Organization). 2014b. *Drug Resistant TB: Surveillance and Response, 2014*. http://www.who.int/tb/publications/global_report/gtbr14_supplement_web_v3.pdf.

WHO (World Health Organization). 2014c. "Latent Tuberculosis Infection Fact Sheet." http://www.who.int/tb/challenges/ltbi_factsheet_2014.pdf.

WHO (World Health Organization). 2014d. *The Use of Delamanid in the Treatment of Multidrug-Resistant Tuberculosis: Interim Policy Guidance* (Geneva: WHO)

WHO (World Health Organization). 2015. *The End TB Strategy* (Geneva: WHO).

WHO (World Health Organization). 2016a. *Global Tuberculosis Report—2016* (Geneva: WHO).

WHO (World Health Organization). 2016b. *Guidance for Managing Ethical Issues in Infectious Disease Outbreaks* (Geneva: WHO).

WHO (World Health Organization). 2016c. "Multidrug Resistant Tuberculosis—2016 Fact Sheet." http://www.who.int/tb/challenges/mdr/mdr_tb_factsheet.pdf.

WHO (World Health Organization). 2017a. *Ethics Guidance for the Implementation of the End TB Strategy* (Geneva: WHO).

WHO (World Health Organization). 2017b. "Tuberculosis - Factsheet No. 104." http://www.who.int/mediacentre/factsheets/fs104/en/.

Further Reading

Coker, R. 2000. *From Chaos to Coercion: Detention and the Control of Tuberculosis* (New York: St. Martin's Press).

Coleman, C. H., Selgelid, M. J., Reis, A., Reichman, L. B., and Jaramillo, E. 2012. "The Role of Informed Consent in Tuberculosis Testing and Screening." *European Respiratory Journal* 39(5): 1057–1059.

Horner, J. 2016. "From Exceptional to Liminal Subjects: Reconciling Tensions in the Politics of Tuberculosis and Migration." *Journal of Bioethical Inquiry* 13(1): 65–73.

Reis, A., and Jaramillo, E. 2011. "Why Ethics Matters in Tuberculosis Prevention, Care and Control." *International Journal of Tuberculosis and Lung Disease* 15(Suppl. 2): S3–S5.

Selgelid, M. J., and Reichman, L. 2011. "Ethical Issues in Tuberculosis Diagnosis and Treatment" *International Journal of Tuberculosis and Lung Disease* 15(Suppl. 2): S9–S13.

Smith, M. J., and Silva, D. S. 2015. "Ethics for Pandemics beyond Influenza: Ebola, Drug-Resistant Tuberculosis, and Anticipating Future Ethical Challenges in Pandemic Preparedness and Response." *Monash Bioethics Review* 33(2–3): 130–147.

Upshur, R. E. G. 2009. "What Does It Mean to 'Know' a Disease? The Tragedy of XDR-TB." In *Public Health Ethics and Practice*, edited by S. Peckham and A. Hann, 51–64 (Cambridge: Polity Press).

CHAPTER 40

CONTROL OF MOSQUITO-BORNE ILLNESSES: A CHALLENGE TO PUBLIC HEALTH ETHICS

LAURA GREISMAN, BARBARA KOENIG, AND MICHELE BARRY

Introduction

Mosquito-borne illnesses kill approximately 725,000 people each year, making mosquitoes the deadliest species on earth (Zielinski, 2016). Globally, since vector-borne diseases tend to thrive where housing conditions are poor and water is unsafe or inadequately sanitized, these illnesses disproportionately affect people living in poverty (WHO, 2014).

With increasing public health threats from emerging and reemerging mosquito-borne infections, including malaria, Zika, dengue, chikungunya, and yellow fever, the World Health Organization (WHO) has recommended strengthening measures for mosquito control. The WHO Vector Control Advisory Group recommends that mosquito control programs have an integrated approach, target the entire mosquito life cycle, and achieve meaningful community engagement (WHO, 2016). Yet achieving all three of these recommendations, and doing so ethically, raises many challenges.

Challenges to implementing successful mosquito control programs include issues that arise in public health interventions for other communicable diseases. For example, surveillance activities necessary for monitoring and addressing communicable diseases raise concerns about privacy. Moreover, there is no easy solution to ensure that the costs of public health activities are fairly distributed, especially when the disease disproportionately affects the poor.

Other, more specific ethical issues result from the particular characteristics of the vector-control approach to mosquito-borne illnesses: from taking an integrated approach, which means mobilizing action across various sectors of society, to targeting interventions across the entire mosquito life cycle, which results in unavoidable environmental impacts. These two features, when taken together, make evident that vector-control interventions have the potential for affecting many people, internationally as well as intergenerationally. As if the ethical challenge was not daunting enough, the emerging nature of many mosquito-borne diseases, such as Zika, encourage the adoption of new technologies and novel interventions, such as genetic modification of the host organism, which introduces a larger degree of uncertainty to activities with already high stakes. These facts, not simply conflicts of values, underscore the need for meaningful community engagement, through mechanisms that are attentive to procedural justice.

This chapter discusses ethical issues related to the implementation of interventions for mosquito-borne illnesses. The first section catalogs key ethical issues related to surveillance activities and describes three examples of public health interventions. The examples are the provision of insecticide-treated nets (ITNs), the spraying of aerial pesticides, and the introduction of genetically modified mosquitoes. These examples are intended to be illustrative, rather than exhaustive, and are organized by increasing level of ethical complexity. In the second section, Zika virus disease (ZVD) will be highlighted as a case example, in order to discuss more specific ethical challenges in depth. Because of the threat Zika poses to developing fetuses, implications for reproductive rights will be discussed.

Ethics and Public Health Interventions Targeting Mosquito-Borne Illnesses

Contemporary public health interventions for mosquito control are varied and can target several stages of the mosquito life cycle. This section begins with an overview of the ethical concerns related to surveillance activities. Following that, the three public health activities presented are notable for two ethically salient reasons. First, the interventions are presented in order according to increasing levels of uncertainty regarding their effectiveness. For instance, while the benefits and risks of insecticide-treated nets (ITNs) are well understood, the long-term impacts of genetically modified mosquitoes are still unclear. Second, the interventions have effects whose reach in time and space vary. As will be seen, ITNs have effects that are both geographically and temporally local, while the introduction of genetically modified mosquitoes has effects that are geographically and temporally far-reaching. As the uncertainty and scope of an intervention's impact increase, so does its ethical complexity.

Surveillance

Before mosquito and disease control programs can be implemented, public health officials must define both the population at risk and the scope of the mosquito-borne public health threat. Surveillance is the process of collecting, analyzing, and interpreting data related to disease activity (WHO, 2006). One goal of surveillance is to collect and analyze information in order to allow for early warning of disease outbreaks (Collman and Robinson, 2011). In the context of mosquito-borne illnesses, surveillance involves collecting information on the human burden of mosquito-borne disease, as well as, later, documenting the effectiveness of control efforts through specific individual- and community-level interventions.

Surveillance activities highlight several ethical challenges. Data collected to monitor disease outbreaks may include sensitive, individually identifiable information (Collman and Robinson, 2011). The Zika epidemic provides an example in which surveillance activities are highly sensitive, primarily targeting pregnant women and their offspring. The unique ethical challenges in ZVD surveillance are explored further in the case study below. While surveillance activities serve a valuable role in public health data collection, they also have a potential negative economic impact on communities, as identified local outbreaks can quickly cripple local tourism-based economies.

Surveillance also raises concerns regarding distributive justice. Low-resource areas frequently lack the infrastructure for adequate surveillance. Failure to quickly identify and monitor an outbreak can result in delays in case finding and efforts to limit spread. In contrast, places that have existing demographic surveillance systems may be able to quickly respond to emerging disease threats (Baiden, Hodgson, and Binka, 2006). Lack of infrastructure and human resources to support a surveillance system puts low resource settings at particularly high risk of harm in the case of epidemic spread of disease.

Provision of Insecticide-Treated Nets

Perhaps the most straightforward way to control mosquito-borne illnesses is to prevent mosquito bites (WHO, 2016). ITNs, when used properly, are a cost-effective way to reduce the burden of mosquito-borne illnesses, providing protection both to individuals using them and to the population by reducing the overall burden of disease in the community (Lengeler, 2004). ITNs are an example of a mosquito control intervention provided at the individual and household levels. Despite the almost certain individual- and community-level benefits, there is much debate as to whether bed nets should be provided for free to families who cannot afford even subsidized netting, and, if they should, which stakeholders should pay for the nets (Curtis et al., 2003). Resource constraints ever-present in low- and middle-income countries have led some to argue against identifying ITNs as a public good, since doing so would place the burden on the communities and local governments affected by mosquito-borne illnesses such as malaria to provide these nets. Others, though, have argued that the cost of providing these nets would not be a large burden for the global community as a whole (Curtis et al., 2003). This lack of consensus requires ethical deliberation. Adding to the ethical tension over the provision of bed nets is the fact that they are an intervention dependent on human behavior to use them, and to use them as intended. In some villages along Lake Victoria, for example, the malaria bed nets are being used for fishing and drying fish (Minakawa et al., 2008). Even when an intervention is well understood and its effects are locally contained, the need for collective action and the fair distribution of costs present an ethical challenge.

Spraying of Aerial Pesticides

Another approach to controlling mosquito-borne illnesses involves eliminating the mosquitoes themselves through interventions that impact large geographical areas. In the 1940s, multiple large-scale mosquito control programs achieved near elimination of *Aedes* mosquitoes in several South American countries (Bolivia, Ecuador, Paraguay, Peru, and Columbia), modeled after the initial campaigns of insecticide spraying which originated in Cuba and Brazil in the early 1900s (Dick et al. 2012). However, these programs ultimately proved to be unsustainable. Insufficient funding, combined with rapid population growth, urbanization, and poor sanitation, resulted in the reemergence and proliferation of *Aedes* mosquitoes throughout the region, as well as a subsequent explosion of mosquito-borne illness in the second half of the twentieth century. The control of mosquito-borne illnesses through vector control remains a priority. Community pesticide spraying is a strategy endorsed by the WHO for control of adult mosquito populations during emergency situations (Beyond Pesticides/National Coalition Against the Misuse of Pesticides, 2002). During outbreaks, the US Centers for Disease Control and Prevention (CDC) endorses the use of spraying, because of its ability to treat large areas very quickly (CDC, 2017).

The benefits of spraying do not come without long-term human and environmental health risks. Synthetic pyrethroids and organophosphates, the two most commonly used sprayed pesticides, have been linked to multiple medical problems, including birth defects, cancer, and chronic dermatologic and respiratory health problems. Infants, children, pregnant women, the elderly, and immunocompromised persons are at highest risk for pesticide-related adverse health outcomes (Beyond Pesticides/National Coalition Against the Misuse of Pesticides, 2002). In addition to individual health risks, there is concern that insecticide spraying may have major unintended environmental impacts, including encouraging mosquito resistance and harming other insect species. For example, in South Carolina, millions of local bees were killed following aerial spraying of insecticides intended for mosquito control (Domonoske, 2016). The elimination of mosquitoes themselves may also be problematic for the ecological health of the environment (Willott, 2004).

Balancing the risks and benefits of insecticide spraying is challenging, as the health and environmental consequences associated with exposure to insecticides must be weighed against the short-term benefits of reducing the adult mosquito population and thereby lowering the burden of mosquito-borne illnesses (Nuffield Council on Bioethics, 2016). Moreover, a reasonable attempt must be made to mitigate risk. Special attention must also be paid to whether the communities with the highest likelihood of being exposed to the risks of pesticide use are vulnerable in any other socially salient ways (Brulle and Pellow, 2006; Northridge et al., 2003). Additionally, pesticides can have transgenerational effects (Kabasenche and Skinner, 2014). Specifically, DDT has been shown to induce germline mutations in people who have been exposed to it, which can lead to increased risk of certain diseases in progeny of future generations who were never exposed to the pesticide (Kabasenche and Skinner, 2014). Further complicating matters, pesticide spraying is undertaken at the community level, and individual consent typically cannot feasibly be obtained.

In order to gauge whether pesticide spraying is an ethically acceptable intervention in a community, there should be carefully planned community engagement through outreach that is transparent, fully communicates risks and benefits, and builds public trust. Guidelines must be developed to ensure public notification in advance of spraying, education about avoiding exposure, and post-spraying surveillance for adverse health outcomes. Lessons can be learned from successful handling of localized outbreaks such as the West Nile outbreak of 1999 in New York City. The New York City Department of Health led an integrated public health response that included the use of pesticide spraying for adult mosquito control with a concurrent large-scale public education campaign to disseminate information on the outbreak and personal safety information on pesticide use (Fine and Layton, 2001).

Introduction of Genetically Modified Mosquitoes

The emergence of new disease threats can prompt the adoption of new technologies that support public health goals. There is significant interest in disease control strategies involving the genetic modification of mosquitoes. Genetic modification of mosquitoes has been performed successfully in the past, consisting of the release of chemically sterilized male mosquitoes intended to outcompete other males and produce no viable offspring. Using this technique, mosquitoes resistant to dengue virus transmission were developed in the 1990s (Olson et al., 1996). Currently, Oxitec, a British biotechnology company, has begun releasing genetically modified self-limiting *Aedes* mosquitoes in Brazil to combat the Zika outbreak (Oxitec, 2016). Oxitec's program releases genetically modified male *Aedes* mosquitoes to mate with female mosquitoes and produce offspring that cannot themselves reproduce, thereby reducing the mosquito population over time (Oxitec, 2016).

Though a promising vector-control strategy, there are many ethical issues surrounding the use of genetically modified organisms (Macer, 2003; Nuffield Council on Bioethics, 2016). Importantly, the potential environmental impact of genetically modified (GM) mosquitoes is poorly understood (Jamrozik et al., 2015). There is also concern that the expense of creating GM mosquitoes may not be sustainable, particularly in low-resource countries. While controversial, this strategy shows promise in that it is effective, showing a reduction of mosquito larvae by 82 percent in areas of Brazil where this technology was used against Zika-carrying *Aedes*, and it targets a particular species in a method that is nontoxic and avoids the use of pesticide (Oxitec, 2016). In addition, strategies making use of CRISPR/Cas9 technology for "gene drives," which may allow scientists to alter certain mosquito traits such as offspring sterility, have spawned intense concern about the risks of "hijacking evolution" (Zielinski, 2016). While gene drive technology has the potential to create mosquitoes unable to carry diseases such as malaria or dengue, the WHO has recommended that further field trials and risk assessments be completed to evaluate the true impact on disease transmission (WHO, 2016).

As more research is completed on the efficacy of GM mosquito control strategies, public health agencies face additional ethical challenges. First, it is essential to determine the potential short- and long-term effects of GM mosquitoes on the ecosystems in areas of use. Second, community education and engagement will be important; it may be unethical to leave decisions regarding the release of GM organisms to a small group of scientists without public input, and success will likely only be achieved with community acceptance and community involvement in implementation. Nevertheless, while public governance of science is an accepted norm, in the face of epidemic disease, public health agencies must also weigh the potential community health and safety benefits of immediate action against the risks associated with waiting for community governance and oversight.

The need for these community governance structures is further underscored by the fact that interventions such as the introduction of GM mosquitoes, perhaps even more so than pesticide spraying, have potential environmental impacts that are both little understood and persistent over time. Determining which risks are acceptable is no easy task and requires the serious consideration of competing values. As a result, there is much room for reasonable disagreement. Implementing fair procedures for decision-making is one way for public health organizations to act in accordance with community interests and values.

Case Study: Zika Virus

Zika virus is a flavivirus that was first discovered in 1947 in the Zika Forest in Uganda. Despite multiple case reports, Zika virus remained relatively quiescent until 2014, when health workers in Brazil noticed an increase in babies born with microcephaly that corresponded with the rapid spread of ZVD from the Pacific islands to Brazil and throughout Latin America and the Caribbean. This outbreak prompted escalation from a public health emergency in Brazil to a WHO-proclaimed Public Health Emergency of International Concern (PHEIC) in February 2016. The WHO estimates that Zika virus has now infected several million people in the Americas. The majority of adults infected with Zika virus are asymptomatic. Those who do develop symptoms typically have a self-limited course of acute low-grade febrile illness with rash, arthritis or arthralgia, eye infections, eye pain, aches, headache, swelling, and vomiting (Petersen et al., 2016). Zika infection has been linked with more severe outcomes, including Guillain-Barré syndrome in some infected adults, as well as adverse fetal outcomes such as severe microcephaly and fetal demise (Petersen et al., 2016).

During the initial Zika outbreak of 2015–2016, the Brazilian government implemented mandatory reporting of cases of Zika-related microcephaly, arguing that it was in the public's best interest to determine if there was truly an association between Zika virus infection during pregnancy and microcephaly (Nuffield Council on Bioethics, 2016). Surveillance in ZVD highlights unique ethical challenges, given that surveillance efforts are targeted at pregnant women and their offspring, as well as the sensitive nature of the disease outcome. Failure to adequately protect the privacy of this data can result in breaches in confidentiality that could harm individuals or communities. The "Fair Information Practice Principles" outlines internationally recognized guidelines to ensure appropriate handling of personal information for surveillance (Collman and Robinson, 2011). Public health agencies should ensure that surveillance programs align with these guidelines. One noteworthy guideline requires officials to ensure the accuracy of the data they collect, noting that the collection of sensitive information should be done in a way that serves the intended purpose. Other requirements include promptly notifying individuals of the personal information that will be collected, obtaining consent whenever possible, and ensuring data security (Collman and Robinson, 2011).

Surveillance may also involve mandatory reporting of cases or clinical outcomes associated with particular mosquito-borne illnesses, sometimes without patient authorization. Public health agencies justify mandatory case finding and reporting based on the likelihood of benefit to the population (Lee, Heilig, and White, 2012), as was the case with ZVD. The need to prioritize public health over individual privacy has led some to stress the need for ethical oversight of surveillance activities (Fairchild and Bayer, 2004). Yet mandated reporting entails an imposition on individual autonomy that warrants the public's demand for justification. Indeed, if mandatory physician reporting had not been implemented in the case of ZVD, there would likely have been substantial delays in establishing a causal link between Zika infection during pregnancy and adverse fetal outcomes.

Although mosquitoes will bite without prejudice of income, mosquito populations flourish in the poor urban slums where inadequate access to public services, sanitation, and clean piped water disproportionately affect those of poorer socioeconomic backgrounds. It is not surprising that the majority of cases of reported microcephaly in Brazil have been among infants of low-income women with poor access to prenatal care or reproductive health services (Watts, 2016). Brazilian Ministry of Health data show that Bahia and Pernambuco—two of the most impoverished states in Brazil—have been disproportionately affected by Zika-related microcephaly (UNFPA, 2016). Without access to contraception or family planning, women in these regions faced considerable challenges in taking the advice of government and public health agencies to "delay pregnancy," and they were at risk for new stigma and victim blaming when they became pregnant during the outbreak. Access to other disease prevention measures, such as insect repellent, window screens, and air conditioning, was also financially out of reach for most women. Government and public health agencies must continue to be mindful of the inequitable distribution of mosquito-borne illnesses and implement interventions to help those communities disproportionately affected. In Brazil, the United Nations Population Fund (UNFPA) is partnering with state and municipal officials to improve access to reproductive health services, including contraception and antenatal care, specifically focusing on ensuring access for women of low socioeconomic status living in poor Northeast states with a high burden of Zika virus (UNFPA, 2016).

Puerto Rico promoted greater access to protective interventions for low-income individuals by addressing price gauging, with fixed prices for condoms, insect repellants, and window screens (Gostin and Hodge, 2016). Despite the novelty of ZVD, the familiar challenge of ensuring universal access to resources that prevent the spread of disease will remain so long as mosquito-borne illnesses remain diseases of the poor.

Unknown Safety of Insect Repellants during Pregnancy

Sometimes, to examine the appropriateness of using a public health intervention, there is a need to gather more evidence about its effect or safety. Use of insect repellants containing diethyltoluamide (DEET) is a highly effective means of preventing mosquito bites, and is strongly recommended to avoid Zika virus infection. DEET is recommended for use in pregnant women, with trial data suggesting that it is safe for women and fetuses when used in the second and third trimesters of pregnancy (McGready et al., 2001). However, there are no studies on the use of DEET in the first trimester, when fetal development may be particularly affected by exposure to chemicals and pharmaceuticals (Johansson et al., 2016). Currently, the WHO and other public health agencies are waging an aggressive campaign urging the use of DEET in any trimester as a preventive measure against Zika. This poses an ethical challenge, as public health agencies have an obligation to determine the safety of DEET use in the first trimester of pregnancy if they are to recommend its use. However, at present, given the substantial risk of microcephaly and fetal demise with Zika-affected pregnancies, encouraging use of DEET is warranted when weighed against the unknown potential risks of DEET use in the first trimester of pregnancy. Nevertheless, longitudinal studies on the impact of DEET use in pregnancy would be valuable.

Reducing the Number of Births

The intersection of Zika virus and women's reproductive rights raises a myriad of ethical challenges. ZVD poses the highest health risk to pregnant women, thus triggering unique public health efforts directed at limiting the exposure of developing fetuses to the virus, primarily through a call to delay pregnancy. Notably, the increasing incidence of Zika-related microcephaly prompted governments in several high-burden countries (Brazil,

Colombia, Ecuador, Jamaica, and El Salvador) to issue controversial and unprecedented public health recommendations, initially urging women living in Zika-affected countries to delay pregnancy for six months to two years (Garsd, 2016). Guidelines as of August 2017 from the WHO and CDC have been revised to recommend delaying conception two months for women and six months for men after potential Zika exposure in an endemic area. While some have argued that calls for delaying pregnancy were justified (Dias, 2016), reproductive rights advocates are deeply concerned that governments made such recommendations in countries where women often have little control over their reproductive health and are subject to high rates of sexual violence.

Research suggests that between 50 and 60 percent of pregnancies in several Latin American countries and in the Caribbean countries (Wilkinson, 2016), and up to 90 percent of pregnancies in El Salvador (Katz, 2016), are unplanned. Some have argued that if a government makes recommendations regarding the timing of pregnancy, there is a responsibility to ensure that all women have access to free or low-cost sexual education, efficacious contraception, and access to abortion services. Indeed, the United Nations High Commissioner for Human Rights, Zeid Ra'ad Al Hussein, called for health systems strengthening to ensure comprehensive sexual and reproductive health services for all women that includes contraception, maternal health care, and safe abortions (OHCHR, 2016).

Preventing Zika-associated fetal complications is further complicated by religious and cultural traditions instantiated in laws prohibiting abortion or severely limiting contraception. Significantly, Pope Francis echoed messages from public health agencies and governments, declaring that delaying pregnancy is permissible in areas affected by Zika (Grant, 2016), and that contraception, in this context, may be the "lesser evil" in cases of serious danger (Wooden, 2016). The pope's clear message of support received praise, given that many women make decisions about their reproductive health based on religious beliefs rather than messages from public health agencies.

The Zika epidemic has sparked international debate about the availability of pregnancy termination worldwide (Garsd, 2016). Pregnant women in Latin America face some of the most restrictive abortion laws in the world. Three countries (the Dominican Republic, El Salvador, and Nicaragua) prohibit abortion completely, and six countries (Guatemala, Haiti, Honduras, Paraguay, Suriname, and Venezuela) provide access to abortion only in the event that it might save the life of the pregnant woman (Kates, Michaud, and Valentine, 2016). A conservative congressman from Brazil proposed a law that would imprison a woman for over four years for aborting a fetus with microcephaly (Sandy, 2016). There is concern that many women in these settings will seek illegal and unsafe abortions.

By intersecting with reproductive rights, the recommendations to delay pregnancy raise even more complex ethical challenges and tensions. The goal of preventing microcephaly by actively discouraging pregnancy conflicts with a respect for reproductive rights. Public health and government agencies must recognize that the women most impacted by ZVD do not have meaningful access to contraceptives or prenatal care. Women who do not have the means to prevent pregnancy may suffer new stigma of victim blaming if they have children born with congenital Zika syndrome. Simultaneously, an intention to respect individual reproductive rights by providing access to abortion may come into conflict with an obligation to respect local cultural values and laws that outlaw abortion. Striking a balance between all three of these ethical goals cannot and should not be done in the absence of meaningful community engagement.

Conclusion

Mosquito-borne illnesses pose a significant public health threat. Given the substantial morbidity and mortality resulting from these infections, as well as the social, economic, and ecological costs, public health agencies and governments must make a renewed commitment to mosquito control. Community engagement and acceptance of mosquito control interventions is essential. In the setting of a fast-paced epidemic, such as the Zika outbreak, it may be justifiable to mandate data collection for disease registries and to call for price fixing for mosquito repellant and screens to ensure equitable access. There must also be an emphasis on further research into the short- and long-term ecological impacts of genetic modification of organisms and mosquito eradication. When more evidence is available to help guide practice, it is essential to re-evaluate interventions in the context of public choice, distributive justice, autonomy, and privacy.

The challenges posed by the Zika epidemic surrounding women's reproductive health autonomy, access to sexual education, efficacious contraception, safe abortions, and prenatal care must serve as a call to action to affect change in an international health system that lacks the necessary infrastructure to provide basic services. As globalization and urbanization continue, it is essential to remember that mosquito-borne illnesses are primarily diseases of the poor. Strengthening countrywide health systems and improving access to clean water and sanitation, screens, netting, low-cost primary health care, immunization, and contraception not only are likely to be effective for controlling mosquito-borne diseases—they are also ethical imperatives.

References

Baiden, F., Hodgson, A., and Binka, F. N. 2006. "Demographic Surveillance Sites and Emerging Challenges in International Health." *Bulletin of the World Health Organization* 84(3): 163.

Beyond Pesticides/National Coalition Against the Misuse of Pesticides. 2002. "Public Health Mosquito Management Strategy." *Pesticides and You* 22(2): 14–23. https://www.beyondpesticides.org/assets/media/documents/infoservices/pesticidesandyou/Summer%2002%20vol.%2022%20no.%202.pdf.

Brulle, Robert J., and Pellow, D. N. 2006. "Environmental Justice: Human Health and Environmental Inequalities." *Annual Review of Public Health* 27: 103–124.

CDC (US Centers for Disease Control and Prevention). 2017. "Information on Aerial Spraying." https://www.cdc.gov/westnile/vectorcontrol/aerial-spraying.html.

Collman, J., and Robinson, A. 2011. "Designing Ethical Practice in Biosurveillance: The Project Argus Doctrine." In *Infectious Disease Informatics and Biosurveillance*, edited by D. Zeng, H. Chen, D. Bies, W. B. Lober, and M. Thurmond, 23–44 (Boston: Springer).

Curtis, C., Maxwell, C., Lemnge, M., Kilama W. L., Steketee R.W., Hawley W. A., et al. 2003. "Scaling-Up Coverage with Insecticide-Treated Nets against Malaria in Africa: Who Should Pay?" *Lancet Infectious Diseases* 3: 304–307.

Dias, M. 2016. "Ethics of Public Health Messaging Abroad: Are the Recent Zika-Related Recommendations of Various Health Agencies Unjustified Paternalism or Sound Public Health Guidance?" *Voices in Bioethics*, March 22. http://www.voicesinbioethics.net/opeds/2016/03/22/ethics-of-public-health-messaging-abroad-are-the-recent-zika-related-recommendations-of-various-health-agencies-unjustified-paternalism-or-sound-public-health-guidance.

Dick, O. B., San Martín, J. L., Montoya, R. H., del Diego, J., Zambrano, B., and Dayan, G. H. 2012. "The History of Dengue Outbreaks in the Americas." *American Journal of Tropical Medicine and Hygiene* 87(4): 584–593.

Domonoske C. 2016. "S.C. County Sprays for Mosquitoes but Accidentally Takes Out Millions of Bees." NPR, September 2. http://www.npr.org/sections/thetwo-way/2016/09/02/492404411/s-c-county-sprays-for-mosquitoes-but-accidentally-takes-out-millions-of-bees.

Fairchild, A. L., and Bayer, R. 2004. "Ethics and the Conduct of Public Health Surveillance." *Science* 303(5658): 631–632.

Fine, A., and Layton, M. 2001. "Lessons from the West Nile Viral Encephalitis Outbreak in New York City, 1999: Implications for Bioterrorism Preparedness." *Clinical Infectious Diseases* 32(2): 277–282. https://academic.oup.com/cid/article/32/2/277/320355/Lessons-from-the-West-Nile-Viral-Encephalitis.

Garsd, J. 2016. "Zika Virus Isn't the First Disease to Spark a Debate about Abortion." NPR, *Goats and Soda Blog*, January 31. http://www.npr.org/sections/goatsandsoda/2016/01/31/464750384/zika-virus-isnt-the-first-disease-to-spark-a-debate-about-abortion.

Gostin, L., and Hodge, J. 2016. "Is the United States Prepared for a Major Zika Virus Outbreak?" *JAMA Opinion* 315(22): 2395–2396. https://jamanetwork.com/journals/jama/fullarticle/2514046.

Grant, M. S. 2016. "Zika Virus Alters Catholic Church Policy on Contraception?" *Huffington Post*, January 25. http://www.huffingtonpost.com/melissa-s-grant/zika-virus-alters-catholic-church-policy-on-contraception_b_9301410.html.

Johansson, M. A., Mier-y-Teran-Romero, L. Reefhuis, J. Gilboa, S. M., Hills, S. L. 2016. "Zika and the Risk of Microcephaly." *New England Journal of Medicine* 375: 1–4. doi:10.1056/NEJMp1605367.

Kabasenche, W. P., and Skinner, M. K. 2014. "DDT, Epigenetic Harm, and Transgenerational Environmental Justice." *Environmental Health* 13(1): 62. https://www.ncbi.nlm.nih.gov/pmc/articles/PMC4124473/.

Kates, J., Michaud, J., and Valentine, A. 2016. "Zika Virus: The Challenge for Women." Henry J. Kaiser Family Foundation, April 15. http://www.kff.org/global-health-policy/perspective/zika-virus-the-challenge-for-women/.

Katz, J. 2016. "The Dilemma of Zika: Pregnancy Warnings Rise in a Region Lacking Contraception." *STAT News*, February 1. https://www.statnews.com/2016/02/01/zika-pregnancy-warnings-latin-america/.

Lee, L. M., Heilig, C. M., and White, A. 2012. "Ethical Justification for Conducting Public Health Surveillance without Patient Consent." *American Journal of Public Health* 102(1): 38–44.

Lengeler C. 2004. "Insecticide-Treated Bed Nets and Curtains for Preventing Malaria." *Cochrane Database Systemic Review* 2004(2): CD000363.

Macer, D. 2003. *Ethical, Legal and Social Issues of Genetically Modified Disease Vectors in Public Health* (Geneva: UNDP/World Bank/WHO Special Programme for Research & Training in Tropical Diseases).

McGready, R. Hamilton, K. A., Simpson, T. C., Luxemburger, C., Edwards, R., Looareesuwan, S., et al. 2001. "Safety of the Insect Repellent *N, N-Diethyl-M-Toluamide* (DEET) in Pregnancy." *American Journal of Tropical Medicine and Hygiene* 65(4): 285–289.

Minakawa, N., Dida, G. O., Sonye, G. O., Futami, K., and Kaneko, S. 2008. "Unforeseen Misuses of Bed Nets in Fishing Villages along Lake Victoria." *Malaria Journal* 7: 165. doi:10.1186/1475-2875-7-165.

Northridge, M. E., Stover, G. N., Rosenthal, J. E., and Sherard, D. 2003. "Environmental Equity and Health: Understanding Complexity and Moving Forward." *American Journal of Public Health* 93(2): 209–214.

Nuffield Council on Bioethics. 2016. "Zika: Ethical Considerations." Briefing Note, February 9. http://nuffieldbioethics.org/wp-content/uploads/NCOB-briefing-note-zika-ethical-considerations.pdf.

OHCHR (Office of the High Commissioner for Human Rights of the United Nations). 2016. "Upholding Women's Human Rights Essential to Zika Response—Zeid." News release, February 5. http://www.ohchr.org/EN/NewsEvents/Pages/DisplayNews.aspx?NewsID=17014&LangID=E.

Olson K. E., Higgs, S., Gaines, P. J., Powers, A. M., Davis, B. S., Kamrud, K. I., et al. 1996 "Genetically Engineered Resistance in Mosquitoes to Dengue Virus Transmission." *Science* 272: 884–886.

Oxitec. 2016. "Expansion of Oxitec's Vector Control Solution in Brazil Attacking Source of Zika Virus and Dengue Fever after Positive Program Results." Intrexon/Oxitec Press Release, January 19. https://www.prnewswire.com/news-releases/expansion-of-oxitecs-vector-control-solution-in-brazil-attacking-source-of-zika-virus-and-dengue-fever-after-positive-program-results-300206021.html.

Petersen, R. L., Jamieson, D. J., Powers, A. M., and Honein, M. A. 2016. "Zika Virus." *New England Journal of Medicine* 374: 1552–1563.

Sandy, M. 2016 "Brazilian Legislators Look to Increase Abortion Penalties in the Wake of the Zika Outbreak." *Time*, February 22. http://time.com/4230975/brazil-abortion-laws-zika-outbreak/.

UNFPA (United Nations Population Fund). 2016. "Poverty, Inequality at the Heart of the Zika Outbreak." News Release, July 21. http://www.unfpa.org/news/poverty-inequality-heart-zika-outbreak.

Watts, J. 2016. "Brazil's Sprawling Favelas Bear the Brunt of the Zika Epidemic." *Guardian*, February 7. http://www.theguardian.com/world/2016/feb/07/brazil-rich-zika-virus-poor.

WHO (World Health Organization). 2006. "Communicable Disease Surveillance and Response Systems: Guide to Monitoring and Evaluating." http://www.who.int/csr/resources/publications/surveillance/WHO_CDS_EPR_LYO_2006_2/en/.

WHO (World Health Organization). 2014. "A Global Brief on Vector-Borne Diseases." http://www.who.int/campaigns/world-health-day/2014/global-brief/en/.

WHO (World Health Organization). 2016. "Mosquito Control: Can it Stop Zika at Source?" http://www.who.int/emergencies/zika-virus/articles/mosquito-control/en/.

Wilkinson, D. 2016. "Should We Prevent Zika Microcephaly Using Birth Control?" *Practical Ethics Blog*. http://blog.practicalethics.ox.ac.uk/2016/02/zika/.

Willott, Elizabeth. 2004. "Restoring Nature, without Mosquitoes?" *Restoration Ecology* 12(2): 147–153.

Wooden, C. 2016. "In Zika Outbreak, Contraceptives May be 'Lesser Evil,' Pope Says." Catholic News Service, February 19. http://www.catholicnews.com/services/englishnews/2016/in-zika-outbreak-contraceptives-may-be-lesser-evil-pope-says.cfm.

Zielinski, A. 2016. "The Ethical Risks of Engineering Mosquitoes into Extinction to Stop Zika." *Think Progress*, February 24. https://thinkprogress.org/the-ethical-risks-of-engineering-mosquitoes-into-extinction-to-stop-zika-88e45e538d25/.

Further Reading

EPA (US Environmental Protection Agency). 2012. "Joint Statement on Mosquito Control in the United States from the U.S. Environmental Protection Agency (EPA) and the U.S. Centers for Disease Control and Prevention (CDC)." https://www.epa.gov/mosquito-control/joint-statement-mosquito-control-united-states.

Fauci, A. S., and Morens, D. M. 2016. "Zika Virus in the Americas—Yet Another Arbovirus Threat." *New England Journal of Medicine* 374: 601–604.

Jamrozik E., de la Fuente-Núñez, V., Reis, A., Ringwald, P., and Selgelid, M. J. 2015. "Ethical Aspects of Malaria Control and Research." *Malaria Journal* 14:518. https://malariajournal.biomedcentral.com/articles/10.1186/s12936-015-1042-3.

Musso, D., Cao-Lormeau, V. M., and Gubler, D. J. 2015 "Zika Virus: Following the Path of Dengue and Chikungunya?" *Lancet* 386: 243–244.

Omer, S., and Beigi, R. 2016. "Pregnancy in the Time of Zika: Addressing Barriers for Developing Vaccines and Other Measures for Pregnant Women." *JAMA* 315(12): 1227–1228.

Salam, A. P., Rojek, A., Dunning, J., and Horby, P. W. 2017. "Clinical Trials of Therapeutics for the Prevention of Congenital Zika Virus Disease: Challenges and Potential Solutions Clinical Trials of Therapeutics to Prevent Congenital ZIKV Disease." *Annals of Internal Medicine* 166(10): 725–732.

Tavares, M. P., and Foster, A. M. 2016. "Emergency Contraception in a Public Health Emergency: Exploring Pharmacy Availability in Brazil." *Contraception* 94(2): 109–114. doi:10.1016/j.contraception.2016.04.006.

CHAPTER 41

GLOBAL HIV/AIDS PREVENTION AND TREATMENT: PUBLIC HEALTH ETHICS CONSIDERATIONS

MARK BARNES AND DEVIN ALEXANDER COHEN

Introduction

DESPITE intensified treatment efforts over the past four decades, an estimated 21.9 million people worldwide living with human immunodeficiency virus (HIV) or acquired immunodeficiency syndrome (AIDS) lack access to affordable antiretroviral treatments (ARVs or ARTs) (UNAIDS, 2015). A number of factors, including meager health care infrastructure and availability, costs of drugs and care, and suboptimal public health prevention efforts, have affected HIV/AIDS care programs, but one of the most enduring barriers worldwide between individuals with HIV/AIDS and treatment has been the stigma associated with these conditions (Turan and Nyblade, 2013). For instance, one study conducted in Botswana and Zambia found that "stigma against HIV-positive persons and fear of discrimination were the key reasons for the low uptake of voluntary counseling and testing to prevent mother-to-child transmission of the virus" (Asante, 2007). Stigma is inherent to a disease that may be transmitted in the most intimate social relationships and may result in death (Bayer, 1989). Indeed, early access to voluntary HIV/AIDS antibody testing in the 1980s was greatly inhibited by fear (especially among men who have sex with men) of being labeled "HIV-positive" and even targeted for hate crimes, since it had become, in the words of one public health scholar, "open season on gays" in many American cities (Bayer, 1989, 101–102).

Since the early 1980s, public health officials have struggled with balancing the rights of people with HIV/AIDS with the protection of uninfected populations. The conflict between personal autonomy and protecting public health is clear enough in the context of contagious disease outbreak and control (Francis et al., 2006; Beauchamp and Childress, 2013), but the ethics of an appropriate sociopolitical response are not so clear. How should a state "get into the business of modifying human behavior, even if it does so to improve health" (Lalonde, 1975, 36)? How is the balance between paternalism (active intervention) and sovereignty (autonomous rule over one's body) best struck, and what social and public health considerations should affect the equation?

This chapter will explore the historical developments in global HIV/AIDS prevention and treatment, and the ethical implications of public health responses thereto, by considering three stages of the epidemic: (i) the period when proven HIV/AIDS treatment options were unavailable, (ii) the time at which safe and effective antiretroviral regimens were developed and made publicly available, and (iii) current efforts for slowing the global spread of HIV/AIDS. The focus throughout will be on social developments affecting government policy with regard to the behavior of people living with HIV/AIDS.

Testing Absent Effective Treatment: The 1980s

In 1981, the US Centers for Disease Control and Prevention (CDC) reported the appearance of two conditions in male, homosexual communities: *Pneumocystis carinii*, a rare form of pneumonia, and *Kaposi's sarcoma*, a rare cancer labeled at the time as "gay-related immune deficiency" (Engel, 2006). The public immediately identified these as part of a "gay" disease, and from 1982 to 1985, hate crimes against men who have sex with men (MSM) tripled in the United States (Engel, 2006, 45). In Haiti, where some believed the epidemic originated, public officials raided gay bars and expelled tourists who frequented businesses known to cater to an MSM clientele (Smallman, 2007). The CDC, recognizing this new syndrome as a sexually transmitted, blood-borne disease (Bayer and Oppenheimer, 2000), fed into public perception that certain demographic groups were the source of the outbreak by designating homosexuality, heroin addiction, hemophilia, and Haitian descent (the "4H Club") as primary "risk factors" for HIV infection (PBS, 2006).

As public stigma associated with HIV/AIDS spread, infection rates among MSM rose—in 1986, some epidemiologists estimated that at least 50 percent of gay men in New York and San Francisco were infected with HIV (Bayer, 1989, 12)—and public health officials were faced with the challenge of bending the infection curve in a discriminatory sociopolitical environment. In New York and San Francisco, regulators took a protectionist approach, shuttering bathhouses that had been openly frequented by MSMs for sexual encounters, focusing on infection-containment for an entire at-risk population in the absence of antibody testing. Advocacy groups objected that the closures focused on social institutions rather than the need to alter MSM attitudes toward safe sex, forcing affected populations underground. Many in the gay community considered such action particularly draconian, considering not all MSM carried the infection and the role of bathhouses in the gay community in facilitating sex in a safe environment (Engel, 2006).

The focus on disease spread in gay communities overlooked the growing incidence in heterosexual communities and across additional at-risk social demographics (Bayer and Oppenheimer, 2000). Many in the United States blamed the sudden rise of infections in the heterosexual community on intravenous drug use by "deviants." Others demonized prostitution for bringing the epidemic to previously "untainted" demographics. Nonetheless, infection rates rose across heterosexual communities, which proved slow to react, particularly with regard to the growing incidence in women (Engel, 2006). In fact, the CDC did not address the risk posed to females by their male partners until 1983 (Bayer and Oppenheimer, 2000), failed to classify a significant number of "unexplained" AIDS cases as involving transmission to or from women until 1986 (Simmons, Farmer, and Shoepf, 2011), and did not revise its case definition of the disease to include opportunistic infections for women until 1993 (Connors, 2011). Further, federal officials initially refused to allow female participation in clinical trials during the development of ARTs in the mid-to-late 1980s (Engel, 2006; Bayer and Oppenheimer, 2000). Globally, women faced substantial barriers to recognition as at-risk communities, given widespread subordination and oppression at the hands of patriarchies (Smallman, 2007).

Early in the epidemic, African and Latin American populations, facing high rates of poverty and intravenous drug use, reported HIV/AIDS cases in disproportionate numbers relative to the general population (Bayer and Oppenheimer, 2000; Engel, 2006). As with women, these populations were further disadvantaged in access to clinical trials for promising treatments. In addition, African American communities generally maintained greater cultural discomfort with male homosexual activities than other communities. This often dissuaded African American MSM from disclosing their sexual activities to friends, family, and physicians, and it deterred traditional community institutions—especially organized religious institutions—from directly confronting the impact of HIV/AIDS on their parishioners and members (Engel, 2006). Accordingly, African American communities had even less access to HIV/AIDS education and treatment than many other populations in the United States throughout the 1980s.

In the early-to-mid-1980s, the universal prognosis for HIV-infected individuals was bleak. Although HIV advocacy groups organized nationally on behalf of impacted communities to inform federal HIV/AIDS policy and lobby for research funding (HHS, 2015), the science required for safe and effective treatment remained years away. Patient access to education and palliative health care services was further inhibited by rising stigmatization within the medical community itself, as physicians turned away HIV/AIDS patients out of fear for their own safety (Daniels, 2006), expressed antipathy toward affected populations (especially MSM) (Bayer and Oppenheimer, 2000), and feared that their presence in a clinic or office would deter other patients from coming to the same places for care, which provoked controversy over medical ethics obligations in the context of an epidemic disease (Daniels, 2006; Smallman, 2007). Furthermore, HIV-infected physicians reportedly hid their own conditions from patients and peers, fearing reprisals, ultimately giving rise to state-level disclosure requirements amid enormous policy controversy (Fein, 1997; Barnes et al., 1990; Engel, 2006).

Following the development and prevalent availability of HIV antibody testing, the CDC encouraged voluntary screening for all Americans deemed "at-risk" for HIV/AIDS. The CDC initially deemed the following populations "at-risk": homosexual and bisexual men, present or past injection drug abusers, persons with clinical laboratory evidence of HIV infection, persons born in countries where heterosexual transmission was believed to play a major role in the spread of AIDS, male and female prostitutes, sex partners of infected persons or persons at increased risk, all persons with hemophilia who had received clotting factor products, and newborn infants of high-risk or infected mothers (Bayer, 1989).

The potential public health impact of widespread voluntary testing was great: theoretically, by identifying HIV-infected individuals, officials could determine next steps for education and prevent further spread. However, encouraging voluntary testing for HIV when no effective treatments were available proved difficult, particularly as the accuracy of early tests was questioned (Bayer, 1989). Without effective treatments, national implementation of voluntary testing primarily benefited the interests of epidemiologic surveillance and accurate targeting of prevention resources. But the *individual* who tested positive on an HIV antibody test received no direct personal health benefit beyond behavior modification suggestions designed to protect his or her partners (Fox et al., 1987). Opponents of voluntary testing particularly feared how health officials would utilize positive results. These fears were heightened by the fact that homosexuality was illegal in over twenty states, and intravenous drug use in all states, in the mid-1980s. Nonetheless, in order to facilitate contact tracing, some states implemented laws requiring clinicians to report to the government all cases in which patients tested positive for HIV (Bayer, 1989).

Contact tracing informed individuals of previous sexual or needle sharing contact with HIV-infected individuals. The benefits of HIV testing in combination with contact tracing were primarily two-fold: a personal benefit of health counseling for HIV-infected individuals (particularly those feeling helpless about the uncertainty of their potential conditions), and a social benefit of encouraging actions that could reduce the risk of HIV transmission to others. More broadly, contact tracing entailed a key role for physicians reporting HIV-infected test results for the benefit of at-risk partners. In theory, contact tracing could be used to identify a large number of HIV-infected and at-risk individuals, raising a core policy question: What would a government do with this information? Proposed legislative limitations on personal autonomy, including domestic calls for quarantine (Engel, 2006) or exclusion from various settings such as physician's offices and even schools, fueled adamant opposition to contact tracing in at-risk communities. While the promotion of *voluntary* partner notification grew in acceptance among the affected, mandatory contact tracing (and HIV testing and partner notification laws) was viewed as a substantial threat to civil liberties, particularly in light of the ongoing discrimination (Engel, 2006; Bayer, 1989).

In response to fears related to mandatory contact tracing, anonymous testing sites arose nationwide. To protect privacy, some HIV testing sites even accepted pseudonyms, highlighting the underlying intent to benefit the patient directly (Bayer, 1989). Anonymity insulated HIV-infected individuals from state reporting requirements, contact tracing, and risk of further stigma (Bayer, 1989). As a public health response, anonymous testing relied on individuals learning of their HIV infection voluntarily and then curbing high-risk behaviors and personally approaching potentially infected contacts, representing a model of epidemic control that de-emphasized coercive public health measures in favor of private voluntarism.

Meanwhile, international responses to the HIV/AIDS epidemic during the 1980s varied greatly. Cuba, for instance, implemented quarantines for HIV-infected individuals and widespread mandatory HIV testing. By 1989, Cuba had tested more than 75 percent of the population over the age of fifteen. Despite backlash by international human rights groups, Cuban *sanitoria* housing HIV-infected individuals reportedly offered residents "free medical care, access to medications, additional food rations, their salaries, and better living conditions than other Cubans" (Smallman, 2007, 40). Whether the underlying justification for the *sanitoria* (separating infected individuals from the uninfected population while providing allegedly adequate health and compensation) may arguably be defensible from a public health perspective, these quarantines removed residents from their families and communities, even when those persons avoided unsafe sexual or needle-sharing contact with others. The policy effectively created a de facto prison primarily for MSM, women, intravenous drug users, and populations on the margins of society. The ethical constraints of Cuba's HIV/AIDS response were loosened later in the epidemic, when the Cuban government shifted from mandatory quarantine to "voluntary" confinement in *sanitoria* (Smallman, 2007, 48–49). While it was reported that Cuba's response to the epidemic proved highly effective, some have doubted the validity of statistics released by the Cuban government (Engel, 2006; Solomon, 2003; Voice of America, 1992; Smallman, 2007).

Conversely, South Africa's initial public health response to HIV/AIDS was focused on voluntarism, and later on prevention education. The nation's initial response was impeded by a president who challenged the causal link between HIV and AIDS. The South African government required supplemental clinical trials for treatments already proven safe and effective abroad, and political leaders failed to make necessary investments into a declining health care infrastructure (Selgelid, 2006; Iliffe, 2006; Patterson, 2006). Accordingly, HIV-infected South Africans relied on public organizations and social advocacy movements for much-needed assistance. Lacking crucial support from the leadership of the predominant national political force, the African National Congress, South Africa was disadvantaged compared to other African nations, at a time when, in 2005, the country had the largest population of HIV-infected individuals of any nation worldwide (Selgelid, 2006).

Although South Africa continues to face one of the world's largest HIV epidemics, advocacy groups, and even the South African government, have more recently made great strides toward lowering infection rates and treating infected persons. South Africa now has the largest antiretroviral program in the world, and it invests more than $1 billion annually in its HIV/AIDS programs, which has resulted in significant decreases in mother-to-child HIV transmission since 2001 (AVERT, 2016a; AIDSMap, 2016). Because of the high prevalence of HIV and the relatively high level of health system infrastructure compared to other countries in the region, South Africa has become a favored locale for prevention studies and HIV vaccine research (SouthAfricaInfo, 2014; Senthilingam, 2016), and the South African government has acknowledged, through concrete policy changes, that the uninfected population is best protected through aggressive treatment of HIV-infected individuals. Accordingly, South Africa has expressly moved away from the regressive public health policies of the late 1980s and has recognized the capacity of HIV/AIDS to impact all demographics, regardless of race or gender (Iliffe, 2006).

AZT and HAART: The 1990s and 2000s

Global public health responses to HIV/AIDS were facilitated by the availability of effective antiretroviral drugs, the first of which—zidovudine, commonly known as AZT—was approved by the US Food and Drug Administration (FDA) in 1990 (HHS, 2015). However, the FDA's stringent criteria for use, and Burroughs-Wellcome's $10,000/year price tag on the drug, initially created significant barriers to access (Bayer and Oppenheimer, 2000). HIV/AIDS advocates, having successfully fought for an expedited approval process for AZT and a formal compassionate use program for patients seeking access to the medication prior to FDA approval, played a key role in ensuring broad accessibility to the first pharmaceutical breakthrough in the HIV/AIDS epidemic by effectively advocating for affordable pricing practices and additional federal research funding (Engel, 2006; NIH 2016).

After a landmark study, "ACTG 076," was stopped early when it demonstrated that giving AZT to HIV-infected pregnant women could dramatically reduce the chance of their babies being infected, a new set of questions arose, including whether HIV screening should be mandatory in pregnancy in order to identify who could be given this preventive intervention. In 1995 the CDC recommended that all pregnant women undergo voluntary testing (CDC, 2006). While recognizing the need to protect newborns from the virulent disease, pregnant women grappled with maintaining autonomy over their bodies and conditions (Iliffe, 2006; Gollub, 1999). Activists feared that women would be forced both to be tested and to take AZT solely for the benefit of their children and without regard to their own health status (Bayer and Oppenheimer, 2000), particularly in light of clinical uncertainty as to AZT's ability to prolong the lives of symptomatic individuals

(Bayer and Oppenheimer, 2000). These fears were exacerbated by reports of AZT's toxic side effects (Bayer and Oppenheimer, 2000).

The FDA's approval of the first protease inhibitor in 1995 ushered in the era of highly active antiretroviral therapy (HAART) (HHS, 2015). HAART was a combination therapy that significantly extended and improved quality of life, with substantially fewer toxic side effects than those of AZT (Engel, 2006). By 1996 the FDA had also approved the first HIV home testing kit (HHS, 2015). The availability of newly approved safe and effective HIV/AIDS treatments, in addition to accessible testing, fundamentally reoriented the public health response to the HIV/AIDS outbreak. Public health officials could now request voluntary testing of at-risk populations with a focus on individual benefit in addition to social utility. The ethical constraints of encouraging voluntary testing of HIV-infected pregnant women became less rigid, as HAART offered a safe and effective treatment regimen to the mother and newborn alike—although most prenatal voluntary testing messages remained focused on the welfare of newborns.

Political demands for mandatory testing for purposes of treatment intervention and screening/exclusion continued into and throughout the 1990s. The advent of mandatory HIV testing and "opt-out" approaches to HIV testing (with consent assumed unless the patient affirmatively chooses otherwise), made anonymous HIV testing sites that had grown in popularity in the mid-to-late 1980s even more appealing for some. Mandatory testing laws in Canada (requiring mandatory testing for those over the age of fifteen requesting permanent residency; see Bisaillon, 2010), United States (mandating testing for prospective immigrants, the armed forces, and individual health, life, and disability insurance policies; see Iliffe, 2006), and Africa (requiring premarital HIV screening in certain nations; see Chattu, 2014), reflected a growing international trend toward mandatory testing in certain situations, despite the World Health Organization's opposition to such required screening (Iliffe, 2006).

HIV testing, even when not required, became more routinized after the advent of safe and effective treatments. In 2006 the CDC recommended "opt-out" HIV screening for all patients in health care settings where diagnostic and screening tests are regularly available and for pregnant women (CDC, 2006). By moving from an "opt-in" to an "opt-out" approach of HIV testing, much in line with its standard position for other diseases, the CDC aimed to protect a degree of personal autonomy while promoting both individual and societal welfare by allowing people to know their HIV-infected status, seek life-extending treatment, and refrain from high-risk behaviors (Beauchamp and Childress, 2013). Routinized opt-out testing approaches also increased fairness, provided an effective safeguard against physicians stereotyping their patients and only screening high-risk populations for HIV/AIDS.

Despite the proven efficacy of opt-out screening, and its being seen in some circles as a reasonable ethics "compromise" between encouraging testing while still allowing refusal, some criticized the approach for its lack of explicit and individualized informed consent. According to one AIDS activist, opt-out testing is "not informed consent, and it is not even consent, [but rather an attempt] to ram HIV testing down people's throats without their [permission]" (Bayer and Fairchild, 2006, 649). Opt-out proponents, however, view opt-in consent as unduly troublesome. They argue that routine opt-out testing permits physicians to spend their limited time with patients discussing other important health needs, rather than reciting a list of legal jargon required for opt-in consent, and offers the only practical option with physician-patient interactions becoming increasingly shorter.

Contact tracing remained a contentious policy debate beginning in the 1980s and continuing into the 1990s. Most US states and territories have implemented mandatory name reporting to the government for people who test HIV-positive (Kaiser Family Foundation, 2015). Some states require the state health department to notify an HIV-infected individual's sexual and needle-sharing partners of his or her condition, known as "partner notification" (New York State Department of Health, 2013), while others rely on treating physicians to exercise discretion in notification (Maryland AIDS Administration, 2007). Furthermore, health departments receiving federal funding through the Ryan White program must show good faith efforts to notify persons placed at risk by HIV-infected patients. Under the current reporting regimes, these public health policies impose a direct obligation on physicians to facilitate partner notification, subject to the American Medical Association's code of ethics (and, in certain jurisdictions, insulating physicians from associated liability).

Today: Global HIV/AIDS Treatment and Prevention

Having effective treatments for HIV has required a global approach focusing on populations in which HIV is prevalent, health care utilization and access is low, medical infrastructure is poor, and resources are limited. At the same time, the global health burden of HIV continues to grow: it is estimated that 34 million people worldwide are currently living with HIV, but only 8 million of the 14.8 million people eligible for ARV treatment under current guidelines receive it (Hayes et al., 2014).

Global access to ART is a prerequisite to effective HIV/AIDS outreach. While pharmaceutical pricing practices have posed barriers to access to effective treatments, some manufacturers have made accommodations in response to competitive market developments. In the early-to-mid-1990s, for example, Glaxo-Wellcome (now GlaxoSmithKline) substantially lowered the price of AZT for pregnant women in low-income countries, following the release of a study from Thailand indicating that a shorter and cheaper course of the drug curbed mother-to-child transmission rates (Iliffe, 2006). Other large drug manufacturers, including nevirapine's manufacturer, Boehringer Ingelheim, responded similarly after advocacy groups and public health agencies publicly chastised the industry for pricing practices (Iliffe, 2006; Kaiser Health News, 2007).

International generic competition further facilitated global access to ART. The most notable international generic HIV/AIDS treatment entered the market in 2001 when Cipla, an Indian generic manufacturer, began to sell its HAART triple therapy for $350 per patient per year, immediately before the UN General Assembly established the Global Fund to Fight AIDS, Tuberculosis and Malaria (GFATM) to facilitate treatment for the HIV-infected in low- and middle-income countries (LMICs) (Iliffe, 2006). Cipla's success paved the way for other countries, such as Brazil and Thailand, to authorize generic manufacturing for the benefit of particularly impoverished at-risk populations (Interagency Coalition on AIDS and Development, 2001).

Effective advocacy greatly enhanced global access to ART. Many advocacy groups, such as Treatment Action Campaign in South Africa, the Gay Men's Health Crisis, and ACT-UP, protested pharmaceutical pricing practices, highlighting the resulting barrier to care and the role of US patents in hindering international generic development and availability (Simmons, Connors, and Farmer, 2011). In addition, advocates pressured pharmaceutical companies to lower the prices of their patented drugs in resource-poor countries. As a result, Merck discounted two of its AIDS treatments by 90 percent in sub-Saharan Africa, and GlaxoSmithKline reduced the price of three HIV/AIDS drugs by 80 percent in sixty-three countries, in 2001 (Interagency Coalition on AIDS and Development, 2001).

International donor funds were also formed to support HIV/AIDS prevention and treatment worldwide, spearheaded by the US President's Emergency Plan for AIDS Relief (PEPFAR) and GFATM (Patterson, 2006). By 2014 the world had invested approximately $20.2 billion in the HIV/AIDS response in LMICs (UNAIDS, 2015; FDA, 2009), and between 2009 and 2014, 84 of 121 LMICs receiving international support increased their domestic spending on HIV/AIDS prevention and treatment (UNAIDS, 2015).

With the increased global availability of HAART, public health researchers have focused on studying methods to prevent the global spread of HIV/AIDS, particularly in Africa, which remains the continent hardest hit by the epidemic. Prevention studies acknowledge the essential role of both treatment and education in preventing HIV transmission and have recognized the epidemic's particular impact on women. One US National Institutes of Health (NIH) HIV Prevention Network (HPTN) study found "BufferGel" to be an effective method for preventing male-to-female transmission, reducing HIV acquisition by 30 percent in female study participants (Karim et al., 2011). Another study in South Africa and Zimbabwe determined that the use of multiple contraceptives, rather than condoms alone, did not reduce the incidence of HIV in study participants (Padian et al., 2007). In contrast, an interventional study in South Africa showed that women engaged in sexual activity utilizing a dapivirine vaginal ring were 65 percent less likely to contract HIV than those not using the ring (AIDS2016, 2016). A key prevention study in men confirmed that male circumcision significantly reduces the risk of HIV in at-risk men (Gray et al., 2007).

More recently, the "PopART Study" (HPTN 071) reviewed the effect of combination prevention strategies in Zambia and South Africa (Hayes et al., 2014). Although follow-up ended in all study populations in mid-2018, primary results will not be available until 2019. Researchers believe that the study could reveal whether combination prevention and treatment interventions can be delivered to scale, the population-level impact of such interventions, and potential adverse effects (including sexual risk disinhibition and increased stigma). The three-year trial was launched in twenty-one African communities (with a total population of approximately 1.2 million people) to test whether new HIV infections can be significantly reduced by flooding communities with multiple opportunities for testing, including home-based testing, and immediately placing all who have tested positive into ART regardless of immune status (Hayes, 2014; HIV Prevention Trials Network, 2018). Scientists hypothesize that HIV incidence will drop by over 60 percent relative to incidence in the control group that receives only standard-of-care public health prevention, testing, and ART availability (Cori et al., 2014).

Positive prevention study findings do not ensure widespread implementation. Acceptance of novel prevention strategies requires adequate government funding and ongoing support by nongovernmental organizations (NGOs) and/or donor agencies, which are often stretched thin for resources. They require on-the-ground health care professionals, workforce, institutional knowledge, and infrastructures capable of administering counseling and care. Certain local traditions may, in some cases, pose challenges to implementing new prevention strategies. For instance, a woman's role in a number of societies is that of caregiver and wife, which could deprive her of the sense of agency more prevalent in many Western cultures. As such, at-risk women may be limited in their opportunities to seek medical advice and remain subject to the sexual wishes of their spouses. Similarly, a number of African communities are reluctant to participate in medical procedures or treatments proven to prevent HIV/AIDS, such a circumcision, based upon historical practices, despite developing scientific findings as to the efficacy of such prevention methods (Timberg, 2007).

Finally, implementation of new prevention strategies is greatly encumbered by discrimination against particularly stigmatized groups. For instance, African men who have sex with men continue to face tremendous stigma and barriers to access to care; some African countries outlaw homosexual practices altogether. Such laws make it difficult, if not impossible, for some men to seek care without risking marginalization, fines, or imprisonment (OutRight Action International, 2007; AVERT, 2016b).

Conclusion

The public health response to the HIV/AIDS epidemic has consistently been characterized by health officials focusing initially on those they believed to be at-risk populations, and only later recognizing the disease's impact across social and cultural divides. Indeed, HIV/AIDS has never been only a "gay" problem, but rather a slowly unfolding transnational public health crisis. The development of AZT and then HAART broadened the public health response to HIV/AIDS beyond epidemiological surveillance and behavioral modification, offering regulators a key treatment resource for facing the crisis head-on. Antiretroviral treatment (ART) has provided a direct clinical avenue for reducing transmission rates, as treatments have become increasingly affordable in LMICs. The continued efforts of global health groups, advocacy organizations, and local governments, however, are required to ensure that prevention research implementation keeps pace with the growing availability of ARTs and future treatment developments.

References

AIDSMap. 2016. "South Africa Has Driven Mother-to-Child HIV Transmission Down to 4%." NAM AIDSMap, July 20. http://www.aidsmap.com/South-Africa-has-driven-mother-to-child-HIV-transmission-down-to-4/page/3073056/.

AIDS2016. 2016. "Study Results Provide Critical New Data to Guide HIV Prevention and Treatment Efforts for Women and Girls." Press Release, July 18. http://www.aids2016.org/Media-Centre/The-Latest/Press-Releases/ArticleID/56/Study-results-provide-critical-new-data-to-guide-HIV-prevention-and-treatment-efforts-for-women-and-girls.

Asante, A. D. 2007. "Scaling Up HIV Prevention: Why Routine or Mandatory Testing Is Not Feasible for Sub-Saharan Africa." *Bulletin of the World Health Organization* 85(8): 64–646. http://www.who.int/bulletin/volumes/85/8/06-037671/en/.

AVERT. 2016a. "HIV and AIDS in South Africa." http://www.avert.org/professionals/hiv-around-world/sub-saharan-africa/south-africa.

AVERT. 2016b. "Homophobia and HIV." http://www.avert.org/professionals/hiv-social-issues/homophobia.

Barnes, M., Rango, N. A., Burke, G. R., and Chiarello, L. 1990. "The HIV-Infected Health Care Professional: Employment Policies and Public Health," *Journal of Law, Medicine and Health Care* 18(4): 311–330.

Bayer, R. 1989. *Private Acts, Social Consequences: AIDS and the Politics of Public Health* (New York: Free Press).

Bayer, R., and Fairchild, A. L. 2006. "Changing the Paradigm for HIV—the End of Exceptionalism." *New England Journal of Medicine* 355(7): 647–649. http://www.nejm.org/doi/pdf/10.1056/NEJMp068153.

Bayer, R., and Oppenheimer, G. M. 2000. *AIDS Doctors: Voices from the Epidemic; An Oral History* (New York: Oxford University Press).

Beauchamp, T. L., and Childress, J. F. 2013. *Principles of Biomedical Ethics*. 7th ed. (New York: Oxford University Press).

Bisaillon, L. M. 2010. "Human Rights Consequences of Mandatory HIV Screening Policy of Newcomers to Canada." *Health and Human Rights in Practice* 12(2): 119–234. http://www.hhrjournal.org/wp-content/uploads/sites/13/2013/07/12-Bisaillon.pdf.

CDC (US Centers for Disease Control and Prevention). 2006. *Revised Recommendations for HIV Testing of Adults, Adolescents, and Pregnant Women*. http://www.cdc.gov/mmwr/preview/mmwrhtml/rr5514a1.htm.

Chattu, V. J. 2014. "Global Health & HIV/AIDS—A Critical Debate on Mandatory HIV Testing Policy." *Journal of Human Virology and Retrovirology* 1(2): 00011. doi:10.15406/jhvrv.2014.01.00011.

Connors, M. 2011. "Sex, Drugs, and Structural Violence: Unraveling the Epidemic Among Poor Women in the United States." In *Women, Poverty, and AIDS*, edited by J. Simmons, M. Connors, and P. Farmer (Monroe, Maine: Common Courage Press).

Cori, A., Ayles, H., Beyers, N., Schaap, A., Floyd, S., Sabapathy, K., et al. 2014. "HPTN 071 (PopART): A Cluster-Randomized Trial of The Population Impact of an HIV Combination Prevention Intervention Including Universal Testing and Treatment: Mathematical Model." *PloS One* 9(1): e84511. https://www.ncbi.nlm.nih.gov/pmc/articles/PMC3893126/.

Daniels, N. 2006. "Duty to Treat or Right to Refuse?" In *Ethics and Infectious Disease*, edited by M. J. Selgelid, M. P. Battin, and C. B. Smith, 148–152 (Malden, Mass.: Blackwell).

Engel, J. 2006. *The Epidemic: A Global History of AIDS* (New York: HarperCollins).

FDA (US Food and Drug Administration). 2009. "FDA Marks 100th HIV/AIDS Drug Authorized for Purchase Under PEPFAR." http://www.worldpharmanews.com/fda/963-fda-marks-100th-hivaids-drug-authorized-for-purchase-under-pepfar

Fein, E. B. 1997. "Medical Workers with H.I.V. Keep Silent, Fearing Reprisals." *New York Times*, December 21. http://www.nytimes.com/1997/12/21/nyregion/medical-workers-with-hiv-keep-silent-fearing-reprisals.html.

Fox, R., Odaka, N. J., Brookmeyer, R., and Polk, B. F. 1987. "Effect of HIV Antibody Disclosure on Subsequent Sexual Activity in Homosexual Men." *AIDS* 1(4): 241–246.

Francis, L. P., Battin, M. P., Jacobson, J. A., Smith, C. B., and Botkin, J. R. 2006. "How Infectious Diseases Got Left Out—And What This Omission Might Have Meant for Bioethics." In *Ethics and Infectious Disease*, edited by M. J. Selgelid, M. P. Battin, and C. B. Smith, 48–63 (Malden, Mass.: Blackwell).

Gollub, E. L. 1999. "Human Rights Is a US Problem, Too: The Case of Women and HIV." *American Journal of Public Health* 89(10): 1479–1482. https://www.ncbi.nlm.nih.gov/pmc/articles/PMC1508808/pdf/amjph00010-0021.pdf.

Gray, R. H., Kigozi, G., Serwadda, D., Makumbi, F., Watya, S., Nalugoda, F., et al. 2007. "Male Circumcision for HIV Prevention in Men in Rakai, Uganda: A Randomised Trial." *Lancet* 369(9562): 657–666.

Hayes, R., Ayles, H., Beyers, N., Sabapathy, K., Floyd, S., Shanaube, K., et al. 2014. "HPTN 071 (PopART): Rationale and Design Of A Cluster-Randomised Trial of the Population Impact of an HIV Combination Prevention Intervention Including Universal Testing and Treatment—A Study Protocol for a Cluster Randomised Trial." *Trials* 15(1): 57.

HHS (US Department of Health and Human Services). 2015. "A Timeline of AIDS." https://www.hiv.gov/hiv-basics/overview/history/hiv-and-aids-timeline.

HIV Prevention Trials Network. 2018. "HPTN 071—the PopART Study." Study Summary. https://www.hptn.org/research/studies/hptn071#block-views-block-study-detail-block-block-2-3.

Iliffe, J. 2006. *The African AIDS Epidemic: A History* (Oxford: James Currey).

Interagency Coalition on AIDS and Development. 2001. *Access to HIV/AIDS Treatment in Developing Countries*. White Paper. http://www.icad-cisd.com/index.php?option=com_jotloader&section=files&task=download&cid=29_b634c8eece9cd639a1e734c793f7051c&Itemid=260&lang=en.

Johnson, D. 1990. "Ryan White Dies of AIDS at 18; His Struggle Helped Pierce Myths." *New York Times*, April 9. http://www.nytimes.com/1990/04/09/obituaries/ryan-white-dies-of-aids-at-18-his-struggle-helped-pierce-myths.html.

Kaiser Family Foundation. 2015. "HIV Testing in the United States." Fact Sheet, June 24. http://kff.org/hivaids/fact-sheet/hiv-testing-in-the-united-states/.

Kaiser Health News. 2007. "Boehringer To Reduce Price of Antiretroviral Nevirapine in Low-, Middle-Income Countries, Official Says." *Morning Briefing*, May 16. http://khn.org/morning-breakout/dr00044932/.

Kakimoto, K. 2008. "Response to Opt-Out Approach to Prevent Mother-to-Child Transmission of HIV." *Bulletin of the World Health Organization* 86(3). https://www.ncbi.nlm.nih.gov/pmc/articles/PMC2647403/

Karim, S. S. A., Richardson, B. A., Ramjee, G., Hoffman, I. F., Chirenje, Z. M., Taha, T., et al. 2011. "Safety and Effectiveness of BufferGel and 0.5% PRO2000 Gel for the Prevention of HIV Infection in Women." *AIDS* 25(7): 957.

Lin, L., and Liang, B. 2005. "HIV and Health Law: Striking the Balance between Legal Mandates and Medical Ethics." *American Medical Association Journal of Ethics* 7(10). http://journalofethics.ama-assn.org/2005/10/hlaw1-0510.html.

Lalonde, M. 1975. *A New Perspective on Health of Canadians: A Working Document* (Ottawa: Information Canada).

Maryland AIDS Administration. 2007. "Important Changes in HIV/AIDS Reporting: Memorandum." Maryland Department of Health and Mental Hygiene, April 24. http://phpa.dhmh.maryland.gov/IDEHASharedDocuments/what-to-report/Notice%20to%20Health%20Officers.pdf.

New York State Department of Health. 2013. "HIV Reporting and Partner Notification Questions and Answers." https://www.health.ny.gov/diseases/aids/providers/regulations/reporting_and_notification/question_answer.htm.

NIH (National Institutes of Health) 2016. "NIH Expands Investment in HIV Cure Research." Press Release, July 13. https://www.nih.gov/news-events/news-releases/nih-expands-investment-hiv-cure-research.

OutRight Action International. 2007. "Africa: IGLHRC's New Study Reveals How Anti-Gay Discrimination Fuels HIV/AIDS Crisis in Africa." Press Release, March 1. https://www.outrightinternational.org/content/africa-iglhrcs-new-study-reveals-how-anti-gay-discrimination-fuels-hivaids-crisis-africa.

Padian, N. S., van der Straten, A., Ramjee, G., Chipato, T., de Bruyn, G., Blanchard, K., et al. 2007. "Diaphragm and Lubricant Gel for Prevention of HIV Acquisition in Southern African Women: A Randomised Controlled Trial." *Lancet* 370(9583): 251–261

Patterson, A. S. 2006. *The Politics of AIDS in Africa* (Boulder, Colo.: Lynne Rienner).

PBS (Public Broadcasting Service). 2006. "Haiti: The High Price of Stigma." *PBS Frontline*, May 30. http://www.pbs.org/wgbh/pages/frontline/aids/countries/ht.html.

Selgelid, M. J. 2006. "Ethics and Infectious Disease." In *Ethics and Infectious Disease*, edited by M. J. Selgelid, M. P. Battin, and C. B. Smith, 3–19 (Malden, Mass.: Blackwell).

Selgelid, M. J., Battin, M. P., and Smith, C. B., eds. 2006. *Ethics and Infectious Disease* (Malden, Mass.: Blackwell).

Senthilingam, M. 2016. "New HIV Vaccine to Be Trialled in South Africa." CNN, July 19. http://www.cnn.com/2016/07/19/health/hiv-vaccine-go-ahead-aids-conference/.

Simmons, J., Connors, M., and Farmer, P. 2011. *Women, Poverty, and AIDS* (Monroe, Maine: Common Courage Press).

Simmons, J., Farmer, P., and Shoepf, B. G. 2011. "A Global Perspective." In *Women, Poverty, and AIDS*, edited by J. Simmons, M. Connors, and P. Farmer, 39–90 (Monroe, Maine: Common Courage Press).

Smallman, S. 2007. *The AIDS Pandemic in Latin America* (Chapel Hill: University of North Carolina Press).

Solomon, L. 2003. "Fidel Castro's Dupes." *Capitalism Magazine*, May 13. http://capitalismmagazine.com/2003/05/fidel-castros-dupes/.

SouthAfricaInfo. 2014. "South African Study 'Opens New Possibilities for Curing HIV.'" March 3. http://www.brandsouthafrica.com/investment-immigration/science-technology/hiv-030314.

Timberg, C. 2007. "HIV Loosens Tribe's Resistance to Circumcision." *Washington Post*, September 7. http://www.washingtonpost.com/wp-dyn/content/article/2007/09/06/AR2007090602760.html.

Turan, J. M., and Nyblade, L. 2013. "HIV-Related Stigma as a Barrier to Achievement of Global PMTCT and Maternal Health Goals: A Review of the Evidence." *AIDS and Behavior* 17(7): 2528–2539.

UNAIDS. 2015. "Fact Sheet: 2014 Statistics." http://www.unaids.org/en/resources/campaigns/HowAIDSchangedeverything/factsheet.

Voice of America. 1992. *Cuba Annual Report: 1989*. United States Information Agency, Office of Research and Policy, Radio Marti Program (New York: Transaction Publishers).

SECTION NINE

NONCOMMUNICABLE DISEASES

CHAPTER 42

AN OVERVIEW OF ETHICS, PUBLIC HEALTH, AND NONCOMMUNICABLE DISEASES

BRENDAN SALONER

Introduction

THE twentieth century marked a transition in the global burden of disease. Thanks to medical and public health advances in areas like sanitation, vaccination, and antibiotics, babies who might have perished in an earlier era from diseases like dysentery were now surviving into adulthood (Wilkinson, 1994). From 1900 to 2004, average life expectancy at birth in the United States increased from fifty to seventy-five years. Comparable gains were experienced in other developed countries (McKeown, 2009). This "epidemiological transition" has been hailed as a public health triumph, and the accompanying gains in life expectancy have been rightfully celebrated. In the march toward longevity, the next frontier is conquering noncommunicable diseases (NCDs).

Important progress has been made in reducing the burden of NCDs. One of the most important public health success stories of the last fifty years has been a marked decrease in smoking in the developed world, resulting in a reduction in lung cancer and other associated illnesses (Jha et al., 2013; Cutler, 2008). Since the mid-1990s, cardiovascular disease mortality has also declined across the developed world, as has mortality associated with many types of cancer (Moran et al., 2014; Cao et al., 2017). The contributors to these reductions likely reflect successful prevention campaigns (e.g., reducing occupational carcinogenic exposures), health education, and advances in clinical medicine (e.g., improved surgical techniques to increase survival after stroke) (Feigin et al., 2014; Ezzati and Riboli, 2013).

Successes notwithstanding, reasons for concern remain. In the United States, overall life expectancy gains have not only slowed recently, they have actually reversed. In 2015, US life expectancy decreased for the first time since 1993 (Xu et al., 2016). The decrease reflected bad news on many fronts—including an increase in deaths related to heart disease, drug addiction and alcoholism, and injuries. The apparent recalcitrance of chronic diseases has called into question the ability of traditional public health measures to address risk factors such as unhealthy neighborhoods, junk foods, drugs and alcohol, and environmental pollutants. These challenges are not unique to the "privileged" industrialized world, as lower- and middle-income countries are contending with the health consequences of Western lifestyles—for example, nearly 80 percent of all smokers globally now live outside higher-income countries (WHO, 2017).

This section of *The Oxford Handbook of Public Health Ethics* addresses the ethical tensions arising from public health efforts to reduce the burden of NCDs. While clinical medicine can treat the exacerbations of NCDs, social and economic environments shape the policy decisions and individual choices most associated with them. This raises several questions that frame the chapters in this section. First, when should governments enact regulations to protect the public's health? Second, when should public health focus on individual behavioral change versus structural changes (e.g., changes in food systems that might prevent cancer or diabetes)? Third, when should public health seek to maximize health gains versus advancing the well-being of more marginalized or disadvantaged groups? Finally, how should responses to different NCDs be balanced against other social investments, including those focused on communicable diseases?

Chapter Overviews

As public health seeks to shape health-related behaviors, the role of social context is emerging as a key factor. In countries like the United States, smoking rates have dramatically decreased in the last fifty years due to a combination of public health education and policy changes such as increased taxation and bans on smoking in public spaces (Garrett et al., 2011), and yet there remains a sizeable, disproportionately poor, and vulnerable population that continues to smoke. In "Tobacco as a Matter of Public Health: Ethical Issues," Kristin Voigt draws on a health equity perspective to argue that public health responses to tobacco must grapple with the socioeconomic gradients that underlie health disparities attributable to tobacco. For example, the decision to smoke reflects a variety of environmental factors, including social stressors and norms that may be more prevalent in disadvantaged communities. Campaigns to "denormalize" smoking are one powerful way to shift society's attitudes to smoking, and yet these campaigns may come at the expense of marginalizing already disadvantaged groups.

The public health ethics around smoking have been largely framed by third-party harms, such as the environmental smoking risks posed to nonsmokers in the presence of smokers. It is ethically more straightforward to prevent a smoking behavior in order to protect the health of a third party (who often did not choose to be exposed to tobacco) than to intervene in order to protect the smoker's own health, a person (it is argued) who chose to smoke. However, arguments framed in terms of third-party harms have their limits. Intervening to protect the smoker's own health requires a level of paternalism. Voigt argues that concerns about paternalism can be answered through approaches that place constraints on choice, but without entirely removing people's right to choose. For example, if people are required to obtain a smoking license, they may be may be prompted to more fully take account of future health risks during the process of obtaining a license—risks that they would irrationally discount under normal conditions.

Tobacco control also requires balancing the interests of current smokers against individuals who have not yet initiated smoking (the "at risk" population). Outright smoking bans may be too punitive for current smokers—especially given the addictive nature of tobacco—even though they pose significant benefit to the at-risk population. Proposals such as a "tobacco-free generation," which prevent people born after a certain year from purchasing cigarettes, can help to move toward a society in which tobacco use is phased out among younger cohorts without completely cutting off tobacco for current smokers. Similar tensions arise when considering marketing, which is particularly influential to prospective smokers. Although there are recognized commercial free speech rights, from a normative perspective these rights should be balanced against the more significant harms associated with encouraging new smoking behavior.

Alcohol and other drugs (AODs) represent another important frontier in the public health campaign against NCDs. Substance use and misuse contribute to the global burden of disease not only through its own impact on morbidity and mortality, but also as a distal contributor to other chronic diseases such as depression and diabetes. In the United States, some contend that a surge in drug overdoses since the mid-1990s is contributing to reversals in life expectancy among many demographic groups (Case and Deaton, 2015). In "Alcohol and Other Drugs: Public Health Ethics Issues," Brendan Saloner argues that there are reasons to believe that many of the negative health consequences of AODs use can be averted, if not outright prevented, through targeted public health interventions. A public health–oriented approach to AODs recommends intervention on multiple pathways.

Saloner argues that there is broad scientific consensus about many risk factors that contribute to harmful AOD use and about effective interventions. However, political and social pressures make it difficult to enact many evidence-based policies across domains such as law enforcement, taxation (for alcohol and legalized drugs), treatment, and harm reduction programs such as needle exchange. Public support is divided because of disagreement about the causes of harmful AOD use—is it attributable to personal choice and responsibility, or to genetics and environmental factors that the individual cannot control? As such, those believing AOD use is significantly the result of individual choice question whether public spending is warranted. It is also divided because the public is uncomfortable with approaches that might signal tolerance for behaviors that are illegal and which many consider to be inherently wrong. As a result, there may be resistance from both policymakers and the public to certain public health approaches to address them, despite scientific evidence supporting them. However, public attitudes can change. With marijuana, for example, Saloner contends that careful, well-evaluated legalization programs may be better than prohibition, but that a more laissez-faire approach (like the current approach to alcohol in many countries) will be more harmful than beneficial.

Many of the questions that frame medical and public health approaches to NCDs in the developed world are emerging in developing countries, but under much more limited resource constraints. As Hayley MacGregor illustrates in "Global Public Health, Noncommunicable Diseases, and Ethics," responding to NCDs in developing countries has been a long-running struggle. The international aid community has historically been more oriented to communicable diseases, which are less likely to be branded "diseases of affluence." Yet, as MacGregor argues, the relationship between socioeconomic status and risk of an NCD is complex in developing countries. Poor diet, lack of physical activity, and other environmental stressors increasingly afflict poor families. These families are least able to withstand the economic impact of a disease that bankrupts the family and debilitates working adults. Although there is a sound argument that addressing NCDs is a powerful tool for promoting economic development, this requires a shift in perspective. Ethically, it is also controversial because it argues in favor of considering nonhealth factors in disease prioritization decisions.

In an increasingly globalized world, changes in health behaviors are closely linked to the influence of multinational food, alcohol, and tobacco companies. These companies operate within regulatory frameworks that make these products inexpensive and pervasive in many countries. MacGregor argues that, ethically, health impacts should be at the forefront of debates about how to make globalization work for people in low- and middle-income countries. She also asserts that there is a basis for taxes on products that contribute to NCDs, including sugar-sweetened beverages. While these taxes are considered a greater burden for the poor, the health benefits to developing countries are substantial and compelling (as evidenced by recent studies of such taxes in Mexico) (Colchero et al., 2017). As in higher-income countries, the frontier of public health intervention in low- and middle-income countries will be around defining how, and under what conditions, health ministries and other actors should shape the choices that affect risk of NCD disease and disability. There is a need for approaches that view regulations enacted at a point in time as affecting a lifetime of choices, and providing options that will provide people with access to the tools to lead healthier lives in the future.

Cancer, the second-leading cause of death in the United States (after heart disease) (CDC, 2017), presents another case where an ethical public health response requires intervention on several tracks, including modifying social determinants and inequitable access to quality health care. Despite real progress in increasing life expectancy of people with cancer, disparities in cancer burden observed in the United States are persistent. In "Treating Cancer as a Public Health Ethics Issue," Yonaira M. Rivera and Otis W. Brawley diagnose the shortcomings of current approaches to cancer prevention and treatment as stemming from a relatively weak public health infrastructure combined with a health system that does not adequately disseminate and reward evidence-based care.

Symptoms of this fragmented approach are evident in the simultaneous undertreatment of cancer in some populations (including cases where cancer might have been prevented entirely) and the use of low-value or even harmful treatments in other groups. Making progress on cancer requires creating an initiative that can systematically screen patients, offer comprehensive education on effective treatment, and provide such treatment in a timely manner. As the authors argue, underserved patients are sometimes offered screening and education without follow-up access to services—compounding the injustice of unequal access with a system that creates unrealized expectations.

As Rivera and Brawley argue, a major challenge in producing better outcomes in cancer is resisting the impulse to do more. Being more targeted in several key respects could shield patients from potential risks (e.g., the non-negligible risks of screenings and biopsies). Patients may be mistrustful of the intentions of clinicians, health system planners, or even public health officials who argue for doing less, particularly among historically marginalized populations that have long been denied access to effective treatments. Better public health communication about cancer might help the public to recognize when they would benefit from certain services, and when they may be better served by doing less. However, the public has a relatively limited understanding of cancer's etiology and treatment. Not all entities communicating about cancer are credible—as the authors point out, pharmaceutical companies may be filling the information void with messages that provide an overly optimistic presentation of cancer drug therapies.

Conclusion

The chapters in this section of *The Oxford Handbook of Public Health Ethics* illustrate that much of the future disease burden attributable to NCDs can be prevented—both through policy changes and individual behavior modifications—and that public health provides sound principles for making progress through a variety of interventions. However, public health programs, in the traditional sense, also have their limits. Many of the conditions that lead to an excess burden of NCDs reflect an inequitable distribution of resources and a lack of economic development. Changing these structural conditions requires social investments and may take years to realize. Reducing structural inequality increases opportunity for the most disadvantaged, and addressing NCDs adds to these justice-based arguments. A fairer future may be a healthier one, and a healthier future may be a fairer one.

References

Cao, B., Bray, F., Beltrán-Sánchez, H., Ginsburg, O., Soneji, S., and Soerjomataram, I. 2017. "Benchmarking Life Expectancy and Cancer Mortality: Global Comparison with Cardiovascular Disease 1981–2010." *BMJ* 357(June): j2765. doi:10.1136/bmj.j2765.

Case, A., and Deaton, A. 2015. "Rising Morbidity and Mortality in Midlife among White Non-Hispanic Americans in the 21st Century." Working Paper (Princeton University, Woodrow Wilson School of Public and International Affairs, Research Program in Development Studies). http://econpapers.repec.org/paper/prirpdevs/15078.full.pdf.htm.

CDC (Centers for Disease Control and Prevention). 2017. "Deaths and Mortality." https://www.cdc.gov/nchs/fastats/deaths.htm.

Colchero, M. A., Rivera-Dommarco, J., Popkin, B. M. and Ng, S. W. 2017. "In Mexico, Evidence of Sustained Consumer Response Two Years after Implementing a Sugar-Sweetened Beverage Tax." *Health Affairs (Project Hope)* 36(3): 564–571. doi:10.1377/hlthaff.2016.1231.

Cutler, D. M. 2008. "Are We Finally Winning the War on Cancer?" *Journal of Economic Perspectives: A Journal of the American Economic Association* 22(4): 3–26.

Ezzati, M., and Riboli, E. 2013. "Behavioral and Dietary Risk Factors for Noncommunicable Diseases." *New England Journal of Medicine* 369(10): 954–964.

Feigin, V. L., Forouzanfar, M. H., Krishnamurthi, R., Mensah, G. A., Connor, M. Bennett, D. A., et al. 2014. "Global and Regional Burden of Stroke during 1990–2010: Findings from the Global Burden of Disease Study 2010." *Lancet* 383(9913): 245–254.

Garrett, B., Dube, S., Trosclair, A., Caraballo, R., and Pechacek, T. 2011. *Cigarette Smoking—United States, 1965–2008*. (Atlanta, Ga.: Centers for Disease Control and Prevention). https://www.cdc.gov/mmwr/preview/mmwrhtml/su6001a24.htm.

Jha, P., Ramasundarahettige, C., Landsman, V., Rostron, B., Thun, M., Anderson, R. N., et al. 2013. "21st-Century Hazards of Smoking and Benefits of Cessation in the United States." *New England Journal of Medicine* 368(4): 341–350. doi:10.1056/NEJMsa1211128.

McKeown, R. E. 2009. "The Epidemiologic Transition: Changing Patterns of Mortality and Population Dynamics." *American Journal of Lifestyle Medicine* 3(Suppl. 1): 19S–26S. doi:10.1177/1559827609335350.

Moran, A. E., Forouzanfar, M. H., Roth, G., Mensah, G., Ezzati, M., Murray, C. J. L., et al. 2014. "Temporal Trends in Ischemic Heart Disease Mortality in 21 World Regions, 1980–2010: The Global Burden of Disease 2010 Study." *Circulation* 129(14): 1483–1492. doi:10.1161/CIRCULATIONAHA.113.004042.

WHO (World Health Organization). 2017. "Tobacco." http://www.who.int/mediacentre/factsheets/fs339/en/.

Wilkinson, R. G. 1994. "The Epidemiological Transition: From Material Scarcity to Social Disadvantage?" *Daedalus* 123(4): 61–77.

Xu, J., Murphy, S. L., Kochanek, K. D. and Arias, E. 2016. *Mortality in the United States, 2015* (Atlanta, Ga.: Centers for Disease Control and Prevention).

CHAPTER 43

TOBACCO AS A MATTER OF PUBLIC HEALTH: ETHICAL ISSUES

KRISTIN VOIGT

Introduction

Tobacco control raises many challenging normative questions. This chapter focuses on normative issues that arise at the population level, particularly with respect to the anti-smoking strategies policymakers might pursue and the reasons and justifications underlying them. It first sets out several background factors that shape the debate about these issues. The chapter then discusses different grounds on which state and public health actors might seek to restrict tobacco consumption. Lastly, the chapter considers normative issues arising in relation to specific anti-smoking strategies.

Background

Tobacco and Its Health Effects

Tobacco has been identified as the most significant health risk factor in high-income countries and the second-leading health risk factor globally, causing an estimated 6.3 percent of the world's disease burden (Lim et al., 2012). Globally, it causes about 5 to 6 million deaths annually (Jha, 2011). For the twenty-first century, a total of 1 billion deaths are predicted, with about half of them occurring in persons under the age of seventy (Jha, 2011; Jha and Peto, 2014).

Long-time smokers face significantly increased risks for conditions such as lung and other cancers and heart disease. Significant differences in mortality rates between never-smokers and smokers become evident from middle age onwards, and the life span of long-term smokers is estimated to be ten to eleven years shorter than that of never-smokers (Doll et al., 2004; Pirie et al., 2013). Smoking has also been linked to a variety of nonfatal conditions, such as asthma and tuberculosis (ASH, 2015). For lifelong, heavy smokers, studies estimate the risk of developing lung cancer over the course of one's life to be up to 25 percent, compared to 0.2 to 1 percent for never-smokers (Brennan et al., 2006). Cessation can mitigate some of these effects. For example, those who quit smoking before the age of thirty have a life expectancy that is almost the same as that of never-smokers (Pirie et al., 2013; Jha et al., 2013).

Tobacco smoke contains a wide range of chemicals, many of which have been identified as posing health risks. Nicotine, because of its addictiveness, is crucial in maintaining smoking behaviors over time (Jarvis, 2004; Benowitz, 2010). As discussed in this chapter, questions about the addictiveness of nicotine and its influence on individual autonomy have played an important role in the normative debate. The direct health risks posed by nicotine, however, are less clear. While nicotine is toxic, the doses contained in cigarettes have traditionally not been considered problematic in themselves. However, the increasing use of electronic cigarettes has been accompanied by greater attention on nicotine as potentially having problematic health consequences when used long-term (Grana, Benowitz, and Glantz, 2014; for discussion about how nicotine has been viewed within the public health community, especially within the context of electronic cigarettes, see Bell and Keane, 2012).

Tobacco as a Global Issue

Across the World Health Organization regions (WHO, 2018), the highest smoking rates can be found in the European Region (29 percent) while the lowest is in the African Region (8 percent). These figures obscure significant variations by gender. Among men, smoking prevalence is highest (46 percent) in the Western Pacific Region (which includes countries such as China, Japan, Australia, and Malaysia); for women, it is highest in the European Region (20 percent) (WHO, 2011). Most of the deaths that tobacco is estimated to cause in the twenty-first century are expected to occur in low- and middle-income countries (Jha, 2011). Efforts by the tobacco industry to recruit nonsmokers in these countries, especially women and adolescents (Gilmore et al., 2015), and increases in smoking rates in many developing countries (Bilano et al., 2015) heighten these concerns. It is crucial, therefore, to approach tobacco as a global issue.

Inequality: Smoking and Disadvantage

An important factor for any normative discussion of tobacco is the close link between tobacco and various kinds of disadvantage. First, smoking is associated with poverty, low education, and other indicators of social class and socioeconomic status. As already mentioned, smoking is increasingly common in low- and middle-income countries. Within industrialized countries, smoking rates tend to be higher in low-income and less educated groups. In the United Kingdom, for example, the smoking rate in managerial and professional occupations is 16 percent, but it reaches 30 percent in manual and routine (i.e. semi- and unskilled) occupations (Lader, 2008). In many low- and middle-income countries, similar associations between education level and smoking have been found (Di Cesare et al., 2013). This makes smoking a major contributor to social inequalities in health outcomes; it is estimated that, in the United Kingdom, it causes about half of the socioeconomic status (SES) difference in death rates (Hiscock et al., 2012).

Research also points to differences in smoking norms across communities. For example, research from deprived neighborhoods in Scotland suggests that smoking is "the norm," that much socializing happens around smoking, and that people in these communities overestimate smoking rates (Wiltshire et al., 2003; MacAskill et al., 2002; Stead et al., 2001). This also gives a very different meaning to cessation, which can be experienced as a break from peer group norms (Chamberlain and O'Neill, 2007; MacAskill et al., 2002). A New Zealand study also raised concern about "smoking islands": communities in which smoking is regarded as a form of resistance to dominant anti-smoking norms (Thompson, Pearce, and Barnett, 2007). Smoking has been associated with additional forms of disadvantage, other than SES, such as sexual and gender minority status (Antin, Lipperman-Kreda, and Hunt, 2015) and poor mental health (Schroeder and Morris, 2010). Finally, social perceptions of smoking and smokers have become increasingly negative (Stuber, Galea, and Link, 2008; Graham, 2011), exposing smokers to negative attitudes, stigmatization, and differential treatment (e.g., nonsmoker hiring policies, which exclude smokers from employment; see Voigt, 2012b; Schmidt, Voigt, and Emanuel, 2013; Asch, Muller, and Volpp, 2013; Houle and Siegel, 2009).

These considerations have led many commentators to urge a social justice perspective in connection with tobacco control (Healton and Nelson, 2004; Voigt, 2010; Breton and Sherlaw, 2011). This includes, in particular, a recognition of how socioeconomic inequalities contribute to unequal smoking rates (Voigt, 2010) and, in turn, a debate about the extent to which inequalities that result from unequal smoking rates should be considered a problem of social justice (Roemer, 1993; Segall, 2010). A social justice perspective may also recommend greater sensitivity to the impact of different anti-smoking strategies on different social groups (Breton and Sherlaw, 2011).

Normative Grounds for Government Attempts to Reduce Tobacco Consumption

On what grounds might it be legitimate, or perhaps even required, for governments and state actors to introduce policies to reduce tobacco consumption? Here the focus is on two particularly salient goals: protecting smokers and protecting third parties. The discussion will also touch on equality considerations, where appropriate.

Protecting Smokers

While the protection of smokers is often recognized as an important goal in arguments around tobacco control, interference with individuals' choices for their own good is often considered disrespectful of individuals and as unduly limiting their freedom. The question of what degree of paternalism might be acceptable in public health is, of course, central to public health ethics. Importantly, paternalistic motivation does not *necessarily* make a policy problematic, and further analysis will be required to determine whether or not such a policy is justified, all things considered (Wilson, 2011). Moreover, as proponents of strategies that seek to protect smokers from harm have argued, there may be reason to think that smoking choices are less than fully autonomous, making interference less paternalistic than it might be in the case of other choices. For example, Robert Goodin's argument focuses on the addictiveness of smoking, combined with the often very young age at which smokers become addicted to tobacco, which means that smokers often did not make an informed choice about becoming smokers. This, he argues, makes interference with such choices less problematic than other kinds of paternalistic interventions (Goodin, 1989). He also argues that smoking choices often lack endorsement by smokers themselves: while they, at one level, "prefer" to smoke, they typically would prefer not to have that preference. Interfering with unendorsed preferences, he argues, and making people act in accordance with those preferences that they themselves endorse (even if they do not currently act on them), is a justified instance of paternalism (Goodin, 1991). More recently, Sarah Conly (2012) has argued that the susceptibility of individuals' decision-making to cognitive biases gives us reason to interfere with smoking choices, possibly to the point of a complete ban of cigarettes.

These arguments seek, in different ways, to make the paternalism implicit in interfering with smokers' choices more acceptable. Of course, such arguments are going to hold little sway for those who consider it a fundamental right to act in ways that might harm oneself (so long as third parties remain unaffected), even where various factors will detract from fully autonomous decision-making. This raises broader concerns about the legitimacy of government interference with risky choices and behaviors, and about the degree of paternalism that might be acceptable in tobacco control (as in other public health contexts) (Flanigan, 2016). Some commentators have sought to establish that smoking choices are more autonomous than is often assumed in the philosophical literature (Shapiro, 1994). A somewhat different approach is to emphasize that even where anti-smoking policies interfere with autonomous choices, the costs of such interference are likely to be outweighed by the health and well-being losses that restrictive tobacco policies could avert (Grill and Voigt, 2016). The association of smoking with various forms of disadvantage also suggests that paternalistic policies can lead to more egalitarian outcomes: in a context where individuals are not equally positioned to abstain from smoking, paternalistic policies can help prevent smoking-related inequalities (Voigt, 2015a; Grill and Voigt, 2016).

Protecting Third Parties

Many prominent arguments in the tobacco control debate have focused not on the harm to smokers, but instead on the harms of smoking to third parties. This has especially been the case with respect to arguments for restrictions on where people can smoke, many of which rely on concerns about the risks associated with exposure to environmental tobacco smoke (Colgrove, Bayer, and Bachynski, 2011).

While such arguments can appeal to widely accepted ideas such as the harm principle (roughly, that individuals have the right to harm themselves but not to harm others), they are not straightforward. While many arguments emphasize that there is no risk-free exposure to secondhand smoke (e.g., HHS, 2006), this does not by itself establish the case for restrictions. Many activities, such as driving a car, involve risks to others, but we generally do not think that any amount of such risks can *by itself* justify restrictive policies; any such justification would involve an assessment of the severity of the risks involved and the benefits derived from the activity. Building the case for smoking bans on the basis of the harms of secondhand smoke must involve an assessment of the harms involved in different contexts (e.g., smoking in cars vs. smoking outdoors), the implications of a ban on smokers, and an argument that the harms are sufficiently great to justify restrictions on smokers. Relatedly, it is important to recognize the limitations these arguments face. Not all anti-smoking policies can be justified on the basis of third-party harms; for example, it has been argued that such arguments are insufficient to establish the case for outdoor smoking bans (Bayer and Bachynski, 2013).

Ethical Issues Arising in Relation to Specific Strategies for Preventing Tobacco-Related Harms

The preceding paragraphs describe the context for the debate about normative issues around smoking, and they also consider some relevant fundamental philosophical questions. The following paragraphs take on issues that arise in relation to specific strategies to reduce tobacco consumption (either by encouraging current smokers to smoke less or quit, or by preventing the uptake of smoking by current nonsmokers) and/or to protect third parties from the effects of smoking.

Restrictions on Use

Perhaps the most common policy strategy to address smoking-related harms has been to restrict where people are allowed to smoke. While such policies can be driven by concern for third parties who, in the absence of protections, would be exposed to environmental tobacco smoke, they can also pursue the goal of reducing smokers' own risks, as smoking bans can increase smokers' incentives to quit or to smoke less. While bans on smoking in enclosed public spaces have become the standard in many countries, a recent debate has focused on whether such bans should be extended to open spaces, such as parks and beaches (Colgrove, Bayer, and Bachynski, 2011; Chapman, 2000, 2015; Bayer and Bachynski, 2013).

Given the associations between smoking and various form of disadvantage, there have been concerns about how smoking bans might affect particularly vulnerable populations, such as when smoking is banned in prisons (Butler et al., 2007) or mental health facilities (Jochelson, 2006). At the same time, this approach may present an important opportunity to ensure cessation among vulnerable populations, especially when concerns about enforced cessation can be alleviated through cessation aids (Williams, 2008).

Restrictions on Sale

A different set of policies restrict the sale of cigarettes, for example by implementing restrictions on sale to children or on the sale of individual cigarettes. These policies, which primarily seek to protect children from harms that they may not yet be in a position to fully understand, are generally considered appropriate and ethically uncontroversial. There have also been proposals to make cigarettes available only for those who have previously purchased a smoking license (Halliday, 2016; Chapman, 2012). Such proposals seek to strike a compromise. On the one hand, they are not overly restrictive and respect people's right to take certain health risks. On the other hand, they help to address concerns that smokers are acting on preferences that are driven by an irrational level of time discounting (giving too little weight to their future well-being relative to immediate pleasures or benefits), as well as the concern that smoking choices are not endorsed by many smokers themselves. Imposing significant costs before cigarettes can be purchased can make smokers more sensitive to the long-term risks of smoking and/or endorsed preferences about smoking. Licenses do involve a restriction on individuals' liberties, but proponents argue that these restrictions are not necessarily greater than they are for other types of interventions, such as taxes (Halliday, 2016).

Perhaps the most radical restriction on sale is to prohibit cigarette sales entirely. While such restrictions were attempted in the United States between 1890 and 1927 (Proctor, 2013), the only country to currently ban cigarette sales altogether is Bhutan (Ugen, 2003). In the tobacco control community, the idea of slowly phasing in a complete ban on cigarettes is gaining traction, for example in the form of a "tobacco-free generation" proposal, where cigarettes will be available only to people born before a certain date, leading, over time, to a situation where no one will be able to legally purchase cigarettes (Berrick, 2013; Walters and Barnsley, 2015; Proctor, 2013; Daynard, 2009; Malone, McDaniel, and Smith, 2014). In 2014, the Tasmanian Parliament debated the introduction of such legislation (Walters and Barnsley, 2015; Berrick, 2013). By allowing current smokers to continue to smoke while at the same time preventing young people from becoming smokers in the first place, such proposals are thought to be less susceptible to illicit markets than a complete ban on tobacco (Walters and Barnsley, 2015). Philosophers, too, have considered such proposals. While for those who insist on the impermissibility of infringing on people's right to smoke, tobacco bans may be overly restrictive, arguments for such bans have been made—on the grounds that smokers' choices are irrational (Conly, 2012), not endorsed by smokers themselves (Goodin, 1991), or because of the well-being losses such a ban could avert (Grill and Voigt, 2016).

An important concern is the protection of future generations, for whom an effective tobacco ban would remove the possibility of becoming smokers in the first place. For current generations, however, and particularly for current smokers, the impact of these kinds of proposals on different smokers, both in terms of health and in terms of well-being more broadly understood, is an open question. While such a ban could lead to particularly significant gains for the disadvantaged, who, as discussed above, have significantly higher smoking rates, there is also the concern that the disadvantaged may find cessation particularly difficult and burdensome, and that additional strategies must be employed to reduce such burdens (Gostin, 2014; Grill and Voigt, 2016).

Marketing Restrictions

Marketing restrictions focus on how and where tobacco can be marketed. They can include requirements to include health warnings on tobacco packaging and advertisements. Some countries also require so-called graphic warning labels that not only describe particular health risks but provide photographs depicting conditions associated with smoking (for examples, see Hammond, 2011). Graphic warning labels have been criticized for their potential to contribute to negative and stigmatizing perceptions of smokers (Haines-Saah, Bell, and Dennis, 2015).

Other types of marketing restrictions include bans on advertisements on print media, TV, and billboards; bans on tobacco companies sponsoring sports teams; and "plain packaging" legislation, which requires all cigarettes to be sold in white packaging, without company logos or brand design. Such restrictions are often seen as crucial in preventing the tobacco industry from glamorizing cigarettes and as an extension of more traditional marketing restrictions. The extent to which such restrictions are implemented varies across the world (Mackay and Eriksen, 2015).

Restrictions on marketing are sometimes challenged as a violation of free speech, especially in the United States, where commercial speech is given a relatively high level of legal protection (Bayer and Kelly, 2010). How much protection commercial speech should be granted in principle, how concerns for free commercial speech should be weighed against public health concerns, and how such questions might be resolved in relation to tobacco marketing in particular, raise complex questions about freedom of expression and the grounds on which this freedom might be restricted. Freedom of expression is generally not considered an absolute right, and the case for its protection must be weighed against the costs of such protection. Moreover, commercial speech seems less closely connected to the basic interests that freedom of expression seeks to protect than is the case for many other forms of speech, such as political expression, making restrictions easier to justify (Cohen, 1993). While "more speech" (e.g., educational messages or social marketing) may seem like an appealing alternative to restrictions, governments cannot match the amount of resources tobacco companies invest into marketing.

Equality considerations can provide another reason for marketing restrictions. Such restrictions can prevent industry activities that target disadvantaged groups, such as industry efforts in low-income countries where restrictions on tobacco are low (Brandt, 2007; Gilmore et al., 2015), placing advertising disproportionately in low-income and ethnic minority neighborhoods (Barbeau et al., 2005; Yerger, Przewoznik, and Malone, 2007), and devising marketing strategies with particular appeal to those on low incomes, the homeless, and those with mental health problems (Apollonio and Malone, 2005; Healton and Nelson, 2004; MacAskill et al., 2002).

Price Policies and Taxation

Tobacco taxation is another way in which governments have sought to reduce tobacco consumption. Taxation has the advantage of providing a disincentive to smoke without being overly restrictive. It has also been recommended as the most cost-effective tobacco control intervention (Shibuya et al., 2003). Taxation, however, raises egalitarian concerns. Proponents argue that taxation is very effective, including (unlike many other interventions) among disadvantaged groups; some studies suggest that it is one of the few interventions that can in fact reduce inequalities in smoking rates (Hill et al., 2014). Thus, while tobacco taxation is a regressive tax, it has also been referred to as "progressive" public health policy to indicate that it will benefit lower-income groups more than higher-income groups to the extent that the former are more sensitive to price changes (Warner, 2000). Such arguments, however, rely on aggregate outcomes and obscure the concern that many people will not be able to quit in response to price increases. These smokers will not see any health benefits from taxation, but they will end up paying a higher proportion of their income on tobacco (Voigt, 2010).

Incentives

There has been an increasing interest in incentives as a means to effect changes in health behaviors, including smoking. While some commentators are skeptical of incentives that seek to change more complex behaviors such as smoking (Jochelson, 2007), there has been some evidence to suggest that financial incentives could increase cessation rates (Volpp et al., 2009). Particular attention has been paid to whether incentives could be effective among disadvantaged groups. Some incentive schemes have targeted disadvantaged populations; for example, a recent scheme offered pregnant women in deprived communities supermarket vouchers for not smoking (Radley et al., 2013). Such schemes also have the advantage of not restricting individuals' options. However, incentive schemes raise problems. Particularly relevant here is the concern that incentives are more accessible for those with better opportunities for quitting, thus creating unfair inequalities (Voigt, 2012a), and that incentive schemes could propagate stigmatizing messages about disadvantaged groups (Voigt, 2017; Popay, 2008), for example by reinforcing perceptions that the poor are irresponsible or too weak-willed to quit on their own.

Cessation Aids

Providing assistance for cessation has also been a central tenet of tobacco control. This includes counseling for patients during medical appointments, "quit lines," and cessation aids such as nicotine patches and gums and other medications. There is also an ongoing and highly polarized debate about electronic cigarettes, which deliver nicotine in the form of a vapor and are seen by some experts as a possible cessation device (though the evidence on this is as yet uncertain; for discussion of some of the normative issues around electronic cigarettes, see van der Eijk, 2016; Voigt, 2015b).

Cessation aids could also be particularly important because of unequal cessation rates across different social groups. Even though the desire to quit and the number of cessation attempts are similar across different social groups, people from lower-income groups are less likely to succeed (Kotz and West, 2009). One normative question here is whether cessation aids should be provided for free or at highly reduced cost—perhaps only to disadvantaged smokers (Healton and Nelson, 2004), or to all smokers, as is the case in the United Kingdom—so as to address financial barriers to their use.

Education and Cessation Advice

Education campaigns seek to underscore the risks of smoking and provide information and advice on cessation. Such campaigns may seem innocuous because they do not involve restrictions on individuals' liberties. Moreover, there are concerns that lower-income and less-educated groups may not be as well informed about the risks as higher-income groups, both in industrialized (Stein et al., 2007; Rutten et al., 2008) and developing countries (Abdullah and Husten, 2004; Jha and Chaloupka, 1999). Education campaigns could help close these knowledge gaps. At the same time, however, not all education campaigns are equally well placed to benefit smokers from low-SES backgrounds and may, therefore, contribute to unequal quit rates among different social groups (Niederdeppe et al., 2008).

Denormalization and Stigma

Many campaigns go beyond the provision of information and aim to "denormalize" smoking; that is, they seek to shape social norms around smoking and/or perceptions of smokers, particularly in relation to perceptions about how common and how desirable smoking is (Lavack, 2001). Different kinds of interventions may (advertently or inadvertently) further denormalization, including several of those already discussed here, such as marketing restrictions, public health messages that depict smoking as disgusting or irresponsible, and smoking bans that make smoking less visible and communicate to smokers that their smoking is socially unacceptable (Voigt, 2013). The rationale of denormalization strategies is primarily to motivate smokers to quit by making its social perception increasingly negative (Kim and Shanahan, 2003).

Denormalization is considered by many a crucial factor in the significant reductions in smoking rates seen over the past few decades, and it is often a central component of comprehensive tobacco control strategies. While there have been attempts to support claims about the effectiveness of denormalization in bringing down smoking rates (Hammond et al., 2006; Kim and Shanahan, 2003; Alamar and Glantz, 2006), the complexity of the mechanisms involved makes this hypothesis difficult to test empirically.

At the same time, many commentators have worried that denormalization strategies stigmatize smokers (Kim and Shanahan, 2003; Bell, McCullough, et al., 2010; Bell, Salmon, et al. 2010). Such stigmatization may violate principles of equal and respectful treatment and thus be problematic in itself (Voigt, 2015b). It may also have negative effects on those stigmatized, for example by making them more secretive about their smoking, and thus losing out on cessation advice and support (Stuber and Galea, 2009). These concerns are compounded by the fact that smoking is associated with other kinds of stigmatized characteristics, such as poverty and poor mental health. While for some commentators, these implications mean that stigmatizing forms of denormalization are wholly unacceptable, others have argued that, at least in principle, the negative effects of stigmatization could be outweighed by the health gains to which it could lead (Bayer, 2008).

A related denormalization approach targets the tobacco industry (Lavack, 2001; Thrasher et al., 2006). Tobacco industry denormalization approaches have been employed, for example, in the "Truth" campaign, which sought to highlight the tobacco industry's reliance on deception regarding the health risks associated with smoking (Healton, 2001). Such campaigns avoid some of the problematic aspects of denormalization campaigns by shifting the focus away from smokers and toward corporations (Voigt, 2013).

Conclusion

This chapter began by highlighting several features of tobacco that should inform the discussion of tobacco as a public health issue. It then discussed some of the normative grounds on which state actors might seek to reduce smoking rates and normative concerns about particular anti-smoking strategies.

To what extent can a discussion of the normative issues around tobacco control be instructive for other areas of public health? Because tobacco has been recognized as a health problem for longer than other health risk factors, such as poor nutrition and lack of physical exercise, and because of the success of policy interventions in achieving substantial reductions in smoking rates, there have been attempts to apply insights from tobacco to other public health concerns. By the same token, arguments in support of restrictive policy approaches to tobacco are often seen as the beginning of a slippery slope that ends with bans on other potentially harmful substances, such as sugar or fatty foods. However, it is important to resist the urge to apply normative arguments made in the context of tobacco to other health problems without considering the combination of features that distinguish tobacco from other substances—in particular the addictiveness of nicotine, the very significant risks for long-term users, and the disproportionately high smoking rates among the disadvantaged. While many normative problems surrounding tobacco are also highly relevant to other health risk factors, it is crucial that the arguments be made on their own terms and in light of the specific characteristics of the risk factor in question. While the normative debate about tobacco can be instructive in many ways, it does not permit straightforward conclusions about other public health issues and the permissible or desirable strategies to address them.

Acknowledgments

I would like to thank Joanna Cohen, Nancy Kass, and Brendan Saloner for their helpful comments on earlier versions of this chapter.

References

Abdullah, A., and Husten, C. 2004. "Promotion of Smoking Cessation in Developing Countries: A Framework for Urgent Public Health Interventions." *Thorax* 59(7): 623–630. doi:10.1136/thx.2003.018820.

Alamar, B., and Glantz, S. 2006. "Effect of Increased Social Unacceptability of Cigarette Smoking on Reduction in Cigarette Consumption." *American Journal of Public Health* 96(8): 1359–1363. doi:10.2105/AJPH.2005.069617.

Antin, T. M., Lipperman-Kreda, S., and Hunt, G. 2015. "Tobacco Denormalization as a Public Health Strategy: Implications for Sexual and Gender Minorities." *American Journal of Public Health* 105(12): 2426–2429. doi:10.2105/AJPH.2015.302806.

Apollonio, D., and Malone, R. 2005. "Marketing to the Marginalised: Tobacco Industry Targeting of the Homeless and Mentally Ill." *Tobacco Control* 14(6): 409–415. doi:10.1136/tc.2005.011890.

Asch, D., Muller, R., and Volpp, K. 2013. "Conflicts and Compromises in Not Hiring Smokers." *New England Journal of Medicine* 368(15): 1371–1373. doi:10.1056/NEJMp1303632.

ASH (Action on Smoking and Health). 2015. "Smoking Statistics: Illness and Death." http://ash.org.uk/files/documents/ASH_107.pdf.

Barbeau, E. M., Wolin, K. Y., Naumova, E. N., and Balbach, E. 2005. "Tobacco Advertising in Communities: Associations with Race and Class." *Preventive Medicine* 40(1): 16–22. doi:10.1016/j.ypmed.2004.04.056.

Bayer, R. 2008. "Stigma and the Ethics of Public Health: Not Can but Should We." *Social Science and Medicine* 67(3): 463–472. doi:10.1016/j.socscimed.2008.03.017.

Bayer, R., and Bachynski, K. 2013. "Banning Smoking in Parks and on Beaches: Science, Policy, and the Politics of Denormalization." *Health Affairs* 32(7): 1291–1298. doi:10.1377/hlthaff.2012.1022.

Bayer, R., and Kelly, M. 2010. "Tobacco Control and Free Speech—An American Dilemma." *New England Journal of Medicine* 362(4): 281–283.

Bell, K., and Keane, H. 2012. "Nicotine Control: E-Cigarettes, Smoking and Addiction." *International Journal of Drug Policy* 23(3): 242–247. doi:10.1016/j.drugpo.2012.01.006.

Bell, K., McCullough, L., Salmon, A., and Bell, J., 2010. "'Every Space Is Claimed': Smokers' Experiences of Tobacco Denormalisation." *Sociology of Health and Illness* 32(6): 1–16. doi:10.1111/j.1467-9566.2010.01251.x.

Bell, K., Salmon, A., Bowers, M., Bell, J., and McCullough, L., 2010. "Smoking, Stigma and Tobacco Denormalization: Further Reflections on the Use of Stigma as a Public Health Tool." *Social Science and Medicine* 70(6): 795–799.

Benowitz, N. 2010. "Nicotine Addiction." *New England Journal of Medicine* 362(24): 2295–2303. doi:10.1056/NEJMra0809890.

Berrick, A. 2013. "The Tobacco-Free Generation Proposal." *Tobacco Control* 22(1): i22–i26. doi:10.1136/tobaccocontrol-2012-050865.

Bilano, V., Gilmour, S., Moffiet, T., d'Espaignet, E. T., Stevens, G. A., Commar, A., et al. 2015. "Global Trends and Projections for Tobacco Use, 1990–2025: An Analysis of Smoking Indicators from the WHO Comprehensive Information Systems for Tobacco Control." *Lancet* 385(9972): 966–976. doi:10.1016/S0140-6736(15)60264-1.

Brandt, A. 2007. *The Cigarette Century: The Rise, Fall, and Deadly Persistence of the Product That Defined America* (New York: Basic Books).

Brennan, P., Crispo, A., Zaridze, D., Szeszenia-Dabrowska, N., Rudnai, P., Lissowska, J., et al. 2006. "High Cumulative Risk of Lung Cancer Death among Smokers and Nonsmokers in Central and Eastern Europe." *American Journal of Epidemiology* 164(12): 1233–1241. doi:10.1093/aje/kwj340.

Breton, E., and Sherlaw, W. 2011. "Examining Tobacco Control Strategies and Aims through a Social Justice Lens: An Application of Sen's Capability Approach." *Public Health Ethics* 4(2): 149–159. doi:10.1093/phe/phr022.

Butler, T., Richmond, R., Belcher, J., Wilhelm, K., and Wodak, A. 2007. "Should Smoking Be Banned in Prisons?" *Tobacco Control* 16(5): 291–293. doi:10.1136/tc.2007.021600.

Chamberlain, K., and O'Neill, D. 2007. "Understanding Social Class Differences in Health: A Qualitative Analysis of Smokers' Health Beliefs." *Psychology and Health* 13(6): 1105–1119. doi:10.1080/08870449808407453.

Chapman, S. 2000. "Banning Smoking Outdoors Is Seldom Ethically Justifiable." *Tobacco Control* 9(1): 95–97. doi:10.1136/tc.9.1.95.

Chapman, S. 2012. "The Case for a Smoker's License." *PLOS Medicine* 9(11): e1001342. doi:10.1371/journal.pmed.1001342.

Chapman, S. 2015. "Is a Smoking Ban in UK Parks and Outdoor Spaces a Good Idea? No." *British Medical Journal* 350(25): h958. doi:10.1136/bmj.h958.

Cohen, J. 1993. "Freedom of Expression." *Philosophy and Public Affairs* 22(3): 207–263.

Colgrove, J., Bayer, R., and Bachynski, K. 2011. "Nowhere Left to Hide? The Banishment of Smoking from Public Spaces." *New England Journal of Medicine* 364(25): 2375–2377. doi:10.1056/NEJMp1104637.

Conly, S. 2012. *Against Autonomy: Justifying Coercive Paternalism* (New York: Cambridge University Press).

Daynard, R. 2009. "Doing the Unthinkable (and Saving Millions of Lives)." *Tobacco Control* 18(1): 2–3. doi:10.1136/tc.2008.028308.

Di Cesare, M., Khang, Y. H., Asaria, P., Blakely, T., Cowan, M. J., Farzadfar, F., et al. 2013. "Inequalities in Non-communicable Diseases and Effective Responses." *Lancet* 381(9866): 585–597. doi:10.1016/S0140-6736(12)61851-0.

Doll, R., Peto, R., Boreham, J., and Sutherland, I. 2004. "Mortality in Relation to Smoking: 50 Years' Observations on Male British Doctors." *British Medical Journal* 328(7455). doi:10.1136/bmj.38142.554479.AE.

Flanigan, J. 2016. "Double Standards and Arguments for Tobacco Regulation." *Journal of Medical Ethics* 42(5): 305–311. doi:10.1136/medethics-2016-103528.

Gilmore, A., Fooks, G., Drope, J., Bialous, S. A., and Jackson, R. R. 2015. "Exposing and Addressing Tobacco Industry Conduct in Low-Income and Middle-Income Countries." *Lancet* 385(9972): 1029–1043.

Goodin, R. 1989. "The Ethics of Smoking." *Ethics* 99(3): 574–624.

Goodin, R. 1991. "Permissible Paternalism: In Defense of the Nanny State." *The Responsive Community* 1(3): 42–51. https://doi.org/10.2307/23600633?ref=no-x-route:11070e6d8136473b8543727d9e511602.

Gostin, L. 2014. "Tobacco Endgame: The Poverty Conundrum." *Hastings Center Report* 44(3): 10–11. doi:10.1002/hast.307.

Graham, H. 2011. "Smoking, Stigma and Social Class." *Journal of Social Policy* 41(1): 83–99. doi:10.1017/S004727941100033X.

Grana, R., Benowitz, N., and Glantz, S. 2014. "E-Cigarettes: A Scientific Review." *Circulation* 129(19): 1972–1986. doi:10.1161/CIRCULATIONAHA.114.007667.

Grill, K., and Voigt, K. 2016. "The Case for Banning Cigarettes." *Journal of Medical Ethics* 42(5): 293–301.

Haines-Saah, R., Bell, K., and Dennis, S. 2015. "A Qualitative Content Analysis of Cigarette Health Warning Labels in Australia, Canada, the United Kingdom, and the United States." *American Journal of Public Health* 105(2): e61–e69. doi:10.2105/AJPH.2014.302362.

Halliday, D. 2016. "The Ethics of a Smoking Licence." *Journal of Medical Ethics* 42(5): 278–284. doi:10.1136/medethics-2013-101347.

Hammond, D. 2011. "Health Warning Messages on Tobacco Products: A Review." *Tobacco Control* 20 (5): 327–337.

Hammond, D., Fong, G. T., Zanna, M. P., Thrasher, J. F., and Borland, R. 2006. "Tobacco Denormalization and Industry Beliefs among Smokers from Four Countries." *American Journal of Preventive Medicine* 31(3): 225–232.

Healton, C. 2001. "Who's Afraid of the Truth?" *American Journal of Public Health* 91(4): 554–558.

Healton, C., and Nelson, K. 2004. "Reversal of Misfortune: Viewing Tobacco as a Social Justice Issue." *American Journal of Public Health* 94(2): 186–191.

HHS (US Department of Health and Human Services). 2006. *The Health Consequences of Involuntary Exposure to Tobacco Smoke: A Report of the Surgeon General* (Atlanta, Ga.: HHS).

Hill, S., Amos, A., Clifford, D., and Platt, S. 2014. "Impact of Tobacco Control Interventions on Socioeconomic Inequalities in Smoking: Review of the Evidence." *Tobacco Control* 23(2): e89–e97. doi:10.1136/tobaccocontrol-2013-051110.

Hiscock, R., Bauld, L., Amos, A., and Platt, S. 2012. "Smoking and Socioeconomic Status in England: The Rise of the Never Smoker and the Disadvantaged Smoker." *Journal of Public Health* 34(3): 390–396. doi:10.1093/pubmed/fds012.

Houle, B., and Siegel, M. 2009. "Smoker-Free Workplace Policies: Developing a Model of Public Health Consequences of Workplace Policies Barring Employment to Smokers." *Tobacco Control* 18(1): 64–69. doi:10.1136/tc.2008.026229.

Jarvis, M. 2004. "Why People Smoke." *British Medical Journal* 328(7434): 277. doi:10.1136/bmj.328.7434.277.

Jha, P. 2011. "Avoidable Deaths from Smoking: A Global Perspective." *Public Health Reviews* 33(2): 569–600.

Jha, P., and Chaloupka, F. 1999. *Curbing the Epidemic: Governments and the Economics of Tobacco Control* (Washington, D.C.: World Bank).

Jha, P., and Peto, R. 2014. "Global Effects of Smoking, of Quitting, and of Taxing Tobacco." *New England Journal of Medicine* 370(1): 60–68. doi:10.1056/NEJMra1308383.

Jha, P., Ramasundarahettige, C., Landsman, V., Rostron, B., Thun, M., Anderson, R. N., et al. 2013. "21st-Century Hazards of Smoking and Benefits of Cessation in the United States." *New England Journal of Medicine* 368(4): 341–350. doi:10.1056/NEJMsa1211128.

Jochelson, K. 2006. "Smoke-Free Legislation and Mental Health Units: The Challenges Ahead." *British Journal of Psychiatry* 189(6): 479–480. doi:10.1192/bjp.bp.106.029942.

Jochelson, K. 2007. *Paying the Patient: Improving Health Using Financial Incentives* (London: King's Fund).

Kim, S., and Shanahan, J. 2003. "Stigmatizing Smokers: Public Sentiment toward Cigarette Smoking and Its Relationship to Smoking Behaviors." *Journal of Health Communication* 8(4): 343–367.

Kotz, D., and West, R. 2009. "Explaining the Social Gradient in Smoking Cessation: It's Not in the Trying, but in the Succeeding." *Tobacco Control* 18(1): 43–46. doi:10.1136/tc.2008.025981.

Lader, D. 2008. *General Household Survey: Smoking and Drinking Among Adults, 2007* (Newport, UK: Office for National Statistics).

Lavack, A. 2001. *Tobacco Industry Denormalization Campaigns: A Review and Evaluation.* Report prepared for Health Canada.

Lim, S. S., Vos, T., Flaxman, A. D., Danaei, G., Shibuya, K., Adair-Rohani, H., et al. 2012. "A Comparative Risk Assessment of Burden of Disease and Injury Attributable to 67 Risk Factors and Risk Factor Clusters in 21 Regions, 1990–2010: A Systematic Analysis for the Global Burden of Disease Study 2010." *Lancet* 380(9859): 2224–2260. doi:10.1016/S0140-6736(12)61766-8.

MacAskill, S., Stead, M., MacKintosh, A.M., and Hastings, G. 2002. "'You Cannae Just Take Cigarettes Away from Somebody and No' Gie Them Something Back': Can Social Marketing Help Solve the Problem of Low-Income Smoking?" *Social Marketing Quarterly* 8(1): 19–34.

Mackay, J., and Eriksen, M. 2015. *The Tobacco Atlas*. 5th ed. (Atlanta, Ga.: American Cancer Society).

Malone, R., McDaniel, P., and Smith, E. 2014. "It Is Time to Plan the Tobacco Endgame." *British Medical Journal* 348(11): g1453. doi:10.1136/bmj.g1453.

Niederdeppe, J., Kuang, X., Crock, B., and Skelton, A. 2008. "Media Campaigns to Promote Smoking Cessation among Socioeconomically Disadvantaged Populations: What Do We Know, What Do We Need to Learn, and What Should We Do Now?" *Social Science and Medicine* 67(9): 1343–1355.

Pirie, K., Peto, R., Reeves, G. K., Green, J., Beral, V., and Million Women Study Collaborators. 2013. "The 21st Century Hazards of Smoking and Benefits of Stopping: A Prospective Study of One Million Women in the UK." *Lancet* 381(9861): 133–141. doi:10.1016/S0140-6736(12)61720-6.

Popay, J. 2008. "Should Disadvantaged People Be Paid to Take Care of Their Health? No." *British Medical Journal* 337(594). doi:10.1136/bmj.a594.

Proctor, R. 2013. "Why Ban the Sale of Cigarettes? The Case for Abolition." *Tobacco Control* 22(1): i27–i30. doi:10.1136/tobaccocontrol-2012-050811.

Radley, A., Ballard, P., Eadie, D., MacAskill, S., Donnelly, L., and Tappin, D. 2013. "Give It Up for Baby: Outcomes and Factors Influencing Uptake of a Pilot Smoking Cessation Incentive Scheme for Pregnant Women." *BMC Public Health* 13(1): 343. doi:10.1186/1471-2458-13-343.

Roemer, J. 1993. "A Pragmatic Theory of Responsibility for the Egalitarian Planner." *Philosophy and Public Affairs* 22(2): 146–166. https://doi.org/10.2307/2265444?ref=no-x-route:f214e1ca7702b3ebcdd96d1e0dc9c8d1.

Rutten, L. J. F., Augustson, E. M., Moser, R. P., Beckjord, E. B., and Hesse, B.W. 2008. "Smoking Knowledge and Behavior in the United States: Sociodemographic, Smoking Status, and Geographic Patterns." *Nicotine & Tobacco Research* 10(10): 1559–1570, doi:10.1080/14622200802325873.

Schmidt, H., Voigt, K., and Emanuel, E. 2013. "The Ethics of Not Hiring Smokers." *New England Journal of Medicine* 368(15): 1369–1371.

Schroeder, S., and Morris, C. 2010. "Confronting a Neglected Epidemic: Tobacco Cessation for Persons with Mental Illnesses and Substance Abuse Problems." *Annual Review of Public Health* 31(1): 297–314. doi:10.1146/annurev.publhealth.012809.103701.

Segall, S. 2010. *Health, Luck, and Justice* (Princeton, N.J.: Princeton University Press).

Shapiro, D. 1994. "Smoking Tobacco: Irrationality, Addiction, and Paternalism." *Public Affairs Quarterly* 8(2): 187–203.

Shibuya, K., Ciecierski, C., Guindon, E., Bettcher, D. W., Evans, D. B., and Murray, C. J. 2003. "WHO Framework Convention on Tobacco Control: Development of an Evidence Based Global Public Health Treaty." *British Medical Journal* 327(7407): 154–157.

Stead, M., MacAskill, S., MacKintosh, A. M., Reece, J., and Eadie, D. 2001. "'It's as If You're Locked In': Qualitative Explanations for Area Effects on Smoking in Disadvantaged Communities." *Health & Place* 7(4): 333–343.

Stein, K., Zhao, L., Crammer, C., and Gansler, T. 2007. "Prevalence and Sociodemographic Correlates of Beliefs Regarding Cancer Risks." *Cancer* 110(5): 1139–1148. doi:10.1002/cncr.22880.

Stuber, J., and Galea, S. 2009. "Who Conceals Their Smoking Status from Their Health Care Provider?" *Nicotine & Tobacco Research* 11(3): 303–307.

Stuber, J., Galea. S., and Link, B. 2008. "Smoking and the Emergence of a Stigmatized Social Status." *Social Science and Medicine* 67(3): 420–430.

Thompson, L., Pearce, J., and Barnett, J. 2007. "Moralising Geographies: Stigma, Smoking Islands and Responsible Subjects." *Area* 39(4): 508–517.

Thrasher, J. F., Niederdeppe, J. D., Jackson, C., and Farrelly, M. C. 2006. "Using Anti-tobacco Industry Messages to Prevent Smoking among High-Risk Adolescents." *Health Education Research* 21(3): 325–337. doi:10.1093/her/cyl001.

Ugen, S. 2003. "Bhutan: The World's Most Advanced Tobacco Control Nation?" *Tobacco Control* 12(4) (2003): 431. doi:10.1136/tc.12.4.431.

van der Eijk, Y. 2016. "Ethics of Tobacco Harm Reduction from a Liberal Perspective." *Journal of Medical Ethics* 42(5): 273–277.

Voigt, K. 2010. "Smoking and Social Justice." *Public Health Ethics* 3(2): 91–106. doi:10.1093/phe/phq006.

Voigt, K. 2012a. "Incentives, Health Promotion and Equality." *Health Economics, Policy and Law* 7(3): 263–283. doi:10.1017/S1744133110000277.

Voigt, K. 2012b. "Nonsmoker and 'Nonnicotine' Hiring Policies: The Implications of Employment Restrictions for Tobacco Control." *American Journal of Public Health* 102(11): 2013–2018.

Voigt, K. 2013. "'If You Smoke, You Stink.' Denormalisation Strategies for the Improvement of Health-Related Behaviours: The Case of Tobacco." In *Ethics in Public Health and Health Policy: Concepts, Methods, Case Studies*, edited by D. Strech, I. Hirschberg, and G. Marckmann, 47–61 (Amsterdam: Springer Netherlands). doi:10.1007/978-94-007-6374-6_4.

Voigt, K. 2015a. "Paternalism and Equality." In *New Perspectives on Paternalism and Health Care*, edited by T. Schramme, 87–100 (Amsterdam: Springer).

Voigt, K. 2015b. "Smoking Norms and the Regulation of E-Cigarettes." *American Journal of Public Health* 105(10): 1967–1972.

Voigt, K. 2017. "Too Poor to Say No? Health Incentives for Disadvantaged Populations." *Journal of Medical Ethics* 43(3): 162–166.

Volpp, K. G., Troxel, A. B., Pauly, M. V., Glick, H. A., Puig, A., Asch, D. A., et al. 2009. "A Randomized, Controlled Trial of Financial Incentives for Smoking Cessation." *New England Journal of Medicine* 360(7): 699–709. doi:10.1056/NEJMsa0806819.

Walters, H., and Barnsley, K. 2015. "Tobacco-Free Generation Legislation." *Medical Journal of Australia* 202(10): 509–510. doi:10.5694/mja15.00416,

Warner, K. 2000. "The Economics of Tobacco: Myths and Realities." *Tobacco Control* 9(1): 78–89. doi:10.1136/tc.9.1.78.

WHO (World Health Organization). 2011. *Global Status Report on Noncommunicable Diseases 2010* (Geneva: WHO). http://www.who.int/nmh/publications/ncd_report2010/en/.

WHO (World Health Organization). 2018. "WHO Regional Offices." http://www.who.int/about/regions/en/.

Williams, J. 2008. "Eliminating Tobacco Use in Mental Health Facilities: Patients' Rights, Public Health, and Policy Issues." *Journal of the American Medical Association* 299(5): 571–573. doi:10.1111/j.1525-1497.2006.00357.x.

Wilson, J. 2011. "Why It's Time to Stop Worrying about Paternalism in Health Policy." *Public Health Ethics* 4(3): 269–279.

Wiltshire, S., Bancroft, A., Parry, O., and Amos, A. 2003. "'I Came Back Here and Started Smoking Again': Perceptions and Experiences of Quitting among Disadvantaged Smokers." *Health Education Research* 18(3): 292–303. doi:10.1093/her/cyf031.

Yerger, V., Przewoznik, J., and Malone, R. 2007. "Racialized Geography, Corporate Activity, and Health Disparities: Tobacco Industry Targeting of Inner Cities." *Journal of Health Care for the Poor and Underserved* 18(1): 10–38. doi:10.1353/hpu.2007.0120.

CHAPTER 44

ALCOHOL AND OTHER DRUGS: PUBLIC HEALTH ETHICS ISSUES

BRENDAN SALONER

INTRODUCTION

THE consumption of alcohol and other drugs (AODs) generates widespread health harms. Alcohol alone contributes 4.6 percent of the global burden of disease (Rehm et al., 2009), and illicit drugs contribute an additional 0.8 percent (Degenhardt et al., 2013). In the United States, drug overdoses (mainly due to opioids) are now the leading cause of injury death (Levi, Segal, and Kohn, 2012), and they are growing. Overdose deaths have been rising in other countries as well (Martins et al., 2015). AODs also contribute to, or exacerbate, health conditions such as cancer. Harder to quantify is the emotional anguish related to harmful AOD use, which affects people using substances as well as their families and communities. For example, children raised by individuals with a serious drug or alcohol problem are at elevated risk for educational and health problems (Lander, Howsare, and Byrne, 2013). Heavy AOD use also contributes to unemployment, homelessness, criminal activity, and poverty (Kasunic and Lee, 2014).

This chapter reviews the ethics of public health approaches designed to reduce the harmful effects of AOD use. These efforts take many forms, including preventing harmful use, reducing the adverse consequences of harmful use, encouraging treatment utilization, and changing the social conditions that give rise to harmful use. Public health approaches extend beyond traditional prevention campaigns or treatment programs to include regulatory policy, criminal justice programs, and social services. This wide reach produces tensions regarding the appropriate scope of public health intervention, especially when such programs encroach on personal choice or privacy.

The chapter examines the normative foundations for public health intervention in AOD use, and then focuses on two types of ethics concerns: those related to the appropriate goals of public health, and those related to the means used to pursue those goals. These concerns prompt key ethical questions, such as the following: What is society's responsibility to prevent, mitigate, or eliminate harms related to AODs? What burdens can reasonably be imposed on society and on affected individuals in pursuit of these goals?

The chapter will begin by providing an epidemiologic overview of AOD use and presenting broad ethical perspectives. It will then focus on justice-based concerns as they relate to prevention and treatment programs, law enforcement, harm reduction, and legalization. While the primary focus is on the United States, the discussion has relevance to other developed countries as well. Perspectives on AOD policy in low- and middle-income countries can be found elsewhere (WHO, 2014; Degenhardt and Hall, 2012).

The Epidemiology of Harmful AOD Use

About 8.1 percent of US adults have a current AOD disorder, based on criteria from the *Diagnostic and Statistical Manual of Mental Disorders* (CBHSQ, 2015). The large majority (two-thirds) of these individuals have a problem solely with alcohol rather than illicit drugs. An even larger population engages in harmful behaviors that may not meet clinical criteria for a disorder, such as misuse of prescription medications or occasional binge drinking (CBHSQ, 2015). The burden of harmful AOD use is more prevalent among men and, with a few exceptions, among individuals of lower socioeconomic status (Compton et al., 2007). Mental illness prevalence is higher among individuals with an AOD disorder (Compton et al., 2007). A common misconception is that minority populations use AODs more often than do whites; in fact, rates are comparable or lower among minority populations, but they are disproportionately likely to be arrested or incarcerated due to an AOD-related offense (Cook and Alegría, 2015).

Why Averting Harmful AOD Use Promotes Justice

Because of the negative effects of AODs on health and well-being, most accounts of justice support the importance of averting harmful AOD use (the emphasis on *harmful* is important, because some forms of AOD use may be neutral or, in fact, provide health benefits). John Rawls (1999, 2001) has argued that a just society would incorporate a principle of fair equality of opportunity, which ensures that people from disadvantaged backgrounds are able to pursue opportunities on equal terms with equally talented people from more advantaged backgrounds. Extending this account, Norman Daniels (2008) argues that fair equality of opportunity requires the use of social resources to meet health needs, since failing to meet these needs would lead to unequal opportunity stemming from disease or disability. Health needs may be met by health care or by interventions addressing social determinants of health such as housing and nutrition (Daniels, Kennedy, and Kawachi, 2004). Amartya Sen (1980, 1993) has argued that a just society should be ultimately concerned with a fair distribution of individual capabilities, or the range of things that a person can "be or do." Similarly, Powers and Faden (2006) argue that public health intervention helps provide a basis for a more just society in part by achieving a level of wellness that enables people to be active and included as participants.

Harmful AOD use diminishes people's ability to participate in valued activities and to pursue opportunities in normatively important ways. First, it increases the risk of premature death and chronic illness (Whiteford et al. 2013), thus shortening the time individuals have to pursue life projects, while also causing physical limitations that may interfere with meaningful activities and self-care. Second, intoxication and addiction impair the capacity of individuals to exert self-control, make decisions, and express their preferences. Impulsive choices—such as stealing from family to support an addiction—may contradict people's own deep desires (e.g., the desire to maintain healthy relationships). Third, harmful AOD use often leads to conditions of social disadvantage and marginalization (Room, 2005), which can reduce the ability of individuals to sustain themselves financially and to maintain valued social connections.

AOD use not only affects those using the substance. A pedestrian may be fatally struck by a drunk driver. Family members are harmed when a family breadwinner loses his or her employment due to addiction. Widely diffused harms include medical spending and losses in economic activity due to reduced productivity.

As described below, harmful AOD use can be prevented or mitigated, which can improve individuals' capabilities and prospects of pursuing opportunities. To the extent that justice requires improving individuals' capabilities and prospects, individuals who would benefit from policies that reduce AOD harms—either caused by their own or others' use—have a justice-based claim to social assistance. Efforts to avert harms from AODs include preventing people from initiating harmful use, treating harmful use once it arises, enforcing laws that keep others safe, and creating a legal environment that supports public health goals.

The Role of Personal Responsibility

Arguments framed in terms of personal responsibility contend that harmful AOD use is to some extent voluntary, and that this voluntariness limits individual claims to social assistance. Hard-line versions of this argument would argue that society should not "bail out" individuals who make unwise choices, even when the stakes are life or death (Miller, 2016). Others argue that while society should not entirely abandon those suffering from addiction, it may take personal choice into account when deciding how to confront addiction or prioritize scarce public health resources (Satel and Lilienfeld, 2014).

In a classic argument, Richard J. Arneson (1989, 2004) distinguishes inequalities arising from the "natural lottery" and those arising from personal preferences or choices, judging inequalities due to choices to be acceptable. For luck egalitarians such as Arneson, justice only requires ameliorating disadvantages that stem from unchosen bad luck (such as having a congenital disability that requires use of a wheelchair), but does not require societal amelioration of disadvantages that result from individuals' judgments, preferences, or free choices.

If the luck egalitarian position argues that assistance is limited for diseases or injuries that occur because of lifestyle free choice (Roemer, 1993, 1995), this raises into question the degree to which AOD use is voluntary and to which individuals can control whether their use will harm themselves or others. Related, even if initiating AOD use is voluntary, becoming addicted surely limits free choice and, on some accounts, calls into question whether this limited choice also limits personal responsibility.

Resolving these questions in practice is murky because many (but not all) key risk factors for AOD use are outside of individuals' control. Low-resource neighborhoods and poverty increase risk factors for harmful AOD use and increase the stakes of harmful use (such as incarceration or job loss) (Caton et al., 2005; Fergusson, Horwood, and Woodward, 2001; Alexandre and French, 2004). Much of the variance in risk of addiction can also be explained by genetic factors; in studies of twins adopted into different family environments, shared genetics accounted for as much as 60 percent of the risk of developing alcoholism (Kendler et al., 1992; Prescott and Kendler, 1999). Finally, as mentioned earlier, addiction is an illness characterized by a loss of personal control. A growing body of research in psychology and behavioral economics emphasizes that addiction may be literally irrational—in the presence of intense cravings, individual decision-making may be substantially dominated by a "hot" reactive self rather than a "cool" deliberative and reasoning self (Kalivas and Volkow, 2005; Everitt and Robbins, 2005; Hyman, Malenka, and Nestler, 2006). Thus, even if it were determined that there is some element of personal choice in initiating AOD use, people who have addictions may have diminished control over when, and how much, they use.

Fully withholding assistance to those harmed by AOD through their own choices may seem overly harsh, or indeed counter to principles of justice such as social solidarity. Following Shlomi Segall (2010), some luck egalitarians may adopt a pluralistic view that does not entirely withdraw support from those with AOD-related disadvantage, but rather assumes that personal responsibility is one of several bases that can be used to determine resource allocation, and could therefore assign less (but at least some) priority to people who are harmed through their own choices.

Prevention through Screening, Education, and Awareness

Preventing harmful AOD use can take many forms—including taxation, broad-based social programs, and other drug control policies (described further in subsequent sections)—but the focus in this section is on prevention through educational and awareness campaigns. For an intervention to be ethically justified, it should be (among other things) effective (Childress et al., 2002). Many prevention campaigns, however, have been shown to be ineffective. For example, the DARE (Drug Abuse Resistance Education) campaign aimed at US school children had little positive effect on preventing AOD initiation (Pan and Bai, 2009). By contrast, other prevention strategies have shown effectiveness, including programs to build psychological skills such as resilience to resist harmful use (Griffin and Botvin, 2010).

Screening, often used as a means of identifying individuals to receive education or other prevention programs, poses its own ethical challenges. One challenge is that screening—outside of the doctor-patient relationship—can intrude into individual privacy. For example, workplace screening may involve collecting information on illegal behaviors that could raise concerns of bodily privacy (to obtain urine or blood samples) or informational privacy. In some cases, such screening can result in dismissal from a job. Finding ways to implement screening in settings where individuals may benefit while assuring necessary privacy is a critical challenge. Relatedly, there are challenges to making participation in prevention programs confidential, especially when these programs occur in workplaces or schools. Individuals may also be reluctant to participate in prevention programs if their status as "high risk" is visible to others. While these concerns may be mitigated in practice, concerns about privacy and stigma could constrain how policymakers target high-risk populations.

Treatment

Most people with current AOD disorders do not receive treatment (CBHSQ, 2015). While a large segment of people recover without any treatment ("spontaneous remission"), treatment can be a highly effective tool for reducing harmful use (Price, Risk, and Spitznagel, 2001). Indeed, some have demonstrated that treatment can "pay for itself," with every dollar invested in treatment resulting in several dollars of reduced social spending (Ettner et al., 2006). However, treatment programs are difficult for many people to access and are largely disconnected from the medical system, a legacy of the historical marginalization of treatment. Outside of medically oriented programs, many people access treatment through self-help programs or the criminal justice system (Smith and Strashny, 2013).

Many individuals in treatment are legally required to participate, which also raises ethical concerns. First, individuals in court-ordered programs have constrained treatment choices compared to other medical patients. However, coerced treatment has been justified on the basis that most individuals with severe addiction would like help achieving sobriety, but need an extra "nudge" to stay committed to a program. Receiving treatment in an outpatient program is less disruptive, and ultimately more productive, than the alternative of incarceration. Second, physicians who care for patients legally coerced into treatment can be asked to report on a person's progress and to divulge sensitive information about drug use, such as the results of urinalysis drug screens. Physicians must ordinarily obtain patient consent to cooperate with law enforcement before initiating care, but the ability to obtain truly free consent can be limited since that consent is obtained under coerced conditions (i.e., where the alternative is jail). In extraordinary circumstances, where obtaining consent may be impossible (e.g., a patient with drug-induced psychosis), some treatment may be justified in order to reduce risk to the patient or to others.

There are also deep philosophical disagreements about *how* best to help individuals with harmful AOD use. These disagreements concern not only scientific debates about which treatments are effective, but also about whether it is appropriate to focus on the character of a person in recovery. "Tough love" treatment programs, in which patients are asked to inform upon, and sometimes punish, fellow patients who deviate from rules, were once popular, but they have now fallen into disrepute. Self-help programs are much less controversial, but some people object to the perspective that people are powerless in the face of their "disease" and must submit to a higher power to overcome addiction. These ideas are not grounded in the medical understanding of addiction, but they may nevertheless be valuable to some people (Humphreys et al., 2004). On the other end of the spectrum, methadone maintenance for opioid use disorder—which has very strong medical evidence—is rejected by many in the self-help community as an addiction by other means (Stancliff et al., 2002). Individuals in methadone maintenance do become physically dependent upon methadone (an opioid), but such treatment is appropriately described as "normalizing" because it helps individuals to maintain functioning and reduces cravings for harmful drugs like heroin. Since restoring normal functioning is a key goal of treatment, this trade-off should be viewed as more than acceptable.

Coercion and Law Enforcement

The United States' legal response to AOD use has led to an increase in imprisonment, the most significant restriction of liberty. The rise in imprisonment is a direct consequence of the "War on Drugs," with a surge in incarceration, including mandatory sentences for possession of small quantities of drugs, since the 1970s (Chanenson and Berman, 2007). Incarceration has serious and wide-reaching negative health consequences. African Americans in particular are at substantially greater risk of imprisonment (Western and Pettit, 2010). Prison is bad for the health of the prisoner (increasing the risk of infectious diseases and mental health problems) and often bad for the health of the prisoner's family (Massoglia, 2008; Turney, 2014; Schnittker et al., 2015). The racial disparities resulting from mass incarceration, on their own, raise questions about the fairness of criminal justice policies (Alexander, 2010).

The many health harms of incarceration raise questions about whether there is any public health justification for incarcerating people for low-level AOD offenses (as distinct from those who distribute drugs). Renewed calls for decriminalizing drug possession are motivated by a desire to reduce the ill effects of incarceration. It is important to note that decriminalization—reducing or eliminating criminal sanctions for drug possession—is different from legalization (discussed further below). For example, marijuana has been decriminalized in twenty-one US states (as of 2016) (NCSL, 2016), but it is illegal to possess marijuana in most of these states. Countries such as Portugal have decriminalized harder drugs. Keeping people out of correctional settings and mitigating the harmful effects of a criminal record are positive effects of decriminalization.

However, there are legitimate concerns about increasing the scope of decriminalization—including normalizing the use of illegal drugs and reducing deterrence. Decriminalization also may eliminate the legal enforcement that leads many people to receive treatment. Many AOD users on their own will not be motivated to seek treatment for their harmful drug use, and individuals in coerced treatment are more likely than others to complete treatment (Saloner and Cook, 2013). That said, coerced treatment involves deprivations of liberty and may not be cost-effective when delivered in a broad, untargeted manner (Kleiman, Caulkins, and Hawken, 2011). One promising model for coerced treatment involves programs that place offenders into programs with swift and certain criminal sanctions for violating drug-testing requirements, but that limit jail time to short periods (such as weekends) for violators. Those successfully meeting sobriety benchmarks can receive reduced judicial supervision, until they are finally released from the program. This model has been successfully implemented in Hawaii (the HOPE program) (Hawken and Kleiman, 2009) and in South Dakota for drunk drivers (the 24/7 program) (Kilmer et al., 2013). Such approaches are ethically appealing because they involve a more delicate and contextually specific use of incarceration while preserving individuals' ability to pursue meaningful lives outside of the criminal justice system.

Harm Reduction

Harm reduction encompasses a broad range of approaches to reducing the harmful effects of AOD use and may overlap with the goals of treatment. The most visible and controversial strategies include needle exchange programs, safe consumption sites, and supervised administration of clinical-grade heroin (now provided on a limited basis in Switzerland, Canada, and other countries).

Other programs that permit AOD use among people participating in employment or housing programs are also controversial. The more moderate examples are "work first" and "housing first" policies that do not require individuals to be abstinent to participate in subsidized housing or employment programs (Collins et al., 2012). Many of these approaches have been shown to be effective (Lurie et al., 1993; Padgett, Gulcur, and Tsemberis, 2006). On the other end of the continuum, Amsterdam has a program that employs individuals with alcohol use disorders to work as street sweepers and pays them in beer (Holligan, 2014). Such a program is ostensibly justified in that it reduces idleness in this group, provides them with a sense of self-worth, and may substitute beer for other even more harmful alcoholic beverages, but the effectiveness of such approaches is not well-evaluated.

In whatever form they take, harm reduction efforts can be justified on straightforward consequentialist terms—providing these programs increases the well-being of AOD-using individuals, and society more broadly, by preventing the bad health outcomes that accompany AOD use (without necessarily reducing substance use). These programs, it is argued, have little downside, since they improve the well-being of people who are not otherwise willing or able to fully abstain from use. If someone is not prepared to stop injecting heroin, their health trajectory can still be improved by ensuring that they have access to safe needles and to naloxone, the medication to reverse an overdose. To reduce stigma and increase acceptance, harm reduction programs often deliberately refrain from making any moral judgments about the "badness" of AOD use, although most are deliberately linked with treatment programs and provide education about treatment. Nonetheless, making commitments to quitting is not a requirement of harm reduction. Moreover, harm reduction programs can have secondary benefits through reduced disease transmission and prevention of other harms to others, and thus may advance other justice-based concerns.

One objection to harm reduction is that it creates conditions that enable continued AOD use and do not necessarily improve an individual's productivity or quality of life. By reducing the health costs of using drugs—such as blood-borne infections or the risk of overdose—one concern about harm reduction is that it neutralizes risks that otherwise encourage quitting (MacCoun, 1998). Harm reduction could also reduce the perceived harms of initiating drug use for children and adolescents to the extent that harm reduction normalizes the behavior. There is some evidence that this may be true for marijuana decriminalization (Pacula, 2010), but research is scarce for "harder" drugs. Moreover, harm reduction as provided in public health interventions generally includes counseling and referral to treatment programs. Even if concerns about normalization were well founded, the government—and affected individuals themselves—arguably has a strong interest in reducing the harmful social ills related to illegal drugs, especially in reducing the transmission of human immunodeficiency virus (HIV), hepatitis C virus, and other costly infectious diseases, and harm reduction could be integrated with treatment to foster long-term health improvement.

Some people may object that harm reduction is problematic despite its potential to improve health. On this view, social programs (especially those funded with government resources) have a duty not only to promote health, but also to represent the values of a good society, including respect for the law and concern for individual dignity. This public role is incompatible with harm reduction programs, which, it is argued, do not go far enough in rejecting behaviors that diminish individual dignity or condone criminality. This view presupposes both that there exists a sufficiently well-developed conception of public morality to draw a bright line between acceptable and unacceptable practices, and that the government has a more compelling interest in advancing that public morality than it does in protecting the public's health (Keane, 2003). In response, it might be argued that public sentiment is contaminated by prejudices that make it unreliable—for example, lesser criticism of alcohol compared with other drugs is interwoven with racial and socioeconomic biases, and does not necessarily reflect clear or objective moral standards.

Legalization, Taxation, and Regulation

Long seen as a utopian (or dystopian) fantasy, drug legalization is no longer hypothetical. As of this writing, growing, selling, and consuming marijuana for recreational purposes is permitted by eight US States and the District of Columbia and is legal for medical purposes in most states, though it remains illegal under federal law. Many arguments are raised in favor of legalizing at least some drugs: legalization provides a framework for regulating the safety and supply of drugs, imposing age requirements for buyers, maintaining standards for purity and potency, mitigating violence in illicit markets, and the collection of revenue through taxes, which can be used to fund treatment programs.

Legalization can encourage use and misuse of AODs, however. While prohibition of alcohol in the United States was a complete failure, alcohol also provides a cautionary tale about the dangers of low taxes and a weak regulatory framework. Despite clear evidence that advertising increases demand among underage consumers (Saffer and Dave, 2006), marketing restrictions have remained weak. Taxes on alcohol products are low relative to the costs their misuse imposes on society (Kleiman, Caulkins, and Hawken, 2011), and the most harmful products are the least expensive. Moreover, there are well-known problems of enforcement, including rogue retailers that continue to sell to underage buyers. Such concerns could be abated, but not entirely avoided, with higher taxes and greater enforcement. However, the regulatory frameworks guiding legalization are not substantially guided by public health evidence, as other stakeholder groups and industries eager to profit play an important role in maintaining an environment with easy access.

Legalization thus requires balancing very different harms and benefits. As mentioned, one purported benefit of legalization is that it enables greater control over price, supply, safety, and access than exists in illicit markets. The health benefits of regulation could be varied and include reducing environmental harms that arise through illegal cultivation, curbing street-level violence, and discouraging heavy use through quantity or place of sale restrictions. Health benefits aside, many see legalization as desirable because it gives more people something that they want—just as responsible adults experience pleasure from consuming cocktails, there are welfare gains to allowing responsible adults to engage in moderate marijuana use. How to weigh these benefits against the compelling interest in protecting the most vulnerable—children, people with a propensity for addiction, and those residing in communities that will be adversely affected by legalization—is unlikely to be a settled question on many theories of justice. In the absence of a clear answer from the standpoint of justice, there is value in pursuing some cautious and controlled experiments in legalization, but these experiments should be evaluated with strong monitoring of unintended health consequences.

Conclusion

Much to the disappointment of temperance crusaders, there will almost certainly never be a future free of AOD use. AOD use is deeply embedded in current social practices, and drugs and alcohol are a source of great pleasure for many individuals. This chapter has surveyed a variety of approaches that could be used to either constrain the spread of harmful use or treat individuals with AOD use problems.

Most strategies involve some regulation of individual choices, and rarely is the government able to remain entirely neutral in its approach to determining which AODs are permitted. This is not a new problem. For example, governments have, for some time, expressed a greater tolerance toward alcohol and its associated harms than toward other addictive substances. The public health perspective is valuable within these debates because it draws policymakers' attention toward the objective impact of different AODs on population health, and particularly on the health of vulnerable subgroups. Public health research also demonstrates the dangers that come with stigmatizing addiction or the unintended consequences of driving certain behaviors underground. Though health impacts alone will not resolve social debates, public health provides one of several valuable voices in a fractious and impassioned public discourse.

Acknowledgments

Excellent and extensive comments were provided by Nancy Kass, Govind Persad, and Kenneth Stoller. Christian Morales provided additional excellent comments and editorial assistance. Any errors or omissions are the author's sole responsibility.

References

Alexander, M. 2010. *The New Jim Crow: Mass Incarceration in the Age of Colorblindness* (New York: The New Press).

Alexandre, P. K., and French, M. T. 2004. "Further Evidence on the Labor Market Effects of Addiction: Chronic Drug Use and Employment in Metropolitan Miami." *Contemporary Economic Policy* 22(3): 382–393.

Arneson, R. J. 1989. "Equality and Equal Opportunity for Welfare." *Philosophical Studies* 56(1): 77–93.

Arneson, R. J. 2004. "Luck Egalitarianism Interpreted and Defended." *Philosophical Topics* 32(1–2): 1–20.

Caton, C. L. M., Dominguez, B., Schanzer, B., Hasin, D. S., Shrout, P. E., Felix, A., et al. 2005. "Risk Factors for Long-Term Homelessness: Findings from a Longitudinal Study of First-Time Homeless Single Adults." *American Journal of Public Health* 95(10): 1753–1759.

CBHSQ (Center for Behavioral Health Statistics and Quality). 2015. "2014 National Survey on Drug Use and Health: Detailed Tables" (Rockville, MD: Substance Abuse and Mental Health Services Administration). https://www.samhsa.gov/data/sites/default/files/NSDUH-DetTabs2014/NSDUH-DetTabs2014.pdf.

Chanenson, S. L., and Berman, D. A. 2007. "Federal Cocaine Sentencing in Transition." *Federal Sentencing Reporter* 19(5): 291–296.

Childress, J. F., Faden, R. R., Gaare, R. D., Gostin, L. O., Kahn, J., Bonnie, R. J., et al. 2002. "Public Health Ethics: Mapping the Terrain." *Journal of Law, Medicine and Ethics* 30(2): 170–178.

Collins, S. E., Malone, D. K., Clifasefi, S. L., Ginzler, J. A., Garner, M. D., Burlingham, B., et al. 2012. "Project-Based Housing First for Chronically Homeless Individuals with Alcohol Problems: Within-Subjects Analyses of 2-Year Alcohol Trajectories." *American Journal of Public Health* 102(3): 511–519.

Compton, W. M., Thomas, Y. F., Stinson, F. S., and Grant, B. F. 2007. "Prevalence, Correlates, Disability, and Comorbidity of *DSM-IV* Drug Abuse and Dependence in the United States: Results from the National Epidemiologic Survey on Alcohol and Related Conditions." *Archives of General Psychiatry* 64(5): 566–576.

Cook, B. L., and Alegría, M. 2015. "Racial-Ethnic Disparities in Substance Abuse Treatment: The Role of Criminal History and Socioeconomic Status." *Psychiatric Services* 62(11): 1273–1281.

Daniels, N. 2008. "What Is the Special Moral Importance of Health?" In *Just Health: Meeting Health Needs Fairly*, 29–78 (New York: Cambridge University Press).

Daniels, N., Kennedy, B., and Kawachi, I. 2004. "Health and Inequality, or, Why Justice Is Good for Our Health." In *Public Health, Ethics, and Equity*, edited by S. Anand, F. Peter, and A. Sen, 63–91 (Oxford: Oxford University Press).

Degenhardt, L., and Hall, W. 2012. "Extent of Illicit Drug Use and Dependence, and Their Contribution to the Global Burden of Disease." *Lancet* 379(9810): 55–70.

Degenhardt, L., Whiteford, H. A., Ferrari, A. J., Baxter, A. J., Charlson, F. J., Hall, W. D., et al. 2013. "Global Burden of Disease Attributable to Illicit Drug Use and Dependence: Findings from the Global Burden of Disease Study 2010." *Lancet* 382(9904): 1564–1574.

Ettner, S. L., Huang, D., Evans, E., Ash, D. R., Hardy, M., Jourabchi, M., et al. 2006. "Benefit–Cost in the California Treatment Outcome Project: Does Substance Abuse Treatment 'Pay for Itself'?" *Health Services Research* 41(1): 192–213.

Everitt, B. J., and Robbins, T. W. 2005. "Neural Systems of Reinforcement for Drug Addiction: From Actions to Habits to Compulsion." *Nature Neuroscience* 8(11): 1481–1489.

Fergusson, D. M., Horwood, L. J., and Woodward, L. J. 2001. "Unemployment and Psychosocial Adjustment in Young Adults: Causation or Selection?" *Social Science and Medicine* 53(3): 305–320.

Griffin, K. W., and Botvin, G. J. 2010. "Evidence-Based Interventions for Preventing Substance Use Disorders in Adolescents." *Child and Adolescent Psychiatric Clinics of North America* 19(3): 505–526.

Hawken, A., and Kleiman, M. 2009. *Managing Drug Involved Probationers with Swift and Certain Sanctions: Evaluating Hawaii's Hope: Executive Summary* (Washington, D.C.: National Criminal Justice Reference Services).

Holligan, A. 2014. "Amsterdam Alcoholics Paid in Beer for Collecting Litter." BBC News Online, January 6. http://www.bbc.com/news/world-europe-25548061.

Humphreys, K., Wing, S., McCarty, D., Chappel, J., Gallant, L., Haberle, B., et al. 2004. "Self-Help Organizations for Alcohol and Drug Problems: Toward Evidence-Based Practice and Policy." *Journal of Substance Abuse Treatment* 26(3): 151–158.

Hyman, S. E., Malenka, R. C., and Nestler, E. J. 2006. "Neural Mechanisms of Addiction: The Role of Reward-Related Learning and Memory." *Annual Review of Neuroscience* 29: 565–598.

Kalivas, P. W., and Volkow, N. D. 2005. "The Neural Basis of Addiction: A Pathology of Motivation and Choice." *American Journal of Psychiatry* 162(8): 1403–1413.

Kasunic, A., and Lee, M. A. C. 2014. "Societal Burden of Substance Abuse." *International Public Health Journal* 6(3): 269.

Keane, H. 2003. "Critiques of Harm Reduction, Morality and the Promise of Human Rights." *International Journal of Drug Policy* 14(3): 227–232.

Kendler, K. S., Heath, A. C., Neale, M. C., Kessler, R. C., and Eaves, L. J. 1992. "A Population-Based Twin Study of Alcoholism in Women." *JAMA* 268(14): 1877–1882.

Kilmer, B., Nicosia, N., Heaton, P., and Midgette, G. 2013. "Efficacy of Frequent Monitoring with Swift, Certain, and Modest Sanctions for Violations: Insights from South Dakota's 24/7 Sobriety Project." *American Journal of Public Health* 103(1): e37–e43.

Kleiman, M. A. R., Caulkins, J. P., and Hawken, A. 2011. *Drugs and Drug Policy: What Everyone Needs to Know* (Oxford: Oxford University Press).

Lander, L., Howsare, J., and Byrne, M. 2013. "The Impact of Substance Use Disorders on Families and Children: From Theory to Practice." *Social Work in Public Health* 28(3–4): 194–205.

Levi, J., Segal, L. M., and Kohn, D. 2012. *The Facts Hurt: A State-by-State Injury Prevention Policy Report* (Washington, D.C.: Trust for America's Health).

Lurie, P., Reingold, A. L., Bowser, B., Chen, D., Foley, J., Guydish, J., et al. 1993. *The Public Health Impact of Needle Exchange Programs in the United States and Abroad: Summary, Conclusions and Recommendations* (Atlanta: Centers for Disease Control and Prevention). https://stacks.cdc.gov/view/cdc/11203.

MacCoun, R. J. 1998. "Toward a Psychology of Harm Reduction." *American Psychologist* 53(11): 1199.

Martins, S. S., Sampson, L., Cerdá, M., and Galea, S. 2015. "Worldwide Prevalence and Trends in Unintentional Drug Overdose: A Systematic Review of the Literature." *American Journal of Public Health* 105(11): e29-e49.

Massoglia, M. 2008. "Incarceration as Exposure: The Prison, Infectious Disease, and Other Stress-Related Illnesses." *Journal of Health and Social Behavior* 49(1): 56–71.

Miller, K. 2016. "Lepage Vetoes Bill Aimed at Increasing Access to Overdose." *Portland Press Herald*, April 20. http://www.pressherald.com/2016/04/20/lepage-vetoes-bill-aimed-at-increasing-access-to-heroin-anti-overdose-drug/. Accessed February 20, 2018.

NCSL (National Conference of State Legislatures). 2016. "Marijuana Overview" (Washington, D.C.: NCSL). http://www.ncsl.org/research/civil-and-criminal-justice/marijuana-overview.aspx.

Pacula, R. L. 2010. *Examining the Impact of Marijuana Legalization on Marijuana Consumption*. Working Paper 770 (Santa Monica, Calif.: RAND Corporation). https://www.rand.org/pubs/working_papers/WR770.html.

Padgett, D. K., Gulcur, L., and Tsemberis, S. 2006. "Housing First Services for People Who Are Homeless with Co-occurring Serious Mental Illness and Substance Abuse." *Research on Social Work Practice* 16(1): 74–83.

Pan, W., and Bai, H. 2009. "A Multivariate Approach to a Meta-Analytic Review of the Effectiveness of the D.A.R.E. Program." *International Journal of Environmental Research and Public Health* 6(1): 267–277.

Powers, M., and Faden, R. 2006. *Social Justice: The Moral Foundations of Public Health and Health Policy* (Oxford: Oxford University Press).

Prescott, C. A., and Kendler, K. S. 1999. "Genetic and Environmental Contributions to Alcohol Abuse and Dependence in a Population-Based Sample of Male Twins." *American Journal of Psychiatry* 156(1): 34–40.

Price, R. K., Risk, N. K., and Spitznagel, E. L. 2001. "Remission from Drug Abuse over a 25-Year Period: Patterns of Remission and Treatment Use." *American Journal of Public Health* 91(7): 1107.

Rawls, J. 1999. *A Theory of Justice*. Rev. ed. (Cambridge, Mass.: Harvard University Press).

Rawls, J. 2001. *Justice as Fairness: A Restatement* (Cambridge, Mass.: Harvard University Press).

Rehm, J., Mathers, C., Popova, S., Thavorncharoensap, M., Teerawattananon, Y. and Patra, J. 2009. "Global Burden of Disease and Injury and Economic Cost Attributable to Alcohol Use and Alcohol-Use Disorders." *Lancet* 373(9682): 2223–2233.

Roemer, J. E. 1993. "A Pragmatic Theory of Responsibility for the Egalitarian Planner." *Philosophy & Public Affairs* 22(2): 146–166.

Roemer, J. E. 1995. "Equality and Responsibility." *Boston Review* 20(2): 3–7.

Room, R. 2005. "Stigma, Social Inequality and Alcohol and Drug Use." *Drug and Alcohol Review* 24(2): 143–155.

Saffer, H., and Dave, D. 2006. "Alcohol Advertising and Alcohol Consumption by Adolescents." *Health Economics* 15(6): 617–637.

Saloner, B., and Cook, B. L. 2013. "Blacks and Hispanics Are Less Likely Than Whites to Complete Addiction Treatment, Largely Due to Socioeconomic Factors." *Health Affairs* 32(1): 135–145.

Satel, S., and Lilienfeld, S. O. 2014. "Addiction and the Brain-Disease Fallacy." *Frontiers in Psychiatry* 4: 141.

Schnittker, J., Uggen, C., Shannon, S. K., and McElrath, S. 2015. "The Institutional Effects of Incarceration: Spillovers from Criminal Justice to Health Care." *Milbank Quarterly* 93(3): 516–560.

Segall, S. 2010. *Health, Luck, and Justice* (Princeton, N.J.: Princeton University Press).

Sen, A. 1980. "Equality of What?" In *The Tanner Lecture on Human Values*. Vol. I, 197–220 (Cambridge: Cambridge University Press).

Sen A. 1993. "Capability and Well-Being." In *The Quality of Life*, edited by M. C. Nussbaum and A. Sen, A., 30–53 (Oxford: Clarendon Press).

Smith, K., and Strashny, A. 2013. "Characteristics of Criminal Justice System Referrals Discharged from Substance Abuse Treatment and Facilities with Specially Designed Criminal Justice Programs." in *The CBHSQ Report* (Rockville, Md.: Substance Abuse and Mental Health Services Administration). https://www.ncbi.nlm.nih.gov/books/NBK362073/.

Stancliff, S., Myers, M. J. E., Steiner, S. and Drucker, E. 2002. "Beliefs about Methadone in an Inner-City Methadone Clinic." *Journal of Urban Health* 79(4): 571–578.

Turney, K. 2014. "Stress Proliferation across Generations? Examining the Relationship between Parental Incarceration and Childhood Health." *Journal of Health and Social Behavior* 55(3): 302–319.

Western, B., and Pettit, B. 2010. "Incarceration and Social Inequality." *Daedalus* 139(3): 8–19.

Whiteford, H. A., Degenhardt, L., Rehm, J., Baxter, A. J., Ferrari, A. J., Erskine, H. E., et al. 2013. "Global Burden of Disease Attributable to Mental and Substance Use Disorders: Findings from the Global Burden of Disease Study 2010." *Lancet* 382(9904): 1575–1586.

WHO (World Health Organization). 2014. *Global Status Report on Alcohol and Health* (Geneva: WHO). http://www.who.int/substance_abuse/activities/gsrah/en/.

CHAPTER 45

GLOBAL PUBLIC HEALTH, NONCOMMUNICABLE DISEASES, AND ETHICS

HAYLEY MACGREGOR

INTRODUCTION

THIS chapter reviews global issues in primary and secondary prevention of noncommunicable diseases (NCDs). Within an overall consideration of health justice, it reflects on two areas for ethical attention: questions of disease prioritization, and questions of individual responsibility. It is only relatively recently that NCDs have claimed more attention and come to be framed as a "global" issue by international health actors in terms of recognizing them as a growing and significant health problem in low- and middle-income countries (LMICs) (Horton, 2007). The World Health Organization (WHO) has been active for some time in pressing for greater concern, but other central players in international development, such as the World Bank and the United Nations Development Programme, have also released key reports calling for action and assisted in raising the attention of governments to problematize the issue (Reubi, Herrick, and Brown, 2016).

Noncommunicable diseases are conventionally defined as conditions that are not transmitted from person to person. They tend to be of long duration, and as such are labeled "chronic" due to their slow progression and the fact that they often affect people for the remainder of their lifetimes. While there might be treatments, there currently are no cures for most of these illnesses. The WHO has indicated four main types of NCD: cardiovascular diseases, cancers, chronic respiratory diseases, and diabetes. According to the WHO, these four types account for 82 percent of the 38 million annual deaths worldwide that are attributable to NCDs (WHO, 2016). The bracketing of these conditions as the main NCDs has drawn a range of critical opinion. It excludes, for instance, other chronic conditions such as mental illnesses, which have significance in terms of morbidity globally (Prince et al., 2007), and also in terms of coexistence of different illnesses, or multiple morbidities (Remais et al., 2012). The WHO's justification for the categorization of the four main types of NCD is to link these to a common set of modifiable risk factors that are labelled "behavioral" and are implicated in increased risk of illness and death: tobacco use, physical inactivity, unhealthy diet, and harmful alcohol usage (WHO, 2005).

It is important to note that there are other diseases that meet the criteria of being non-infectious and chronic, and indeed there are communicable diseases that can also become "chronic lifelong conditions" (van Olmen et al., 2011). Human immunodeficiency virus (HIV) infection is a case in point: it becomes a chronic disease with treatment, and indeed associations have been identified with NCD risk (see, for example, Carr, 2003). Thus, the value of a rigid category distinction between infectious and noncommunicable disease is increasingly questioned. For example, research has revealed connections between infections and the etiology of conditions such as cancers that have been classified as noncommunicable, and there is a need to better understand these direct interactions, especially in countries with a dual disease burden (Remais et al., 2012). However, the distinction persists.

Long considered a problem primarily for high-income countries of the "Global North," concerns have grown that the NCD burden has been increasing worldwide and in (LMICs), especially since the mid-1990s (Murray and Lopez, 1996; Murray et al., 2013). It has been argued that global burden of disease studies have played a significant role in revealing NCDs as an issue in the Global South in epidemiological terms, and in drawing public health attention to the changing global distribution of disease. However, political attention to the issue and the consequences of such shifts has lagged behind (Reubi, Herrick, and Brown, 2016). The WHO now claims that NCDs disproportionately affect LMICs, and that approximately 75 percent of NCD deaths annually—28 million deaths—occur in LMICs (WHO, 2016). In 2012 the WHO director-general noted that people in LMICs have up to four times the risk of death and disability from NCDs than those in high-income countries (WHO, 2012). The proportion of deaths globally from NCDs is greater than from HIV, tuberculosis, and malaria combined (WHO, 2005). Only in the African Region are communicable diseases and maternal, perinatal, and nutritional conditions still the most common causes of death, and the double burden of communicable and noncommunicable disease is becoming a significant challenge (UN, 2011a). The increase in the proportionate contribution of NCDs to the global disease burden can partly be attributed to improvements in combating infectious disease and maternal and child health (MCH) problems. The increase in NCDs has also increased the overall burden of chronic lifelong conditions (infectious and noncommunicable) globally, which has significant implications for countries where health systems were set up to focus primarily on acute disease and MCH (Atun et al., 2013).

Until relatively recently, concern about the rising burden of NCDs in LMICs was not reflected to a large extent in global health goals, spending priorities, or policy implementation (Horton, 2007; Alleyne et al. 2013; Stuckler and Basu, 2013). In some donor agencies, until a few years ago, such illnesses were still explicitly considered as an issue primarily for rich countries and their health systems. NCDs did not feature in the Millennium Development Goals of 2000, which specifically named other disease categories for priority attention. However, the United Nations summit on NCDs in 2011—only the second ever to be devoted to health—marked an effort to consolidate it as an issue of concern for LMICs, requiring more urgent global attention and action. A recent shift to redress this inattention is discernable in donor and research funding agencies, and a reduction of premature death from NCDs is a target of the Sustainable Development Goals adopted in September 2015 (WHO, 2015). The WHO Global Action Plan for the Prevention and Control of NCDs (2013–2020) aims for a 25 percent relative reduction in premature mortality from the organization's four main types of NCD by 2025 (WHO, 2017).

A framing of NCDs as a global issue has become common in accounts of the extension of the problem of NCDs to LMICs. Indeed "globalization" is routinely underscored as a key driver of the rising disease burden, alongside determinants such as population aging and urbanization (see, for example, WHO, 2005). In particular, the infiltration across the globe of the processed and fast food, soft drink, and tobacco industries are cited alongside urbanization to point to significant changes in food systems, diets, and patterns of food preparation, as well as more sedentary lifestyles. In some accounts, "globalization" is at times portrayed as a negative force directly driving ill health from NCDs. The impacts on health of widening global inequalities that have accompanied these large-scale processes of change have received less attention—increasingly these diseases are also linked to poverty and socioeconomic disparity associated with economic globalization (Narayan, Ali, and Koplan, 2010). It thus seems simplistic to portray the association between "global" drivers and disease factors such as obesity as a unidirectional, simple causal relationship (Goryakin et al., 2015). A sweeping evocation of globalization as the causal factor for a rising burden of NCDs can thus override more nuanced accounts of the factors contributing to changing disease burdens and a consideration of political-economy and the contexts and local environments in which these changes and diseases are experienced.

As the global prevalence of noncommunicable disease rises, it is pertinent to consider the ethical issues associated with framings of the disease burden and the priorities for primary and secondary prevention responses, especially in low-resource settings. These issues will be addressed in this chapter under two broad areas: firstly, prioritization and resource allocation; and secondly, questions of responsibility with respect to prevention measures. I focus on the tension between an emphasis on individual-level action and a systems approach that pays attention to broader structural factors, global and national inequalities, health system drivers, and sociopolitical determinants of NCDs.

Prioritization and Resource Allocation: NCDs as a Development Issue

Ethical debates about how to prioritize NCDs in LMICs revolve around questions of who is affected, what causes these diseases, and what effects these diseases have on the productivity and well-being of people in these countries. Justice-based arguments for giving priority to NCDs depend on the empirical claim that ameliorating them would increase health equity. Others go further, arguing that addressing NCDs is a key to promoting equity in other domains, pointing to the role that the NCD burden places on the economic prospects of the most disadvantaged (Anand, Peter, and Sen, 2006).

The prioritization of NCDs, as opposed to other disease areas (such as infections, undernutrition, or MCH), has attracted divergent views with respect to decisions about resource allocation for research funding and donor budgets at the international level. Setting resource priorities for NCDs requires balancing the needs of NCDs relative to meeting needs for preventing communicable diseases and MCH. One approach to setting health priorities would be to compare the disability-adjusted life years (DALYs) that are averted by scaling up programs to address NCDs versus other diseases. However, priority-setting by burden of disease has drawn criticism, not least for measuring the problem rather than examining solutions, for making value-based assumptions about health and well-being that cannot necessarily be taken as universals, and for sidelining considerations such as equity (Mooney and Wiseman, 2000; Anand and Hanson, 1998). Disease burden is not sufficient to account for broader factors that complicate the ability to make simple decisions on prioritization. For instance, a parameter such as cost-effectiveness can provide one of several criteria for disease prioritization, and must be balanced by considerations of equity (Johri and Norheim, 2012). A study examining potential NCD programs in Mexico found that while there was wide variation in effectiveness, many programs would provide excellent cost-effectiveness ratios (Salomon et al., 2012).

One factor that may not be immediately appreciated simply by comparing health gains from NCD programs versus other health programs is the extent to which NCD programs might uniquely advance economic "development." Several rationales could be explored for investing in NCDs, but I focus in some detail on the relationship between NCDs and poverty, as it is pertinent and significant in LMIC settings. The "development" case for prioritization of NCDs makes an ethical argument linked to the impoverishment of vulnerable households by the occurrence of disease. This argument was articulated strongly in 2011 when the United Nations General Assembly held a high-level meeting on noncommunicable disease. At that time, Secretary-General Ban Ki-moon declared NCDs a key development issue affecting the well-being, longevity, and financial security of poor people (UN, 2011b). Thus, the particular discursive framing around NCDs as a development issue was foregrounded in the political positioning for greater recognition (Reubi, Herrick, and Brown, 2016). The declaration that followed the summit traced this argument for NCDs as an issue for development attention, outlining the links between poverty and NCDs. The declaration emphasized the greater impact of such illnesses on poor households, both on account of catastrophic health expenditure in the face of an illness exacerbation and ongoing expenditure from household incomes due to the chronic nature of illnesses and the need for care. This argument underscores the view that the effects of living with an NCD are greater for poor people, and particularly for people in countries with weak health systems and public sector health financing mechanisms. If people have to pay out of pocket for health care, this can quickly lead to a downward spiral into deeper poverty.

A second, related argument to give greater priority to NCDs points to the indirect impact of NCD on countries' economic productivity (see, for example, Yach, Stuckler, and Brownell, 2006). This argument assumes that taking nonhealth factors into account in health resource allocation is fair and consistent with providing the greatest amount of good in society. Others, however, argue that medical care is a "separate sphere" where resource allocation should be limited to preventing illness and treating disease (Brock, 2003). These arguments also depend upon data suggesting that NCDs in LMICs are associated with earlier progression to disability and mortality (Murray et al., 2013). Poor access to quality health care can lead to inadequate treatment of NCDs and earlier development of serious sequelae (Bhojani et al., 2014). This can cause incapacity of economically active members of households, or a working person might stop earning to care for a relative. The high cost to hospital care and social care systems of untreated NCDs is a further societal-level impact that provides a rationale for investing in primary and secondary prevention of NCDs.

Despite the 2011 United Nations meeting, no "Global Fund" to combat NCDs was established, in contrast to the UN high-level meeting on HIV several years earlier. An exclusion of NCDs from funding agendas until more recently seemed partly to derive from the misconception that these were "diseases of affluence," associated with greed, not need (Narayan, Ali, and Koplan, 2010). This view led to the conclusion that NCDs are thus not "diseases of poverty." Setting aside ethical questions about whether the "poorest of the poor" are the most legitimate recipients of health funding, and whether this is justifiable in terms of redressing other inequalities, the complex manifestations of NCDs when considered from a global and national perspective suggests that simple attempts to categorize people based on their deservingness of interventions can lead to problematic generalizations. A paucity of fine-grained epidemiological data from LMICs compared to high-income settings on the nature of the NCD burden, and disaggregated data to reveal the relationship between prevalence and socioeconomic status, has also prevented clear conclusions.

Thus, for example, data from Bangladesh clearly show that the proportion of deaths due to NCDs has increased in the rural demographic surveillance site there (Matlab Health and Demographic Surveillance System) over the past three decades, and that the proportion of deaths due to communicable diseases has dropped (Chowdhury et al., 2013). The 2011 Bangladesh Urban Health Survey found a higher prevalence of hypertension and diabetes in the higher wealth quintiles, but the lower wealth quintiles were not unaffected (NIPORT, Mitra and Associates, and ICF International, 2013). A different picture has emerged from the analysis done by Lloyd-Sherlock et al. (2014), using publicly available data from the WHO Study on Global Aging and Adult Health, in China, Ghana, India, Mexico, South Africa, and the Russian Federation. These findings conclude that hypertension affects poorer groups as much as the rich, if not more. Other studies (e.g., Dinsa et al., 2012; Capingana et al., 2013; Hosseinpoor et al., 2012) analyzing data on socioeconomic status (SES) and NCDs suggest that patterns vary for different conditions and for their associated risk factors. The literature on obesity, for example, also shows a complex relationship with income. Increasingly, malnutrition is understood as encompassing over- and undernutrition, as well as nutrient and calorie depletion. These two conditions can coexist in the same household as a "double burden" of malnutrition (Haddad, Cameron, and Barnett, 2014; Shrimpton and Rokx, 2013).

Another reason why securing NCD funding may seem less urgent is that NCDs tend to have a more insidious course, and the benefits of interventions might not be as immediately evident as those for infectious conditions with acute and swift consequences. As noted, epidemiological data on prevalence and measures such as DALYs may reveal the scale and nature of the burden of NCDs. However, since there is not dramatic evidence of death in the public eye, such as can be associated with epidemic-prone infectious diseases, NCDs might seem less apparent to the public. This reflects a known bias that can skew resource allocation away from large, dispersed harms affecting many unknown people ("statistical victims") in favor of more concentrated risk among fewer people ("identified victims"). Ethicists have debated whether it is just to give priority to identified victims, especially where more good can be done helping the widely dispersed (Daniels, 2012). A further reason to account for the fact that NCDs have not received significant attention could relate to the fact that infectious diseases and MCH problems have not been "solved" in LMICs, and indeed high-income countries have not solved the NCD problem. Others have drawn attention to the fact that there has not been the same level of activism for NCDs as there has been for infectious conditions like HIV. Although different disease-specific advocacy organizations came together to form the NCD Alliance, there has not been the same degree of cohesion, and involvement of pharmaceutical interests has been a complicating factor (Stuckler and Basu, 2013; Reubi, Herrick, and Brown, 2016).

Issues of Responsibility in the Framing of NCDs and Prevention Responses

A second ethical issue related to how NCDs might be framed refers to assumptions about the role of personal responsibility in disease etiology. Such assumptions can be significant in terms of what primary and secondary prevention responses are implemented.

Should personal responsibility be included in health considerations? An argument can be made that, given that the four main NCDs have been linked to individual behavioral factors, that people should be held accountable for their behavior. If individual choice is responsible for the burden of NCDs, then one might claim that less societal priority should be provided for such illnesses. However, an argument could be made that, even if some diseases reflect choice, a just society should place greater emphasis on preventing avoidable inequality than on assigning blame (Wikler, 2002). Furthermore, the drivers of NCDs are complex and linked to structural predictors, and not merely to individual behaviors. In fact, the behavior of an individual might be considerably less relevant, as in the example of disease risk of metabolic syndrome linked to early-life nutrition (Barker, 1990). Moreover, the ability of people to do something about their NCD risk or to prevent progression of disease is likewise restrained by their resources and environment, which includes political and sociocultural factors over which they might have limited agency. This suggests that "choice" is not the sole or most salient factor to consider, given that unhealthy environments are perpetuated (particularly for people of lower socioeconomic status), which implies some reciprocal responsibility to address the health problems that ensue.

This point about the relevance of structural predictors for NCD prevalence is illustrated by considering the situation of those living in urban areas in the Global South. The share of the poor living in urban areas is rising, and a third of urban dwellers live in low-income urban settlements (Mitlin and Satterthwaite, 2013). Such contexts often do not enable physical activity. People have limited cooking space and rely on unhealthy, pre-prepared street food. The broader food environment is likely to make healthy lifestyle choices difficult or unaffordable. When considering the "global" dimensions of NCDs and the factors driving disease, it is thus important to go beyond a focus on behavior and also bear in mind these broader structural factors, as well as the "conditions of life" (Whyte, 2012). Moreover, where alternative choices may be available, cultural and socioeconomic factors can militate against adoption of the proposed changes.

The medical approach to prevention of NCDs, particularly conditions included in the WHO's four main types of NCD, has tended to focus on individual-level risk factors for developing disease. This has led to considerable emphasis on individual behavioral change. An approach that frames noncommunicable diseases primarily as "diseases of lifestyle" (e.g., linked to inactivity, poor diet, or smoking) and a matter of individual-level health risk factors has been powerful in shaping debates about appropriate prevention responses. Such an approach has also been influential in the design of "risk communication" and of models of care aimed at encouraging secondary prevention, such as those based upon notions of individual responsibility for self-management of these illnesses. In some cases, these suggestions for self-management include attempts to think creatively about ways of addressing chronic lifelong conditions in the context of low levels of human resources for health (e.g., van Olmen et al., 2011). However, care needs to be taken that models based on patient "responsibility" do not slip into punitive regimes that assume personal negligence and culpability, and that emphasize responsibility above a right to receive equal levels of care (MacGregor et al., 2016).

Adequate health financing mechanisms and efforts toward universal health coverage to address the "health system determinants" of NCDs can also greatly assist those with chronic illness to afford measures to prevent disease progression (Kontis et al., 2017). More effort could be given to assessing innovative social protection programs that link to the health sector (Roelen and Davies, 2014). In some countries, social grants for chronic illness have been discussed as a form of social protection entitlement for those with a diagnosed chronic illness where certain lifestyle changes that are expensive can have a significant impact on disease progression (Schneider et al., 2011).

Not all public health responses have been focused on individual behavior, and there is growing attention on societal influences, with a policy focus on the food, infrastructure, and health system environment. A comprehensive view of responses would be to see responsibility for public health action on NCDs dispersed to several levels, including national governments, health professionals, and individuals, in a "whole-of-government and whole-of-society" response (UN, 2011a). In the United States, for example, the Centers for Disease Control and Prevention (CDC) argues for "winnable battles" for high impact, population-level measures, including measures to address nutrition, obesity, and physical activity levels through environmental strategies to improve the public's health (CDC, 2017). Some LMICs have attempted national-level regulation of the food industry, such as through limitations to salt and fat contents of processed foods, or measures such as the much discussed "sugar tax" on sugar-sweetened beverages to address obesity. Findings have been emerging from such a measure in Mexico which indicate that this area remains one for lively debate (see, for example, Nakhimovsky et al., 2016; Colchero et al., 2016). There is an argument that population-level measures such as soda or fat taxes could place a greater burden on particular groups, such as people who are poor. Food luxuries might become harder for them to afford, thus limiting their choices. On the positive side, it could be argued that the health benefits that would arise outweigh the burdens (Brownell and Frieden, 2009). Debates about who should bear the cost of these measures continue. It could be argued, however, that the public health urgency is great enough, and the population-level gains potentially large enough, to justify such measures, even if poor people bear a higher cost.

The policy domain of strategic regulation of key industries requires more research to evaluate the potential for unintended consequences and ensure greater efficacy. Narayan, Ali, and Koplan (2010, 1196) call for a "respectful partnership" of different actors to spearhead measures to control NCDs, but they also point to widening global inequalities and note that "[c]urrent political and economic incentives favor industry and other interest groups at the expense of health." A similar point has been made by Stuckler, Basu, and McKee (2011) regarding the interests and incentives of big multinationals. They contend that the pharmaceutical industry has a lot to gain from exploiting discourse about a rising burden of NCDs, as well as promoting the extension of drug use in "at risk" categories of people. These challenges all need to be considered in responses to NCDs at national and global levels.

Conclusion

This chapter has highlighted factors related to the global burden of NCD, poverty, and inequality that are relevant to justice. Existing data confirm that NCDs are highly prevalent in LMICs. The link between NCDs and poverty is also clear from emerging data, which, along with arguments that NCDs add a further financial burden on poor households, create even deeper justice concerns. Moreover, NCDs are linked to structural drivers at least as much as to individual behaviors, and the ability of people to take action with respect to their NCD risk is constrained by their resources and environment.

Simple attempts to categorize people based on their deservingness of prevention and treatment can lead to problematic generalizations. Given that debates are happening in the presence of inadequate data and inadequate health systems, it is likely that all current responses will be flawed and imperfect. This points to the need for building up a wider evidence base and capacity to address these challenges.

From the perspective of justice, addressing NCDs will require a deeper engagement with political factors and with the social determinants of health. Broader considerations of social justice require us to see the NCD burden against the backdrop of social and economic inequality, at global, national, and local scales. Given the reality that the resources for allocation are often limited with respect to discussions of funding or provision in LMICs, it is inevitable that assessments of historical and current inequalities and assessments of means and levels of access to safety nets affect how particular groups are identified for the allocation of resources. An ethical account of public health approaches to NCDs would need to balance the competing demands that come from populations that have claims based on redressing historical inequalities—such as unjust access to affordable health—with current pressing health needs. In the context of limited resources, a further approach would be to consider packages of minimally adequate care from the state. Where multiple inequalities exist, there are likely to be trade-offs of equity and justice that have to be weighed. An understanding of the complexity of the ethical issues at stake is key to achieving more just responses for primary and secondary prevention of NCDs.

References

Alleyne, G., Binagwaho, A., Haine, A., Jahan, S., Nugent, R., Rojhani, A., et al. 2013. "Embedding Non-communicable Diseases in the Post-2015 Development Agenda." *Lancet* 381(9866): 566–574.

Anand, S., and Hanson, K. 1998. "DALYs: Efficiency versus Equity." *World Development* 26(2): 307–310.

Anand, S., Peter, F., and Sen, A., eds. 2006. *Public Health, Ethics and Equity* (Oxford: Oxford University Press).

Atun, R., Jaffar, S., Nishtar, S., Knaul, F. M., Barreto, M. L., Nyirenda, M., et al. 2013. "Improving Responsiveness of Health Systems to Non-communicable Diseases." *Lancet* 381(9867): 690–697.

Barker, D. J. 1990. "The Fetal and Infant Origins of Adult Disease." *BMJ* 301(6761): 1111.

Bhojani, U., Devedasan, N., Mishra, A., De Henauw, S., Kolsteren, P., and Criel, B. 2014. "Health System Challenges in Organizing Quality Diabetes Care for Urban Poor in South India." *PLoS One* 9(9): e106522.

Brock, D. W. 2003. "Separate Spheres and Indirect Benefits." *Cost Effectiveness and Resource Allocation* 1: 4. https://www.ncbi.nlm.nih.gov/pmc/articles/PMC156023/.

Brownell, K. D., and Frieden, T. R. 2009. "Ounces of Prevention: The Public Policy Case for Taxes on Sugared Beverages." *New England Journal of Medicine* 360(18): 1805–1808.

Capingana, D. P., Magalhães, P., Silva, A. B., Gonçalves, M. A., Baldo, M. P., Rodrigues, S. L., et al. 2013. "Prevalence of Cardiovascular Risk Factors and Socioeconomic Level among Public-Sector Workers in Angola." *BMC Public Health* 13(1): 1–9.

Carr, A. 2003. Cardiovascular Risk Factors in HIV-Infected Patients. *Journal of Acquired Immune Deficiency Syndrome* 34: S73–S78.

CDC (Centers for Disease Control and Prevention). 2017. "Nutrition, Physical Activity, and Obesity." https://www.cdc.gov/winnablebattles/obesity/index.html.

Chowdhury, A. M. R., Bhuiya, A., Chowdhury, M. E., Rasheed, S., Hussain, Z., and Chen, L. C. 2013. "The Bangladesh Paradox: Exceptional Health Achievement Despite Economic Poverty." *Lancet* 382(9906): 1734–1745.

Colchero, M. A., Popkin, B., Rivera, J., and Ng, S. W. 2016. "Beverage Purchases from Stores in Mexico under the Excise Tax on Sugar Sweetened Beverages: Observational Study." *British Medical Journal* 352: h6704. https://www.bmj.com/content/352/bmj.h6704.

Daniels, N. 2012. "Reasonable Disagreement about Identified vs. Statistical Victims." *Hastings Center Report* 42(1): 35–45.

Dinsa, G. D., Goryakin, Y., Fumagalli, E., and Suhrcke, M. 2012. "Obesity and Socioeconomic Status in Developing Countries: A Systematic Review." *Obesity Reviews* 13(11): 1067–1079.

Goryakin, Y., Lobstein, T., James, W. P. T., and Suhrcke, M. 2015. "The Impact of Economic, Political and Social Globalization on Overweight and Obesity in the 56 Low and Middle Income Countries." *Social Science & Medicine* 133: 67–76.

Haddad, L., Cameron L., and Barnett, I. 2014. "The Double Burden of Malnutrition in SE Asia and the Pacific: Priorities, Policies and Politics." *Health Policy Plan* 30(9): 1193–1206.

Horton, R. 2007. "Chronic Diseases: The Case for Urgent Global Action." *Lancet* 370 (9603): 1881–1882.

Hosseinpoor, A. R., Bergen, N., Mendis, S., Harper, S., Verdes, E., Kunst, A., et al. 2012. "Socioeconomic Inequality in the Prevalence of Noncommunicable Diseases in Low- and Middle-Income Countries: Results from the World Health Survey." *BMC Public Health* 12(1): 474.

Johri, M., and Norheim, O. F. 2012. "Can Cost-Effectiveness Analysis Integrate Concerns for Equity? Systematic Review." *International Journal of Technology Assessment in Health Care* 28(2): 125–132.

Kontis, V., Bennett, J. E., Mathers, C. D., Li, G., Foreman, K., and Ezzati, M. 2017. "Future Life Expectancy in 35 Industrialised Countries: Projections with a Bayesian Model Ensemble." *Lancet* 389(10076): 1323–1335.

Lloyd-Sherlock, P., Beard, J., Minicuci, N., Ebrahim, S., and Chatterji, S. 2014. "Hypertension among Older Adults in Low- and Middle-Income Countries: Prevalence, Awareness and Control." *International Journal of Epidemiology* 43(1): 116–128.

MacGregor, H., McKenzie, A., Jacobs, T., and Ullauri, A. 2016. *Analysis of Factors Affecting the Scale Up and Roll Out of Adherence Clubs in the Cape Town Metro* (Cape Town: Western Cape Department of Health and City of Cape Town).

Mitlin, D., and Satterthwaite, D. 2013. *Urban Poverty in the Global South: Scale and Nature* (Abingdon, UK: Routledge).

Mooney, G., and Wiseman, V. 2000. "Burden of Disease and Priority Setting." *Health Economics* 9: 369–372.

Murray, C. J. L., Ezzati, M., Flaxman, A. D., Lim, S., Lozano, R., Michaud, C., et al. 2013. "GBD 2010: Design, Definitions, and Metrics." *Lancet* 380(9859): 2063–2066.

Murray, C. J. L., and Lopez, A. D. 1996. *The Global Burden of Disease: A Comprehensive Assessment of Mortality and Disability from Diseases, Injuries, and Risk Factors in 1990 and Projected to 2020* (Geneva: World Health Organization).

Nakhimovsky, S. S., Feigl, A. B., Avila, C., O'Sullivan, G., Macgregor-Skinner, E., and Spranca, M. 2016. "Taxes on Sugar-Sweetened Beverages to Reduce Overweight and Obesity in Middle-Income Countries: A Systematic Review." *PLoS One* 11(9): e0163358.

Narayan, K. M., Ali, M. K., and Koplan, J. P. 2010. "Global Noncommunicable Diseases—Where Worlds Meet." *New England Journal of Medicine* 363: 1196–1198.

NIPORT (National Institute of Population Research and Training), Mitra and Associates, and ICF International. 2013. *Bangladesh Demographic and Health Survey 2011* (Dhaka, Bangladesh, and Calverton, Md.: NIPORT/Mitra and Associates/ICF International).

Prince, M., Patel, V., Saxena, S., Maj, M., Maselko, J., Phillips, M.R., et al. 2007. "No Health without Mental Health." *Lancet* 370(9590): 859–877.

Remais, J. V., Zeng, G., Li, G., Tian, L., and Engelgau, M. M. 2012. "Convergence of Non-communicable and Infectious Diseases in Low- and Middle-Income Countries." *International Journal of Epidemiology* 42(1): 221–227.

Reubi, D., Herrick, C., and Brown, T. 2016. "The Politics of Non-communicable Diseases in the Global South." *Health and Place* 39:179–187.

Roelen, K., and Davies, M. 2014. "NCD-Sensitive Social Protection." In *Non-communicable Disease and Development: Future Pathways*, edited by H. MacGregor, S. Lally, G. Bloom, M. Davies, S. Henson, A. Mejía Acosta, et al., IDS Evidence Report 100 (Brighton, UK: IDS).

Salomon, J. A., Carvalho, N., Gutiérrez-Delgado, C. Orozco, R. Mancuso, A. Hogan, D. R., et al. 2012. "Intervention Strategies to Reduce the Burden of Non-communicable Diseases in Mexico: Cost Effectiveness Analysis." *BMJ* 344:e355

Schneider, M., Waliuya, W., Barrett, S., Musanje, J., and Swartz, L. 2011. "'Because I Am Disabled I Should Get a Grant': Including Disability in Social Protection Programmes." Paper presented at the International Conference on Social Protection for Social Justice, 13–15 April 2011 (Brighton, UK: Institute of Development Studies).

Shrimpton, R., and Rokx, C. 2013. *The Double Burden of Malnutrition: A Review of Global Evidence*. Health, Nutrition and Population (HNP) Discussion Paper (Washington D.C.: World Bank).

Stuckler, D., and Basu, S. 2013. "Malignant Neglect: The Failure to Address the Need to Prevent Premature Non-communicable Disease Morbidity and Mortality." *PLoS Medicine* 10(6): e1001466.

Stuckler, D., Basu, S., and McKee, M. 2011. "Commentary: UN High Level Meeting on Non-communicable Diseases: An Opportunity for Whom?" *British Medical Journal* 343: d5336.

UN (United Nations). 2011a. *Political Declaration of the High-Level Meeting of the General Assembly on the Prevention and Control of Non-communicable Diseases* (New York: UN).

UN (United Nations). 2011b. *Prevention and Control of Non-communicable Diseases: Report of the Secretary-General. Sixty-Sixth Session, Follow-up to the Outcome of the Millennium Summit* (Geneva: UN). https://www.un.org/ga/search/view_doc.asp?symbol=A/66/83&Lang=E.

van Olmen, J., Ku, G. M., Bermejo, R., Kegels, G., Hermann, K., and Van Damme, W. 2011. "The Growing Caseload of Chronic Life-Long Conditions Calls for a Move towards Full Self-Management in Low-Income Countries." *Globalization and Health* 7: 38.

WHO (World Health Organization). 2005. *Preventing Chronic Disease: A Vital Investment* (Geneva: World Health Organization).

WHO (World Health Organization). 2012. "World Health Day 2012—Good Health Adds Life to Years." http://www.who.int/mediacentre/news/releases/2012/whd_20120403/en/

WHO (World Health Organization). 2015. "NCD and the Sustainable Development Goals." http://www.who.int/global-coordination-mechanism/ncd-themes/sustainable-development-goals/en/.

WHO (World Health Organization). 2016. “Noncommunicable Diseases.” http://www.who.int/mediacentre/factsheets/fs355/en/.

WHO (World Health Organization). 2017. *Global Action Plan for the Prevention and Control of NCDs 2013–2020* (Geneva: World Health Organization). http://www.who.int/nmh/publications/ncd-action-plan/en/.

Whyte, S. R. 2012. “Chronicity and Control: Framing ‘Non-communicable Diseases’ in Africa.” *Anthropology and Medicine* 19(1): 63–74. http://cms.ku.dk/samf-sites/antro-sites/antropologi-inst/english/staff/pubdet/?id=357a52d9-c2da-42b8-a17c-d4ac7fb2bfd8.

Wikler, D. 2002. “Personal and Social Responsibility for Health.” *Ethics and International Affairs* 16(2): 47–55.

Yach, D., Stuckler, D., and Brownell, K. D. 2006. “Epidemiologic and Economic Consequences of the Global Epidemics of Obesity and Diabetes.” *Nature* 12: 62–66.

CHAPTER 46

TREATING CANCER AS A PUBLIC HEALTH ETHICS ISSUE

YONAIRA M. RIVERA AND OTIS W. BRAWLEY

INTRODUCTION

CANCER is a group of diseases that together constitute the second-leading cause of death in the United States (Siegel, Miller, and Jemal, 2017). Approximately 600,000 Americans die from the disease annually. The lifetime risk of cancer death is 19 percent for American women and 23 percent for American men, and it is estimated that 38 percent of all American women and 42 percent of all American men will be diagnosed with cancer in their lifetime (Siegel, Miller, and Jemal, 2016).

In the United States, the most commonly diagnosed cancers are of the breast, prostate, lung, and colon and rectum, which together account for more than half of all cancers diagnosed annually and nearly half of all cancer deaths. While most cancer incidence and mortality rates are in decline, the incidence of melanoma, liver, and thyroid cancers is increasing, as are mortality rates for liver cancer (Siegel, Miller, and Jemal, 2017).

There was a 26 percent reduction in overall age-adjusted cancer death rates in the United States from 1991 to 2014. Most of the decline was due to tobacco control, followed by improvements in treatment and screening. However, even with such a decline in mortality, cancer is expected to surpass heart disease and become the leading cause of death among Americans by 2030. It has already surpassed cardiovascular disease in the populations of twenty-one states (Siegel, Miller, and Jemal, 2016) and in certain racial and ethnic minority groups (CDC, 2017a, 2017b). It is estimated that at least 45.1 percent of all cancer deaths in 2014 were attributed to known risk factors. The most common causes of cancer death were tobacco use (29.6 percent) and the combination of obesity, high caloric intake, alcohol, and lack of exercise (15.8 percent) (Islami et al., 2018).

Making continued progress on cancer requires broad changes to public health and medicine. While there are many ethical challenges related to alleviating the public health burden of cancer, this chapter considers three. First, there are a number of ethical issues raised by questions of social justice, health disparities, and the overall cancer burden in the United States. They include disparities in cancer prevention and outcomes due to social and structural inequalities, an underinvestment in public health infrastructure, high variability in both screening and treatment patterns, and poor subject/patient engagement in decision-making related to health. Second, a number of ethics issues emerge in cancer screening, a core prevention strategy for cancer. Pervasive public health ethics questions include how much data needs to be in place to support efficacy of screening programs before they should be implemented, and what the obligation is to provide access to care when screening detects a problem. Finally, cancer highlights the tension between protecting clinician judgment and respecting and enhancing patient autonomy. The focus of this chapter is the United States, but many of the issues raised are relevant to other high-income countries.

Disparities, Social Justice, and Cancer in the United States

There are significant racial, ethnic, socioeconomic, and geographic disparities in cancer incidence and mortality in the United States. African American adults, for example, have higher overall cancer incidence and mortality rates compared to other racial/ethnic groups (NCI, 2008). Although Latinos, Asian Americans, Pacific Islanders, and Native Americans have lower overall incidence and mortality rates, certain subgroups have extremely high rates of certain cancers. For example, Latinos in the United States have a higher incidence of liver, cervical, and stomach cancers. Among Asians there is higher incidence and mortality from liver cancer; Southeast Asians, in particular, have a disproportionately high cervical cancer incidence and mortality rate (Siegel, Miller, and Jemal, 2017). Cancer mortality is also higher among Americans with less education, compared to those with a college education. There also are state-by-state differences in cancer mortality related to socioeconomic status (Ma et al., 2018).

The cornerstone of public health interventions to prevent cancer among diverse communities involves community or public education to promote healthy behaviors. Even then, there is an ethical challenge to assure all populations are respected and targeted with truthful, fact-based messaging that respects language, culture, and medical experience. These challenges are particularly relevant in persuasive messages used by public health campaigns to educate at-risk populations about cancer prevention, some of which appeal to fear or disgust (Guttman and Salmon, 2004). For example, some anti-tobacco campaigns rely on scary images to present smoking in a negative, unappealing light.

Similarly, human papillomavirus (HPV) vaccine campaigns may utilize guilt to persuade parents to vaccinate their children as a way to prevent HPV-related cancers. In such scenarios, it is important to consider how such strong appeals may be perceived by the intended audience, as they may create unnecessary fears or concerns, particularly if statements are based on tentative data (Guttman and Salmon, 2004). While there may be a limited role for such provocative messaging, more positive messaging should be adopted when feasible and likely to be effective.

Other disparities reflect inequalities in insurance status and education level (Ward et al., 2004), which in turn affect access to preventive and therapeutic care. Educational attainment, for example, has been strongly and inversely associated with all-cancer mortality (Albano et al., 2007), and not having insurance is correlated with poorer survival in every stage of colon and breast cancer, regardless of racial or ethnic background (Ward et al., 2008). Uninsured patients with stage 1 colon cancer have inferior five-year survival rates compared to insured patients with more advanced stage 2 disease (Ward et al., 2008). The implementation of the Patient Protection and Affordable Care Act (also known as Obamacare, or the ACA) has provided increased access to care and is reducing disparities in some populations. However, some states have chosen not to expand their Medicaid programs in line with the ACA (Robbins et al., 2015), creating greater state-by-state disparities in cancer and other diseases.

Debates about resource allocation for cancer often concern tradeoffs between efficiency (a utilitarian criterion) and equity (an egalitarian criterion). In public health, the utilitarian approach is achieved by reducing the greatest amount of burden of disease, often described as preventing the most disability-adjusted life years (DALYs) within a social budget. This approach is more concerned with aggregate well-being than distributive outcomes. By contrast, the egalitarian approach is concerned with how resource allocation decisions affect those most disadvantaged, and how resource allocation can narrow equity gaps (Faden and Powers, 2008; Buchanan, 2008).

In particular, commitments to equity motivate policies to alleviate disparities. Many disparities in cancer incidence and mortality can be attributed to inequities in the distribution of resources for screening and treatment, especially across socioeconomic groups. Specific justice questions concern the distribution of government funds for cancer prevention programs and educational efforts, as well as how decisions are made to tailor programs to populations with a high burden of cancer. For example, a poor community that lives adjacent to a waste-producing plant experiences compounded inequities both in its heightened exposure to carcinogens and in its typically worse access to preventive and therapeutic care.

Equity in Community Interventions

Issues of equity also arise in the context of community interventions focused on prevention. As noted, preventive interventions depend on changing behaviors that contribute to nearly half of cancer deaths (between about 5 and 10 percent of all cancers are hereditary) (Siegel, Miller, and Jemal, 2017). However, the ability to meaningfully alter these behaviors may also reflect inequality in resources across racial and socioeconomic groups. For example, the lack of available recreation spaces or crime fears in the inner city prevent physical activity, which is important in preventing disease.

Resource inequalities also affect the sustainability and reach of interventions aimed at empowering and educating individuals. Social justice issues are raised when programs for vulnerable populations are introduced without consideration of their sustainability. Cancer prevention, for example, is often realized by utilizing community health educators (CHEs) to reach populations and deliver cancer prevention information. Despite the success of CHEs in empowering communities to partake in cancer prevention and screening efforts, many of these programs are funded through time-bound mechanisms (Spencer, Gunter, and Palmisano, 2010), making funding the most influential barrier to program longevity (Koskan et al., 2013). This also limits programs that rigorously train future CHEs.

Another justice concern is disseminating health information to communities with limited access to the services or resources advocated. For example, genetic screening for cancer is recommended in certain situations (NCI, 2013); and yet access to genetic testing has been severely limited in nonwhite populations and among those with less income or education (Underhill et al., 2017). Furthermore, educating a community about a service that is not actually available to that community can evoke distress. Nonetheless, increasing knowledge and awareness of these services may play a role in community mobilization and subsequent efforts to make these services accessible and affordable.

Equity and Cancer Treatment

Finally, cancer treatment is also affected by justice and resource allocation questions. Despite the fact that multiple treatment options will often exist for a given type of cancer, there is rarely broader societal dialogue—outside of conversations between patients, their families, and clinicians—about how to effectively meet treatment needs within resource constraints. A cost-benefit or cost-effectiveness approach, favored by utilitarians, would emphasize improving average patient outcomes within the available societal budget. This perspective has some legitimacy, given the dearth of available resources and the rising costs of cancer treatment. Because this approach maximizes *average* population outcomes, it gives no emphasis to the distribution of these outcomes or the moral relevance of privileging care to more disadvantaged groups in the name of justice, even when more costly than providing care to a more privileged subpopulation (Sulmasy, 2007). Even if a utilitarian approach were desirable, there is no consistency in which cancer therapies are available across insurance plans or health care systems. This can impede individuals with less comprehensive health insurance from receiving access to all reasonable cancer therapies (Sulmasy, 2007).

In addition, while the leading government and private cancer organizations have come together to recommend a roadmap for cancer research relevant to health disparities (Polite et al., 2017), and while there are some financing policies relevant to cancer at the local, state, and national government levels, there is no comprehensive framework that strives for equity in cancer treatment. This can be compounded by a market-based health care system that attempts to control costs through cost-sharing and other mechanisms that result in more disadvantaged patients being unable to afford these treatments (Sulmasy, 2007). Cancer care is expensive; in fact, cancer care costs are the leading cause of bankruptcy in the United States (Ramsey et al., 2016). Even among the insured, high copayments prevent substantial numbers of Americans from getting needed cancer treatment or counseling regarding diet or smoking (Altice et al., 2016). High costs cause substantial numbers of people to forego preventive therapies and needed treatment, and in turn can further increase health disparities (Sulmasy, 2007).

Ethics and Cancer Screening

A subset of cancer prevention efforts aims specifically to promote cancer screening. In cancer screening, asymptomatic individuals are tested to identify those who might have either early disease or early markers indicative of a risk of developing a particular cancer. Examples of markers include colon polyps or cervical dysplasia. The intent is to intervene to prevent cancer or cure the disease.

Before implementing a screening program, the population-level benefits and risks of screening must be considered. In 1968, Wilson and Jungner published what have become the accepted criteria for appropriate screening. Among these ten guidelines are that the condition screened for should be an important health problem, facilities for diagnosis and treatment should be available, there should be a suitable test or exam for the disease, the test should be acceptable to the target population, and the cost of finding a case should be economically balanced in relation to global possible expenditure (Wilson and Jungner, 1968). The guidelines, however, are not always followed. Further, widespread screening for certain tumors has been introduced without prior evaluation of benefit and harm. This occurred, for example, in lung cancer screening with chest X-ray in the 1960s, neuroblastoma screening in children with a test for urine catecholamines in the 1980s, and prostate cancer screening with prostate-specific antigen in the 1990s (Welch and Albertsen, 2009). Cancer screening can carry significant risks. Among them are false positive findings, followed by invasive, and often expensive, follow-up tests and the physical and psychological harm that can result. The use of screening when not justified can also divert scarce resources from more valuable public health programs—an important justice concern.

Today, cancer screening is available for cancers of the breast, cervix, prostate, lung, colon, and rectum. A number of US organizations issue screening guidelines, including the American Cancer Society (ACS, 2017); the National Comprehensive Cancer Network (NCCN, 2017); the US Preventive Services Task Force (USPSTF), which issues federal government recommendations (USPSTF, 2018a); and some disease-specific professional organizations. Guidelines are needed because of the limitations of the tests and treatments. For lung, prostate, and breast cancer in certain ages, many guidelines suggest "shared decision-making," where patients and physicians jointly consider the benefits and risks of a test before deciding to undertake it (Sandman and Munthe, 2009).

Despite the importance and promise of cancer screening, both the lay public and many medical professionals do not understand its limitations (Woloshin et al., 2012). Misplaced optimism about the value of screening tools is common among clinicians. Many clinicians do not understand the operating characteristics of a screening test, such as sensitivity, specificity, and positive predictive value, or the number of individuals needed to screen and/or treat to save one life. Some clinicians argue for or advise a screening test when experts deem the test inappropriate. In such a scenario, oversight from health systems and public health agencies may be needed to deliver accurate information and guidance about when to screen, even if doing so reduces physician discretion.

Screening programs can also raise questions of equity. Among medically underserved communities, there may be a lack of resources and infrastructure to get appropriate diagnostic testing if a cancer screening test comes back positive (Underhill et al., 2017). Disadvantaged communities are often slower to gain access to beneficial new medical technologies (Goldman and Lakdawalla, 2005). For example, there were no black-white mortality disparities in breast and colon cancers until the early 1980s, when beneficial screening and treatment became available. Once screening and treatment were introduced, white mortality rates began declining faster than black mortality rates (DeLancey et al., 2008).

Screening also raises questions regarding the amount of supporting evidence that should exist before a test is widely publicized and implemented. Many organizations recommended a monthly breast self-exam for women until several clinical trials showed it to be ineffective. Yet some local and national cancer programs and initiatives continue to promote it as a way to empower individuals to be cognizant of changes in their body. This tension still permeates educational campaigns and programs that want to continue to send a message that taking control and doing something about cancer prevention is important; however, this comes amid mounting evidence that monthly breast self-exams have not been proven to improve cancer survival rates, translating into false positives, false negatives, and unnecessary costs and procedures (Brody, 2012). Similar issues have been raised regarding prostate cancer screening with prostate-specific antigen (PSA) testing (Van der Kwast and Roobol, 2017). Widely recommended for almost two decades, increasing questions have been raised about a number of factors—including overdiagnosis leading to unnecessary treatment. While still recommended at many leading medical centers, the American Cancer Society and the USPSTF now recommend more limited application, guided by informed decision-making (ACS, 2017; USPSTF, 2018b).

The growing availability of genetic testing also raises questions in the context of cancer screening and ethics. One important concern, relevant to all screening programs, is the degree to which inadequate or incorrect information may lead to potentially inappropriate treatment decisions. A recent study, for example, highlighted that half of surveyed women with newly diagnosed breast cancer undergoing bilateral mastectomy after genetic testing did not have mutations linked to an increase in risk of a hereditary cancer. Instead, they had variants of uncertain significance (VUS), which are often harmless (Kurian et al., 2017). This example brings forth issues related to unnecessary costs and inconvenience of treatment, and highlights the problem of relying on providers who do not have appropriate training to interpret genetic test results in light of limited clinical guidelines.

Autonomy and Medical Paternalism

Within the broader debate about cancer care lies a question about how much care can be standardized using guidelines that would apply to clinically similar patients. Yet patient preferences are important and should be respected. An ongoing ethical tension in cancer care concerns how to balance respect for autonomy with paternalism, whether from a physician or a public health authority. This tension can be seen in how individuals are approached along several decision points in the care continuum, such as the promotion of prevention and screening programs, or decisions about treatment. Autonomy, which appeals to the importance of choice and individual freedom, highlights an individual's capacity to make his or her own decisions about care (Beauchamp, 2003). Respect for autonomy is an important core principle in medicine. However, respecting patient autonomy can create tension with professional opinion and knowledge. Medical paternalism will sometimes aim to increase the clinical benefit to a patient at the risk of limiting patient autonomy (Beauchamp, 2003). The field has shifted toward providing greater patient autonomy since the advent of bioethics and patients' rights movements in the 1970s (Angelos and Bennett, 2001), but some patients want to defer decision-making to their doctors (Rosenbaum, 2015).

While strongly paternalistic approaches that relinquish a competent patient's decision-making powers altogether are viewed negatively in bioethics, other attenuated forms of paternalism may be more acceptable and, indeed, appropriate. Some have praised informed and shared decision-making as a way to improve patient autonomy and empower individuals to take control over their health (Sandman and Munthe, 2009). This view has been challenged by those who worry that patients may not have the ability to think through all the options and make the best decision for themselves (Merz and Fischhoff, 1990). This paternalistic approach argues that patients may not be in the right frame of mind to make a treatment decision, given the contradictory empirical evidence at hand, and instead might make decisions based on emotions and heuristics.

Relatedly, Rebecca Kukla has suggested something called "conscientious autonomy" as a potential bridge between self-driven and expert-driven decision-making: "We need to remember that trust and deference to experts and authorities is not irrational.... Indeed, good, responsible epistemic practices in the mundane world require that we intelligently delegate authority and defer to experts" (Kukla, 2005, 40).

Given their technical training, it is common for health care providers to know more about a disease and its treatment than lay patients, and at times this translates to a paternalistic approach to care delivery, whereby the provider determines what treatment the patient receives. It is important that providers convey balanced information regarding the risks and benefits of available treatment options. Furthermore, patients must be given the option of accepting or refusing therapy; a health care provider who does not respect a patient's right to refuse therapy is violating patient autonomy.

More recently, the concept of *libertarian paternalism* has achieved increased attention. Libertarian paternalism attempts to balance respect for patient autonomy with paternalistic "nudges" to help patients make what are paternalistically thought to be better decisions (Aggarwal, Davies, and Sullivan, 2014). Here, a provider may assist a patient in making a decision by presenting a reasonable menu of options, but offering as the default option the one the health care provider believes is likely provide the greatest clinical benefit. Although nudging seemingly serves as a compromise between putting forward experts' views about best options and ultimately patient decision-making, it can be prone to abuse. The physician who too strongly wants a patient to consent to an intervention may not provide a balanced view of the benefits and risks. Although the physician may be motivated by what she or he believes is the patient's best interest (Groll, 2014), there are times when financial conflicts or concerns may steer how options are presented. This minimization of autonomy inhibits the patient's ability to engage in his or her cancer care. In such cases, when there is a true disagreement, it is best that a third party—such as a hospital ethics committee—become involved.

When there is uncertainty about the best approach to prevent or treat cancer, prudent public health professionals, as well as medical providers, must do their best to identify what evidence is available, while acknowledging that the balance of risks and benefits is not entirely understood. An example of this arises in lung cancer screening, where screening guidelines from multiple organizations recommend informed and/or shared decision-making between patients and providers (CMS, 2015). Similarly, in patients with a family history of colorectal, ovarian, or other hereditary cancers, recommendations point to discussing risks and benefits with clinicians.

While patient autonomy may be of crucial importance in contexts of genuine uncertainty in the delivery of cancer care, there may be a lesser role for autonomy when patients want treatments for which there is no evidence, or when evidence points against it (e.g., whole body screening). In these scenarios, a more paternalistic approach may be justifiable, particularly when leading public health agencies have taken a clear stand on the issue. Regardless, there is a need to erect policy frameworks that emphasize to patients and practitioners alike that uncertainty should be acknowledged when it exists in a practice based on evidence.

Moving Forward

Questions of social justice, ethics, and cancer screening, and the right balance between paternalism and autonomy, continue to emerge in relation to public health policy in cancer prevention, screening, and treatment. Policymakers, health care institutions, and others responsible for and influencing delivery of quality, affordable cancer care must identify ways to reduce social inequalities while also striving to improve the evidence base for prevention and treatment decisions for both individuals and populations. This mandate is only heightened by the rapidly changing nature of cancer research and practice, as seen in the case of genetic testing and other emerging modalities.

Most cancer is preventable through personal behavior change, and yet these behaviors are undergirded by structural norms and barriers that significantly increase the risk of cancer in disadvantaged populations. Indeed, factors such as poverty, poor access to screening, greater likelihood to initiate smoking, lack of transportation, racism, socioeconomic discrimination, and other factors highlight the social dimension of cancer incidence and public health response (Link and Phelan, 1995). An ongoing question for public health remains how best to use limited resources to protect and increase access to preventive and therapeutic care for underserved communities, including in the context of reducing morbidity and mortality from cancer. Utilitarian approaches provide some general guideposts for how to allocate resources in cost-effective ways. Yet concerns about equity indicate that cost-effectiveness must be considered alongside other factors. Certain cancer prevention, screening, and treatment strategies will not diffuse to all communities unless there is an explicit commitment to ensuring equitable access, highlighting the importance of targeted attention to reduce cancer health disparities in the name of promoting both good outcomes and social justice.

References

ACS (American Cancer Society). 2017. "American Cancer Society Guidelines for the Early Detection of Cancer." https://www.cancer.org/healthy/find-cancer-early/cancer-screening-guidelines/american-cancer-society-guidelines-for-the-early-detection-of-cancer.html.

Aggarwal, A., Davies, J., and Sullivan R. 2014. "'Nudge' in the Clinical Consultation—An Acceptable Form of Medical Paternalism?" *BMC Medical Ethics* 15(1): 31. https://bmcmedethics.biomedcentral.com/articles/10.1186/1472-6939-15-31.

Albano, J. D., Ward, E., Jemal, A., Anderson, R., Cokkinides, V. E., Murray, T., et al. 2007. "Cancer Mortality in the United States by Education Level and Race." *Journal of the National Cancer Institute* 99(18): 1384–1394.

Altice, C. K., Banegas, M. P., Tucker-Seeley, R. D., and Yabroff, K. R. 2016. "Financial Hardships Experienced by Cancer Survivors: A Systematic Review." *JNCI: Journal of the National Cancer Institute* 109(2). https://academic.oup.com/jnci/article/109/2/djw205/2905657.

Angelos, P., and Bennett, C. L. 2001. "Communication: From Paternalism to Shared Decision Making." *Oncology News International* 10(2). http://www.cancernetwork.com/articles/communication-paternalism-shared-decision-making.

Beauchamp, T. L. 2003. "Methods and Principles in Biomedical Ethics." *Journal of Medical Ethics* 29(5): 269–274.

Brody, H. 2012. "From an Ethics of Rationing to an Ethics of Waste Avoidance." *New England Journal of Medicine* 366(21): 1949–1951.

Buchanan, D. R. 2008. "Autonomy, Paternalism, and Justice: Ethical Priorities in Public Health." *American Journal of Public Health* 98(1): (2008): 15–21.

CDC (Centers for Disease Control and Prevention). 2017a. "Health of Asian or Pacific Islander Population" (Atlanta: National Center for Health Statistics). https://www.cdc.gov/nchs/fastats/asian-health.htm.

CDC (Centers for Disease Control and Prevention). 2017b. "Health of Hispanic or Latino Population" (Atlanta: National Center for Health Statistics). https://www.cdc.gov/nchs/fastats/hispanic-health.htm.

CMS (Centers for Medicare and Medicaid Services). 2015. "Decision Memo for Screening for Lung Cancer with Low Dose Computed Tomography (LDCT) (CAG-00439N)." https://www.cms.gov/medicare-coverage-database/details/nca-decision-memo.aspx?NCAId=274.

DeLancey, J. O. L., Thun, M. J., Jemal, A., and Ward, E. M. 2008. "Recent Trends in Black-White Disparities in Cancer Mortality." *Cancer Epidemiology and Prevention Biomarkers* 17(11): 2908–2912.

Faden, R. R., and Powers, M. 2008. "Health Inequities and Social Justice." *Bundesgesundheitsblatt-Gesundheitsforschung-Gesundheitsschutz* 51(2): 51–157.

Goldman, D. P., and Lakdawalla, D. N. 2005. "A Theory of Health Disparities and Medical Technology." *Contributions in Economic Analysis and Policy* 4(1).

Groll, D. 2014. "Medical Paternalism—Part 1." *Philosophy Compass* 9(3): 186–193.

Guttman, N., and Salmon, C. T. 2004. "Guilt, Fear, Stigma and Knowledge Gaps: Ethical Issues in Public Health Communication Interventions." *Bioethics* 18(6): 531–552.

Islami, F., Goding Sauer, A., Miller, K. D., Siegel, R. L., Fedewa, S.A., Jacobs, E.J., et al. 2018. "Proportion and Number of Cancer Cases and Deaths Attributable to Potentially Modifiable Risk Factors in the United States." *CA: A Cancer Journal for Clinicians* 68(1): 31–54. doi:10.3322/caac.21440/full.

Koskan, A., Friedman, D. B., Messias, D. K. H., Brandt, H. M., and Walsemann, K. 2013. "Sustainability of Promotora Initiatives: Program Planners' Perspectives." *Journal of Public Health Management and Practice* 19(5): E1.

Kukla, R. 2005. "Conscientious Autonomy: Displacing Decisions in Health Care." *Hastings Center Report* 35(2): 34–44.

Kurian, A. W., Li, Y., Hamilton, A. S., Ward, K. C., Hawley, S. T., Morrow, M., et al. 2017. "Gaps in Incorporating Germline Genetic Testing into Treatment Decision-Making for Early-Stage Breast Cancer." *Journal of Clinical Oncology* 35(20): 2232–2239.

Link, B. G., and Phelan, J. 1995. "Social Conditions as Fundamental Causes of Disease." In "Extra Issue: Forty Years of Medical Sociology: The State of the Art and Directions for the Future." *Journal of Health and Social Behavior* 35: 80–94.

Ma, J., Siegel, R. L., Ward, E. M., and Jemal, A. 2018. "State-Level Educational Disparities in Mortality in the United States, 2010–2014." *Preventive Medicine* 106: 53–59. https://www.sciencedirect.com/science/article/pii/S0091743517303547.

Merz, J. F., and Fischhoff, B. 1990. "Informed Consent Does Not Mean Rational Consent: Cognitive Limitations on Decision-Making." *Journal of Legal Medicine* 11(3): 321–350.

NCCN (National Comprehensive Cancer Network). 2017. "Guidelines for Detection, Prevention and Risk Reduction." https://www.nccn.org/professionals/physician_gls/default.aspx#detection.

NCI (National Cancer Institute). 2008. "Cancer Health Disparities." https://www.cancer.gov/about-nci/organization/crchd/cancer-health-disparities-fact-sheet#q4.

NCI (National Cancer Institute). 2013. "Genetic Testing for Hereditary Cancer Syndromes." https://www.cancer.gov/about-cancer/causes-prevention/genetics/genetic-testing-fact-sheet#q4.

Polite, B. N., Adams-Campbell, L. L., Brawley, O. W., Bickell, N., Carethers, J. M., Flowers, C. R., et al. 2017. "Charting the Future of Cancer Health Disparities Research: A Position Statement from the American Association for Cancer Research, the American Cancer Society, the American Society of Clinical Oncology, and the National Cancer Institute." *CA: A Cancer Journal for Clinicians* 67(5): 353–361.

Ramsey, S. D., Bansal, A., Fedorenko, C. R., Blough, D.K., Overstreet, K. A., et al. 2016. "Financial Insolvency as a Risk Factor for Early Mortality Among Patients With Cancer." *Journal of Clinical Oncology* 34(9): 980–986.

Robbins, A. S., Han, X., Ward, E. M., Simard, E. P., Zheng, Z., and Jemal, A., 2015. "Association between the Affordable Care Act Dependent Coverage Expansion and Cervical Cancer Stage and Treatment in Young Women." *JAMA* 314(20): 2189–2191.

Rosenbaum, L. 2015. "The Paternalism Preference—Choosing Unshared Decision Making." *New England Journal of Medicine* 373(7): 589–592.

Sandman, L., and Munthe, C. 2009. "Shared Decision-Making and Patient Autonomy." *Theoretical Medicine and Bioethics* 30(4): 289–310.

Siegel, R. L., Miller, K. D., and Jemal, A. 2016. "Cancer Statistics, 2016." *CA: A Cancer Journal for Clinicians* 66(1): 7–30.

Siegel, R. L., Miller, K. D., and Jemal, A. 2017. "Cancer Statistics, 2017." *CA: A Cancer Journal for Clinicians* 67(1): 7–30.

Spencer, M. S., Gunter, K. E., and Palmisano, G. 2010. "Community Health Workers and Their Value to Social work." *Social Work* 55(2): 169–180.

Sulmasy, D. P. 2007. "Cancer Care, Money, and the Value of Life: Whose Justice? Which Rationality?" *Journal of Clinical Oncology* 25(2): 217–222.

Underhill, M. L., Blonquist, T. M., Habin, K., Lundquist, D., Shannon, K., Robinson, K., et al. 2017. "A State-Wide Initiative to Promote Genetic Testing in an Underserved Population." *Cancer Medicine* 6(7): 1837–1844.

USPSTF (US Preventive Services Task Force). 2018a. ""Search Recommendations: Cancer Screening." https://www.uspreventiveservicestaskforce.org/BrowseRec/Search?s=cancer+screening.

USPSTF (US Preventive Services Task Force). 2018b. Final Recommendation Statement: Prostate Cancer: Screening. https://www.uspreventiveservicestaskforce.org/Page/Document/UpdateSummaryFinal/prostate-cancer-screening1?ds=1&s=prostate.

Van der Kwast, T. H., and Roobol, M. J. 2017. "Prostate Cancer: Draft USPSTF 2017 Recommendation on PSA Testing: A Sea-Change?" *Nature Reviews Urology* 14(8): 457.

Ward, E., Halpern, M., Schrag, N., Cokkinides, V., DeSantis, C., Bandi, P., et al. 2008. "Association of Insurance with Cancer Care Utilization and Outcomes." *CA: A Cancer Journal for Clinicians* 58(1): 9–31.

Ward, E., Jemal, A., Cokkinides, V., Singh, G. K., Cardinez, C., Ghafoor, A., et al. 2004. "Cancer Disparities by Race/Ethnicity and Socioeconomic Status." *CA: A Cancer Journal for Clinicians* 54(2): 78–93.

Welch, H. G., and Albertsen, P. C. 2009. "Prostate Cancer Diagnosis and Treatment after the Introduction of Prostate-Specific Antigen Screening: 1986–2005." *Journal of the National Cancer Institute* 101(19): 1325–1329.

Wilson, J. M. G., and Jungner, G. 1968. *Principles and Practice of Screening for Disease* (Geneva: World Health Organization). http://apps.who.int/iris/handle/10665/37650.

Woloshin, S., Schwartz, L. M., Black, W. C., and Kramer, B. S. 2012. "Cancer Screening Campaigns—Getting Past Uninformative Persuasion." *New England Journal of Medicine* 367(18): 1677–1679.

SECTION TEN

FOOD, WATER, AND NUTRITION

CHAPTER 47

AN OVERVIEW OF ETHICAL ISSUES IN FOOD, WATER, AND NUTRITION IN PUBLIC HEALTH

CLAIRE DAVIS AND JESSICA FANZO

Introduction

Food and water are essential to public health, as well as to the development and sustainability of nations and the planet. Yet climate change, an expanding global population, and an increasingly globalized, geopolitical world present ethical challenges to ensuring the availability of these resources. Today, more than ever before, there is a need to take stock of the critical assets that allow human societies to thrive.

Food and Nutrition

As major contributors to the health status of populations, food and nutrition play an important role in addressing the global burden of malnutrition. Through food and diets, nutrition ensures that nutrient needs are met to sustain a healthy life. The ramifications of malnutrition have a direct impact on human health and well-being. From a child suffering cognitive impairment as a result of stunting to the many countries grappling with obesity epidemics and rising rates of noncommunicable disease, food is a key component in establishing positive health outcomes.

Malnutrition

Malnutrition affects every country, whether developing or developed, and it presents a considerable challenge for governments around the world. Different types of malnutrition can coexist in the same country, community, or household, and even at the individual level. Globally, one person in three today is malnourished (Development Initiatives, 2017). The UN aims to end hunger and all forms of malnutrition by 2030, but if current trends continue, one person in two could be malnourished by then (GloPan, 2016).

Food security has been defined as a state in which "all people at all times have physical, social and economic access to sufficient, safe and nutritious food to meet their dietary needs and food preferences for an active and healthy life" (FAO, 2009, 1). The causes of malnutrition are complex, though access to food that meets the Food and Agriculture Organization of the United Nations' (FAO's) definition is a core issue. Other causes include immediate if chronic problems, such as disease burden, as well as more systemic factors, such as political or social issues that prevent or hinder equal distribution of food resources (HLPE, 2017).

Undernutrition

Globally, 815 million people are undernourished, despite progress made during recent decades (FAO et al., 2017). The number of people who are undernourished globally will likely increase because of the 2017 famine crisis, in which Nigeria, Somalia, South Sudan, and Yemen are at risk of or are facing famines. Undernutrition is most prevalent among impoverished groups that lack food security. The most vulnerable are unborn children, infants and children under five, women of reproductive age, and older persons. The consequences of undernourishment are lifelong and intergenerational, potentially leading to negative impacts on child growth and development, quality of life, resistance to infection, and survival (HLPE, 2017).

Chronic food insecurity at the household, community, or larger societal level is often at the core of undernutrition. Food insecurity may occur as a result of socioeconomic pressure, urban or rural residence, or disruption due to civil instability and conflict. "Hidden" forms of undernutrition that result from insufficient levels of energy, protein, and micronutrients are less apparent than instances of severe "wasting" undernourishment, though "hidden" undernourishment is more common.

Undernutrition is the main form of malnutrition among children under five, though this is decreasing (Black et al., 2013; WHO, 2017b). Still, it is the underlying cause of approximately 45 percent of deaths among this age group, mainly in low- and middle-income countries (LMICs) (WHO, 2017a). The burden of stunting, or chronic undernutrition, in children under the age of five is significant. In 2017, nearly 151 million children under the age of five (22.2 percent) worldwide were stunted. Globally, 50 million children under the age of five (7.5 percent) suffered from wasting or were moderately acutely malnourished, and 16 million suffered from severe wasting. Nearly all of these children resided in Africa and Asia (Development Initiatives, 2018; UNICEF, WHO, and World Bank, 2017).

Overweight and Obesity

Overweight and obesity affect almost every country in the world and are rapidly rising in all age groups. Globally, obesity has nearly tripled since 1975 (WHO, 2017b). The greatest burdens are experienced by high-income countries and countries experiencing a nutrition transition, a process in which diets shift from traditional staple foods to processed foods (Popkin, Adair, and Ng, 2012). This dietary change, coupled with increasingly sedentary lifestyles, has fueled a global increase in the risk of noncommunicable diseases, which represent the leading causes of adult morbidity and mortality (Gakidou et al., 2017).

Overweight and obesity represent the main burden of malnutrition for adults. The WHO (2017b) estimates that overweight and obesity are now responsible for more deaths than undernutrition. It is estimated that 2 billion adults suffer from overweight and obesity (38.9%), while 462 million adults are underweight (Development Initiatives, 2018; WHO, 2017a; WHO, 2017b; Ng et al., 2014).

Children are also increasingly at risk of being overweight or obese. Over 38 million children under the age of five (5.6 percent) were overweight or obese in 2017, compared to 30 million in 2000. Overweight and obesity now affect young children in developing countries, with 20 million overweight children in Asia and 10 million in Africa (Development Initiatives, 2018; UNICEF, WHO, and World Bank, 2017).

WATER

As is the case with food, water is integral to human health and well-being. The essential nature of water is interwoven with that of food: water is needed for drinking, cooking, and personal hygiene, as well as for agricultural production. As such, it is also central to addressing the global burden of malnutrition.

In contrast to food, however, there is no clear definition or internationally agreed upon framework for water security. In some contexts, water insecurity is understood in relation to the "institutional and governance aspect of access to water" (Lopez-Gunn, De Stefano, and Llamas, 2012, 90). Elsewhere, it is defined by a lack of physical infrastructure and storage (Lopez-Gunn, De Stefano, and Llamas, 2012).

Although the global community has yet to agree on a universal definition of water security, millions of people around the world experience the daily realities of going without clean water. Approximately 844 million people worldwide—or one in ten—do not have clean water (WHO and UNICEF, 2017). At the current rate of progress, clean drinking water for all those living in LMICs will not be achieved until 2039 (WHO and UNICEF, 2017).

Burdens on Health and Nutrition

The lack of clean water threatens health and nutrition through both direct and indirect pathways. Each year, approximately 3.4 million people die from water-related disease as a result of unsafe drinking water and poor sanitation (WHO, 2001). As with diet-related mortality, the greatest burden of ill-health is in developing countries, where 97 percent of annual water-related mortality occurs because of inadequate public health infrastructure (CDC, 2016).

Many of these disease burdens, such as stunting, intestinal helminths, and diarrhea, lead to negative effects on nutritional status. Water, sanitation, and hygiene (WASH) play a fundamental role in improving nutritional outcomes. Indeed, 50 percent of malnutrition is associated with repeated diarrhea or intestinal worm infections resulting from WASH inadequacies (WHO, 2008).

A lack of safe water close to home has many indirect effects on nutrition. In such conditions, people are often left with no choice but to drink unsafe water from unprotected sources. WASH interventions—including solar disinfection of water, provision of soap, and improvement of water quality—have been identified as having an impact on stunting reductions in children under five years of age, although further research is needed to better elucidate these connections (Dangour et al., 2013).

Human health and nutrition is also dependent on agricultural production, which carries complex implications for water. Agriculture is reliant on water; indeed, it uses 70 percent of all available freshwater worldwide (World Bank, 2007). However, agriculture is also a major source of pollution, comprising the largest source of water pollution in developed nations (World Bank, 2007). In addressing the relationship between agriculture and water, the health of future generations is also at stake. Protecting natural resources such as water and land now will ensure that there will be clean water and food for the world's growing population.

Public Health Ethics

The ethical concerns and implications of food, nutrition, and water have resonance for both planetary well-being and human health. The health of our species is intertwined with that of our environment: humanity cannot survive without enough food and water to nourish the world's people, but the planet's resources are suffering from the ramifications of a changing climate. Food and water also hold a special status: they are essential to survival, but their inherent benefits lie in their consumption. Given that human health and nutrition thus relies on an ongoing cycle of depletion and replenishment of these resources, there is a unique moral need to ensure that food and water are constantly available (Thompson, 2010).

By 2050 there will be an estimated 9 billion people sharing the globe, with the greatest growth in urban centers and the world's poorest countries (UN, 2015). The current population of 7 billion uses nearly 40 percent of the world's land and 70 percent of its freshwater supply to produce its food (UNEP, 2010). In turn, agricultural production is a major driver of climate change, contributing over one-quarter of all greenhouse gas emissions (Vermeulen, Campbell, and Ingram, 2012). Food, nutrition, and water are essential for human health, but their practical applications are rife with ethical quandaries.

Some of the most significant public health ethics issues arising in food, water, and nutrition have been selected for close examination: the three chapters of *The Oxford Handbook of Public Health's* food, water, and nutrition section scrutinize issues related to water security, malnutrition, and obesity prevention. They are briefly summarized below.

In "Water, Justice, and Public Health," Madison Powers delves into the threats posed to water security by both traditional and more contemporary challenges. He presents the reader with a framework for understanding the connection between water and public health that elucidates the fundamental human right to water and sanitation. With this framework of justice and water as a backdrop, Powers explores the health implications of access to water and sanitation, as well as ethical issues posed by the management and global commodification of water resources.

Jessica Fanzo presents an analysis of malnutrition that spans time and space in "Malnutrition, Public Health, and Ethics." Addressing the full spectrum of malnutrition, from stunting and wasting to overweight and obesity, Fanzo illustrates the importance of nutrition within the public health context. She examines intergenerational issues of justice and inequities of diets around the world as part of the chapter's focus on disease burdens associated with malnutrition.

Anne Barnhill's chapter, "Obesity Prevention and Promotion of Good Nutrition: Public Health Ethics Issues," continues the theme of food and nutrition, as Barnhill provides a deeper analysis of overweight and obesity. As overweight and obesity rates rise around the world, so too do related disease burdens and mortality risks. In addition to the human health costs, Barnhill considers the financial costs of overweight and obesity in her discussion of the public health community's efforts to encourage healthy eating. The chapter highlights how obesity prevention efforts raise ethical concerns about stigma and moral blame, as well as individual choice and market regulation.

As these three chapters illustrate, the ethical implications of food, water, and nutrition are tied to justice, equity, and fairness. These concerns span the continuum of time, as justice must be broadly envisioned across generations. The same holds true for geography, as the dietary choices of those in high-income countries carry tangible repercussions for the quality of life of people in low-income countries. In short, justice cannot be constrained to one time and place. Stigma and blame are components of this discussion, as are the concepts of individual choice and market regulation. These ethical issues, which all too often hinge upon poverty and power, must be clarified and addressed to ensure justice in the context of policies affecting food and water.

Poverty, exploitation, and social injustice are at the root of food and water insecurity. These larger systemic issues, which ultimately give rise to the health burdens resulting from food and water insecurity, must be addressed through a comprehensive approach that addresses inequities. As Lopez-Gunn, De Stefano, and Llamas, (2012) argue, insecurity cannot be addressed solely through technical solutions. Instead, government and the development community must employ approaches that address how ethical values and political will affect food and water resources, and how these constraints ultimately influence malnutrition and burdens related to water, sanitation, and hygiene.

Conclusion

Amartya Sen (1982, 459) said "there is no such thing as an apolitical food problem." The same can be said for water. The governance and power issues associated with these resources are rife with ethical complexity. Ensuring human health requires that we foster the well-being of our growing population and our planet, a task that is both seemingly insurmountable and of paramount importance, and one that requires us to both consider and act upon the ethical implications of how we engage with food, nutrition, and water.

References

Black, R. E., Victora, C. G., Walker, S. P., Bhutta, Z. A., Christian, P., de Onis, M., et al. 2013. "Maternal and Child Undernutrition and Overweight in Low-Income and Middle-Income Countries." *Lancet* 382(9890): 427–451.

CDC (Centers for Disease Control and Prevention). 2016. "Global Water, Sanitation, & Hygiene (WASH)" (Atlanta, Ga.: CDC). http://www.cdc.gov/healthywater/global/wash_statistics.html.

Dangour, A. D., Watson, L., Cumming, O., Boisson, S., Velleman, Y., Cavill, S., et al. 2013. "Interventions to Improve Water Quality and Supply, Sanitation and Hygiene Practices, and Their Effects on the Nutritional Status of Children." *Cochrane Database of Systematic Reviews* 8: CD009382. https://www.cochranelibrary.com/cdsr/doi/10.1002/14651858.CD009382.pub2/full.

Development Initiatives. 2017. *Global Nutrition Report 2017: Nourishing the SDGs* (Bristol, UK: Development Initiatives).

Development Initiatives. 2018. *2018 Global Nutrition Report: Shining a Light to Spur Action on Nutrition* (Bristol, UK: Development Initiatives).

FAO (Food and Agriculture Organization of the United Nations). 2009. "World Summit on Food Security: Declaration of the World Summit on Food Security" (Rome: FAO).

FAO (Food and Agriculture Organization of the United Nations), IFAD (International Fund for Agricultural Development), UNICEF (United Nations Children's Fund), WFP (World

Food Programme), and WHO (World Health Organization). 2017. *The State of Food Security and Nutrition in the World 2017: Building Resilience for Peace and Food Security* (Rome: FAO).

GloPan (Global Panel on Agriculture and Food Systems for Nutrition). 2016. *Food Systems and Diets: Facing the Challenges of the 21st Century*. Foresight Report (London: GloPan). https://www.glopan.org/sites/default/files/Downloads/Foresight%20Report.pdf.

Gakidou, E., Afshin, A., Abajobir, A. A., Abate, K. H., Abbafati, C., Abbas, K. M., et al. 2017. "Global, Regional, and National Comparative Risk Assessment of 84 Behavioural, Environmental and Occupational, and Metabolic Risks or Clusters of Risks, 1990–2016: A Systematic Analysis for the Global Burden of Disease Study 2016." *Lancet* 390 (10100): 1345–1422.

HLPE (High Level Panel of Experts on Food Security and Nutrition). 2017. *Nutrition and Food Systems* (Rome: Committee on World Food Security).

Lopez-Gunn, E., De Stefano, L. and Llamas, M. R. 2012. "The Role of Ethics in Water and Food Security: Balancing Utilitarian and Intangible Values." *Water Policy* 14(Suppl. 1): 89–105.

Ng, M., Fleming, T., Robinson, M., Thomson, B., Graetz, N., Margono, C., et al. 2014. "Global, Regional, and National Prevalence of Overweight and Obesity in Children and Adults during 1980–2013: A Systematic Analysis for the Global Burden of Disease Study 2013." *Lancet* 384(9945): 766–781. https://www.ncbi.nlm.nih.gov/pmc/articles/PMC4624264/.

Popkin, B. M., Adair, L. S., and Ng, S. W. 2012. "Global Nutrition Transition and the Pandemic of Obesity in Developing Countries." *Nutrition Reviews* 70(1): 3–21.

Sen, A. 1982. "The Food Problem: Theory and Policy." *Third World Quarterly* 4(3): 447–459.

Thompson P. B. 2010. "Food Aid and the Famine Relief Argument (Brief Return)." *Journal of Agricultural and Environmental Ethics* 23: 209–227.

UN (United Nations). 2015. *World Urbanization Prospects: The 2014 Revision ST/ESA/SER.A/366* (Geneva: Department of Economic and Social Affairs, Population Division).

UNEP (United Nations Environment Programme). 2010. *Assessing the Environmental Impacts of Production and Consumption* (Nairobi, Kenya: UNEP). http://www.resourcepanel.org/reports/assessing-environmental-impacts-consumption-and-production.

UNICEF (United Nations Children's Fund), WHO (World Health Organization), and the World Bank. 2017. *Group Joint Child Malnutrition Estimates: Key Findings of the 2017 Edition* (New York: UNICEF). https://www.who.int/nutgrowthdb/jme_brochoure2017.pdf?ua=1

Vermeulen, S. J., Campbell, B. M. and Ingram, J. S. 2012. "Climate Change and Food Systems." *Annual Review of Environment and Resources* 37(1). https://www.annualreviews.org/doi/abs/10.1146/annurev-environ-020411-130608.

WHO (World Health Organization). 2001. *Water for Health—Taking Charge* (Geneva: WHO). http://www.who.int/water_sanitation_health/wwdreport.pdf?ua=1.

WHO (World Health Organization). 2008. *Safer Water, Better Health, Costs, Benefits and Sustainability of Interventions to Protect and Promote Health* (Geneva: WHO).

WHO (World Health Organization). 2017a. "Malnutrition Fact Sheet." http://www.who.int/mediacentre/factsheets/malnutrition/en/.

WHO (World Health Organization). 2017b. "Obesity and Overweight: Fact Sheet No. 311." http://www.who.int/mediacentre/factsheets/fs311/en/.

WHO (World Health Organization) and UNICEF (United Nations Children's Fund). 2017. *Progress on Drinking Water, Sanitation and Hygiene: 2017 Update and SDG Baselines* (Geneva: WHO).

World Bank. 2007. *World Development Report 2008: Agriculture for Development* (Washington, D.C.: World Bank Group).

CHAPTER 48

WATER, JUSTICE, AND PUBLIC HEALTH

MADISON POWERS

Introduction

SECURE access to clean water is central within many discussions of public health ethics. The task of this chapter is threefold. The first section, "Water and Theoretical Approaches to Public Health Ethics," surveys two complementary philosophical frameworks that address water resource management issues and their relation to public health. Theories of social justice and human rights that provide the normative focus of this chapter share a commitment to health as a core element of human well-being, which is foundational to the requirements of justice.

The second section, "Scarcity and the Problem of Common-Pool Resources," describes the health implications of how access to water and sanitation services are managed along with competing demands. The discussion highlights the extent to which principles of hydrology, together with demographic trends and land use patterns, make the task of integrated water resource management a particular kind of moral problem. In most circumstances, secure access to clean water and sanitation requires some entity to manage a common-pool resource, which requires choices among competing uses over an increasingly wide geographic region. The upshot is that the highly consequential choices of water managers become more complicated and ethically contested as competition for progressively scarce resources intensifies.

The third section, "Global Commodification, Governance, and Control over Resources," addresses ethical issues posed by the global commodification of water; in particular, it looks at the mechanisms and emerging patterns of control and institutions of governance. Globalization introduces new controversies about the kinds of institutional arrangements best suited for ensuring distributive fairness and promoting water security for all current users, including the global poor, and for future generations.

Water and Theoretical Approaches to Public Health Ethics

Secure access to clean water and water for other purposes is an important concern within contemporary theories of social justice. Such theories assume that a just society is one that provides favorable social conditions and sufficient resources for the secure realization of the most important elements of well-being for its members. This approach involves a two-step argument.

The first task is the identification of the core elements of well-being that anyone should want, whatever else they would want as part of a decent or dignified human life (Nussbaum, 2000; Powers and Faden, 2006). Social justice accordingly involves the arrangement of a society's major institutions and social practices in order to secure sufficient levels of well-being across each of the core elements for each member of that society. Health, including the preservation of life and the reduction of premature morbidity, is widely recognized as a core element of human well-being that just social institutions have the responsibility to protect and promote (Powers and Faden, 2006; Griffin, 2008; Ruger, 2010; Venkatapuram, 2011; Liao, 2015).

The second step places the practical focus on identifying the *necessary social conditions* and the *essential resources* that are required for realizing the basic core elements for well-being for all members of a society. Chief among the necessary social conditions are institutional arrangements that effectively combat structurally entrenched forms of disadvantage, including unfair mechanisms of political control that benefit some segments of society at the expense of others. The moral objection is that these arrangements systematically disfavor vulnerable social groups and the occupants of marginalized and disempowered social positions, and thus undermine their prospects for realizing sufficient levels of health and other core elements of well-being.

Resources are deemed "essential if they are indispensable for survival" (De Schutter and Pistor, 2016, 5). While the precise list of resources of such strategic moral importance is subject to disagreement at the margins, most theories agree that water, food, and shelter are essential resources that trigger a heightened degree of moral concern because of their indispensable role in preserving life and protecting health quality (Daniels, 2008; Rawls, 2001). Theories of social justice therefore emphasize the importance of a social guarantee for the provision of clean water and sanitation services, along with water for food and the preservation of the ecological prerequisites for sustainable access to such services across generations (Powers and Faden, 2006; Venkatapuram, 2011).

Philosophical discussions of human rights also emphasize the special strategic importance of water resources for human well-being, in particular for health. The task of specifying human rights claims involves a two-stage argument that is similar in format to theories of social justice. Interest-based theories of human rights begin with a conception of the core elements of the right holder's well-being, which are of overriding importance to every human being (Raz, 1986; Tasioulas, 2015). Typically, human rights are described as the minimum demands of justice. They are the most basic claims or entitlements that all individuals have against the major institutions of any organized society (Shue, 1996; Nickel, 2007).

The second step of the argument is the identification of the "object" of human rights—what the right is a *claim to*—by reference to the various resources and social conditions that are indispensable to the fulfillment of those rights (Raz, 2015; Liao and Etinson, 2012). Thus, a human right grounded in a universal moral interest in health consists of claims to specific objects, such as access to basic health care and primary public health services, along with a public guarantee of the social infrastructure necessary for the provision of clean water and sanitation services for direct personal use and water suitable to the production of food (Nickel, 2007; Risse, 2014).

Human rights theory has been especially prominent in international conversations regarding water policy ever since clean drinking water and sanitation were declared to be a human right in the Dublin Statement on Water and Sustainable Development in 1992 (World Meteorological Organization, 1992). In 2010 the United Nations (UN) declared "the right to safe and clean drinking water and sanitation as a human right that is essential for the full enjoyment of life and all human rights" (UNGA, 2010).

Social structural theories of justice have been particularly influential in some domestic contexts, and they complement human rights approaches. Both approaches emphasize the indispensability of effective public institutions that have the requisite organizational capacity and adhere to principles of fair access to sufficient clean water and sanitation services and other vital uses for everyone, now and for future generations.

The public health rationale for social guarantees of clean water and sanitation as a requirement of justice is well known (Barlow, 2013). Approximately 3.4 million people die annually from water-related diseases (WHO, 2001). Of those who die each year from lack of access to safe drinking water and adequate sanitation, 1.4 million are children (UNICEF, 2004). More than 2.4 billion people lack improved sanitation (WHO/UNICEF JMP, 2015). For at least 1.8 billion people, the primary source of drinking water is contaminated by human waste (Bain et al., 2014). The global burden of waterborne disease is unevenly distributed. Approximately 97 percent of deaths related to inadequate water sanitation occur in developing countries where the public health infrastructure is weak (CDC, 2016).

Access to water for drinking, cooking, and personal hygiene is thus a big part of the health-related rationale for both human rights and principles of social justice. Water is an important resource for sanitation in securing health and overall well-being. The absence of adequate sanitation facilities and infrastructure results in a heavy burden of disease (e.g., stunting, intestinal helminths, diarrhea) and has an established impact on privacy, dignity, and physical safety for girls and women (WHO/UNICEF JMP, 2015).

While much of the human rights literature focuses on clean water for drinking and sanitation, water also matters from a public health perspective because it is needed for food production that sustains life and ensures proper nutrition (UN CESCR, 2002). Agriculture looms large in this discussion because it accounts for approximately 70 percent of all freshwater withdrawals worldwide, and among the developed nations it is the largest source of water pollution (World Bank, 2007).

Scarcity and the Problem of Common-Pool Resources

Indispensability for health, scarcity, and barriers to access give water its acute moral salience. In simple economic terms, scarcity is defined as the condition in which demand for water—from all sectors, including individuals, agriculture, and manufacturing—exceeds the available supply. In addition, a problem that has come into sharper focus over the last few decades is physical scarcity occurring in places other than arid and desert regions. Physical scarcity is the condition in which there is simply not enough water available to meet the needs of the inhabitants of a region. However, in less developed countries and poor regions of developed countries, poverty and inadequate institutional capital investment remain among the most important factors in the lack of water resources sufficient to meet demand. A UN Development Programme report concluded that "[t]he scarcity at the heart of the global water crisis is rooted in power, poverty and inequality and not in physical availability" (UNDP, 2006, 2).

Physical scarcity nonetheless complicates matters, especially in regions where infrastructure is inadequate and poverty impedes access for many people. At a landmark United Nations conference at Mar del Plata, Argentina, in 1977, the focus was upon the previously counterintuitive notion that water is becoming physically scarce in many regions of the world as a result of disruptions of the hydrologic cycle, in part because of changes in the built environment (UN, 1977). Water scarcity came to be recognized as a common-pool resource problem.

A common-pool resource is one in which availability in sufficient quantity and quality to meet the demands of each person and for a multiplicity of purposes depends on the activities of all who draw upon that resource. In response to an understanding of regional water availability as a joint function of growing physical scarcity, poverty and other durable impediments to access, and the necessity of allocating among competing uses, conference participants endorsed the idea of integrated water resources management (IWRM).

The scope of the management task, properly done, is breathtaking. A managing entity has to preside over water storage, treatment, and recycling. It has to regulate a variety of types of agricultural and industrial activities, and balance competing uses. It has to exercise some control over suburban sprawl, industrial siting, and land use matters that implicate traditional ideas of private land rights. It has to adjudicate between the interests of those living upstream and those living downstream in a river basin, and ensure that the water in aquifers and rivers is not too polluted for use for water supply, industrial production, agricultural use, or for the protection of biodiversity, wetlands, and aquatic systems in rivers (Falkenmark, 2001).

The enormous ethical implications of IWRM soon became clear. There was a dawning recognition of the potential for proper water management to touch upon nearly every aspect of individual decision-making and collective social organization. Indeed, the most widely cited definitions of IWRM encompass many of the normative dimensions at stake. The Global Water Partnership definition is as follows: "IWRM is a process which promotes the coordinated development of water, land, and related resources, in order to maximize the resultant economic social and welfare in an equitable manner without compromising the sustainability of vital ecosystems" (GWP, 2000).

The GWP summarizes the ethical significance of this definition by noting three distinct, frequently competing goals. The goal of economic efficiency is rooted in the value of economic growth and development, the goal of equity is a matter of adjudicating fairly between the competing claims of current users, and the goal of sustainability refers to the underlying health of ecosystems that assures availability of adequate resources to future generations.

A major impetus for IWRM was a fundamental change in the scientific consensus among hydrologists. The long-standing assumption of stationarity—the idea that interannual hydrologic variability fluctuates within an overall envelope of stability—was abandoned (Postel, Daily, and Ehrlich, 1996). It gradually became clear from longitudinal data sets that historical patterns of physical availability throughout the world were changing, sometimes rapidly, and that the amount of physically available freshwater was in widespread decline (Milly et al., 2008).

The causes of decline in available freshwater are complex and interactive (Vörösmarty et al., 2010). The initial models focused on the immediate consequences of the built environment, such as cities, large dams and other alterations of rivers, and cleared forests. The construction of cities and extended areas of hardscape (concrete and asphalt), along with the destruction of watersheds, wetlands, and forests, leads to more runoff into oceans. Consequently, there is less absorption into surface waters and aquifers. Surface water levels and aquifer reserves also exert interactive influence, with declining aquifers reducing the replacement rates of surface waters and the decreased capture of rainwater in bodies of surface water then resulting in slower recharge rates for aquifers (Glennon, 2009).

Demographic changes are another factor. Population growth and the concentration of populations in urban areas result in an accelerated rate of withdrawal of water from all sources. These include rainwater, surface water sources such as lakes and rivers, and groundwater stored in aquifers below the surface. The high-demand problem is not confined to the populous urban areas of the developed world. High-demand water users are becoming more geographically concentrated in regions that cannot sustain demand levels because of a combination of physical scarcity and insufficient financial resources to provide water and sanitation services to the population, especially in megacities (McDonald et al., 2014).

In addition, not all types of water are equally renewable, and not all uses of water have the same effects on watersheds. Water used for industrial purposes and large-scale agriculture can be so heavily polluted that it becomes unsuitable for drinking or bathing, and some types of pollution are less amenable to conventional treatment processes (Hoffman, 2009).

The combined problems stemming from economic scarcity and physical scarcity are now widely seen as global issues, and although heavily concentrated in India and China, no region of the world is unaffected. Current estimates are that by 2025, 1.8 billion people will experience absolute water scarcity and as much as two-thirds of the world will experience water stress (UN-Water, 2017).

Absolute water scarcity is defined as a condition in which individuals have insufficient access to safe and affordable water to satisfy their needs for drinking, washing, or their livelihoods for a significant period of time. *Water stress* is defined as a condition of intermittent insufficiency. However, estimates of the shortfall in water availability are bound up with a number of empirical and normative assumptions, and these assumptions reflect the interdependence between economic and physical scarcity. Whether an area qualifies as "water scarce" depends on how people's needs are defined and whether per capita use will increase, as it has in developed and developing countries. It also depends on whether the requirements for preservation of water ecosystems are taken into account and whether the long-term trend of increasingly water-intensive agricultural and industrial processes will continue, as well as whether and what kind of pricing mechanisms will be adopted in order to restrain overuse (Rijsberman, 1994). All of these judgments are normatively laden social choices. They extend far beyond any technocratic vision of sound fiscal management.

Perhaps unsurprisingly, there is considerable overlap between areas now most affected by economic scarcity and many of the regions at greatest risk for worsening physical scarcity. Cited below are some of the key facts that illuminate the unequal global burden of water scarcity.

Accessible surface water is diminishing. Over 1.4 billion people currently live in river basins where the use of water exceeds minimum replacement levels, leading to the dewatering of rivers (World Bank, 2005). Widely cited estimates show an expected increase of people living in river basins under severe surface water stress from 1.6 billion in 2000 to 3.9 billion by 2050. That is roughly 40 percent of the anticipated world population of 9.7 billion people (OECD, 2012). New research shows that areas affected disproportionately are large population centers of the developing world, with more than 40 percent of some of the world's great cities supplied by surface water expected to be vulnerable to severe shortages and drought by 2040 (Padowski and Gorelick, 2014).

Up to 2 billion people who depend on winter snow to deliver their summer water could see shortages by 2060 as upland and mountain snowpack continue to dwindle (Mankin et al., 2015). Among the worst affected are the predominantly poor inhabitants of the Tien Shan located in China, Kazakhstan, Kyrgyzstan, and Uzbekistan. About half of the mountain's glacier volume in that region could be depleted by the 2050s (Farinotti et al., 2015).

More than half of the world's population is experiencing groundwater depletion below recharge rates, mostly due to industrial agriculture, overgrazing, and deforestation. Aquifer withdrawals are predicted to increase by 50 percent by 2025 in developing countries, and 18 percent in developed countries (UNEP, 2007). This trend is significant because aquifers account for 35 percent of human water use worldwide. Recent satellite studies confirm that nearly a third of the world's thirty-seven largest aquifers are being drained more quickly than they are being replenished, and the main impact is in the poor, densely populated regions of northwestern India, Pakistan, and northern Africa (Richey et al., 2015).

Climate change makes these challenges worse. Among the main areas to face greater losses of accessible water are the equatorial regions, which are already among the most water-stressed areas. These areas also tend to be the parts of the world most dependent on rainfall rather than irrigation as the basis for agriculture. Rain-dependent agricultural areas that are at much greater risk of crop failure are the hottest, driest regions of the world.

The disruption of the hydrological cycle due to global warming is likely to hit these regions first and worst (Powers, 2014). The Intergovernmental Panel on Climate Change (IPCC, 2014) predicts yields from rain-dependent agriculture could be down by 50 percent as soon as 2020. Many of the world's poorest are concentrated in Southeast Asia, where some of the world's largest rivers no longer flow to the sea due to glacier decline, which is also attributed in large part to global warming.

The upshot is that the reduced availability of water will not be distributed equally across the globe. Given these geographic patterns of water scarcity, it is no wonder that water resource management discussions at the international level no longer focus solely on the localized challenges addressed by IWRM. Matters of regional water security are bound up with geopolitical issues of national and international security. According to one estimate, there are 276 transnational river basins, and the risk of conflict is significant (Chellamy, 2013).

For example, China has embarked upon a series of roughly 130 dam and water diversion projects. They will alter the course and flow of rivers that pass through ten other countries, affecting 2 billion people. Because China controls the entire Tibetan plateau, where these rivers originate in its vast glaciers, it alone has the power to control the primary water supply for all of Southeast Asia (Christopher, 2013). Some legal and political theorists propose to manage such conflicts by a principle of hydrosolidarity, an aspirational ideal encouraging collaboration among all affected parties in order to achieve fairness between upstream and downstream users and preserve a common asset (Wouters, Vinogradov, and Magsig, 2008). In some contexts, mutual recognition of common interests has resulted in voluntary agreements among riparian users without legal, institutional sanctions and enforcement mechanisms (Ostrom, 1990). However, as the Tibetan plateau situation illustrates, the extent of potential water-based cross-border conflict remains an open question.

Global Commodification, Governance, and Control over Resources

The global poor face new threats to water security, even within regions of the world where physical water scarcity is not severe. The reason is that water is now a valuable global commodity, attracting foreign investment in water-rich, cash-poor nations and potentially making economic access to water for the poor more difficult. Here again, the root of the problem lies in "power, poverty and inequality." Three types of water-intensive foreign investment, domestic forays into global commodity markets, and other interventions in domestic resource policy have provoked the most ethical controversy.

First, multinational corporations have off-shored many of the most water-intensive and most water-contaminating manufacturing activities (Richter et al., 2013). The off-shoring occurs on both the front end of the production process and, again, on the back end with the disposal of toxic wastes at the end of the life cycle of consumer and industrial products (Pellow, 2007; Keyi, 2014). In many developing countries, off-shoring at both ends of the lifecycle of consumer goods is facilitated by the fact that environmental regulation is lax. The result is that the social costs of water pollution is "externalized"—imposed on society at large or on nearby landowners and individuals who suffer the adverse health effects of pollution, far away from most of the affluent consumers, who enjoy the benefits of these products without bearing the environmental health burdens of their production (Kuehr, 2016). Many human rights and nongovernmental organizations are particularly critical of the World Bank's role in encouraging the trend toward massive deregulation that exacerbates the risk of severe environmental health externalities, especially in countries run by autocrats, where economic development is prioritized over the protection of health and the environment (GRAIN, 2013).

In addition, most developing countries impose few restrictions on the quantity of water used. For example, both domestic and foreign-based soda and bottled water companies are allowed to extract massive quantities of water for virtually no cost beyond the purchase price of the adjacent land. The problem is that water ownership rights throughout much of the world are established according to the "law of capture" or "rule of prior appropriation." Legal rights to water from rivers and lakes is granted to whomever is first to divert it for their own use, as long as they put it to some beneficial use, no matter how much they extract (FAO, 2006).

Second, multinational agribusiness conglomerates are locating water-intensive agricultural facilities in developing countries. Land with an adequate supply of water is an asset of crucial importance for agriculture, especially for water-intensive, large-scale industrial agricultural enterprises (Klare, 2012). Critics have dubbed it the "land and water grab" (Kugelman and Levenstein, 2013). Although it is too early to assess its ultimate scale and impact, massive foreign investment in large tracts of land has occurred in many water-rich, economically desperate countries, where land is extraordinarily cheap by developed world standards (World Bank, 2010).

Often, agricultural land is purchased or leased under long-term contracts that provide little or no compensation to the host nation, other than the vague, unenforceable promise to stimulate economic development (GRAIN, 2013; CHRGJ, 2010). Foreign investment in agricultural land is further incentivized by lax environmental regulation and the lack of adequate legal titling of traditional lands sufficient to protect the holders of traditional land and water claims (Knight et al., 2012). Knowledgeable critics point to the consequences of purchases or leases of land. Water is diverted from use for local agriculture and the satisfaction of basic human needs, only to be abandoned once the nutrients have been depleted and nearby rivers polluted from chemical fertilizer run-off

(De Schutter, 2011; Schiffman, 2013; Robertson and Pinstrup-Anderson, 2010; HRW, 2012). The upshot is that the benefits of large-scale global land and water acquisition go primarily to the global affluent, while the environmental health consequences of degraded water quality are shifted to the poorest, most vulnerable regions of the world in exchange for dubious economic benefits (Dean, Lovely, and Wan, 2009).

Third, foreign investors and transnational water management corporations have taken over the operation of municipal water and sanitation services, and, in some cases, taken control over all water resources within large river basin areas. The initial rationale for privatization focused on the special expertise of private management corporations and the prospect of obtaining greater efficiencies than publicly controlled facilities achieve. The aim was to replace state-subsidized services with more cost-sensitive pricing mechanisms (Scheierling, 2016). The effects have been debated by way of competing case studies, with cases being cited where access by the poor has expanded and cases where access has been lost (Barlow, 2007; Segerfeldt, 2005). However, even the World Bank's own internal analysis concluded that "there is no statistically significant difference between the efficiency performance of public and private operators in this sector" (Estache, Perelman, and Trujillo, 2005).

Privatization arrangements initially arose as a byproduct of World Bank lending policies that made them a condition of loans, but now they have the backing of an array of international organizations based in the developed nations that are home to the multinational investors. As the privatization movement retains its allure among global economic elites, it increasingly relies on a new rationale. The argument is that many national governments have too much sovereign debt and not enough tax revenue to fund the necessary infrastructure improvements. They point to infrastructure that is needed to fulfill the sixth of seventeen Sustainable Development Goal (SDGs), which establishes ambitious targets for ensuring universal and equitable access to water and sanitation services, greater water efficiency, and the protection and restoration of water-related ecosystems (UN, 2017). Cost estimates for achieving these targets range between $74 billion to $116 billion annually (World Bank, 2016). The UN Conference on Trade and Development estimates the seventeen SDGs overall will require between $3.3 trillion and $4.5 trillion a year to implement (UNCTAD, 2014). Many countries lack the resources.

Moreover, the new privatization argument is bolstered by the prediction that the investment shortfall is unlikely to be made up from donations from developed nations. A recent report survey shows that aid donors pledged to spend $54 billion in aid for water and sanitation between 2002 and 2010 but only released $37 billion (WaterAid and Development Initiatives, 2012). Even the full $54 billion donated over nine years is but a drop in the bucket. A recent OECD (2015) analysis confirms what developing nations already know about pledges of foreign assistance of any sort: massive shortfalls between promised aid and received donations are the norm.

The conclusion of this new argument for privatization is that there is simply no alternative, and that the best option involves public-private partnerships (PPPs), widely encouraged by the World Bank and various nongovernmental organizations (NGOs) representing the interests of developed nations. PPPs get their capital from global hedge fund and pension fund investors. The investors create profit-driven private corporations that acquire public utilities, like water, and they fill the governing boards with representatives of these funds (*Bretton Woods Observer*, 2015). Instead of promising management expertise that will yield greater efficiencies, the new rationale offers the prospect of much-needed capital for infrastructure.

The problem with the "no-alternative" argument is that it ignores two issues of structural injustice that contributed to the infrastructural shortfall. The first problem is the morally tainted origin of the sovereign debt. Decades of international lending practices by the IMF and World Bank imposed onerous austerity conditions that deprived debtor states of their capacity to undertake public welfare programs, leaving them with a choice between privatization of essential services or their elimination (Stiglitz, 2007). The second problem is tax competition, the process by which countries compete for foreign registration of corporate headquarters, luring them with tax breaks and subsidies. In response to competitive pressures, nations cut corporate taxes dramatically, inaugurating a race to the bottom, depriving themselves and other countries of the revenues necessary to fund essential services (Dietsch, 2015).

Critics also argue that PPPs and the water privatization approach generally raise serious ethical questions about the kinds of decisions that should be subject to collective democratic decision-making (Bachvarova, 2013). The problem is that the governing body has a strict fiduciary duty to shareholders, and often a very attenuated accountability to ratepayers, because they insist on management contracts that give them wide policy discretion, without the usual mechanisms of review of public utility oversight boards (Romero, 2015; Alexander, 2014). The point of such criticisms is that there is far more at stake than efficient management. When multinational corporations assume authority over vital resources, they pre-empt the moral judgments of those communities affected by such policies on decisions about fees, subsidies for the poor, and long-term investment for the sake of future generations (Kishimoto, Lobina, and Petitjean, 2015). More generally, critics object that PPPs are emblematic of a larger and more insidious global trend toward de-democratization of the public sphere, where the interests of hypermobile capital bypass democratically accountable collective decision-making (Brown, 2015).

Conclusion

Threats to water security, and ultimately to public health, take various forms. Traditional challenges posed by poverty and economic scarcity are conjoined with physical scarcity. The need for management of whole river basins highlights the competing social values and ethical decisions that transcend concerns about efficient management. Even the task of democratic decision-making regarding collective goals is being put to the test. Transboundary rivers pose problems that go beyond the scope of authority of any political jurisdiction, and the transformation of water into a global commodity puts global capital in competition with sovereign nations to determine the future of water resources. Threats to water security in every instance are rooted in "power, poverty and inequality."

References

Alexander, N. 2014. *The Emerging Multi-polar World Order* (Washington, D.C.: Heinrich Böll Stiftung). http://us.boell.org/2014/12/03/emerging-multi-polar-world-order.

Bachvarova, M. 2013. "Non-domination's Role in the Theorizing of Global Justice." *Journal of Global Ethics* 9(2): 173–185.

Bain, R., Cronk, R., Hossain, R., Bonjour, S., Onda, K., Wright, J., et al. 2014. "Global Assessment of Exposure to Faecal Contamination through Drinking Water Based on a Systematic Review." *Tropical Medicine and International Health* 19(8): 917–927.

Barlow, M. 2007. *Blue Covenant: The Global Water Crisis and the Coming Battle for the Right to Water* (London: New Press).

Barlow, M. 2013. *Blue Future: Protecting Water for People and the Planet Forever* (London: New Press).

Bretton Woods Observer. 2015. "Throwing Evidence to the Wind? The World Bank Continues Pushing PPPs." *Bretton Woods Observer: A Quarterly Critical Review of Developments at the World Bank and IMF*, Autumn: 1–2.

Brown, W. 2015. *Undoing the Demos: Neoliberalism's Stealth Revolution* (New York: Zone Books).

CDC (Centers for Disease Control and Prevention). 2016. "Global Water, Sanitation, and Hygiene." http://www.cdc.gov/healthywater/global/wash_statistics.html.

CESCR (United Nations Committee on Economic, Social and Cultural Rights). 2002. "General Comment No. 15: The Right to Water and Sanitation."

Chellamy, B. 2013. *Water, Peace, and War: Confronting the Global Water Crisis* (Lanham, Md.: Rowman and Littlefield).

CHRGJ (Center for Human Rights and Global Justice). 2010. *Foreign Land Deals and Human Rights: Case Studies on Agricultural and Biofuel Investment* (New York: NYU School of Law).

Christopher, M. 2013. *Water Wars: The Brahmaputra River and Sino-Indian Relations*. Case Study (Newport, R.I.: US Naval War College, Center on Irregular Warfare and Armed Groups). https://digital-commons.usnwc.edu/cgi/viewcontent.cgi?referer=https://www.google.com/&httpsredir=1&article=1007&context=ciwag-case-studies.

Daniels, N. 2008. *Just Health* (Cambridge: Cambridge University Press).

Dean, J., Lovely, M., and Wan, H. 2009. "Are Foreign Investors Attracted to Weak Environmental Regulations? Evaluating the Evidence from China." *Journal of Development Economics* 90: 1–13.

De Schutter, O. 2011. "How Not to Think of Land-Grabbing: Three Critiques of Large-Scale Investments in Farmland." *Journal of Peasant Studies* 38(2): 249–279.

De Schutter, O., and Pistor, K. 2016. "Introduction: Toward Voice and Reflexivity." *In Governing Access to Essential Resources*, edited by K. Pistor and O. De Schutter, 3–45 (New York: Columbia University Press).

Dietsch, P. 2015. *Catching Capital: The Ethics of Tax Competition* (New York: Oxford University Press).

Estache, A., Perelman, S., and Trujillo, L. 2005. "Infrastructure Performance and Reform in Developing and Transition Economies: Evidence from a Survey of Productivity Measures." Policy Research Working Paper 3514 (Washington, D.C.: World Bank). https://openknowledge.worldbank.org/bitstream/handle/10986/8844/wps3514.pdf?sequence=1.

Falkenmark, M. 2001. "The Greatest Water Problem: The Inability to Link Environmental Security, Water Security and Food Security." *International Journal of Water Resources Development* 17(4): 539–554.

FAO (Food and Agriculture Organization of the United Nations). 2006. *Modern Water Rights: Theory and Practice* (Rome: FAO). ftp://ftp.fao.org/docrep/fao/010/a0864e/a0864e00.pdf.

Farinotti, D., Longuevergne, L., Moholdt, G., Duethmann, D., Mölg, T., Bolch, T., et al. 2015. "Substantial Glacier Mass Loss in the Tien Shan over the Past 50 Years." *Nature Geoscience* (Advance Online Publication, August 17). doi:10.1038/ngeo2513.

Glennon, R. 2009. *Unquenchable: America's Water Crisis and What to Do about It* (Washington, D.C.: Island Press).

GRAIN. 2013. "The G8 and Land Grabs in Africa." https://www.grain.org/article/entries/4663-the-g8-and-land-grabs-in-africa.

Griffin, J. 2008. *On Human Rights* (Oxford: Oxford University Press).

GWP (Global Water Partnership). 2000. *Integrated Water Resources Management* (Stockholm, Sweden: GWP).

Hoffman, S. J. 2009. *Planet Water: Investing in the World's Most Valuable Resource* (Hoboken, N.J.: John Wiley & Sons).

HRW (Human Rights Watch). 2012. *"Waiting Here for Death": Forced Displacement and "Villagization" in Ethiopia's Gambella Region* (Washington, D.C.: HRW). https://reliefweb.int/report/ethiopia/%E2%80%9Cwaiting-here-death%E2%80%9D-forced-displacement-and-%E2%80%98villagization%E2%80%99-ethiopia%E2%80%99s-gambella.

IPCC (Intergovernmental Panel on Climate Change). 2014. *Climate Change 2014: Impacts, Adaptation, and Vulnerability (Summary for Policymakers)*. https://www.ipcc.ch/pdf/assessment-report/ar5/wg2/ar5_wgII_spm_en.pdf.

Keyi, S. 2014. "China's Poisonous Waterways." *New York Times*, SR4. https://www.nytimes.com/2014/04/05/opinion/chinas-poisonous-waterways.html.

Kishimoto, S., Lobina, E., and Petitjean, O., eds. 2015. *Our Public Water Future: The Global Experience with Remunicipalisation* (London: Public Services International Research Unit).

Klare, K. 2012. *The Race for What's Left: The Global Scramble for the World's Last Resources.* (New York: Picador).

Knight, R., Adoko, J., Siakor, S. K., Salomao, A., Auma, T., Kaba, A., et al. 2012. *Protecting Community Lands and Resources: Evidence from Liberia, Mozambique and Uganda* (Washington, D.C., and Rome: Namati and International Development Law Organization). http://namati.org/wp-content/uploads/2012/06/protecting_community_lands_resources_inter_FW.pdf.

Kuehr, R., ed. 2016. *Solving the E-Waste Problem: Guiding Principles to Develop E-Waste Management Systems and Legislation* (New York: United Nations University). http://world-loop.org/wp-content/uploads/2016/01/Step_WP_WEEE-systems-and-legislation_final.pdf.

Kugelman, M., and Levenstein, S. L., eds. 2013. *The Global Farms Race: Land Grabs, Agricultural Investment, and the Scramble for Food Security* (Washington, D.C.: Island Press).

Liao, S. M. 2015. "Human Rights as Fundamental Conditions for a Good Life." In *Philosophical Foundations of Human Rights*, edited by R. Cruft, M. Liao, and M. Renzo, 79–100 (Oxford: Oxford University Press).

Liao, S. M., and Etinson, A. 2012. "Political and Naturalistic Conceptions of Human Rights: A False Polemic?" *Journal of Moral Philosophy* 9: 327–352.

Mankin, J. S., Viviroli, D., Singh, D., Hoekstra, A.Y., and Diffenbaugh, N. S. 2015. "The Potential for Snow to Supply Human Water Demand in the Present and Future." *Environmental Research Letters* 10(11). doi:10.1088/1748-9326/10/11/114016.

McDonald, R. I., Weber, K., Padowski, J., Flörke, M., Schneider, C., Green, P. A., et al. 2014. "Water on an Urban Planet: Urbanization and the Reach of Urban Water Infrastructure." *Global Environmental Change* 27: 96–105.

Milly, P. C. D., Julio, B., Malin, F., Robert, M., Zbigniew, W., Dennis, P., et al. 2008. "Stationarity Is Dead: Whither Water Management?" *Science* 319: 573–574.

Nickel, J. 2007. *Making Sense of Human Rights*. 2nd ed. (Malden, Mass.: Blackwell).

Nussbaum, M. 2000. *Women and Human Development: The Capabilities Approach* (Cambridge: Cambridge University Press).

OECD (Organisation for Economic Co-operation and Development). 2012. *OECD Environmental Outlook to 2050: The Consequences of Inaction* (Paris: OECD Publishing). doi:10.1787/9789264122246-en.

OECD (Organisation for Economic Co-operation and Development). 2015. *2014 Global Outlook on Aid: Results of the 2014 DAC Survey on Donors' Spending Plans and Prospects for Improving Aid Predictability* (Paris: OECD Publishing). http://www.oecd.org/dac/aid-architecture/GlobalOutlookAid-web.pdf.

Ostrom, E. 1990. *Governing the Commons* (Cambridge: Cambridge University Press).

Padowski, J., and Gorelick, S. 2014. "Global Analysis of Urban Surface Water Supply Vulnerability." *Environmental Research Letters* 9(10): 104004. doi:10.1088/1748-9326/9/10/104004.

Pellow, D. N. 2007. *Resisting Global Toxics: Transnational Movements for Environmental Justice* (Cambridge, Mass.: MIT Press).

Postel, S. L., Daily, G. C., and Ehrlich, P. R. 1996. "Human Appropriation of Renewable Fresh Water." *Science* 271(5250): 785–788.

Powers, M. 2014. "Moral Responsibility for Climate Change." In *Routledge Companion to Bioethics*, edited by J. Arras, E. Fenton, and R. Kukla, 133–146 (New York: Routledge).

Powers, M., and Faden, R. 2006. *Social Justice: The Moral Foundations of Public Health and Health Policy* (New York: Oxford University Press).

Rawls, J. 2001. *Justice as Fairness: A Restatement* (Cambridge, Mass.: Harvard University Press), 171–176.

Raz, J. 1986. *The Morality of Freedom* (Oxford: Clarendon Press).

Raz, J. 2015. "Human Rights in the Emerging World Order." In *Philosophical Foundations of Human Rights*, edited by R. Cruft, M. Liao, and M. Renzo, 217–231 (Oxford: Oxford University Press).

Richey, A. S., Thomas, B. F., Lo, M. H., Reager, J. T., Famiglietti, J. S., Voss, K., et al. 2015. "Quantifying Renewable Groundwater Stress with GRACE." *Water Resources Research* 51: 5217–5238. doi:10.1002/2015WR017349.

Richter, B. D., Abell, D., Bacha, E., Brauman, K., Calos, S., Cohn, A., et al. 2013. "Tapped Out: How Can Cities Secure Their Water Future?" *Water Policy* 15(3): 335–363. doi:10.2166/wp.2013.105.

Rijsberman, F. R. 1994. "Water Scarcity: Fact or Fiction?" Paper presented at the 4th International Crop Science Congress. http://www.cropscience.org.au/icsc2004/plenary/1/1994_rijsbermanf.htm.

Risse, M. 2014. "The Human Right to Water and Common Ownership of the Earth." *Journal of Political Philosophy* 22(2): 178–203.

Robertson, B., and Pinstrup-Anderson, P. 2010. "Global Land Acquisition: Neo-colonialism or Development Opportunity." *Food Security* 2: 271–283.

Romero, M. J. 2015. *What Lies Beneath?: A Critical Assessment of PPPs and Their Impact on Sustainable Development* (European Network on Debt and Development). http://eurodad.org/files/pdf/559e6c832c087.pdf.

Ruger, J. P. 2010. *Health and Social Justice* (Oxford: Oxford University Press).

Scheierling, S. M., ed. 2016. "Special Issue: Contributions to the International Water Resource Economics Consortium 11th Annual Meeting." *Water Resources and Economics* 13: 1–74.

Schiffman, R. 2013. "Hunger, Food Security, and the African Land Grab." *Ethics and International Affairs* 27(3): 239–249.

Shue, H. 1996. *Basic Rights: Subsistence, Affluence, and U.S. Foreign Policy*. 2nd ed. (Princeton, N.J.: Princeton University Press).

Segerfeldt, F. 2005. *Water for Sale: How Business and the Market Can Resolve the World's Water Crisis* (Washington, D.C.: Cato Institute).

Stiglitz, J. 2007. *Making Globalization Work* (New York: W. W. Norton).

Tasioulas, J. 2015. "On the Foundations of Human Rights." In *Philosophical Foundations of Human Rights*, edited by R. Cruft, M. Liao, and M. Renzo, 45–70 (Oxford: Oxford University Press).

UN (United Nations). 1977. *Report of the United Nations Water Conference, Mar del Plata, 14–25 March, 1977* (New York: United Nations).

UN (United Nations). 2017. "The Global Goals for Sustainable Development, Goal #6: Clean Water and Sanitation." https://www.un.org/sustainabledevelopment/water-and-sanitation/.

UN CESCR (United Nations Committee on Economic, Social and Cultural Rights). 2002. "General Comment No. 15, The Right to Water and Sanitation."

UNCTAD (United Nations Conference on Trade and Development). 2014. *World Investment Report 2014: Investing in the SDGs: An Action Plan* (Geneva: United Nations). http://unctad.org/en/PublicationsLibrary/wir2014_en.pdf.

UNDP (United Nations Development Programme). 2006. *Human Development Report 2006: Beyond Scarcity: Power, Poverty and the Global Water Crisis* (New York: Palgrave Macmillan). http://hdr.undp.org/en/reports/global/hdr2006/chapters/.

UNEP (United Nations Environment Programme). 2007. *Global Environment Outlook: Environment for Development (GEO-4)* (Valletta, Malta: Progress Press).

UNGA (United Nations General Assembly). 2010. Resolution 64/292, The Human Right to Water and Sanitation.

UNICEF (United Nations Children's Fund). 2004. *The State of the World's Children 2005* (New York: UNICEF). https://www.unicef.org/publications/index_24432.html.

UN-Water (United Nations Water). 2017. "Statistics." http://www.unwater.org/water-facts/.

Venkatapuram, S. 2011. *Health Justice* (Cambridge: Polity Press).

Vörösmarty, C. J., McIntyre, P. B., Gessner, M. O., Dudgeon, D., Prusevich, A., Green, P., et al. 2010. "Global Threats to Human Water Security and River Biodiversity." *Nature* 467: 555–561.

WaterAid and Development Initiatives. 2012. *Addressing the Shortfall* (London: WaterAid). http://www.wateraid.org/what-we-do/our-approach/research-and-publications/view-publication?id=61e34b58-cb09-4d28-afda-2fd35fe2097b.

WHO (World Health Organization). 2001. *Water for Health: Taking Charge* (Geneva: WHO). http://www.who.int/water_sanitation_health/wwdreport.pdf?ua=1

WHO/UNICEF JMP (World Health Organization/United Nations Children's Fund Joint Monitoring Programme on Water Supply and Sanitation). 2015. *Progress on Sanitation and Drinking Water: 2015 Update and MDG Assessment* (Geneva: WHO). http://www.wssinfo.org/.

World Bank. 2005. *Human Development Report: Equity and Development 2006* (Washington, D.C.: World Bank).

World Bank. 2007. *World Development Report 2008: Agriculture for Development* (Washington, D.C.: World Bank Group).

World Bank. 2010. *Protecting Land Rights is Key to Large-Scale Land Acquisitions* (Washington, D.C.: World Bank).
World Bank. 2016. *The Costs of Meeting the 2030 Sustainable Development Goal Targets on Drinking Water, Sanitation, and Hygiene* (Washington, D.C.: World Bank). http://www.worldbank.org/en/topic/water/publication/the-costs-of-meeting-the-2030-sustainable-development-goal-targets-on-drinking-water-sanitation-and-hygiene.
World Meteorological Organization. 1992. "Dublin Statement on Water and Sustainable Development." http://www.wmo.int/pages/prog/hwrp/documents/english/icwedece.html.
Wouters, P., Vinogradov, S., and Magsig, B.-O. 2008. "Water Security, Hydrosolidarity, and International Law: A River Runs through It..." *Yearbook of International Environmental Law* 19(1): 97–134.

Further Reading

2030 Water Resources Group. 2017. "Who We Are—2030WRG." https://www.2030wrg.org/who-we-are/mission-vision/.
Global Goals for Sustainable Development. "The Global Goals for Sustainable Development, Goal #6." http://www.globalgoals.org/global-goals/clean-water-sanitation/.
Global Infrastructure Initiative. http://www.globalinfrastructureinitiative.com/
Leadership Group on Water Security in Asia. 2009. *Asia's Next Challenge: Securing the Region's Water Future* (Washington, D.C.: Leadership Group on Water Security in Asia).
Naficy, S. E. 2016. "The Human Right to Water." Corporate Accountability International blog. https://www.stopcorporateabuse.org/human-right-water
Olleta, A. 2007. "The World Bank's Influence on Water Privatisation in Argentina." International Environmental Law Research Centre (IELRC) paper. https://www.scribd.com/document/41895453/The-World-Bank-Influence-in-Water-Privatisation-in-Argentina.
Pistor, K., and De Schutter, O. 2016. *Governing Access to Essential Resources* (New York: Columbia University Press).
UN (United Nations). 2008. *Making the Law Work for Everyone*, Vol. 1: *Report of the Commission on the Legal Empowerment of the Poor* (New York: Commission on Legal Empowerment of the Poor and United Nations Development Programme). https://www.un.org/ruleoflaw/files/Making_the_Law_Work_for_Everyone.pdf.

CHAPTER 49

MALNUTRITION, PUBLIC HEALTH, AND ETHICS

JESSICA FANZO

Introduction

THERE are numerous challenges involved in addressing the various forms of malnutrition around the world. This chapter will highlight some key ethical issues that arise in addressing the multiple burdens of malnutrition in food and public health systems and the stakeholders that interact within these systems. Following a brief discussion of the landscape of malnutrition, the chapter will focus on ethical issues that society presently faces in addressing the burden of malnutrition, including the complexities of working multisectorally, the responsibility of addressing both chronic malnutrition and overweight and obesity, and the convergence and divergence in addressing acute malnutrition. The chapter then looks to the past, focusing on the "blame" placed on mothers for affecting the health of their offspring through their past exposures. The final section looks to the future and examines intergenerational justice issues related to how people's dietary decisions affect the planet and the most vulnerable.

The Landscape of Malnutrition

Defining the Different Forms of Malnutrition

Nutrition is an essential component of human health, as it is the basis of ensuring that nutrient needs, acquired through diets, are sufficiently met to sustain a healthy life. Approximately 45 percent of mortality of young children can be attributed to undernutrition (Pelletier et al., 1994). Diets are also the leading risk factor for adult morbidity and mortality due to noncommunicable diseases such as cardiovascular disease and stroke (Forouzanfar et al., 2015).

There are two overarching biological manifestations of malnutrition that can occur when nutrient needs are not met: undernutrition, which can manifest as either acute or chronic, and overweight and obesity. The causes of these two biological burdens are complex and can involve immediate causes, such as inadequate diets associated with macro- and micronutrient deficiencies, as well as communicable and noncommunicable disease burden. Underlying causes include women's status; functioning health and food systems; the environment, which includes sanitation, hygiene, and the natural environment; education and knowledge; and the political economy. These all play an important role in the manifestations of optimal nutrition (Acosta and Fanzo, 2012; Reinhardt and Fanzo, 2014; UNICEF, WHO, and World Bank, 2015).

Undernutrition: The Burden of Stunting and Wasting

Chronic malnutrition is defined as a form of growth failure that causes both physical and cognitive delays in growth and development. Compared to children who have been given ideal opportunities to grow and develop, a chronically malnourished child will be challenged to attain the same height, will likely not develop the same cognitive ability, and will have a higher risk of poor health outcomes throughout life (Reinhardt and Fanzo, 2014).

One manifestation of chronic malnutrition is stunting, a complex biological outcome that manifests within a child's body. Stunting, also known as linear growth failure, is defined as the inability to attain potential height for a particular age, and it is the most common measurement used to identify chronic malnutrition. Although stunting in children under five years of age has declined globally from 40 to 23 percent since 1990 (Black et al., 2013; UNICEF, WHO, and World Bank, 2017), an estimated 155 million children remain moderately or severely stunted (UNICEF, WHO, and World Bank, 2017). One could argue that a child who is stunted will never achieve the human capability of pursuing a "dignified and minimally flourishing life," as Martha Nussbaum (2011, 35) has eloquently described it. Optimal nutrition provides for life; emotions; bodily health and integrity; and senses, imagination, and thought.

Acute malnutrition, most often demonstrated by wasting, is frequently seen in temporary or cyclical settings such as emergencies, seasonal variations, and highly infectious disease environments, and it is accompanied by a high risk of mortality. Fifteen percent of all child deaths are attributed to acute malnutrition, and unless provided with appropriate treatment, the fatality rate among children who are severely malnourished is eight times that of normal children (Bergeron and Castleman, 2012). Wasting is measured in children under five as weight for height. Wasting has decreased 11 percent since 1990 (Black et al., 2013), but 50 million children still suffer from it (UNICEF, WHO, and World Bank, 2017), and this figure is likely to rise in the context of climate change and conflict (FAO, 2017).

Deficiencies of essential vitamins and minerals (e.g., micronutrients such as iron, zinc, vitamin A, folate, iodine) continue to be widespread and have significant adverse effects on child survival and development, as well as on the health of adolescent girls and women. To date, while measuring the micronutrient status of populations poses challenges, there are an estimated 2 billion people with some form of micronutrient deficiency (IFPRI, 2016).

Overweight and Obesity and Noncommunicable Diseases

Currently, a staggering 2.1 billion people suffer from overweight and obesity globally (Ng et al., 2014), and an estimated 42 million children under five years of age are overweight. Two-thirds of these children reside in low- and middle-income countries (LMICs) (Black et al., 2013; UNICEF, WHO, and World Bank, 2017). Overweight and obesity are increasing around the world (IFPRI, 2015).

These growing rates of overweight and obesity worldwide are linked to a rise in noncommunicable diseases (NCDs)—life-threatening conditions that are overburdening health systems—as overweight and obesity are major risk factors for NCDs. Like overweight and obesity, NCDs—mainly cancer, cardiovascular disease, chronic respiratory diseases, and diabetes—are increasing among populations almost everywhere. NCDs are currently the most common causes of death and disability worldwide, accounting for 68 percent of global mortality, or two out of every three deaths. Seventy-five percent of these deaths occur in LMICs (WHO, 2014). Cardiovascular disease (CVD) alone is a significant cause of premature death and the primary driver of morbidity for all NCDs, including in LMICs (Zoghbi et al., 2014). Thirty percent of NCD-related deaths in LMICs occur before the age of sixty (the productive age bracket), as compared to 13 percent in high-income countries (HICs) (Harikrishnan et al., 2014; WHO, 2010). One can argue that the higher death tolls found in LMICs are associated with poorly functioning health systems as well changing diets and lifestyles.

Why Nutrition Matters for Public Health

In connection with a rise in obesity and NCDs, society is facing unprecedented changes in demography, epidemiology, and dietary transitions globally, regionally, and within nations that have significant impacts on nutrition and health outcomes. Diets are transitioning because of globalization, urbanization, and income growth. In some low-income countries (LICs), many of the poor eat grain- or tuber-dominated diets that are low in micronutrients, because this is what is accessible and affordable in rural places or urban slums. As household incomes rise, the consumption of both healthy and unhealthy foods generally increases. High-income households tend to rely less on staple grains and more on animal-source foods (including red and processed meats), fruits and vegetables, and foods high in sugar, salt, and saturated and trans fats, such as highly processed and packaged foods and sugar-sweetened beverages (Monteiro et al., 2004; Monteiro et al., 2013; Popkin, Adair, and Ng, 2012).

How does society begin to make a dent in the multiple burdens of malnutrition, including changes to diets and their subsequent health outcomes? Functioning, connected, and resilient public health and food systems are important contributors toward positive change. If food systems are insufficient or not functioning, effects on health can be deleterious. A food system that incorporates nutrition goals can improve the health of communities across the life cycle through positive changes in the way food is produced, processed, packaged, labeled, distributed, marketed, consumed, and disposed of (Pinstrup-Andersen, 2012). Similarly, the health sector should take responsibility for emphasizing, supporting, and ensuring the physical and mental health of food producers and consumers (Hawkes and Ruel, 2006).

Reacting in the Present: A Moral Obligation to Act

Beneficence: Justifying Priorities

What should be prioritized in addressing malnutrition, and what priority strategy is most important for public health in the immediate and long term? Many would argue that hunger and undernutrition should be a top priority, since it is the moral obligation of governments to ensure that their citizens do not go hungry and that children have the best chance of survival and growth in their early lives. Undernutrition is often framed as not being the fault of the individual, but rather a failure of the state or of international cooperation. In contrast, many see overweight and obesity as the fault of the individual and of people's inability to make rational food choices. In the United States, policy approaches to target overweight and obesity reflect larger societal views on personal responsibility and autonomy, though this perspective neglects the causal factors involved in overnutrition (Gostin, 2010).

Addressing the divergent forms of malnutrition is complex: both undernutrition and overweight and obesity require the engagement of multiple sectors and disciplines to reduce their respective burdens and ensure sustained change. Countries with significant levels of low birth weight and stunting are sensitive to the consequences of changing diets and activity patterns (Adair et al., 2013). At the same time, trends in obesity are crippling some of the poorest countries, even as they are still reeling from undernutrition, micronutrient deficiencies, and infectious diseases (Popkin, Adair, and Ng, 2012). Many countries struggle to deal with multiple forms of malnutrition at the same time (IFPRI, 2016).

While there is a moral imperative to ensure that no one goes hungry under the "right to food" mandate, prioritizing one form of mlanutrition over another may not be possible, because the causes and consequences of all these burdens are interwoven. The idea would be to ensure that every approach provides a public health benefit for individuals and weighs the beneficence of priorities as well as the burdens of alternative priority settings. But the question remains: Who has the responsibility to ensure that everyone realizes the right to better nutrition?

Everybody's Business, Nobody's Responsibility: Cooperation across Sectors to Address Stunting

The causes of chronic undernutrition are multidimensional, which creates many challenges in understanding the condition and finding solutions through interventions and policies (Fanzo and Pronyk, 2011). There is no single root cause of chronic malnutrition (UNICEF, WHO, and World Bank 2015). To ensure improvements in nutrition, multi-sectoral approaches are essential (Alderman et al., 2013). Addressing the burden of stunting is inextricably linked to wider progress in achieving the globally agreed-upon Sustainable Development Goals and the overall transformation and development of nations. Significant gains will hinge on concurrent steps to reduce poverty, improve access to education, empower women and girls, and facilitate access to basic infrastructure. Working on multiple fronts simultaneously has the potential to leverage synergies and catalyze gains that extend beyond those achieved through sector-specific programs working in isolation (Fanzo and Pronyk, 2011).

The heightened global awareness of nutrition points to the need for development institutions and governments to better understand the linkages between multiple sectors and nutrition. There is a need for coordination between multiple sectors and a variety of stakeholders in governments, nongovernmental organizations (NGOs), civil society, the United Nations (UN), the donor community, farmer and producer organizations, and the agribusiness, food, and beverage industries (Nisbett et al., 2014; Fanzo, 2015). The interconnections between national and international institutions that work on tackling malnutrition are complicated, with many different players that count nutrition and food security as part of their core directive (Nisbett et al., 2014).

Since 2005 or so, there has been a more substantive, unified advocacy response to ensure nutrition is a development priority—momentum spurred in part by many international organizations and governments partnering to draw greater investments and attention to nutrition. International organizations are prioritizing investments in nutrition programming and complementing them with increased governance and management of national multisectoral nutrition policies and strategies (SUN, 2013). With nutrition becoming increasingly recognized at the highest political levels, a collective and coordinated response by the international community, through multilateral mechanisms as well as bilateral channels, is an implied acknowledgment that food and nutrition security represents a global public good (Page, 2013).

Allocation Decisions to Address Malnutrition and Convergence of Actions

The different manifestations of chronic and acute malnutrition have led to academic and programmatic specialization, as well as competition (Bergeron and Castleman, 2012). Yet the manifestations of acute and chronic malnutrition often coexist in the same locations and under similar circumstances, such as seasonal variation, poverty, humanitarian crises, urban slums, or neglected rural places. There is very little convergence in working together on double-duty screening methods, service provisions, program implementation, or funding.

Allocation decisions are often framed as a blatant choice between addressing underlying causes and chronic forms of malnutrition versus the more immediate causes and acute forms of malnutrition, with acute situations receiving the bulk of funding. These decisions are highly debated in the nutrition community, which is often then split into two major groups of practitioners that use different programmatic models to address malnutrition and compete for precious resources (Menon and Stoltzfus, 2012).

This division puts excessive pressure on governments to determine where and how they should act, and with whom they should align. In the absence of a consensus among experts, governments may lack the epistemic basis they need to fulfill their moral obligations (Fanzo, 2015). This debate arguably undermines the development of integrated efforts that build resilience due to the reinforced divergence in thought and action that comes from focusing on single topics or approaches, rather than providing a more comprehensive view to addressing the manifestations of malnutrition (Menon and Stolzfus, 2012; Fanzo, 2015).

The Growing NCD Burden on Society's Watch

Obesity has a complex etiology. It is not caused by one factor in isolation, and therefore the most effective interventions will be multisectoral. While many see overweight and obesity as the fault of the individual and of people's irrational food choices, this is not necessarily true, as there are other factors that play a significant role (Gostin, 2010). The food industry, and policies such as agriculture subsidies and trade policies—to name just a few factors—all have a significant influence on dietary choices, and on the ability of various populations to access healthy food. There is an extensive literature demonstrating that the food environment—particularly at home, work, and school—influences health-related behaviors and health outcomes (Macintyre, Ellaway, and Cummins, 2002; Gittelsohn et al., 2009), and that this environment is increasingly obesogenic (Swinburn et al., 2011). Developmental programming plays a key role in obesity in adult life, which is discussed more fully in the next section.

Although overweight and obesity are major risk factors of NCDs, very few governments in LMICs recognize the issue and are taking action. A systematic policy review by Lachat et al. (2014) showed that in LMICs, where the burden of NCDs is high and rising, the gap between policy and burden is substantial. The review showed that although NCD strategies were found for 47 percent of LMICs (54 of 116), only a minority provided specific actions to promote healthier diets and physical activity.

During the era of the Millennium Development Goals (MDGs), which ended in 2015, NCDs and overweight and obesity increased, slowly and insidiously, among populations almost everywhere. The overweight/obesity and diet-related NCD burden was substantively ignored during the MDG era. That has changed, however, as the new Sustainable Development Goals (SDGs) have been ushered in. Childhood overweight is a global tracking indicator of SDG2 (Zero Hunger) and a NCD reduction target is embedded in SDG3 (Good Health and Well-Being). However, there is no target or indicator to track overweight and obesity in adults, which is a missed opportunity (Fanzo, 2016).

Learning from the Past: The Unknown Behaviors of Genes

Epigenetics and the Fetal Origins Hypothesis: A Double Fate

The causes of undernutrition and overweight and obesity are similar and intertwined in many ways. Stunted growth in early life increases the risk of being overweight later in life. Similarly, factors such as poverty and lack of knowledge about adequate diets can be exacerbated by inappropriate marketing of unhealthy foods and beverages to children, which potentially leads to undernutrition as well as overweight and obesity (Popkin, Adair, and Ng, 2012). In addition to environmental factors, epigenetics may influence dietary patterns by creating links to the food-social experience of prior generations.

In addition to the health behaviors of adults, such as smoking, exercise, and diet, there are also earlier environmental factors that may affect the well-being of the fetus and have repercussions into adult life that may include obesity and NCD risk. There has been growing evidence linking low birth weight (LBW) to an increased risk for both cardiovascular disease and diabetes (Barker et al., 2002; Barker, 2006). Poor weight gain in the first two years of life and stunting in children and adults have also been correlated with adult diseases (Victora et al., 2008).

Nutrition and disease potential can also be influenced by epigenetics, which refers to the dynamic chemical modifications to DNA that occur (Esteller, 2008). In particular, altered maternal nutrition, including both undernutrition and maternal obesity, has been shown to lead to transgenerational transmission of metabolic disorders, such as NCDs, to the fetus and in the early-life period (Vickers, 2014; Aiken and Ozaane, 2013). Human studies have demonstrated an epigenetic link between alterations in the early-life environment and increased susceptibility to obesity and related metabolic disorders in later life (Wadhwa et al., 2009; Adair et al., 2013). Ongoing epigenetics research and research in the origins of health and disease offer opportunities to explain how the social environment, physical place, and resources available to people have enduring effects on their health.

Exposure to specific foods is seen as a point of potential intervention in the long-term health of individuals and populations. It is thought that the diet in prenatal and early postnatal life impacts obesity later in life, as well as adult-onset diseases such as diabetes and heart disease. Nutrition and food are among many environmental factors that can induce epigenetic changes in the organisms that are directly exposed, and in subsequent generations that inherit epigenetic traits (Kaushik and Anderson, 2016).

Not all nutrition-sensitive postnatal interventions have wholly positive outcomes such as energy-dense food safety nets and therapeutic foods. The current focus of some of these interventions is to improve weight gain among children born small for gestational age, or those who suffer from severe malnutrition. However, "rapid growth" during infancy is sometimes associated with increased risk of obesity, insulin resistance, and elevated blood pressure in childhood and adulthood (Ong and Loos, 2006). It is still not clear whether benefits of these interventions, which promote faster growth in LMICs, outweigh the possible long-term risks into adulthood (Adair et al., 2013).

Nonmaleficence and Justice: Framing the Science of Epigenetics

Epigenetics raises issues of intergenerational justice and responsibility. Though not widespread, the tendency to frame the emerging epigenetic science as a way of holding mothers culpable for their offspring's later disease risk is troubling (Winett, Wulf, and Wallack, 2016). The unintended consequences of "mother blame" or "community blame" for the fetal origins of disease could present ethical concerns, as opposed to understanding the disease burden through multiple factors beyond just individual decision-making to social, political, economic, and physical environments.

Looking to the Future: Do People Have the Right to Eat Wrongly?

The Inequities of Diets around the World

Both the types of foods people eat and the demand for new diets are in rapid transition. As countries get wealthier, the demand for animal-source foods, sugars, oils, and fats increases. As incomes rise, people spend less of their income on diets, and diets change toward more luxury foods and fewer staple grain foods. These transitions are driving a new demand for certain types of foods that are grown, processed, and consumed in particular ways (Keats and Wiggins, 2014; Khoury et al., 2014; Reardon, Timmer, and Minten, 2012). As countries accumulate wealth, their citizens are shifting from plant-based diets rich in fruits, vegetables, and legumes to highly refined foods, meats, and dairy products, with the exception of a few poor countries that cannot afford such a shift (Popkin, Adair, and Ng, 2012; Wilkinson, 2009; Hawkes and Popkin, 2015). It should be noted that there are profound inequities, both globally and within countries, with respect to access to and affordability of nutritious foods. There is no ethically simple way to reconcile these competing demands in the face of growing economies, international trade, globalization, and urbanization (FAO, 2013).

One example of this inequity is with animal-source foods (ASFs). Although many countries are shifting from plant-based diets to more ASFs (Keats and Wiggins, 2014; Zeisel and Da Costa, 2009), access to ASFs by the poorest remains limited in both availability and accessibility. This limitation affects health because ASFs provide nutrients that are more difficult to obtain in adequate quantities from plant-source foods alone (Dewey and Adu-Afarwuah, 2008; Black et al., 2013). Deficiencies of these nutrients lead to serious conditions, such as anemia, blindness, and even mortality. In contrast, overconsumption of processed meats and ASFs high in saturated fats contributes to increased risk of obesity and NCDs (You and Henneberg, 2016; Bouvard et al., 2015). The benefits of ASF consumption are nuanced: for vulnerable populations, ASFs can provide essential nutrients that are otherwise hard to obtain, but for others, consumption of these foods needs to be limited to mitigate the risk of obesity and NCDs.

Justice: Those Who Suffer the Consequences of Diet Choices

The decision of what to eat is inextricably linked to the ethics of how that choice affects environmental sustainability and human well-being. The increased demand for certain resource-intensive foods, such as beef, has serious ramifications for both climate change and human health (Mearns and Norton, 2010). The production of foods from animal sources is resource-intensive and is the major contributor to greenhouse gas emissions from the agricultural sector (Walker et al., 2005; Garnett, 2009). Overconsumption of meat and an escalating demand for livestock have created ethical conflicts over ensuring animal welfare and limiting demands on the environment (Stokstad, 2010).

If certain resource-intensive foods are considered critically important for human health, then their distribution and access must be made equitable—an existing imbalance that needs to be addressed. There are also low-resource alternative sources that should be considered in filling nutrient gaps for all countries. These foods, such as farmed fish, mollusks, insects, and protein-rich plant food, make significant contributions to nutrition, while leaving a smaller footprint on the planet.

The dietary choices of people in high-income countries (HICs) have significant ramifications for less wealthy populations. The energy-intensive lifestyles and diets of those in HICs are significant anthropogenic contributors to climate change. However, economically poor households are likely to experience a disproportionate burden of the impacts of climate change (Olsson et al., 2014). The food security of those households will most likely not improve under climate variability, and diets will actually deteriorate along with nutrition outcomes. Those who are wealthier will suffer less, even though their choices have far-reaching consequences. Society must address the questions of justice that are central to the increasingly globalized nature of food choices.

From environmental and food security justice perspectives, addressing these ethical issues requires concerted efforts to reduce consumption of animal products in high-income countries, and to discourage consumption in growing economies with populations that are finally wealthy enough to increase meat and dairy in their diets. Some have argued that a 30 percent reduction in production and adult consumption levels of animal-source foods would meet national greenhouse gas emission targets and would simultaneously reduce years of life lost from heart disease by 15 percent (Wilkinson, 2009). The question remains of how to encourage such changes in a way that does not infringe on personal liberties.

Conclusion

Addressing all forms of malnutrition, along with the causes and consequences of dietary and lifestyle choices, requires more accountability. How does society achieve meaningful accountability—and accountability to whom and for what? While some would argue it is clear that people need to be thinking "intergenerationally" about their decisions because of the effects on future risks, others argue that there are many more pressing issues, and that prioritizing requires trade-offs. Still others would argue that there is a moral obligation to address undernutrition immediately, especially acute malnutrition in humanitarian situations, and think later about development, epigenetics, and dietary impacts on future planetary and human health. Society has a moral obligation to consider these concerns across different time frames, because these issues mattered in the past, they matter now, and they will matter in the future.

References

Acosta, A. M., and Fanzo, J. 2012. "Fighting Maternal and Child Malnutrition: Analysing the Political and Institutional Determinants of Delivering a National Multisectoral Response in Six Countries. A Synthesis Paper." Report prepared for DFID (Sussex, UK: Institute of Development Studies).

Adair, L. S., Fall, C. H., Osmond, C., Stein, A. D., Martorell, R., Ramirez-Zea, M., et al. 2013. "Associations of Linear Growth and Relative Weight Gain during Early Life with Adult

Health and Human Capital in Countries of Low and Middle Income: Findings from Five Birth Cohort Studies." *Lancet* 382(9891): 525–534.

Aiken, C. E., and Ozanne, S. E. 2013. "Transgenerational Developmental Programming." *Human Reproduction Update* 20(1):63–75. http://dx.doi.org/10.1093/humupd/dmt043.

Alderman, H. H., Elder, L. K., Goyal, A., Herforth, A. W., Hoberg, Y. T., Marini, A., et al. 2013. *Improving Nutrition through Multisectoral Approaches* (Washington, D.C.: World Bank Group). http://documents.worldbank.org/curated/en/625661468329649726/Improving-nutrition-through-multisectoral-approaches.

Barker, D. J. 2006. "Adult Consequences of Fetal Growth Restriction." *Clinical Obstetrics and Gynecology*, 49(2): 270–283.

Barker, D. J., Eriksson, J. G., Forsén, T., and Osmond, C. 2002. "Fetal Origins of Adult Disease: Strength of Effects and Biological Basis." *International Journal of Epidemiology* 31(6): 1235–1239.

Bergeron, G., and Castleman, T. 2012. "Program Responses to Acute and Chronic Malnutrition: Divergences and Convergences." *Advances in Nutrition: An International Review Journal* 3(2): 242–249.

Black, R. E., Victora, C. G., Walker, S. P., Bhutta, Z. A., Christian, P., De Onis, M., et al. 2013. "Maternal and Child Undernutrition and Overweight in Low-Income and Middle-Income Countries." *Lancet* 382(9890): 427–451.

Bouvard, V., Loomis, D., Guyton, K. Z., Grosse, Y., Ghissassi, F. E., Benbrahim-Tallaa, L., et al. 2015. "International Agency for Research on Cancer Monograph Working Group Carcinogenicity of Consumption of Red and Processed Meat." *Lancet Oncology* 16(16): 1599–1600. http://dx.doi.org/10.1016/S1470-2045(15)00444-1.

Dewey, K. G., and Adu-Afarwuah, S. 2008. "Systematic Review of the Efficacy and Effectiveness of Complementary Feeding Interventions in Developing Countries." *Maternal and Child Nutrition* 4(Suppl. 1): 24–85.

Esteller, M. 2008. "Epigenetics in Cancer." *New England Journal of Medicine* 358(11): 1148–1159.

Garnett, T. 2009. "Livestock-Related Greenhouse Gas Emissions: Impacts and Options for Policy Makers." *Environmental Science & Policy* 12(4): 491–503.

Fanzo, J. 2015. "Ethical Issues for Human Nutrition in the Context of Global Food Security and Sustainable Development." *Global Food Security* 7(2015): 15–23.

Fanzo, J. 2016. "Non-communicable Diseases, Food Systems and the Sustainable Development Goals." *Sight and Life* 30(1): 34.

Fanzo, J., and Pronyk, P. M. 2011. "A Review of Global Progress toward the Millennium Development Goal 1 Hunger Target." *Food and Nutrition Bulletin* 32(2): 144–158.

FAO (Food and Agriculture Organization of the United Nations). 2013. *The State of Food and Agriculture* (Rome, FAO). http://www.fao.org/publications/sofa/the-state-of-food-and-agriculture/en/.

FAO (Food and Agriculture Organization of the United Nations). 2017. *The State of Food Security and Nutrition* (Rome, FAO).

Forouzanfar, M. H., Alexander, L., Anderson, H. R., Bachman, V. F., Biryukov, S., Brauer, M., et al. 2015. "Global, Regional, and National Comparative Risk Assessment of 79 Behavioural, Environmental and Occupational, and Metabolic Risks or Clusters of Risks in 188 Countries, 1990–2013: A Systematic Analysis for the Global Burden of Disease Study 2013." *Lancet* 386(10010): 2287–2323.

Gittelsohn, J., Song, H. J., Suratkar, S., Kumar, M. B., Henry, E. G., Sharma, S., et al. 2009. "An Urban Food Store Intervention Positively Affects Food-Related Psychosocial Variables and Food Behaviors." *Health Education and Behavior* 37(3): 390–402.

Gostin, L.O., ed. 2010. *Public Health Law and Ethics: A Reader* (Berkeley: University of California Press).

Harikrishnan, S., Leeder, S., Huffman, M. M., Jeemon, P., and Prabhakaran, D. 2014. *A Race against Time: The Challenge of Cardiovascular Disease in Developing Economies* (New Delhi, India: Centre for Chronic Disease Control). http://www.ccdcindia.org/wp-content/uploads/2015/12/A-RACE-AGAINST-TIME.pdf.

Hawkes, C., and Popkin, B. M. 2015. "Can the Sustainable Development Goals Reduce the Burden of Nutrition-Related Non-communicable Diseases without Truly Addressing Major Food System Reforms?" *BMC Medicine* 13(1): 143.

Hawkes, C., and Ruel, M. T. 2006. *Overview: Understanding the Links between Agriculture and Health; Focus 2020* (Washington, D.C.: International Food Policy Research Institute).

IFPRI (International Food Policy Research Institute). 2015. *Global Nutrition Report 2015* (Washington, D.C.: IFPRI).

IFPRI (International Food Policy Research Institute). 2016. *Global Nutrition Report 2016* (Washington, D.C.: IFPRI).

Kaushik, P., and Anderson, J. T. 2016. "Obesity: Epigenetic Aspects." *Biomolecular Concepts* 7(3): 145–155.

Keats, S., and Wiggins, S. 2014. *Future Diets: Implications for Agriculture and Food Prices* (London: Overseas Development Institute).

Khoury, C. K., Bjorkman, A. D., Dempewolf, H., Ramirez-Villegas, J., Guarino, L., Jarvis, A., et al. 2014. "Increasing Homogeneity in Global Food Supplies and the Implications for Food Security." *Proceedings of the National Academy of Sciences* 111(11): 4001–4006.

Lachat, C., Nago, E., Roberfroid, D., Holdsworth, M., Smit, K., Kinabo, J., et al. 2014. "Developing a Sustainable Nutrition Research Agenda in Sub-Saharan Africa—Findings from the SUNRAY Project." *PLoS Medicine* 11(1): e1001593.

Macintyre, S., Ellaway, A., and Cummins, S. 2002. "Place Effects on Health: How Can We Conceptualise, Operationalise and Measure Them?" *Social Science and Medicine* 55(1): 125–139.

Mearns, R., and Norton, A., eds. 2010. *Social Dimensions of Climate Change: Equity and Vulnerability in a Warming World* (Washington, D.C.: World Bank Group).

Menon, P., and Stoltzfus, R. J. 2012. "Building Convergence in Science, Programs, and Policy Actions on Child Undernutrition: Symposium Rationale and Overview." *Advances in Nutrition: An International Review Journal* 3(2): 224–226.

Monteiro, C. A., Moubarac, J. C., Cannon, G., Ng, S. W., and Popkin, B. 2013. Ultra-Processed Products Are Becoming Dominant in the Global Food System. *Obesity Reviews* 14(S2): 21–28.

Monteiro, C. A., Moura, E. C., Conde, W. L., and Popkin, B. M. 2004. Socioeconomic Status and Obesity in Adult Populations of Developing Countries: A Review. *Bulletin of the World Health Organization* 82(12): 940–946.

Ng, M., Fleming, T., Robinson, M., Thomson, B., Graetz, N., Margono, C., et al. 2014. "Global, Regional, and National Prevalence of Overweight and Obesity in Children and Adults during 1980–2013: A Systematic Analysis for the Global Burden of Disease Study 2013." *Lancet* 384(9945): 766–781.

Nisbett, N., Gillespie, S., Haddad, L., and Harris, J. 2014. "Why Worry about the Politics of Childhood Undernutrition?" *World Development* 64: 420–433.

Nussbaum, M. C. 2011. *Creating Capabilities* (Cambridge, Mass.: Harvard University Press).

Olsson, L., Opondo, M., Tschakert, P., Agrawal, A., Eriksen, S.H., Ma, S., et al. 2014. "Livelihoods and Poverty." In *Climate Change 2014: Impacts, Adaptation, and Vulnerability. Part A: Global and Sectoral Aspects. Contribution of Working Group II to the Fifth Assessment*

Report of the Intergovernmental Panel on Climate Change, edited by C. B. Field, V. R. Barros, D. J. Dokken, K. J. Mach, M. D. Mastrandrea, T. E. Bilir, et al., 793–832. (Cambridge: Cambridge University Press).

Ong, K. K., and Loos, R. J. F. 2006. "Rapid Infancy Weight Gain and Subsequent Obesity: Systematic Reviews and Hopeful Suggestions." *Acta Paediatrica* 95(8): 904–908.

Page, H. 2013. *Global Governance and Food Security as Global Public Good* (New York: NYU Center on International Cooperation).

Pelletier, D. L., Frongillo, E. A., Jr., Shroeder, D. G., and Habicht, J. P. 1994. "A Methodology for Estimating the Contribution of Malnutrition to Child Mortality in Developing Countries." *Journal of Nutrition* 124(10): 2106S.

Pinstrup-Andersen, P. 2012. "The Food System and Its Interaction with Human Health and Nutrition." In *Reshaping Agriculture for Nutrition and Health*, edited by S. Fan and R. Pandya-Lorch, 21 (Washington, D.C.: International Food Policy Research Institute).

Popkin, B. M., Adair, L. S., and Ng, S. H. 2012. "Global Nutrition Transition and the Pandemic of Obesity in Developing Countries." *Nutrition Reviews* 70(1): 3–21.

Reardon, T., Timmer, C. P., and Minten, B. 2012. "Supermarket Revolution in Asia and Emerging Development Strategies to Include Small Farmers." *Proceedings of the National Academy of Sciences* 109(31): 12332–12337.

Reinhardt, K., and Fanzo, J. 2014. "Addressing Chronic Malnutrition through Multi-sectoral, Sustainable Approaches: A Review of the Causes and Consequences." *Frontiers in Nutrition* 1: 13.

SUN (Scaling Up Nutrition). 2013. *Progress Report* (Geneva: CFS).

Stokstad, E. 2010. "Could Less Meat Mean More Food?" *Science* 327(5967): 810–811.

Swinburn, B. A., Sacks, G., Hall, K. D., McPherson, K., Finegood, D. T., Moodie, M. L., et al. 2011. "The Global Obesity Pandemic: Shaped by Global Drivers and Local Environments." *Lancet* 378(9793): 804–814.

UNICEF (United Nations Children's Fund), WHO (World Health Organization), and World Bank. 2015. *UNICEF-WHO-World Bank Joint Child Malnutrition Estimates* (New York: UNICEF).

UNICEF (United Nations Children's Fund), WHO (World Health Organization), and World Bank. 2017. *UNICEF-WHO-World Bank Joint Child Malnutrition Estimates* (New York: UNICEF).

Vickers, M. H. 2014. "Early Life Nutrition, Epigenetics and Programming of Later Life Disease." *Nutrients* 6(6): 2165–2178.

Victora, C. G., Adair, L., Fall, C., Hallal, P. C., Martorell, R., Richter, L., et al. 2008. "Maternal and Child Undernutrition: Consequences for Adult Health and Human Capital." *Lancet* 371(9609): 340–357.

Wadhwa, P. D., Buss, C., Entringer, S., and Swanson, J. M. 2009. "Developmental Origins of Health and Disease: Brief History of the Approach and Current Focus on Epigenetic Mechanisms." *Seminars in Reproductive Medicine* 27(5): 358–368.

Walker, P., Rhubart-Berg, P., McKenzie, S., Kelling, K. and Lawrence, R. S. 2005. "Public Health Implications of Meat Production and Consumption. *Public Health Nutrition* 8(4): 348–356.

Wilkinson, J. 2009. "The Globalization of Agribusiness and Developing World Food Systems." *Monthly Review* 61(4): 38.

Winett, L. B., Wulf, A. B., and Wallack, L. 2016. "Framing Strategies to Avoid Mother-Blame in Communicating the Origins of Chronic Disease." *American Journal of Public Health* 106(8): 1369–1373.

WHO (World Health Organization). 2010. *Global Status Report on Noncommunicable Diseases 2010* (Geneva: WHO).

WHO (World Health Organization). 2014. *Global Status Report on Noncommunicable Diseases 2014* (Geneva: WHO).

You, W., and Henneberg, M. 2016. "Meat Consumption Providing a Surplus Energy in Modern Diet Contributes to Obesity Prevalence: An Ecological Analysis." *BMC Nutrition* 2(1): 1.

Zeisel, S. H., and Da Costa, K.-A. 2009. "Choline: An Essential Nutrient for Public Health." *Nutrition Reviews* 67(11): 615–623.

Zoghbi, W. A., Duncan, T., Antman, E., Barbosa, M., Champagne, B., Chen, D., et al. 2014. "Sustainable Development Goals and the Future of Cardiovascular Health: A Statement from the Global Cardiovascular Disease Taskforce." *Journal of the American Heart Association* 3(5): e000504.

Further Reading

Barker, D. J., Godfrey, K. M., Gluckman, P. D., Harding, J. E., Owens, J. A., and Robinson, J. S. 1993. "Fetal Nutrition and Cardiovascular Disease in Adult Life." *Lancet* 341(8850): 938–941.

Carletto, G., Ruel, M., Winters, P. and Zezza, A. 2015. "Farm-Level Pathways to Improved Nutritional Status: Introduction to the Special Issue." *Journal of Development Studies* 41(8): 945–957.

Field, J. O. 1987. "Multisectoral Nutrition Planning: A Post-mortem." *Food Policy* 12(1): 15–28.

Godfray, H. C. J., Beddington, J. R., Crute, I. R., Haddad, L., Lawrence, D., Muir, J. F., et al. 2010. "Food Security: The Challenge of Feeding 9 Billion People." *Science*, 327(5967): 812–818.

Harris, J. L., Pomeranz, J. L., Lobstein, T., and Brownell, K. D. 2009. "A Crisis in the Marketplace: How Food Marketing Contributes to Childhood Obesity and What Can Be Done." *Annual Review of Public Health* 30: 211–225.

HLPE (High Level Panel of Experts on Food Security and Nutrition). 2017. *Nutrition and Food systems* (Rome: Committee on World Food Security).

Levine, R., and Kuczynski, D. 2009. *Global Nutrition Institutions: Is There an Appetite for Change?* (Washington, D.C.: Center for Global Development).

Rothstein, M. A., Cai, Y., and Marchant, G. E. 2009. "The Ghost in Our Genes: Legal and Ethical Implications of Epigenetics." *Health Matrix* 19(1): 1.

Van Huis, A., Van Itterbeeck, J., Klunder, H., Mertens, E., Halloran, A., Muir, G., et al. 2013. *Edible Insects: Future Prospects for Food and Feed Security* (New York: Food and Agriculture Organization of the United Nations).

Wallack, L., and Thornburg, K. 2016. "Developmental Origins, Epigenetics, and Equity: Moving Upstream." *Maternal and Child Health Journal* 20(5): 935–940.

CHAPTER 50

OBESITY PREVENTION AND PROMOTION OF GOOD NUTRITION: PUBLIC HEALTH ETHICS ISSUES

ANNE BARNHILL

INTRODUCTION

RECENT decades have seen sharp increases in overweight and obesity worldwide (Ng et al., 2014). According to public health organizations and experts, these high rates of overweight and obesity have significant consequences for public health, increasing the risk for diet-related disease and causing an estimated 3.4 million deaths worldwide in 2010 (Lim et al., 2013). Along with the human cost—in terms of illness and early death—obesity and diet-related disease have significant financial costs (Finkelstein et al., 2009). To many researchers and policymakers, this "obesity epidemic" demands a comprehensive response by public health and the global community more generally (IOM and CAPOP, 2012; WHO, 2013). Yet some aspects of the public health response to obesity have generated ethical controversy. This chapter introduces obesity prevention and then discusses some ethical concerns with efforts to foster healthy eating. Though obesity prevention encompasses both efforts to increase physical activity and to promote healthy eating, this chapter focuses on the latter efforts because they have generated more controversy.

Explanations of Unhealthy Eating and Obesity

Researchers have created complex models of eating behavior (e.g., Afshin et al.'s (2014) "barriers and opportunities for healthy eating," or Story et al.'s (2008) "ecological framework depicting the multiple influences on what people eat") that identify a wide variety of influences on eating behavior. These influences include facets of the individual, aspects of the community environment, social and cultural influences, policies, and basic structural features of societies. According to many such models and frameworks, individual behavior should be understood in the context of local food environments, which are situated within larger systems. These larger systems include national and international policies and rules, as well as structural features of societies, such as economic systems or health care systems.

Some features of local food environments identified as influencing eating include pervasive and low-cost packaged food and fast food; aggressive marketing that makes these foods desirable and socially normative; and the lesser availability and higher cost of healthier foods such as fruits, vegetables, and whole grains (Afshin et al., 2014; Story et al., 2008; Schwartz and Brownell, 2007). For example, Schwartz and Brownell (2007, 79–80) give a vivid description of the food environment as a "toxic environment":

> Driving down the highway, we see dozens of drive through windows at fast food restaurants, billboards with advertisements for inexpensive snacks, and soft drinks at drugstores, and when we stop for gas, shelf after shelf of high-fat and high-sugar snacks at gas station mini marts.... A variety of good tasting snacks and meals are now highly visible and accessible for most Americans, and there is also evidence that since the 1970's, portion sizes have gotten larger, and far exceed federal guidelines. These foods are also extremely convenient compared with home made meals, fast food and packaged foods are easier to obtain and ready to eat immediately, as they require little preparation .... Another layer of the toxic environment that promotes the consumption of unhealthful foods is their heavy promotion by the food industry.

This "toxic environment" interacts with human biology and psychology to create obesity, according to Schwartz and Brownell.

Moving out from the local environment, there are broader systems, policies, and social forces cited as creating local food environments and causing obesity. These include rising incomes in developing countries, which lead to dietary shifts toward energy-dense and less healthy foods in those countries, also known as the "nutrition transition" (Popkin, Adair, and Ng, 2012); lifestyles that discourage physical activity, encouraged by technological advances and transportation and zoning policy, such as policies that encourage commuting by car rather than public transportation or bicycle (Lang and Rayner, 2007); agricultural policies, such as subsidies for corn and soy that have led to an excess of cheap corn and soy, which are used in sugary and high-fat processed foods;

technological advances in food processing and distribution that have increased the availability of convenient, high-calorie foods (Finkelstein and Zuckerman, 2008); and so on. Some scholars offer even "bigger picture" explanations of obesity, arguing that neoliberalism—the political economic system emphasizing free market capitalism and a minimal state—contributes to increasing rates of obesity, in part because it encourages seeing consumer choice as a right, and thus seeing government regulation of the food marketplace as illegitimate (Guthman and DuPuis, 2006; Wilkerson, 2010).

Obesity Prevention Efforts

As the previous chapter, "Malnutrition, Public Health, and Ethics," discussed, there are multiple influences on unhealthy eating and obesity that occur at multiple levels. Accordingly, efforts to promote healthy diets target these multiple levels. A contrast is sometimes drawn between *individual-focused* approaches and *environment-focused* approaches (Roberto et al., 2015; Brownell et al., 2010; Kirkland, 2011), but in fact multiple kinds of obesity efforts can be distinguished, including efforts focused on changing how individuals interact with their environments, such as individual weight-loss interventions; policies that directly change local food environments, such as opening more grocery stores in underserved neighborhoods; policies affecting the food supply and food marketplace, such as agricultural subsidies, or regulations limiting the amount of sodium or trans-fat packaged foods; and policies addressing broader social and economic factors that influence health, such as policies that increase access to health care, improve public transportation, and reduce poverty.

Although these approaches are distinct, they are not mutually exclusive and could be pursued simultaneously. Indeed, given the complexity of obesity, it is likely that complementary approaches are required. For example, the World Cancer Research Fund International's NOURISHING framework identifies ten focal policy areas for healthy eating and the prevention of diet-related disease (WCRF, 2016). These include policies focused on behavior change; policies focused on changing the food environment, such as restrictions on advertising, as well as subsidies and taxes to change consumer choices; and policies focused on food system change, such as incentivizing the production of healthier foods.

Given the limited effectiveness of individual-focused efforts, such as nutrition education or weight-loss interventions, researchers and advocates commonly claim that such efforts are not sufficient and need to be supplemented or replaced with environment-focused interventions, as the NOURISHING framework does (Story et al., 2008; Schwartz and Brownell, 2007; Roberto et al., 2015). But some scholars go farther, arguing that, given the limited effectiveness of obesity prevention efforts in general, the public policy focus should be on policies addressing broader social and economic factors that influence health, policies accomplishing multiple goals at once, and *not* policies focusing on obesity prevention per se (Williams, 2015). For example, Garrath Williams (2015) points to the mixed and disappointing evidence on community-level obesity prevention efforts. He suggests that the public policy focus should *not* be on wider implementation of community-level efforts, but rather on public policies that address broader social and economic factors that influence health. Julie Guthman (2011) and Anna Kirkland (2011) also call for a shift in attention from efforts to change the food environment to broader social policies, such as policies that increase access to health care and transportation.

Despite these critical voices, expert recommendations remain focused on addressing obesity directly. They typically highlight the need to change food environments and the composition of products available in the marketplace, as well as encouraging individual behavior change (WHO, 2013; IOM and CAPOP, 2012; Roberto et al., 2015).

Ethical Concerns with Obesity Efforts

Obesity prevention and healthy eating efforts raise a range of ethical issues. For example, ten Have et al. (2013, 305) identify eight potential ethical pitfalls with obesity prevention efforts: these efforts may negatively affect "physical health, psychosocial well-being, equality, informed choice, social and cultural values, privacy and the attribution of responsibilities and liberty."

The remainder of this chapter discusses a few of these ethical pitfalls. Along the way, some ethical arguments *for* obesity prevention are also discussed.

Justice, Equality, and Fairness

One set of ethical concerns centers on justice, equity, and fairness. First, consider high-income countries. Some argue that the higher rate of overweight/obesity and diet-related diseases among some racial/ethnic minority groups and lower-income populations is an equity and justice issue, and that there is thus a justice-based ethical reason to focus preventive efforts on these groups (Kumanyika, 2005). Obesity prevention efforts that provide resources or increase food access—such as efforts to increase food access for low-income populations and in underserved areas—address multiple justice-based concerns. Not only do these efforts address health disparities, they also address disparities in food access that are seen as a separate and important justice issue. Access to healthy, culturally appropriate food is seen as an important resource; inadequate access is seen as a failure of distributive justice; and increased food access is a central goal of the food justice movement (Alkon and Agyeman, 2011; Szende, 2015). Inadequate food access is also seen as the result of other injustices, such as institutional racism (Szende, 2015).

When society turns to obesity efforts that restrict or disincentivize options, or that penalize certain behaviors, quite different justice-based and fairness-based arguments are made. Financial disincentives, such as taxes on sugary drinks, or higher health insurance premiums for employees who do not participate in employer wellness programs to promote healthy eating and physical activity, are objected to as regressive (that is, they take a larger percentage of the income of low-income people), and as unfair or inequitable for that reason (Barry, Niederdeppe, and Gollust, 2013). Some object to the perceived inequity of "targeting" low-income and minority groups with efforts that may not be welcome and that smack of "micromanaging" their personal choices (Kirkland, 2011; Barnhill and King, 2013). In response, others argue that disadvantaged groups have the most to gain from taxes on sugary drinks, because they have higher rates of obesity. Thus, far from being regressive and unfair, these efforts can disproportionately *benefit* disadvantaged groups (Barry, Niederdeppe, and Gollust, 2013).

Turning to low- and middle-income countries, there is a complex relationship between disadvantage and diet-related disease. Some, but not all, risk factors and diet-related diseases are more prevalent in lower-income populations (Di Cesare et al., 2013). This raises a distinct equity question: As increasing attention is put on reducing the global burden of diet-related illness, will this burden be reduced in an equitable way (Di Cesare et al., 2013; Schmidt and Barnhill, 2015)? Will scarce resources in low- and middle-income countries be spent disproportionately on prevention and treatment for better-off, middle-class populations that have more political power? Some have argued that there is an ethical demand to focus prevention on the most disadvantaged populations in these countries (Schmidt and Barnhill, 2015).

Stigma and Moral Blame

A second set of ethical pitfalls with obesity efforts concerns stigma, responsibility, and moral blame. Scholars and activists have criticized the public conversation about obesity as characterized by negative moral judgments of overweight people, including the view that they are lazy or lack self-control (Puhl and Heuer, 2010); the "belittling" view that overweight people are victims of their environments and do not exercise their agency (Guthman, 2007; Kirkland, 2011); and the inappropriate attribution of responsibility and moral blame to overweight people for being overweight, when in fact overweight has environmental and social causes, and thus is not something individuals cause and not something that individuals should be morally blamed for or held liable for. Some discussions of obesity and responsibility combine distinct kinds of responsibility that, as a matter of ethical reasoning, ought to be distinguished, such as causal responsibility (e.g., whether individuals caused their overweight, or whether it was caused by external factors), role responsibility (e.g., whether it is the individual's role to ensure healthy eating, or whether this is society's job, or both), blameworthiness (e.g., whether people deserves moral blame for their eating habits or body weight, and whether the food industry deserves moral blame for its actions), and liability (e.g., whether people should be held liable for the higher costs associated with eating behavior or weight, for example by paying taxes on junk food or paying higher health insurance premiums if they are overweight). Wikler (1987) offers a helpful discussion of distinct notions of responsibility at play in discussions of health.

Some scholars question whether public concern with obesity and diet-related disease derives primarily from concern for public health, or whether it instead reflects something else, such as bias against overweight and obese people, moral judgments about people who are overweight or obese, or an aesthetic preference for thinness. A related argument is that public concern with obesity is an instance of "moral panic," in which groups or behaviors seen as deviant come to be seen as a threat to society, typically involving an exaggeration of risks. (Campos, 2006; Guthman, 2007).

Some specific obesity prevention efforts have also been called stigmatizing, such as public information campaigns meant to evoke guilt, shame, scorn, and other negative emotions (Kliff, 2012; Abu-Odeh, 2014; Fairchild, Bayer, and Colgrove, 2015). Researchers have argued that stigmatization is counterproductive in reducing obesity (Goldberg and Puhl, 2013). Stigma increases stress and unhealthy eating, reduces the quality of care provided to overweight people, and reduces their utilization of health care (Puhl and Heuer, 2010). Stigmatizing obesity efforts also runs the risk of exacerbating background discrimination against people who are overweight and obese. The consensus among ethicists is that the stigmatization of overweight and obesity is counterproductive and ethically inappropriate, though there may be some vagueness about what stigma in fact is. "Stigma" and "stigmatization" are used by some authors to refer to a specific kind of social sanction that is severe and all-encompassing, involving a loss of status, shame, and self-punishment. But other authors and researchers use these terms more loosely so that they refer to public disapproval, social marginalization, self-directed shame, and other related phenomena (Bayer, 2008a; Bayer, 2008b; Burris, 2008). A useful definition comes from Andrew Courtwright (2013, 78), who states that "for an institution to stigmatize a health related characteristic or behavior involves changing norms about the desirability of the activity, marking the bearers of the trait, and excluding them from the broader community, a process that can, but does not necessarily, create a spoiled social identity."

Choice, Paternalism, and Regulation of the Marketplace

A third set of ethical concerns with healthy eating and obesity efforts focuses on choice, paternalism, and government regulation of the marketplace. Recommended obesity policies typically include increased regulation of the food industry, such as reformulating, taxing, or banning products and placing restrictions on food marketing. These regulations are sometimes framed as protecting consumers from a food industry that not only imperils health but also undermines consumer autonomy by misleading, deceiving, manipulating, or exploiting consumers (Nestle and Ludwig, 2010; Frieden, 2013; Roberto et al., 2015; Farley, 2015). Public resistance to these aggressive regulations is sometimes explained as the result of industry influence, with the industry working behind the scenes to shape public opinion (Nestle, 2007; Frieden, 2013; Farley, 2015;

Aaron and Siegel, 2017; Kearns, Schmidt, and Glantz, 2016). But this resistance should not be dismissed without careful examination, because it reflects long-standing ethical objections to government paternalism.

Governmental efforts to promote healthier eating are sometimes derided as instances of the "nanny state." This complaint reveals philosophical objections to paternalistic policies that interfere with individuals' choices or actions in an effort to improve those individuals' welfare, such as policies banning the sale of certain products like large sugary drinks or food made with trans fats (Dworkin, 2017). Paternalistic policies are objected to as counterproductive—since individuals are better placed than the government to know and to promote their own welfare—and as violating individual autonomy (Feinberg, 1986; Dworkin, 1972; Mill, 2002), though theorists disagree about when paternalistic interference amounts to a problematic violation of individual autonomy, and when it is ethically inappropriate, all things considered (Feinberg, 1986; Conly, 2013). Paternalism is also objected to as degrading, demeaning, failing to treat people as equals, or assuming that people value health more than they actually do (Conly, 2013; Noë, 2012; Pugh, 2014).

In the context of obesity efforts, increasing evidence from behavioral economics that humans are prone to cognitive biases and are "systematically irrational" casts doubt on a human ability to make food choices that promote welfare (Sunstein, 2014; Thaler and Sunstein, 2008). In response to the autonomy objection, Sarah Conly (2013, 2014) has argued that paternalistic policies that prevent irrational eating, such as limits on portion sizes in restaurants, can be ethically justifiable even though they violate autonomy; such policies respect the person by helping one accomplish long-term goals of staying healthy and living a long life—goals that virtually everyone has, according to Conly.

Some theorists argue that autonomy and self-determination must be distinguished from unfettered choice, and that unfettered choice is not necessary for autonomy or self-determination, and in fact can undermine them (such as when people choose unhealthy lifestyles). Being able to exercise control over our lives and determine the shape of our lives requires some level of health; thus, choice-limiting public health policies may promote long-term autonomy or self-determination (Conly, 2013).

Taking a step back, some argue that obesity efforts that limit choice should not even be seen as *paternalistic* policies, because their ultimate aim is not just to increase individual welfare, but also to reduce the social costs of poor health and advance the common good (Bayer and Moreno, 1986; Gostin and Gostin, 2009). Illness has social costs, and some ethicists have argued that healthy eating policies should be seen not as policies aimed at improving each citizen's health in order to increase that citizen's own welfare, but as policies aiming to improve each citizen's health in order to reduce the social costs of illness and advance the common good (Gostin and Gostin, 2009). Relatedly, the health costs associated with diet-related illnesses are sometimes framed as externalities that are unfairly imposed on others by those whose eating behavior is unhealthy; on this line of thought, healthy eating efforts are seen as ways to reduce these unfair burdens, not just as efforts to help the targeted individuals themselves.

As an alternative to choice-limiting policies and efforts, Richard Thaler and Cass Sunstein (2008) propose *libertarian paternalism*, or efforts to change people's behavior in ways that will improve their welfare, but without blocking any choices or attaching significant costs to any choices. Examples include "nudges" like putting healthy food first in a cafeteria line, since people are more likely to choose the food that comes first (Thaler and Sunstein, 2008). Though libertarian paternalism does not limit choice, it has still faced many of the same objections made to choice-limiting paternalistic policies. For example, criticisms include that the government will not succeed in making people better off by using nudges, since the government is not well placed to know what is good for us (Sunstein, 2014). Nudging has also been criticized as being demeaning or disrespectful, or as not respecting autonomy, because it does not treat people as rational agents capable of making good decisions for themselves (Hausman and Welch, 2010; Waldron, 2014). Nudging has also been criticized as overly controlling or manipulative (Saghai, 2013; Waldron, 2014).

Conclusion

The existing ethical conversation captures many ethical dimensions of obesity prevention efforts, including the fairness of policies, their stigmatizing potential, and the ethics of limiting choice. Are these efforts fair? Do they make the distribution of food, health, and opportunities to be healthy more equitable and more just, or less equitable and less just? Do these efforts stigmatize people in counterproductive or unethical ways? Is "obesity epidemic" discourse problematic because of the assumptions or moral judgments latent in it? Do some obesity efforts limit individual choice in ethically inappropriate ways, or is this choice limitation ethically justifiable as a way to protect individuals from industry influence and help them achieve their own ends?

This ethical conversation would be enriched it if more fully incorporated a discussion of the *value of eating* (Barnhill et al., 2014). Food provides sustenance, comfort, hedonic pleasure, and aesthetic pleasure to individuals. Sharing food is a foundational experience in virtually all kinds of human relationships and social groups. Patterns of eating express personal and group identities (Anderson, 2014; Rozin and Siegal, 2003; Guptill, Copelton, and Lucal, 2013). In short, eating—even unhealthy eating—has social meaning and value for individuals and groups (Resnik, 2010; Barnhill et al., 2014).

Conversely, healthy eating can have disvalue. Efforts to adopt healthier eating patterns can have a range of costs for individuals and families, include psychological costs (e.g., stress, discouragement), social costs (e.g., changing dietary patterns can cause tension with family members who don't like the changes), and economic costs (e.g., spending more money on food, or spending more time cooking) (Devine and Barnhill, 2017). A vivid portrayal of these costs comes from a study of mothers' experiences making home-cooked meals, with 150 mothers of different incomes levels and racial/ethnic backgrounds (Bowen, Elliott, and Brenton, 2014). For these mothers, making home-cooked meals could take time away from other valuable experiences, such as helping a child with her homework. It also required a predictable work schedule, which not all have, and it required foresight and planning. Making home-cooked meals also had discernible personal and social costs: "We rarely observed a meal in which at least one family member didn't complain about the food they were served," the researchers reported (Bowen, Elliott, and Brenton, 2014, 24).

A discussion of value is already included, in a limited way, in discussions of healthy eating efforts. Commentators have noted that these efforts promote health—a valuable state—at the expense of pleasure and convenience, which are ways that some consumers find unhealthy foods valuable. But a broader examination of the ways in which eating has value and disvalue would enrich the ethical conversation, clarifying what is really at stake for individuals and groups when public health experts try to change their eating habits.

A more detailed understanding of the value of unhealthy eating could also help us design healthy eating efforts that preserve the social and personal value of unhealthy eating experiences while making these experiences healthier. An example would be a policy that incrementally changes how children's birthdays are celebrated at school, replacing sweets with healthier foods as the means of celebration (Barnhill et al., 2014). If we understand what people find valuable and disvaluable about unhealthy eating, we'll have more luck designing policies that improve unhealthy eating experiences while retaining their value. Such policies may be more likely to be successful at changing behavior, more likely to garner public support, and less likely to trigger ethical complaints.

References

Aaron, D. G., and Siegel, M. B. 2017. "Sponsorship of National Health Organizations by Two Major Soda Companies." *American Journal of Preventive Medicine* 52(1): 20–30.

Abu-Odeh, D. 2014. "Fat Stigma and Public Health: A Theoretical Framework and Ethical Analysis." *Kennedy Institute of Ethics Journal* 24(3): 247–265.

Afshin, A., Micha, R., Khatibzadeh, S., Schmidt, L. A., and Mozaffarian, D. 2014. "Dietary Policies to Reduce Noncommunicable Diseases." In *The Handbook of Global Health Policy*, edited by G. W. Brown, G. Yamey, and S. Wamala, 177–193 (Chichester, UK: John Wiley & Sons). doi:10.1002/9781118509623.ch9.

Alkon, A. H., and Agyeman, J. 2011. *Cultivating Food Justice: Race, Class, and Sustainability* (Cambridge, Mass.: MIT Press).

Anderson, E. N. 2014. *Everyone Eats: Understanding Food and Culture* (New York: NYU Press).

Barnhill, A., and King, K. F. 2013. "Evaluating Equity Critiques in Food Policy: The Case of Sugar-Sweetened Beverages." *Journal of Law, Medicine & Ethics* 41(1): 301–309.

Barnhill, A., King, K. F., Kass, N., and Faden, R. 2014. "The Value of Unhealthy Eating and the Ethics of Healthy Eating Policies." *Kennedy Institute of Ethics Journal* 24(3): 187–217.

Barry, C. L., Niederdeppe, J., and Gollust, S. E. 2013. "Taxes on Sugar-Sweetened Beverages: Results from a 2011 National Public Opinion Survey." *American Journal of Preventive Medicine* 44(2): 158–163.

Bayer R. 2008a. "Stigma and The Ethics of Public Health: Not Can We but Should We." *Social Science and Medicine* 67(3): 463–472.

Bayer, R. 2008b. "What Means This Thing Called Stigma? A Response to Burris." *Social Science and Medicine* 67(3): 476–477.

Bayer, R., and Moreno, J. D. 1986. "Health Promotion: Ethical and Social Dilemmas of Government Policy." *Health Affairs* 5(2): 72–85.

Bowen, S., Elliott, S., and Brenton, J. 2014. "The Joy of Cooking?" *Contexts* 13(3): 20–25.

Brownell, K. D., Kersh, R., Ludwig, D. S., Post, R. C., Puhl, R. M., Schwartz, M. B., et al. 2010. "Personal Responsibility and Obesity: A Constructive Approach to a Controversial Issue." *Health Affairs* 29(3): 379–387.

Burris, S. 2008. "Stigma, Ethics and Policy: A Commentary on Bayer's "Stigma and the Ethics of Public Health: Not Can We but Should We." *Social Science and Medicine* 67(3): 473–475.

Campos, P. 2006. "Fat and the Politics of Fear." *Health at Every Size* 20(3): 133.

Conly, S. 2013. *Against Autonomy: Justifying Coercive Paternalism* (Cambridge: Cambridge University Press).

Conly, S. 2014. "Against Autonomy: Justifying Coercive Paternalism." *Journal of Medical Ethics* 40(5): 349–351.

Courtwright, A. 2013. "Stigmatization and Public Health Ethics." *Bioethics* 27(2): 74–80.

Devine, C. M., and Barnhill, A. 2017. "The Ethical and Public Health Importance of Unintended Consequences: The Case of Behavioral Weight Loss Interventions." *Public Health Ethics* (Online First, December 20). doi:10.1093/phe/phx026.

Di Cesare, M., Khang, Y. H., Asaria, P., Blakely, T., Cowan, M. J., Farzadfar, F., et al. 2013. "Inequalities in Non-communicable Diseases and Effective Responses." *Lancet* 381(9866): 585–597.

Dworkin, G. 1972. "Paternalism." *Monist* 56(1): 64–84.

Dworkin, G. 2017. "Paternalism." In *The Stanford Encyclopedia of Philosophy* (Stanford, Calif.: Stanford University). Article first published 2002; revised 2017. https://plato.stanford.edu/archives/spr2017/entries/paternalism/.

Fairchild, A. L., Bayer, R., and Colgrove, J. 2015. "Risky Business: New York City's Experience with Fear-Based Public Health Campaigns." *Health Affairs* 34(5): 844–851.

Farley, T. A. 2015. "The Problem with Focusing on Childhood Obesity." *New York Times*, December 18. https://www.nytimes.com/2015/12/18/opinion/the-problem-with-focusing-on-childhood-obesity.html.

Feinberg, J. 1986. *Harm to Self* (New York: Oxford University Press).

Finkelstein, E. A., Trogdon, J. G., Cohen, J. W., and Dietz, W. 2009. "Annual Medical Spending Attributable to Obesity: Payer- and Service-Specific Estimates." *Health Affairs* 28(5): w822–w831.

Finkelstein, E. A., and Zuckerman, L. 2008. *The Fattening of America: How the Economy Makes Us Fat, If It Matters, and What to Do about It* (Hoboken, N.J.: John Wiley & Sons).

Frieden, T. R. 2013. "Government's Role in Protecting Health and Safety." *New England Journal of Medicine* 368(20): 1857–1859.

Goldberg, D. S., and Puhl, R. M. 2013. "Obesity Stigma: A Failed and Ethically Dubious Strategy." *Hastings Center Report* 43(3): 5–6.

Gostin, L. O., and Gostin, K. G. 2009. "A Broader Liberty: J. S. Mill, Paternalism and the Public's Health." *Public Health* 123(3): 214–221.

Guptill, A. E., Copelton, D. A., and Lucal, B. 2013. *Food and Society: Principles and Paradoxes* (Hoboken, N.J.: John Wiley & Sons).

Guthman, J. 2007. "Can't Stomach It: How Michael Pollan et al. Made Me Want to Eat Cheetos." *Gastronomica* 7(3): 75–79.

Guthman, J. 2011. *Weighing in: Obesity, Food Justice, and the Limits of Capitalism* (Berkeley: University of California Press).

Guthman J., and DuPuis, M. 2006. "Embodying Neoliberalism: Economy, Culture, and the Politics of Fat." *Environment and Planning D: Society and Space* 24(3): 427–448. doi:10.1068/d3904.

Hausman, D. M., and Welch, B. 2010. "Debate: To Nudge or Not to Nudge." *Journal of Political Philosophy* 18(1): 123–136.

IOM (Institute of Medicine), and CAPOP (Committee on Accelerating Progress in Obesity Prevention). 2012. *Accelerating Progress in Obesity Prevention: Solving the Weight of the Nation* (Washington, D.C.: National Academies Press).

Kearns, C. E., Schmidt, L. A., and Glantz, S. A. 2016. "Sugar Industry and Coronary Heart Disease Research: A Historical Analysis of Internal Industry Documents." *JAMA Internal Medicine* 176(11): 1680–1685.

Kirkland, A. 2011. "The Environmental Account of Obesity: A Case for Feminist Skepticism." *Signs* 36(2): 463–485.

Kliff, S. 2012. "Georgia's Shocking Anti-Obesity Ad Campaign." *Washington Post Blogs*, January 3. https://www.washingtonpost.com/blogs/wonkblog/post/georgias-shocking-anti-obesity-ad-campaign/2012/01/03/gIQAZB8HYP_blog.html.

Kumanyika, S. 2005. "Obesity, Health Disparities, and Prevention Paradigms: Hard Questions and Hard Choices." *Preventing Chronic Disease* 2(4): 1.

Lang, T., and Rayner, G. 2007. "Overcoming Policy Cacophony on Obesity: An Ecological Public Health Framework for Policymakers." *Obesity Reviews* 8(Suppl. 1): 165–181.

Lim, S. S., Vos, T., Flaxman, A. D., Danaei, G., Shibuya, K., Adair-Rohani, H., et al. 2013. "A Comparative Risk Assessment of Burden of Disease and Injury Attributable to 67 Risk Factors and Risk Factor Clusters in 21 Regions, 1990–2010: A Systematic Analysis for the Global Burden of Disease Study 2010." *Lancet* 380(9859): 2224–2260.

Mill, J. S. 2002. *On Liberty* (Mineola, N.Y.: Dover).

Nestle, M. 2007. *Food Politics: How the Food Industry Influences Nutrition and Health* (Berkeley: University of California Press).

Nestle, M., and Ludwig, D. S. 2010. "Front-of-Package Food Labels: Public Health or Propaganda?" *JAMA* 303(8): 771–772.

Ng, M., Fleming, T., Robinson, M., Thomson, B., Graetz, N., Margono, C., et al. 2014. "Global, Regional, and National Prevalence of Overweight and Obesity in Children and Adults during 1980–2013: A Systematic Analysis for the Global Burden of Disease Study 2013." *Lancet* 384(9945): 766–781.

Noë, A. 2012. "The Value in Sweet Drinks?" *Cosmos and Culture* (blog), National Public Radio, September 24. http://www.npr.org/blogs/13.7/2012/09/24/161277720/the-value-in-sweet-drinks.

Popkin, B. M., Adair, L. S., and Ng, S. W. 2012. "Global Nutrition Transition and the Pandemic of Obesity in Developing Countries." *Nutrition Reviews* 70(1): 3–21.

Pugh, J. 2014. "Coercive Paternalism and Back-Door Perfectionism." *Journal of Medical Ethics* 40(5): 350–351.

Puhl, R. M., and Heuer, C. A. 2010. "Obesity Stigma: Important Considerations for Public Health." *American Journal of Public Health* 100(6): 1019–1028.

Resnik, D. 2010. "Trans Fat Bans and Human Freedom." *American Journal of Bioethics* 10(3): 29.

Roberto, C. A., Swinburn, B., Hawkes, C., Huang, T. T., Costa, S. A., Ashe, M., et al. 2015. "Patchy Progress on Obesity Prevention: Emerging Examples, Entrenched Barriers, and New Thinking." *Lancet* 385(9985): 2400–2409.

Rozin, P., and Siegal, M. 2003. "Vegemite as a Marker of National Identity." *Gastronomica* 3(4): 63–67.

Saghai, Y. 2013. "Salvaging the Concept of Nudge." *Journal of Medical Ethics* 39(8): 487–493.

Schmidt, H., and Barnhill, A. 2015. "Equity and Noncommunicable Disease Reduction under the Sustainable Development Goals." *PLoS Medicine* 12(9): e1001872.

Schwartz, M. B., and Brownell, K. D. 2007. "Actions Necessary to Prevent Childhood Obesity: Creating the Climate for Change." *Journal of Law, Medicine & Ethics* 35(1): 78–89.

Story, M., Kaphingst, K. M., Robinson-O'Brien, R., and Glanz, K. 2008. "Creating Healthy Food and Eating Environments: Policy and Environmental Approaches." *Annual Review of Public Health* 29: 253–272.

Sunstein, C. R. 2014. *Why Nudge?: The Politics of Libertarian Paternalism* (New Haven, Conn.: Yale University Press).

Szende, I. 2015. "Food Deserts, Justice and the Distributive Paradigm." In *Just Food: Philosophy, Justice and Food*, edited by J. M. Dieterle, 57–67 (London: Rowman and Littlefield International).

ten Have, M., Van Der Heide, A., Mackenbach, J. P., and De Beaufort, I. D. 2013. "An Ethical Framework for the Prevention of Overweight and Obesity: A Tool for Thinking through a Programme's Ethical Aspects." *European Journal of Public Health* 23(2): 299–305.

Thaler, R.H., and Sunstein, C. 2008. *Nudge: Improving Decisions about Health, Wealth, and Happiness* (New Haven, Conn.: Yale University Press).

Waldron, J. 2014. "It's All for Your Own Good." *New York Review of Books*, October 9. http://www.nybooks.com/articles/2014/10/09/cass-sunstein-its-all-your-own-good/.

WCRF (World Cancer Research Fund International). 2016. NOURISHING Framework. http://www.wcrf.org/int/policy/nourishing-framework.

WHO (World Health Organization). 2013. *Global Action Plan for the Prevention and Control of Non-Communicable Diseases 2013–2020* (Geneva: World Health Organization).

Wikler, D. 1987. "Who Should Be Blamed for Being Sick?" *Health Education and Behavior* 14(1): 11–25.

Wilkerson, A. 2010. "'Obesity,' the Transnational Plate, and the Thin Contract." *Radical Philosophy Review* 13(1): 43–67. doi:10.5840/radphilrev20101314.

Williams, G. 2015. "The IDEFICS Intervention: What Can We Learn for Public Policy?" *Obesity Reviews* 16(Suppl. 2): 151–161.

SECTION ELEVEN

INJURIES

CHAPTER 51

AN OVERVIEW OF THE ETHICS OF INJURY IN PUBLIC HEALTH

ADNAN A. HYDER

Introduction

OVER 4.6 million people die from injuries globally each year, making injuries one of the leading causes of death and disability around the world (IHME, 2016). The majority of these deaths occur in low- and middle-income countries (LMICs), where 90 percent of the world's population reside and vulnerable populations abound (Gosselin et al., 2009). While injuries affect people of all ages, genders, and socioeconomic status, the poor are more at risk, especially in LMICs (Hyder and Peden, 2003). In LMICs, unmitigated risk factors dominate, exposures to risks predominate, investments in safety are low, and access to quality care is variable. As a result, addressing the burden of injuries in LMICs is critical to reducing the burden of injuries globally.

Global health investments are currently not optimally directed toward injury prevention, and international health organizations are not primarily focusing on injuries (Lopez, 2008; Stuckler et al., 2008). Stimulating this area of attention requires that the public health community prioritize critical assessments of injury burden and risk factors, test and evaluate known interventions, and develop new interventions for application in those settings, with particular attention to LMICs. Such efforts have implications for human subjects in research, international collaborations, vulnerable populations, and legal interventions. Public health work in injury and trauma[1] thus invokes ethics issues that are both similar to other public health work and also specific to this area. Because public health attention and analyses of these ethics issues have been somewhat limited, they require further elaboration and reflection from those working in the fields of public health, injury prevention, biomedical ethics, and global health.

Types of Ethics Issues

Injuries can be intentional (involving an intent to cause damage), such as homicides, suicides, or assaults; or unintentional (without the intent to cause physical damage), such as road traffic injuries, falls, or burns (Norton, Hyder, and Butchart, 2011). Few papers in the literature have discussed the ethics of injury prevention and control, especially in LMICs. Some have focused on research, while others present a more general ethics approach to public health. For example, Elana Newman, Elizabeth Risch, and Nancy Kassam-Adams (2006) reviewed the ethics of trauma-related research focusing on post-traumatic stress disorder (PTSD), psychiatric stress, and psychological distress; they discuss research on such victims and promote a "flexible" approach that "counters assumptions and biases" (29) against the victims. Public health ethics issues around injury prevention and control are both varied and complex. Some of them relate to gaps in public health programs, others to deeper equity issues, and others to global health challenges. A few examples are presented below.

Interventions, such as helmets for motorcycle riders, poison control centers, and smoke alarms, have been implemented in high-income countries (HICs) for some time, but have not been widely tested in LMICs. Can they be tested ethically in a new context? How does this relate to background inequities, especially in a low-income context?

Vulnerable groups can be defined with respect to the distribution and impact of specific injuries. For example, in the field of road traffic injuries, "vulnerable road users" are defined as pedestrians, motorcyclists, and bicyclists. First, their vulnerability is defined by their socioeconomic status, which is assumed to be lower than car owners, especially in an LMIC context (those who use a bicycle or walk by choice are assumed to be a smaller proportion of people on the road). Second, their vulnerability is related to their exposure to the risk of road traffic injuries as they traverse the road with no physical structure between them and other vehicles. Third, this vulnerability is further magnified, since access to urgent care and medical treatment is often determined both by economic and social status. Therefore, a public health ethics analysis questions why such vulnerable populations are not protected and how public health programs can ensure their protection in a timely and effective manner, with attention to the fact that high-income countries have implemented these interventions for many years.

As mentioned above, both the magnitude and nature of the burden of injuries are greater in LMICs. Thus, public health action and research are greatly needed to address the problem and define appropriate solutions. Excluding populations in such countries from research, for example, would be a serious justice issue if the people who need the most benefit are not part of either programs or research. However, their vulnerability means that both general protections for all human subjects and special protections are needed to ensure that such actions are relevant and provide benefit.

Elihu D. Richter and colleagues (2001) analyzed a case study of a public-sector decision to increase speeds on interurban roads in Israel, and they claim that such a policy change was unethical. They report that the increase in speed limits, in the face of significant evidence to the contrary, led to a predictable increase in deaths and crashes along specific roads in Israel;

and that, in the absence of pre-hoc decision guidelines to stop the change in the speed limit, the decision amounted to "unfettered human experimentation" (Richter et al, 2001, 129). Such analysis reveals two critical questions: Can the promulgation of public sector laws be considered "experimental," and do they require the principles of ethics as a guideline?

The principle of autonomy requires implementation of informed consent to ensure that participation in public health programs by people is both voluntary and based on good information. In injury prevention and control, the application of informed consent can be challenging in specific circumstances. For example, subjects may not know they are being observed as part of injury programs—this can happen in contexts of observations of large numbers of human subjects for actions or safety devices that are clearly visible. The best examples come from the field of road traffic injury research, such as observations of how many motorcycle riders wear a helmet at a junction, red light, or gas station, or monitoring the speed of vehicles as they pass a fixed point or intersection. In these cases, the individuals do not know they are part of a monitoring process; however, the methods are minimally intrusive. Another example of challenging circumstances around consent arises in the field of emergency care. Injured patients may arrive at an emergency room unconscious and need to be registered in a quality assurance database, or injuries may be so severe that, despite consciousness, it is neither timely nor appropriate to take consent. Many experts indicate that adults exposed to even severe injury or trauma can give informed consent, but this is a point of debate within the ethics field (Fontes, 2004; Rosenstein, 2004).

Injuries often occur within a social context where either the causation of the injury or its consequences are a source of social stigma. Acid burns to women, usually on the face, and injuries that lead to visible disabilities often result not only in physical incapacitation, but also in negative social responses. Work on these types of injuries carries with it special risks—people might be put at risk for more stigma, reliving unpleasant experiences (referred to as "distress"), and further exacerbating their trauma. Thus, ethically, special precautions must be taken, including assuring privacy, provision of acute care if needed, referral to mental health services, and ancillary care.

An important issue in injury prevention and control involves those injuries that are intentional and have the potential to involve medico-legal issues. Any form of intentional injury caused by violence—homicides, suicides, assaults, violence against women, child abuse—puts victims at high risk of further injury and legal proceedings and has to be addressed carefully. Special ethical guidelines already exist for responding to some of these types of injuries—such as violence against women—while public health specialists need to use special ethical precautions to protect people enrolled in preventive or curative programs for these types of injuries.

Chapter Overviews

The overall goal of this volume's dedicated section on injuries in public health is to highlight ethics issues emerging from the study of those areas globally, with special attention to LMICs. The specific objectives of this section are to explore ethics issues in injury prevention and control; define a set of ethics issues within international injury work, especially in LMICs; and provide an initial analysis around the nature of these ethics issues, their specificity, and potential pathways for addressing them. The section addresses public health ethics issues overall for injuries, but also provides examples when work on specific injury types raises ethical concerns. While the section predominantly focuses on the ethics of public health programs, examples of ethics issues in research are also provided. This section does not discuss ethical issues pertaining to the distribution of injuries or risk factors, or equity issues in the distribution of global resources for injury prevention.

The two chapters that follow on unintentional and intentional injuries, respectively, explore issues like those identified above in the context of both types of injury and timeline of injury. In "Preventing Unintentional Injuries: Ethical Considerations in Public Health," Shanthi Ameratunga, Monique Jonas, and Danilo Blank explore public health ethics issues relating to unintentional injuries—those injuries that occur without intent, such as road traffic injuries, burns, drowning, poisoning, or falls. The authors introduce the notion of the ethics of prevention and the role of the state in such programs, including concerns for equity and justice. The need for prevention, especially to control risks for injury, while also managing potential conflicts with autonomy is addressed by the authors. They discuss the application of the harm principle and provide a pathway for consideration of the public health ethics issues for any proposed injury program.

In "Violence and Public Health Ethics," Omrana Pasha, Myra Hyder, and Adnan Hyder define some of the key public health ethics issues in the prevention, control, and management of violence and intentional injuries such as homicides, suicides, interpersonal violence, and sexual violence. The authors raise ethical issues in considering the roles of public health in addressing the victims and perpetrators of violence, consider key ethics issues in collecting data on these types of intentional injuries, and provide examples of how ethical and legal issues merge in considering violence as a public health problem.

Conclusion

This section of *The Oxford Handbook of Public Health Ethics* presents a set of key public health ethics issues arising in the arena of injuries—for one of the first times to our knowledge—which represents an innovation in the literature. The high burden of death and disability from injuries globally, with dominance in LMICs, together with the relative neglect in global health investments, makes this an important area for both intellectual discourse and public health action. It is hoped that the content in this section provides a significant step forward in promoting active consideration of key ethics issues—including autonomy and justice—as national and global efforts to prevent and control injuries move ahead.

Note

1. Although the term *injury* has been used in the general literature synonymously with *trauma*, *injury* is the comprehensive term and includes, for example, road traffic injury as well as drowning and poisoning. The term *trauma* can be classified as a subset of injury, encompassing, in contrast, only visible physical injuries (excluding poisoning, for example).

References

Fontes, L. A. 2004. "Ethics in Violence against Women Research: The Sensitive, the Dangerous, and the Overlooked." *Ethics and Behavior* 14(2): 141–174. doi:10.1207/s15327019eb1402_4.

Gosselin, R. A., Spiegel, D. A., Coughlin, R., and Zirkle, L. G. 2009. "Injuries: The Neglected Burden in Developing Countries." *Bulletin of the World Health Organization* 87(4): 246–246a.

Hyder, A. A., and Peden, M. 2003. "Inequality and Road-Traffic Injuries: Call for Action." *Lancet* 362(9401): 2034–2035. doi:10.1016/S0140-6736(03)15145-8.

IHME (Institute for Health Metrics and Evaluation). 2016. "Global Burden of Disease Study—GBD Compare." Web tool (Seattle: Institute for Health Metrics and Evaluation). http://ihmeuw.org/4jep.

Lopez, A. 2008. "Health and Health-Research Priorities: Has WHO Got It Right?" *Lancet* 372(9649): 1525–1527. doi:10.1016/S0140-6736(08)61632-3.

Newman, E., Risch, E., and Kassam-Adams, N. 2006. "Ethical Issues in Trauma-Related Research: A Review." *Journal of Empirical Research on Human Research Ethics* 1(3): 29–46. doi:10.1525/jer.2006.1.3.29.

Norton, R., Hyder, A. A., and Butchart, A. 2011. "Unintentional Injuries and Violence." In *Global Health: Diseases, Programs, Systems, and Policies*, 3rd ed., edited by M. H. Merson, R. E. Black, and A. Mills, 407–436 (Sudbury, Mass.: Jones and Bartlett).

Richter, E. D., Barach, P., Berman, T., Ben-David, G., and Weinberger, Z. 2001. "Extending the Boundaries of the Declaration of Helsinki: A Case Study of an Unethical Experiment in a Non-Medical Setting." *Journal of Medical Ethics* 27: 126–129.

Rosenstein, D. L. 2004. "Decision-Making Capacity and Disaster Research." *Journal of Traumatic Stress* 17(5): 373–381. doi:10.1023/B:JOTS.0000048950.36359.a2.

Stuckler, D., King, L., Robinson, H., and McKee, M. 2008. "WHO's Budgetary Allocations and Burden of Disease: A Comparative Analysis." *Lancet* 372(9649): 1563–1569. doi:10.1016/S0140-6736(08)61656-6.

CHAPTER 52

PREVENTING UNINTENTIONAL INJURIES: ETHICAL CONSIDERATIONS IN PUBLIC HEALTH

SHANTHI AMERATUNGA,
MONIQUE JONAS, AND DANILO BLANK

"It is necessary that the weakness of the powerless is transformed into a force capable of announcing justice. For this to happen, a total denouncement of fatalism is necessary. We are transformative beings and not beings for accommodation."

Paulo Freire, *Pedagogy of the Heart* (Freire, 1997, 6)

Introduction

THE Latin origin of the word *injury* refers to an injustice (Baker, 1997)—a principle at the core of deliberations in public health and ethics. Globally, in 2013 an estimated 973 million people sustained injuries requiring health care, and 4.8 million died as a consequence of these injuries (Haagsma et al., 2016). Almost 90 percent of these deaths occurred in low- and middle-income countries, imposing disastrous and burdensome developmental consequences on people in fragile economies (Alonge, Khan, and Hyder, 2016; Norton and Kobusingye, 2013; Seedat et al., 2009).

Unintentional injuries account for approximately 69 percent of deaths and 72 percent of disability-adjusted life years related to injury, common mechanisms being road crashes, falls, and drowning (Norton and Kobusingye, 2013). While the defining feature of unintentional injuries is that they are not premeditated or deliberately inflicted, operationalizing this distinction can be problematic and is not always helpful. Even jurisdictions with robust coronial reviews acknowledge inconsistencies in available information to classify the intent of an injury death (Dodds et al., 2014). A rigid distinction based on intent can also undermine the benefits of an integrated approach to injury prevention (Cohen et al., 2003; Langley, 2008). Furthermore, it has been argued that associating the notion of unintentional injury with the term *accident* may convey an impression of fatalism, weakening the public health tenet that most injuries are predictable, and therefore preventable (Blank and Xiang, 2014; Davis and Pless, 2001; Langley, 1988; Pless and Hagel, 2005). As Norman Daniels (2008) appropriately points out in more general terms, viewing health conditions as the products of bad luck fosters a reluctance to apply principles of justice to them and supports risk acceptance and nonintervention on the part of the state.

Beyond terminology, two interlinked concepts are at the core of debates about the role of the state in preventing unintentional injuries. The first relates to social justice, or the responsibility of states to prevent harm in a just society. The second relates to autonomy, and the extent to which it is deemed permissible to limit personal freedoms to prevent harm. In this chapter, we critique arguments relating to these concepts and explore how the framework developed by Nancy E. Kass (2001) to assess the justifiability of a public health intervention could assist injury prevention.

Responsibility and Unintentional Injury

Attributions of moral responsibility are common in injury prevention discourse. The claim that states should take measures to prevent injuries from occurring within their territory implies that injury prevention is a responsibility of the state as the body charged with protecting the welfare of its people. Thus, the occurrence of injuries can be considered relevantly attributable to the state, and the state can be held accountable for injury prevention (Shoemaker, 2011). This claim is open to contestation.

First, it could be argued that unintentional injuries are, by definition, unintentional, and that "accidents" occur despite, rather than because of, human intention. We can control, so the argument goes, the actions that we intend, and we are responsible for our intentional acts (Glannon, 1995). But we cannot control, or be responsible for, actions we do not intend. This reasoning could lead us to accept that "bad things" happen and avoid preoccupation with what might go wrong.

There are several problems with this line of argument. The first relates to the claim that moral responsibility is limited to intentional acts. If this were true, individuals would not be responsible for their omissions, or for reckless or careless behavior. But it is sometimes proper to attribute responsibility for an act omitted, a risk taken, or a state of affairs brought about, even if it is not the intended result of an intentional act (Daniels, 2008). We hold people responsible for fulfilling obligations or satisfying norms the demands of which often go beyond having a given set of intentions. Role obligations involving care for others exemplify this. Parents, for example, can be held responsible for harm to children resulting from negligence, not intent. Drivers who drink alcohol and drive, or who fall asleep at the wheel, are responsible for any harm they cause to others. While intentions are relevant to responsibility, responsibility encompasses more than intentions. It can require certain actions to be taken, or certain states of affairs to be brought about.

Another flaw with this line of argument lies in the implicit connection drawn between responsibility and blame. There is a reluctance to blame people for outcomes that are substantially beyond their control. Such reluctance is strongest at the micro level: responsibility for specific events that result in unintentional injury. The argument outlined above is most relevant to this level. Beyond this, however, questions arise about the context in which the event occurred and factors that elevated or reduced risk. These structural, macro-level questions capture considerations that render an event beyond an individual's control. Features such as the layout or quality of the road upon which the driver speeds, the conditions for obtaining a driver's license, the availability of public transport, road lighting, and safety features in cars can all affect whether a crash occurs and whether an injury results (Hosking et al., 2011; McClure et al., 2016; McMichael, 1999; Runyan, 2015). These contextual contributors are typically outside an individual's control. But that does not mean that they are uncontrollable by their very nature. They are precisely the kind of things that states, under certain conditions (such as access to sufficient resources) can address. Establishing that individual responsibility should be tempered by recognition of the limitations of individual control does not absolve the state of responsibility. Rather, it should encourage consideration of whether there is a role for the state, and therefore a shift of responsibility to systems within control of the state.

The most proximal causes of injuries are often individual actions. This offers the starting point for another argument against state action; one based upon deterrence. It posits that responsibility for an outcome lies largely with the person or persons who contributed the most to its occurring. One reason to maintain this stance, despite multiple contributory causes, is to incentivize good choices. If responsibility tracks the choices that contribute most directly to an outcome, individuals have reason to take choices seriously. So, the argument concludes, injury prevention should focus on individual decision-making.

This line of argument assumes that if the state takes responsibility for preventing injuries, individual responsibility will be correspondingly diminished. Given that there are often multiple causes of events, some outside the individual's control, why should we be concerned by diminishment of inflated attributions of responsibility to the individual? One reason might be that, even if the attribution of full responsibility to an individual is somewhat artificial, it is a useful artifice, in that it encourages people to take care to avoid causing injury—more care than they may otherwise take. So there may be good consequentialist reasons to emphasize individual responsibility in injury prevention.

Of course, the success of this argument rests on the facts of the matter. However, determining what influences risk-taking is not straightforward. Evidence can be variously interpreted, and interpretations are sometimes ideologically driven. As evident in the voluminous literature over decades, there is vociferous debate regarding whether regulations requiring bicycle helmet use do or do not reduce risk, because helmets (and compliance with safety regulations) reduce the sense of vulnerability, leading to riskier cycling behavior (Gamble and Walker, 2016; Pless, 2016; Wilde, Robertson, and Pless, 2002). The debate hinges on the concept of "risk homeostasis"—the idea that there is a fixed level of risk that people accept, and that if environmental risk is perceptibly reduced, behavioral risk correspondingly increases (Wilde, 1982). Proponents and detractors attribute diametrically opposing levels of importance to the arguably weak evidence for risk homeostasis in nonexperimental conditions (Wilde, Robertson, and Pless, 2002). The main purpose of such explorations of responsibility is to identify the best opportunities for interventions addressing injuries—from the individual to the state.

Injury Prevention as a Matter of Justice

So far, we have presented and critiqued two arguments against state involvement in injury prevention. There are other compelling arguments in favor of state involvement. Following John Rawls, Daniels's account of distributive justice requires state action to ensure that citizens have equal access to the opportunities typically available in that society, or the "normal opportunity range" (Daniels, 2008). Disease and disability impair access to many opportunities. Thus, justice requires that the state concern itself not only with ensuring fair access to health care and public health provisions, but also that it contribute to a fair distribution of the social determinants of health (Solar and Irwin, 2010). The state's role in injury prevention is thus connected with its obligation, owed to each citizen, to take reasonable measures to ensure equal access to the normal opportunity range.

Several aspects of this approach are noteworthy. Firstly, Daniels accepts that the normal opportunity range is society-dependent. What opportunities are available and valued differ among societies. Thus, the normal opportunity range is relativized to each society. While this approach recognizes both the realities of wealth distribution between nations, along with the entitlement of each society to develop its own characteristic way of life, it can be accused of too readily accepting a problematic status quo. Secondly, while the Rawlsian approach provides a plausible basis for establishing the state's role in injury prevention and provides a starting point for reasoning about resource allocation, it does not offer a comprehensive account of how to allocate resources or what measures are permissible in meeting health-related needs.[1]

Other prominent accounts of distributive justice in health, such as Amartya Sen and Martha Nussbaum's capabilities approach (Nussbaum, 1996, 2000; Sen, 1993), support a role for the state in ensuring access to those all-purpose means that enable quality of life. State involvement in injury prevention is required by such accounts, although details of how to allocate resources between this and other state responsibilities, and what mechanisms for injury prevention are preferable, are typically absent (Taylor et al., 2016). Finer-grained decision-making must supplement general theory. These decisions will be challenged not only by doubt about the legitimacy of state involvement in injury prevention, but also by concerns about interference in zones of personal freedom.

Personal Freedom and Injury Prevention

State efforts to reduce and prevent injury often provoke deep disagreement. Legislative measures prohibiting or requiring certain acts based on harm prevention are perhaps most controversial. What some see as sensible measures that prudent people would take voluntarily, others regard as abhorrent infractions upon personal freedom, illustrated by the fierce, now almost forgotten, objections attending the passage of laws requiring seatbelt use in many jurisdictions. Many object in principle to being told what to do by their government, detecting in such measures a lack of respect for the capacity and choices of citizens. Injury prevention strategies that limit individual choice are often seen as paternalistic. Those who place a higher value upon free choice than upon welfare find paternalistic policies objectionable, because, in legislating behaviors, the state tells individuals what to do, as though they are unable to make such decisions for themselves (Radoilska, 2009). Thus, not only is individual choice limited, but individuals are perceived to be treated disrespectfully by paternalist lawmakers.

Unquestionably, decision-making in public health is fraught, dynamic, contested on the grounds of reasonableness, and not always predicated on irrefutable scientific evidence (Gostin and Powers, 2006; McGinnis et al., 2009). Yet legislation of individual behavior is not universally rejected. Some supporters emphasize that such laws can reduce claims upon collective health resources, and thus regard them as justified by social cost minimization rather than harm prevention (Gostin and Gostin, 2009). Others, attending to values such as welfare, community, and solidarity, reject the primacy accorded to individual choice (Bayer and Fairchild, 2004; Beauchamp, 1985; Jochelson, 2006) and question the reality of the ideal of fully informed, autonomous choice valorized by libertarians and other critics of paternalism. Psychology and behavioral economics have revealed common heuristics and biases in human reasoning that give cause to doubt that human choice and behavior are consistently considered and autonomous (Tversky and Kahneman, 1974). It is also problematic to assume, as objectors to paternalistic injury prevention measures seem to, that an absence of legal requirement equates to a neutral choice environment. Especially in societies in which legal instruments control some risks, individual risk assessments can be informed—sometimes misleadingly—by an absence of legal control.

Richard Thaler and Cass Sunstein draw upon studies of human reasoning and decision-making to argue for an approach to many policy problems, which they call "libertarian paternalism" (Thaler, 2008). Their approach has been employed in injury prevention; for example, a campaign in Montana designed to increase seatbelt use drew upon the "norms principle"—the heuristic by which our own behavior is heavily influenced by our beliefs about what others do. In other words, we tend to want to conform. That campaign ran the slogan "Most of Us Wear Seatbelts" (Linkenbach and Perkins, 2003). Seatbelt use was reported to have increased substantially, although the effect waned with time (Blumenthal-Barby and Burroughs, 2012; Linkenbach and Perkins, 2003). This approach, referred to as "nudging," is seen as a way of enabling people to make better choices: choices that they themselves regard as better, but which are difficult to make without environmental support because of weak will or the everyday challenges of reasoning. The underlying idea is that our choices or actions do not always closely correlate with our autonomous will, and that respecting autonomy permits, and perhaps even requires, the state to design situations that favor health-promoting choices without cutting off other options. Advocates of this approach emphasize its balanced advancement of autonomy and welfare: unlike old-fashioned paternalism, it preserves choice, but without abandoning individuals to their own folly.

Several governments have enthusiastically embraced the possibilities of nudging, but the approach is open to a number of criticisms. Some maintain that, despite Thaler and Sunstein's depiction (Thaler, 2008), nudging is essentially a form of paternalism proper. Although some nudges do not target the agent's welfare (for instance, those which encourage prosocial choices), they succeed by effectively cutting off options, even if choice is ostensibly preserved (Hausman and Welch, 2010). Critics such as Hausman and Welch (2010) warn that although nudging seems less problematic than openly coercive forms of paternalism, its invisibility renders it a greater threat to free choice.

The Harm Principle and Injury Prevention

In comparison to the controversy surrounding paternalistic state action to prevent injuries, there is considerable acceptance of the state's role in preventing third-party harm. John Stuart Mill's harm principle permits state constraint of personal freedom where necessary to prevent harm to others (Mill, 1975). For Millian liberals, individual freedom is valuable for its own sake, and is also a necessary condition to secure other valuable goods, such as welfare and societal progress. Because, in Isaiah Berlin's words, "freedom for the wolves has often meant death for the sheep" (Berlin, 1969, xlv), the state has a role in reducing the exposure of individuals to harms inflicted by others.

The harm principle is prominent in discussions of public health, including injury prevention (Nuffield Council on Bioethics, 2007). Measures that may be too controversial to gain political traction when framed as prevention of harm to individuals are often acceptable when their prevention of third-party harm is emphasized. Consumer product safety regulations, playground safety standards, installing barriers to control access to water, building codes to reduce risks of earthquake-related collapse or fire-related injuries, laws mandating the placement of window guards to prevent falls from high-rise buildings, and blood alcohol restrictions for drivers are examples of this. Although there is widespread agreement that third-party harm prevention is a legitimate state concern, there is often controversy about whether a given measure is necessary to prevent harm, or whether the constraints on freedom it entails is proportionate to the third party harm it may prevent (Feinberg, 1987).

Beyond this, the established liberal framework, with its focus upon individual rights, is increasingly seen as inadequate to deal with the essentially collective interests at the heart of public health. Reorientation, supplementation, or even abandonment of the harm principle may be required to capture the collective nature of both harm-producing actions and the health-relevant goods harmed thereby (Hardin, 1968). While the notion that state regulation of personal choice to prevent third-party harm is typically accepted by communitarian commentators, the harm principle's other main plank—that agents should be free from intervention in actions that do not harm others—is subject to critique. Collective action problems are not easily managed by the harm principle. Public goods such as accessible pavements and roads with unimpeded lines of visibility can be threatened by apparently harmless acts that can, under given conditions, pose a health risk. Even more fundamentally, the focus upon the micro-level individual actions and their effects is seen by some as obscuring collective interests and the values—such as solidarity, trust, reciprocity, and relational autonomy—associated with them (Baylis, Kenny, and Sherwin, 2008; Jennings, 2009).

Putting Ethics into Practice

Given the preceding account, supporters and objectors submit a range of moral arguments in relation to public health interventions, including injury prevention. Consequently, several frameworks have been developed to assist practitioners in evaluating the ethical risks that public health measures can typically produce (Childress et al., 2002; Kass, 2001; Marckmann et al., 2015; Nuffield Council on Bioethics, 2007; Tannahill, 2008). We employ the tool developed by Kass (2001) to illustrate how a systematic analysis of ethical implications can help to discuss, debate, develop, and evaluate robust public health approaches to preventing unintentional injuries.

What Are the Public Health Goals of the Proposed Program?

Kass emphasizes that the goal of a public health intervention should be specified in terms of reduced mortality, morbidity, and disability, rather than merely targeted changes in intermediary factors (e.g., improved knowledge, attitudes, and behaviors). She also recommends considering the health gains from social programs outside conventional realms of public health. This is of relevance to injury prevention, where poverty reduction, improved living conditions, safer working conditions, and access to stronger engagement of marginalized groups in developing public policy are highly salient, equity-focused interventions. This emphasis aligns closely with the recommendations of the World Health Organization (WHO) Commission on Social Determinants of Health (2008; see also Sadana and Blas, 2013) and Tom Frieden's Health Impact Pyramid (Mack et al., 2015), where interventions addressing socioeconomic factors and controlling the relative deprivation that increases exposure to environmental hazards are postulated to have the greatest population impact.

How Effective Is the Program in Achieving Its Stated Goals?

This question focuses on the assumptions underlying specified public health goals. Many educational programs that aim to change awareness and behaviors of child pedestrians or novice drivers do not necessarily result in reductions in injury, despite favorable effects on intermediary factors such as changes in attitudes (Duperrex, Roberts, and Bunn, 2002; Roberts, Kwan, and Cochrane Injuries Group Driver Education Review, 2001). Foreshadowing the next step in the tool, Kass argues that the strength of the evidence should be that much greater when the burdens posed by a program are more substantial. The paradoxical gaps in data from less-resourced settings where injuries are disproportionately greater are particularly challenging in this context. Consequently, initiatives like the Bloomberg Philanthropies Global Road Safety program (Hyder et al., 2012) focus on enhancing research capacity alongside evaluations of promising interventions in low- and middle-income countries.

What Are the Known or Potential Burdens of the Program?

The societal burdens posed directly or indirectly by public health initiatives can include costs; infringements of personal freedom; and risks to privacy and confidentiality, liberty, and self-determination. Even educational interventions, which are usually voluntary and impose fewer burdens (cf. more coercive approaches, such as legislation and mandatory building codes and product standards) can be deemed paternalistic, manipulative, or coercive. These could also require burdensome measures to achieve effective implementation, result in inequitable outcomes due to required levels of literacy or access to services, and stigmatize groups profiled or targeted in media campaigns or messages. A deficit analysis problematizing individuals shifts the blame from unsafe environments in which people live to the victims involved.

Can Burdens Be Minimized? Are There Alternative Approaches?

If the public health program is deemed to impose any burdens, this step challenges us to consider the least coercive and invasive approach, without "greatly reducing" the effectiveness of the program. Alternatively, we can consider how the program could be modified to minimize the burden or unwanted consequence. This requires sufficient data on perceived and actual burdens, as well as a commitment to modify the program, if required, based on the information gathered. Injury prevention programs developed by or in partnership with indigenous communities often have attributes of mainstream interventions that have been modified to reduce risks of stigmatization and increase acceptability, thereby enhancing the intended outcome (Cullen et al., 2016).

In many countries with high rates of drowning, adverse living conditions make the task of constant vigilant parental supervision of young children particularly burdensome. Village-based supervised child-care programs in Bangladesh and Cambodia are increasingly recognized as reducing drowning risks, providing other health co-benefits, and mitigating the demands on impoverished families (WHO, 2014).

Is the Program Implemented Fairly?

Drawing on the principle of distributive justice, Kass argues that public health programs have an imperative to reduce societal inequalities, especially where these relate to health outcomes, and ensure a fair distribution of benefits, burdens, and harms. This does not mean that programs or resources necessarily have to be allocated equally across populations; rather, unequal distributions require support using a clear, justifiable rationale and data. For example, programs that subsidize or provide smoke alarms at no cost for low-income families could be construed as stereotyping these families as particularly needy or dependent. However, the argument in support typically relates to the risks of fire-related injuries in the absence of a functional smoke alarm. This aligns with principles proposed by Rawls and Daniels, among other philosophers, who propose a positive dimension to unequal resource allocation to address prevalent inequities in the structural determinants of health.

How Can the Benefits and Burdens of a Program Be Fairly Balanced?

The notion of balance in this step requires attention to procedural justice (i.e., a fair and democratic process to consider differing perspectives and settle disagreements). We agree with Catriona Mackenzie and others who discuss the notion of relational autonomy that concerns about social justice must be central to a reasonable conception of individual autonomy (Baylis, Kenny, and Sherwin, 2008). However, consensus on this point is unlikely, and the overall aim would be to determine which public health functions are justifiable, while acknowledging that some infringements of privacy and other burdens would be inevitable. Negotiating on these points is challenging, given the time, opportunities, and processes required for meaningful consultation, and the remarkable imbalances in power and political clout that can shape the nature of the discourse. Divergent views on what constitutes threats to freedom and liberty are common, especially from industries resisting what is deemed undue regulation. This is evident in challenges from the car manufacturing industry in the 1970s in the wake of increasing pressure to improve vehicle safety standards (Nader, 1972), and in more recent push-backs from the alcohol industry to harm reduction policies seen as a threat to sales and profits (Moodie et al., 2013).

Conclusion

Reflecting on the multiple competing standpoints involved, it is heartening to note the increasing acknowledgement that realizing noticeable reductions in the injury burden requires social change, and that this involves systemic interventions deeply rooted in empowered communities working through institutions that define the forms and functions of society (McClure et al., 2016; Mohan and Tiwari, 2000). Such comprehensive action considers individual and communal responsibilities in injury causation as a whole, taking into account the often thin boundary between violence and unintended harm. This imperative, in a field where a commitment to social justice is a core value, requires more robust political commitment and resources than are evident to date.

Note

1. Daniels, in collaboration with James Sabin, has developed an account of procedural justice, known as Accountability for Reasonableness (A4R), in recognition of ethical and political theory's inability to generate substantive conclusions about resource allocation that are both unambiguous and uncontroversial. A4R is proposed to foster allocation decisions that command respect on the basis of the fair process by which they were reached, even when the conclusions are not universally endorsed (Daniels and Sabin, 1997, 1998).

References

Alonge, O., Khan, U. R., and Hyder, A. A. 2016. "Our Shrinking Globe: Implications for Child Unintentional Injuries." *Pediatric Clinics of North America* 63(1): 167–181.

Baker, S. P. 1997. "Advances and Adventures in Trauma Prevention." *Journal of Trauma, Injury, Infection, and Critical Care* 42 (3): 369–373.

Bayer, R., and Fairchild, A. L. 2004. "The Genesis of Public Health Ethics." *Bioethics* 18(6): 473–492.

Baylis, F., Kenny, N. P., and Sherwin, S. 2008. "A Relational Account of Public Health Ethics." *Public Health Ethics* 1(3): 196–209.

Beauchamp, D. E. 1985. "Community: The Neglected Tradition of Public Health." *Hastings Center Report* 15(6): 28–36.

Berlin, I. 1969. *Four Essays on Liberty* (Oxford: Oxford University Press).

Blank, D., and Xiang, H. 2014. "Will the Final Battle Not Be between Good and Evil, but Rather Injuriologists and Accidentologists?" *Injury Prevention* 21(3): 211–212.

Blumenthal-Barby, J. S., and Burroughs, H. 2012. "Seeking Better Health Care Outcomes: The Ethics of Using the 'Nudge.'" *American Journal of Bioethics* 12(2): 1–10.

Childress, J. F., Faden, R. R., Gaare, R. D., Gostin, L. O., Kahn, J., Bonnie, R. J., et al. 2002. "Public Health Ethics: Mapping the Terrain." *Journal of Law, Medicine & Ethics* 30(2): 170–178.

Cohen, L., Miller, T., Sheppard, M. A., Gordon, E., Gantz, T., and Atnafou, R. 2003. "Bridging the Gap: Bringing Together Intentional and Unintentional Injury Prevention Efforts to Improve Health and Well Being." *Journal of Safety Research* 34(5): 473–483.

Commission on Social Determinants of Health. 2008. *Closing the Gap in a Generation: Health Equity through Action on the Social Determinants of Health: Final Report of the Commission on Social Determinants of Health* (Geneva: World Health Organization). http://www.who.int/social_determinants/thecommission/finalreport/en/.

Cullen, P., Clapham, K., Byrne, J., Hunter, K., Rogers, K., Senserrick, T., et al. 2016. "Implementation of a Driver Licensing Support Program in Three Aboriginal Communities: A Brief Report from a Pilot Program." *Health Promotion Journal of Australia* 27(2): 167–169.

Daniels, N. 2008. *Just Health: Meeting Health Needs Fairly* (New York: Cambridge University Press).

Daniels, N., and Sabin, J. 1997. "Limits to Health Care: Fair Procedures, Democratic Deliberation, and the Legitimacy Problem for Insurers." *Philosophy & Public Affairs* 26(4): 303–350.

Daniels, N., and Sabin, J. 1998. "The Ethics of Accountability in Managed Care Reform." *Health Affairs* 17(5): 50–64.

Davis, R. M., and Pless, B. 2001. "BMJ Bans 'Accidents.'" *BMJ* 322(7298): 1320–1321.

Dodds, L., Robinson, K. M., Daking, L., and Paul, L. 2014. "The Concept of 'Intent' within Australian Coronial Data: Factors Affecting the National Coronial Information System's Classification of Mortality Attributable to Intentional Self-Harm." *Health Information Management Journal* 43(3): 13–22.

Duperrex, O., Roberts, I., and Bunn, F. 2002. "Safety Education of Pedestrians for Injury Prevention." *Cochrane Database of Systematic Reviews* 2: CD001531. https://www.cochranelibrary.com/cdsr/doi/10.1002/14651858.CD001531/epdf/abstract.

Feinberg, J. 1987. *The Moral Limits of the Criminal Law*, vol. 1: *Harm to Others* (New York: Oxford University Press).

Freire, P. 1997. *Pedagogy of the Heart* (New York: Continuum).

Gamble, T., and Walker, I. 2016. "Wearing a Bicycle Helmet Can Increase Risk Taking and Sensation Seeking in Adults." *Psychological Science* 27(2): 289–294.

Glannon, W. 1995. "Responsibility and the Principle of Possible Action." *Journal of Philosophy* 92(5): 261–274.

Gostin, L. O., and Gostin, K. G. 2009. "A Broader Liberty: J. S. Mill, Paternalism and the Public's Health." *Public Health* 123(3): 214–221.

Gostin, L. O., and Powers, M. 2006. "What Does Social Justice Require for the Public's Health? Public Health Ethics and Policy Imperatives." *Health Affairs* 25(4): 1053–1060.

Haagsma, J. A., Graetz, N., Bolliger, I., Naghavi, M., Higashi, H., Mullany, E. C., et al. 2016. "The Global Burden of Injury: Incidence, Mortality, Disability-Adjusted Life Years and Time Trends from the Global Burden of Disease Study 2013." *Injury Prevention* 22(1): 3–18.

Hardin, G. 1968. "The Tragedy of the Commons: The Population Problem Has No Technical Solution; It Requires a Fundamental Extension in Morality." *Science* 162(3859): 1243–1248.

Hausman, D. N., and Welch, B. 2010. "Debate: To Nudge or Not to Nudge." *Journal of Political Philosophy* 18(1): 123–136.

Hosking, J., Ameratunga, S., Morton, S., and Blank, D. 2011. "A Life Course Approach to Injury Prevention: A 'Lens and Telescope' Conceptual Model." *BMC Public Health* 11: 695.

Hyder, A. A., Allen, K. A., Di Pietro, G., Adriazola, C. A., Sobel, R., Larson, K., et al. 2012. "Addressing the Implementation Gap in Global Road Safety: Exploring Features of an Effective Response and Introducing a 10-Country Program." *American Journal of Public Health* 102(6): 1061–1067.

Jennings, B. 2009. "Public Health and Liberty: Beyond the Millian Paradigm." *Public Health Ethics* 2(2): 123–134.

Jochelson, K. 2006. "Nanny or Steward? The Role of Government in Public Health." *Public Health* 120(12): 1149–1155.

Kass, N. E. 2001. "An Ethics Framework for Public Health." *American Journal of Public Health* 91(11): 1776–1782.

Langley, J. D. 1988. "The Need to Discontinue the Use of the Term 'Accident' When Referring to Unintentional Injury Events." *Accident Analysis and Prevention* 20(1): 1–8.

Langley, J. D. 2008. "WHO and CDC Nomenclature." *Injury Prevention* 14(5): 342.

Linkenbach, J., and Perkins, H. W. 2003. "Most of Us Wear Seatbelts: The Process and Outcomes of a 3-Year Statewide Adult Seatbelt Campaign in Montana." Paper presented at the National Conference on the Social Norms Model, Boston, Mass., July 17, 2003. http://www.socialnormsresources.org/casestudies/montanaseatbelt.php.

Mack, K. A., Liller, K. D., Baldwin, G., and Sleet, D. 2015. "Preventing Unintentional Injuries in the Home Using the Health Impact Pyramid." *Health Education & Behavior* 42(Suppl. 1): 115S-122S.

Marckmann, G., Schmidt, H., Sofaer, N., and Strech, D. 2015. "Putting Public Health Ethics into Practice: A Systematic Framework." *Frontiers in Public Health* 3: 23. https://www.ncbi.nlm.nih.gov/pmc/articles/PMC4319377/.

McClure, R. J., Mack, K., Wilkins, N., and Davey, T. M. 2016. "Injury Prevention as Social Change." *Injury Prevention* 22(3): 226–229.

McGinnis, J. M., Hattis, D. B., Steinzor, R., and Olden, K. 2009. "Scientific Issues in Environmental Health Decision Making." In *Environmental Health Sciences Decision Making: Risk Management, Evidence and Ethics: Workshop Summary*, edited by Y. Coble, C. Coussens, and K. Quinn (Washington, D.C.: Institute of Medicine).

McMichael, A. J. 1999. "Prisoners of the Proximate: Loosening the Constraints on Epidemiology in an Age of Change." *American Journal of Epidemiology* 149(10): 887–897.

Mill, J. S. 1975. *On Liberty* (New York: Norton).

Mohan, D., and Tiwari, G. 2000. *Injury Prevention and Control* (New York: Taylor & Francis).

Moodie, R., Stuckler, D., Monteiro, C., Sheron, N., Neal, B., Thamarangsi, T., et al. 2013. "Profits and Pandemics: Prevention of Harmful Effects of Tobacco, Alcohol, and Ultra-Processed Food and Drink Industries." *Lancet* 381(9867): 670–679.

Nader, R. 1972. *Unsafe at Any Speed: The Designed-In Dangers of the American Automobile* (New York: Grossman).

Norton, R., and Kobusingye, O. 2013. "Injuries." *New England Journal of Medicine* 368(18): 1723–1730.

Nuffield Council on Bioethics. 2007. *Public Health: Ethical Issues* (London: Nuffield Council on Bioethics).

Nussbaum, M. C. 1996. "Human Functioning and Social Justice: In Defense of Aristotelian Essentialism." *Political Theory* 20(2): 202–246.

Nussbaum, M. C. 2000. *Women and Human Development the Capabilities Approach* (New York: Cambridge University Press).

Pless, I. B. 2016. "Risk Compensation: Revisited and Rebutted." *Safety* 2(3): 16. doi:10.3390/safety2030016.

Pless, I. B., and Hagel, B. E. 2005. "Injury Prevention: A Glossary of Terms." *Journal of Epidemiology & Community Health* 59(3): 182–185.

Radoilska, L. 2009. "Public Health Ethics and Liberalism." *Public Health Ethics* 2(2): 135–145.

Roberts, I., Kwan, I., and Cochrane Injuries Group Driver Education Review. 2001. "School-Based Driver Education for the Prevention of Traffic Crashes." *Cochrane Database of Systematic Reviews* 3: CD003201. https://www.cochranelibrary.com/cdsr/doi/10.1002/14651858.CD003201/full.

Runyan, C. W. 2015. "Using the Haddon Matrix: Introducing the Third Dimension." *Injury Prevention* 21(2): 126–130.

Sadana, R., and Blas, E. 2013. "What Can Public Health Programs Do to Improve Health Equity?" *Public Health Reports* 128(Suppl. 3): 12–20.

Seedat, M., Van Niekerk, A., Jewkes, R., Suffla, S., and Ratele, K. 2009. "Violence and Injuries in South Africa: Prioritising an Agenda for Prevention." *Lancet* 374(9694): 1011–1022.

Sen, A. 1993. "Capability and Well-Being." In *The Quality of Life*, edited by M. Nussbaum, and A. Sen, 30–53 (Oxford: Clarendon Press).

Shoemaker, D. 2011. "Answerability and Accountability: Towards a Wider Theory of Moral Responsibility." *Ethics* 121(3): 602–632.

Solar, O., and Irwin, A. 2010. "A Conceptual Framework for Action on the Social Determinants of Health." Social Determinants of Health Discussion Paper 2 (Policy and Practice) (Geneva: World Health Organization).

Tannahill, A. 2008. "Beyond Evidence—to Ethics: A Decision-Making Framework for Health Promotion, Public Health and Health Improvement." *Health Promotion International* 23(4): 380–390.

Taylor, L. A., Tan, A. X., Coyle, C. E., Ndumele, C., Rogan, E., Canavan, M., et al. 2016. "Leveraging the Social Determinants of Health: What Works?" *PLoS ONE* 11(8): e0160217.

Thaler, R. H. 2008. *Nudge: Improving Decisions about Health, Wealth, and Happiness* (New Haven, Conn.: Yale University Press).

Tversky, A., and Kahneman, D. 1974. "Judgment under Uncertainty: Heuristics and Biases." *Science* 185(4157): 1124–1131.

WHO (World Health Organization). 2014. *Global Report on Drowning: Preventing a Leading Killer* (Geneva: World Health Organization).

Wilde, G. J. S. 1982. "The Theory of Risk Homeostasis: Implications for Safety and Health." *Risk Analysis* 2(4): 209–225.

Wilde, G. J. S., Robertson, L., and Pless, B. 2002. "For and Against: Does Risk Homeostasis Theory Have Implications for Road Safety?" *British Medical Journal* 324(7346): 1149–1152.

CHAPTER 53

VIOLENCE AND PUBLIC HEALTH ETHICS

OMRANA PASHA, MYRA F. HYDER, AND ADNAN A. HYDER

Understanding Violence through a Public Health Lens

The World Health Organization (WHO) has defined violence as the "intentional use of physical force or power... that either results in or has a high likelihood of resulting in injury, death, psychological harm, maldevelopment or deprivation" (WHO, 2002). The WHO has developed a typology of violence based on the victim-perpetrator relationship: self-directed violence, interpersonal violence, and collective violence, represented in Figure 53.1.

This chapter builds on previous work (Kass, 2004; Thomas et al., 2002) and focuses on the ethics of public health practice as related to self-directed and interpersonal violence. *Self-directed violence* encompasses a range of behaviors, including acts of fatal and non-fatal suicidal behavior, as well as behaviors for which the intention is not to kill oneself but rather to harm, as in self-mutilation. Suicidal ideation (i.e., thinking about, considering, or planning for suicide) is often included in this definition because of its association with self-directed violence (Crosby, Ortega, and Melanson, 2011). *Interpersonal violence* is further categorized by the relationship between the victim and perpetrator, who may be an intimate partner, family member, acquaintance, or stranger. It may also be characterized by the victim's age or sex (e.g., violence against children, adolescents, women, and elderly persons), or by the nature of the violence (e.g., physical, sexual, psychological, or deprivation/neglect). By contrast, *collective violence* is defined as the instrumental use of violence by people identifying themselves as a group against another group to achieve political, economic, or social objectives. While the practice of public health within the context of collective violence is a pressing concern, it is beyond the scope of this chapter.

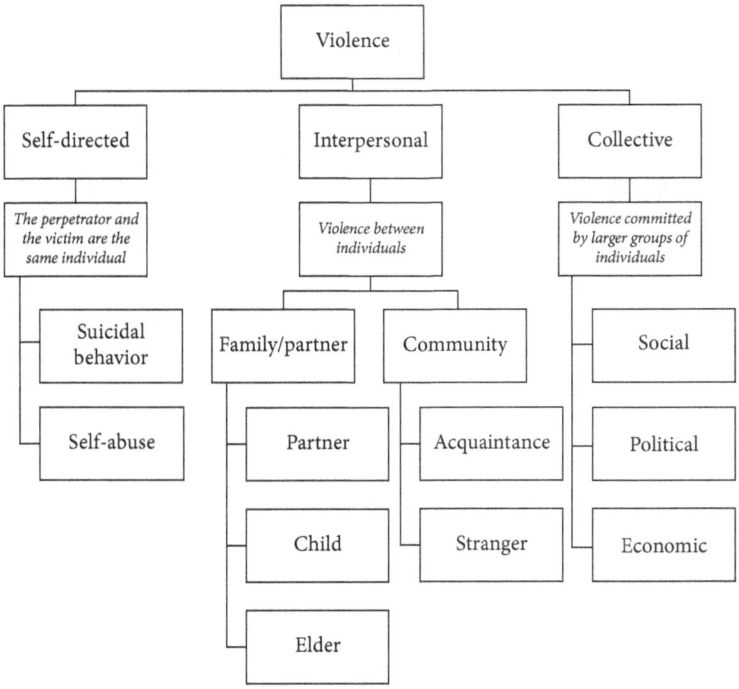

FIGURE 53.1 A typology of violence (adapted from WHO 2002).

In this chapter, we first discuss the impact of violence on public health and the role of public health practitioners in addressing violence. We then review fundamental ethical principles and current guidelines for public health workers to address violence, and examine some ethical challenges for research and programs dealing with interpersonal and self-directed violence. We conclude by suggesting a way forward for the ethical practice of public health regarding violence.

The Impact of Violence on the Public's Health

Rates of self-directed violence differ by geography, by demographic characteristics, and by individual vulnerability, including mental health status. An estimated 800,000 suicide deaths occur each year (Lozano et al., 2012). In 2015 suicide was one of the three leading causes of death globally among people aged fifteen to twenty-nine, and the seventeenth leading cause of death among all ages. Globally, the age-standardized rate of suicide death is 14 per 100,000, with the highest rates seen among people aged over seventy (29.3 per 100,000) and those between the ages of fifty and sixty-nine (18.5 per 100,000) (Lozano et al., 2012). Suicide attempts are twenty times more common than suicide fatality (WHO, 2014), and rates of nonsuicidal self-injury are even higher: 4–6 percent of people have deliberately self-injured at least once (Weber et al., 2013).

Interpersonal violence is the fourth-leading cause of death and leads to substantial disability among youth aged ten to twenty-nine, accounting for 200,000 deaths annually (WHO, 2014). Reliable global estimates of child maltreatment are scarce; however, one in four adults reports having been physically abused during childhood (Stoltenborgh et al., 2013). Physical and sexual violence against women is similarly pervasive, as one in three women reports being abused during her lifetime (WHO, 2013). Violence against elderly persons is increasingly recognized to be a problem, with estimates of one in six of people above sixty years of age experiencing some form of abuse (Yon et al., 2017).

Knowledge of the burden of violence, its risk factors, and effective interventions has increased exponentially. In many high-income countries, this increased knowledge has resulted in significant declines in violence-related mortality and morbidity. By contrast, in many low- and middle-income countries (LMICs), rates of violence are twice as high, and there is an imperative to rapidly advance a violence prevention agenda that recognizes the unique ethical challenges faced by LMICs, examples of which are discussed in this chapter.

Preventing and Responding to Violence: The Role of Public Health

According to the WHO *Global Plan of Action* (2016a), national health care systems should provide services to those affected by violence, gather data to assess the magnitude of the problem, provide and evaluate interventions, develop intersectoral links, and engage in advocacy and training to address and prevent violence (see Figure 53.2).

Provision of Health Care for Victims of Violence

National health systems have a key role to play in the multisectoral response to violence. They provide appropriate clinical care to address the outcomes of violence, treatment of physical injuries, and management of mental health effects seen in victims of violence (García-Moreno et al., 2015). There is a dearth of evidence of effective health care interventions for violence prevention, especially for resource-poor settings; however, there is a consensus that health care professionals should identify patients experiencing violence and provide supportive care as well as referral to other services (US Preventive Services Task Force, 2013). Health care systems can contribute to violence prevention or recurrence and mitigation of the consequences, in addition to urgent and ongoing care.

Examples of the roles that health care professionals play in managing violence and its impact include identifying cases where injuries are a result of violence (Concialdi and Read, 2016), assessment of individual risk of violence or preventive screening for violence

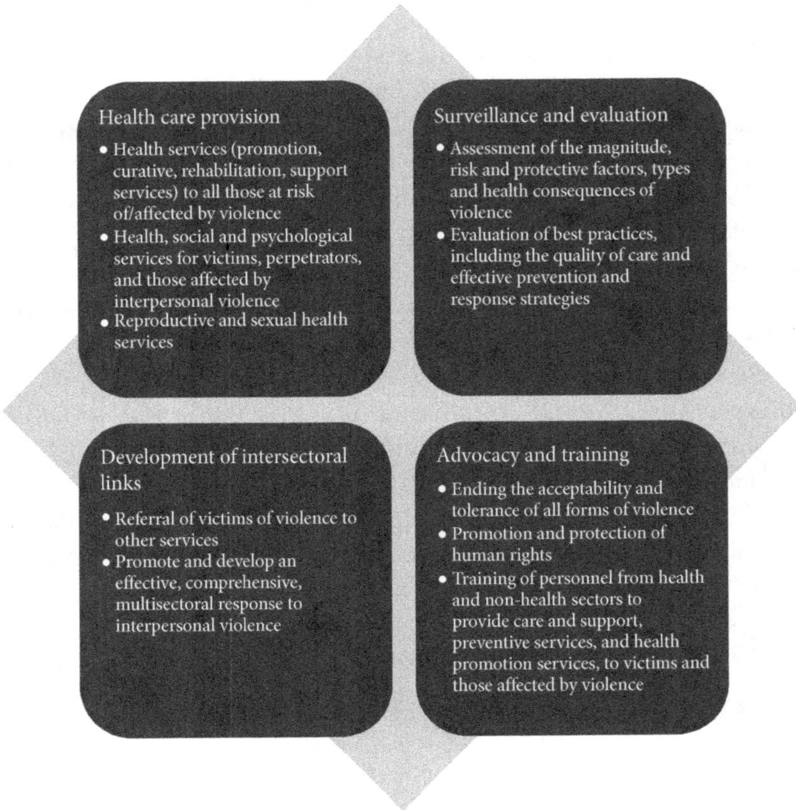
Health care provision
• Health services (promotion, curative, rehabilitation, support services) to all those at risk of/affected by violence
• Health, social and psychological services for victims, perpetrators, and those affected by interpersonal violence
• Reproductive and sexual health services
Surveillance and evaluation
• Assessment of the magnitude, risk and protective factors, types and health consequences of violence
• Evaluation of best practices, including the quality of care and effective prevention and response strategies
Development of intersectoral links
• Referral of victims of violence to other services
• Promote and develop an effective, comprehensive, multisectoral response to interpersonal violence
Advocacy and training
• Ending the acceptability and tolerance of all forms of violence
• Promotion and protection of human rights
• Training of personnel from health and non-health sectors to provide care and support, preventive services, and health promotion services, to victims and those affected by violence

FIGURE 53.2 The role of national health systems in addressing violence (adapted from the Resolution of the 67th World Health Assembly, May 2016).

(US Preventive Services Task Force, 2013), and gathering forensic evidence (ACEP, 2013). In the context of self-directed violence, for example, screening for suicide risk among populations assessed to be at high likelihood for suicide is also carried out by health care personnel (Walrath et al., 2015).

Development of Intersectoral Links

Intersectoral collaboration is necessary for the success of efforts to mitigate and prevent violence. The health system ought to work closely with social services, education systems, local communities, policymakers, and law enforcement in a collaborative and meaningful way to effectively address violence. National legislative mechanisms also play a critical role in violence prevention in any country (WHO, 2002).

At the most basic and individual level, this linkage involves referring victims of interpersonal violence by health care workers to protective services such as alternative living arrangements, social services, access to mental health care, and legal support if possible and desired by the individual (WHO, 2009), as well as appropriate collection and preservation of forensic evidence by health care personnel in cases of violence, particularly sexual violence (Foresman-Capuzzi, 2014). However, a more robust collaborative process is necessary to address violence at the population level. An example of this is the WHO Regional Office for Europe's plan to reduce the prevalence of child maltreatment by implementing preventive programs that address risk and protective factors, including social determinants (WHO/Europe, 2014). Specifically, the plan calls for addressing the causes of maltreatment through coordinated and sustained efforts in multiple sectors (health, education, employment, welfare, justice, housing, trade and industry, media and communications, and nongovernmental organizations) as well as health systems.

In the context of suicide, the current link between health and other sectors, such as national legislatures and the community at large, centers on issues of access to adequate and consistent mental health care, perceived causes of suicide (i.e., underlying mental illness or social conditions), widespread social stigmatization, and most societies' overarching desire to prevent suicide (Ho, 2014).

Surveillance and Evaluation

National public health authorities ought to conduct surveillance to collect accurate, timely, and comprehensive data to better understand and prevent the occurrence of violence. Monitoring the occurrence and nature of violent deaths and injuries, ensuring that data are disseminated routinely and expeditiously, and applying these data to develop, implement, and evaluate programs and strategies to reduce and prevent violence are all integral parts of an effective surveillance mechanism. An example of surveillance for violence is the Canadian Incidence Study of Reported Child Abuse and Neglect (CIS), which gathers information across provinces and territories, each of which functions under its own legislation for child welfare. The CIS is the longest-standing national surveillance mechanism for violence against children, bringing together disparate reporting mechanisms and establishing standard definitions for types of child maltreatment (Tonmyr, 2015). Despite these strengths, this passive surveillance mechanism represents only those cases that are reported to child welfare agencies; therefore, there is likely underreporting of cases (Tonmyr et al., 2010).

Advocacy and Training

The global public health community has taken a lead in raising awareness of the impact of violence and has advanced the agenda of violence prevention through advocacy mechanisms focusing on international human rights treaties as well as civil and political rights, such as the Convention on the Elimination of All Forms of Discrimination against Women (CEDAW) (Schopper, Lormand, and Waxweiler, 2006). Other activities at this level include the development of technical guidelines, policy papers, and research to support violence prevention programs and advocate for increased investment in violence prevention (WHO, 2002).

At the country level, advocacy and capacity development spans legislative and policy standards, allocation of adequate resources, strengthening systems that prevent and respond to violence, and changing social and cultural norms that tolerate violence. The WHO *Global Status Report on Violence Prevention 2014* outlines the status of violence prevention activities across the globe (Mikton et al., 2016). More than two-thirds of countries have national action plans to address child maltreatment and intimate partner or sexual violence; however, these plans are unlikely to be informed by data. Almost 60 percent of countries do not have reliable data on violence-related mortality, and even fewer have information specific enough to inform programming. Additionally, fewer than half of all countries report implementation of large-scale, evidence-based interventions for violence prevention. Even more concerning is the dearth of effective legislative recourse for victims of violence in many countries. Despite a growing evidential basis for addressing violence as a public health issue and widespread adoption of international commitments to violence prevention, countries need to do more to reduce the occurrence and impact of violence (Mikton et al., 2016). With this background in mind, we will now provide a summary of ethical principles used in the context of public health and public health response. We will then describe specific ethical challenges in the context of interpersonal violence, linking how these principles can provide some guidance for the challenges described.

Ethical Principles for Public Health

Beauchamp and Childress (2012) outline four ethical principles applicable to all of biomedicine: beneficence, nonmaleficence, respect for autonomy, and justice. *Beneficence* involves evaluating positive impacts of health actions and balancing the benefits against risks, whereas *nonmaleficence* means understanding, reducing, and avoiding any negative effects of interventions. *Respect for autonomy* requires respecting the rights of individuals and communities to determine their own course of action and support for independent decision-making. *Justice* is the ethical duty to promote and act with fairness. It generally includes both a distributive component (for example, the equitable distribution of resources for health, or distribution of the opportunity to be healthy) and a procedural component (having fair procedures in place to resolve disagreements or set priorities among competing demands).

Yet within public health, how the above four principles are specified, and which ethical demands are given priority, is important. Because public health seeks to maximize the health of entire populations as opposed to only individuals, public health ethics frameworks seek to assure that policies and programs that aim to improve the health of the public do so with minimal infringement to liberty and with privileged attention to justice (Childress et al., 2002). Public health ethics asks public health professionals to identify population-wide priorities for health, consider the effectiveness and benefits of programs or policies in achieving these public health priorities, maximize benefits over harms (utility), justify that the public health activities will minimize morbidity or mortality, pose the least infringement to autonomy rights as possible, and maintain privacy and confidentiality as well as public trust (Kass, 2001; Childress et al., 2002). In addition, particularly since public health outcomes are correlated with social justice and equity outcomes, attention to justice is a core commitment of public health. This requires ensuring that populations are not inadvertently targeted, that unjust conditions are rectified, and that, ultimately, procedural justice (participation of the public, local communities, and affected groups through transparency processes) is in place to resolve disagreements (Kass, 2001; Childress et al., 2002).

Ultimately, most areas of public health—including how best to design screening or vaccination programs; how to organize data collection, surveillance, or disease and injury reporting; how best to allocate scarce resources; and when to have more coercive and regulatory measures implemented in the name of improving the public's health—raise ethics issues, and attention to effectiveness, least infringement, necessity, and fair distribution and procedures becomes essential. Indeed, the last decades have seen an increasing focus on ethical issues inherent in the practice of public health (Dawson, 2009, 2011; Peckham and Hann, 2010; Faden and Shebaya, 2016; Goldberg, 2017).

The next section highlights key ethics challenges, particularly in the area of interpersonal violence as a public health issue, including surveillance and data gathering related to violence, screening programs for violence, and public health interventions to address violence.

Ethical Challenges in Addressing Interpersonal Violence

Data suggest that the prevalence of violence is higher among those with lower incomes; nonetheless, it remains a critical public health problem for adults of all income levels (Breiding, Chen, and Black, 2014). Often, it is advocated that efforts to combat violence focus on low-income and minority groups (APA, 2009). While the rationale for such an approach is understandable, there is a risk of reinforcing classist, racist, and inaccurate presuppositions that individuals in these populations are uniquely predisposed to act violently (Greaves et al., 1995). In the United States, low-income, urban communities that are largely populated by minorities experience a greater law enforcement presence in response to violence, increasing the likelihood of police-involved violence with each encounter and perpetuating a cycle of violence (Obasogie and Newman, 2017). In LMICs, urban space is increasingly organized in response to crime and violence and to a lack of confidence in the state's provision of security. This isolation perpetuates a fear of the "Other" and contributes to the social, economic, and political fragmentation of cities (Moser, 2004). In such contexts, violence cannot be viewed in isolation; it is necessary to understand these phenomena in their broader sociological context of inequality, deprivation, and insecurity (Kruijt, 2007).

Gathering Information for Surveillance, Evaluation, and Research to Address Violence

The collection, holding, and dissemination of data related to violence may pose risks to both those who report the information and those who collect it (Lee and Renzetti, 1990; Fontes, 2014). This necessitates maintaining high standards to ensure confidentiality in research studies and any other data collection related to violence. While there is little empirical evidence that participants in research on violence are at greater risk of harm than any other research participants (Sikweyiya and Jewkes, 2011), the potential risk of individual harm, risks to those involved in gathering data, and a broader concern of risks to a community or identity are all important considerations. Concerns about confidentiality emerge not only from breaches of confidentiality of data already collected, but also from how data gathering activities are conducted (WHO, 2001). Further, there can be risks associated with having names on a list or registry of those impacted by violence.

An example of the latter from an LMIC context is the Hudood Ordinances that became part of Pakistan's penal code in 1979, enforcing severe punishments for adultery. In combination with Pakistan's 1984 Law of Evidence, the law requires four Muslim men of good character to come forward as witnesses to verify a woman's claim of rape. In cases where there are no witnesses, police reports of rape are treated as a confession of adultery, and the victims have been subject to punishment (Rathore, 2015). In such a setting, the identification of sexually abused women by public health programs is especially dangerous. There is the potential that public health workers who have knowledge of the identity of a rape victim may be compelled to testify to this information in legal proceedings against the woman for the illegal act of adultery, or *zina*.

Existing guidelines, which have been applied to gathering data for the purpose of surveillance, evaluation, research, and screening for violence, seek to reduce the risk of harm to victims of violence. The WHO's safety guidelines for the conduct of research on violence against women (WHO, 2001, 2016b) include guidance for informed consent, privacy, and confidentiality, as well as direction on staff recruitment and training to prioritize the safety of participants and research teams. Identifying victims of violence and including them in data collection, the nature and site of the interaction between the respondent and the data collector, and methods of eliciting information must be carefully structured to minimize the risks of data collection, from those of being observed answering questions to those associated with having names on a list or in a database. For example, decisions about whether interviews should be conducted at the respondent's home or another place should balance the preferences and safety of the respondent against the potential loss of confidentiality (Rosenbaum et al., 2006; Fraga, 2016).

The WHO guidelines also address the potential for psychological harm to research or surveillance participants due to the nature of the inquiry, such as recalling traumatic experiences (WHO, 2016b). Careful selection and specialized, extensive training of those responsible for collecting information on violence may improve the quality of data collected and reduce the risk of traumatizing the respondents (Cyr and Lamb, 2009), as well as knowing how to respond and what referral resources must be in place if a respondent becomes upset. Some best practices include the use of open-ended prompts, while minimizing option-posing, suggestive questions that often feel riskier or harmful to respondents (Cyr and Lamb, 2009).

Appropriate interpretation of findings from both research and programmatic data to help formulate policies to prevent violence and mitigate against its harm is also important. As noted in the WHO's Intervention Research Recommendation G, "dissemination of results... should avoid stigmatizing or exacerbating risks faced by... vulnerable populations" (WHO, 2016b, 20). For example, the classic US 1990 National Family Violence Survey determined that women were as likely to report having used physical violence against their male partners as vice versa (Straus and Gelles, 1990). However, most acts of violence committed by women were defensive in nature, men were much more likely to perpetrate sexual abuse and coercive control than women, and the likelihood of injury to men was much smaller than that to women (Swan et al., 2008). Without this detail, data from the original study might be cited as exculpatory in trials of violence against women. Selective utilization of data is a challenge across all domains of policymaking; however, public health workers have a responsibility to uphold the integrity of data findings and, in doing so, guard against making the problem of violence worse.

While we recognize that measurement of the occurrence of violence and evaluation of interventions for violence are important steps in establishing evidence-based programs for violence prevention (WHO, 2014), data gathering on violence also should include attempts to measure the harm experienced by respondents as a product of the data gathering process itself. Assessment of the risks associated with data gathering for victims of violence will continue to contribute to the development of evidence-based standards for research and surveillance for this population. As we advocate for ethical public health surveillance to address violence as a public health issue, this raises the issue of individual versus communal benefit. Surveillance must be in the context of functioning systems that also respond to such cases of violence individually; the absence of such systems (or functioning systems) does not outright mean the inability for effective surveillance, but rather should lead to the linking of programs with efforts to ensure provision of selected services.

Addressing Violence through the Health System

The WHO (2014) has recognized victim identification, care, and support programs that reduce future harm to those affected by violence as one of the seven evidence-based "best buys" for violence prevention programs. As such, there are several key sets of recommendations for screening and identifying those at risk for, or affected by, violence (US Preventive Services Task Force, 2013; WHO, 2014), as well as those at risk of committing violence (Betz and Wintemute, 2015). Violence screening programs should be carefully tailored to the appropriate context, yet many of the providers in LMIC sites in which violence screening is advocated (e.g., antenatal clinics) are likely to lack the training, skills, and time to provide counseling for intimate partner violence. Furthermore, these resource-constrained settings may lack subsequent support mechanisms for victims of violence, such as welfare benefits, social services, alternative living arrangements, or effective legal mechanisms. In LMICs, workers who identify someone as having experienced interpersonal violence may have no options but to send them back to their abusive homes or neighborhoods.

In this instance, it is essential to articulate *who* benefits from screening or identification of those affected by violence. While information about violence can play a crucial role in advocacy efforts, the benefits to individuals screened or identified are not clear. At a minimum, providers should be trained to respond with some amount of counseling and to provide support for those who remain in abusive situations, even if no additional services are locally available (Friedman, 2016).

Many existing interventions for reducing violence, such as family counseling, require the involvement of other members of the victim's family or community, and may even involve the perpetrator of the violence. Akin to individual counseling, considering the wishes of the victim is paramount; those experiencing or at risk of violence should have the opportunity to make informed decisions about the inclusion of other individuals in their family or community.

Ethical Challenges in Addressing Suicide

Suicide is an area of public health that often draws increased attention. Ethics challenges arise in the process of assessment and management of individuals' suicide risk, delivery of interventions with a risk of adverse events, and balancing considerations of autonomy and safety. The WHO (2012) has advocated for the inclusion of questions on suicidal behaviors in population-based surveys as part of a strategy to improve case registration and when conducting research for suicide prevention. Studies have attempted to address the fear that inquiries about suicidal ideation may increase self-harm. Those studies so far suggest that asking about suicide does not bring about such an increase, although less is known about the impact of such questions in large-scale survey settings (Dazzi et al., 2014). As in all public health surveillance and research, if screening tools identify people at risk, appropriate referral is a minimum requirement, and in cases where imminent risk of harm is uncovered, public health professionals may need to ensure that emergency treatment is immediately available (as discussed in WHO guidelines).

The potential exclusion of those at heightened risk for suicide from participation in research due to concerns about the severity of their condition and the imminence of death can be problematic (Zimmerman et al., 2015). Suicide risk ought not constitute a barrier to participation in trials for interventions on mental health, in the same way that those at risk for death due to physical illness (e.g., end-stage cancer) are increasingly included in clinical trials. It is ethically imperative that opportunities to participate in research be equally distributed and accessible to all, including those with mental health issues, various ethnic or cultural backgrounds, or overlapping marginalizing identities. This is particularly the case for research studies that hold the prospect of direct benefit for an individual or community of individuals in need of public health attention and intervention. One of the constraints in research in this regard is the potential challenge to researchers in cases where participation is unable to prevent suicide-related harm, as of course will happen for much of medical research (IOM, 2002).

Another ethical dilemma occurs when respect for individual autonomy clashes with paternalism, or the need to provide the best care to further the well-being of patients (Kelly and Dale, 2011); this challenge emerges when those at imminent risk of self-harm refuse further treatment. In programs involving suicidal individuals, it is important to inform them and, when involved, their families about the possibility of involuntary hospitalization in case of imminent suicide risk. For example, seeking informed consent for treatment involving individuals at high risk of suicide due to compromised mental status, cognitive deficits, and impaired ability to judge reality (e.g., people with schizophrenia) poses a set of particularly difficult ethical challenges, and yet it is essential to appreciate that mental health challenges and suicide are deeply correlated (Appleby et al., 2001). Public health practitioners are required to balance risks and benefits of interventions, including involuntary treatment in the context of the importance of autonomy. The involvement of a legally acceptable representative or a patient advocate to provide consent when such involvement is appropriate, and the need for an informed consent process tailored to the participant's capacity to understand (including the provision of adequate time for the participant to assimilate the informed consent process), are important considerations. For public health practitioners, the major practical ethical challenge remains the necessity of referral to care for those identified to be at risk of self-harm and the provision of emergent care for those at imminent risk of suicide. Specifically, in the context of preventing self-harm, paternalism can be justified and individual decision-making might be overridden.

Finally, public health models of suicide examine questions of the degree to which suicide is the result of individual factors versus social determinants. According to Scott Fitzpatrick (2018, 181), "[b]ecause many of the causes of suicide extend beyond individual behavior to the population level (for example, injustice, discrimination, mental illness) and relate to membership of various social groups and communities (for example, Indigenous; lesbian, gay, bisexual, transgender, intersex, queer; those in the criminal justice system) they can also be addressed through population-based strategies." This model underscores the need, consistent with a public health approach, to also examine and intervene on social determinants in making progress toward suicide prevention.

Conclusion

It is essential that the global health community fully understand the ethical issues of public health interventions around violence. These have been defined for different types of violence, including interpersonal and self-directed violence. Despite recent efforts by the WHO and violence prevention professionals, many governments and the wider community fail to recognize that injuries caused by intentional behavior are no *accident*, that violence does not *just happen*, and that we can prevent these conditions in an ethical and meaningful way. Of course, it is critical not only to identify the determinants of violence, but also to be thoughtful about the ethics challenges that emerge in collecting data about them, as well as those that arise in addressing them.

References

ACEP (American College of Emergency Physicians). 2013. *Evaluation and Management of the Sexually Assaulted or Sexually Abused Patient*. E-book. 2nd ed. (Dallas: ACEP). http://www.evawintl.org/library/DocumentLibraryHandler.ashx?id=413.

APA (American Psychological Association). 2009. *Effective Strategies to Support Positive Parenting in Community Health Centers: Report of the Working Group on Child Maltreatment Prevention in Community Health Centers* (Washington, D.C.: APA). https://www.apa.org/pi/prevent-violence/resources/positive-parenting.pdf.

Appleby, L., Shaw, J., Sherratt, J., Robinson, J., and McDonnell, R. 2001. *Safety First: Five-Year Report of the National Confidential Inquiry into Homicides and Suicides by People with a Mental Illness* (London: Department of Health).

Beauchamp, L. T., and Childress, J. F. 2012. *Principles of Biomedical Ethics*. 7th ed. (New York: Oxford University Press).

Betz, M. E., and Wintemute, G. J. 2015. "Physician Counseling on Firearm Safety: A New Kind of Cultural Competence." *JAMA* 314(5): 449–450.

Breiding, M. J., Chen, J., and Black, M. C. 2014. *Intimate Partner Violence in the United States—2010* (Atlanta: Centers for Disease Control and Prevention, National Center for Injury Prevention and Control). https://stacks.cdc.gov/view/cdc/21961.

Childress, J. F., Faden, R. R., Gaare, R. D., Gostin, L. O., Kahn, J., Bonnie, R. J., et al. 2002. "Public Health Ethics: Mapping the Terrain." *Journal of Law, Medicine & Ethics* 30(2): 170–178.

Concialdi, M., and Read, S. 2016. "Child Abuse Neglect: Mandatory Reporting for EMS Providers. What to Look For, What to Report and How." *EMS World* 45(5): 52–55.

Crosby, A. E., Ortega, L., and Melanson, C. 2011. *Self-Directed Violence Surveillance: Uniform Definitions and Recommended Data Elements, Version 1.0* (Atlanta: Centers for Disease Control and Prevention, National Center for Injury Prevention and Control). https://www.cdc.gov/violenceprevention/pdf/self-directed-violence-a.pdf.

Cyr, M., and Lamb, M. E. 2009. "Assessing the Effectiveness of the NICHD Investigative Interview Protocol When Interviewing French-Speaking Alleged Victims of Child Sexual Abuse in Quebec." *Child Abuse and Neglect* 33(5): 257–268.

Dazzi, T., Gribble, R., Wessely, S., and Fear, N. T. 2014. "Does Asking about Suicide and Related Behaviours Induce Suicidal Ideation? What Is the Evidence?" *Psychological Medicine* 44 (16): 3361–3363.

Dawson, A. 2009. "Transparency, Accountability and Vaccination Policy." *Journal of Medical Ethics* 35(5): 274.

Dawson, A. 2011. "Public Health Ethics and the Justification of HIV Screening." *American Journal of Bioethics* 11(4): 48–49.

Faden, R., and Shebaya, S. 2016. "Public Health Ethics." In *The Stanford Encyclopedia of Philosophy*, edited by Edward N. Zalta (Stanford, Calif.: Metaphysics Research Lab, Stanford University). https://plato.stanford.edu/archives/win2016/entries/publichealth-ethics/.

Fitzpatrick, S. J. 2018. "Reshaping the Ethics of Suicide Prevention: Responsibility, Inequality and Action on the Social Determinants of Suicide." *Public Health Ethics* 11(2):179–190.

Fontes, L. A. 2014. "Ethics in Violence against Women Research: The Sensitive, the Dangerous, and the Overlooked." *Ethics and Behavior* 14(2): 141–174.

Foresman-Capuzzi, J. 2014. "CSI and U: Collection and Preservation of Evidence in the Emergency Department." *Journal of Emergency Nursing* 40(3):229–236.

Fraga, S. 2016. "Methodological and Ethical Challenges in Violence Research." *Porto Biomedical Journal* 1(2): 77–80.

Friedman, M. 2016. "Domestic Violence against Women and Autonomy." In *Applied Ethics: A Multicultural Approach*, edited by L. May and J. B. Delston, 314–325. (New York: Routledge).

García-Moreno, C., Hegarty, K., d'Oliveira, A.F.L., Koziol-McLain, J., Colombini, M., and Feder, G. 2015. "The Health-Systems Response to Violence against Women." *Lancet* 385: 1567–1579.

Goldberg, D. S. 2017. *Public Health Ethics and the Social Determinants of Health* (Cham, Switzerland: Springer International).

Greaves, L., Wylie, A., Champagne, C., Karch, L., Lapp, R., Lee, J., et al. 1995. "Women and Violence: Feminist Practice and Quantitative Method." In *Changing Methods: Feminists Transforming Practice*, edited by S. Burt and L. Code, 301–325 (Toronto: University of Toronto Press).

Ho, A. O. 2014. "Suicide: Rationality and Responsibility for Life." *Canadian Journal of Psychiatry* 59(3): 141–147.

IOM (Institute of Medicine). 2002. *Reducing Suicide: A National Imperative* (Washington, D.C.: National Academies Press). doi:10.17226/10398.

Kass, N. E. 2001. "An Ethics Framework for Public Health." *American Journal of Public Health* 91(11): 1776–1782.

Kass, N. E. 2004. "Public Health Ethics: From Foundations and Frameworks to Justice and Global Public Health." *Journal of Law, Medicine & Ethics* 32(2): 232–242.

Kelly, C., and Dale, E. 2011. "Ethical Perspectives on Suicide and Suicide Prevention." *Advances in Psychiatric Treatment* 17(3): 214–219.

Kruijt, D. 2007. *Fractured Cities: Social Exclusion, Urban Violence and Contested Spaces in Latin America* (London: Zed Books).

Lee, R. M., and Renzetti, C. M. 1990. "The Problems of Researching Sensitive Topics: An Overview and Introduction." *American Behavioral Scientist* 33(5): 510–528.

Lozano, R., Naghavi M., Foreman K., Lim S., Shibuya K., Aboyans V., et al. 2012. "Global and Regional Mortality from 235 Causes of Death for 20 Age Groups in 1990 and 2010: A Systematic Analysis for the Global Burden of Disease Study 2010." *Lancet* 380(9859): 2095–2128.

Mikton, C. R., Butchart, A., Dahlberg, L. L., and Krug, E. G. 2016. "Global Status Report on Violence Prevention 2014." *American Journal of Preventive Medicine* 50(5): 652–659.

Moser, C. O. 2004. "Urban Violence and Insecurity: An Introductory Roadmap." *Environment and Urbanization* 16(2): 3–16.

Obasogie, O. K., and Newman, Z. 2017. "Police Violence, Use of Force Policies, and Public Health." *American Journal of Law and Medicine* 43(2–3): 279–295.

Peckham, S., and Hann, A. 2010. Public Health Ethics and Practice (Bristol, UK: Policy Press).

Rathore, M. A. 2015. "Women's Rights in Pakistan: The Zina Ordinance and the Need for Reform." School of Public Policy Capstones 38. https://scholarworks.umass.edu/cppa_capstones/38.

Rosenbaum, A., Rabenhorst, M. M., Reddy, M. K., Fleming, M. T., and Howells, N. L. 2006. "A Comparison of Methods for Collecting Self-Report Data on Sensitive Topics." *Violence and Victims* 21(4): 461–471.

Schopper, D., Lormand, J. D., and Waxweiler, R., ed. 2006. *Developing Policies to Prevent Injuries and Violence: Guidelines for Policy-Makers and Planners* (Geneva: World Health Organization).

Sikweyiya, Y., and Jewkes, R. 2011. "Perceptions about Safety and Risks in Gender-Based Violence Research: Implications for the Ethics Review Process." *Culture, Health and Sexuality* 13(9): 1091–1102.

Stoltenborgh, M., Bakermans-Kranenburg, M. J., van Ijzendoorn, M. H., and Alink, L. R. 2013. "Cultural-Geographical Differences in the Occurrence of Child Physical Abuse? A Meta-analysis of Global Prevalence." *International Journal of Psychology* 48(2): 81–94.

Straus, M. A., and Gelles, R. J. 1990. *Physical Violence in American Families: Risk Factors and Adaptations to Violence in 8,145 Families* (New Brunswick, N.J.: Transaction).

Swan, S. C., Gambon, L. J., Caldwell, J. E., Sullivan, T. P., and Snow, D. L. 2008. "A Review of Research on Women's Use of Violence with Male Intimate Partners." *Violence and Victims* 23(3): 301–314.

Thomas, J. C., Sage, M., Dillenberg, J., and Guillory J. V. 2002. "A Code of Ethics for Public Health." *American Journal of Public Health* 92(7): 1057–1059.

Tonmyr, L. 2015. "The Canadian Incidence Study of Reported Child Abuse and Neglect: A Partnership." *Health Promotion and Chronic Disease Prevention in Canada* 35(8–9): 117–118.

Tonmyr, L., Li, Y. A., Williams, G., Scott, D., and Jack, S. M. 2010. "Patterns of Reporting by Health Care and Nonhealth Care Professionals to Child Protection Services in Canada." *Paediatrics and Child Health* 15(8): e25–e32.

US Preventive Services Task Force. 2013. *Screening for Intimate Partner Violence and Abuse of Elderly and Vulnerable Adults* (Rockville, Md.: U.S. Department of Health and Human Services, Agency for Healthcare Research and Quality).

Walrath, C., Garraza, L. G., Reid, H., Goldston, D. B., and McKeon, R. 2015. "Impact of the Garrett Lee Smith Youth Suicide Prevention Program on Suicide Mortality." *American Journal of Public Health* 105(5): 986–993.

Weber, N. S., Fisher, J. A., Cowan, D. N., Postolache, T. T., Larsen, R. A., and Niebuhr, D. W. 2013. "Descriptive Epidemiology and Underlying Psychiatric Disorders among Hospitalizations with Self-Directed Violence." *PLoS ONE* 8(3): e59818.

WHO (World Health Organization). 2001. *Putting Women First: Ethical and Safety Recommendations for Research on Domestic Violence Against Women* (Geneva: WHO Department of Gender, Women and Health). http://www.who.int/gender/violence/womenfirtseng.pdf.

WHO (World Health Organization). 2002. *The World Report on Violence and Health* (Geneva: WHO). http://apps.who.int/iris/bitstream/10665/42495/1/9241545615_eng.pdf.

WHO (World Health Organization). 2009. *Reducing Violence through Victim Identification, Care and Support Programmes* (Geneva: WHO). http://www.who.int/violence_injury_prevention/violence/programmes.pdf

WHO (World Health Organization). 2013. *Global and Regional Estimates of Violence against Women: Prevalence and Health Effects of Intimate Partner Violence and Non-Partner Sexual Violence* (Geneva: WHO). https://www.who.int/reproductivehealth/publications/violence/9789241564625/en/.

WHO (World Health Organization). 2014. *Preventing Suicide: A Global Imperative* (Geneva: WHO). http://www.who.int/mental_health/suicide-prevention/world_report_2014/en/.

WHO (World Health Organization). 2016a. *Global Plan of Action to Strengthen the Role of the Health System in Addressing Interpersonal Violence, in Particular Against Women and Girls, and Against Children* (Geneva: WHO). http://www.who.int/topics/violence/UNFPA-GAP2-violence.pdf.

WHO (World Health Organization). 2016b. *Ethical and Safety Recommendations for Intervention Research on Violence against Women* (Geneva: WHO). http://preventgbvafrica.org/wp-content/uploads/2014/10/VAW_Research_Ethics_Safety_9_3_14.pdf.

WHO/Europe (World Health Organization Regional Office for Europe). 2014. *Investing in Children: The European Child Maltreatment Prevention Action Plan 2015–2020* (Copenhagen, Denmark: World Health Organization/Europe). http://www.euro.who.int/__data/assets/pdf_file/0009/253728/64wd13e_InvestChildMaltreat_140439.pdf.

Yon, Y., Mikton, C. R., Gassoumis, Z. D., and Wilber, K. H. 2017. "Elder Abuse Prevalence in Community Settings: A Systematic Review and Meta-analysis." *Lancet Global Health* 5(2): e147–e156.

Zimmerman, M., Clark, H. L., Multach, M. D., Walsh, E., Rosenstein, L. K., and Gazarian, D. 2015. "Have Treatment Studies of Depression Become Even Less Generalizable? A Review of the Inclusion and Exclusion Criteria Used in Placebo-Controlled Antidepressant Efficacy Trials Published during the Past 20 Years." *Mayo Clinic Proceedings* 90(9): 1180–1186.

Further Reading

US Preventive Services Task Force. 2014. *Screening for Suicide Risk in Adolescents, Adults, and Older Adults in Primary Care* (Rockville, Md.: US Department of Health and Human Services, Agency for Healthcare Research and Quality). https://www.uspreventiveservicestaskforce.org/Home/GetFileByID/1899.

WHO (World Health Organization). 2012. *Public Health Action for the Prevention of Suicide* (Geneva: WHO). http://apps.who.int/iris/bitstream/handle/10665/75166/9789241503570_eng.pdf.

SECTION TWELVE

GENETICS

CHAPTER 54

AN OVERVIEW OF ETHICS AND PUBLIC HEALTH GENETICS

DEBRA J. H. MATHEWS

Introduction

Although public health genetics can trace its roots back to the eugenics movement of the early twentieth century and the start of newborn screening in the 1960s, it emerged as a field in the late 1990s and grew up in parallel with and driven by the Human Genome Project (HGP). Public health genetics (more commonly referred to as "community genetics" in Europe) can be described as "the application of advances in genetics and molecular biotechnology to improving public health and preventing disease" (Austin, Peyser, and Khoury, 2000, 82). While the work of public health genetics had been ongoing for some time, both in the United States and internationally (for example, the World Health Organization had screening and counseling programs for beta thalassemia in the 1980s [Modell and Kuliev, 1998]), a cohesive field took time to emerge. A key event in the birth of the field—perhaps its US birth announcement—came in 1997 when the US Centers for Disease Control and Prevention (CDC) established the Office of Genetics and Disease Prevention, now known as the Office of Public Health Genomics (CDC, 2018). The timing of this birth makes enormous sense, given that large-scale sequencing of the human genome as part of the HGP began in 1996, although a completed first draft was not published until 2003. The genomic data provided by the HGP fueled the field of public health genetics. Gilbert Omenn commented in 2000 that the prospect of a decoded human genome would launch a "golden age for the public health sciences" (Omenn, 2000, 1).

Shortly before the establishment of the Office of Genetics and Disease Prevention, Muin Khoury (who would become the head of that office) and colleagues laid out the current and potential role of genetics in executing the core functions of public health

(Khoury and the Genetics Working Group, 1996), as defined by the Institute of Medicine (IOM, 1988). These core functions of public health include assessment, policy development, and assurance of health services, onto which Khoury and colleagues mapped, respectively, activities such as epidemiological studies of disease-environment interactions, policy regarding deployment of particular genetic tests for disease prevention, and development of public health genetic programs such as the addition of newborn screening tests. The authors also noted that studies of the ethical, legal, and social implications of these interventions would be required prior to deployment. Throughout the development of the field of public health genetics, there has been a focus on the ethical issues raised by the application of genetics and genomics to improving population health.

In 1998, at the First Annual Conference on Genetics and Public Health, held in Atlanta, Georgia, many of the ethical challenges raised by the chapters in this section of *The Oxford Handbook of Public Health Ethics* were discussed. (In fact, two chapter authors were presenters at the meeting—Gail Geller and Eric Juengst; see also Khoury et al., 1998). That same year, the journal *Community Genetics* launched in Europe. The first issue focused largely on genetic testing, but it also highlighted the importance of attention to ethical, legal, and social issues. The editor cautioned that in our pursuit of the benefits of community genetics/public health genetics, "we should not bargain on ethical principles of autonomy, doing good and not harm, justice, and providing equal access and solidarity" (ten Kate, 1998, 2).

In 2000 a "mini-symposium" on public health genetics highlighted the range of issues that the emerging field was confronting, including nutrition and genetics, population screening for hemochromatosis, ecogenetics (the relationship of genetic variation to risks from environmental exposures), behavioral genetics, and host-pathogen interactions, as well as research and training in ethical, legal, and social implications of public health genetics. Importantly, many of the challenges and research questions discussed, studied, or forecast then are still with us today.

Since the late 1990s, as technology has become more powerful, less expensive, and more accessible, public health genomics has gained traction internationally. The World Health Organization's Human Genomics in Global Health Initiative now has collaborating partners in Brazil, Cuba, India, Jordan, and beyond (WHO, 2018). With such technological improvements and increased international reach, we are finally coming to a sufficient understanding of parts of the human genome to allow researchers to better address the kinds of questions raised twenty years ago.

Chapter Overviews

This section of *The Oxford Handbook of Public Health Ethics* is dedicated to the examination of ethics and public health genetics. The section's chapters are arranged in roughly chronological order, from public health genetics' past, to the present challenges faced by the field, and, finally, largely looking to the future. The chapters are introduced below.

Eugenics

In "Eugenics and Public Health: Historical Connections and Ethical Implications," Paul Lombardo looks back at the early relationship between public health and genetics in America. As Lombardo writes, many in the public health field are unaware of the historical relationship between genetics, eugenics, and public health. This history is important to remember, not only because it has shaped genetic practice, but also because many of the questions and concerns raised by this shared history remain with us today. As Lombardo notes, both eugenics and public health emphasized population-based solutions for health problems and saw a role for the state in accomplishing their goals.

The term *eugenics* was coined by Francis Galton in 1883 (Galton, 1883, 17), and it came to describe a science that "promised an improvement in future generations by selective encouragement of childbirth for productive, healthy members of society, along with simultaneous discouragement of parenthood among the chronically ill, the disabled, and others who depended upon public welfare" (Lombardo, this volume). While there was certainly resistance to eugenics from some in public health, there was also profound overlap among prominent figures in these fields, including multiple eugenicists who served as president of the American Public Health Association, and as faculty at leading schools of public health in the United States. However, perhaps the greatest US public health impact came not from those professional or academic intersections, but rather from the passage of eugenic health laws in US states. For example, "eugenic marriage laws" mandated premarital testing and imposed certain restrictions, using arguments from disease prevention and, sometimes, "race betterment." These laws went on to include sterilization and anti-miscegenation laws, and eventually restrictions on immigration, in an effort to "protect our racial stock" (Knox, 1915). As Lombardo writes, these eugenic laws with public health rationales "violated expectations of autonomy, equal treatment, and justice by often targeting the most vulnerable—the poor, the disabled, and sexual and racial minorities—as the objects of eugenic reform" (Lombardo, this volume). While Lombardo notes that "historical similarities are not moral equivalents" (Pernick, 1997, 1770), he cautions that society must be careful not to repeat the mistakes and transgressions of the past as we again embrace the power of genomics in service of public health.

Newborn Screening

In "Newborn Screening in the United States: Ethical Issues," Michelle Huckaby Lewis and Jeffrey R. Botkin discuss the topic of newborn screening, perhaps the largest and most familiar contemporary public health genetics program. Begun in the 1960s with a test for phenylketonuria (PKU) developed by Dr. Robert Guthrie, the vast majority of babies born each year in the United States have their blood spotted onto Guthrie cards shortly after birth. State-administered screening programs test the blood for a range of markers that indicate the presence (or increased risk) of disease. The original goal of newborn screening was to identify babies with disease so that treatment could be initiated before the disease caused permanent damage. While newborn screening has been a tremendously successful public health program, it remains controversial due to details of both the testing and post-testing storage and use.

Though newborn screening began with one simple screen for an abnormal presence of phenylalanine metabolites in the blood, new technology has enabled a dramatic increase in the number and type of conditions that can be detected. For example, new technology (tandem mass spectrometry) in the 1990s made possible the simultaneous identification of dozens of metabolic conditions. Unlike PKU, some of these newly identifiable conditions were poorly understood and could not be readily treated. Over time, tremendous variability developed across US state programs, such that babies in different states received very different testing (e.g., screening for two conditions versus dozens). Efforts at standardization were met with controversy, largely due to the dramatic increase in the number of recommended screening tests, expansion beyond the public health mission, and lack of attention to the associated ethical issues (Botkin et al., 2006).

One such ethical issue relates to parental consent. Parental consent is generally not required for newborn screening and historically has not been required for the retention and secondary use of de-identified blood spots. However, the expansion beyond the public health mission, changes in risks associated with secondary use, and public perceptions of such uses make "the question of how to allocate decision-making authority for newborn screening among parents, states, and physicians less clear" (Lewis and Botkin, this volume) It is worth noting that the controversy surrounding the storage and use of blood spots for research reflects a broader conversation regarding the benefits, harms, and acceptability of using leftover clinical samples for biomedical research.

Biobanking

The practice of biobanking is discussed in "Public Health Genomics, Biobanking, and Ethics" by Karen Meagher, R. Jean Cadigan, Gail E. Henderson, and Eric T. Juengst. As human biospecimens and data are increasingly being collected into large-scale biobanks, a parallel evolution is taking place in the relationship between biobanks and those whose samples and data are being collected, stored, and used. These biobanks are often designed for translational genomic research or health care quality improvement, but are facing increasing calls for use in public health surveillance and intervention (Khoury and Evans, 2015; Aswini and Varun, 2010). Further, just as the decreasing cost and increasing accessibility of large-scale genetic testing, including whole genome sequencing, will challenge the paradigm of newborn screening, so will it transform biobank research.

Meagher et al. examine three case studies that illustrate such challenges: the MyCode Community Health Initiative at the Geisinger Health System (GHS), the GeneScreen research project using the Kaiser Permanente Northwest Research Biobank (KPNW-RB), and the US Precision Medicine Initiative (PMI) *All of Us* Research Program Biobank at Mayo Clinic. As noted by Meagher et al., "At the intersection of biobanking and public health, researchers, biobank curators, and participants face challenges when implementing confidentiality protections, informed consent method and scope, community engagement, and return and disposition of results. Each of the three cases demonstrates shifting contexts in these regards, as research increasingly has translational implications, resulting in a mix of research, clinical, and public health purposes" (Meagher et al., this volume).

However, these contexts have different cultures, norms, and moral traditions, and implementing their goals using the same resource (biobank) or blurring the lines between these contexts comes with both benefits and risks. For example, stripping identifying information (taking, for a moment, the current regulatory stance that DNA and genomic data are not inherently identifying) from biospecimens may be an important step to help protect confidentiality in the context of research, but this protection for the research context eliminates the option of returning clinically useful results to biospecimen contributors. If a biobank is built for clinical purposes, which require maintaining identifying information and facilitating return of results, the standards for informed consent and the necessary privacy and confidentiality measures will be a poor fit for public health purposes. These current and near-term ethical challenges must be addressed, and how they are addressed will help shape future directions.

Infectious Disease

In "Genetic Epidemiology, Infectious Disease, and Public Health Ethics," Priya Duggal, Gail Geller, and Andrea Sutherland explore some of the ethical challenges ahead that will be raised by the application of genomics to the study, prevention, and control of infectious disease, including challenges related to the kind of blurring between contexts noted by Meagher et al. Existing and emerging genomic technologies have the potential to enhance and shape our ability to reduce the global burden of infectious disease, including helping us better understand infectious disease pathology; develop, improve, or re-engineer diagnostic, vaccines, and therapies; and improve public health interventions (e.g., source and contact tracing). As noted by Duggal, Geller, and Sutherland (this volume), there is also "growing evidence that *host* genetic factors, and the interaction between host, vector and pathogen, influence variability in infection rates, immune responses," and a range of other factors shaping an individual's response to infectious disease and medical countermeasures.

Infectious diseases are incredibly diverse both in their interactions with humans and in the constellation of ethical issues raised by our study of and combat with them. While there is a tremendous body of literature exploring the ethical, legal, and social implications of genomics related to Mendelian and complex disease, and much of this can be applied to infectious disease, the literature focused on ethics, genomics, and infectious disease is in its infancy (Geller et al., 2014). Duggal, Geller, and Sutherland use three examples to explore the kinds of ethical issues we should anticipate in this context: inequities in HIV morbidity and mortality (inequities that exist and may be exacerbated by genomic approaches to public health interventions), personalized vaccines (e.g., adjustments made to which vaccine or doses to deliver, or policies about whom to vaccinate upon identification of a genetic disposition to vaccine-related adverse events), and triage during epidemics (e.g., prioritizing or deprioritizing those with certain genotypes that predict likelihood or severity of infection for access to scarce resources). As this science progresses, more ethical issues will emerge that we did not anticipate and that are not yet represented in the literature discussing the ethical, legal and social issues raised by genetics. As noted by the authors, we must extract what lessons we can from related ethical, legal, and social issues from the past; continue to systematically forecast any issues that might arise; and assess those that are confronted in the future.

Conclusion

Although public health genetics and genomics is still a relatively young field, it is poised to take an increasingly important role in global public health. As the cost of genomic testing and sequencing has decreased and small, portable testing devices have been developed, the range and scale of uses and possible scale have expanded from the kinds of screening programs that the World Health Organization and others have been engaged in for decades, to the kinds of infectious disease–oriented efforts described and anticipated by Duggal, Geller, and Sutherland. While practitioners of public health have long been sensitive to the ethical tensions inherent in their work, the growing infusion of genomics requires attention to new ethical dimensions, many of which are familiar to those in genomics but new to public health, and some of which will be novel and are yet to be identified, understood, and addressed.

References

Aswini, Y. B., and Varun, S. 2010. "Genetics in Public Health: Rarely Explored." *Indian Journal of Human Genetics* 16(2): 47–54.

Austin, M. A., Peyser, P. A., and Khoury, M. J. 2000. "The Interface of Genetics and Public Health: Research and Educational Challenges." *Annual Review of Public Health* 21: 81–99.

Botkin, J. R., Clayton, E. W., Fost, N. C., Burke, W., Murray, T. H., Baily, M. A., et al. 2006. "Newborn Screening Technology: Proceed with Caution." *Pediatrics* 117(5): 1793–1799.

CDC (Centers for Disease Control and Prevention). 2018. "About Us—Genomics." https://www.cdc.gov/genomics/about/achievements.htm.

Galton, F. 1883. *Inquiries into Human Faculty and its Development* (London: Macmillan).

Geller, G., Dvoskin, R., Thio, C. L., Duggal, P., Lewis, M. H., Bailey, T. C., et al. 2014. "Genomics and Infectious Disease: A Call to Identify the Ethical, Legal and Social Implications for Public Health and Clinical Practice." *Genome Medicine* 6(11): 106. https://genomemedicine.biomedcentral.com/articles/10.1186/s13073-014-0106-2.

IOM (Institute of Medicine). 1988. *The Future of Public Health* (Washington, D.C.: National Academy Press).

Khoury, M. J., and Evans, J. P. 2015. "A Public Health Perspective on a National Precision Medicine Cohort: Balancing Long-Term Knowledge Generation with Early Health Benefit." *JAMA* 313(21): 2117–2118.

Khoury, M. J., and the Genetics Working Group. 1996. "From Genes to Public Health: The Applications of Genetic Technology in Disease Prevention." *American Journal of Public Health* 86(12): 1717–1722.

Khoury, M. J., Puryear, M., Thomson, E., and Bryan, J. 1998. "Translating Advances in Human Genetics into Disease Prevention and Health Promotion." *Community Genetics* 1: 93–108.

Knox, H. A. 1915. "Measuring Human Intelligence: A Progressive Series of Standardized Tests Used by the Public Health Service to Protect Our Racial Stock." *Scientific American* 112: 52–58.

Modell, B., and Kuliev, A. 1998. "The History of Community Genetics: The Contribution of the Haemoglobin Disorders." *Community Genetics* 1: 3–11.

Omenn, G. S. 2000. "Public Health Genetics: An Emerging Interdisciplinary Field for the Post-Genomic Era." *Annual Review of Public Health* 21: 1–13.

Pernick, M. 1997. "Eugenics and Public Health in American History." *American Journal of Public Health* 87(11): 1767–1772.

ten Kate, L. P. 1998. "Editorial." *Community Genetics* 1:1–2.

WHO (World Health Organization). 2018. "About WHO's Human Genomics in Global Health Initiative." http://www.who.int/genomics/about/en/.

CHAPTER 55

EUGENICS AND PUBLIC HEALTH: HISTORICAL CONNECTIONS AND ETHICAL IMPLICATIONS

PAUL LOMBARDO

Introduction

Although the historical literature on eugenics has proliferated since 1980, there has been only limited inquiry into the linkages between the field of public health and the field of eugenics (some notable exceptions are Pernick, 1997; Stern, 2005; Fairchild, 2003). This history has not made its way into many texts in public health, and people in the field are often unaware of these connections. These linkages may seem counterintuitive, because we generally identify public health with environmental interventions, from improving sanitation to battling infectious disease, while we think of eugenics as a dark "pseudo-science" that was completely dedicated to manipulating heredity. In fact, the history is more complex than these assumptions might suggest. This chapter details some points of connection between the two fields and explores the ethical significance of that history.

In the first decades of the twentieth century in the United States, three fields of scientific and medical study emerged that promised to provide new tools with which to understand societal problems and improve the lives of citizens: public health, genetics, and eugenics. Both the public health movement and the eugenics movement called for governmental action, as they consciously focused on re-engineering both the physical world and social relations within it. Eventually, both public health practice and eugenic policy would incorporate genetic thinking as one means of accomplishing the progress their proponents hoped would characterize a modern world.

Each of these areas of inquiry raised ethical questions about the role of the state in combating disease and related social problems, and about the boundaries surrounding individual choice when the common good was at stake. This chapter focuses on how, early in the last century, the public health movement found points of accommodation and cooperation with the fledgling eugenics movement.

Eugenics

The English gentleman Francis Galton coined the term *eugenics* in 1883, giving a new name to the commonplace idea that control of reproduction could be a prerogative of societies and governments. To Galton, eugenics was "the study of agencies under social control that may improve or impair the racial qualities of future generations, whether physically or mentally" (Galton, 1883, 17). In time, reflecting the Greek roots of the word, eugenics became known as the "well-born" science, or the discipline of "better breeding." It promised an improvement in future generations by selective encouragement of childbirth for productive, healthy members of society, along with the simultaneous discouragement of parenthood among the chronically ill, the disabled, and others who depended upon public welfare.

Galton was also a pioneer in the field of biostatistics, and eugenics developed a quantitative emphasis in tandem with the vital statistics movement in public health. When Gregor Mendel's experiments in heredity and the "laws" they posited were rediscovered, eugenicists in the United States looked to them as tools they could use alongside statistics to develop a more thorough understanding of genetics.

Public health and eugenics matured simultaneously, and leaders in the two fields shared three key ideas: prevention, efficiency, and progress. Both fields held that halting disease spread by prevention was more efficient than working to discover a cure to apply person by person. To the public health community, a vaccine to prevent disease inception was better than a medicine to treat disease. Eugenicists considered expenditures on hospitals and asylums to care for the ill to be less efficient than controlling reproduction among those thought likely to have children who would populate those institutions. Eugenicists promoted the idea that crime, poverty, disease, and the suffering they generated could be eradicated, along with the notion that as societal quality improved, the burden of taxes paid to combat negative conditions would be diminished. They urged public health methods in this endeavor; namely, to segregate people from the general population, and isolate them in institutions so they could not spread disease or breed. In the literature of both public health and eugenics, prevention and efficiency joined progress, a general faith in the ability of human ingenuity to design and manage a better world, where social problems would eventually be conquered.

The hope that surrounded eugenics in its early years attracted most geneticists as that science was in its infancy. Public health physicians also saw eugenics as a practical application of the insights of their own field. While many people involved with genetic science or public health eventually rejected the class and racial bigotry and the repressive state measures that came to characterize the public eugenics movement in the United States, most did not reject the basic premise of eugenics: that efficient prevention of social problems was a necessary condition for social progress.

The Promise of Eugenics: Population Health

Unlike medicine more generally, the public health movement emphasized population-based solutions for health problems, rather than a focus on individual patients, and eugenics had a similar focus. Galton (1889, 35) himself had said that "the science of heredity is concerned with large populations rather than with individuals." The medical educator Harvey Jordan (1912, 396–399) predicted that in light of eugenics and the "general change from individualism to collectivism," all medicine would eventually be transformed to public health, and all physicians from "doctors of private diseases" to "guardians of the public health." Medicine would become "a science of the prevention of weakness and morbidity; their permanent not temporary cure, their racial eradication rather than their personal palliation" (Jordan, 1912, 396–399).

But early public health advocates often clashed with the eugenicists. The more radical eugenicists voiced chilling prescriptions for those who burdened society. Of the unemployable, the economist Frank W. Taussig (1911, 300) complained that it was too soon "to chloroform them once for all." He predicted a future in which the "feeble minded,... those saturated with alcohol or tainted with hereditary disease,... [i]rretrievable criminals and tramps" could "simply be stamped out" (Taussig, 1911, 300). Charles B. Davenport, the most famous of US eugenicists, launched his career in the field by questioning the role of philanthropy and public health. Rather than spend "tens of millions... to bolster up the weak and alleviate the suffering of the sick," argued Davenport, why not spend a similar amount to "redeem mankind from vice, imbecility and suffering" through eugenics (Davenport, 1910, 34–35)?

Davenport's allies thought that social interventions like charity interrupted natural processes such as disease and could thwart the workings of evolution. The harshest critics of public health argued that programs for vaccination and sanitation did nothing but delay the inevitable demise of inferior organisms not fit to live in a state of nature. Said one such critic: "Death is the normal process of elimination in the social organism;... in prolonging the lives of defectives we are tampering with the function of the social kidneys" (Cole, 1914, 503). As late as 1936, some critics of traditional public health interventions saw little eugenic value in public health practices (Allan, 1936).

But many public health advocates eventually developed an accommodation with eugenicists. They recognized the quandary: public health prevention might alleviate disease but rescue those whom nature might otherwise destroy. The problem could be solved by attention to heredity. While future generations were not threatened by a "genetically defective" person today, if that same person had children, generational decline would continue. Attending to heredity projected public health prevention into the future mode. The prominent geneticist Herbert Spence Jennings (1927, 45, 47) stated, "The *only* remedy is to stop the propagation of bearers of defective genes. The public health worker must take this fact seriously; a burden of responsibility is placed on him; he *must* become genetically minded, eugenically minded."

As the historian Martin Pernick (1997, 1769) has noted, "eugenics and public health could cooperate, rather than competing." The goal of public health and eugenics was population health, or the common good rather than the welfare of any individual. The clearest measure of cooperation between the two fields was in the passage of health laws based on eugenic premises.

Eugenic Laws

The expansive reach of public health law is justified by the government's "police power," the inherent authority to adopt laws to protect health, welfare, and morals, and an exception to the usual expectation that states should not interfere with the property rights or the liberty and bodily integrity of citizens. Among all other health law, public health law holds a unique position by using interventions not merely offered to patients, but mandated by government. It often invokes the ancient legal maxim *salus populi suprema lex*, "the health of the people is the highest good" (Freund, 1904, iii). Advocates within the eugenics movement made their most enduring mark through the passage of laws. Those laws were often the result of focusing on the same goals that were articulated by leaders in the public health movement.

Since protections of the US Constitution often place boundaries between the prerogatives of government and the rights of individuals, the most dramatic features of public health law resemble martial law—law that is available in time of war, or when the social structure is so severely threatened by catastrophic events such as civil disorder, epidemics, or natural disasters that the usual deference to individual rights can be set aside. Public health interventions like mandatory vaccination, seizure of property, and orders of quarantine interrupt the usual expectations of citizens but are justified as means that prevent more substantial imminent harms to the general populace.

The earliest eugenic laws prohibited the issuance of marriage licenses to the "defective." These laws were designed to reduce the number of children who would inherit the problematic physical, mental, and moral shortcomings their parents exhibited. A Connecticut statute outlawed marriage among people suffering from epilepsy. It was upheld with arguments that echoed public health principles placing the common good over individual liberty. According to the Connecticut Supreme Court, "Laws of this kind may be regarded as an expression of the conviction of modern society that disease is largely preventable by proper precautions,...even at the cost of narrowing what in former days was regarded as the proper domain of individual right" (*Gould v. Gould*, 78 Conn. 242, 61 A. 604 [Conn. 1905]).

A later group of statutes mandated medical testing for sexually transmitted infections, like syphilis, prior to marriage. Widely supported in the public health community, these laws were uniformly known as the "eugenic marriage laws." Critics attacked their fundamental premises, arguing that infectious diseases were not inherited. But supporters believed that disease susceptibility as well as propensities to unhealthy and immoral behavior were inherited. Eugenic-minded public health supporters also pointed to the effect of the laws, which they hoped would prevent the birth of innocent children who would die prematurely or be burdened with disease.

A Louisiana health officer applauded the introduction of laws to regulate marriage. In the future, he said, "science will give positive data as to the fit and the unfit, and the state will put forth its strong arm for race betterment" (Dowling, 1915, 1143–1144). Analyzing the history of such laws years later, a former chief of the Division of Venereal Disease of the US Public Health Service confirmed the eugenic bases of early marriage laws: "Certain principles of eugenics sponsored by the national office of the American Eugenics Society gained wider acceptance. Those principles stressed the importance of health examinations and waiting periods between application for and issuance of marriage licenses [... and] advocated restricted marriages of the unfit" (Shafer, 1954, 488).

The next wave of eugenic laws focused on sexual sterilization, a procedure that could make the shortcomings of marriage restriction irrelevant. Sterilization would ensure, using a more efficient means, that unfit children would not be born. The state of Indiana passed the first sterilization law in 1907, and over the next twenty years a dozen other states inscribed eugenics into state health laws. Though some critics condemned both the effectiveness of sterilization laws in decreasing inherited disease and the intrusion on bodily integrity they required, their objections were mooted when the US Supreme Court endorsed eugenical surgery in the 1927 case of *Buck v. Bell* (274 U.S. 200 [1927]). In that case, Justice Oliver Wendell Holmes Jr. announced the constitutional validity of Virginia's law, and left an opinion that contained a shorthand credo for many sterilization devotees: "Three generations of imbeciles are enough" (*Buck v. Bell*). Holmes's opinion incorporated a reference to the premier public health precedent of the century, *Jacobson v. Massachusetts* (197 U.S. 11 [1905]), which upheld the constitutionality of mandatory vaccination in the face of a smallpox epidemic. "The principle that sustains compulsory vaccination," said Holmes, "is broad enough to cover cutting the fallopian tubes" (*Buck v. Bell*).

"Racial integrity" legislation that prohibited interracial marriage was also part of the eugenic program. Public health physicians issued vital statistics reports with instructions on the legal requirements to track births and deaths according to the race of the participants, and to refuse marriage licenses to people of different races (Plecker, 1924). Eugenic laws to prohibit "pollution" of white bloodlines by race mixing were adopted in the majority of states. The quantitative, statistical emphasis of eugenics meshed easily with the increasing collection of vital statistics by states, yielding a bureaucratic tool to ensure racial separation for eugenic purposes.

As early as 1912, public health leaders joined with eugenicists to screen travelers to Ellis Island for "feeblemindedness," along with other purportedly hereditary conditions. Public health officers received training in eugenics at Charles Davenport's nearby Eugenics Record Office in Cold Spring Harbor, New York. Public Health Service physicians proudly announced how IQ tests would be enlisted in the Ellis Island screening process to identify "mental enfeeblement" and "protect our racial stock" (Knox, 1915). Representatives of the Immigration Restriction League used the language of public health sanitation to justify their push for restricting some nationalities from migrating to America: "Just as we isolate bacterial invasions, . . . so we can compel an inferior race to remain in its native habitat," said one immigration restrictionist (Hall, 1919, 126). This type of eugenic advocacy was important to the passage of the Immigration Act of 1924, which abruptly limited the flow of Italians and Jews from Europe to America for most of the twentieth century. In each of these cases, a public health rationale was used as the foundation for laws to curtail the liberties of marginal groups, even though the scientific basis for those laws was always questionable and their impact on public health was negligible.

Leaders in Eugenics and Public Health

Advocates for an expanded national role for public health proposed legislation to the US Congress in 1897 that recited openly eugenic goals when they called for the collection of statistics related to marriages. Those studies would identify people "liable to produce physically and mentally defective offspring" and provide "information leading to race improvement through better marriage selection" ("Bill to Establish," 1897, 1194). In the twentieth century, the newly named Public Health Service continued eugenic advocacy. Officers of the Service supported the conclusion that social problems could be cured by eugenic interventions and argued that "eugenics is a science. It is a fact, not a fad" (Rucker, 1915, 219). They supported programs to eradicate disease-carrying parasites, and felt equally qualified to comment on the danger of "human parasites" (Rucker, 1917, 228).

Early in his tenure as Surgeon General (1912–1920), Dr. Rupert Blue announced his support for eugenic laws. He favored health certificates for both men and women in advance of marriage, as well as laws that would allow the compulsory sterilization of "defectives" ("Wants Law for Health Certificates," 1913, 29). Enlisting three of his staff physicians, Blue authorized "the most approved line of investigation known to the modern science of eugenics," for one would-be bridegroom ("Eugenic Examination," 1913). The doctors unanimously decided to award him a eugenic marriage certificate ("Officially Recognize Eugenics," 1913). Blue's administration also initiated a daily column that ran in general newspapers called *Uncle Sam, M.D.* The column discussed the importance of heredity to health and recited some of the key conclusions of eugenics: that "defective persons breed defective persons," and that knowledge of heredity will enable "prevention of the creation of degenerate and insane persons, on the one hand, and normal, efficient people, on the other" ("Uncle Sam, M.D.," 1919). Blue was a member of the Eugenics Committee of the American Genetics Association, and he represented that organization at an international eugenics congress ("Membership: The Eugenics Committee," 1914; International Eugenics Committee, 1914). He also presided over the program of eugenic examinations undertaken at Ellis Island to screen out "defective" immigrants (Hrdlička 1919, 127).

Hugh Cumming followed Blue as Surgeon General (1920–1936). Cumming sat on the advisory council of the American Eugenics Society and in 1921 helped organize the Second International Eugenics Congress (1920–1921). He published articles explaining the relationship between eugenics and preventive medicine (e.g., Cumming, 1928).

In 1931 Cumming joined other eugenicists who had become president of the American Public Health Association (APHA). Indiana's first in the nation 1907 eugenic sterilization law was a project of public health reformer John N. Hurty, president of the APHA in 1912. William A. Evans, Commissioner of Health in Chicago, was a professor of public health at Northwestern University and APHA president in 1917. Evans wrote a syndicated column for the *Chicago Tribune* entitled "How to Keep Well" that kept readers up to date on eugenic publications and regularly "answered questions on hygiene, sanitation and prevention of disease," including eugenics (see, for example, "How to Keep Well," 1913). Mazyck P. Ravenel edited the *American Journal of Public Health* and was APHA president in 1921. He repeatedly invoked eugenic family studies and urged more attention to eugenic prevention (e.g., Ravenel, 1924). Among the many other leaders in public health and eugenics was William Welch, founder of the Johns Hopkins School of Hygiene and Public Health and vice-chairman of the Scientific Board of the Eugenics Record Office in 1910.

The Shadow of the Holocaust

The primary eugenic goals—to eliminate disease, crime, and poverty by managing heredity and infusing law with science—comprised a hopeful program that included a future of healthy babies and the promise of prosperity. This hopeful side of eugenics generated much of its attraction not only for the public health world, but for most Americans as well. Retrospective ethical analyses of eugenics have focused on how eugenic policies used the stigma of disease, medically coercive practices, racial and ethnic bigotry, and policies of exclusion and discrimination as the means to meet eugenic goals. We associate eugenics with fear, hatred, and racism because the campaign to remake the United States as a eugenic nation relied on those strategies to pass eugenic legislation, and focused that legislation in patently discriminatory ways. Eugenic laws violated expectations of autonomy, equal treatment, and justice by often targeting the most vulnerable—the poor, the disabled, and sexual and racial minorities—as the objects of eugenic reform.

We also associate eugenics with Nazism, and some commentators still assert that eugenics fell out of favor because its ideology had fueled the Holocaust. But such claims ignore the fact that laws restricting marriage among people with disabilities or people of different races, laws mandating premarital health screening, laws that allowed for coerced sterilization, and laws designed to restrict immigration by specific ethnic groups—all adopted in the United States early in the twentieth century—remained in force decades after news of Nazi horrors, and some endured into the twenty-first century. An accurate ethical analysis of eugenics must go beyond Nazi analogies and focus on both the goals of eugenics and the means that were used in an attempt to achieve those goals in the United States, Germany, and around the world. Ethical analysis reveals that the police power, via public health law, is always open to abuse. The history of public health law demonstrates that it has been abused, particularly against society's most disfavored and most vulnerable members (Willrich, 2011). This theme also describes the history of eugenics in America, which for a time intersected with the history of public health.

Ethical Problems with Eugenics

At this remove, one could argue that one basic premise of eugenics is not in itself objectionable: Who would argue with a plan to lower the incidence of morbidity or stave off, even for a time, inevitable mortality? But it is impossible to ignore the twentieth-century record of coercion and discrimination by officials and agencies of government in the name of eugenics. Reverting to categories that attempt to separate eugenics into activities one might consider innocuous from those that are clearly objectionable, such as "positive" versus "negative" eugenics, or "voluntary" versus "authoritarian" eugenics, does not erase the pejorative impact of the term itself. Any idea one labels as "eugenics" is tainted by the stain of history and condemned.

There are four reasons for this response. In its most notorious incarnations, eugenics (1) embraced a program focused on changing the population, and the program was designed to be carried out via coercive governmental involvement sanctioned by law; (2) explicitly endorsed a simplistic model of biological determinism that medicalized social problems, such as crime and poverty along with every manner of disease, and argued that these conditions were passed down predictably from parent to child and could be eradicated by medical science; (3) involved measures, including physical detention, social segregation, and surgical sterilization, that intruded upon what we now think of as fundamental human rights, such as the right of bodily integrity and the right of privacy in reproductive decision-making; and (4) rested upon transparent devaluing and stigmatization of specific groups, most notably those with disabilities or ill health, who were often explicitly targeted or disproportionally impacted by policies that were manifestly unjust in application.

In the American context, these features of eugenics were combined with the inherent power of coercion implicit in public health law, yielding an ethically toxic result. A retrospective assessment of the legacy of public health eugenics suggests that caution is in order when plans are proposed for managing population health through reproductive interventions. We cannot afford to forget that it is difficult, if not impossible, to eliminate all potential for abuse by government agencies clothed in the police power.

Issues in Public Health Ethics Today: A New Eugenics?

The term *eugenics* again became popular about twenty-five years ago as news of the Human Genome Project grew. Sensational and often irresponsible speculations filled the popular media about the potentially genetic basis for crime or the potential for "super babies." The expansion of legally mandated newborn screening or encouragement to use prenatal genetic diagnostics has suggested to some that a new eugenics may be afoot, pursuing those same ends and consequently devaluing people by labeling them with the diseases they endure, or characterizing them by the disabilities they embody. Other concerns have been raised about the difficulty of maintaining confidentiality in growing genetic databases that may be accessed by public health officials (see, "Public Health Genomics, Biobanking, and Ethics," this volume). Finally, some worry that a disproportionate reliance on research in public health genetics may deter researchers, as it did during the eugenics era, from the environmental interventions that traditionally characterized public health efforts.

By the 1990s, the word *eugenics* had become commonplace in critiques of the new reproductive technologies. But can the term be applied accurately to these technologies? Some technologies would not be considered eugenic if the word is used in its classic sense to signal "well-born." Procedures like intracytoplasmic sperm injection (ICSI) allow people who would otherwise not reproduce to pass on a genetic legacy of infertility. To those who historically embraced the label of "eugenicist," ICSI would have been considered dysgenic—the opposite of eugenic.

Technologies like preimplantation genetic diagnosis (PGD) allow choices in favor of or against specific conditions in an embryo, and thus share "morally relevant" characteristics with classical eugenic motives (Iltis, 2016). Some commentators see pro-natal policies like tax credits for additional children, or newborn screening for untreatable disorders, as eugenic (Mehlman, 2011). Others focus upon unequal access to artificial reproductive technologies among the poor or disabled, likening that trend to eugenics (Daar, 2017).

A proposal to sterilize welfare-receiving mothers, a specific ethnic group, or disabled people as a means to a healthier society and lower taxes would meet all the criteria that we associate with the historic abuses of eugenics, but no official policy exists at this time in support of such steps. We are left to analyze less obviously direct parallels between today's genetic practices and past eugenic schemes. Our analysis must include the cautionary note that "historical similarities are not moral equivalents" (Pernick, 1997). But we have not outgrown interethnic bigotry, and we still see regular evidence that contempt for the poor, the sick, or those with disabilities is part of our public moral landscape. We would be well advised also to remember that the same sentiments exist today that motivated people earlier in the twentieth century to use science and the power of public health to segregate themselves from the diseased and the different, and to argue that such separation would improve the lot of human beings.

How we use public health science to pursue a hoped-for healthy future, and whether our pursuit partakes of the dehumanizing features of the earlier eugenics movement, will determine whether the fields of public health and genetics can disentangle their legacy from that of the most egregious violations of human rights in the name of eugenics.

References

Allan, W. 1936. "The Relationship of Eugenics to Public Health." *Eugenical News* 21:73.

"Bill to Establish a Department of Public Health and to Define Its Duties, A." 1897. *American Journal of Public Health & Nation's Health* 28:1191–1194.

Cole, L. J. 1914. "The Relation of Philanthropy and Medicine to Race Betterment." In *Proceedings of the First National Congress on Race Betterment*, 503 (Battle Creek, Mich.: Race Betterment Foundation).

Cumming, H. S. 1928. "The Progress of Medicine." *Washington Post*, January 8.

Daar, J. 2017. *The New Eugenics: Selective Breeding in an Era of Reproductive Technologies* (New Haven, Conn.: Yale University Press).

Davenport, C. B. 1910. *Eugenics: The Science of Human Improvement by Better Breeding* (New York: Holt).

Dowling, O. 1915. "The Marriage Health Certificate, A Deeply Rooted Social Problem." *Journal of the American Public Health Association* 5:1139–1145.

"Eugenic Examination Gets First Certificate." 1913. *Lincoln Star* (NE).

Fairchild, A. L. 2003. *Science at the Borders: Immigrant Medical Inspection and the Shaping of the Modern Industrial Labor Force* (Baltimore, Md.: Johns Hopkins University Press).

Freund, E. 1904. *The Police Power: Public Policy and Constitutional Rights* (Chicago: Callaghan).

Galton, F. 1883. *Inquiries into Human Faculty and its Development* (London: Macmillan).

Galton, F. 1889. *Natural Inheritance* (London: Macmillan).

Hall, P. 1919. "Immigration Restriction and World Eugenics," *Journal of Heredity* 10: 25–27.

"How to Keep Well." 1913. *Courier Journal* (Louisville, Ky.): 2.

Hrdlička, A. 1919. *Physical Anthropology* (Philadelphia: Wistar Institute).

Iltis, A.S. 2016. "Prenatal Screening and Prenatal Diagnosis: Contemporary Practices in Light of the Past." *Journal of Medical Ethics* 42(6): 334–339.

"International Eugenics Committee." 1914. *Journal of Heredity* 5(8): 340.

Jennings, H. S. 1927. "Public Health and Race Progress—Are They Compatible?" *Science* 66:45–50.

Jordan, H. E. 1912. "The Place of Eugenics in the Medical Curriculum." In *Problems in Eugenics: Papers Communicated to the First International Eugenics Congress*, 396–399 (London: Eugenics Education Society).

Knox, H. A. 1915. "Measuring Human Intelligence: A Progressive Series of Standardized Tests Used by the Public Health Service to Protect Our Racial Stock." *Scientific American* 112: 52–58.

Mehlman, M. J. 2011. "Modern Eugenics and the Law." In *A Century of Eugenics in America*, edited by P. Lombardo (Bloomington: Indiana University Press).

"Membership: The Eugenics Committee." 1914. *Journal of Heredity* 5(8): 340.

"Officially Recognize Eugenics." 1913. *New Castle Herald* (Penn.), 4.

Pernick, M. 1997. "Eugenics and Public Health in American History." *American Journal of Public Health* 87(11): 1767–1772.

Plecker, W. A. 1924. "The New Virginia Law to Protect Racial Integrity." *Virginia Health Bulletin* 16: 1.

Ravenel, M. P. 1924. "Evolution and Preventive Medicine." *American Journal of Public Health* 14(12): 1016–1019.

Rucker, W. C. 1915. "More Eugenic Laws." *Journal of Heredity* 6: 219–226.

Rucker, W. C. 1917. "A Program of Public Health for Cities." *American Journal of Public Health* 7: 225–234.

"Second International Eugenics Congress." 1921. *Eugenics Review* 12–13(1920–1921): 253.

Shafer, J. K. 1954. "Premarital Health Examination Legislation: History and Analysis." *Public Health Report* 69: 487–493.

Stern, A. M. 2005. *Eugenic Nation: Faults and Frontiers of Better Breeding in Modern America* (Berkeley: University of California Press).

Taussig, F. W. 1911. *Principles of Economics* (New York: Macmillan).

"Uncle Sam, M.D." 1919. *Index Journal* (Greenwood, S.C.), 4.

"Wants Law for Health Certificates from Persons Entering Into Marriage." 1913. *Day Book* 2(255): 29.

Willrich, M. 2011. *Pox: An American History* (New York: Penguin).

CHAPTER 56

NEWBORN SCREENING IN THE UNITED STATES: ETHICAL ISSUES

MICHELLE HUCKABY LEWIS AND
JEFFREY R. BOTKIN

INTRODUCTION

NEWBORN screening is a public health program designed to identify and treat infants with certain conditions prior to the onset of symptoms in order to ameliorate or prevent disability and/or death. Shortly after birth, blood obtained from an infant's heel is placed on a filter card and sent to a laboratory to test for biochemical and genetic markers for certain endocrine, metabolic, genetic, and infectious disorders. Newborn screening tests are used to identify infants who may be at increased risk for certain diseases so that these infants can be referred for diagnostic testing and, if necessary, treatment.

In the United States, newborn screening programs are operated by the state departments of health in all fifty states plus the District of Columbia. Almost all of the four million infants born in the United States each year undergo newborn screening, and approximately 12,500 infants are identified yearly with a newborn screening condition (CDC, 2012).

Despite this success, newborn screening has been controversial for three reasons. First, new technology has made possible the identification of a greater number of conditions. For many of these conditions, the natural history and benefit of treatment are not well understood. The determination of what conditions should be targeted is a constant challenge for state newborn screening programs. Second, there have been high-profile controversies over the retention and secondary use of residual blood samples left over after the screening tests are complete (Lewis, 2014). Third, newborn screening is mandated by state law in virtually all states; parental consent is not required although most states allow parents to opt out for religious or philosophical reasons. This chapter explores key ethical issues that newborn screening programs currently face and may face in the future.

The Development of Newborn Screening in the United States

Newborn screening began as a blood test performed shortly after birth to prevent the intellectual disability caused by untreated phenylketonuria (PKU), a rare, hereditary, metabolic disorder in which affected individuals cannot process the protein phenylalanine. Once a patient with PKU becomes symptomatic, irreversible brain damage has already occurred.

In 1960, Dr. Robert Guthrie developed a bacterial inhibition assay to detect elevated blood phenylalanine levels before the onset of symptoms. This discovery enabled the identification of affected individuals prior to the onset of symptoms so that they could be treated, thereby preventing the devastating consequences of this disease (Guthrie, 1992). By 1973, forty-three states had enacted legislation to screen newborns for PKU (AAP/HRSA Newborn Screening Task Force, 2000).

Expansion of Newborn Screening

Over time, new technology has made possible the simultaneous detection of increasing numbers of rare conditions using the same newborn screening filter cards that are used to detect PKU. The early evolution of state newborn screening programs occurred by the addition of a single, treatable condition, one at a time, to state newborn screening panels based on the premise that early identification and treatment would improve the health outcomes of affected infants. The development of tandem mass spectrometry (tandem MS/MS) technology in the 1990s challenged this paradigm. The use of the tandem MS/MS technology allowed the simultaneous identification of dozens of metabolic conditions—some of which were poorly understood, and some with no available treatment—using the same newborn screening filter cards that were used to detect PKU. Within a short period, most screening programs within the United States began to use tandem MS/MS as the principal tool for newborn screening analysis (Crowe, 2008).

In 1999, an American Academy of Pediatrics Task Force report commissioned by the US Department of Health and Human Services (HHS) noted that states varied widely with respect to the number of conditions included in their mandatory screening panels and in the mechanism for determining which tests should be included in the panels. Some states required screening for as few as two conditions, while other states required screening for more than forty.

While these inconsistencies in practice reflected differences in community values, public health technical capabilities, and political and economic realities, the practical effect of these inconsistencies was that infants across the country did not "have equal access to newborn screening and its potential to prevent morbidity and mortality" (AAP/HRSA Newborn Screening Task Force, 2000, 399). The Task Force called for a more uniform national policy for the selection of newborn screening tests.

In response to this recommendation, in 2002, the American College of Medical Genetics (ACMG) was commissioned to develop a uniform panel of conditions for screening. The subsequent 2006 ACMG report assigned conditions to one of three categories: (1) core panel, (2) secondary targets (conditions that are part of the differential diagnosis of a core panel condition), or (3) not appropriate for newborn screening. Of the eighty-four conditions considered, the ACMG report identified twenty-nine conditions as primary targets for newborn screening and an additional twenty-five conditions that could be identified in the course of screening for core panel conditions. Thirty conditions were determined to be inappropriate for newborn screening. The ACMG report recommended that both core panel conditions and secondary target conditions be included on state newborn screening panels, a significant expansion in the number of conditions targeted by newborn screening (ACMG, 2006).

The ACMG report was controversial. Some commentators argued that it would be unethical not to expand newborn screening for serious, potentially treatable conditions despite the lack of data on the efficacy of screening (Howell, 2006). Others advocated a more cautious approach, citing the lack of sufficient research about the impact of screening (Botkin et al., 2006). This debate raised legitimate questions about whether it is ethically appropriate to screen newborns for a large number of poorly understood conditions via a mandatory, state-based public health program.

Although the ACMG report acknowledged that the benefit to the child being screened should be the overriding consideration, an additional criterion for consideration was the benefit to the family and society of early identification of the condition. This broader definition of "benefit" was used to justify inclusion of conditions on the core panel for which there was only anecdotal evidence of effective treatment. The report cited the potential benefit of obtaining genetic information that could establish that others in the family may be at genetic risk of disease, the ability to inform subsequent reproductive decisions for the child's parents, and the possibility of shortening the diagnostic odyssey as important factors that also should be considered. These considerations beyond direct benefit to the infant tended to lower the bar for inclusion of new tests on the recommended panel.

The methodology used to develop the ACMG recommendations was criticized for its failure to address key ethical issues, including the implications of mandating tests with uncertain results (Botkin et al., 2006). Critics of the recommendations suggested that instead of adopting the recommendations on a population-wide level, state programs move forward under a research paradigm to evaluate the risks and benefits of early detection by newborn screening (Botkin et al., 2006).

Despite these criticisms, the Advisory Committee on Heritable Disorders and Genetic Diseases in Newborns and Children (the Advisory Committee) adopted the ACMG panel as its Recommended Uniform Screening Panel (RUSP), and these recommendations were endorsed by the Secretary of HHS (Sebelius, 2010). The Advisory Committee is a federal advisory committee created to provide evidence-based recommendations for including (or excluding) conditions on the RUSP. The RUSP establishes a standardized list of disorders that are recommended by the Advisory Committee, but individual state departments of health operate newborn screening programs. Each state decides which disorders will be included on its newborn screening panel, and states continue to vary with respect to the mechanism by which new conditions are added to the panels and the level of evidence required to make these decisions. By 2008 almost all of the states had added the twenty-nine core conditions to the state newborn screening panel, and most states had begun screening for a majority of the secondary target conditions (President's Council on Bioethics, 2008). The Advisory Committee subsequently has recommended additional conditions for inclusion on the RUSP.

Future of Newborn Screening

The debate about the circumstances under which it is appropriate to add new conditions to state newborn screening panels has continued unabated. The New York experience is one example in which disease advocates successfully lobbied for inclusion of a condition on a state newborn screening panel despite the lack of clear evidence to support its inclusion. In 2006, in response to parental advocacy, the New York legislature voted to add Krabbe disease to the state panel, even though it was not included on the RUSP. In 2010, the Advisory Committee declined to add Krabbe disease to the RUSP, citing insufficient evidence regarding the benefits and harms of treatment of this disease (Kemper et al., 2010).

The argument that conditions should not be added to state panels without sufficient evidence has been countered by the view that identification of infants with rare conditions for which there currently is no available treatment will allow those children to participate in research on innovative therapies that may prevent the morbidity or mortality associated with that disease (Alexander and Van Dyck, 2006). However, this justification arguably is beyond the scope of the public health mission of newborn screening.

The prospect of conducting genomic sequencing as part of newborn screening further complicates this debate. In 2013 the US National Institutes of Health (NIH) provided grants totaling $25 million to four institutions to "explore the implications, challenges, and opportunities associated with the possible use of genomic sequence information in the newborn period" (NIH, 2012). These grants were intended to stimulate research to expand the scale of data available for analysis in the newborn period and to advance our understanding of specific disorders identifiable via newborn screening through DNA-based analysis. Despite the enthusiasm for this technology, state newborn screening programs and the US health care delivery system are not equipped with sufficient personnel to interpret sequence variants and provide appropriate clinical follow-up to the infants who would be identified as at increased risk of disease on such a large scale (Botkin and Rothwell, 2016).

Moreover, while genomic sequencing in the newborn period could produce results that might be of direct, immediate benefit to the health of the infant, other types of results with varying importance to the health of the child will be discovered for many newborns. If genomic sequencing were incorporated into newborn screening, state newborn screening programs would have to decide which results would be returned to infants' families. In 2013, the ACMG published a list of fifty-six genes (revised to fifty-nine genes in 2016) that are highly associated with serious health conditions, for which we have treatment or prevention strategies, and for which we have sensitive and specific tests (Green et al., 2013). The ACMG recommended that, when sequencing is done for any clinical indication, the laboratory should look for variants in these fifty-nine genes. Many of these conditions are adult-onset diseases, such as breast or colon cancer, adding a whole new paradigm to the newborn screening enterprise. Although the ACMG specifically excluded newborn screening in its recommendations, research to evaluate the return of results of genomic sequencing in the newborn period currently is underway, as noted above.

In the past, genetic testing for adult-onset conditions has not been deemed to be in a child's best interests, in part because testing in childhood precludes an individual from being able to make his or her own choice about whether to undergo testing for that condition in the future. The ACMG recommendation is inconsistent with this principle, but advocates of this practice have argued that it would be unethical not to look for this information and provide it to parents who might be at increased risk but otherwise would have no reason to undergo genetic testing themselves. In this situation, the ethical duties of clinicians to inform and educate parents and other family members who also may be affected is unclear, but counseling adult family members, including parents, about their increased genetic risk for adult-onset conditions is clearly beyond the scope of the public health mission of newborn screening.

Implementation of the ACMG recommendation in the newborn screening context would place tremendous strain on newborn screening programs. Current estimates are that one of the ACMG variants will be found in about 2 percent of those undergoing genome sequencing. If sequencing were performed on 4 million infants per year, 80,000 infants per year would be identified with a finding, compared with the 12,500 infants identified through newborn screening each year under the current paradigm. Under this new scenario, screening for the ACMG conditions could become the primary focus of newborn screening programs and draw programs far beyond their public health mission.

A second set of questions would arise over the disclosure of carrier results to families. Carriers are heterozygous for an autosomal recessive condition and are usually asymptomatic. However, if two carriers reproduce, there is a 25 percent chance with each pregnancy that an affected child will be born. Therefore, knowledge about carrier status can be helpful to adults of reproductive age. Several current newborn screening tests, such as those for cystic fibrosis and sickle cell disease, identify carriers, and most state programs alert parents when their child is identified as a carrier. Although carrier screening results in newborn screening have been disclosed for several decades, whether children identified as carriers through newborn screening programs use this information when they reach reproductive age has not been determined.

It has been estimated that each individual carries between 50 and 100 variants classified as disease causing; therefore, it is likely that if sequencing is used in the context of newborn screening, a high percentage, if not all, of newborns will be identified as a carrier for one or more conditions, many of which will be quite rare at the population level (1000 Genomes Project Consortium, 2010). The value of this information to newborns is questionable, particularly because adults of reproductive age can obtain carrier screening when considering or during pregnancy. Due to these considerations and others, several groups have stated that the use of genome sequencing as a screening tool in newborn screening programs is premature at best (Botkin et al., 2015; Johnston et al., 2018).

The continued variation between states regarding the operation of state newborn screening programs also raises distributive justice concerns. First, state newborn screening panels continue to screen for different numbers of conditions despite the creation of the RUSP. These differences mean that babies born in different states are screened for different conditions and therefore do not share equally in the potential benefits of newborn screening. Second, states vary with respect to the follow-up and treatment provided for infants identified with rare conditions through newborn screening (Botkin, Anderson, and Rothwell, 2012). In states that provide screening but not treatment for a particular condition, families may be unable to afford treatment, and affected infants may not benefit from screening. Third, when DNA-based analysis techniques are used, the selection of variants for molecular panel testing can exacerbate disparities if the variants chosen are not reflective of a genetically diverse and ethnically admixed population. The use of this technology can be problematic if the panels were designed prior to sufficient study of the mutation spectrum of nonwhite populations. In that case, the use of these panels would have limited value in diverse populations (Pique et al., 2017).

The Retention and Secondary Research Use of Residual Newborn Screening Dried Blood Samples

More blood is collected on the filter card than typically is needed. As a result, a small quantity of the blood sample often remains unused after completion of newborn screening testing. Residual newborn screening dried blood samples (DBS) can be used for newborn screening program operations, such as quality assurance and quality control, public health surveillance, and public health and biomedical research (Olney et al., 2006). Since newborn screening is performed on almost all of the babies born in the United States, DBS can be a tremendous source of population-level data.

Due to the mandatory nature of newborn screening, parents typically are provided limited education about the screening and the policies related to the retention and secondary use of DBS. Historically, parental consent was not required for the retention and secondary use of de-identified DBS because the samples were not considered human subjects for purposes of the federal human subjects research regulations. Nevertheless, the retention and secondary research use of de-identified DBS without explicit parental consent has been controversial. Whether explicit parental consent should be required to retain de-identified DBS and use them for secondary research, or, alternatively, whether parents should be informed about a state's retention and use policy and then be given the option to refuse, has been a subject of debate.

Parental concerns about the retention and secondary use of de-identified DBS without consent led to litigation against the state departments of health in Texas (*Beleno v. Texas Dept. of State Health Services*, U.S. District Court, Western District of Texas, No. SA09CA0188 [2009]), Minnesota (*Bearder v. State*, 806 N.W.2d 766 [2011]), and Indiana (*Doe v. VanNess*, Marion County Superior Court, No. 49D011409CT031 [2014]). In the Texas and Indiana litigation, the parents claimed that the state's retention and secondary use of DBS without parental consent violated constitutional privacy rights. In the Minnesota litigation, the parents claimed that the state violated the genetic privacy provisions of the state Government Data Practices Act.

The Texas litigation was settled, and the Texas legislature passed new legislation that requires parental consent for the secondary research use of DBS. The Indiana lawsuit was dismissed. The Minnesota Supreme Court held that DBS could be used for newborn screening program operations without consent, but any other secondary use would require parental consent. As a result of the litigation, millions of archived DBS and decades' worth of newborn screening data were destroyed (Lewis, 2015).

In 2014, the U.S. Congress passed the Newborn Screening Saves Lives Reauthorization Act (Reauthorization Act) to extend federal programs that assist states with the improvement and expansion of state newborn screening programs (Newborn Screening Saves Lives Reauthorization Act, Pub. L., 2014, 113–240). This law also required that DBS be considered human subjects for purposes of federal human subjects research regulations; therefore, parental consent was required for the use of DBS in federally funded research whether or not the samples were retained with identifiers. The Reauthorization Act also anticipated updated human subjects research regulations, and the provision that required that DBS be treated as human subjects and therefore subject to informed consent requirements for secondary research use was only to be in effect until the new, updated regulations were promulgated.

Ultimately, the final version of the regulation retained the old (pre-Reauthorization Act) provisions that require informed consent only for the use of identifiable blood or tissue samples, with no exceptions for DBS. However, parental consent is required in states, such as Texas, Minnesota, and Michigan, in which state law requires parental consent for the secondary research use of DBS. This controversy illustrates a larger tension in biomedical science between the value of residual clinical samples for research purposes and the public expectation that patients will be informed and offered choice regarding the research use of their biospecimens.

Should Newborn Screening Be Mandatory?

The original justification for newborn screening was the prevention of the devastating consequences of untreated PKU. Newborn screening was considered a public health initiative, and the goal to protect the health of infants was imperative. The need for informed consent prior to the performance of medical procedures did not become entrenched in American law until the 1970s. When newborn screening programs were becoming routinized, the question of whether to obtain parental permission for newborn screening did not receive broad consideration. Today, most states require newborn screening, and states vary regarding whether parents are permitted to refuse the screening (Lewis, 2014).

The increasing pressure to add tests for conditions for which effective treatment is unavailable, coupled with the controversy surrounding the retention and secondary use of DBS, makes the question of how to allocate decision-making authority for newborn screening among parents, states, and physicians less clear. The original justification for mandating newborn screening was the identification and timely treatment of infants with rare disorders in order to prevent the morbidity and mortality of disease. Some have argued that since the mission of newborn screening programs has expanded beyond the immediate health benefit of the infant to include broader benefits to the family and society, the original justification is no longer sufficient to warrant mandatory screening (Ross, 2011). Opponents of informed consent requirements for newborn screening argue that it is unethical to risk missing even one child with a treatable condition and that ethical arguments notwithstanding, logistical considerations, including the fact that there is no budget for training health care providers to provide informed consent or financial support for their time to do so, make informed consent impractical, if not impossible (Paul, 1999).

The relevant professional societies differ with respect to the optimal nature of the consent and refusal process. The American Academy of Pediatrics and the American College of Medical Genetics and Genomics "support the mandatory offering of newborn screening for all children," and recommend that "parents should have the option of refusing the procedure" (AAP Committee on Bioethics, Committee on Genetics, and ACMG Social, Ethical, and Legal Issues Committee, 2013, 621). The American Society for Human Genetics supports improved parental education about newborn screening, but it "does not advocate a change in most state programs that mandate screening but permit parental refusals" (Botkin et al., 2015, 13).

If protection of newborns remains our primary concern, then all newborns should be screened. Nevertheless, it is possible to respect the wishes of parents with regard to less treatable disorders and research participation and still achieve the goals of testing all newborns for the more treatable disorders. A shared decision-making model, in which screening is mandatory for treatable conditions and parental consent is required to screen for less treatable conditions and for participation in research, would be one mechanism to achieve the dual goals of protection of the infant's health and respect for parental autonomy. Such a two-tiered approach would require significant changes in the operation of state newborn screening programs, both at the level in which newborn screening samples are obtained and in the laboratories in which screening is performed.

Conclusion

The controversy related to DBS highlights the need for improved parental education about newborn screening and related issues. Parents must be better educated about the newborn screening process and given a role in decision-making regarding discoveries about the genetic makeup of their children. It is important that this education process includes information about the potential research use of DBS in states where DBS are retained for this purpose. The overarching goal should be to educate parents and the public about the purposes of newborn screening programs and how the information obtained will be used.

Newborn screening programs have prevented needless suffering by thousands of infants and their families. In the future, these same programs have the potential to address more conditions that cause disability and suffering for children and families. Newborn screening programs will continue to evolve, but the primary public health mission of protecting the health of children should remain paramount.

References

1000 Genomes Project Consortium. 2010. "A Map of Human Genome Variation from Population-Scale Sequencing." *Nature* 476 (7319): 1061–1073.

AAP (American Academy of Pediatrics) Committee on Bioethics, Committee on Genetics, and ACMG (American College of Medical Genetics and Genomics) Social, Ethical, and Legal Issues Committee. 2013. "Ethical and Policy Issues in Genetic Testing and Screening of Children." *Pediatrics* 131(3): 620–622.

AAP (American Academy of Pediatrics)/HRSA (Health Resources and Services Administration) Newborn Screening Task Force. 2000. "Serving the Family from Birth to the Medical

Home: Newborn Screening: a Blueprint for the Future—A Call for a National Agenda on State Newborn Screening Programs." *Pediatrics* 106(2, pt. 2): 389–422.

ACMG (American College of Medical Genetics and Genomics). 2006. "Newborn Screening: Toward a Uniform Screening Panel and System." *Genetics in Medicine* 8: 1S–252S.

Alexander, D., and Van Dyck, P. 2006. "A Vision of the Future of Newborn Screening." *Pediatrics* 117(5, pt. 2): S350–354.

Botkin, J. R., Anderson, R., and Rothwell, E. 2012. "Expanded Newborn Screening: Contemporary Challenges to the *Parens Patriae* Doctrine and the Use of Public Resources." In *Medicine and Social Justice: Essays on the Distribution of Health Care*, edited by R. Rhodes, M. P. Battin, and A. Silvers (Oxford: Oxford University Press).

Botkin, J. R., Belmont, J. W., Berg, J. S., Berkman, B. E., Bombard, Y., Holm, I. A., et al. 2015. "ASHG Statement: Points to Consider: Ethical, Legal, and Psychosocial Implications of Genetic Testing in Children and Adolescents." *American Journal of Human Genetics* 97(1): 6–21.

Botkin, J. R., Clayton, E. W., Fost, N. C., Burke, W., Murray, T. H., Baily, M. A., et al. 2006. "Newborn Screening Technology: Proceed with Caution." *Pediatrics* 117(5): 1793–1799.

Botkin, J. R., and Rothwell, E. 2016. "Whole Genome Sequencing and Newborn Screening." *Current Genetic Medicine Reports* 4(1): 1–6.

CDC (US Centers for Disease Control and Prevention). 2012. "CDC Grand Rounds: Newborn Screening and Improved Outcomes." *MMWR* 61(21): 390–393.

Crowe, S. 2008. "A Brief History of Newborn Screening in the United States." Staff Discussion Paper, President's Council on Bioethics. http://bioethics.georgetown.edu/pcbe/background/newborn_screening_crowe.html.

Green, R. C., Berg, J. S., Grody, W. W., Kalia, S. S., Korf, B. R., Martin, C. L., et al. 2013. "ACMG Recommendations for Reporting of Incidental Findings in Clinical Exome and Genome Sequencing." *Genetics in Medicine* 15(7): 565–574.

Guthrie, R. 1992. "The Origin of Newborn Screening." *Screening* 1: 5–15.

Howell, R. R. 2006. "We Need Expanded Newborn Screening." *Pediatrics* 1117(5): 1800–1805.

Johnston, J., Lantos, J. D., Goldenberg, A., Chen, F., Parens, E., Koenig, B. A., members of the NSIGHT Ethics and Policy Advisory Board. 2018. "Sequencing Newborns: A Call for Nuanced Use of Genomic Technologies." *The Hastings Center Report* 14 Aug. 2018. https://doi.org/10.1002/hast.874.

Kemper, A. R., Knapp, A. A., Green, N. S., Comeau, A. M., Metterville, D. R., and Perrin, J. M. 2010. "Weighing the Evidence for Newborn Screening for Early-Infantile Krabbe Disease." *Genetics in Medicine* 12(9): 539–543.

Lewis, M. H. 2014. "Newborn Screening Controversy: Past, Present, and Future." *JAMA Pediatrics* 168(3): 199–200.

Lewis, M. H. 2015. "Lessons from the Residual Newborn Screening Dried Blood Spot Litigation." *Journal of Law Medicine and Ethics* S43(1): 32–35.

NIH (National Institutes of Health). 2012. *Genomic Sequencing and Newborn Screening Disorders Request for Applications* (Bethesda, Md.: NIH). https://grants.nih.gov/grants/guide/rfa-files/RFA-HD-13-010.html.

Olney, R. S., Moore, C. A., Ojodu, J. A., Lindegren, M. L., and Hannon, W. H. 2006. "Storage and Use of Residual Dried Blood Spots from State Newborn Screening Programs." *Journal of Pediatrics* 148(5): 618–622.

Paul, D. 1999. "Contesting Consent: The Challenge to Compulsory Neonatal Screening for PKU." *Perspectives in Biology and Medicine* 42(2): 207–219.

Pique, L., Graham, S., Pearl, M., Kharrazi, M., and Schrijver, I. 2017. "Cystic Fibrosis Newborn Screening Programs: Implications of the CFTR Variant Spectrum in Nonwhite Patients." *Genetics in Medicine* 19: 36–44.

President's Council on Bioethics. 2008. *The Changing Moral Focus of Newborn Screening* (Washington, D.C.: President's Council on Bioethics). https://bioethicsarchive.georgetown.edu/pcbe/reports/newborn_screening/.

Ross, L. F. 2011. "Mandatory versus Voluntary Consent for Newborn Screening?" *Kennedy Institute of Ethics Journal* 20(4): 299–328.

Sebelius, K. 2010. "Letter to R. Rodney Howell, M.D." https://www.hrsa.gov/sites/default/files/hrsa/advisory-committees/heritable-disorders/reports-recommendations/response-rusp-2010052.pdf.

CHAPTER 57

PUBLIC HEALTH GENOMICS, BIOBANKING, AND ETHICS

KAREN M. MEAGHER, R. JEAN CADIGAN, GAIL E. HENDERSON, AND ERIC T. JUENGST

Introduction

Public health genomics, defined as the use of genomics to improve population health by reducing morbidity and mortality, has been galvanized by new genomic sequencing technologies that facilitate discovery of deleterious variants among many individuals. Advances in next-generation sequencing have yielded methods capable of handling samples at a larger scale and with lower costs—less than $1,000 to sequence a human genome (van Dijk et al., 2014). These advances have also facilitated diversification of scientific applications, with genomics combining with the population health sciences to yield potential health gains through the promise of preventive genomic sequencing.

As translational genomic research moves to this larger scale, *biobanks*, defined as professionally curated collections of biospecimens and associated data stored for future research use, are becoming critical research resources (e.g., Henderson, Cadigan, et al., 2013). Storage of biospecimens has gradually increased in complexity over the last century, building vast systems for detailed curation of data sets. Greater biobanking sophistication has developed alongside an increasing number of population-based biobanks and a rise in biobanking consortia, partly in response to the need for larger numbers of samples for use in genome-wide associations studies (De Souza and Greenspan, 2013; Qi and Franks, 2016). Large sample sizes and careful curation are also needed for a further understanding of complex diseases through epidemiological study designs such as case-control and cohort studies (Burton et al., 2013; Olson et al., 2014). Increasingly, researchers advocate using biobanks to support population surveillance and preventive genomic screening interventions within the biobank cohorts (Khoury and Evans, 2015; Aswini and Varun, 2010). This chapter explores the ethical, social, and policy issues that public health uses of research biobanks raise for those responsible for their design and governance.

Contemporary bioethics typically distinguishes the domains of clinical ethics, research ethics, and public health ethics, in order to reflect the different moral traditions that animate practice in these spheres. In the biobank context, however, these domains overlap dramatically (Wolf et al., 2018). For researchers, health systems managers, and the curators of large-scale biobanks that use specimens and data for public health genomics, it can be quite unclear which moral tradition should govern biobanking policies and practices.

Three contemporary genomic research projects illustrate the kinds of public health uses that might be proposed for biobanks and the logistical and ethical challenges such uses may encounter. In these cases, the professionals involved face ethical questions at the intersections of research, clinical, or public health ethics. When health systems and health information managers, for example, seek to use patient data from biobanks to continuously improve delivery of patient care, they must reconcile the rules governing biobanks developed for research purposes with the exigencies of clinical practice (Alzu'bi, Zhou, and Waltzlaf, 2014; Rahimzadeh and Bartlett, 2014). Curators of research biobanks must also grapple with the ethical implications of generating research information that increasingly carries health implications for individual participants (Wolf et al., 2012; Bledsoe et al., 2012). And just as the lines between research and clinical practice are being blurred in new ways, public health genomics raises questions about when and how to approach emerging health implications for populations as well as individuals. Watson and Barnes (2011) previously argued that classification of biobanks helps to ensure appreciation of their diversity. It is important to be mindful of such classifications as projects, findings, and implications extend beyond the context of a biobank's original design.

The cases described here, all based in the United States, are the MyCode Community Health Initiative at the Geisinger Health System (GHS), the GeneScreen research project using the Kaiser Permanente Northwest Biobank (KP-NWBB), and the US Precision Medicine Initiative (PMI) *All of Us* Research Program Biobank at Mayo Clinic. Taken together, these projects highlight ethical and policy considerations that will need to be anticipated and addressed as research biobanks are used for public health genomics.

Case Studies

The Geisinger MyCode Community Health Initiative

GHS is an integrated health system. In 2007 it launched the MyCode Community Health Initiative to collect and store samples of patients' blood, serum, and DNA linked to the electronic health record (EHR). As a "learning health system," GHS seeks to rapidly integrate research findings that derive from and bear directly on clinical practice (IOM, 2007; Carey et al., 2016). MyCode predominately recruits patients and obtains opt-in consent during face-to-face patient visits to GHS clinics (online consent has recently been added). The consent rate is more than 85 percent of those approached (Carey et al., 2016). MyCode has over 150,000 participants, including both adults and children, and adds approximately 1,000 participants per week (Murray, 2016). In 2017 MyCode announced plans to expand beyond GHS, aiming to scale up the research program in other health care systems (Sylvester, 2017).

Because MyCode's collection is designed as both a health care tool for Geisinger patients and a research resource, it anticipates a number of features that would also characterize public health uses of such collections. For example, through its partnership with Regeneron Pharmaceuticals, MyCode sequences all the samples in its biobank, providing an opportunity for preventive genomic screening of every biobank contributor. In 2013 the American College of Medical Genetics and Genomics (ACMG) put forward a list of fifty-six (fifty-nine as of 2017) medically actionable genes to be opportunistically examined whenever genomic sequencing is performed for clinical reasons (Green et al., 2013; Kalia et al., 2017). With the advent of these guidelines and the routine sequencing of all MyCode samples, the protocol and consent forms were changed to make the return of medically actionable findings to participants and their clinicians, and their deposit into the patients' EHR, a routine feature of participation (Carey et al., 2016). This change to the consent form was instituted after focus groups revealed strong support for return of actionable research results in the interest of clinical benefits. As a result, all MyCode participants are now screened for seventy-six genes related to twenty-seven conditions, the bulk of which are the ACMG recommended list.

Thus, while MyCode was originally established as a research biobank, implementation of this return of results program resembles the essential features of a public health screening program: universal screening of participants to identify increased disease risk across the biobank's population, with no individual participant selection of the targets of screening or the disposition of results (Murray, 2017). As of November 2018, results have been returned to 1,044 participants, their clinicians, and EHRs, with gene variants primarily related to cancer and cardiovascular disease (Geisinger MyCode Community Health Initiative, 2018). A significant proportion of these participants would not have met the threshold for clinical genetic testing (based on family history) and were not symptomatic, thus reinforcing the potential importance of such preventive genomics findings (Murray, 2016, slide 30). MyCode does not return negative findings (Carey et al., 2016), so participants who have not been given a positive result do not know whether their DNA has yet been screened (Geisinger MyCode Community Health Initiative, 2017). MyCode may be considered a "large-scale pilot" of a public health genomic screening program (Murray, 2017), and its organization and scale will offer critical insights, particularly regarding population prevalence, penetrance, and actionability of gene variants (Buchanan et al., 2018).

GeneScreen KP-NWBB

GeneScreen is a US government-funded (through the National Institutes of Health [NIH]) preventive screening research project launched in early 2016 to assess the harms and benefits of targeted sequencing of seventeen genes related to eleven medically actionable genetic conditions (all also on the MyCode list) (Adams et al., 2016). In recruiting adults who are not selected because of any suspected increased risk of genetic conditions, it resembles MyCode's approach. In GeneScreen, adults were recruited from a University of North Carolina (UNC) medicine clinic and the KP-NWBB. Recruitment letters invited recipients to a website that provided educational material and offered online consent. Those who joined were asked to take a survey regarding their personal and family health and their attitudes and knowledge about genetics and genetic testing. The consent rate at KP-NWBB, which resembles MyCode in recruitment through a biobank, was higher than via the UNC clinic population (30 percent vs. 16 percent). We will focus here on the KP-NWBB component.

Like MyCode, participants joining GeneScreen KP-NWBB agreed to have medically actionable findings placed in their EHRs and disclosed to their clinicians. However, MyCode promotes research with investigators from inside and outside the institution, while GeneScreen is a self-contained research project. GeneScreen KP-NWBB included investigation of the use of online education and consent, decision-making regarding participation, and the responses to both negative and positive screening results (Cadigan, Butterfield, et al., 2017). From a public health genomics perspective, GeneScreen KP-NWBB provides an example of an investigation of the harms and benefits of public health genomic screening—an ELSI (ethical, legal, and social implications) project that could be modified and scaled up throughout a biobank or used to inform similar interventions in other cohorts (e.g., Sankar and Parker, 2016).

Precision Medicine Initiative *All of Us* Research Program Biobank at the Mayo Clinic

The PMI Biobank at the Mayo Clinic is the centralized repository for the *All of Us* Research Program (Gallagher, 2016). The biobank will store, curate, and make available to researchers more than 35 million biospecimens collected from the one million *All of Us* volunteers (who join through a national network of hospital- and drug-store-based recruitment sites). The goal is to facilitate study of individual differences in health and disease by combining research using biospecimens with information provided by participants such as lifestyle self-report, medication history, EHRs, and real-time mobile health technology (NIH, 2015, 2016).

Initial operational plans for *All of Us* envisioned individual control over the disposition of contributed samples beyond either MyCode or GeneScreen (Hudson, Lifton, and

Patrick-Lake, 2015), potentially compromising its public health uses. The original vision was that participants would be free to choose whether and which individual or collective research results they would like to receive. Moreover, unlike either MyCode or GeneScreen, the PMI Working Group recommended that participant data *not* be treated as clinical data, and research results not be automatically shared with participants' physicians, entered into participants' EHRs, or surveilled for findings with clinical implications (Hudson, Lifton, and Patrick-Lake, 2015). The responsibility for linking research results to clinical expertise initially lay with individual participants, although program-facilitated clinical communication or care is still under discussion.

The richness of the data collected about each contributor means that, in some instances, the cohort cannot be "de-identified" or "anonymized," making mass screening interventions feasible. As a result, leaders in public health genomics have already highlighted the potential use of the PMI Biobank for preventive genomic screening (Khoury and Evans, 2015). At one *All of Us* Return of Results workshop, attendees addressed the variety of decisions that will need to be made if the program moves toward "active return," when researchers or qualified clinical experts contact participants directly, in contrast to plans for participant-driven "passive access" through electronic portals (Ozenberger, 2017).

Granting PMI Biobank contributors greater latitude reflects the participatory vision that informs the PMI overall (Hudson, Lifton, and Patrick-Lake, 2015). Placing individual participant empowerment at the heart of the PMI was an important and effective strategy for garnering public and political support for the initiative in an era of widespread distrust of the federal government and the health care system (Blasimme and Vayena, 2016). As NIH director Francis Collins stated, "What we're doing with the PMI cohort *is intersecting in a synergistic way with other fundamental changes in medicine and research to empower Americans to live healthier lives*" (Collins, 2015, emphasis added). Nonetheless, the effects of this individualized control on any public health uses of the Biobank have yet to be assessed.

Four Issues Brought to Light by Case Analysis

At the intersection of biobanking and public health, researchers, biobank curators, and participants face challenges when implementing confidentiality protections, informed consent method and scope, community engagement, and return and disposition of results. Each of the three cases demonstrates shifting contexts in these regards, as research increasingly has translational implications, resulting in a mix of research, clinical, and public health purposes (see Table 57.1).

Table 57.1 Public Health Genomics and Biobank Case Studies: Four Key Features for Comparison

	Confidentiality protections	Informed consent		Engagement	Results and disposition of results	
Case study	Samples identifiable	Consent method	Consent (broad or specific)	Community engagement*	Return of results	Medical record deposit
MyCode	Yes	In person and Online	Broad	Yes	Positive results from screening of 76 genes	Yes
GeneScreen KP-NWBB	Yes	Online	Broad to KP-NWBB, Specific to GeneScreen	ABC governs biobank use, CAB created for GeneScreen	Positive and negative results from screening of 17 genes	Yes
PMI *All of Us*	Tier-dependent	Online	Broad	Yes	TBD	No

*Engagement with participants in the project's associated biobank; CAB: Community Advisory Board.

Confidentiality and Sample Identifiability

Biospecimens alone are not currently considered identifiable, and despite considerable debate, regulatory categories designate research involving unidentified biospecimens as not covered by human subject regulations (HHS, 2018, §101(b)(4); Rothwell et al., 2015). However, in order to return results, it is essential to maintain the link to participants' identities, thus meeting the regulatory definition of "human subjects research" (HHS, 2018, §102(f)), and triggering the same rights and protections for biobank participants as participants in clinical trials of new drugs: that is, the right to informed consent, the right to withdraw (samples and data) from research, and protections against unauthorized access to their samples, data, and research results.

Because the uses to which biospecimens will be put might not be determined at the moment of their collection, it can be challenging to identify and implement protections for participants that are also consonant with public health, clinical, or research professional norms. In effect, whenever the return of results is embraced in pursuit of public health goals or as a fiduciary clinical obligation in conjunction with biobank research, the practical need for identifiability simultaneously activates the full panoply of ethical requirements for research with human volunteers. This practical necessity of identifiability triggers the cascade of other policy issues that complicate the management of biobanks. Public health considerations might also suggest a need to consider questions of "group confidentiality" in addition to individual confidentiality, and unless the context is rendered with greater clarity, it might not be obvious which set of concerns should govern biobank policies or various actors' conduct (Alpert, 2000; Goodman and Meslin, 2014).

Tensions can result between the ethical support *for* a certain organization of data when it facilitates a public health mission to promote health, and ethical cautions *against* that same organizational scheme in research if it places research participants' confidentiality at greater risk (Goodman and Meslin, 2014). Offering greater data protection often suggests removing individual identifying information from data, while facilitating return of individual results involves maintaining a link to identifiable individuals. *All of Us* attempts to manage this tension using tiers of data sets, with all tiers requiring researcher verification and research ethics training, and the most public tier stripped of "obvious" identifiers (Proffitt, 2017). Simultaneously, a centralized approach to data storage is meant to allow the *All of Us* program to mediate re-contact while acknowledging the ambitious nature of such return: "This bidirectional exchange with participants—is something that is really innovative.... A few have done it, but certainly not on this scale of potentially at least [a] million people" (Josh Denny, *All of Us* Research Program Data and Research Center, cited in Proffitt, 2017). Meanwhile, that "bidirectional" vision is encountering hiccups from the participant side: early testing of PMI consent forms revealed that approximately 20 percent would not agree to share their EHRs with researchers, which would limit researchers' access to information about exposure, phenotype, and family history (Pittman, 2017).

Informed Consent

Informed consent for research traditionally requires explicit description of the reasons for specimen and data collection, the potential risks and benefits associated with their use, the specification of future users and uses, a stated duration of research activity, and the opportunity to withdraw participation (HHS, 1998). When the purpose of a collection is for future and typically unspecified use by researchers who may or may not be known to the biobank at the time of collection, ensuring that consent is informed is challenging. Despite this, many researchers, biobankers, and regulatory officials are now pushing to obtain broad consent for all future uses of specimens. Additionally, deposit of positive genomic research findings into EHRs, such as is done in MyCode and GeneScreen, precludes some opportunity to withdraw, since it is nearly impossible to remove results from EHRs (Prince et al., 2015). A 2012 national survey of 456 US biobanks examined biobank policies and practices, including informed consent practices (Henderson, Cadigan, et al., 2013). Biobanks address these issues in different ways, including opt-in consent to sample storage, an option broadly consenting to biospecimen use in future research, "narrower" or more specific forms of consent, or some combination of these alternatives (Henderson, Cadigan, et al., 2013). Different approaches to informed consent in biobanking research are illustrated by the three cases. While the KP-NWBB used broad consent for the biobank, additional specific consent was sought for the preventive genomic sequencing in GeneScreen. MyCode and KP-NWBB's broad opt-in consent practices reflect what the majority of biobanks surveyed have used. The PMI *All of Us* Research Program will also use broad, opt-in consent, with possible additional consent sought as the program develops.

Projects like GeneScreen and MyCode take initial steps toward the possibility of extending the public health benefits of genomic screening to different life stages (Evans et al., 2013), and the public health genomics community holds out similar hopes for the PMI (Khoury and Galea, 2016). In contrast to other forms of public health prevention, like newborn screening, it is harder to justify bypassing informed consent (Jones and Bayer, 2007). The three cases described here are precursors to public health interventions, designed as research projects operating with some type of informed consent—either to the project itself or to participation in the biobank from which samples were acquired.

Engagement

GeneScreen and MyCode return genetic findings deemed medically actionable, justified by application of public health screening criteria (e.g., if an acceptable medical treatment or prevention can be applied, and its application will make a difference in morbidity or mortality). Acceptability of such preventive screening is an important component of evaluating the harms and benefits of screening. Public trust in health institutions is often necessary for the success of population health campaigns. Similarly, trust in research institutions can make or break rates of participation, which is of concern to biobanks whose utility depends on size and diversity of collections. Efforts to engage communities to assess acceptability and foster trust can be accomplished by community advisory boards, focus groups, or deliberative democracy, and each of these approaches has strengths and limitations (Simon, Newbury, and L'heureux, 2011; Koenig, 2014). Previous studies of biobanking practices reveal considerable reliance on community advisory boards (CABs) and other forms of community engagement (Henderson, Edwards, et al., 2013; Haldeman et al., 2014).

Each of the three cases demonstrates different efforts to engage with communities. MyCode did extensive investigations of the Geisinger population, including focus groups and follow-up evaluations (Carey et al., 2016). This donor engagement model to elicit views on screening for actionable genes was not employed with KP-NWBB, which primarily relied on the GeneScreen website and surveys to ensure adequate understanding. An Advisory for Biospecimen Committee (ABC) governs research use of Northwest regional specimen resources (Kaiser Permanente, 2015). In addition, GeneScreen researchers developed a study-specific CAB, composed of ten individuals representing various community organizations, and which considered questions such as the target age for recruitment and whether individuals with no insurance should be eligible. As the PMI Working Group advised, a desire for highly interactive participant representation is infused throughout the *All of Us* plans, including participant engagement in observational self-reports, co-design of studies, mediated access to data, contribution to quality control, and receipt of aggregate and/or individual results (Hudson, Lifton, and Patrick-Lake, 2015). The engaged vision of participation is also expected to facilitate the *All of Us*'s population health emphasis, shifting attention "away from a disease focus to a focus on all members of the public" (Hudson, Lifton, and Patrick-Lake, 2015, 41).

Return and Disposition of Individual Results: Policies and Practices

Many scholars interested in the ethical and legal concerns of biobanking argue that biobanks have a responsibility to return individual results to participants who indicate they want them (e.g., Holm et al., 2014; Wolf et al., 2012). Each of the three cases has returned, or will return, some genetic information to participants (see Table 57.1). However, the criteria used to determine medical actionability is itself contested, and as understanding about genes and their relationships to disease improves, determinations of medical actionability will also change (Lázaro-Muñoz et al., 2017). For example, ACMG's latest recommendation of return of findings in clinical exome and genome sequencing added four genes to its list and, somewhat disconcertingly, removed one gene (Kalia et al., 2017). In addition, as clinical and public health translational research gets closer to improving diagnosis, treatment, or intervention on the basis of genetic information, contributors to biobanks increasingly are viewed not only as research participants, but also as patients and target populations. This thus raises the question of whether genetic test results with health implications discovered in a research context should be transferred to a clinical record, and if so, by whom (Prince et al., 2015).

Both KP-NWBB and MyCode join a minority of biobanks that are returning individual results to contributors (Cadigan, Edwards, et al., 2017) and, even more unusually, depositing these findings directly into patients' EHRs. The PMI Working Group recommended that basic health information (e.g., serum cholesterol) be returned to individual participants and recommended working with laboratories certified as complying with the Clinical Laboratory Improvement Amendments (CLIA) requirements that assure analytic validity of results (Hudson, Lifton, and Patrick-Lake, 2015). In stark contrast with MyCode and GeneScreen, however, the PMI did not initially plan to automatically place actionable findings in patient EHRs, and it has no clear means to do so, given the many clinical recruitment sites and diaspora of research labs that are supposed to contribute to and use its central biobank (Hudson, Lifton, and Patrick-Lake, 2015). Interestingly, as the norms of clinical and public health ethics continue to influence the implementation of *All of Us*, this position may already be changing (as mentioned above, and as recently discussed at the *All of Us* Research Program meeting; see, e.g., Ozenberger, 2017), which could present the *All of Us* Biobank with substantial logistical challenges.

These cases also raise future issues for translational genomic research that makes use of biobanks. A distinct trade-off exists between the privacy risks of sustaining identifiable data and the possible health benefits of returning results to affected individuals.

There are also impending questions about follow-up and clinical care. As participants become patients, to what extent do research obligations include facilitating a transition to clinical care? Must health systems managers anticipate which preventive and ameliorative interventions are covered by insurance before recruiting participants or returning results (Prince, 2015)? The answers to these questions are especially important for public health genomics, as gains in population health will evaporate if there are significant barriers to accessing care.

Conclusion

Biobanking research fosters advances in genetics, extending benefits along a translational pathway from bench to bedside, and even beyond to population health. The cases presented here represent the initial period of exploring the potential promise of public health genomics (Khoury and Galea, 2016). As MyCode anticipates, a learning health approach to genomic testing promises greater effectiveness and efficiency in the provision of health care. GeneScreen explores the possibility of reducing morbidity and mortality through genetic or genomic population screening of asymptomatic adults. *All of Us* pursues a vision of precision translation at both clinical and public health levels of intervention, in part through development of sophisticated risk stratification and health outcome prediction models. As a national research initiative, *All of Us* also seeks inclusion of diverse participants in hopes of remedying current representational limits of genomic research—a goal that also speaks to the possibility for public health genomics to address health disparities (Khoury, 2013).

Some of the ethical questions and social implications raised by these possibilities concern the design of biobanks as research, clinical, and/or public health entities. Researchers, biobank curators, and health systems managers must grapple with how smoothly we might be able to move information generated in one context to another. Greater seamlessness will facilitate innovation and could help protect research participants whose health needs are uncovered during the course of research, but it also risks blurring the historical boundaries between contexts.

Whether moving genetic findings more seamlessly between research and clinical contexts exacerbates or improves participant-patient understanding might depend on how such communication takes place. The MyCode project demonstrates that successful communication strategies must reach health care providers and clearly communicate to members of the public when they are transitioning from being regarded as research participants, clinical patients, or members of general populations. GeneScreen and MyCode have established a base of evidence for understanding why screening might be valuable to patients when family history alone has not warranted referral to genetic testing. *All of Us* demonstrates that both public biobanks and the public health uses to which they give rise are subject to existing research and clinical ethical norms. The three cases examined here suggest a nascent path forward for devising best practices in public health genomic biobanking, demonstrating both initial progress and a continued need for ELSI studies of this intriguing intersection.

Acknowledgments

We would like to thank Michael F. Murray for his comments on an earlier draft of this paper. Support for the preparation of this article was provided by the U.S. National Human Genome Research Institute (NHGRI), Grants NIH 2P50 HG004488 (G. Henderson, principal investigator). The authors have no other relevant affiliations or financial involvement with any organization with a financial interest in or financial conflict with the subject matter discussed in the manuscript.

References

Adams, M. C., Evans, J. P., Henderson, G. E., and Berg, J. S. 2016. "The Promise and Peril of Genomic Screening in the General Population." *Genetics in Medicine* 18(6): 593–599.

Alpert, S. A. 2000. "Privacy and the Analysis of Stored Tissues." In *Research Involving Human Biological Materials: Ethical Issues and Policy Guidance*, vol. 2: *Commissioned Papers*, A-1. (Rockville, Md.: National Bioethics Advisory Commission).

Alzu'bi, A., Zhou, L., and Waltzlaf, V. 2014. "Personal Genomic Information Management and Personalized Medicine: Challenges, Current Solutions, and Roles of HIM Professionals." *Perspectives in Health Information Management* 11:1c.

Aswini, Y. B., and Varun, S. 2010. "Genetics in Public Health: Rarely Explored." *Indian Journal of Human Genetics* 16(2): 47–54.

Blasimme, A., and Vayena, E. 2016. "'Tailored-to-You': Public Engagement and the Political Legitimation of Precision Medicine." *Perspectives in Biology and Medicine* 59(2): 172–188.

Bledsoe, M. J., Grizzle, W. E., Clark, B. J., and Zeps, N. 2012. "Practical Implementation Issues and Challenges for Biobanks in the Return of Individual Research Results." *Genetics in Medicine* 14(4): 478–483.

Buchanan, A. H., Manickam, K., Meyer, M. N., Wagner, J. K., Hallquist, M. L. G., Williams, J. L., et al. 2018. "Early Cancer Diagnoses through BRCA1/2 Screening of Unselected Adult Biobank Participants." *Genetics in Medicine* 20(5): 554558.

Burton, H., Chowdhury, S., Dent, T., Hall, A., Pashayan, N., and Pharoah, P. 2013. "Public Health Implications from COGS and Potential Risk Stratification and Screening." *Nature Genetics* 45(4): 349–351.

Cadigan, R. J., Butterfield, R., Rini, C., Waltz, M., Kuczynski, K. J., Meussig, K., et al. 2017. "Online Education and e-Consent for GeneScreen, a Preventive Genomic Screening Study." *Public Health Genomics* 20(4): 235–246.

Cadigan, R. J., Edwards, T. P., Lassiter, D., Davis, A. M., and Henderson, G. E. 2017. "'Forward Thinking' in U.S. Biobanking." *Genetic Testing and Molecular Biomarkers* 21(3): 148–154.

Carey, D. J., Fetterolf, S. N., Davis, F. D., Faucett, W. A., Kirchner, H. L., Mirshahi, U., et al. 2016. "The Geisinger MyCode Community Health Initiative: An Electronic Health Record-Linked Biobank for Precision Medicine Research." *Genetics in Medicine* 18(9): 906–913.

Collins, F. S. 2015. "Building the Precision Medicine Initiative National Research Cohort: The Time is Now." Letter from the Director, September 26 (Bethesda, Md.: National Institutes of Health) https://www.nih.gov/about-nih/who-we-are/nih-director/statements/building-precision-medicine-initiative-national-research-cohort-time-now.

De Souza, Y. G., and Greenspan, J. S. 2013. "Biobanking Past, Present, and Future: Responsibilities and Benefits." *AIDS* 27(3): 303–312.

Evans, J. P., Berg, J. S., Olshan, A. F., Magnuson, T., and Rimer, B. K. 2013. "We Screen Newborns, Don't We? Realizing the Promise of Public Health Genomics." *Genetics in Medicine* 15(5): 332–335.

Gallagher, C. 2016. "Mayo Clinic to Be Home of National Precision Medicine Initiative (PMI) Cohort Program Biobank." News Release, May 26 (Rochester, Minn.: Mayo Clinic). http://newsnetwork.mayoclinic.org/discussion/mayo-clinic-to-be-home-of-national-precision-medicine-initiative-pmi-cohort-program-biobank.

Geisinger MyCode Community Health Initiative. 2017. "MyCode Consent Form." -https://emerge.mc.vanderbilt.edu/wp-content/uploads/2017/08/MyCode-Main-Consent-Version-30-_Geisinger.pdf.

Geisinger MyCode Community Health Initiative. November 1, 2018. "MyCode Results Reported." https://www.geisinger.org/-/media/OneGeisinger/pdfs/ghs/research/mycode/gsc-nov-2018.pdf.

Goodman, K. W., and Meslin, E. M. 2014. "Ethics, Information Technology, and Public Health: Duties and Challenges in Computational Epidemiology." In *Public Health Informatics and Information Systems*, edited by J. A. Magnuson and P.C. Fu, 191–209. (London: Springer-Verlag).

Green, R. C., Berg, J. S., Grody, W. W., Kalia, S. S., Korf, B. R., Martin, C. L., et al. 2013. "ACMG Recommendations for Reporting Incidental Findings in Clinical Exome and Genome Sequencing." *Genetics in Medicine* 15(7): 565–574.

Haldeman, K. M., Cadigan, R. J., Davis, A., Goldenberg, A., Henderson, G. E., Lassiter, D., et al. 2014. "Community Engagement in US Biobanking: Multiplicity of Meaning and Method." *Public Health Genomics* 17(2): 84–94.

Henderson, G. E., Cadigan, R. J., Edwards, T. P., Conlon, I., Nelson, A. G., Evans, J. P., et al. 2013. "Characterizing Biobank Organizations in the U.S.: Results From a National Survey." *Genome Medicine* 5(1): 3.

Henderson, G. E., Edwards, T. P., Cadigan, R. J., Davis, A. M., Zimmer, C., Conlon, I., et al. 2013. "Stewardship Practices of U.S. Biobanks." *Science Translational Medicine* 5(215): 215cm7.

HHS (US Department of Health and Human Services). 1998. "Informed Consent Checklist." https://www.hhs.gov/ohrp/regulations-and-policy/guidance/checklists/index.html.

HHS (US Department of Health and Human Services). 2018. "Basic HHS Policy for Protection of Human Research Subjects - 45 CFR 46 §101." https://www.hhs.gov/ohrp/regulations-and-policy/regulations/45-cfr-46/index.html#46.101

Holm, I. A., Savage, S. K., Green, R. C., Juengst, E. T., McGuire, A., Kornetsky, S., et al. 2014. "Guidelines for Return of Research Results from Pediatric Genomic Studies: Deliberations of the Boston Children's Hospital Gene Partnership Informed Cohort Oversight Board." *Genetics in Medicine* 16(7): 547–552.

Hudson, K., Lifton, R., and Patrick-Lake, B. 2015. *The Precision Medicine Initiative (PMI) Cohort Program: Building a Research Foundation for 21st Century Medicine* (Bethesda, Md.: National Institutes of Health).

IOM (Institute of Medicine). 2007. *The Learning Healthcare System: Workshop Summary* (Washington, D.C.: The National Academies Press).

Jones, M. M., and Bayer, R. 2007. "Paternalism and Its Discontents: Motorcycle Helmet Laws, Libertarian Values, and Public Health." *American Journal of Public Health* 97(2): 208–217.

Kalia, S. S., Adelman, K., Bale, S. J., Chung, W. K., Eng, C., Evans, J. P., et al. 2017. "Recommendations for Reporting of Secondary Findings in Clinical Exome and Genome Sequencing, 2016 Update (ACMG SF v2.0): A Policy Statement of the American College of Medical Genetics and Genomics." *Genetics in Medicine* 19(2): 249–255.

Kaiser Permanente. 2015. Biospecimen Resources, Kaiser Permanente Northwest. https://research.kpchr.org/About/Capabilities/Biospecimen-Resources.

Khoury, M. J. 2013. "Why We Can't Wait: A Public Health Approach to Health Disparities in Genomic Medicine." *Centers for Disease Control and Prevention: Genomics and Health Impact Blog*, June 27. https://blogs.cdc.gov/genomics/2013/06/27/why-we-cant-wait/.

Khoury, M. J., and Evans, J. P. 2015. "A Public Health Perspective on a National Precision Medicine Cohort: Balancing Long-Term Knowledge Generation with Early Health Benefit." *JAMA* 313(21): 2117–2118.

Khoury M. J., and Galea, S. 2016. "Will Precision Medicine Improve Population Health?" *JAMA* 316(13): 1357–1358.

Koenig, B. A. 2014. "Have We Asked Too Much of Consent?" *Hastings Center Report* 44(4): 33–34.

Lázaro-Muñoz, G., Conley, J. M., Davis, A. M., Prince, A. E. R., and Cadigan, R. J. 2017. "Which Results to Return: Subjective Judgments in Selecting Medically Actionable Genes." *Genetic Testing and Molecular Biomarkers* 21(3): 184–194.

Murray, M. F. 2016. "Screening 100,000 Unselected Adults with Whole Exome Sequencing." Presentation, North Carolina Medical Genetics Association, Chapel Hill, N.C., October 28, 2016.

Murray, M. F. 2017. Personal communication, February 14.

NIH (National Institutes of Health). 2015. "Precision Medicine Initiative Cohort Program Biobank (U24)." https://grants.nih.gov/grants/guide/rfa-files/RFA-PM-16-004.html.

NIH (National Institutes of Health). 2016. "NIH Funds Biobank to Support Precision Medicine Initiative Cohort Program." https://www.nih.gov/news-events/news-releases/nih-funds-biobank-support-precision-medicine-initiative-cohort-program.

Olson, J. E., Bielinski, S. J., Ryu, E., Winkler, E. M., Takahashi, P. Y., Patha, J., et al. 2014. "Biobanks and Personalized Medicine." *Clinical Genetics* 86(1): 50–55.

Ozenberger, B. 2017. "Workshop Goals/Key Questions." Presentation, Return of Genetic Results in the *All of Us* Research Program, Bethesda, Md., March 6–7, 2017.

Pittman, D. 2017. "Precision Medicine Initiative Hits a Snag." *Politico Morning eHealth*, October 10. https://www.politico.com/tipsheets/morning-ehealth/2017/10/10/precision-medicine-initiative-hits-a-snag-222722.

Prince, A. E. 2015. "Prevention for Those Who Can Pay: Insurance Reimbursement of Genetic-Based Preventive Interventions in the Liminal State between Health and Disease." *Journal of Law and the Biosciences* 2(2): 365–395.

Prince, A. E., Conley, J. M., Davis, A. M., Lázaro-Muñoz, G., and Cadigan, R. J. 2015. "Automatic Placement of Genomic Research Results in Medical Records: Do Researchers Have a Duty? Should Participants Have a Choice?" *Journal of Law, Medicine & Ethics* 43(4): 827–842.

Proffitt, A. 2017. "Josh Denny on the *All of Us* Research Program, Data Management on a National Scale." *Bio IT World*, November 6. http://www.bio-itworld.com/2017/11/06/josh-denny-on-the-all-of-us-research-program-data-management-on-a-national-scale.aspx.

Qi, L., and Franks, P. W. 2016. "Nutrigenetics of Type 2 Diabetes." In *The Genetics of Type 2 Diabetes and Related Traits: Biology, Physiology and Translation*, edited by J. C. Florez, 539–560 (Boston, Mass.: Springer).

Rahimzadeh, V., and Bartlett, G. 2014. "Genetics and Primary Care: Where Are We Headed?" *Journal of Translational Medicine* 12: 238.

Rothwell, E., Maschke, K. J., Botkin, J. R., Goldenberg, A., Murray, T. H., and Rivera, S. M. 2015. "Biobanking Research and Human Subjects Protections: Perspectives of IRB Leaders." *IRB: Ethics & Human Research* 37(2): 8–13.

Sankar, P. L., and Parker, L. S. 2016. "The Precision Medicine Initiative's *All of Us* Research Program: An Agenda for Research on its Ethical, Legal, and Social Issues." *Genetics in Medicine* 19(7): 743–750.

Simon, C. M., Newbury, E., and L'heureux, J. 2011. "Protecting Participants, Promoting Progress: Public Perspectives on Community Advisory Boards (CABs) in Biobanking." *Journal of Empirical Research on Human Research Ethics* 6(3): 19–30.

Sylvester, J. 2017. "Geisinger Goes National with Genetic Research Program." *Daily Item* (Sunbury, Penn.), November 14. http://www.dailyitem.com/news/local_news/geisinger-goes-national-with-genetic-research-program/article_d58e3869-103a-5399-aa35-1575344f42a8.html.

van Dijk, E. L., Auger, H., Jaszczyszyn, Y., and Thermes, C. 2014. "Ten Years of Next-Generation Sequencing Technology." *Trends in Genetics 30* (9): 418–426.

Watson, P. H., and Barnes, R. O. 2011. "A Proposed Schema for Classifying Human Research Biobanks." *Biopreservation and Biobanking* 9(4): 327–333.

Wolf, S. M., Amendola, L. M., Berg, J. S., Chung, W. K., Clayton, E. W., Green, R. C., et al. 2018. "Navigating the Research-Clinical Interface in Genomic Medicine: Analysis from the CSER Consortium." *Genetics in Medicine* 20(5): 545–553.

Wolf, S. M., Crock, B. N., Van Ness, B., Lawrenz, F., Kahn, J. P., Beskow, L. M., et al. 2012. "Managing Incidental Findings and Research Results in Genomic Research Involving Biobanks and Archived Data Sets." *Genetics in Medicine* 14(4): 361–384.

CHAPTER 58

GENETIC EPIDEMIOLOGY, INFECTIOUS DISEASE, AND PUBLIC HEALTH ETHICS

PRIYA DUGGAL, GAIL GELLER, AND ANDREA SUTHERLAND

The Danger of Infectious Disease and the Opportunity of Genomics

Genomic information offers the opportunity for greater "personalized" prevention and treatment (Pashayan et al., 2013) of infectious diseases, as well as new tools for addressing epidemics and newly emerging pathogens (Malik, 2013). Scientific advances in genomics can elucidate infectious disease pathology, immunology, and vaccinology; augment research and development of preventive and therapeutic measures; and enhance the efficiency of public health interventions and policies (Eisen and MacCullum, 2009; Telenti, 2004; Trautmann and Sekaly, 2011; Omenn, 2000; Pang, 2002; Yan, 2010, 203–220; Yang et al., 2008; Brusic and August, 2004). Such developments would mitigate the burden of infectious diseases, which contribute to significant morbidity and mortality worldwide (WHO, 2012). Infectious agents can cause illnesses that are acute (e.g., influenza), chronic (e.g., hepatitis B), have significant sequelae (e.g., meningococcal), or generate new epidemics (e.g., Ebola, Zika). While the disease burden is highest in low-income countries, new emerging and antibiotic-resistant infectious diseases threaten public health globally (Roca et al., 2015). Even for infectious diseases that have vaccines or treatments, preventive and therapeutic measures can be highly burdensome, variably effective, prohibitively expensive, or difficult to access for large portions of the population globally. Each infectious disease brings ethical dilemmas, ranging from resource allocation and contact tracing, to preventive and therapeutic care provision, to clinical trials—all of which could benefit from vector, pathogen, and host genomic scientific knowledge and application.

To control the spread of vector-borne diseases like malaria and dengue, genome editing tools are being used for the precise deletion of functional genes or insertion of toxic genes in vector mosquitoes (Reegan et al., 2017). Genomics also has been critical in pathogen identification (e.g., SARS) (Yeh et al., 2004). Rapid and large-scale sequencing provides stronger and more accurate evidence than was previously possible for source and contact tracing and is widely applied for surveillance and outbreak management (Gilmour et al., 2013), as was done in the 2014–2015 measles outbreak in Disneyland and the 2014–2016 Ebola epidemic in West Africa (Gire et al., 2014; Vogel, 2014). Additionally, pathogen genomics has focused on improved precision for the diagnosis of microbial infection, identifying transmission, understanding emerging drug resistance, and identifying targets for new therapeutics and vaccines.

There is growing evidence that *host* genetic factors, and the interaction between host, vector, and pathogen, influence variability in infection rates, immune responses (Eisen and MacCullum, 2009; Poland et al., 2013), susceptibility (Withrock et al., 2015), disease progression and severity (Keynan, Malik, and Fowke, 2013; Srivastava et al., 2009), and response to preventive and therapeutic interventions (Petrizzo et al., 2012; Kaslow, McNicholl, and Hill, 2008; Mentzer et al., 2015; Pittman et al., 2016; Liang et al., 2014; Al-Qahtani et al., 2013; Zeng, 2014; Jiang et al., 2013; Zhang et al., 2010; Liu et al., 2011; Kirk et al., 2005; Mbarek et al., 2011; Sonneveld et al., 2012; Ovsyannikova, Jacobson, and Poland, 2004; Buonaguro et al., 2011; Nohynek et al., 2012; Mentzer et al., 2015; Pan et al., 2014; Jilg and Chung, 2013; Png et al., 2011; Hennig et al., 2008). Genome-wide association studies have identified several favorable host variants: the *IL28B* genotype, which predisposes individuals to spontaneously clear the hepatitis C virus (HCV); and the *CCR5Δ32* genotype, which is protective against human immunodeficiency virus (HIV) infection (Dean et al., 1996; Livingstone, 1964; Mann et al., 1992; Mira et al., 2004; Ge et al., 2009; Thomas et al., 2009). Moreover, genetic information about the pathogen can influence its impact on the host. For example, differences in HIV subtype have been shown to have marked differences in disease progression in Kenya and Uganda (Baeten et al., 2007; Kiwanuka et al., 2008; Kiwanuka et al., 2010). In the United States, HIV-1 subtype B–infected hemophiliacs, those with lower viral replication capacity, had a survival advantage relative to those with higher replication capacity (Barbour et al., 2004). Differences in the specificity of a virus for a particular host tissue (called viral tropism) are associated with speed of disease progression, although it is unclear if it is the cause or consequence (Hunt et al., 2006; Briz et al., 2008). Genomic research is making important contributions to our understanding of infectious disease pathogenesis and immune response, and to future vaccine development and treatment strategies (Trautmann and Sekaly, 2011; Yang et al., 2008; Mentzer et al., 2015; Ovsyannikova, Jacobson, and Poland, 2004; Dandekar and Dandekar, 2010; Hill, 2001; Ozdemir, Faraj, and Knoppers, 2011; Ozdemir et al., 2011; Poland et al., 2007; Chapman and Hill, 2012).

This chapter explores the ethical, legal, and social implications (ELSI) of applying advances in genomics to public health prevention and control of infectious diseases. It starts with a brief description of the historical connection between infectious disease control and the prevention of genetic diseases. It then describes insights gleaned from ELSI research on the application of genomics to complex diseases and their relevance to infectious disease, drawing on three examples that highlight different ethical issues: inequities in HIV, personalized vaccines, and triage during epidemics. Throughout, the chapter incorporates considerations for future research and policy.

Historical Connections between Infectious and Genetic Disease Control

Ethical and policy questions stemming from the progressive fusing of genetic and epidemiological measures have long, rich traditions. Historically, case reporting, isolation and quarantine, contact tracing, and behavioral regulation and oversight developed as the cornerstones of infectious disease control (Fairchild, Bayer, and Colgrove, 2007; Mooney, 2015) and faced the bioethical conflict of autonomy versus the greater public health benefits. With advances in medical genetics, a generation of physicians began to apply genetics to public health methods of disease control, starting with preventing the birth of individuals with hereditary diseases (Comfort, 2012; also see, "Eugenics and Public Health: Historical Connections and Ethical Implications," this volume) and shifting to the recognition that "complex diseases" result from the interaction between multiple genes and the environment. Although infectious disease surveillance might appear to be the epitome of one-size-fits-all medicine, it is now recognized that there is individual variability in susceptibility, transmission, and disease severity. The concept of "precision medicine" (White House, 2017; Jameson and Longo, 2015; Collins and Varmus, 2015) is evolving to broader considerations of "precision public health" (Hood and Flores, 2012; Khoury et al., 2012), which will have applications to infectious diseases. In short, in the genomic era, infectious disease surveillance may enhance research capabilities and target individuals for prevention and treatment to optimize infection control, and to prevent either horizontal or vertical transmission. This complex, integrative, and multidisciplinary approach to public health will require informed bioethical considerations that mediate between numerous pairs (or poles) of social and medical values, including autonomy versus public health surveillance; liberty versus disease control measures; privacy versus the duty not to harm others; and the responsibilities of patients to themselves, to their families, and to society.

ELSI Considerations for Genomics, Infectious Disease, and Public Health

Many insights relevant to infectious disease can be discerned from the more than twenty years of ELSI research on genomics applications in complex diseases (McEwen et al., 2014). Pertinent issues include the reliability, validity, confidentiality, and disclosure of genetic information. Clinical next-generation sequencing and the increasing number of large biobanks raise issues of the interpretation of data, data storage, data sharing, informed consent, incidental findings and return of results, and identifiability and privacy (Pinxten and Howard, 2014; Ross, Rothstein, and Clayton, 2013; Tabor et al., 2011; Kaye, 2012; McGuire et al., 2011; Wolf, 2013; Wolf et al., 2008, 2012; Meltzer, 2006; McGuire and Beskow, 2010; Bunnik et al., 2013).

However, a number of factors unique to infectious disease underscore the importance of identifying novel ELSI issues that might emerge from the application of genomics in this context (Geller et al., 2014). Importantly, the nature of disease transmission and susceptibility differs, with implications for who is at increased risk. Infectious diseases are most often transmitted horizontally (not directly through family members), based on exposure (air, sexual, vector) to related or unrelated individuals. Horizontal transmission is ethically problematic because those exposed are often unaware of their risk. In addition, potential benefits or harms of disease interventions (i.e., vaccine policy) accrue to the entire population, in keeping with the goals of public health. But there are well-described ethical tensions between the goals and implementation of personalized medicine and those of public health. Existing literature on the ethical, legal, and policy issues in infectious disease describes the potential for stigmatization of individuals or subpopulations, the challenge of balancing individual interests (e.g., privacy, autonomy, freedom of movement) against risks of harms to others and to public health, and obligations on the part of employers or health professionals (Gostin, Bayer, and Fairchild, 2003; Battin et al., 2009).

There has been some discussion of the ELSI issues involved in using pathogen genomic sequencing for source and contact tracing (Rump and Woonink, 2012; Rump et al., 2013; Bubela and Yanow, 2012; Luheshi et al., 2015). Human genetic markers could lead to identification of people at a higher risk for contracting or spreading a disease. People can be "super-spreaders" (infected hosts who infect disproportionately more secondary contacts) due to a biological predisposition to shed high levels of infectious particles, not limiting their risk behaviors, or continued shedding post-recovery. The ability of pathogen sequencing to identify a human source of infection creates potential questions of blame and legal liability, stigmatization, and risks to privacy (Rump and Woonink, 2012; Rump et al., 2013).

The significance of genomic information, and its application, may generate specific ELSI concerns, including imbalance in health-related risks and potential benefits to individuals and populations; protection of privacy and confidentiality of personal information; challenges to autonomy, choice, and limitations on liberty; social and behavioral impacts of genomic information on individuals, family members, and others; and equitable distribution of scarce resources. Although these issues are in no way unique to infectious diseases, they need to be considered as part of development in practice and policy as scientific understanding of the role of genomics in infectious disease management advances (Geller et al., 2014). Genotypic information may exacerbate the inherent tension between the goals of personalized medicine (to tailor prevention and treatment to individuals) and those of public health (to maximize wellness for entire populations), giving rise to inequitable distribution of benefits and harms among specific subgroups of the population and adding an additional layer to the perennial tension between individual and population interests in public health.

Ethical challenges often arise when there is a gap in the time between the identification of a problem and the capacity to mitigate it. That is the case with genomic discoveries and infectious diseases; those at either increased risk of contracting or transmitting infection or those who are more or less likely to respond to interventions might be identified before there are safe and effective interventions to offer, or before risk-mitigation policies can be adopted. Another significant ethical challenge results from the variability in predictive value of genotypic information and how variable risk can complicate risk management policy, cost-benefit analyses, allocation of scarce resources, and considerations of privacy and autonomy.

Cost-Benefit Analyses

Cost-benefit analysis and overall predicted impact on morbidity and mortality might influence the ethical justifiability of preventive interventions targeted at individuals and populations (Pittman et al., 2016). Investing in the research to identify genetic variants, and to ensure individuals are screened, raises questions about cost, efficient use of limited resources, and moral duties. Vaccines are used for many infectious diseases, but the scientific knowledge about individual variation of efficacy/immunogenicity and safety/reactogenicity of these vaccines is limited. Vaccines or other public health measures that work for the majority of the community and result in positive public health, such as reduction of morbidity and mortality, have been accepted. However, the ability to identify a genetic predisposition for adverse events or immunogenomic markers that predict immunogenicity following vaccination might provide an opportunity for immunization programs to screen and thus limit adverse outcomes or immune failures in a subset of individuals. However, if the genetic markers are not absolutely predictive, or if the adverse event was not severe, this may cause undue concern, decrease vaccination rates, and in the end not be cost-effective. In light of the large public investment in and strong support for vaccines from state and federal authorities, it is not clear how immunization programs ought to consider the moral and policy arguments related to screening for genetic risk factors.

Allocation of Scarce Resources

Disparities in access to treatments and prevention can be a result of financial, educational, sociocultural, geographical, or environmental barriers. When circumstances, such as a pandemic, create demands for resources that exceed supply, decision-making about the distribution and allocation of resources may be influenced by genetic information. Tailored drugs or vaccines might be developed and produced for at-risk genetic ("orphan") subgroups or, contrary to social justice, for those who can pay. It remains to be seen what the implications would be for health insurance coverage and public financing of interventions if they vary by genotype. The extent to which infectious disease genomics will be translated into benefits for public health will likely be largely influenced by the allocation of resources for research and development efforts. Research that is likely to have the greatest global benefits might not be given funding priority by those countries with the greatest resources. Differences in regional investments in genomic science and technology will have important implications for equitable distribution of benefits and public health impact (OECD, 2013, 7–9).

Privacy, Autonomy, and Choice

In the context of infectious disease management, individual rights and liberties such as autonomous decision—making, freedom of choice and action, privacy, and the right to personal information can conflict with public health priorities. Whereas public health programs may target people or subgroups with particular risk factors, the possibility to ascertain (or to require reporting of) otherwise unobservable genetic risk factors may complicate issues of protection of personal information, privacy, and autonomy.

Considerations of privacy and autonomy are being challenged by genetic sequencing technologies that will likely contribute to our understanding of host genomics in the context of infectious disease. The growing literature on the ethical implications of sequencing has focused on privacy, data sharing, return of results and the management of incidental findings, and best practices for obtaining informed consent (Pinxten and Howard, 2014; Ross, Rothstein, and Clayton, 2013; Tabor et al., 2011; Kaye, 2012; McGuire et al., 2011; Wolf, 2013; Wolf et al., 2008, 2012; Meltzer, 2006; McGuire and Beskow, 2010; Bunnik et al., 2013). Informed consent policies and practices for sequencing information will need to consider (1) whether the information that people have in the context of infectious disease is different in morally relevant ways from chronic disease, and (2) whether the processes for disclosing information about host genomics should vary in different parts of the world.

It is important to consider ways in which individual genotyping could be used or mandated, and how this genetic information could affect personal liberties. Individual genomic data might be consulted when decisions about prevention and control are considered, such as determining which subpopulations should be screened and which vaccine formulation is appropriate. Genomic data about individuals and groups might be consulted during disease outbreaks, in planning for public health programs, or in developing new or assessing existing public health policies: Where are the genomic clusters or hotspots for infection; where should vaccines be deployed most urgently; which therapies should be offered to which genomic populations; and where should treatment programs, isolation policies, mandatory vaccination, or public health control programs be implemented to halt the spread of infections? Genetic markers of infectivity or likelihood of being a "super-spreader" could be used to justify quarantine and isolation policies, with the concomitant implications for individual liberty. The value placed on individual autonomy varies in different cultures, so the primacy that it receives in the context of public health planning and decision-making, and the role of informed consent, might be different in different countries (Geller et al., 2014; Knoppers, Zawati, and Kirby, 2012; Rotimi and Marshall, 2010).

In the United States, the legal and policy paradigm in genomics places a high value on privacy, which can conflict with the public health framework in which individual rights can be overridden for the benefit of others (Gerard, Hayes, and Rothstein, 2002). Federal and state genetic privacy legislation protects patients from discrimination based on their genetic profile. But it is unlikely that the potential benefit of the utilization of genomic information in the diagnosis, treatment and/or prevention of infectious disease was considered when these laws were enacted. Specific individuals may be better suited to work in high-risk job placements during an infectious disease outbreak because they are more likely to have a protective response to a vaccine, or because their genotype makes them less likely to develop severe infection (Geller et al., 2014). Alternatively, others might have a variant associated with increased risk of severe infection. In both situations, the provisions of the Genetic Information Nondiscrimination Act of 2008 (GINA, a US law addressing aspects of genetic discrimination in employment and insurance contexts) may limit the ability to use genetic information to determine which employees would be best suited to high-risk job placements in case of an infectious disease outbreak. Furthermore, this may increase liability for injuries from vaccines in individuals whose genotype is associated with greater susceptibility to adverse reactions following vaccination. Additionally, those who are found to be at increased risk for adverse events might be exempted from mandatory vaccine laws, potentially affecting herd immunity.

More recent advances in genetic sequencing technologies present even greater challenges for law and policy development because of the rapidity with which the science is changing. As knowledge of the role of pathogen and host genomic factors in the treatment and control of infectious disease expands, evaluating the current legal framework to determine which current genetic privacy laws—both state and federal—may hinder or facilitate the ability to use genetic information to protect the health of both individuals and the general public is critical. The next sections explore some of these ELSI issues in the context of three specific examples.

Health Disparities, Inequities, and Vulnerabilities in Infectious Disease

There are significant racial and ethnic disparities in infectious disease morbidity and mortality (Callinan et al., 2013; Adekoya, 2007; Christensen et al., 2009). For example, in the United States, the burden of HIV/AIDS is highest among African American, Latino, and other racial/ethnic minorities (CDC, 2012), and case rates of tuberculosis are disproportionately high in African Americans and American Indian/Alaska Natives (Bloss et al., 2011; CDC, 2012). Racial and ethnic disparities were also evident during the 2009–2010 influenza A (H1N1) virus pandemic, when rates of H1N1-related hospitalizations, complications, and deaths disproportionally affected African Americans, people of Hispanic race/ethnicity, and American Indian/Alaska Natives (Callinan et al., 2013).

Although social determinants of health such as poverty and limited and/or delayed access to care are often the major factors contributing to these health disparities, host genotypic variation also plays a role. For example, known protective variants for HIV and HCV (CCR5Δ32 and IL28B, respectively) have a lower allele frequency in those with African ancestry (Huang et al., 1996; Duggal et al., 2013). The relative absence of this protective effect in a subgroup of the population that is already stigmatized exacerbates the health disparities in disease prevalence in the United States.

Compounding the risk of stigma for these marginalized populations is ongoing research on pathogen genomics and phylogenetic sequencing that can compromise privacy by associating particular strains of the virus with particular individuals and social networks (Rump and Woonink, 2012; Rump et al., 2013; Bubela and Yanow, 2012). In addition, HIV phylogenetic analysis has been used to identify the direction of transmission from one person to another. Although this is useful for targeting interventions, it has also resulted in criminal liability cases. This is problematic in several African countries, where behaviors associated with HIV transmission are illegal. The Ethics Working Group of the Phylogenetics and Networks for Generalized HIV Epidemics in Africa consortium (PANGEA-HIV) is working to combat the adverse consequences of collecting large samples of viral sequence data among key populations of Africa (Coltart et al., 2018; Pillay et al., 2007; Pillay et al., 2015).

Increasingly, collections of biospecimens from patient populations, study cohorts, and research trials, are being stored for potential future use (see, "Public Health Genomics, Biobanking, and Ethics," this volume). Among the areas of increasing research interest is information related to the impact of genetics on infections and the course of infectious diseases. Particular ethical challenges could arise when DNA or tissue samples from specific communities are collected and banked, particularly if those populations are already vulnerable. Research may also reveal health information about an entire group, risking discrimination and stigmatization of that group. Therefore, it is necessary to consider consequences for the group—not simply for the individual—when planning appropriate policies, best practices, and informed consent processes.

Public Health Impact of Personalizing Vaccines

Vaccine policies involve balancing considerations of individuals versus communities and will become more complex when applying genomics to infectious diseases. The nascent field of "vaccinomics"—the application of genomics to understanding individual or subpopulation variation in immunogenic responses to vaccines—could be used to apply a systems biology approach to vaccinology to assist in the elucidation of the genetic determinants and variability of immune responses to vaccines (Poland et al., 2007). The immunogenomic differences among individuals could inform policy and planning for public health vaccination programs and public health response to pandemics.

This enhanced understanding may include the assessment of the safety and effectiveness of vaccines, thereby potentially guiding future vaccine policy development (Poland, Ovsyannikova, and Jacobson, 2008). Vaccines could be targeted for those most likely to have a protective response induced by immunization, or those least likely to have adverse events. The ability to predict and quantify an individual's response to vaccination based upon immunogenomics could enhance vaccine safety by facilitating causality assessments of adverse reactions after vaccination. For example, a recent discovery points to a gene variant associated with a significantly increased risk of febrile seizure following vaccination for measles, mumps, and rubella (Feenstra et al., 2014); however, febrile seizures are rare and usually benign, raising questions about the usefulness of screening. As another example, the AS03 adjuvanted pandemic 2009 influenza A/H1N1 vaccine was associated with an increased risk of narcolepsy among children, with differences in the risk estimates for associations between different countries due, in part, to differences in the prevalence of the HLA-subtype DQB1*602 (Partinen et al., 2014). The identification of this HLA-subtype assisted causality assessment and has potential implications for vaccine development, clinical practice, and vaccination programs. In addition, research has identified genetic predictors of the immune response to several infectious diseases (Pulendran, 2009; Poland et al., 2013; Mentzer et al., 2015).

However, vaccines and genomic research are highly polarized among the public and stakeholders, including the vaccine research community, and vaccinomic science carries the potential for both positive and negative consequences (Ozdemir, Faraj, and Knoppers, 2011). The history of compulsory vaccination provides an important example of resistance to coercive public health measures, based on a range of beliefs, including religious, ethical, and libertarian objections (Colgrove, 2006; Durbach, 2004; Greenough, 1995). With advances in vaccinomic research, mandatory vaccination policies (e.g., California SB277 [2015]) may need to be reconsidered based on genetic factors that influence vaccination risk or efficacy. Identifying subpopulations at increased risk of adverse events may lead to policies *not* to immunize these subpopulations, thereby reducing community protection, assuming the vaccines would be effective in these subpopulations. Alternatively, identification of a genetic basis for an increased risk of adverse reaction to vaccination, even if the adverse reaction is extremely rare, may lead to increased vaccine refusals and could provide the anti-vaccination movement with scientific justification to promote resistance to immunization more generally. However, vaccines are only one means of preventing and controlling infectious diseases. Additional strategies are necessary, particularly during an epidemic of a highly virulent infectious disease.

Emerging Infectious Disease Epidemics

Highly virulent, infectious diseases continue to pose public health threats worldwide. The prevention and control of such diseases involve significant ELSI and policy challenges that may be influenced by genomic discoveries. For example, the 2014–2016 Ebola outbreak illustrates the enormous public health challenges surrounding a highly infectious, high-mortality disease outbreak for which there is currently no approved prevention or treatment other than supportive care. It is known that risk of transmission is high in the case of direct contact with bodily fluids of symptomatic individuals, and that in an epidemic situation, where access to adequate health care is poor, the case fatality rate among those with symptomatic infection is extremely high. People exposed to Ebola show phenotypic variability in susceptibility to infection and disease severity. Thus, it is likely that human genetic variation may contribute to individual immunity and infectivity. Additionally, it is not known who may remain infected with subclinical disease, but some early evidence suggests this may occur; therefore, the range of infectivity and virulence of Ebola is unknown (Leroy et al., 2000).

If scientists identify genetic variants that are associated with an increased likelihood of contracting Ebola, spreading it, having more severe disease, or responding to treatment, an ethical tension would arise between screening at-risk groups (patients or health care workers) for these variants and using the genomic information to influence a range of decisions. For example, in the absence of effective interventions and sufficient facilities to treat all infected patients, genetic information could be used to triage patients at greatest risk of severe disease to receive care first. Or perhaps health care workers could be screened in order to alter precautionary practices based on their genotype. These and other ethical challenges need to be considered when designing and conducting genomic research on host factors and host-pathogen interactions for acute, emerging infectious diseases.

In recognition that public health preparedness requires ethics preparedness, the Presidential Commission for the Study of Bioethical Issues created a set of policy recommendations to facilitate a proactive response to public health epidemics. The commission's report, *Ethics and Ebola* (Presidential Commission for the Study of

Bioethical Issues, 2015), articulates lessons from the US response to the epidemic in western Africa for ethics preparedness in future public health emergencies, and examines ethical dimensions of restrictive public health measures, the use of placebos for treatment and vaccine trials, and the collection and sharing of biospecimens for future research. Traditional public health response to these outbreaks, such as contact tracing, isolation, follow up, and/or quarantine, may not be contested, but how best to implement these measures is often far from clear. In addition to these traditional infection control measures, attention must be paid to the rapid development and testing of preventive and infectious disease control interventions, including the application of host and pathogen genomics, in the context of an outbreak. For example, in cases where affected individuals refuse to provide names of their contacts, pathogen genomics enables a more precise type of contact tracing, raising ethical concerns about privacy and discrimination.

Conclusion

While the science of genomics in the context of infectious disease is still in its infancy, and it is too early to identify all of the potential ELSI issues that may emerge from it, such considerations should factor into the development of policy recommendations for public health strategies to prevent and control infectious disease, both domestically and internationally (Geller et al., 2014; Pang, 2013). Attention to ELSI issues could also guide research questions and decisions about public investments in science. This would contribute to the ongoing systematic effort to provide an evidence base for the utility, priority, and ethical acceptability of genomic applications in infectious disease (Burke et al., 2010; Malogajski et al., 2013).

References

Adekoya, N. 2007. "Medicaid/State Children's Health Insurance Program Patients and Infectious Diseases Treated in Emergency Departments: US 2003." *Public Health Reports* 122(4): 513–520.

Al-Qahtani, A., Khalak, H. G., Alkuraya, F. S., Al-Hamoudy, W., Alswat, K., Balwi, M. A. A., et al. 2013. "Genome-Wide Association Study of Chronic Hepatitis B Virus Infection Reveals a Novel Candidate Risk Allele on 11q22.3." *Journal of Medical Genetics* 50(11): 725–732.

Baeten, J. M., Chohan, B., Lavreys, L., Chohan, V., McClelland, R. S., Certain, L., et al. 2007. "HIV-1 Subtype D Infection Is Associated with Faster Disease Progression Than Subtype A in Spite of Similar Plasma HIV-1 Loads." *Journal of Infectious Disease* 195(8): 1177–1180.

Barbour, J. D., Hecht, F. M., Wrin, T., Segal M. R., Ramstead, C. A., Liegler, T. J., et al. 2004. "Higher CD4+ T Cell Counts Associated with Low Viral Pol Replication Capacity among Treatment-Naive Adults in Early HIV-1 Infection." *Journal of Infectious Disease* 190(2): 251–256.

Battin, M., Francis, L., Jacobson, J., and Smith, C. 2009. "Seeing Infectious Disease as Central." In *The Patient as Victim and Vector: Ethics and Infectious Disease*, 3–13 (Oxford: Oxford Scholarship Online). http://www.oxfordscholarship.com/view/10.1093/acprof:oso/9780195335842.001.0001/acprof-9780195335842-chapter-1.

Bloss, E., Holtz, T. H., Jereb, J., Redd, J. T., Podewils, L. J., Cheek, J. E., et al. 2011. "Tuberculosis in Indigenous Peoples in the U.S., 2003–2008." *Public Health Reports* 126(5): 677–689.

Briz, V., Poveda, E., González, M. del M., Martín-Carbonero, L., González-González, R., and Soriano, V. 2008. "Impact of Antiretroviral Therapy on Viral Tropism in HIV-Infected Patients Followed Longitudinally for Over 5 Years." *Journal of Antimicrobial Chemotherapy* 61(2): 405–410.

Brusic, V., and August, J. T. 2004. "The Changing Field of Vaccine Development in the Genomics Era." *Pharmacogenomics* 5(6): 597–600.

Bubela, T., and Yanow, S. 2012 "Molecular Typing Technology: A Legal Perspective." *Public Health Ethics* 5(3): 317–320.

Bunnik, E. M., de Jong, A., Nijsingh, N., and de Wert, G. M. W. R. 2013 "The New Genetics and Informed Consent: Differentiating Choice to Preserve Autonomy." *Bioethics* 27(6): 348–355.

Buonaguro, L., Wang, E., Tornesello, M. L., Buonaguro, F. M., and Marincola, F. M. 2011. "Systems Biology Applied to Vaccine and Immunotherapy Development." *BMC Systems Biology* 5(1): 146.

Burke, W., Burton, H., Hall, A. E., Karmali, M., Khoury, M. J., Knoppers, B., et al. 2010. "Extending the Reach of Public Health Genomics: What Should Be the Agenda for Public Health in an Era of Genome-Based and 'Personalized' Medicine?" *Genetics in Medicine* 12(12): 785–791.

Callinan, L., Holman, R., Esposito, D., and McDonald, M. 2013. "Racial/Ethnic Disparities in Infectious Disease Hospitalizations in Arizona." *Journal of Health Disparities* 6(2): 50–71.

CDC (Centers for Disease Control and Prevention). 2012. "Trends in Tuberculosis—United States, 2011." *Morbidity and Mortality Weekly Report* 61(11): 181–185.

Chapman, S. J., and Hill, A. V. S. 2012. "Human Genetic Susceptibility to Infectious Disease." *Nature Reviews Genetics* 13(3): 175–188.

Christensen, K. L. Y., Holman, R. C., Steiner, C. A., Sejvar, J. J., Stoll, B. J., and Schonberger, L.B. 2009. "Infectious Disease Hospitalizations in the United States." *Clinical Infectious Diseases* 49(7): 1025–1035.

Colgrove, J. 2006. *State of Immunity: The Politics of Vaccination in Twentieth-Century America* (Berkeley: University of California Press).

Collins, F., and Varmus, H. 2015. "A New Initiative on Precision Medicine." *New England Journal of Medicine* 372: 793–795.

Coltart, C. E. M., Hoppe, A., Parker, M., Dawson, L., Amon, J. J., Simwinga, M., et al. 2018. "Ethical Considerations in HIV Phylogenetic Research. *Lancet HIV* 5(11): e656–e666

Comfort, N. 2012. *The Science of Human Perfection* (New Haven, Conn.: Yale University Press).

Dandekar, T., and Dandekar, G. 2010. "Pharmacogenomic Strategies against Microbial Resistance: From Bright to Bleak to Innovative." *Pharmacogenomics* 11(9): 1193–1196.

Dean, M., Carrington, M., Winkler, C., Huttley, G. A., Smith, M. W., Allikmets, R., et al. 1996. "Genetic Restriction of HIV-1 Infection and Progression to AIDS by a Deletion Allele of the CKR5 Structural Gene." *Science* 273(5283): 1856–1862.

Duggal, P., Thio, C. L., Wojcik, G. L., Goedert, J. J., Mangia, A., Latanich, R., et al. 2013. "Genome-Wide Association Study of Spontaneous Resolution of Hepatitis C Virus Infection: Data from Multiple Cohorts." *Annals of Internal Medicine* 158(4): 235–245.

Durbach, N. 2004. *Bodily Matters: The Anti-Vaccination Movement in England, 1853–1907* (Durham, N.C.: Duke University Press).

Eisen, J. A., and MacCullum, C. J. 2009. "Genomics of Emerging Infectious Disease: A *PLoS* Collection." *PLoS Biology* 7(10).

Fairchild, A. L., Bayer, R., and Colgrove, J. 2007. *Searching Eyes: Privacy, the State, and Disease Surveillance in America* (Berkeley: University of California Press).

Feenstra, B., Pasternak, B., Geller, F., Carstensen, L., Wang, T., Huang, F., et al. 2014. "Common Variants Associated with General and MMR Vaccine-Related Febrile Seizures." *Nature Genetics* 46(12): 1274–1282.

Ge, D., Fellay, J., Thompson, A. J., Simon, J. S., Shianna, K. V., Urban, T. J., et al. 2009. "Genetic Variation in IL28B Predicts Hepatitis C Treatment-Induced Viral Clearance." *Nature* 461(7262): 399–401.

Geller, G., Dvoskin, R., Thio, C. L., Duggal, P., Lewis, M. H., Bailey, T. C., et al. 2014. "Genomics and Infectious Disease: A Call to Identify the Ethical, Legal and Social Implications for Public Health and Clinical Practice." *Genome Medicine* 6(11): 106. https://genomemedicine.biomedcentral.com/articles/10.1186/s13073-014-0106-2.

Gerard, S., Hayes, M., and Rothstein, M. A. 2002 "On the Edge of Tomorrow: Fitting Genomics into Public Health Policy." *Journal of Law, Medicine & Ethics* 30: 173.

Gilmour, M. W., Graham, M., Reimer, A., and Van Domselaar, G. 2013. "Public Health Genomics and the New Molecular Epidemiology of Bacterial Pathogens." *Public Health Genomics* 16(1–2): 25–30.

Gire, S. K., Goba, A., Andersen, K. G., Sealfon, R. S. G., Park, D. J., Kanneh, L., et al. 2014. "Genomic Surveillance Elucidates Ebola Virus Origin and Transmission during the 2014 Outbreak." *Science* 345(6202): 1369–1372.

Gostin, L., Bayer, R., and Fairchild, A. 2003. "Ethical and Legal Challenges Posed by Severe Acute Respiratory Syndrome: Implications for the Control of Severe Infectious Disease Threats." *JAMA* 290(24): 3229–3237.

Greenough, P. 1995. "Global Immunization and Culture: Compliance and Resistance in Large-Scale Public Health Campaigns." *Social Science Medicine* 41(5): 605–607.

Hennig, B. J., Fielding, K., Broxholme, J., Diatta, M., Mendy, M., Moore, C., et al. 2008. "Host Genetic Factors and Vaccine-Induced Immunity to Hepatitis B Virus Infection." *PLoS ONE* 3(3): e1898.

Hill, A. V. S. 2001. "The Genomics and Genetics of Human Infectious Disease Susceptibility." *Annual Review of Genomics and Human Genetics* 2(1): 373–400.

Hood, L., and Flores, M. 2012. "A Personal View on Systems Medicine and the Emergence of Proactive P4 Medicine: Predictive, Preventive, Personalized and Participatory." *New Biotechnology* 29(6): 613–624.

Huang, Y., Paxton, W. A., Wolinsky, S. M., Neumann, A. U., Zhang, L., He, T., et al. 1996. "The Role of a Mutant CCR5 Allele in HIV-1 Transmission and Disease Progression." *Nature Medicine* 2(11): 1240–1243.

Hunt, P. W., Harrigan, P. R., Huang, W., Bates, M., Williamson, D. W., McCune, J. M., et al. 2006. "Prevalence of CXCR4 Tropism among Antiretroviral-Treated HIV-1–Infected Patients with Detectable Viremia." *Journal of Infectious Diseases* 194(7): 926–930.

Jameson, J. L., and Longo, D. L. 2015. "Precision Medicine—Personalized, Problematic, and Promising." *New England Journal of Medicine* 372(23): 2229–2234.

Jiang, D.-K., Sun, J., Cao, G., Liu, Y., Lin, D., Gao, Y.-Z., et al. 2013. "Genetic Variants in STAT4 and HLA-DQ Genes Confer Risk of Hepatitis B Virus-Related Hepatocellular Carcinoma." *Nature Genetics* 45(1): 72–75.

Jilg, N., and Chung, R. T. 2013. "One More Piece in the Interleukin 28B Gene Puzzle? The Case of Hepatitis B." *Hepatology* 57(3): 870–872.

Kaslow, R. A., McNicholl, J., and Hill, A. V. S., eds. 2008. *Genetic Susceptibility to Infectious Diseases* (New York: Oxford University Press).

Kaye, J. 2012. "The Tension between Data Sharing and the Protection of Privacy in Genomics Research." *Annual Review of Genomics and Human Genetics* 13: 415–431.

Keynan, Y., Malik, S., and Fowke, K. R. 2013. "The Role of Polymorphisms in Host Immune Genes in Determining the Severity of Respiratory Illness Caused By Pandemic H1N1 Influenza." *Public Health Genomics* 16(1–2): 9–16.

Khoury, M. J., Gwinn, M. L., Glasgow, R. E., and Kramer, B. S. 2012. "A Population Approach to Precision Medicine." *American Journal of Preventative Medicine* 42(6): 639–645.

Kirk, G. D., Turner, P. C., Gong, Y., Lesi, O. A., Mendy, M., Goedert, J. J., et al. 2005. "Hepatocellular Carcinoma and Polymorphisms in Carcinogen-Metabolizing and DNA Repair Enzymes in a Population with Aflatoxin Exposure and Hepatitis B Virus Endemicity." *Cancer Epidemiology Biomarkers and Prevention* 14(2): 373–379.

Kiwanuka, N., Laeyendecker, O., Robb, M., Kigozi, G., Arroyo, M., McCutchan, F., et al. 2008. "Effect of Human Immunodeficiency Virus Type 1 (HIV-1) Subtype on Disease Progression in Persons From Rakai, Uganda, with Incident HIV-1 Infection." *Journal of Infectious Diseases* 197(5): 707–713.

Kiwanuka, N., Robb, M., Laeyendecker, O., Kigozi, G., Wabwire-Mangen, F., Makumbi, F. E., et al. 2010. "HIV-1 Viral Subtype Differences in the Rate of CD4+ T-cell Decline among HIV Seroincident Antiretroviral Naive Persons in Rakai District, Uganda." *JAIDS: Journal of Acquired Immune Deficiency Syndromes* 4(2): 180–184.

Knoppers, B. M., Zawati, M. H., and Kirby, E. S. 2012. "Sampling Populations of Humans across the World: ELSI Issues." *Annual Review of Genomics and Human Genetics* 13: 395–413.

Leroy, E., Baize, S., Volchkov, V., Fisher-Hoch, S., Georges-Courbot, M.-C., Lansoud-Soukate, J., et al. 2000. "Human Asymptomatic Ebola Infection and Strong Inflammatory Response." *Lancet* 355(9222): 2210–2215.

Liang, B., Guo, Y., Li, Y., and Kong, H. 2014. "Association between IL-10 Gene Polymorphisms and Susceptibility of Tuberculosis: Evidence Based on a Meta-Analysis." *PLoS ONE* 9(2): e88448.

Liu, L., Li, J., Yao, J., Yu, J., Zhang, J., Ning, Q., et al. 2011. "A Genome-Wide Association Study with DNA Pooling Identifies the Variant rs11866328 in the GRIN2A Gene That Affects Disease Progression of Chronic HBV Infection." *Viral Immunology* 24(5): 397–402.

Livingstone, F. B. 1964. "Aspects of the Population Dynamics of the Abnormal Hemoglobin and Glucose-6-Phosphate Dehydrogenase Deficiency Genes." *American Journal of Human Genetics* 16(4): 435–450.

Malik, S. 2013. "Genomics Research: The Underpinning of Infectious Disease Prevention and Control Strategies." *Public Health Genomics* 16(1–2): 3.

Malogajski, J., Brankovic, I., Verweij, S. P., Ambrosino, E., van Agtmael, M. A., Brand, A., et al. 2013. "Translational Potential into Health Care of Basic Genomic and Genetic Findings for Human Immunodeficiency Virus, Chlamydia Trachomatis, and Human Papilloma Virus." *BioMed Research International* 2013: e892106.

Mann, D., Carrington, M., O'Donnell, M., Miller, T., and Goedert, J. 1992. "HLA Phenotype Is a Factor in Determining Rate of Disease Progression and Outcome In HIV-1-Infected Individuals." *AIDS Research and Human Retroviruses* 8(8): 1345–1346.

Mbarek, H., Ochi, H., Urabe, Y., Kumar, V., Kubo, M., Hosono, N., et al. 2011. "A Genome-Wide Association Study of Chronic Hepatitis B Identified Novel Risk Locus in a Japanese Population." *Human Molecular Genetics* 20(19): 3884–3892.

McEwen, J. E., Boyer, J. T., Sun, K. Y., Rothenberg, K. H., Lockhart, N. C., and Guyer, M. S. 2014. "The Ethical, Legal, and Social Implications Program of the national Human Genome Research Institute: Reflections on an Ongoing Experiment." *Annual Review of Genomics and Human Genetics* 15(1): 481–505.

McGuire, A. L., Basford, M., Dressler, L. G., Fullerton, S. M., Koenig, B. A., Li, R., et al. 2011. "Ethical and Practical Challenges of Sharing Data from Genome-Wide Association Studies: The eMERGE Consortium Experience." *Genome Research* 21(7): 1001–1007.

McGuire, A. L., and Beskow, L. M. 2010. "Informed Consent in Genomics and Genetic Research." *Annual Review of Genomics and Human Genetics* 11: 361–381.

Meltzer, L. A. 2006. "Undesirable Implications of Disclosing Individual Genetic Results to Research Participants." *American Journal of Bioethics* 6(6): 28–30.

Mentzer, A. J., O'Connor, D., Pollard, A. J., and Hill, A. V. S. 2015. "Searching for the Human Genetic Factors Standing in the Way of Universally Effective Vaccines." *Philosophical Transactions of the Royal Society B* 370: 20140341.

Mira, M. T., Alcaïs, A., Nguyen, V. T., Moraes, M. O., Di Flumeri, C., Vu, H. T., et al. 2004. "Susceptibility to Leprosy is Associated with PARK2 and PACRG." *Nature* 427(6975): 636–640.

Mooney, G. 2015. *Intrusive Interventions: Public Health, Domestic Space, and Infectious Disease Surveillance in England, 1840–1914* (Rochester, N.Y.: University of Rochester Press).

Nohynek, H., Jokinen, J., Partinen, M., Vaarala, O., Kirjavainen, T., Sundman, J., et al. 2012. "AS03 Adjuvanted AH1N1 Vaccine Associated with an Abrupt Increase in the Incidence of Childhood Narcolepsy in Finland." *PLoS ONE* 7(3): e33536.

OECD (Organisation for Economic Co-operation and Development). 2013. "Public Health in an Age of Genomics." OECD Science, Technology and Industry Policy Paper No. 8 (Paris: OECD Publishing). https://www.oecd-ilibrary.org/science-and-technology/public-health-in-an-age-of-genomics_5k424rdzj3bx-en.

Omenn, G. S. 2000. "Public Health Genetics: An Emerging Interdisciplinary Field for the Post-genomic Era." *Annual Review of Genomics and Human Genetics* 21(1): 1–13.

Ovsyannikova, I. G., Jacobson, R. M., and Poland, G. A. 2004. "Variation in Vaccine Response in Normal Populations." *Pharmacogenomics* 5(4): 417–427.

Ozdemir, V., Faraj, S. A., and Knoppers, B. M. 2011. "Steering Vaccinomics Innovations with Anticipatory Governance and Participatory Foresight." *OMICS: A Journal of Integrative Biology* 15(9): 637–646.

Ozdemir, V., Pang, T., Knoppers, B. M., Avard, D., Faraj, S. A., Zawati, M. H., et al. 2011. "Vaccines of the 21st Century and Vaccinomics: Data-Enabled Science Meets Global Health to Spark Collective Action for Vaccine Innovation." *OMICS: A Journal of Integrative Biology* 15(9): 523–527.

Pan, L., Zhang, L., Zhang, W., Wu, X., Li, Y., Yan, B., et al. 2014. "A Genome-Wide Association Study Identifies Polymorphisms in the HLA-DR Region Associated with Non-response to Hepatitis B Vaccination in Chinese Han Populations." *Human Molecular Genetics* 23(8): 2210–2219.

Pang, T. 2002. "The Impact of Genomics on Global Health." *American Journal of Public Health* 92(7): 1077–1079.

Pang, T. 2013. "Genomics for Public Health Improvement: Relevant International Ethical and Policy Issues around Genome-Wide Association Studies and Biobanks." *Public Health Genomics* 16(1–2): 69–72.

Partinen, M., Kornum, B. R., Plazzi, G., Jennum, P., Julkunen, I., and Vaarala, O. 2014. "Narcolepsy as an Autoimmune Disease: The Role of H1N1 Infection and Vaccination." *Lancet Neurology* 13(6): 600–613.

Pashayan, N., Hall, A., Chowdhury, S., Dent, T., Pharoah, P. D. P., and Burton, H. 2013. "Public Health Genomics and Personalized Prevention: Lessons from the COGS Project." *Journal of Internal Medicine* 274(5): 451–456.

Petrizzo, A., Tornesello, M., Buonaguro, F. M., and Buonaguro, L. 2012. "Immunogenomics Approaches for Vaccine Evaluation." *Journal of Immunotoxicology* 9(3): 236–240.

Luheshi, L., Raza, S., Moorthie, S., Hall, A., Blackburn, L., Rands, C., et al. 2015. *Pathogen Genomics into Practice*. PHG Foundation Report. http://www.phgfoundation.org/report/pathogen-genomics-into-practice.

Pillay, D., Herbeck, J., Cohen, M. S., de Oliveira, T., Fraser, C., Ratmann, O., et al. 2015. "The PANGEA-HIV Consortium: Phylogenetics and Networks for Generalised HIV Epidemics in Africa." *Lancet Infectious Diseases* 15(3): 259–261.

Pillay, D., Rambaut, A., Geretti, A. M., and Brown, A. J. 2007. "HIV Phylogenetics." *BMJ: British Medical Journal* 335(7618): 460–461.

Pinxten, W., and Howard, H. C. 2014. "Ethical Issues Raised by Whole Genome Sequencing." *Best Practice and Research Clinical Gastroenterology* 28(2): 269–279.

Pittman, K. J., Glover, L. C., Wang, L., and Ko, D. C. 2016. "The Legacy of Past Pandemics: Common Human Mutations That Protect against Infectious Disease." *PLoS Pathogens* 12(7): e1005680.

Png, E., Thalamuthu, A., Ong, R. T. H., Snippe, H., Boland, G. J., and Seielstad, M. 2011. "A Genome-Wide Association Study of Hepatitis B Vaccine Response in an Indonesian Population Reveals Multiple Independent Risk Variants in the HLA Region." *Human Molecular Genetics* 20(19): 3893–3898.

Poland, G. A., Kennedy, R. B., McKinney, B. A., Ovsyannikova, I. G., Lambert, N. D., Jacobson, R. M., et al. 2013. "Vaccinomics, Adversomics, and the Immune Response Network Theory: Individualized Vaccinology in the 21st Century." *Seminars in Immunology* 25(2): 89–103.

Poland, G. A., Ovsyannikova, I. G., and Jacobson, R. M. 2008. "Personalized Vaccines: The Emerging Field of Vaccinomics." *Expert Opinion on Biological Therapy* 8(11): 1659–1667.

Poland, G. A., Ovsyannikova, I. G., Jacobson, R. M., and Smith, D. I. 2007. "Heterogeneity in Vaccine Immune Response: The Role of Immunogenetics and the Emerging Field of Vaccinomics." *Clinical Pharmacology and Therapeutics* 82(6): 653–664.

Presidential Commission for the Study of Bioethical Issues. 2015. *Ethics and Ebola: Public Health Planning and Response*. https://bioethicsarchive.georgetown.edu/pcsbi/sites/default/files/Ethics-and-Ebola_PCSBI_508.pdf.

Pulendran, B. 2009. "Learning Immunology from the Yellow Fever Vaccine: Innate Immunity to Systems Vaccinology." *Nature Reviews Immunology* 9(10): 741–774.

Reegan, A. D., Ceasar, S. A., Paulraj, M. G., Ignacimuthu, S., and Al-Dhabi, N. A. 2017. "Current Status of Genome Editing in Vector Mosquitoes: A Review." *Bioscience Trends* 10(6): 424–432.

Roca, I., Akova, M., Baquero, F., Carlet, J., Cavaleri, M., Coenen, S., et al. 2015. "The Global Threat of Antimicrobial Resistance: Science for Intervention." *New Microbes and New Infections* 6: 22–29.

Ross, L. F., Rothstein, M. A., and Clayton, E. W. 2013. "Premature Guidance about Whole-Genome Sequencing." *Personalized Medicine* 10(6): 523–526.

Rotimi, C. N., and Marshall, P. A. 2010. "Tailoring the Process of Informed Consent in Genetic and Genomic Research." *Genome Medicine* 2(3): 20.

Rump, B., Cornelis, C., Woonink, F., and Verweij, M. 2013. "The Need for Ethical Reflection on the Use of Molecular Microbial Characterization in Outbreak Management." *Eurosurveillance* 18(4): 20384.

Rump, B. O., and Woonink, F. 2012. "Ethical Questions Concerning the Use of Molecular Typing Techniques in the Control of Infectious Diseases." *Public Health Ethics* 5(3): 311–313.

Sonneveld, M. J., Wong, V. W.-S., Woltman, A. M., Wong, G. L. H., Cakaloglu, Y., Zeuzem, S., et al. 2012. "Polymorphisms Near IL28B and Serologic Response to Peginterferon in HBeAg-positive Patients with Chronic Hepatitis B." *Gastroenterology* 142(3): 513–520.e1.

Srivastava, B., Błażejewska, P., Heßmann, M., Bruder, D., Geffers, R., Mauel, S., et al. 2009. "Host Genetic Background Strongly Influences the Response to Influenza A Virus Infections." *PLoS ONE* 4(3): e4857.

Tabor, H. K., Berkman, B. E., Hull, S. C., and Bamshad, M. J. 2011. "Genomics Really Gets Personal: How Exome and Whole Genome Sequencing Challenge the Ethical Framework of Human Genetics Research." *American Journal of Medical Genetics Part A* 155(12): 2916–2924.

Telenti, A. 2004. "The Genetic Cohorts: Facing the New Challenges in Infectious Diseases—the HIV Model." *Enfermedades Infecciosas y Microbiología Clínica* 22(6): 337–341.

Thomas, D. L., Thio, C. L., Martin, M. P., Qi, Y., Ge, D., O'Huigin, C., et al. 2009. "Genetic Variation in IL28B and Spontaneous Clearance of Hepatitis C Virus." *Nature* 461(7265): 798–801.

Trautmann, L., and Sekaly, R.-P. 2011. "Solving Vaccine Mysteries: A Systems Biology Perspective." *Nature Immunology* 12(8): 729–731.

Vogel, G. 2014. "Genomes Reveal Start of Ebola Outbreak." *Science* 345(6200): 989–990.

White House. 2017. "The Precision Medicine Initiative, 2016." https://obamawhitehouse.archives.gov/node/333101.

Withrock, I. C., Anderson, S. J., Jefferson, M. A., McCormack, G. R., Mlynarczyk, G. S. A., Nakama, A., et al. 2015. "Genetic Diseases Conferring Resistance to Infectious Diseases." *Genes and Diseases* 2(3): 247–254.

Wolf, S. M. 2013. "Return of Individual Research Results and Incidental Findings: Facing the Challenges of Translational Science." *Annual Review of Genomics and Human Genetics* 14(1): 557–577.

Wolf, S. M., Crock, B. N., Van Ness, B., Lawrenz, F., Kahn, J. P., Beskow, L. M., et al. 2012. "Managing Incidental Findings and Research Results in Genomic Research Involving Biobanks and Archived Data Sets." *Genetics in Medicine* 14(4): 361–384.

Wolf, S. M., Lawrenz, F. P., Nelson, C. A., Kahn, J. P., Cho, M. K., Clayton, E. W., et al. 2008. "Managing Incidental Findings in Human Subjects Research: Analysis and Recommendations." *Journal of Law, Medicine & Ethics* 36(2): 219–248.

WHO (World Health Organization). 2012. "World Health Statistics 2012." http://www.who.int/gho/publications/world_health_statistics/EN_WHS2012_Full.pdf.

Yan, Q., ed. 2010. "Immuno-Informatics and Systems Biology Methods for Personalized Medicine." In *Systems Biology in Drug Discovery and Development, Methods and Protocols*, 203–220. Methods in Molecular Biology 637 (Totowa, N.J.: Humana Press).

Yang, X., Yang, H., Zhou, G., and Zhao, G.-P. 2008. "Infectious Disease in the Genomic Era." *Annual Review of Genomics and Human Genetics* 9(1): 21–48.

Yeh, S. H., Wang, H. Y., Tsai, C. Y., Kao, C. L., Yang, J. Y., Liu, H. W., et al. 2004. "Characterization of Severe Acute Respiratory Syndrome Coronavirus Genomes in Taiwan: Molecular Epidemiology and Genome Evolution." *Proceedings of the National Academy of Sciences* 101(8): 2542–2547.

Zeng, Z. 2014. "Human Genes Involved in Hepatitis B Virus Infection. *World Journal of Gastroenterology* 20(24): 7696–7706.

Zhang, H., Zhai, Y., Hu, Z., Wu, C., Qian, J., Jia, W., et al. 2010. "Genome-Wide Association Study Identifies 1p36.22 as a New Susceptibility Locus for Hepatocellular Carcinoma in Chronic Hepatitis B Virus Carriers." *Nature Genetics* 42(9): 755–758.

SECTION THIRTEEN

ENVIRONMENTAL HEALTH

CHAPTER 59

AN OVERVIEW OF ETHICS AND ENVIRONMENTAL HEALTH

DAVID B. RESNIK

INTRODUCTION

WE often think that protecting the environment and promoting public health go hand-in-hand, and we are usually correct in this assumption. For example, reducing water pollution not only benefits human health, but it also benefits fish and other forms of aquatic life living in streams, rivers, and lakes. Proper disposal of hazardous waste protects people and nonhuman species from harm. However, environmental protection and public health promotion sometimes conflict (Resnik, 2009). For example, building a dam may help to promote public health by ensuring that people have an adequate supply of water for drinking, sanitation, and agriculture. But the dam may damage ecosystems and habitats and threaten various species. Clearing land to build a new hospital may benefit public health by providing residents with access to medical care, but it may also harm the environment by contributing to deforestation. Moreover, the hospital itself may consume a great deal of energy and generate waste, both of which may adversely impact the environment. Pesticides used in agriculture and mosquito control can promote public health by helping to provide food for the world's growing population, but they also pose risks to human health and nonhuman species.

The moral dilemmas related to environmental health ethics go beyond conflicts involving public health and protection of species, habitats, or ecosystems. Other values at stake may include respect for autonomy and human rights, social justice, economic development, animal welfare, sustainability, and obligations to future generations (Resnik, 2012). For example, a new domestic waste disposal center located in a rural part of a county may benefit the whole community at the expense of those living near the center, who may face increased health risks. Enhanced air quality standards may promote public health and protect the environment but also slow economic development. Zoning regulations that attempt to control urban sprawl to facilitate walking and biking can promote public health but interfere with property rights. Zoning regulations that prevent people from building in areas prone to flooding (to minimize the human toll of natural disasters) may also interfere with property rights. Policies designed to protect fetuses from exposures to toxic chemicals may discriminate against women and violate their right to work. A building code that sets high safety standards may protect public health but also make housing unaffordable. Population control policies may help societies control the adverse environmental and public health effects of development and growth but also threaten reproductive rights. Climate change policies raise issues of global justice, because various nations (and communities within nations) may face different economic, social, and health impacts of climate change and bear differential responsibility for causing climate change.

Environmental health ethics lies at the intersection of several different disciplines, including public health ethics, environmental ethics, biomedical ethics, business ethics, and environmental law. It draws on ethical concepts, principles, and theories from these different areas and makes use of facts and empirical data from various scientific disciplines, including toxicology, exposure biology, ecology, climatology, hydrology, medicine, epidemiology, public health, occupational health, and economics (Frumkin, 2010; Resnik, 2012). Environmental health ethics issues range from local concerns, such as waste management and urban development, to national ones, such as air and water quality, to global concerns, such as climate change. Environmental health ethics topics (some of which overlap) include:

- **Regulation of Toxic Substances:** Issues pertaining to the regulation of pesticides and industrial chemicals.
- **Air and Water Pollution:** Issues related to establishing standards for air and water quality.
- **Water Use:** Issues related to water rights and allocating water among different users.
- **Waste Management:** Issues related to managing domestic, agricultural, construction, hazardous, radioactive, medical, sewage, and electronic waste.
- **Agriculture:** Issues related to the use of pesticides, chemical fertilizers, genetically modified (GM) crops, and antibiotics in agriculture.
- **Transgenic Organisms:** Issues related to creating GM organisms for use in agriculture, medicine, and industry.
- **Vector-Borne and Zoonotic Diseases:** Issues related to controlling or preventing diseases carried by mosquitoes, birds, ticks, pigs, and other nonhuman vectors.
- **Antibiotic Use:** Issues related to the proper use of antibiotics in medicine and agriculture to prevent antibiotic resistance.
- **Food Safety:** Issues related to promoting health and safety in food manufacturing, preparation, marketing, and consumption.

- **The Built Environment:** Issues related to environmental and health risks pertaining to structures used for living and working, such as houses, schools, roads, dams, bridges, and cities.
- **Occupational Health:** Issues related to managing health risks at work.
- **Disaster Management:** Issues related to preparing for and responding to natural disasters, such as hurricanes, floods, tornadoes, fires, and earthquakes.
- **Energy Production and Use:** Issues related to acquiring and using different forms of energy, such as coal, oil, natural gas, biofuels, wind energy, and nuclear, solar, and hydroelectric power.
- **Climate Change:** Issues pertaining to minimizing humanity's role in causing global warming and mitigating the effects of climate change on human health and environment.
- **Population Control:** Issues pertaining to controlling population growth, which has widespread impacts on health and the environment.
- **Precaution:** Issues related to taking precautionary measures to prevent harm to public health and the environment in the face of uncertain scientific evidence.
- **Environmental Justice:** Issues related to the distribution of health risks among different human populations living or working in the environment.
- **Environmental Research Ethics:** Issues related to the ethical conduct of environmental health research, such as the ethics of research with human or animal subjects, research integrity (e.g., misconduct, authorship, peer review, conflict of interest), and social responsibility.

Many of these issues overlap and are addressed in chapters in the Environmental Health section of *The Oxford Handbook of Public Health Ethics*, and some are dealt with in chapters in other sections of this volume.

While the notion that environmental health ethics should constitute a field of study in its own right is relatively new, many of the issues that fall within its purview have been discussed for some time (Potter, 1971; Shrader-Frechette, 1991, 2002, 2011; Cranor, 1997, 2011; Pierce and Jameton, 2001; Elliott, 2011; Brown, 2012). Over forty years ago, the scholar credited with first coining the term *bioethics*, Van Rensselaer Potter (1971), conceived of bioethics as fundamentally concerned with environmental issues. Potter argued that medicine and health care should incorporate ecological concepts, and that bioethics should involve a global integration of biology and human values (Whitehouse, 2003). Potter's approach to bioethics soon lost favor, however, as bioethicists began focusing on issues in medical practice and research, such as end-of-life decisions, informed consent, medical paternalism, assisted reproduction, allocation of scarce medical resources, clinical trials, human genetics, confidentiality, and research with vulnerable populations (Whitehouse, 2003). Scholars who focused on environmental issues formed their own discipline (i.e., environmental ethics) and tended to focus on topics not directly related to health care, such as agriculture, sustainability, animal welfare, climate change, and obligations to future generations. Some have suggested that bioethicists should bridge the gap between medical and environmental ethics and reincorporate Potter's vision (Whitehouse, 2003). Renewed interest in environmental and global bioethics reflects this philosophical outlook (Dwyer, 2009; Resnik, 2009).

The methods used to make ethical decisions pertaining to environmental health are similar to those used in other practical ethics disciplines. To make an ethical decision pertaining to environmental health policy or practice, one should strike a reasonable balance among competing values, principles, or interests in light of the relevant facts and information and available options (Kass, 2001; Beauchamp and Childress, 2012; Resnik, 2012). Public policy should include input from various stakeholders, such as government officials, business leaders, and environmental and public health groups, as well as the general public and uniquely impacted communities. Public policy decisions are often made by government agencies and officials who may be influenced by powerful business interests or political organizations. To ensure that environmental health decision-making is fair, publicly accountable, and inclusive, efforts should be made to include populations that lack political or economic power and influence in decision-making (Shrader-Frechette, 2002). Decision-making approaches involving democratic deliberation in open forums can help promote participation of these populations.

Overview of Section Chapters

The five chapters in this section of *The Oxford Handbook of Public Health Ethics* address several important topics in environmental health ethics. In "Industrial Chemicals, Pesticides, Public Health, and Ethics," Elise M. R. Smith and Mark F. Miller address the ethical issues raised by exposures to chemicals and pesticides, including conflicts between public health and the agriculture industry, public health and social justice, and public health and environmental protections. In "Occupational Health and the Built Environment: Ethical Issues," David B. Resnik examines the ethical issues related to health risks people encounter in environments in which they live and work, including property rights, worker rights, environmental justice, economic development, and access to affordable housing. In "Environmental Justice, Ethics, and Public Health," James Dwyer describes how environmental exposures raise issues of justice, explores different approaches to environmental justice, and considers our moral duties to promote environmental justice. In "Energy, Emissions, and Public Health Ethics," Cheryl C. Macpherson considers the ethical issues raised by climate change, including environmental protection versus economic development, national and international justice, and moral responsibility. Lastly, in "Environmental Health Research and Ethics," David B. Resnik considers some of the key ethical issues that arise in environmental health research involving human subjects, including returning individualized research results, protecting privacy and confidentiality, research on environmental interventions, intentional exposure studies, and protecting vulnerable human subjects. Together, the chapters in this section of the *Oxford Handbook* provide the reader with a useful introduction to some of the ethical and policy dilemmas that arise at the intersection of public health and the environment.

Acknowledgments

This research was supported by the Intramural Program of the National Institute of Environmental Health Sciences (NIEHS), National Institutes of Health (NIH). It does not represent the view of the NIEHS, NIH, or US government.

References

Beauchamp, T., and Childress, J. 2012. *Principles of Biomedical Ethics*. 7th ed. (New York: Oxford University Press).

Brown, D. A. 2012. *Climate Change Ethics: Navigating the Perfect Moral Storm* (New York: Routledge).

Cranor, C. 1997. *Regulating Toxic Substances: A Philosophy of Science and the Law* (New York: Oxford University Press).

Cranor, C. 2011. *Legally Poisoned: How the Law Puts Us at Risk for Toxicants* (Cambridge, Mass.: Harvard University Press).

Dwyer, J. 2009. "How to Connect Bioethics and Environmental Ethics: Health, Sustainability, and Justice." *Bioethics* 23(9): 497–502.

Elliott, K. C. 2011. *Is a Little Pollution Good for You? Incorporating Societal Values in Environmental Research* (New York: Oxford University Press).

Frumkin, H., ed. 2010. *Environmental Health: From Global to Local*. 2nd ed. (New York: John Wiley & Sons).

Kass, N. E. 2001. "An Ethics Framework for Public Health." *American Journal of Public Health* 91(11): 1776–1782.

Pierce, J., and Jameton, A. 2001. *The Ethics of Environmentally Responsible Health Care* (New York: Oxford University Press).

Potter, V. R. 1971. *Bioethics: Bridge to the Future* (Englewood Cliffs, N.J.: Prentice-Hall).

Resnik, D. B. 2009. "Human Health and the Environment: In Harmony or in Conflict?" *Health Care Analysis* 17(3): 261–276.

Resnik, D. B. 2012. *Environmental Health Ethics* (Cambridge: Cambridge University Press).

Shrader-Frechette, K. S. 1991. *Risk and Rationality: Philosophical Foundations for Populist Reforms* (Berkeley: University of California Press).

Shrader-Frechette, K. S. 2002. *Environmental Justice: Creating Equity, Reclaiming Democracy* (New York: Oxford University Press).

Shrader-Frechette, K. S. 2011. *Taking Action, Saving Lives: Our Duties to Protect Environmental and Public Health* (New York: Oxford University Press).

Whitehouse, P. J. 2003. "The Rebirth of Bioethics: Extending the Original Formulations of Van Rensselaer Potter." *American Journal of Bioethics* 3(4): W26–W31.

CHAPTER 60

INDUSTRIAL CHEMICALS, PESTICIDES, PUBLIC HEALTH, AND ETHICS

ELISE M. R. SMITH AND MARK F. MILLER

Introduction

Chemical development and material science have revolutionized agriculture, medicine, commerce, transportation, hygiene, and nearly every other aspect of human life. They have advanced research and innovation, contributed to economic growth, and allowed longer high-quality lives for many individuals. However, there is increasing evidence that many industrial chemicals, including those found in consumer products, may adversely impact public health and environmental health. For example, coal burning, waste incineration, pesticide applications, and chlorine bleaching of paper and pulp create byproducts, known as dioxins, that continuously enter ecosystems, bioaccumulate in food chains, and negatively impact health by increasing risks related to cancer, thyroid disorders, immune deficiencies, cardiovascular events, diabetes, reproductive issues, and developmental disorders (Steenland et al., 1999; Schecter et al., 2006).

When chemicals are used in industrial processes or consumer products, they do not always remain in the intended location or substrate, leading to unintended exposures and the potential for adverse effects on public health. Limiting our exposure to industrial chemicals can be challenging, because they are ubiquitous within our environment. These substances are found not just in the air we breathe and the water we drink, but also in our food, drugs, cosmetics, detergents, personal care products, building materials, and solvents—to name but a few examples. No matter how cautious we may be in our personal decision-making, there is often "nowhere to hide" from toxicants (Cranor, 2011a, 16).

This chapter will consider ethical concerns related to public health and the development and use of industrial chemicals; it examines various regulatory approaches, including evidence-based decision-making, risk analysis, a precautionary approach, and international consensus. Also, the chapter will assess specific ethics issues, including food production and pesticides, the influence of economic stability and profit derived from industrial chemicals, conflicts between public health priorities and environmental protections, and health inequities related to the use of industrial chemicals.

Background

Accurately determining the extent to which a chemical poses a health risk to human populations is complicated. Typically, the health risk associated with a chemical derives from a combination of its potential to do harm (the hazard) and the likelihood of and amount of it reaching a biological target (the exposure). Hazards derive from the ability of a chemical to have a specific adverse effect, depicted with dose-response curves. In most cases, the response is proportional to the dose: higher doses produce greater toxicity than lower doses. Adverse effects are then dependent on the amount of chemical exposure, but they are also influenced by exposure route, duration, timing, and individual susceptibilities (e.g., genetics, sex, co-exposures, age). By understanding the dose-response relationship, scientists can identify a No-Observed-Adverse-Effect-Level (NOAEL) for a given chemical. Based on a combined understanding of hazard and exposure, scientists have also developed the concept of a threshold for toxicological concern using linear extrapolation, below which there would be no appreciable risk to human health (Kroes, Kleiner, and Renwick, 2005). Using this threshold, risk assessors and risk managers can incorporate safety factors to set reference doses (RfDs) (i.e., estimates of daily exposure that are assumed to be without adverse health impacts on humans).

While traditional risk assessment methods have proven appropriate for most chemicals with adequate toxicological information, the assumptions of dose-response proportionality and thresholds for response have both come under increased debate in the scientific community for some specific applications (Vandenberg et al., 2012). Endocrine-disrupting chemicals—commonly found in plasticizers and pesticides (e.g., Bisphenol A, DDT)—have been reported to have adverse effects at low levels that are not observed at higher levels (i.e., non-monotonicity). This is of great concern because RfDs based on high-level testing would not necessarily be protective for low-dose exposures. Further, evidence from cancer studies indicates that carcinogens may not have a threshold level within the environmentally relevant range (Asante-Duah, 2017), because even a minute amount of these substances in the body can increase the risk of cancer or mutations that lead to cancer. Known carcinogens include alcoholic beverage consumption, wood dust, benzene, formaldehyde, nickel compounds, solar radiation, and trichloroethylene found in industrial solvents.

Similar to carcinogens, it has also been postulated that there is no safe threshold for certain neurotoxicants. Exposure to neurotoxicants causes neurodevelopmental and neurodegenerative disorders and subclinical brain dysfunction; this may include autism, attention deficit disorder, or cerebral palsy. As an example, it is now widely recognized that lead can cause adverse neurologic effects at exposure levels that only a decade ago were thought to be safe (Caito and Aschner, 2017). Indeed, current research suggests that there may not be a threshold for lead under which adverse effects are not seen. Similarly, as we develop better tools to measure low-level exposures and subtle effects of arsenic, scientists are similarly beginning to question whether there is any safe level of arsenic exposure (Wasserman et al., 2014). As an alternative to the ongoing low-dose extrapolation debate, it may be more useful to focus on avoidable and unavoidable exposure through biomonitoring and promoting levels of toxicants that are "as low as reasonably achievable" (Neumann, 2009, 459).

The use of industrial chemicals has also substantially modified the environmental ecosystem. One of the most problematic issues is the bioaccumulation of chemicals in the environment, especially persistent organic pollutants (POPs). POPs can be found in many synthetic compounds created for pest control (e.g., DDT), industrial applications such as electrical transformers and additives to paints and lubricants (e.g., PCBs), and stain-resistant consumer goods (e.g., PFAS). Because of their durable chemical structures, POPs do not readily degrade within organisms or in the environment and may bioaccumulate in the fatty tissue of humans and wildlife. As a result, they may have harmful impacts on human health and population health. Exposure to POPs has been associated with significant health issues, including certain cancers, reductions in immune response, impaired reproduction, and severe developmental malformations (UNEP, 2009). Further, because POPs are distributed globally, no single government acting alone can protect its citizens or its environment from the risks related to POPs (Adeola, 2004; Carpenter, 2011).

Regulation of Industrial Chemicals

To protect public and environmental health, the US government has enacted numerous laws to govern the production, use, sale, exposure, and disposal of potentially hazardous chemicals. Specific federal laws exist for (1) food and drugs, (2) pesticides, and (3) toxic chemicals. The Federal Food, Drug, and Cosmetic Act (FFDCA) and other laws provide the Food and Drug Administration (FDA) with broad authority to regulate many food products, dietary supplements, food additives, infant formula, prescription and nonprescription drugs, vaccines, medical devices, cosmetics, veterinary feed and drugs, and tobacco products. Complimentary to the FDA efforts, the Environmental Protection Agency (EPA) sets tolerance levels for pesticides in food or as residue on food for human consumption as well as in animal feed (21 U.S.C. § 301).

The Federal Insecticide, Fungicide, and Rodenticide Act (FIFRA) (7 U.S.C. §§ 136–136y) is the primary statute regulating pesticides in the United States, with the goal of protecting applicators, consumers, and the environment. In 1972 FIFRA was significantly revised and strengthened to place the primary burden of proof for safety on pesticide manufacturers; applicants must show that pesticides "will not cause any unreasonable adverse effects on the environment," including any risks to human health and environmental health (7 U.S.C. §§ 136–136y). Animal studies seek to determine the dose at which the chemical has NOAEL; post-market reviews may change or revoke registration if adverse effects are discovered. As part of the premarket registration, the EPA determines allowable uses and dosages based on mechanistic and animal studies submitted by companies, and the application of safety factors to ensure public health protection for vulnerable populations. The Food Quality Protection Act (1996) added more significant protections for infants and children by lowering acceptable levels of toxic chemicals in food residue (codified at 21 U.S.C. § 346(a)). States may also enact additional laws should they opt for stricter controls than those provided federally.

Apart from food, drugs, cosmetics, and pesticides, nearly all other chemicals are regulated under the Toxic Substances Control Act (TSCA), first passed in 1976 and amended in 2016 (15 U.S.C. § 2601 et seq. [1976]).[1] Current TSCA regulations require manufacturers to send premanufacture notification. New toxic chemicals must be registered and may require testing if exposure poses danger or raises concerns. The regulations explicitly require the protection of vulnerable populations (e.g., children, pregnant women), enhance authority to require manufacturer testing for new and existing chemicals, and increase transparency of toxicity data. The present TSCA inventory includes more than 83,000 chemicals, but an early evaluation by EPA estimates only 35,000 in current active usage. To regulate the use of a chemical under TSCA, the EPA must show that scientific evidence supports a finding of "unreasonable risk." While the current iteration of the TSCA provides EPA with authority to conduct chemical evaluations during the registration period (ninety-day review process during premarketing) and supports review and regulation efforts through the collection of listing fees, some scientists believe that there are simply too many chemicals to review, given the resources available to the EPA (Krimsky, 2017).

Other countries have adopted more precautionary approaches to the regulation of chemicals. Specifically, the European Union has developed the Registration, Evaluation, Authorization, and Restriction of Chemicals (REACH) system, wherein the manufacturer and importers must provide sufficient data to demonstrate safety prior to marketing: "no data no market" (European Commission, 2016). The theoretical grounding for this policy is the precautionary principle (PP), which requires "taking preventive action in the face of uncertainty; shifting the burden of proof to the proponents of an activity; exploring a wide range of alternatives to possibly harmful actions; and increasing public participation in decision making" (Kriebel et al., 2001, 871). Regardless of whether one adheres to some form of the precautionary approach, determining an acceptable level of risk remains the key issue in chemical regulation regardless of jurisdiction.

It is logical that countries will adopt different regulatory models tailored to their different needs, priorities, and values within a given jurisdiction. However, chemicals do not adhere or conform to these geographical parameters, and they often have far-reaching consequences, extending internationally and ultimately affecting the balance of the ecosystem worldwide. International consensus, such as the treaty process, has also proven to be an effective approach to address risks associated with a wide range of persistent chemicals. For example, the Stockholm Convention is a global treaty to protect human health and the environment from the harmful effects of POPs (UNEP, 2009). Ratified by more than 150 nations, the Stockholm Convention "requires its parties to take measures to eliminate or reduce the release of POPs into the environment," effectively banning them on a global scale (UNEP, 2009, Overview; UNEP, 2018).

Ethical Issues

Public health promotion often encompasses values related to the health and well-being of populations. Typical examples of public health initiatives include disease control, promotion of healthy lifestyles, providing safe food and water, and the creation of accessible health care systems. Although the use of industrial chemicals has helped in many of these endeavors, they also do sometimes hinder these public health initiatives because of conflicting goals or values. In this next section, we will exemplify how public health goals may be helped or hindered in agricultural development, industrial viability, and profit, as well as in terms of environmental justice.

Public Health versus Agriculture

Although developed countries often have a substantial amount of food production, many resource-limited nations have little to no food security, which exacerbates rates of mortality and morbidity. Although there is a strong moral imperative to use pesticides that promote food security on a global scale to ensure basic nourishment, the use of pesticides has concomitantly created many unintended effects on the environment. This section explores the agricultural methods that have historically had various effects on public health.

Industrialization contributed to a revolution in agriculture models, as the mechanized power and technological innovations of tractors, seed drills, cultivators, and reapers enabled large-scale planting and harvesting. To achieve large-scale efficiency and profits, industrial farming turned to monoculture, producing large crops of one fruit or vegetable or grain. However, reducing the biodiversity of crops also limited their natural resistance, providing the opportunity for weeds, insects, and bacteria to blight entire crops. To counter this problem and ensure high yields, the agriculture industry turned to the development and increased use of pesticides (Davis, 2014). In the early twentieth century, various types of arsenate (e.g., copper, lead, calcium) were commonly used on crops. These chemicals resulted in soil contamination, reduced foliage, and a harmful residue on plants, fruits, and vegetables, which contaminated soil and water on an international scale (Nordstrom, 2002; Bencko and Yan Li Foong, 2017). Progress in finding a replacement for arsenic lagged until the development of DDT.

Used during the Second World War to prevent diseases such as typhus and malaria, DDT also effectively killed mosquitoes, houseflies, body lice, Colorado beetles, and gypsy moths (Davis, 2014). Unfortunately, some insects have developed resistance to DDT over time. In her influential book *Silent Spring*, Rachel Carson (1962) documented the significant negative long-term effects of pesticides (focusing mainly on DDT) on wildlife and humans. Although there was little scientific consensus about the detrimental effects of pesticides at that time, Carson argued that environmental health was imperiled by the use of toxic chemicals driven by corporate greed and corruption. She argued that pesticide use was a moral and urgent matter deserving attention; in so doing, she transferred the "scientific" debate regarding acceptable use of industrial chemicals into the broader public forum that also questioned the right for individuals not to be exposed to chemicals regardless of identified health risks (Murphy, 2018). Subsequently, many countries banned DDT in the 1970s, and in 2001, as mentioned earlier, the United Nations ratified an international treaty at the Stockholm Convention limiting the use of POPs. Nonetheless, the use of various chemicals in industrial agriculture has had a devastating effect on the environment. The ongoing growth of industrial farming continues to erode natural ecosystems, disturbing homeostasis and creating a detrimental amount of nitrogen and phosphorus (namely through algal bloom), which at high levels creates pollutants in water and air, resulting in a detrimental effect on public health to present and future generations (Tilman et al., 2002).

The World Health Organization (WHO) has reported high levels of acute malnutrition in Ethiopia, Kenya, Nigeria, Somalia, Uganda, and Yemen due to food shortages (WHO, 2018). Those shortages not only cause starvation but also weaken the human immune system, thereby rendering populations more susceptible to disease. Agricultural and biotechnological innovation have significantly contributed to increased availability of calories per capita (FAO, 2018). In an effort to increase food production, advances in biotechnology have produced genetically modified organisms (GMOs), some of which include the transfer of insect-resistant genes into plants. Some of these GMO crops actually produce their own pesticides, such as BT toxins. Although the BT toxins were at first deemed to be effective at pest resistance, various insect species have since become resistant to them and other pesticides. Indeed, pesticide resistance is becoming widespread in insects, fungi, mites, weeds, and rodents (Resnik, 2012). The development of pesticide resistance may undermine the gains in food supply that were partly achieved through pesticide use and may further increase food insecurity in an ever-growing world population. Pesticide resistance in certain pests (e.g., mosquitoes) may also increase the incidence of vector-borne diseases, which may result in significant large-scale public health issues.

Intergenerational ethics suggests that future people have the same intrinsic moral value as those currently living, since the only difference is one of temporality (Nolt, 2017). From this perspective, present-day populations have a responsibility to sustain resources for future generations. One could argue, however, that humans are capable of developing technology that will address human and environmental health issues arising in the future, so that science and technological innovation will ultimately prevail. This logic requires a leap of faith and discounts risks to public health and environmental health in the near future. It also begs the question: How much foresight and value should we assign to the well-being of future generations in our current policymaking and decisions regarding industrial chemicals and public health?

Public Health versus Industry and Economic Productivity

While regulation is often necessary to protect human and environmental health against toxic or hazardous chemicals (as in the case of DDT and POPs), overregulation may stifle scientific and industrial development (Resnik, 2012). Industrial wealth and economic growth are often seen as a trade-off to environmental considerations (Wubben, 2000). One may find it ethically sound to prioritize environmentally friendly practices, as they often have a positive effect on environmental protection and sustainability, which are often linked to public health promotion. However, others may prioritize industrial profits that promote economic growth and may result in higher-paying jobs as well as a higher standard of living. Various studies have concluded that economic wealth is an important determinant of public health (Lange and Vollmer, 2017). Interestingly, novel business models have emerged where companies—often referred to as "green" businesses—use corporate social responsibility and environmental stewardship as selling points to enhance profit (Orsato, 2006). Others argue that attention to environmental values may not always support increased profits and so must be seen as having independent and intrinsic value (Figge and Hahn, 2012). Balancing environmental regulation and economic development requires careful consideration of sometimes competing values.

As discussed earlier, to prohibit or regulate the use of a chemical in the United States, it is necessary to demonstrate that it poses an "unreasonable risk." However, evidence of unreasonable risk can only be established through expensive and often time-consuming toxicology studies on animals or epidemiological studies on humans. Tort law provides potential legal avenues for addressing environmental harm. However, injury compensation requires substantial evidence to prove that a specific chemical caused disease or harm (Cranor, 2011b). When an individual or group seeks legal recourse for harm caused by a chemical, all relevant prior studies completed by the industry must be revealed during the early stages of the legal process. Since many toxic chemicals are put on the market with little study of the effects of long-term or repeated exposure, the evidence required to seek a remedy or compensation is virtually nonexistent. Without studies demonstrating that a chemical presents an unreasonable risk, the legal threat to the chemical corporation essentially disappears. This can ultimately benefit a chemical producer in litigation (Cranor, 2011b). In court, the burden of proof lies with the plaintiff, who typically cannot afford the costly and lengthy studies required to produce evidence.

In order to ensure that more research is conducted prior to the marketing of an industrial chemical, some scholars have promoted the notion of a strong precautionary principle. The precautionary principle advocates for greater precaution (often through regulation) commensurate with the level of scientific uncertainty and suggests that stakeholders engaged in the risk-creating activity should assume the legal burden of proof to more effectively mitigate scientific uncertainty (Sachs, 2011). A strong precautionary principle would promote regulation even in cases where there are considerable economic costs. Some have considered that the precautionary principle should include the development of methods to ultimately reduce individual and public health risks and increase public participation regarding decision-making (Hansen, Carlsen, and Tickner, 2007). Public participation may include public hearings and inquiries, public opinion surveys, referendums, consensus conferences, citizen advisory panels, and focus groups (Rowe and Frewer, 2000). Conversely, opponents of the precautionary principle argue that it is impractical and would paralyze or unduly impede every step in the development and implementation of chemicals and their regulations (Sunstein, 2003). Finally, Gary Marchant and Kenneth Mossman (2004) have suggested that the precautionary principle is "arbitrary and capricious," because it has been applied in an inconsistent and ad hoc manner in policy and in courts of law.

Environmental Justice and Susceptible Populations

According to the US EPA (2019), environmental justice generally refers to the "fair treatment and meaningful involvement of all people regardless of race, color, national origin, or income with respect to the development, implementation, and enforcement of environmental laws, regulations, and policies." Although industry and government may be principally responsible for chemicals that pose risks, the individuals or groups—such as children, the elderly, and factory workers—ultimately bear a disproportionate level of environmental risk to health. Public health decisions are typically rooted in consequentialist and utility-based considerations where the preferred ethical choice is the one that brings the lowest mortality and morbidly rates to the population. Recently, however other theoretical justifications have been suggested. This may include liberal or communitarian ethics (Roberts and Reich, 2002). Liberalist approaches to public health generally include greater emphasis on rights to health or health care, based on the argument that they often pave the way to a range of life-supporting opportunities for individuals or groups. Although a liberal ethics theory may seem to counter public health initiatives—such as an individual's right to develop chemicals—a liberalist could also argue that an individual has a right not to be exposed to harmful toxicants that deters their future opportunities. Communitarian ethics is often seen as a more logical match to public health, as it emphasizes the community rather than the individual. By embracing virtues in social order and communal responsibility, a communitarian could argue that given the widespread real or potential public health effect of industrial chemicals, regulatory matters should always be developed in collaboration with citizens that will be affected.

Environmental justice issues have been raised by scholars and activist grassroots movements concerned with the devastating and unfair effect of chemical uses on susceptible groups. There are many examples: a disproportionate amount of off-site commercial water landfill isolates are found in proximity to predominantly African American communities in the United States; laborers in mining and stonework are commonly exposed to crystalline silica asbestos; First Nation communities have significant issues with their proximity to radioactive waste; and victims of Hurricanes Katrina and Rita were temporarily housed in trailers with very high concentrations of formaldehyde (Adams et al., 2011; Bullard and Johnson, 2002; Shrader-Frechette, 2002; Maddalena et al., 2009; Burgard and Lin, 2013).

Research has shown that susceptible populations often have few resources or power to protect themselves; they are often minorities disadvantaged in various ways (e.g., education, income, occupation) (Shrader-Frechette, 2002). Conversely, when there is strength in numbers and public support, patient advocacy organizations representing susceptible populations have at times been successful in influencing decisions for increased research, treatment, and awareness of common illnesses, including cancer, diabetes, mental illness, and cardiovascular disease (Rose, 2013).

There is significant debate in the environmental justice literature surrounding the notion of an individual's ability to "freely consent" to environmental risks. It has been argued that individuals who choose to work in risky environments—e.g., coal miners, farmers, cleaners—should be allowed to do so. The argument rests on the assumption that workers choose their employment and are compensated for their work. Thus, they "freely" accept the occupational and chemical hazards of their jobs, including exposure to hazardous chemicals or byproducts from manufacturing processes. In reality, this scenario of free choice and implicit consent is not entirely accurate. At times, chemical hazards may not be clearly and accurately explained to workers resulting in an inability to assess health risks. Even when health risk information is adequately disclosed, a worker's choices are often extremely limited in a tight labor market. In such an environment, one accepts the available job regardless of the hazards, or one faces unemployment (Shrader-Frechette, 2002). As such, consent is not actually "free." Generally, individuals who have considerable wealth and access to many opportunities do not choose to live or work in environmentally risky conditions.

Public Health versus the Environment

Human health and protection of the environment are often seen as symbiotic—what is good for the environment is also good for human health, and vice versa. However, in some cases, policymakers have prioritized public health to the detriment of environmental protections. For example, certain insects and animals present real threats to crops and may reduce human food sources. The resulting malnutrition can reduce cognitive function and immunity, and also increase the rate of tuberculosis and infectious disease (Chandra, 1992; Levitsky and Strupp, 1995; Cegielski and McMurray, 2004). The use of insecticides and pesticides to control or eliminate insects or animals that harm crops and reduce food stocks could be rationalized as a necessary "evil" to safeguard public health.

Mosquito-borne diseases such as Zika, malaria, dengue fever, and West Nile virus take a heavy toll on human health (Tolle, 2009). In the name of public health, widespread spraying of DDT in the 1950s and 1960s nearly eradicated many pathogens. This example illustrates the serious harm that a well-intended decision in the interest of public health can have on the environment as well as human health (Hemingway et al., 2006). While many countries have adopted better alternatives to extensive chemical spraying (such as the clearing of standing water in close proximity to dense populations which lowers morbidity and mortality, especially for malaria [Alonso et al., 1991]), there remains a significant public health threat worldwide from both pathogens and pesticide use. Although other alternatives for mosquito abatement are being pursued, such as genetically modified disease-resistant mosquitoes (Waltz, 2016), these may also create a negative effect on the ecosystem. Central to the debate about how best to control mosquito-borne diseases is the ethics question about the limits of the right of humans to modify species for their own interests. Should human well-being always be superior to that of the environment?

The applied ethics literature has focused on human rights, human health, human well-being, and human values. These human values have been applied to various decision-making problems regarding environmental protection and environmental health. A very limited few in sociology and ethics advocate for a post-anthropocentric model wherein humans forego traditional anthropocentric privileges to value coexistence with all organisms and promote sustainable and ecological values (Ferrando, 2016). Although some might criticize ecological or post-anthropocentric models as being very ideological and lacking decision-making application and feasibility (Resnik, 2009), they do propose a different approach worthy of further consideration; namely, a world in which humans would not make all decisions based on their own interests and would reprioritize based on what is good for the entire ecosystem. Although this notion may seem radical, it may be worthwhile and instructive to reflect on the values, beauty, and balance that a post-anthropocentric view might offer.

Conclusion

Ethical and regulatory issues linked to agriculture, economic growth, environmental justice, and environmental protections are commonplace. Regulation of the chemical industry ranges from less rigorous risk analysis to the more comprehensive application of precautionary principles. This chapter has outlined some of the conflicting goals and values between public health and the agriculture industry, public health and industrial development, public health and environmental justice, and public health and environmental protections. Greater emphasis on social responsibility and community engagement in scientific development and industrial practices will help support decision-making that better serves not only public health but also environmental and intergenerational health. Finally, we might reflect on the benefits of moving from the current anthropocentric model to a post-anthropocentric standpoint that allows for a balanced and open consideration of more ecological and sustainable options and greater coexistence with other organisms.

Acknowledgment

We thank David B. Resnik and Bruce Androphy for their insightful comments and suggestions regarding this manuscript. Elise M. R. Smith is supported by a collaborative fellowship from the National Institutes of Health (NIH) and the Fonds de Recherche du Québec en Santé (FRQS). The chapter does not represent the view of the NIH, the FRQS, or any governmental institution.

Note

1. Regulation of industrial chemicals is also considered in the Safe Water Drinking Act (42 U.S.C. § 300f) and the Clean Air Act (42 U.S.C. § 7401).

References

Adams, V., Kaufman, S. R., Van Hattum, T., and Moody, S. 2011. "Aging Disaster: Mortality, Vulnerability, and Long-Term Recovery among Katrina Survivors." *Medical Anthropology* 30(3): 247–270.

Adeola, F. O. 2004. "Boon or Bane? The Environmental and Health Impacts of Persistent Organic Pollutants (POPs)." *Human Ecology Review* 11(1): 27–35.

Alonso, P. L., Lindsay, S. W., Armstrong, J. R. M., De Francisco, A., Shenton, F.C., Greenwood, B. M., et al. 1991. "The Effect of Insecticide-Treated Bed Nets on Mortality of Gambian Children." *Lancet* 337(8756): 1499–1502.

Asante-Duah, K. 2017. *Public Health Risk Assessment for Human Exposure to Chemicals* (Washington, D.C.: Springer).

Bencko, V., and Yan Li Foong, F. 2017. "The History of Arsenical Pesticides and Health Risks Related to the Use of Agent Blue." *Annals of Agricultural and Environmental Medicine* 24 (2): 312–316.

Bullard, R. D., and Johnson, G. S. 2002. "Environmentalism and Public Policy: Environmental Justice: Grassroots Activism and Its Impact on Public Policy Decision Making." *Journal of Social Issues* 56(3):555–578.

Burgard, S. A., and Lin, K. Y. 2013. "Bad Jobs, Bad Health? How Work and Working Conditions Contribute to Health Disparities." *American Behavioral Scientist* 57(8): 1105–1127.

Caito, S., and Aschner, M. 2017. "Developmental Neurotoxicity of Lead." In *Neurotoxicity of Metals*, 3–12 (Cham, Switzerland, Springer).

Carpenter, D. O. 2011. "Health Effects of Persistent Organic Pollutants: The Challenge for the Pacific Basin and for the World." *Reviews on Environmental Health* 26(1): 61–69.

Carson, R. 1962. *Silent Spring* (Boston: Houghton Mifflin).

Cegielski, J. P., and McMurray, D. N. 2004. "The Relationship between Malnutrition and Tuberculosis: Evidence from Studies in Humans and Experimental Animals." *International Journal of Tuberculosis and Lung Disease* 8(3): 286–298.

Chandra, R. K. 1992. "Protein-Energy Malnutrition and Immunological Responses." *Journal of Nutrition* 122(3): 597–600.

Cranor, C. F. 2011a. *Legally Poisoned: How the Law Puts Us at Risk from Toxicants* (Cambridge, Mass.: Harvard University Press).

Cranor, C. F. 2011b. *Toxic Torts* (Cambridge, Mass.: Cambridge University Press).

Davis, F. R. 2014. *Banned: A History of Pesticides and the Science of Toxicology* (New Haven, Conn.: Yale University Press).

EPA (US Environmental Protection Agency). 2019. "Environmental Justice." https://www.epa.gov/environmentaljustice.

European Commission. 2016. "Environment - Chemicals - REACH." http://ec.europa.eu/environment/chemicals/reach/reach_en.htm.

FAO (Food and Agriculture Organization of the United Nations). 2018. "Food Supply—Livestock and Fish Primary Equivalent." http://www.fao.org/faostat/en/#data/CL/visualize.

Ferrando, F. 2016. "The Party of the Anthropocene: Post-humanism, Environmentalism and the Post-anthropocentric Paradigm Shift Past the Human: Narrative Ontologies and Ontological Stories: Studies and Research Contributions." *Relations* 4: 159–174.

Figge, F., and Hahn, T. 2012. "Is Green and Profitable Sustainable? Assessing the Trade-Off between Economic and Environmental Aspects." *International Journal of Production Economics* 140(1): 92–102.

Hansen, S. F., Carlsen, L., and Tickner, J. A. 2007. "Chemicals Regulation and Precaution: Does REACH Really Incorporate the Precautionary Principle." *Environmental Science & Policy* 10(5): 395–404.

Hemingway, J., Beaty, B. J., Rowland, M., Scott, T. W., and Sharp, B. L. 2006. "The Innovative Vector Control Consortium: Improved Control of Mosquito-Borne Diseases." *Trends in Parasitology* 22(7): 308–312.

Kriebel, D., Tickner, J., Epstein, P., Lemons, J., Levins, R., Loechler, E. L., et al. 2001. "The Precautionary Principle in Environmental Science." *Environmental Health Perspectives* 109(9): 871–876.

Krimsky, S. 2017. "The Unsteady State and Inertia of Chemical Regulation under the US Toxic Substances Control Act." *PLoS Biology* 15(12): e2002404. https://journals.plos.org/plosbiology/article?id=10.1371/journal.pbio.2002404.

Kroes, R., Kleiner, J., and Renwick, A. 2005. "The Threshold of Toxicological Concern Concept in Risk Assessment." *Toxicological Sciences* 86(2): 226–230.

Lange, S., and Vollmer, S. 2017. "The Effect of Economic Development on Population Health: A Review of the Empirical Evidence" *British Medical Bulletin* 121(1): 47–60.

Levitsky, D. A., and Strupp, B. J. 1995. "Malnutrition and the Brain: Changing Concepts, Changing Concerns." *Journal of Nutrition* 125(Suppl. 8): 2212S–2220S.

Maddalena, R., Russell, M., Sullivan, D. P., and Apte, M. G. 2009. "Formaldehyde and Other Volatile Organic Chemical Emissions in Four FEMA Temporary Housing Units." *Environmental Science & Technology* 43(15): 5626–5632.

Marchant, G. E., and Mossman, K. L. 2004. *Arbitrary and Capricious: The Precautionary Principle in the European Union Courts.* (Washington, D.C.: American Enterprise Institute Press).

Murphy, M. K. 2018. "Scientific Argument without a Scientific Consensus: Rachel Carson's Rhetorical Strategies in the *Silent Spring* Debates." *Argumentation and Advocacy* (Online First, January 23). https://doi.org/10.1080/00028533.2018.1429065.

Neumann, H. G. 2009. "Risk Assessment of Chemical Carcinogens and Thresholds." *Critical Reviews in Toxicology* 39(6): 449–461.

Nolt, J. 2017. "Future Generations in Environmental Ethics." In *The Oxford Handbook of Environmental Ethics*, edited by S. M. Gardiner and A. Thompson (Oxford: Oxford University Press).

Nordstrom, D. K. 2002. "Worldwide Occurrences of Arsenic in Ground Water." *Science* 296(5576): 2143–2145.

Orsato, R. J. 2006. "Competitive Environmental Strategies: When Does It Pay to Be Green?" *California Management Review* 48(2): 127–143.

Resnik, D. B. 2009. "Human Health and the Environment: In Harmony or in Conflict?" *Health Care Analysis* 17(3): 261–276.

Resnik, D. B. 2012. *Environmental Health Ethics* (Cambridge, Mass.: Cambridge University Press).

Roberts, M. J., and Reich, M. R. 2002 "Ethical Analysis in Public Health." *Lancet* 359(9311): 1055–1059.

Rose, S. L. 2013. "Patient Advocacy Organizations: Institutional Conflicts of Interest, Trust, and Trustworthiness." *Journal of Law, Medicine & Ethics* 41(3): 680–687.

Rowe, G., and Frewer, L. J. 2000. "Public Participation Methods: A Framework for Evaluation." *Science, Technology, & Human Values* 25(1): 3–29.

Sachs, N. M. 2011. "Rescuing the Strong Precautionary Principle from Its Critics." *University of Illinois Law Review* 2011: 1285–1338.

Schecter, A., Birnbaum, L., Ryan, J. J., and Constable, J. D. 2006. "Dioxins: An Overview." *Environmental Research* 101(3): 419–428.

Shrader-Frechette K. S. 2002. *Environmental Justice: Creating Equality, Reclaiming Democracy*. (Oxford: Oxford University Press).

Steenland, K., Piacitelli, L., Deddens, J., Fingerhut, M., and Chang, L. I. 1999. "Cancer, Heart Disease, and Diabetes in Workers Exposed to 2,3,7,8-Tetrachlorodibenzo-P-Dioxin." *Journal of the National Cancer Institute* 91(9): 779–786.

Sunstein, C. R. 2003 "Beyond the Precautionary Principle." *University of Pennsylvania Law Review* 151(3):1003–1058.

Tilman, D., Cassman, K. G., Matson, P. A., Naylor, R., and Polasky, S. 2002. "Agricultural Sustainability and Intensive Production Practices." *Nature* 418: 671–677. https://www.nature.com/articles/nature01014.

Tolle, M. A. 2009. "Mosquito-Borne Diseases." *Current Problems in Pediatric and Adolescent Health Care* 39(4): 97–140.

UNEP (United Nations Environment Programme). 2009. The Stockholm Convention on Persistent Organic Pollutants. http://www.pops.int/TheConvention/Overview/tabid/3351/Default.aspx.

UNEP (United Nations Environment Programme). 2018. "Status of Ratifications of the Stockholm Convention." http://chm.pops.int/Countries/StatusofRatifications/PartiesandSignatoires/tabid/4500/Default.asp

Vandenberg, L. N., Colborn, T., Hayes, T. B., Heindel, J. J., Jacobs, D. R., Jr., Lee, D. H., et al. 2012. "Hormones and Endocrine-Disrupting Chemicals: Low-Dose Effects and Nonmonotonic Dose Responses." *Endocrine Reviews* 33(3): 378–455.

Waltz, E. 2016. "US Reviews Plan to Infect Mosquitoes with Bacteria to Stop Disease." *Nature News* 533(7604): 450.

Wasserman, G. A., Liu, X., LoIacono, N. J., Kline, J., Factor-Litvak, P., van Geen, et al. 2014. "A Cross-Sectional Study of Well Water Arsenic and Child IQ in Maine Schoolchildren." *Environmental Health* 13(1): 23.

WHO (World Health Organization). 2018. *Emergencies; Famine and Health* (Geneva: WHO). http://www.who.int/emergencies/humanitarian-emergencies/famine/en/.

Wubben, E. F. M. 2000. *The Dynamics of the Eco-Efficient Economy: Environmental Regulation and Competitive Advantage* (Cheltenham, UK: Edward Elgar).

CHAPTER 61

OCCUPATIONAL HEALTH AND THE BUILT ENVIRONMENT: ETHICAL ISSUES

DAVID B. RESNIK

Introduction

People are often exposed to hazardous environmental agents (e.g., chemicals, toxins, pathogens, allergens) in areas in which they live and work. The design, construction, and location of buildings, bridges, residential communities, waste sites, and workplaces can also impact human health and the environment in various ways. Ethical issues involving conflicts among different stakeholders and basic values sometimes arise in managing these risks. This chapter will address some of these issues.

The built environment can be defined as the environment constructed by human beings for a variety of purposes, such as living, working, shopping, recreating, eating, and attending school. It includes many different types of structures, such as houses, apartments, factories, shopping malls, office buildings, schools, roads, sidewalks, airports, parks, cities, dams, waste sites, sewers, electric power lines, pipelines, suburbs, and cities (Jackson and Kochtitzky, 2009). The built environment plays a key role in supporting human health, as it provides people with basic needs such as shelter, food, water, work, transportation, and so on. However, the built environment can also place human health at risk and harm the (nonhuman) environment (see Box 61.1).

The workplace environment plays an essential role in supporting human health and well-being. Work provides people with important benefits, such as income, self-esteem, life experiences, intellectual or physical challenges, community, comradery, and health insurance. Having a meaningful job is essential to leading a healthy, productive, and rewarding life (Perry and Hu, 2010). Work also benefits society by providing jobs, goods, and services, and by stimulating economic development, but it also poses potential risks for human health and the environment (see Box 61.2).

Box 61.1 Health Risks Associated with the Built Environment

Design. Poorly designed buildings, bridges, roads, tunnels, and other structures can place human life and health at risk. Although safety is part of engineering's professional ethos (Harris et al., 2013), history contains many instances of disasters that resulted from engineering design flaws, such as the failure of Banqiao Reservoir Dam, located on the River Ru in Zhumadian Prefecture in China, which killed an estimated 171,000 people and destroyed 11 million homes in 1975; the collapse of the Hyatt Regency walkway in Kansas City, Missouri, in 1981, which killed 114 people and injured 200; and an explosion at the Chernobyl nuclear power plant in Russia, which killed 30 workers, sickened hundreds of residents initially, and led to increased thyroid cancer in children in the vicinity (Engineering Failures, 2015). Design flaws can also lead to less dramatic adverse outcomes, such as increased pedestrian or automobile accidents (Jackson and Kochtitzky, 2009).

Materials. Materials used in building construction can have adverse impacts on human health. Materials that are not strong enough to bear weight, pressure, or vibrations may collapse or move, possibly injuring or killing residents. Inferior materials used in home construction were a major factor in the enormous death toll (about 250,000 people) in the Haitian earthquake in January 2010. Most of the homes in Haiti were constructed out of brittle and inflexible materials, such as concrete, mud, and sticks, which were unable to resist the 7.0 magnitude quake. In comparison, only 521 people died in an 8.8 magnitude quake that hit Chile in February 2010. Chile had stricter building codes, which required structures to meet earthquake resistance standards (Barrionuevo and Robbins, 2010). Materials may also expose residents to toxic chemicals, such as lead, which interferes with neurological development and learning in children; asbestos, which causes mesothelioma, a rare lung cancer; and formaldehyde, which has been linked to certain types of cancer (Frumkin, 2010). Since the 1970s, the United States has taken steps to ban the use of lead in paint and asbestos in insulation and roofing materials, but formaldehyde, used chiefly to make plywood, remains a concern (National Cancer Institute, 2015). (For further discussion of toxic chemicals, see "Industrial Chemicals, Pesticides, Public Health, and Ethics," this volume).

Maintenance. A well-built and well-designed structure can still be dangerous if it is not properly maintained. The United States' physical infrastructure, which was once the envy of nations around the world, is now in dire need of repair, due to years of neglect (ASCE, 2015). Weathered bridges, overpasses, roads, train tracks, and dams pose a serious safety threat. For example, the collapse of the I-35W bridge in Minneapolis, Minnesota, in 2007, which killed 13 people and injured dozens, has been attributed to neglectful maintenance (Sofge, 2012). Lack of funding has been the main reason for infrastructure neglect. According to one estimate, it will cost $3.6 trillion to repair America's infrastructure (ASCE, 2015).

Location. The location of structures can have a significant impact on health. For example, people who live in areas prone to hurricanes, flooding, tornadoes earthquakes, or forest fires face increased health risks related to these natural disasters (Frumkin, 2010). In some cases, building designs and materials can reduce the impacts of disasters. For example, many homes in areas where tornadoes occur frequently include basements or other safe shelters that offer protection for residents. Homes in areas prone to earthquakes may be constructed to absorb or diffuse vibrations in the earth. Residents of homes located near waste disposal sites, factories, or hog farms may be exposed to toxic chemicals, air or water

(*continued*)

Box 61.1 Continued

pollution, or noxious fumes. People who live in areas where radon gas is present in the soil may need to monitor radon levels to protect themselves from dangerous radiation (Frumkin, 2010).

Organization. The organization of the built environment can have a major impact on health. For example, urban sprawl is a pattern of development characterized by decentralized living and working arrangements over vast areas, with reliance on automobiles for transportation on highways and interconnecting streets (Jackson and Kochtitzky, 2009). Urban sprawl can increase ozone and other forms of air pollution, decrease land available for recreation, and discourage the use of alternative forms of transportation that involve exercise, such as walking and biking. By decreasing opportunities for exercise, urban sprawl can contribute to obesity and its associated health problems, such as diabetes (Jackson and Kochtitzky, 2009). By encouraging reliance on automobiles, urban sprawl can increase carbon dioxide emissions that contribute to global warming, which has a variety of adverse impacts on human health and the environment (Resnik, 2010). Many people also object to urban sprawl on aesthetic grounds (Resnik, 2012).

Box 61.2 Health Risks Associated with the Work Environment

Working Conditions. Some jobs involve inherently dangerous working conditions. For example, firefighters can be harmed or killed by inhaling smoke, coming into contact with fire or extreme heat, getting trapped inside burning buildings, and so on. Coal miners may breathe in dangerous coal dust or noxious fumes, or be trapped or killed in a cave-in. Employers can usually take some steps to manage or mitigate these risks. For example, firefighters can wear protective clothing. Coal mine owners can supply miners with protective gear and can reinforce tunnels to prevent cave-ins. Employers can also implement occupational health and safety programs that provide training in health and safety and treatment for work-related injuries.

Occupational Exposures. Some jobs expose workers to radiation, toxic chemicals, and other dangerous substances. Some examples of potentially harmful exposures include lead (battery plant workers, electronics recycling workers), ionizing radiation (nuclear power plant workers, radiation technicians), pesticides (agricultural workers), toluene (painters, automobile body shop workers, nail salon workers), carbon monoxide (automobile mechanics), benzene (oil refinery workers), coal dust (coal miners), brominated flame retardants (electronics recycling workers), formaldehyde (construction workers), and infectious diseases (health care workers). In many cases, employers can take steps to reduce or mitigate exposures, such as providing employees with protective clothing, monitoring exposures, implementing occupational health and safety programs, and designing the work environment to reduce exposure (e.g., including proper ventilation to minimize inhalation of dangerous chemicals or dust) (Perry and Hu, 2010) (For more on toxic chemicals, see "Industrial Chemicals, Pesticides, Public Health, and Ethics," this volume).

Physical Stress. Some occupations are physically demanding. Examples include construction worker, furniture mover, warehouse worker, factory worker, professional football player, soldier, fire fighter, and farm worker. The physical demands of these and other jobs may result in exhaustion, fatigue, and acute and chronic injuries (e.g., cuts, broken bones, strained muscles, and repetitive motion injuries). Employers can take steps to reduce and mitigate these risks, such as implementing occupational health and safety programs, designing the work flow to minimize physical stress, and providing employees sufficient time off to allow for rest and recovery (Perry and Hu, 2010).

Psychological Stress. Some occupations are psychologically stressful. Examples include health care worker, police officer, fire fighter, K-12 educator, solider, attorney, high-level manager, and social worker. Psychological stress can increase the risk of fatigue, burnout, and mental illness (e.g., anxiety, depression, and substance abuse). Employers can take steps to reduce and mitigate these risks, such as providing employees with counseling, exercise facilities, training in self-care, and adequate vacation time.

Ethical Issues Related to Property Rights

Some of the ethical issues related to managing the health risks of the built and workplace environment involve conflicts between the property rights of individuals or businesses and the welfare of neighbors, employees, communities, or society at large. Property owners may want to use or commercialize their land or buildings without any external government restrictions, such as zoning laws, building codes, land development rules, water use laws, wetlands protections, and so on (Shrader-Frechette, 1988; Resnik, 2010). However, the health of individuals, communities, and society at large may be negatively impacted by how individuals and businesses use and commercialize their property. Consider the following example:

> People who live in a new housing development built near a hog farm want to stop the farmer from raising hogs because they are concerned about the stench and increased risk of respiratory disease caused by the farm. They petition the state to regulate hog farming and sue hog farmers for creating a public nuisance. The hog farmers argue, however, that they were raising hogs long before these housing developments sprung up in rural areas, and that they should be able to continue what had long been a part of their farming tradition. They also argue that they depend on hog farming for their livelihood and that hog farming makes important contributions to the economy.

How should we think about possible limitation on the farmers' rights to use their land? Libertarians, such as Robert Nozick (1974), argue that property is a fundamental right and that restrictions on property rights are justified only to prevent people from infringing on the rights of others. If homeowners choose to live near an already existing hog farm, they are voluntarily accepting this risk, and the farmer's rights to use his land for the hog farm take precedence. Homeowners thus have a cogent argument for preventing a farmer from starting a new hog farm in their neighborhood, because he would be infringing on their property rights, but they have no valid claim against an already existing farm.

One could argue, however, that the libertarian view gives too much weight to property rights. Utilitarians, such as Richard Brandt (1998), offer a perspective on property rights that stands in sharp contrast to libertarianism. According to utilitarians, all rights, including property rights, can be restricted to promote the common good. To determine whether to restrict a right, one needs to ascertain the likely consequences of the restriction for affected stakeholders and society as a whole. For example, a farmer's rights to use his land for a hog farm could be restricted if the social benefits of the restriction are likely to outweigh the harms. Utilitarians would also need to factor in the benefits of not imposing restrictions in their calculus. For example, a hog farm might benefit the local economy by providing jobs and tax revenue, and these benefits would need to be considered in assessing the likely consequences of a particular restriction.

There are some problems with the utilitarian approach to property, however. A well-known objection to utilitarianism is that it does not offer enough protection for individual rights or welfare (Timmons, 2002). In the domain of property rights, utilitarians would favor extensive restrictions on property rights if those restrictions are likely to maximize overall social good. One might argue that property rights deserve more protection than would be provided by a utilitarian approach. Another well-known objection to utilitarianism is that it does not provide a defensible framework for dealing with the distribution of benefits and harms in society (Timmons, 2002). For example, utilitarianists might endorse a property rights scheme that favors wealthy and powerful individuals and businesses at the expense of people of low socioeconomic status (SES) if the scheme is likely to produce more overall good than alternative schemes.

As an alternative to libertarianism and utilitarianism, consider the views of John Rawls (1971), who defended an egalitarian view of property rights that gives consideration to the distribution of benefits and harms in society. According to Rawls, property is a social institution that should conform to principles of justice, including the difference principle, which holds that unequal distributions of basic goods are acceptable only if they are compatible with equality of opportunity and they benefit the least advantaged members of society, such as people of low SES. Since allowing people to have property rights can result in an unequal distributions of goods, property rights may be restricted to promote equality of opportunity or the interests of the least advantaged members of society. To return to the hog farmer example, Rawls could argue that the hog farmer's rights could be restricted insofar as the use of his land interferes with equality of opportunity or harms the least advantaged members of society. If the hog farmer's neighbors are among the least advantaged members of society, then his property right to raise hogs could be restricted to protect his neighbors from harm, under a Rawlsian view. However, a Rawlsian might oppose restrictions on the farmer's right to raise hogs if the people who work for the hog farmer are among the least advantaged members of society, and the neighbors are affluent, since restricting the farmer's rights could take away jobs from poor farmworkers.

One might argue, however, that Rawls's view does not provide enough protection for those rights, because it allows the government to arbitrarily restrict property rights to help the least advantaged members of society. For example, a Rawlsian might endorse a local government's plan to use eminent domain to take private property from a wealthy landowner to build a public skateboard park to benefit the poor. One could argue that this plan would treat the landowner unfairly because he deserves to have control over his land. At the very least, the government would need to have a more compelling reason for taking this land (e.g., to build a public school), and it would need to pay the landowner the fair market value of the land.

Perhaps the best approaches to property rights would combine insight from all three views. One could argue that property rights are important but that they can be restricted for compelling reasons, such as promoting public health and safety, controlled development, or social justice. Property rights should not be restricted arbitrarily, and the burden of proof should fall on those who would impose restrictions (Resnik, 2012).

Ethical Issues Related to the Distribution of Health Risks

Some issues related to managing the health risks associated with the built and workplace environment involve ethical concerns about the distribution of these risks within society. People face different environmental risks, depending on where they live, work, go to school, recreate, travel, and so on. Consider the following example:

> A county is running out of space at its landfill. Last year, voters in the county rejected a motion to ship its waste to another county, so the county needs to find a site for a new landfill. A panel of scientists, civil engineers, sanitation experts, and citizen representatives appointed by the county has identified three potential sites for the new landfill. The first choice for the site is in a rural area in the poorest part of the county. The second choice is also in a sparsely populated rural area but is close to a public school. The third choice is on the edge of an affluent suburban area. People living in the area identified as the first choice learn about the panel's recommendation and circulate a petition opposing the new landfill.

How should the county decide where to locate this landfill? The outcome of this decision will impact the distribution of health risks, since people living near that landfill will face increased health risks. Locating the landfill at the panel's preferred site will increase the health risks of a population that is already economically disadvantaged. Would it be fair to require these people to suffer additional hardships for the benefit of the county? Locating the landfill at the second choice will adversely impact school children, who arguably deserve special protection because they are vulnerable to exploitation and still undergoing growth and development. Locating the landfill at the third site would adversely impact the health of the most people because it would be close to a wealthy suburban area.

The three approaches to distributive justice discussed above would provide different answers to these questions. A utilitarian would favor placement of the landfill in the area that produces the most good/least bad consequences for the most people—most likely the first site. A utilitarian would oppose locating the landfill at the third site (on the edge of the suburbs), since this would adversely impact the health of the most people. A utilitarian would also consider the possible benefits of living near the landfill. For example, the landfill might provide job opportunities for the local population that would offset increased health risks. A Rawlsian would argue that placement of the landfill should not adversely impact the least advantaged members of society, and would, therefore, oppose locating it at the first site, which is the poorest part of the county. A Rawlsian would oppose locating the landfill near the school for similar reasons. A libertarian would have little to say about this particular decision, other than it should respect individual rights. For example, if the preferred site is on private property, the county should negotiate with landowners for the land it intends to use, instead of taking it.

In addition to distributive justice issues, this example also raises issues of procedural justice, or questions about how society should make decisions concerning the distribution of benefits and harms. One could argue that procedural justice requires the county to make its decision based on meaningful input from affected stakeholders, scientific experts, and the public at large (Shrader-Frechette, 2002). Its decision-making process should be democratic, open, transparent, inclusive, and publicly accountable (Gutmann and Thompson, 1998). The county should do more than appoint a panel with experts and citizen representatives; it should also hold community meetings and other activities to solicit public input. It is especially important for the government to solicit input from stakeholders who have low SES or are underrepresented minorities, since members of these groups may not be heard unless their opinions are sought (see "Environmental Justice, Ethics, and Public Health," this volume, for further discussion of environmental justice).

Ethical Issues Related to Occupational Health and Safety Standards

Questions concerning the distribution of risks also arise in developing standards for occupational health and safety. People who work in particular industries face increased health risks (see Box 61.2). Since the beginning of the twentieth century, many countries have adopted occupational health and safety regulations to protect workers from harm. The Occupational Health and Safety Administration (OSHA) develops and enforces standards in the United States. US states may adopt and enforce their own standards as long as they comply with federal standards (Perry and Hu, 2010).

Very often, people who face increased health risks also have low SES and little economic or political power (Perry and Hu, 2010). For example, many nail salon workers are poor immigrants with limited English proficiency. They are exposed to dangerous chemicals, such as dibutyl phthalate, toluene, and formaldehyde, at work, and many have developed illnesses related to these exposures. Nail salon workers may not understand the risks they face (and how to reduce them), or their rights as employees (Nir, 2015). Other workers who may be especially vulnerable to exploitation include migrant workers, adolescent workers, and fast food industry workers. One could argue that providing adequate protections for these workers is a matter of basic fairness.

Health and safety standards that protect workers from harm should be economically feasible. Measures used to maximize occupational health and safety should not be so expensive that they force employers to significantly reduce their operations or go out of business (Cranor, 2011). For example, requiring that workers at battery plants have no exposure to lead would be so expensive that battery companies would go out of business. The benefits of such a policy would not outweigh the costs to the company, its employees, and society. Instead of requiring no lead exposure, OSHA sets acceptable levels of lead exposure for various industries, which take into account the practical and economic realities of the work environment (OSHA, 2015).

Workplace health and safety policies may sometimes conflict with workers' rights to expose themselves to occupational risks. In 1982 a battery manufacturer, Johnson Controls, decided to exclude all fertile women from working in jobs that exposed them to high levels of lead, after discovering that eight women had become pregnant while maintaining dangerous blood levels of lead, despite careful monitoring from the company. Johnson Controls implemented this policy to protect fetuses from harm and avoid legal liability. In 1984 female employees at Johnson Controls brought a class action lawsuit against the company, alleging that its policy discriminated against women. The company asserted a business necessity defense to this allegation, arguing there was no other way to protect fetuses from dangerous lead exposures. The case went all the way to the US Supreme Court, which ruled that the company's fetal protection policy violated the Civil Rights Act of 1964, because it applied only to fertile women, even though men may also cause harm to a fetus if they impregnate a woman while they have dangerous levels of lead in their blood (*International Union, United Auto Workers, et al. v. Johnson Controls, Inc.*, 1991). This important ruling supports the idea that workplace policies designed to protect employees or others from harm should not discriminate on the basis of gender, race, or other characteristics not uniquely linked to health risks. The ruling also affirms a worker's right to decide whether or not to expose oneself to occupational health and safety risks (Bernstein, 1992).

Ethical Issues Related to Housing Standards

Housing standards often reflect a tension between promoting health and safety and affordable housing. One reason why Haiti's 2010 earthquake was more destructive than Chile's in that same year is that Chile had stronger housing standards than Haiti (see Box 61.1). However, increasing housing safety often leads to increased costs, which can reduce the availability of affordable housing and have adverse impacts on the overall economy, as a result of depressing the real estate market (Resnik, 2012). Societies must decide whether the benefits of safe housing standards are worth the costs. When new standards are developed as a result of new scientific research on hazards in the home, older homes may need to be brought up to date. For example, hundreds of thousands of homes in the United States containing lead paint have been remediated since the 1970s as a result of housing standards designed to limit lead exposure in the home. Since people of high SES can more easily afford to pay increased housing prices than people of low SES, regulations that inflate the costs of housing raise issues of social justice because they can exacerbate socioeconomic disparities (Resnik, 2012).

Conclusion

Ethical issues in the built environment and occupational health will continue to emerge as scientists learn more about environmental and health impacts of how people live and work. To address these issues, decision-makers should have access to scientific information concerning the health impacts of the built and workplace environment and should be aware of the basic values at stake. Affected stakeholders, as well as the public at large, should have meaningful input into government decision-making related to these issues.

Acknowledgments

This research was supported by the Intramural Program of the National Institute of Environmental Health Sciences (NIEHS), National Institutes of Health (NIH). It does not represent the view of the NIEHS, NIH, or US government.

References

ASCE (American Society of Civil Engineers). 2015. *2013 Report Card for America's Infrastructure.* http://www.infrastructurereportcard.org/.

Barrionuevo, A. and Robbins, L. 2010. "1.5 Million Displaced after Chilean Quake." *New York Times* February, 28, A1.

Bernstein, A. E. 1992. "*UAW v. Johnson Controls*: A Final Word on Fetal Protection Policies and Their Effect on Women's Rights in Today's Economy." *Hofstra Labor and Employment Law Journal* 9(2): 5. http://scholarlycommons.law.hofstra.edu/hlelj/vol9/iss2/5.

Brandt, R. 1998. *A Theory of the Good and the Right*. Rev. ed. (Amherst, N.Y.: Prometheus Books).

Cranor, C. 2011. *Legally Poisoned: How the Law Puts Us at Risk from Toxicants* (Cambridge, Mass.: Harvard University Press).

Engineering Failures. 2015. "About." http://engineeringfailures.org/

Frumkin, H. 2010. "Healthy Buildings." In *Environmental Health: From Global to Local*, 2nd ed., 689–728 (New York: John Wiley & Sons).

Gutmann A., and Thompson, D. 1998. *Democracy and Disagreement* (Cambridge, Mass.: Harvard University Press).

Harris, C. E., Pritchard, M. S., Rabins, M. J., James, R., and Englehardt, E. 2013. *Engineering Ethics: Cases and Concepts*. 5th ed. (Boston: Wadsworth).

International Union, United Auto Workers, et al. v. Johnson Controls, Inc., 499 U.S. 187 (1991).

Jackson, R., and Kochtitzky, C. 2009. *Creating a Healthy Environment: The Impact of the Built Environment on Public Health* (Atlanta, Ga.: Centers for Disease Control and Prevention). http://www.sprawlwatch.org/health.pdf.

National Cancer Institute. 2015. "Formaldehyde and Cancer Risk." Fact Sheet. http://www.cancer.gov/about-cancer/causes-prevention/risk/substances/formaldehyde/formaldehyde-fact-sheet.

Nir, S. M. 2015. "Cuomo Orders Emergency Measures to Protect Workers at Nail Salons." *New York Times*, May 11, A14.

Nozick, R. 1974. *Anarchy, State, and Utopia* (New York: Basic Books).

OSHA (Occupational Safety and Health Administration). 2015. "Lead." https://www.osha.gov/SLTC/lead/standards.html.

Perry, M., and Hu, H. 2010. "Workplace Health and Safety." In: *Environmental Health: From Global to Local*, 2nd ed., edited by H. Frumkin, 729–767 (New York: John Wiley & Sons).

Rawls, J. 1971. *A Theory of Justice* (Cambridge, Mass.: Harvard University Press).

Resnik, D. B. 2010. "Urban Sprawl, Smart Growth, and Deliberative Democracy." *American Journal of Public Health* 100(10): 1852–1856.

Resnik, D. B. 2012. *Environmental Health Ethics* (Cambridge: Cambridge University Press).

Shrader-Frechette, K. S. 1988. "Agriculture, Ethics, and Restrictions on Property Rights." *Agricultural and Environmental Ethics* 1(1): 21–40.

Shrader-Frechette, K. S. 2002. *Environmental Justice: Creating Equity, Reclaiming Democracy* (New York: Oxford University Press).

Sofge, E. 2012. "The Minnesota Bridge Collapse, 5 Years Later." *Popular Mechanics*, August 1. http://www.popularmechanics.com/technology/infrastructure/a7931/the-minnesota-bridge-collapse-5-years-later-11254114/.

Timmons, M. 2002. *Moral Theory* (Lanham, Md.: Rowman and Littlefield).

CHAPTER 62

ENVIRONMENTAL JUSTICE, ETHICS, AND PUBLIC HEALTH

JAMES DWYER

INTRODUCTION

HUMAN beings build houses, roads, factories, cities, and much more. They also cut down trees, cultivate crops, use antibiotics, burn fossil fuels, and much more. These changes to the built and natural environments have profound effects on human health. Because the effects on people's health prospects are unevenly distributed within societies, between nations, and between generations, environmental changes raise issues of justice. Issues of justice also arise because people's contributions to environmental problems are quite different. Furthermore, issues of justice arise because many people who are affected by environmental problems have not been allowed or empowered to participate meaningfully and equally in decisions that profoundly affect their lives.

This view of environmental justice is broader than the view that the United States Environmental Protection Agency (EPA) uses:

> Environmental justice is the fair treatment and meaningful involvement of all people regardless of race, color, national origin, or income with respect to the development, implementation, and enforcement of environmental laws, regulations, and policies. EPA has this goal for all communities and persons across this nation. It will be achieved when everyone enjoys: the same degree of protection from environmental and health hazards, and equal access to the decision-making process to have a healthy environment in which to live, learn, and work. (EPA, 2018)

The EPA view includes many valuable points, including the emphasis on meaningful involvement and equal access, the concern to protect people equally against health hazards, and the aim to achieve healthy environments for all. But this view is too narrow in several ways. Although it addresses the distribution of health risks, it ignores how these risks vary according to gender, nation of residence, and generation. Although it mentions laws, regulations, and policies, it does not focus attention on institutions, structures, and background conditions (Rawls, 1971; Young, 2011). Although it considers participation and distribution, it ignores altogether issues of justice that arise because of uneven contributions to environmental problems. The EPA's view of environmental justice is too narrow because it reflects a legal model of nondiscrimination rather than a robust model of social justice. This chapter takes a broader view.

Issues of Environmental Justice

While issues of justice about a wide range of environmental problems could be raised, this chapter focuses on waste disposal, air pollution, climate change, and ecological footprints. It aims to show how these environmental problems raise issues of justice, not to settle these issues with a definitive analysis. Later it includes more about the analysis and work that needs to be done to address issues of environmental justice.

Waste Disposal

People produce waste. All of us eat food and excrete waste products. Many of us buy things and throw away plastic, glass, paper, and aluminum. Some of us drive cars and dispose of old tires, and we buy new computers and dispose of old ones. Some of us provide health care and generate medical waste. And many of us depend on industries that produce mining tailings, toxic chemicals, and other dangerous byproducts.

The value, kind, and amount of byproducts have changed over time. Products that were once valued are now considered waste products. Human waste and animal waste were used extensively as manure, but when concentrated animal feed operations produce tons of animal waste, tainted with antibiotics, this waste becomes a cost and a hazard. The kind of waste that some people produce has changed as well. For thousands of years, most waste was organic material that decomposed relatively quickly. Now some waste products remain intact and hazardous for generations. The amount of waste has also increased. By 1990 the average American was producing 4.5 pounds of waste per day, up from 2.7 pounds in 1960 (Rodenbeck, Orloff, and Falk, 2010).

People and corporations have disposed of waste by dumping it into bodies of water, discarding it on land, or burning it. Each method poses health risks and raises issues of justice. A terrible example of the risk of dumping waste into water comes from Minamata Bay, Japan. In 1951 the Chisso Corporation began using mercury sulfate and ferric sulfide as catalysts at its chemical factory in Minamata (Weiss, 1996). Because the factory discharged the wastewater into Minamata Bay, methylmercury accumulated in fish and shellfish (Harada, 1972). Perhaps as many as 10,000 people who ate this seafood developed forms of mercury poisoning. The harm went on for many years while the Chisso Corporation deceived people, obstructed investigations, and avoided responsibility (George, 2001).

The disposal of waste on land also involves health risks and raises issues of justice. The health risks include direct exposure to toxic substances; groundwater contaminated by leachates; gases released by decomposing waste; rats, mice, mosquitoes, and flies that flourish around dumps; and traffic and air pollution from trucks that haul waste. Issues of justice arise around the distribution of these risks, the participation of citizens in decisions, and the factors that contribute to the production of wastes. Indeed, in the United States, the disposal of solid waste led to the modern environmental justice movement (UCCCRJ, 1987).

In the United States, waste sites are disproportionately located in low-income and minority communities (EPA, 2015a). This pattern raises questions about whether it is fair for the larger community to impose the health risks of waste disposal on people who are already disadvantaged. This pattern also raises issues about political power and participation. Although minority communities have often opposed decisions to locate dumps in their communities, they have struggled to get the information they need, to be heard in the decision-making process, and to be treated as political equals. If disadvantaged people and communities had more political power, and if the health costs of waste were included in the cost of production, then producers and cities would have more incentives to reduce the waste stream.

Air Pollution

In December 1952 a disaster struck London. Because the weather was unusually cold, people burned more coal. Because the atmospheric conditions were stagnant, particulate matter and sulfur dioxide remained in the air. As a result of this air pollution, many people became ill and died. Retrospective analyses now estimate that 10,000–12,000 people died from the respiratory and cardiac effects of this air pollution (Bell, Davis, and Fletcher, 2004). When a hurricane or earthquake kills 10,000 people, it is recognized as a major disaster, but air pollution rarely receives the same attention, because the ill effects are often incremental and insidious.

People contribute to air pollution by burning coal, oil, gasoline, charcoal, wood, and other biomass. The combustion of these fuels adds particulate matter, sulfur dioxide, nitrogen oxides, ozone, mercury, and lead to the atmosphere (Bell and Samet, 2010). Particulate matter exacerbates respiratory and cardiac problems. Sulfur dioxide impairs lung function. Nitrogen oxides and ozone increase respiratory problems. Mercury can enter the food chain, bioaccumulate, and cause neurological problems. Lead, which was added to gasoline for many years, can cause cancer and neurological problems.

Although all people breathe air, they are not equally exposed to and affected by air pollution. Although most people burn fuels, they do not equally contribute to and profit from activities that produce air pollution. Although most people care about air quality, they are not equally empowered to participate in key decisions about air pollution. These differences in exposure, susceptibility, contribution, profit, participation, and power raise issues of justice.

Consider air pollution in the United States. Some groups are more exposed or susceptible to air pollution. People who work outdoors are more exposed than people who work indoors. People with asthma are more susceptible to the ill effects of sulfur dioxide and ozone, and children are more susceptible to the ill effects of nitrogen oxides, ozone, lead, and mercury. Race, ethnicity, and income also matter. The EPA's mapping tool shows that five of its six measures of air pollution are disproportionately higher among low-income and minority groups (EPA, 2015a). It is hard to argue that this distribution is fair, especially for the children who are affected.

Consider air pollution in China. A recent study estimated that air pollution in China contributes to about 4,400 deaths per day (Rohde and Muller, 2015). As in the United States, some groups are more exposed to pollution or more susceptible to its ill effects. In addition, some groups profit more. Because air pollution is an externality (Samuelson and Nordhaus, 2009), Chinese corporations benefit from higher profits, some members of the middle-class benefit from economic growth, and consumers outside of China benefit from lower prices. These consumers buy goods at prices that do not reflect the true cost of production. One should recall Thoreau's ([1854] 1995, 28) definition of cost: "the amount of what I will call life which is required to be exchanged for it, immediately or in the long run." Of course, one could argue that Chinese citizens have made a political decision to trade clean air for economic growth, but this argument depends on widespread and meaningful participation in decisions about acceptable levels of pollution.

Climate Change

Human beings are producing, in aggregate, more greenhouse gases than the natural world can absorb and recycle. In 2013, for the first time, the measurement of carbon dioxide at the Mauna Loa Observatory in Hawaii exceeded 400 ppm (NOAA ESRL, 2015). In 1959 the average measurement at the same observatory was 316 ppm, and the preindustrial level was probably about 280 ppm. The net increase in greenhouse gases is changing the earth's climate.

This change poses serious risks to people's health (IPCC, 2007). Heat waves will lead to deaths by thermal stress. Storms will combine with rising sea levels to produce surges that will kill or displace people, damage infrastructure, and compromise farmland. Climate change will also exacerbate a number of infectious diseases, such as diarrhea, malaria, dengue fever, and others (Patz, 2010). The largest health risks may result from the impact of climate change on water resources and food production. Melting glaciers, declining snowpacks, and persistent droughts will impact water resources that are already overdrawn in many areas (WWF, 2014).

Climate change has already affected human health in a serious way. Careful estimates have attributed between 160,000 and 300,000 deaths per year to climate change

(McMichael et al., 2004; Global Humanitarian Forum, 2015). These estimates were based on an increase in average temperature of 0.5°C. It now seems likely that the increase will exceed 2.0°C. Of course, much of the impact on human health still depends on what people and societies do now to reduce emissions and to adapt to changes that are coming.

We are all vulnerable to the health risks posed by climate change, but we are not equally vulnerable. Because greenhouse gases are increasing and portions of those gases remain in the atmosphere for long periods, future generations will be at greater risk. People's vulnerability also depends on their geographical location. People who live at low elevations near coasts, in drought-prone areas, and in cities where the climate is already hot will be at greater risk. People's vulnerability depends, furthermore, on the qualities of the society in which they live. People who live in high-income and well-governed societies will be, in general, less vulnerable to the health risks of climate change, because these societies will have the resources and commitment to protect their citizens. People will also be less vulnerable in communities with high levels of solidarity, civic engagement, and neighborliness (McKibben, 2010). People's vulnerability also depends on their relative position within society. Social determinants, such as power, wealth, income, employment, education, housing, race, and gender, are likely to affect people's vulnerability to the health risks posed by climate change.

The distribution of risk leads to issues of justice, but so do the differing contributions to the problem. Future generations have not contributed any emissions, but they will enter a world filled with all the health risks associated with climate change. Even if we focus on the present generation, we see large differences in emissions between and within countries. Per capita emissions in the United States are twice as high as in Japan, five times as high as in Chile, and fifty times as high as in Ghana (Boden, Marland, and Andres, 2015). But in every country, some people's emissions are unsustainable. About 11 percent of the world's population is responsible for 50 percent of its carbon emissions (Chakravarty et al., 2009).

Ecological Footprints

An *ecological footprint* is a mode of measuring the amount of land and water that people require to provide the resources they use and to absorb the wastes they produce (Wackernagel and Rees, 1996). Since some land can produce more goods or absorb more wastes than other land, an ecological footprint needs to be expressed in a common unit. It is often expressed in global hectares (ghas) of land with average biological productivity. It can also be expressed in the number of "earths" that would be required if everyone used resources and produced wastes at a given level. Since the earth currently has about 1.8 ghas per person, the footprint in earths is the footprint in ghas divided by 1.8.

The global ecological footprint depends on the total population, patterns of consumption and production, the amount of biologically productive land available, and the productivity of that land. For example, consuming vegetables and grains has less impact than consuming beef, since raising cattle often uses large amounts of grain, water, and oil, and also produces large amounts of greenhouse gases (Steinfeld et al., 2006). Because of increases in population, production, and consumption, the global footprint is now about 1.5 earths.

Although the overall global footprint raises important issues of justice between generations, it conceals large differences between and within countries. As a first step toward disaggregating the overall footprint, Table 62.1 lists average footprints in selected countries (Global Footprint Network, 2016).

These averages show large differences between countries, but they conceal large differences between people within the same country. In every country, some people are using resources, producing wastes, and damaging ecosystems at a high and unsustainable rate. In an essay on sustainable development, Kate Raworth (2012, 19) writes, "the biggest source of planetary-boundary stress today is excessive resource consumption by roughly the wealthiest ten percent of the world's population."

Some people will view biocapacity as a commodity to be owned, used, and traded by private individuals, for-profit corporations, and sovereign countries. Other people will argue that many forms of biocapacity—especially the capacity of the oceans and atmosphere to act as carbon sinks—should be treated as a global commons, to which people have an equal right (Singer, 2004). Although the use of ecological footprints as environmental accounting tools will not settle disputed issues of justice, it will help to focus attention on these important issues.

The use of ecological footprints also focuses attention on a crucial ethical task: the need to promote health in ways that recognize the claims of justice and sustainability (Dwyer, 2009). Some societies have done a better job at this ethical task. In the United States, the average life expectancy is about seventy-eight years, but the average ecological footprint is about 4.4 earths. In other words, the United States only attains about eighteen years of life from one earth. In Costa Rica, the average life expectancy is also about seventy-eight years, but the ecological footprint is much less, about 1.5 earths. That is about fifty-two years from one earth. Fortunately, there are many ways that countries could promote health that also reduce environmental impacts.

Table 62.1 Ecological Footprints

Country	Footprint in ghas	Footprint in earths
United Arab Emirates	10.7	5.9
United States	8.0	4.4
Canada	7.0	3.9
Sweden	5.9	3.3
Japan	4.7	2.6
Costa Rica	2.7	1.5
Sierra Leone	1.1	0.6
India	0.9	0.5

Source: Global Footprint Network, 2016.

The Work of Environmental Justice

A sense of justice needs to include a sense of environmental justice: a disposition to treat people fairly with respect to environmental changes and problems. This disposition should lead people to work to address environmental injustices. Depending on the context, this work might take somewhat different forms and have somewhat different aims.

The first, and perhaps most important, form of work aims to show how certain environmental problems or conditions raise issues of justice. At an abstract level, this work tries to show that environmental problems and conditions affect people's life prospects in an uneven, and seemingly unfair, way; that people contribute to environmental problems in an uneven, and seemingly unfair, way; or that people are not empowered to participate in environmental decisions in a meaningful and fair way. For example, the EPA mapping tool shows that eleven of the twelve environmental risks that it measures are higher in minority and low-income communities (EPA, 2015b, 24).

Uneven distributions tend to raise issues of justice, but they do not always settle those issues, because some uneven distributions may turn out to be justified when all things are considered. So the second form of work seeks to articulate, guide, and justify judgments of justice. This work encompasses different approaches. One approach is to articulate features or concerns that are morally salient in making judgments of environmental justice. This chapter has already noted three features: the distribution of risks, the contributions to the problem, and opportunities for participation. Depending on the context and the problem, it may be important to explain more specific features, such as the effects on disadvantaged groups, the benefits that natural environments provide, knowledge of the risks, past contributions, basic rights and liberties, the nature of community-based participatory research, and other features. This work helps people to take morally relevant features into account when making judgments.

Philosophers and other thinkers have often sought to do more than articulate morally salient features or concerns. They have developed a range of approaches to deal with multiple concerns and to address conflicts. Some approaches formulate decision methods (Resnik, 2012; Beauchamp and Childress, 2001). These methods often include strategies, processes, and unranked principles. Other approaches rely on principles that rank values or establish priorities. For example, in *A Theory of Justice*, John Rawls (1971) tries to show why a principle of equal liberty, and a principle of equality of opportunity, should take priority over a principle that governs economic goods. Some philosophers have not been satisfied with ordered principles. They have sought to develop comprehensive theories by which conflicting concerns can be evaluated in commensurate terms. Utilitarianism is a classic example.

It is not my purpose here to evaluate these various approaches, since there is no simple way to overcome disagreements about principles and theories. For example, libertarian thinkers continue to insist that the formal opportunity provided by contracts and markets is sufficient, whereas Rawlsian thinkers continue to emphasize the importance of fair equality of opportunity and the need to correct market failures that result in pollution. Notably, even when people disagree about principles, they sometimes agree about particular judgments and actions (Jonsen and Toulmin, 1990). When there is enough agreement on judgments of justice, it is vitally important to consider ethical issues about responsibility. So the third aspect of work on environmental justice tries to articulate and foster forms of responsibility.

Many discussions of responsibility tend to be rather legalistic. They try to set out the conditions under which it would be right to punish people for acts or to hold them liable for harms. A particular harm is identified in the past; then an individual person is held liable if a clear causal chain connects the harm to the person's actions and if that person was at fault (acted intentionally, recklessly, or negligently). Although this model of responsibility can be applied or extended to some environmental injustices, it doesn't quite fit or illuminate problems with the following features: the harm is a future risk; the victims are not specifiable; the causal chains are not clear; the people and corporations contributing to the problems are acting according to accepted norms and practices.

We need an account of responsibility that illuminates people's responsibility to change accepted practices, background conditions, and structural processes. In her discussion of responsibility for structural injustices, Iris Marion Young (2011, 110) writes:

> The ground of my responsibility lies in the fact that I participate in the structural processes that have unjust outcomes. These processes are ongoing and ought to be transformed so that they are less unjust. Thus I share with others the responsibility to transform these processes to reduce and eliminate the injustice that they cause. My responsibility is essentially shared with others because the harms are produced by many of us acting together within accepted institutions and practices, and because it is not possible for any of us to identify just what in our own actions results in which aspects of the injustice that particular individuals suffer.

Since many structures, institutions, and practices do not adequately account for environmental risks, people need to take responsibility to bring about change. Thus, responsibility, as its etymology suggests, shades into responsiveness (Dwyer, 2013).

To respond more adequately to environmental injustices, many people and institutions will need to change. To further this change is the fourth aspect of the work of environmental justice. It involves both practical and philosophical work. Indeed, John Dewey (1916, 336) writes, "Philosophy is thinking what the known demands of us—what responsive attitude it exacts." And in much of his philosophical work, Dewey tries to show how attitudes, habits, and institutions need to change to respond to current problems and situations.

What does the current environmental situation demand? To respond more adequately, many societies will need to change practices, institutions, structures, and background conditions. For example, market economies that externalize environmental costs and harms will have to change. Maybe it will be possible to tax pollution and decouple economic development from carbon emissions and environmental degradation

(Nordhaus, 2015). But maybe it will be necessary to change deep ideas about what economic development means (Jackson, 2011). I am not sure. But given the analysis presented here, it seems that a just and sustainable future demands much greater equity in terms of carbon emissions, environmental footprints, environmental health risks, and political power.

To respond to environmental injustices, many people will need to change the way they live. Many of us contribute too much to solid waste and air pollution; many of us have environmental footprints that are unsustainable; and 10 percent of us produce about 50 percent of carbon emissions. To address the most serious and urgent environmental injustices will probably require changes in habits of actions, attitudes toward people and nature, and ideas about what is good and just. In other words, the changes will need to include virtues.

The virtue of justice needs to include a sense of environmental justice that is combined with solidarity, respect, responsibility, and a duty to care. People may also need to develop dispositions that are more specifically focused on the environment: concern for sustainability, modesty of consumption, humility with respect to nature, and gratitude for the home that the earth provides. None of these individual and social changes is likely to occur without the active engagement of many citizens and civic groups. And so the work of environmental justice needs to emphasize active citizenship: a courage to confront injustice, a habit of engaging with others, a disposition for advocacy, a sense of the common good, and an understanding that important goods will sometimes conflict. The people who engage in this work need political freedom and ways to overcome the influence of money.

Conclusion

Because many environmental problems are so serious and urgent, public health ethics needs to raise issues of environmental justice, explore what justice demands, address questions of responsibility, and work to change things for the better. But some ethical issues extend beyond human health and environmental justice; they concern how human beings should relate to nonhuman animals, plants, ecosystems, and the whole of nature. The attitudes that we adopt toward nature, the respect we show the earth, the awe we feel for the diversity of life, and the scope of our sense of community—all these are matters of deep ethical concern.

References

Beauchamp, T. L., and Childress, J. F. 2001. *Principles of Biomedical Ethics*. 5th ed. (New York: Oxford University Press).

Bell, M. L., Davis, D. L., and Fletcher, T. 2004. "A Retrospective Assessment of Mortality from the London Smog Episode of 1952: The Role of Influenza and Pollution." *Environmental Health Perspectives* 112: 6–8.

Bell, M. L., and Samet, J. M. 2010. "Air Pollution." In *Environmental Health: From Global to Local*, 2nd ed., edited by H. Frumkin, 387–415 (San Francisco: John Wiley & Sons).

Boden, T., Marland, G., and Andres, B. 2015. "Ranking of the World's Countries by 2007 per capita Fossil-Fuel CO_2 Emission Rates." http://cdiac.ornl.gov/trends/emis/top2007.cap.

Chakravarty, S., Chikkatur, A., de Coninck, H., Pacala, S., Socolow, R., and Tavoni, M. 2009. "Sharing Global CO2 Emission Reductions among One Billion High Emitters." *Proceedings of the National Academy of Sciences* 106(29): 11884–11888. http://www.pnas.org/content/106/29/11884.

Dewey, J. 1916. *Democracy and Education*. In *The Middle Works 1899–1924, Volume 9* (1980) (Carbondale: Southern Illinois University Press).

Dwyer, J. 2009. "How to Connect Bioethics and Environmental Ethics: Health, Sustainability, and Justice." *Bioethics* 23(9): 497–502.

Dwyer, J. 2013. "On Flying to Ethics Conferences: Climate Change and Moral Responsiveness." *International Journal of Feminist Approaches to Bioethics* 6(1): 1–18.

EPA (Environmental Protection Agency). 2018. *Environmental Justice*. http://www3.epa.gov/environmentaljustice/.

EPA (Environmental Protection Agency). 2015a. *EJSCREEN: Environmental Justice Screening and Mapping Tool*. http://www2.epa.gov/ejscreen.

EPA (Environmental Protection Agency). 2015b. *EJSCREEN Technical Documentation*. https://www.epa.gov/sites/production/files/2015-05/documents/ejscreen_technical_document_20150505.pdf.

George, T. S. 2001. *Minamata: Pollution and the Struggle for Democracy in Postwar Japan*. Cambridge, Mass.: Harvard University Press.

Global Footprint Network. 2016. "Footprints for Nations." http://www.footprintnetwork.org/en/index.php/GFN/page/footprint_for_nations/.

Global Humanitarian Forum. 2015. "Climate Change—the Anatomy of a Silent Crisis." http://www.ghf-ge.org/human-impact-report.pdf.

Harada, M. 1972. *Minamata Disease*. Kumamoto, Japan: Iwanami Shoten.

IPCC (Intergovernmental Panel on Climate Change). 2007. *Fourth Assessment Report: Climate Change 2007: Impacts, Adaptation and Vulnerability, Summary for Policymakers*. https://www.ipcc.ch/publications_and_data/ar4/wg2/en/contents.html.

Jackson, T. 2011. *Prosperity without Growth: Economics for a Finite Planet* (New York: Routledge).

Jonsen, A., and Toulmin, S. 1990. *The Abuse of Casuistry: A History of Moral Reasoning* (Berkeley: University of California Press).

McKibben B. 2010. *Eaarth: Making a Life on a Tough New Planet* (New York: Henry Holt).

McMichael, A. J., Campbell-Lendrum, D., Kovats, S., Edwards, S., Wilkinson, P., Wilson, T., et al. 2004. "Global Climate Change." In *Comparative Quantification of Health Risks: Global and Regional Burden of Disease Due to Selected Major Risk Factors*, edited by M. Ezzati, A. D. Lopez, A. Rogers, and C. J. L. Murray, 1543–1649 (Geneva: WHO Press).

NOAA ESRL (National Oceanic and Atmospheric Administration Earth Systems Research Laboratory). 2015. "Trends in Atmospheric Carbon Dioxide 2013." http://www.esrl.noaa.gov/gmd/ccgg/trends/.

Nordhaus, W. 2015. *The Climate Casino: Risk, Uncertainty, and Economics for a Warming World* (New Haven, Conn.: Yale University Press).

Patz, J. 2010. "Climate Change." In *Environmental Health: From Global to Local*, 2nd ed., edited by H. Frumkin, 279–328 (San Francisco: John Wiley and Sons).

Rawls, J. (1971). *A Theory of Justice* (Cambridge, Mass.: Harvard University Press).
Raworth, K. 2012. "A Safe and Just Space for Humanity: Can We Live within the Doughnut?" Oxfam Discussion Paper (Oxford: Oxfam). https://www.oxfam.org/sites/www.oxfam.org/files/file_attachments/dp-a-safe-and-just-space-for-humanity-130212-en_5.pdf.
Resnik, D. B. 2012. *Environmental Health Ethics* (New York: Cambridge University Press).
Rodenbeck, S., Orloff, K., and Falk, H. 2010. "Solid and Hazardous Waste." In *Environmental Health: From Global to Local*, 2nd ed., edited by H. Frumkin, 559–590 (San Francisco: John Wiley & Sons).
Rohde, R. A., and Muller, R. A. 2015. "Air Pollution in China: Mapping of Concentrations and Sources." *PLoS ONE* 10(8). http://journals.plos.org/plosone/article?id=10.1371/journal.pone.0135749.
Samuelson P., and Nordhaus, W. 2009. *Economics*. 19th ed. (New York: McGraw-Hill Education).
Singer, P. 2004. *One World: The Ethics of Globalization*. 2nd ed. (New Haven, Conn.: Yale University Press).
Steinfeld, H., Gerber, P., Wassenaar, T., Castel, V., Rosales, M., and de Haan, C. 2006. *Livestock's Long Shadow: Environmental Issues and Options* (Rome: Food and Agriculture Organization of the United Nations).
Thoreau, H. D. (1854) 1995. *Walden*. Annotated ed. (New York: Houghton Mifflin Company).
UCCCRJ (United Church of Christ Commission for Racial Justice). 1987. *Toxic Wastes and Race in the United States: A National Study on the Racial and Socio-economic Characteristics of Communities Surrounding Hazardous Waste Site* (New York: United Church of Christ).
Wackernagel, M., and Rees, W. 1996. *Our Ecological Footprint* (Gabriola Island, B.C.: New Society Publishers).
Weiss, B. 1996. "Long Ago and Far Away: A Retrospective on the Implications of Minamata." *Neurotoxicology* 17(1): 257–264.
WWF (World Wide Fund for Nature). 2014. *Living Planet Report 2014: Species and Spaces, People and Places* (Gland, Switzerland: World Wide Fund for Nature).
Young, I. M. 2011. *Responsibility for Justice* (New York: Oxford University Press).

CHAPTER 63

ENERGY, EMISSIONS, AND PUBLIC HEALTH ETHICS

CHERYL C. MACPHERSON

INTRODUCTION

A public health ethics concerned with whether and how to respond to conditions that harm health must address the public health impacts of climate change. This chapter reviews evidence that the primary cause of climate change is industrial production and energy use that helps billions of people access water, food, and other goods, but also generates, as byproducts, greenhouse gas emissions, abbreviated herein as "emissions." As emissions concentrate within Earth's finite atmosphere, they cause climate change and harm health by disrupting seasonal weather patterns; average global temperatures and sea levels; and the quality and quantity of water, air, and other resources (Watts et al., 2015; Haines et al., 2007; Resnik, 2012).

Decades of evidence and a range of disciplines ground efforts around the world to reduce the range, severity, frequency, and number of people harmed by emissions (Watts et al., 2015; Patz et al., 2014; Frumkin et al., 2008). Drawing on evidence and ethics, this chapter defines emissions as health determinants with ethical implications, and it discusses how ethically informed policies can help reduce emissions to the benefit of everyone.

CAUSES

Energy used to obtain water, food, and other necessities comes primarily from the petroleum industry. For forty years that industry has contributed the biggest global increases in emissions (Patz et al., 2014), which is accompanied by deforestation that annually destroys 20 million acres of rainforest and generates 20 percent of emissions (Auerbach, 2008). Even successful carbon-neutral strategies are outweighed by emissions produced in meeting demands for energy from growing and socioeconomically developing populations (Haines et al., 2007; UNEP, 2005). This demand reflects global population growth from 2.5 billion in 1950 to 7 billion in 2014, which is expected to reach 9 billion before 2050 (Resnik, 2012, Fig. 9.4). Reducing this growth by making contraception more accessible in low- and middle-income countries (LMICs) would reduce global emissions and improve respiratory health in LMICs, where billions of people routinely burn biomass for household energy (Haines et al., 2007).

Growing populations need more food, along with more energy to produce, package, and transport that food. Industrial food production uses fifty times more petroleum than other approaches to meet those needs, and rising petroleum prices increase pressure to cultivate larger areas of land at lower levels of productivity (Harvey and Pilgrim, 2011). One-third of global land surface is already used for animal production, and meat and dairy consumption are rising significantly, even in LMICs (Popkin, 2009). Reducing animal production would reduce emissions and deforestation, and in wealthy nations it would reduce heart disease by reducing dietary animal fat (Roberts and Stott, 2010).

Globally, the agricultural industry produces about one-third of emissions and uses one-half of all chemical pesticides. Meat production alone causes over half of all soil erosion and antibiotic consumption and 20 percent of water use (Popkin, 2009). Global groundwater withdrawal has risen ten-fold annually since the 1960s, with agricultural use in the United States costing over 1 billion dollars annually, generating 6 percent of India's total emissions, and intensifying needs for water regulations (Rothausen and Conway, 2011). For several reasons, however, water resists regulation (Scott et al., 2011; Resnik, 2012).

By marketing Western products and consumption patterns, globalization increases short-term (i.e., less than one year) socioeconomic gains for industries and governments and drives further demand and production. Globalization also consolidates industrial interests and enhances industry access to, and influence on, government decision-makers regarding how much energy to produce and use, and at what levels of efficiency (Global Policy Forum, 2016). Public interests should be central to such decisions and often parallel shareholder interests in long-term gains and viability, but industries today seem more focused on the short term and market share. Industrial emissions provide short-term benefits but, in the long term, undercut employee health and productivity, damage industrial and other infrastructure and natural resources, and shift consumer spending to essential goods. These impacts should be considered in policymaking involving health, natural resources, and trade.

Impacts

Atmospheric concentrations of carbon dioxide barely changed for millennia but have risen steadily since 1950 (Resnik, 2012, Fig. 9.2). As inadvertent byproducts of energy production and use, emissions challenge determinations about responsibility that are necessary to fair and effective policy. Their harms are documented in thousands of peer-reviewed publications and include altered seasonal weather patterns (Herring et al., 2014) which affect geographic ranges of vectors and disease reservoirs; rates of development, survival, and reproduction for vectors, reservoirs, and pathogens; vector biting behaviors; prevalence of infections; and transmission to humans (Watts et al., 2015; Patz et al., 2014).

Weather changes contribute to outbreaks of meningitis, tick-borne encephalitis, cholera, and mosquito-borne and other illnesses, with substantial costs (Watts et al., 2015; Costello et al., 2009; McMichael et al., 2008). In 2006 an outbreak of mosquito-borne Chikungunya cost India over 5 million US dollars in lost income (Meason and Paterson, 2014). Chikungunya first reached the Western Hemisphere in 2013 in the Caribbean (Fischer and Staples, 2014), with untold costs to health care and lost income and tourism revenue.

Increased frequency and severity of heat waves, floods, droughts, wildfires, and other environmental changes also reduce quality and quantity of food and water, damage ecosystems that support health, and increase morbidity and death (Resnik, 2012). The 700 heat-related deaths annually in the United States between 1999 and 2009 will increase as the annual number of hot days (over 32°C or 90°F) triples by 2050 and increases respiratory and mental illness and substance abuse (Patz et al., 2014). Heat-related disasters usually involve floods that spread waterborne bacterial and viral illnesses and "trigger broad dislocations, often to places ill-prepared for refugees who are overwhelmed by undernutrition and stress" (Patz et al., 2014, 1571). Disaster, dislocation, and refugee conditions raise national security concerns and facilitate infectious disease transmission (Patz et al., 2014; Jarvis et al., 2011; McMichael et al., 2006) and mental illnesses that develop slowly while increasing aggression and suicide (Maughan, Berry, and Davison, 2014).

Over 1 billion people were injured or made ill by water-related disasters between 1992 and 2001 (McMichael et al., 2006). Global water needs will double by 2050 due to development and population growth (UNDP, 2015). Simultaneously, oceans that once absorbed 30 percent of emissions are losing that capacity through acidification and pollution from, among other things, 13,000 pieces of plastic per square kilometer of ocean (UNDP, 2015). Emissions are reducing access to safe water across the United States (Maibach et al., 2008). California's population, now 80 percent larger than in the 1970s, imposed water restrictions due to a severe multiyear drought that began in 2012 (Mann and Gleick, 2015). In April 2017, California's Executive Order B-40-17 declared that having threatened freshwater supplies, devastated agriculture, and harmed fish, animals, and environments, this drought had ended in all but four counties, and that conservation as a way of life will continue through the development of permanent restrictions on wasteful water use (such as hosing sidewalks and driveways) and requirements for reporting water use.

As land is degraded by deforestation, overcultivation, and overgrazing to support growing populations, wind-borne dust polluted with fertilizers and chemicals reduces air quality and increases respiratory illness (WHO, 2015). Rising ozone concentrations significantly increase asthma-related hospitalization and premature death (Kinney, 2008), although millions of respiratory illnesses and premature deaths would be prevented by implementing existing emission-reducing technologies (Frumkin and McMichael, 2008). Meanwhile, mainstream news reports describe poor air quality across Asia as driving a market for unproven filtration systems and canisters of North American air.

The extreme hurricanes Harvey and Irma in the United States in August and September 2017 indicate the growing health and economic dangers of emissions, climate change, and the associated extreme weather. The science and scientists that enabled accurate prediction and tracking of those hurricanes, and facilitated preparations that protected hundreds of thousands of people in their paths, also predict the impacts of emissions on climate change and health. Many American leaders, however, deny that human activities or emissions cause climate change.

Denial

Signed by nearly 200 nations in December 2015, the historic COP21 agreement to reduce global emissions emerged from scientific consensus that emissions harm health, are caused primarily by energy production and use, and can be significantly reduced by slowing production. Denial of the evidence and opposition to regulation are motivated by short-sighted self-interests, misunderstandings of science and peer review, and commitments associated with conservative political affiliations (Valles, 2015; Jamieson, 2014; Evans and Feng, 2013).

Corporately funded denial campaigns designed to polarize dialogue and delay policy responses have been successful and are being expanded (Farrell, 2016; Myers et al., 2015). Denial campaigns communicate authoritatively but misrepresent evidence by, for example, citing evidence of rising regional per capita food production (Zycher, 2015) while ignoring influences of obesity, food waste, and other confounding factors. Denial can sometimes be overcome through dialogue that fosters partnerships aimed at identifying shared political and ethical commitments to health across ideologies, and these commitments may promote a range of health goals, including emission reduction (Gruen and Ruddick, 2009).

Emissions are Health Determinants

The increasingly prevalent and visible harms of emissions deserve attention from everyone concerned with causes of disease, requirements for health, and ethics (Frumkin et al., 2008). Emissions are physical components of our environment, affect health and resources for health, and have ethical implications. Few individuals, communities, or populations have full control over their exposure to hazardous environmental components released into the air, water, or earth by human activities. This challenges fair and ethical management of public health and of environmental health determinants, some of which function at epigenetic levels (Dupras, Ravitsky, and Williams-Jones, 2014; Dupras and Ravitsky, 2016). Because physical environments and their components constitute health determinants (WHO, 2016), emissions are health determinants.

Public health ethics weighs the accuracy, relevance, and implications of evidence; and it uses evidence to elucidate ethical grounds for, and challenges to, public health programs and policies (Faden and Shebaya, 2015). These involve relationships within and between social structures, institutions, governments, and international and other entities, and these influence health and constitute health determinants that affect real people and populations (Macpherson and Akpinar-Elci, 2015; Jennings, 2015).

Relationships create practical and ethical issues and can hinder or enhance the success of public health interventions. Successful smoking reduction policies, for example, alter individual choices and social norms about the acceptability of smoking; this affects tobacco sales, and when sales drop, tobacco companies market more heavily in LMICs lacking such policies, exposing already vulnerable populations to rising rates of lung cancer (Dawson and Verweij, 2015). Policies governing tobacco sales and marketing, and accessibility and quality of tobacco, affect health through relationships between and within various entities.

Relationships

Relationships are central to public health, and public health programs succeed best by using multiple levels of influence involving relationships among individuals, populations, and institutions (Wardrope, 2015). Using this approach, healthy eating programs can position healthy foods prominently and attractively in groceries or restaurants to facilitate individual choice, make healthy choice the default, cultivate temperance as a virtue, connect virtue with health, shift social norms about food, and reinforce all this with social structures (Rozier, 2015). Linking a specific behavior to its impact on others can improve the success of conservation programs (Schultz, 2011), and equally of emission reduction and other health programs.

Relationships form "an intricate web of cooperation and interdependence" with "tremendous significance for health and health care" (Jennings and Dawson, 2015, 37, 33). Public health ethics, like bioethics and medicine, is increasingly attentive to relationships and the environments and institutions in which relationships occur. These determine the impacts of emissions in different geographic regions, their local significance, and the effectiveness of interventions. Emission-related priorities center on air quality in China (Nielsen, 2016), agriculture in India (Gopichandran and Dawson, 2016), zoonotic diseases in Arctic and tropical regions (Macpherson, Bidaisee, and Macpherson, 2016), and drought and floods that disrupt migratory pastoralists in Africa and the Middle East who may misunderstand national and private borders (Metz, 2016).

Individual and collective actions, including emission-producing actions, manifest themselves through relationships. At personal and political levels, individual actions can be morally persuasive and can catalyze collective agreements, because other individuals sometimes emulate actions that protect the commons, like those aiming to reduce emissions (Hourdequin, 2010; Singer, 2011, 235). Individuals and their actions are inseparable from the communities and environments in which they exist, and relational approaches expose systemic patterns of injustice therein that threaten shared interests in health, safety, and survival (Baylis, Kenny, and Sherwin, 2008). Drawing from feminist theory, public health ethics can use relational approaches to illuminate connections between disadvantage and health, stakeholder involvement and power in health systems and processes, and social structures and norms that shape individual abilities to identify and express health-related preferences (Rogers, 2006).

Teasing apart these connections can enhance understandings of and responses to health threats, including emissions. Freedom and solidarity connect with well-being, for example, and are expressed through autonomous actions in here and now "places" in which populations, social structures, and other entities exist and health determinants function (Jennings, 2015; Jennings and Dawson, 2015; Eckenwiler, Straehle, and Chung, 2012). Policies affecting emissions influence health from within these places by shaping individual and collective understandings about, and preferences and capacities for, emission reduction. To succeed, these policies must target these places and relationships within and beyond them. Public health ethics can guard against systemic interests and moral indignation that confuse or mislead policymaking and other interventions, but this requires acknowledging its own internal biases (Schmidt, 2014).

The early bioethicist Van Rensselaer Potter recognized that relationships and interdependencies between living things influence impacts of biomedical and social advances (Potter, 1971, 1–12; ten Have, 2012; Whitehouse, 2002). Drawing from his work in biochemistry and oncology during the socially turbulent 1960s, Potter constructed a "global bioethics" that used humanities and social sciences to deepen understanding and guide medical, scientific, and technological advances in ways that would benefit, rather than undermine, health and survival (Potter, 1971, 1–12). Often overlooked, this relational approach is foundational to bioethics work on health, and particularly emissions (Macpherson, 2016, 202; Macpherson, 2013a; ten Have, 2012; Dawson, 2010).

Ethics

Bioethics is often described as an umbrella encompassing public health ethics, medical and research ethics, and other ethics specialties. Many environmental or climate ethicists, however, do not identify themselves as bioethicists or address health in their work. What seems to be the first publication directly addressing emissions in a mainstream bioethics journal documents health harms associated with the production, transportation, and disposal of latex gloves; and asks whether the harms outweigh the benefits of using latex gloves in health care (Pierce and Kerby, 1999). This question remains salient given their steadily growing use nearly twenty years later.

Despite subsequent attempts to rekindle Potter's bioethics (Whitehouse, 2002, 2003; Whitehouse and Fishman, 2004; ten Have, 2012) and increasingly visible impacts of emissions, climate change remains of peripheral interest within mainstream bioethics (Macpherson, 2013a, 2013b; Dawson, 2010; Dwyer, 2009). Exceptions include its integration into a few bioethics programs in the United States, United Kingdom, and Europe; published reflections prompted by Hurricane Katrina on health determinants that harm those least able to protect themselves and recover (Dwyer, 2005; Moreno, 2005); several peer reviewed articles in the *Kennedy Institute of Ethics Journal, Journal of Bioethical Inquiry*, and elsewhere; and proposals for specialties in ecoethics (Ehrlich, 2009), environmental bioethics (Pierce, 2009), green bioethics (Richie, 2014), and One Bioethics (Thompson and List, 2015) to overcome this disinterest.

One Bioethics aims to prevent or resolve ethical dilemmas like those associated with the 2014 Ebola outbreak by integrating the ethics of "complex issues involving human, animal, and environmental health" into One Health initiatives (Thompson and List, 2015, 98). One Health recognizes that ethics and relationships between humans, animals, and environments are central to the health of each and bear on the management of emerging and other diseases (Capps et al., 2015; Shomaker, Green, and Yandow, 2013).

Even in LMICs, where it is often culturally or economically inappropriate, medical technologies and Western conceptions of autonomy dominate bioethics, but bioethics would have greater relevance to, and better inform, health policy and practice everywhere if it embraced collective concerns (Dawson, 2010; Macpherson, 2013a). Bioethicists and health professionals have professional and civic responsibilities. For bioethicists, these involve public trust in their willingness and ability to inform policymakers and the public about risks and harms to health.

Recognizing emissions as one such harm, some health professionals are accepting this responsibility by making environmental sustainability an ethical priority in their institutions. Accordingly, they are reducing costs and energy use by increasing patient proximity to ambient light and green spaces, because doing so reduces pain, aggression, and fatigue while accelerating recovery and increasing cognition and longevity (Sadler, 2015; Gomez et al., 2013; Sadler et al., 2011). Medical curricula and practice are increasingly responsive to emissions (Walpole et al., 2016; Chivian, 2014; Roberts and Stott, 2010; Macpherson, 2009; Auerbach, 2008). Equally safe but less wasteful procedures for cannulation and intravenous antibiotic preparation are being taught (Bajgoric et al., 2014), and patient compliance and outcomes are improving in conjunction with strategies to reduce medication waste (Maughan, Berry, and Davison, 2014).

Packaging contributes greatly to medical waste. Britain's National Health Service (NHS) produced nearly 6 kilograms of waste per patient per day from 2005 to 2006, while France produced under 2 kilograms, and Germany only 0.4 kilograms, per patient per day (Hutchins and White, 2009). Reprocessing rather than discarding medical devices prevented over 2,000 tons of landfill waste in the United States in 2008, saving hospitals nearly $1.5 million (Kwakye et al., 2010). Health care emissions in the United States, however, were thirty times higher than those of the NHS in 2007 (Richie, 2014). Legal and policy responses to emissions in the United Kingdom are moving the NHS toward carbon neutrality (NHS SDU, 2016).

Large quantities of emissions are produced by all medical institutions and industries because they use large amounts of energy and other resources for routine maintenance, procurement, disposal, and transportation. The assisted reproductive technology (ART) industry and the institutions in which it functions share responsibility for these emissions and may have additional responsibilities, given that their emissions are not produced while caring for patients with medical conditions (Richie, 2014). ART differs from other medical institutions and industries in that it does not treat, cure, or prevent disease; its ethical acceptability is contested by a range of stakeholders; and it increases, consumes, and disposes with the "sole purpose of creating more consuming humans" who will use more energy and resources in the future (Richie, 2014, 5).

Ethically Informed Policy

Ethically informed policies are needed to reduce emissions, adapt to emissions already present, apportion responsibility for their future production, and ensure accountability for present and future production. These policies will require well-defined goals built on strong and objective evidence, multiple targets with sensitivity to local environments and priorities, and resources for implementation and outcome measurement. They are challenged by disagreement about, among other things, how to fairly apportion responsibilities.

Responsibility for emissions is complicated because their sources and quantities vary over time, they are used to obtain both luxuries and necessities like potable water, and the extent to which knowingly producing them imparts obligations to reduce them is debatable (Singer, 2011, 236). Such complexities may be countered by framing emissions as an affront to the natural world, and the need to reduce them as a moral imperative, in order to evoke support across conflicting ideologies (Markowitz and Shariff, 2012). A responsibility to develop empathy for those harmed by emissions in distant places and times can be met by strategically circulating stories from individuals and entities about their experiences to unify and drive responses (Bushell, Colley, and Workman, 2015).

States and industries have moral responsibilities to reduce emissions, and because large-scale emission production violates human rights to life and health, signatories to human rights agreements also have legal responsibilities to do so (Levy and Sidel, 2014; Meason and Paterson, 2014; Singh, 2012). Human rights approaches are applicable because climate change jeopardizes the minimal moral threshold to "life, health and subsistence" through, for example, recurring storm surges and heat waves; they offer advantages over cost benefit analyses, which, in aggregating harms and needs, overlook the most vulnerable, like the elderly or economically disadvantaged; and they can inform policy development regarding the infliction of harm "on others and the role that compensation may play in our decision making," because destroying someone's property or health is a harm, wrong, and rights violation, regardless of whether it is compensated (Caney, 2010, 172). Human rights agreements support using resources to promote health and justice, but their influence is limited by the laws and capacities of states to uphold them (Syrett, 2015; Jennings, 2015; Daniels, 2006).

Globalization and development processes impose moral responsibilities because they elevate emissions and demand for energy, harm health and environments that sustain health, and connect us to future generations (Holland, 2006; Macpherson, 2016, 205–207). Globalization raises ethical questions about whom we, individually and collectively, are morally responsible and accountable to (Verkerk and Lindemann, 2011); and about the size of burdens created by emissions, how to apportion responsibility for creating those burdens, and what to do if that responsibility is not met (Kingston, 2014). What constitute dangerous, fair, and preferred responses to emissions are ethical, rather than scientific, determinations.

Strategy

Ethically grounded policymaking respects diverse stakeholder goals even when these goals conflict with moral convictions of policymakers; it also ranks benefits and burdens fairly; exposes rationales for support, opposition, or neutrality that affect consensus-building; and delineates associated values (Churchill, 2002). Values pervaded the policy goals of former US president George W. Bush, who sought to protect the American way of life by promoting economic growth and emissions despite harms even within the United States (Singer 2011, 229). Had his values been different, he might have pursued this goal through other strategies, like promoting alternative energy. Similarly, development policies that fail by excluding local stakeholders from their design could succeed with different strategies (Ruger, 2015).

Values are apparent in the contrasts between policymaking, which occurs over months, and science, which accumulates evidence, wisdom, and authority over centuries; these values shape scientists' responsibilities to participate in policymaking, clarify implications of evidence, and distinguish between fact- and value-based disagreements (Jamieson, 2014). Dialogue about the harms and benefits of proposed interventions would reduce policymaking conflicts and shift attention from values to evidence in decisions such as whether and when the benefit of reducing mosquito-borne disease outweighs the harms of using DDT, or the harms of deforestation outweigh economic benefits (Resnik, 2012). Such dialogue illuminates environmental differences that affect the fairness of policy goals and strategies (Macpherson, 2013a), and ensures that "reasonable people who disagree can view policies as fair and legitimate" (Daniels, 2006, 26).

Global population growth can be slowed to reduce emissions by improving women's economic and health indicators and access to contraception (Resnik, 2012; Singer, 2011, 209; Haines et al., 2007). Slowing population growth raises contentious questions about reproductive freedom (Resnik, 2012; Callahan, 2009), such as where and when does freedom from overcrowding outweigh freedom to choose how many children to have; is it justifiable to manipulate birthrates or stipulate who may have children; and is it acceptable to provide sex education and with what specific information (Veatch, 1972)?

It would also, however, protect the capacity of social structures to manage dwindling resources and infrastructure (Ehrlich and Harte, 2015). Natural resources that once seemed infinite cannot support 8 billion people living Western lifestyles, so new concepts of growth, development, and well-being are needed, with policies supporting them (Jamieson, 2014; Buchholz, 1998).

Emission-producing activities involve multiple sectors, nations, and stakeholders. Employing a range of targets will help ensure that infrastructure is designed and situated with sensitivity to extreme weather, carbon sinks, and indigenous populations; cost-benefit calculations incorporate the entire cost of producing and consuming a unit of energy; and carbon-neutral technologies receive widespread investment and adoption (Jamieson, 2014). Political and financial commitment to such work depends largely on values and environmental conditions (Macpherson, 2013a), and bioethics capacity to frame and communicate medical risk could be used to enhance related dialogue (Valles, 2015).

The health implications of emissions should be prominent in climate deliberations and policy (Singh, 2012), and also integrated into legal frameworks and governance to improve public health infrastructure and mechanisms (Wiley, 2010). Shortcomings in these worsened Hurricane Katrina's impacts on the most vulnerable in 2005, but bioethicists resisted probing interests in preserving our "fragile and increasingly ailing planet" (Moreno, 2005, W19). With few exceptions, mainstream bioethics continues to resist investigation of collective interests and common goods despite its grounding in the search, across diverse groups and conflicting ideologies, for common values and interests that bear on dynamics between environments and health (Whitehouse, 2003).

Conclusion

Activities involving industrial energy release emissions that cause climate change. Emissions are health determinants that affect individuals and populations through relationships of many sorts, and that impact and harm health differently in different environments. Public health ethics helps advance deliberations about whether, when, and how to reduce health harms and threats, including those of emissions. It can deepen understanding among policymakers and other stakeholders about values that influence policy goals and targets, and help nurture concepts of growth and development that are compatible with the preservation of natural environments that sustain health and wellbeing.

References

Auerbach, P. S. 2008. "Physicians and the Environment." *JAMA* 299(8): 956–958.

Bajgoric, S., Appiah, J., Wass, V., and Shelton, C. 2014. "Sustainability in Clinical Skills Teaching." *The Clinical Teacher* 11(4): 243–246.

Baylis, F., Kenny, N. P., and Sherwin, S. 2008. "A Relational Account of Public Health Ethics." *Public Health Ethics* 1(3): 196–209.

Buchholz, R. A. 1998. "The Ethics of Consumption Activities: A Future Paradigm?" *Journal of Business Ethics* 17(8): 871–882.

Bushell, S., Colley, T., and Workman, M. 2015. "A Unified Narrative for Climate Change." *Nature Climate Change* 5(11): 971–973.

Callahan, D. 2009. "Ethics and Population." *Hastings Center Report* 39(3): 11–13.

Caney, S. 2010. "Climate Change, Human Rights, and Moral Thresholds." In *Climate Ethics: Essential Readings* (New York: Oxford University Press).

Capps, B., Bailey, M. M., Bickford, D., Coker, R., Lederman, Z., Lover, A., et al. 2015. "Introducing One Health to the Ethical Debate about Zoonotic Diseases in Southeast Asia." *Bioethics* 29(8): 588–596.

Chivian, E. 2014. "Why Doctors and their Organisations Must Help Tackle Climate Change: An Essay by Eric Chivian." *BMJ* 348: g2407. http://www.bmj.com/content/348/bmj.g2407.full.

Churchill, L. R. 2002. "What Ethics Can Contribute to Health Policy." In *Ethical Dimensions of Health Policy* (New York: Oxford University Press).

Costello, A., Abbas, M., Allen, A., Ball, S., Bell, S., Bellamy, R., et al. 2009. "Managing the Health Effects of Climate Change." *Lancet* 373(9676): 1693–1733.

Daniels, N. 2006. "Equity and Population Health: Towards a Broader Bioethics Agenda." *Hastings Center Report* 36(4): 22–35.

Dawson, A. 2010. "The Future of Bioethics: Three Dogmas and a Cup of Hemlock." *Bioethics* 24(5): 218–225.

Dawson, A., and Verweij, M. 2015. "Public Health: Beyond the Role of the State." *Public Health Ethics* 8(1): 1–3.

Dupras, C., and Ravitsky, V. 2016. "Epigenetics in the Neoliberal 'Regime of Truth.'" *Hastings Center Report* 46(1): 26–35.

Dupras, C., Ravitsky, V., and Williams-Jones, B. 2014. "Epigenetics and the Environment in Bioethics." *Bioethics* 28(7): 327–334.

Dwyer, J. 2005. "Global Health and Justice." *Bioethics* 19(5–6): 460–475.

Dwyer, J. 2009. "How to Connect Bioethics and Environmental Ethics: Health, Sustainability, and Justice." *Bioethics* 23(9): 497–502.

Eckenwiler, L., Straehle, C., and Chung, R. 2012. "Global Solidarity, Migration and Global Health Inequity." *Bioethics* 26(7): 382–390.

Ehrlich, P. R. 2009. "Ecoethics: Now Central to All Ethics." *Journal of Bioethical Inquiry* 6(4): 417–436.

Ehrlich, P. R., and Harte, J. 2015. "Biophysical Limits, Women's Rights and the Climate Encyclical." *Nature Climate Change* 5(10): 904–905.

Evans, J. H., and Feng, J. 2013. "Conservative Protestantism and Skepticism of Scientists Studying Climate Change." *Climatic Change* 121(4): 595–608.

Faden, R., and Shebaya, S. 2015. "Public Health Ethics." In *The Stanford Encyclopedia of Philosophy*, edited by Edward N. Zalta (Stanford, Calif: Stanford University). http://plato.stanford.edu/archives/spr2015/entries/publichealth-ethics/.

Farrell, J. 2016. "Corporate Funding and Ideological Polarization about Climate Change." *Proceedings of the National Academy of Sciences* 113(1): 92–97.

Fischer, M., and Staples, J. E. 2014. "Notes from the Field: Chikungunya Virus Spreads in the Americas—Caribbean and South America, 2013–2014." *Morbidity and Mortality Weekly Report* 63 (22): 500–501.

Frumkin, H., Hess, J., Luber, G., Malilay, J., and McGeehin, M. 2008. "Climate Change: The Public Health Response." *American Journal of Public Health* 98(3): 435–445.

Frumkin, H., and McMichael, A. J. 2008. "Climate Change and Public Health." *American Journal of Preventive Medicine* 35(5): 403–410.

Global Policy Forum. 2016. "The Privatization of Global Governance: Corporate Influence on the UN." https://www.globalpolicy.org/corporate-influence.html.

Gómez, A., Balsari, S., Nusbaum, J., Heerboth, A. and Lemery, J., 2013. "Perspective: Environment, Biodiversity, and the Education of the Physician of the Future." *Academic Medicine* 88(2): 168–172.

Gopichandran, V., and Dawson, A. 2016. "Ethics and the Impact of Climate Change in South Asia." In *Bioethical Insights into Values and Policy: Climate Change and Health*, edited by C. C. Macpherson, 103–113 (New York: Springer Press).

Gruen, L., and Ruddick, W. 2009. "Biomedical and Environmental Ethics Alliance: Common Causes and Grounds." *Journal of Bioethical Inquiry* 6(4): 457–466.

Haines, A., Smith, K. R., Anderson, D., Epstein, P. R., McMichael, A. J., Roberts, I., et al. 2007. "Policies for Accelerating Access to Clean Energy, Improving Health, Advancing Development, and Mitigating Climate Change." *Lancet* 370(9594): 1264–1281.

Harvey, M., and Pilgrim, S. 2011. "The New Competition for Land: Food, Energy, and Climate Change." *Food Policy* 36: S40–S51.

Herring, S. C., Hoerling, M. P., Peterson, T. C., and Stott, P. A. 2014. "Explaining Extreme Events of 2013 from a Climate Perspective." *Bulletin of the American Meteorological Society* 95(9): S1–S104.

Holland, A. 2006. "Must We Give Up Environmental Ethics?" In *Environmental Ethics and International Policy*, edited by H. ten Have, 119–143 (Paris: UNESCO Publishing).

Hourdequin, M. 2010. "Climate, Collective Action and Individual Ethical Obligations." *Environmental Values* 19(4): 443–464.

Hutchins, D. C. J., and White, S. M. 2009. "Coming Round to Recycling." *BMJ* 338: b609. http://www.bmj.com/content/338/bmj.b609.

Jamieson, D. 2014. *Reason in a Dark Time: Why the Struggle against Climate Change Failed—And What It Means for Our Future* (New York: Oxford University Press).

Jarvis, L., Montgomery, H., Morisetti, N., and Gilmore, I. 2011. "Climate Change, Ill Health, and Conflict." *BMJ* 342: 777–778.

Jennings, B. 2015. "Relational Liberty Revisited: Membership, Solidarity and a Public Health Ethics of Place." *Public Health Ethics* 8(1): 7–17.

Jennings, B., and Dawson, A. 2015. "SOLIDARITY in the Moral Imagination of Bioethics." *Hastings Center Report* 45(5): 31–38.

Kingston, E. 2014. "Climate Change as a Three-Part Ethical Problem: A Response to Jamieson and Gardiner." *Science and Engineering Ethics* 20(4): 1129–1148.

Kinney, P. L. 2008. "Climate Change, Air Quality, and Human Health." *American Journal of Preventive Medicine* 35(5): 459–467.

Kwakye, G., Pronovost, P. J., and Makary, M. A. 2010. "Commentary: A Call to Go Green in Health Care by Reprocessing Medical Equipment." *Academic Medicine* 85(3): 398–400.

Levy, B. S., and Sidel, V. W. 2014. "Collective Violence Caused by Climate Change and How it Threatens Health and Human Rights." *Health and Human Rights International Journal* 16(1): 32–40.

MacPherson, C. C. 2009. "Time for Physicians to Take Action on Climate Change." *Academic Medicine* 84(7): 817.

Macpherson, C. C. 2013a. "Climate Change Is a Bioethics Problem." *Bioethics* 27(6): 305–308.
Macpherson, C. C. 2013b. "Climate Change Matters." *Journal of Medical Ethics* 40: 288–290.
Macpherson, C. C. 2016. "Why Bioethics Should Address Climate Change and How It Might Do So." In *Bioethical Insights into Values and Policy: Climate Change and Health*, edited by C. C. Macpherson, 199–216 (New York: Springer Press).
Macpherson, C. C., and Akpinar-Elci, M. 2015. "Caribbean Heat Threatens Health, Well-Being and the Future of Humanity." *Public Health Ethics* 8(2): 196–208.
Macpherson, C. C., Bidaisee, S., and Macpherson, C. N. L. 2016. "Environmental Harms in Distant Polar Regions and Small Island Developing States." In *Bioethical Insights into Values and Policy: Climate Change and Health*, edited by C. C. Macpherson, 127–142 (New York: Springer Press).
Maibach, E. W., Chadwick, A., McBride, D., Chuk, M., Ebi, K. L., and Balbus, J. 2008. "Climate Change and Local Public Health in the United States: Preparedness, Programs and Perceptions of Local Public Health Department Directors." *PLoS ONE* 3(7): e2838.
Mann, M. E., and Gleick, P. H. 2015. "Climate Change and California Drought in the 21st Century." *Proceedings of the National Academy of Sciences* 112(13): 3858–3859. http://www.pnas.org/content/112/13/3858.
Markowitz, E. M., and Shariff, A. F. 2012. "Climate Change and Moral Judgement." *Nature Climate Change* 2(4): 243–247.
Maughan, D., Berry, H., and Davison, P. 2014. "What Psychiatrists Should Know about Environmental Sustainability and What They Should Be Doing about It." *International Psychiatry* 11(2): 27–30.
McMichael, A. J., Friel, S., Nyong, A., and Corvalan. C. 2008. "Global Environmental Change and Health: Impacts, Inequalities, and the Health Sector." *BMJ* 336: 191. https://www.bmj.com/content/336/7637/191.
McMichael, A. J., Woodruff, R. E., and Hales, S. 2006. "Climate Change and Human Health: Present and Future Risks." *Lancet* 367(9513): 859–869.
Meason, B., and Paterson, R. 2014. "Chikungunya, Climate Change, and Human Rights." *Health and Human Rights* 16(1): 105–112.
Metz, T. 2016. "Climate Change in Africa and the Middle East in Light of Health and Salient Regional Values." In *Bioethical Insights into Values and Policy: Climate Change and Health*, edited by C. C. Macpherson, 115–125 (New York: Springer Press).
Moreno, J. D. 2005. "In the Wake of Katrina: Has 'Bioethics' Failed?" *American Journal of Bioethics* 5(5): W18–W19.
Myers, T. A., Maibach, E. Peters, E., and Leiserowitz, A. 2015. "Simple Messages Help Set the Record Straight about Scientific Agreement on Human-Caused Climate Change: The Results of Two Experiments." *PloS ONE* 10(3): e0120985.
NHS SDU (National Health Service Sustainable Development Unit). 2016. "Health and Care System Carbon Footprint." http://www.sduhealth.org.uk/policy-strategy/reporting/hcs-carbon-footprint.aspx.
Nielsen, L. W. 2016. "Climate Change Vulnerability and Health Impacts in South East Asia and China." In *Bioethical Insights into Values and Policy: Climate Change and Health*, edited by C. C. Macpherson, 89–101 (New York: Springer Press).
Patz, J. A., Frumkin, H., Holloway, T., Vimont, D. J., and Haines, A. 2014. "Climate Change: Challenges and Opportunities for Global Health." *JAMA* 312(15): 1565–1580.
Pierce, C., and Kerby, J. 1999. "The Global Ethics of Latex Gloves: Reflections on Natural Resource Use in Healthcare." *Cambridge Quarterly of Healthcare Ethics* 8(1): 98–107.

Pierce, J. 2009. "Environmental Bioethics: A Manifesto." *Health After Oil*, November 13. https://healthafteroil.wordpress.com/2009/11/13/environmental-bioethics%E2%80%94a-manifesto/.

Popkin, B. M. 2009. "Reducing Meat Consumption Has Multiple Benefits for the World's Health." *Archives of Internal Medicine* 169(6): 543–545.

Potter, V. R. 1971. *Global Bioethics: Bridge to the Future* (Englewood Cliffs, N.J.: Prentice Hall).

Resnik, D. B. 2012. *Environmental Health Ethics* (New York: Cambridge University Press).

Richie, C. 2014. "What Would an Environmentally Sustainable Reproductive Technology Industry Look Like?" *Journal of Medical Ethics* 41(5): 383–387.

Roberts, I., and Stott, R. 2010. "Doctors and Climate Change." *BMJ* 341: c6357.

Rogers, W. A. 2006. "Feminism and Public Health Ethics." *Journal of Medical Ethics* 32(6): 351–354.

Rothausen, S. G. S. A., and Conway, D. 2011. "Greenhouse-Gas Emissions from Energy Use in the Water Sector." *Nature Climate Change* 1(4): 210–219.

Rozier, M. D. 2015. "Structures of Virtue as a Framework for Public Health Ethics." *Public Health Ethics* 9(1): 37–45.

Ruger, J. P. 2015. "Good Medical Ethics, Justice and Provincial Globalism." *Journal of Medical Ethics* 41(1): 103–106.

Sadler, B. L. 2015. "Why Health Care Is Going Green." *Hastings Center Report* 45(4): 51.

Sadler, B. L., Berry, L. L., Guenther, R., Hamilton, D., Hessler, F. A., Merritt, C., et al. 2011. "Fable Hospital 2.0: The Business Case for Building Better Health Care Facilities." *Hastings Center Report* 41(1): 13–23.

Schmidt, V. H. 2014. "Public Health Ethics: Problems and Suggestions." *Public Health Ethics* 8(1): 18–26.

Schultz, P. W. 2011. "Conservation Means Behavior." *Conservation Biology* 25(6): 1080–1083.

Scott, C. A., Pierce, S. A., Pasqualetti, M. J., Jones, A. L., Montz, B. E., and Hoover, J. H. 2011. "Policy and Institutional Dimensions of the Water-Energy Nexus." *Energy Policy* 39(10): 6622–6630.

Shomaker, T. S., Green, E. M., and Yandow, S. M. 2013. "Perspective: One Health; A Compelling Convergence." *Academic Medicine* 88(1): 49–55.

Singer, P. 2011. *Practical Ethics*. 3rd ed. (New York: Cambridge University Press).

Singh, Jerome A. 2012 "Why Human Health and Health Ethics Must Be Central to Climate Change Deliberations." *PLoS Medicine* 9(6): e1001229. doi:10.1371/journal.pmed.1001229.

Syrett, K. 2015. "Comment on Jennings, 'Right Relation and Right Recognition in Public Health Ethics: Thinking through the Republic of Health.'" *Public Health Ethics* 9(2): 180–182.

ten Have, H. A. M. J. 2012. "Potter's Notion of Bioethics." *Kennedy Institute of Ethics Journal* 22(1): 59–82.

Thompson, P. B., and List, M. 2015. "Ebola Needs One Bioethics." *Ethics, Policy & Environment* 18(1): 96–102.

UNDP (United Nations Development Programme). 2015. "Sustainable Development Goals: Life Below Water." http://www.undp.org/content/undp/en/home/sustainable-development-goals/goal-14-life-below-water.html.

UNEP (United Nations Environment Programme). 2005. "CO2 Emissions, Energy Use and Economic Development; Latin America and the Caribbean." http://www.grida.no/search?query=co2+emissions+energy+use+and+economic+development+latin+america+and+the+caribbean.

Valles, S. A. 2015. "Bioethics and the Framing of Climate Change's Health Risks." *Bioethics* 29(5): 334–341.

Veatch, R. M. 1972. "Ethics Population Policy and Population Education." *Social Education* 36(4): 363–368.

Verkerk, M. A., and Lindemann, H. 2011. "Theoretical Resources for a Globalised Bioethics." *Journal of Medical Ethics* 37: 92–96.

Walpole, S. C., Pearson, D., Coad, J., and Barna, S. 2016. "What Do Tomorrow's Doctors Need to Learn about Ecosystems?—A BEME Systematic Review: BEME Guide No. 36." *Medical Teacher* 38(4): 338–352.

Wardrope, A. 2015. "Relational Autonomy and the Ethics of Health Promotion." *Public Health Ethics* 8(1): 50–62.

Watts, N., Adger, W. N., Agnolucci, P., Blackstock, J., Byass, P., Cai, W., et al. 2015. "Health and Climate Change: Policy Responses to Protect Public Health." *Lancet* 386(10006): 1861–1914.

Whitehouse, P. J. 2002. "Van Rensselaer Potter: An Intellectual Memoir." *Cambridge Quarterly of Healthcare Ethics* 11(4): 331–334.

Whitehouse, P. J. 2003. "The Rebirth of Bioethics: Extending the Original Formulations of Van Rensselaer Potter." *American Journal of Bioethics* 3(4): 26–31.

Whitehouse, P. J., and Fishman, J. R. 2004. "Justice and the House of Medicine: The Mortgaging of Ecology and Economics." *American Journal of Bioethics* 4(2): 43–45.

WHO (World Health Organization). 2015. "Climate Change and Human Health: Land Degradation and Desertification." http://www.who.int/globalchange/ecosystems/desert/en/.

WHO (World Health Organization). 2016. "Health Impact Assessment: The Determinants of Health." http://www.who.int/hia/evidence/doh/en/.

Wiley, L. F. 2010. "Mitigation/Adaptation and Health: Health Policymaking in the Global Response to Climate Change and Implications for Other Upstream Determinants." *Journal of Law, Medicine & Ethics* 38(3): 629–639.

Zycher, B. 2015. "The Strange Silence about Climate Policy and the Looming Apocalypse." American Enterprise Institute, *Inside Sources*, September 29. https://www.aei.org/publication/the-strange-silence-about-climate-policy-and-the-looming-apocalypse/.

Further Readings

Gardiner, S., Caney, S., Jamieson, D., and Shue, H., eds. 2010. *Climate Ethics: Essential Readings* (New York: Oxford University Press).

Jamieson, D. 2014. *Reason in a Dark Time: Why the Struggle against Climate Change Failed—And What It Means for Our Future* (New York: Oxford University Press).

Kolstad C., Urama, K., Broome, J., Bruvoll, A., Olvera, M. C., Fullerton, D., et al. 2014. "Social, Economic and Ethical Concepts and Methods." In *Climate Change 2014: Mitigation of Climate Change. Contribution of Working Group III to the Fifth Assessment Report of the Intergovernmental Panel on Climate Change*, edited by O. Edenhofer, R. Pichs-Madruga, Y. Sokona, E. Farahani, S. Kadner, K. Seyboth, et al. (Cambridge: Cambridge University Press). https://www.ipcc.ch/pdf/assessment-report/ar5/wg3/ipcc_wg3_ar5_chapter3.pdf.

Macpherson, C. C., ed. 2016. *Bioethical Insights into Values and Policy: Climate Change and Health* (New York: Springer).

Schor, J. B. 2010. *Plenitude: The New Economics of True Wealth* (New York: Penguin).

CHAPTER 64

ENVIRONMENTAL HEALTH RESEARCH AND ETHICS

DAVID B. RESNIK

Introduction

Scientific research enhances our understanding of the relationship between human health and the environment and aids in the development of interventions or policies that can improve environmental health. Environmental health research raises a number of different ethical issues, ranging from scientific integrity issues to animal and human subjects issues (Resnik, 2012; Shamoo and Resnik, 2015). This chapter will focus on some of the ethical issues that arise in environmental health research involving human participants. Common research designs for conducting environmental health research with human subjects include observational studies (e.g., prospective cohort studies, retrospective case-control studies), interventional studies (e.g., clinical trials), and intentional exposure studies (Resnik, 2012). The chapter will consider some of the ethical issues related to these study designs, as well as some that cut across different designs, such as returning individualized research results, safeguarding privacy and confidentiality, and protecting vulnerable human subjects.

Background on Ethics and Regulations

To understand the ethical issues related to environmental health research with human subjects, it will be useful to understand the ethical and legal standards that apply to research with human participants, which are embodied or reflected in federal regulations (e.g., HHS, 2009, 2017; EPA, 2013), international codes (e.g., ORI, 2019; WMA, 2013), government reports (National Commission, 1979), and agency guidance documents (e.g., OHRP, 2019), a number of which are referenced in the discussion below. These standards embody various ethical principles of research involving human participants, such as sound scientific design, risk minimization, reasonableness of risks, informed consent, and protection of confidentiality and privacy (Emanuel, Wendler, and Grady, 2000). They also require that an independent committee, such an institutional review board (IRB), review and oversee the research.

Cross-Cutting Issues

Returning Individualized Research Results

Environmental health researchers often collect information on participants that they may be interested in receiving, such as the results of clinical examinations or tests, environmental sampling, or genetic/genomic testing. Results may include information that is gathered as part of the study, or they may include information that investigators happen to discover (i.e., incidental findings). In some cases, this information may have a direct bearing on the participant's health. For example, if an investigator discovers that a participant has dangerously high blood pressure, he or she could refer the participant to a physician for treatment. The investigator might even offer emergency treatment to the participant if a problem that requires emergency care is detected and the investigator has the ability to provide that care. In other cases, the information may have no direct relationship to the participant's health and may be difficult to interpret.

Suppose, for example, that researchers are testing environmental samples collected in the home for levels of different flame retardants, but there is no established safe level for a particular retardant. Sharing information about the levels of this retardant in the home with the participant may have little value to the participant and may even lead to needless worry or confusion, especially if the participant has no way of controlling his or her exposure to this chemical (Resnik, 2012). Or suppose that investigators are testing for the presence of a chemical in the home (such as lead) for which there is an established safe level, but they are using a processing laboratory that does not have a good track record of producing accurate and reliable results. If the laboratory incorrectly determines that levels of lead in the samples are safe (false negative), then the participants might fail to take steps to prevent exposure to dangerous levels of lead in the home. If the laboratory incorrectly determines that levels of lead are unsafe (false positive), then the participants might experience needless stress or make a rash decision (such as selling their home). Thus, return of individualized results to participants presents significant ethical dilemmas for environmental health researchers, because providing this information may be beneficial or harmful (Resnik, 2012).

Two divergent views on the return of individualized research results have emerged in the literature. According to the *autonomy approach*, participants should receive all research results that they choose to receive. This approach can benefit participants and promote their ability to make autonomous choices concerning their health or life plans (Fernandez, Kodish, and Weijer, 2003; Brody et al., 2007). Proponents of this approach recommend that the consent form provide participants with information about the results they may choose to receive and when they will be available. The research proposal should include plans to provide participants with guidance on how to understand and use their results, including plans for medical referrals, if appropriate (Brody et al., 2007). To ensure that results are reliable and accurate, testing should be done in certified laboratories or using test kits that have been validated and approved for marketing (President's Commission, 2013).

According to the *harm-avoidance approach*, however, participants should receive only those results that have a well-established practical value, such as information that can be used to prevent or treat disease, or to guide choices concerning reproduction or life plans (Wolf et al., 2008; Resnik, 2011). The obligation to do no harm provides the main justification for this approach, since returning results that have no established practical value may cause participants needless worry and may lead them to make unwise choices, such as selling their home because they wrongly assume that it is unsafe (Resnik, 2011). Another reason why some recommend this approach is that returning results without established practical value increases the costs of the study unnecessarily (Wolf et al., 2008). Bioethicists, scientists, and professional associations continue to debate the merits of different approaches to returning research results (President's Commission, 2013).

An important legal ruling helped establish the legal duty to return research results relevant to preventing or treating disease. During the early 1990s, the Kennedy Krieger Institute (KKI), an affiliate of Johns Hopkins University, conducted a study funded by the US Environmental Protection Agency (EPA) and the Centers for Disease Control and Prevention (CDC) to determine whether less expensive forms of lead abatement are as effective at preventing exposures to lead in the home as full lead abatement. The investigators were interested in learning whether these less expensive forms of lead abatement can significantly reduce exposures, because full lead abatement can be expensive ($10,000 or more per home). Baltimore city leaders were concerned that landlords would abandon their homes to avoid paying the full price of lead abatement, which would have an adverse impact on the community. The study recruited families with young children who were living in homes containing lead paint on interior walls. Homes were randomly assigned to receive $1,650, $3,500, or $6,000–$7,000 worth of lead abatement. The study also included a control group consisting of homes with full lead abatement and another consisting of homes without interior lead paint. Twenty-five families participated in the study—five in each group. Investigators measured levels of lead in the children's blood and in dust, soil, and water samples collected from the homes.

The investigators helped the landlords obtain grants to pay for lead abatement and encouraged them to rent their homes to families with young children. The study included plans to inform the families of dangerous lead levels, but the consent document did not warn families that children might accumulate dangerous levels of lead as a result of continuing to live in a home undergoing lead abatement. Two of the families sued the investigators and KKI, alleging that they were not informed of dangerous lead levels in a timely manner. Viola Hughes, the mother of Ericka Grimes, alleged that she was not informed that her daughter's blood contained dangerous lead levels until nine months after these levels were detected. The court found that the investigators could be sued for negligence on the basis that they had failed to inform the parents of dangerous lead levels in a timely fashion (*Grimes v. Kennedy Krieger Institute*, 2001). Although the legal duty to return clinically useful research results appears to be well established, it is not clear whether researchers have a legal duty to return results that are not clinically useful.

Protecting Privacy and Confidentiality

Environmental health researchers often collect data and samples in homes or workplaces, which raises issues concerning the protection of confidentiality and privacy. For example, researchers conducting a study in the home may inadvertently observe evidence of child or elder abuse/neglect, domestic violence, or illegal activity (such as the sale or possession of illegal drugs). Although investigators have an ethical obligation to protect the confidentiality and privacy of research participants, they have legal and ethical duties to report child or elder abuse. While protecting privacy and confidentiality is important, one might argue that investigators should override this obligation in order to protect vulnerable residents of the home (such as children or frail elderly people) from harm.

Investigators should inform participants of their obligations to report suspected child or elder abuse and establish procedures for research staff to follow when evidence of abuse is discovered. Staff should also be trained in how to collect data and samples in a domestic setting without invading privacy unnecessarily. Likewise, investigators who are collecting data or samples in the workplace may observe violations of health and safety standards, worker harassment/abuse, or other problems. While protecting the employer's confidentiality and privacy is important, investigators may override this obligation in order to protect employees from imminent harm. They should inform employers of any plans to report dangerous conditions that they happen to observe, and also establish procedures for research staff to follow (Resnik, 2012).

Protecting Vulnerable Participants

Environmental health research often includes vulnerable participants, or people who have a compromised ability to provide informed consent or protect their own interests (Levine et al. 2004). Federal research regulations include additional protections for specific classes of vulnerable participants, including children, fetuses, neonates, and prisoners. For example, the regulations limit the risks that children, fetuses, neonates, and prisoners can be exposed to in research that does not benefit them directly (HHS, 2009). The main rationale for special safeguards is that vulnerable subjects have a compromised ability to make autonomous choices concerning their risk exposure, due to their lack of decision-making capacity or susceptibility to coercion or undue influence, and thus need additional protection from harm (Levine et al., 2004).[1] For several decades the US research regulations classified pregnant women as vulnerable subjects, but recent changes have made it clear that fetuses, not pregnant women, are vulnerable (HHS, 2017; Resnik, 2018).

A controversial environmental health research project has raised key issues concerning the protection of vulnerable participants. The Children's Environmental Exposure Research Study (CHEERS) was a research project sponsored by the EPA, the CDC, and the Duvall County (Florida) Health Department, in which investigators planned to observe children's in-home exposures to pesticides and other chemicals. The American Chemistry Council (ACC) also contributed money to the project. The investigators planned to recruit sixty families with children who used high levels of pesticides in their homes, as well as a control group of ten families who used a low level of pesticides or none at all. The investigators planned to visit the homes thirty times over a two-year period. During these three-hour visits, the investigators would collect soil and dust samples and blood and urine from the children. The parents would play an active role in the study by keeping a journal of their pesticide and chemical use and videotaping their children's activities. For their efforts, the parents would receive a free video camera and $970. The investigators planned to inform the parents about safe use of pesticides and inform them of unsafe levels of pesticides (or other chemicals) detected in the home or the children's blood or urine. The families could remain in the study even if they reduced their pesticide use, and they could withdraw at any time without penalty (Resnik and Wing, 2007).

The investigators planned to implement the study in fall of 2004, but they put the study on hold when a public controversy erupted. Critics charged that the study intentionally exposed children to pesticides, targeted low-income minority groups, offered the participants too much money, and was tainted by industry bias. The EPA terminated the study in the spring of 2005 after Senator Barbara Boxer of California threatened to derail Stephen Johnson's nomination as EPA Administrator if the agency did not cancel it (Resnik and Wing, 2007). The charges brought by the critics lacked merit, however. First, the study was an observational study, not an intentional exposure study. The study even included a screening procedure to ensure that parents would not begin using pesticides in order to qualify for the study. After obtaining consent from the parents, the investigators would immediately visit the home to determine their level of pesticide use. If the sample analysis indicated they already used high levels of pesticides, they might qualify for enrollment in this group; if not, they might qualify for the control group.

Second, the study did not target low-income minority groups, as none of the enrollment criteria mentioned race, ethnicity, or income. The main reason for selecting Duvall

County as the research site was that investigators already knew that many residents in the area used high levels of pesticides in the home to deal with roaches, rodents, and other pests. Third, the amount of money offered to the participants may have seemed high, but it would have been less than the federal minimum wage when one considers that the parents would contribute about 150 hours of their time to the study. Fourth, although the ACC helped support the study, it had no role in planning or implementing the project. Still, although the study was scientifically and ethically sound, the investigators could have done more to enhance its public perception by working more closely with members of the local community on recruitment, publicity, and other issues (Resnik and Wing, 2007).

One of the results of the CHEERS controversy is that the EPA adopted human research regulations that prohibit the agency from funding intentional exposure studies involving children or pregnant or nursing women (EPA, 2013). The EPA adopted these rules in response to a congressional mandate that the agency not fund pesticide experiments involving those populations (Resnik, 2007a). One might argue, however, that the EPA went too far in protecting children, fetuses, and infants from harm, because the regulations prohibit the agency from conducting or sponsoring intentional exposures studies that present no more than a minimal risk to participants.[2] For example, children are often exposed to sunscreens and insect repellants in their daily lives. It would be important for promoting children's health to have a better understanding of how these chemicals interact with children's anatomy and physiology at exposure levels that children often encounter, yet the EPA cannot fund such research (Resnik, 2007a). The regulations also prevent the EPA from collaborating with institutions that are conducting controlled trials of medications used to prevent or treat environment-related health problems (such as asthma), because these studies involve intentional exposures (Resnik, 2007a). It is ironic that advocates for children's health, who pressured the EPA into banning intentional exposure studies involving children or pregnant or nursing women, may have inadvertently undermined the health of these groups.

The debate over including children or pregnant or nursing women in intentional exposure studies illustrates a perennial issue related to protecting vulnerable research participants; namely, the dilemma between underprotection and overprotection (Mastroianni and Kahn, 2001). While it is important to protect vulnerable research participants from harm or exploitation, excluding them from studies may adversely impact their interests, because it may prevent researchers from conducting research that can benefit their health. For example, most drugs are prescribed to children and pregnant women on an off-label basis because these groups have been routinely excluded from clinical trials of new drugs (Resnik, 2007a; Schonfeld, 2013). Excluding children and pregnant women from drug studies can prevent researchers and clinicians from obtaining the knowledge that is needed for safe and effective prescribing. Environmental health researchers and the committees that oversee their studies need to carefully consider whether it is appropriate to include or exclude vulnerable participants, taking into account the need to protect these individuals from harm or exploitation and the potential public health benefits of inclusion.

Design-Related Issues

Research on Environmental Interventions

Interventional studies, such as the KKI study, attempt to determine the effectiveness of an intervention in treating, preventing, or mitigating an environmental health problem. In randomized controlled trials (RCTs), participants are randomly assigned to either the group that receives the intervention or a control group. In some cases, the control group may receive a placebo to control for bias due to the placebo effect. While RCTs in clinical medicine study the effectiveness of medical interventions (such as drugs or devices), RCTs in environmental health study the effectiveness of environmental interventions, such as lead or mold remediation, mosquito control, sanitation, or water purification (Allen, Barn, and Lanphear, 2015).

One of the key ethical issues in clinical trial design is whether patients/participants in a control group should ever receive an intervention thought to be ineffective (such as a placebo) when a therapy for the condition is known to be effective. Numerous writers have argued that it is unethical to include placebo control groups in clinical trials when a therapy is known to be effective at treating the condition under investigation, because this trial design violates the physician's obligation to provide optimal medical care for his or her patients. Placebos may only be used when no therapy is known to be effective for a condition (Miller and Weijer, 2007). Others have argued that it can be ethical to include a placebo control group in a clinical trial when a therapy is known to be effective if the participants consent to the study and withholding therapy does not cause them significant, long-term harm (Miller and Brody, 2007). Similar issues arise when patients/participants in a clinical trial are given a therapy thought to be suboptimal when an optimal therapy is available.

In the KKI study, participants in the experimental groups lived in homes that did not receive full lead abatement, even though full lead abatement was known to be effective at preventing lead exposure. Some argued that the study was unethical because the three experimental groups did not receive full lead abatement (Spriggs, 2004). Others argued that the study was ethical because it did not impose significant risks on participants in the experimental groups and it offered them partial lead abatement, which is a significant benefit. The study also benefitted the residents of Baltimore who were living in homes containing interior lead paint because it demonstrated that partial lead abatement can be effective at preventing lead exposure (Buchanan and Miller, 2006).

An important factual issue is whether the participants in the experimental groups were already living in homes with lead paint before the study began, since it appears that some residents moved into the partially abated homes when they joined the study (Nelson, 2001). If the participants in the experimental groups were already living in homes with lead paint, then the study would impose only minimal risks on them (e.g., the risk of the blood draw), since they were already exposed to lead. However, if they moved into homes with lead paint in order to join the study, then this would impose more than minimal risks on participants, since the risks would include the risk of lead exposure. One could argue that the benefits of the study would not outweigh the risks if the participants were not already living in homes with lead paint.

The debate about withholding effective environmental health interventions in controlled experiments parallels, in some ways, the debate about using placebo control groups in clinical trials (Allen, Barn, and Lanphear, 2015). However, it is important to note that clinical trials are different from environmental intervention experiments, because the investigators in clinical trials are typically physicians who have ethical obligations to provide optimal care to their patient/participants, whereas the investigators in environmental intervention studies usually do not have physician-patient relationships with the participants (Resnik, 2012). Nevertheless, one might maintain that environmental health researchers are still obligated to benefit study participants and treat them fairly (Resnik, 2008).

Intentional Exposure Studies

Environmental health researchers sometimes conduct studies in which human participants are intentionally exposed to an environmental agent (such as a chemical or allergen) in order to better understand the health effects of the agent. Although animal experiments, in vitro cell and tissue studies, and human observational studies can produce useful knowledge concerning the health impacts of environmental agents, they often do not provide researchers with precise knowledge concerning human health effects and causal mechanisms. Intentional exposure studies can help close this knowledge gap (Resnik, 2007b). For example, the EPA's National Exposure Research Laboratory conducts research that exposes human participants to air pollutants, such as ozone or diesel exhaust, in a controlled setting. The exposure takes place in a sealed chamber in which participants breathe air with a controlled dose of pollutant. The air in the chamber is safe to breathe for a limited time (Resnik, 2007b). The participants may also be asked to perform activities that involve moderate physical exertion. The investigators collect samples and data before and after the exposure and carefully monitor the participants during the study. Participants usually undergo a bronchoscopy after the exposure to allow investigators to collect tissue from the respiratory tract (Resnik, 2007b).

The main ethical issue pertaining to intentional exposure studies is whether the risks to the participants are acceptable in relation to the expected benefits (Resnik, 2007b; London et al., 2010). While investigators can take steps to minimize risks, participants may still face significant risks in some studies. For example, the main risks of the EPA's air pollution studies are associated with breathing polluted air for a short time and the bronchoscopy. While exposure to polluted air for a short time poses a minimal risk for a healthy volunteer, a bronchoscopy can lead to respiratory irritation, mild bleeding, and, in rare cases, a pneumothorax, a condition in which gas collects around the lungs. However, these problems usually resolve themselves or can be easily treated

(NHLBI, 2012). Proponents of intentional exposure studies argue that they yield valuable information that cannot be obtained by other means. This information can be useful in developing interventions or regulations to protect people from the harmful effects of air pollution (Resnik, 2007b).

Recent controversial intentional exposure studies included a dozen or so experiments conducted by private companies during the 1990s that exposed human participants to small quantities of pesticides (London et al., 2010). In some experiments, the investigators gave the participants a drink laced with pesticides; in others, they placed pesticides on the participants' skin. Following exposure to the chemical, the investigators collected and analyzed the participants' blood and urine to better understand how the body metabolizes and eliminates the chemical. The companies conducted the experiments in order to submit data to the EPA to convince the agency to increase the allowable level of pesticide residue on foods. Private companies and commercial farmers were concerned that the lower levels of allowable pesticide residues mandated by the Food Quality Protection Act of 1996 would be ineffective at controlling weeds and pests.

Critics objected to these experiments on the grounds that they benefitted the pesticide companies but not society. They also argued that the experiments were underpowered—some studies had as few as twenty-five participants—which meant that the experiments might not be able to detect statistically significant adverse effects. Moreover, some of the experiments used company employees as participants, which was potentially coercive (Lockwood, 2004; London et al., 2010). While the majority of commentators agree that most of these particular studies were flawed, some have argued that some types of human pesticide experiments would be acceptable if they meet rigorous scientific and ethical standards. Human pesticide experiments might provide government agencies or health care professionals with information they could use to protect public health (NRC, 2004; Resnik and Portier, 2005).

Conclusion

Environmental health research involving human participants raises ethical issues pertaining to such topics as returning individualized research results, safeguarding privacy and confidentiality, conducting interventional or intentional exposure studies, and protecting vulnerable participants. Environmental health researchers and oversight committees need to be aware of these issues and take appropriate measures to ensure that research meets ethical and scientific standards.

Acknowledgments

This research was supported by the Intramural Program of the National Institute of Environmental Health Sciences (NIEHS), National Institutes of Health (NIH). It does not represent the view of the NIEHS, NIH, or US government.

NOTES

1. US federal regulations have classified pregnant women as vulnerable subjects even though adult women are normally fully capable of making autonomous decisions. Pregnant women are treated as vulnerable subjects due to the vulnerability of the fetus. Regulatory revisions issued in 2017 (and intended to take effect in 2018) remove pregnant women from that classification (HHS, 2017).
2. US federal regulations define *minimal risk* as when "the probability and magnitude of harm or discomfort anticipated in the research are not greater in and of themselves than those ordinarily encountered in daily life or during the performance of routine physical or psychological examinations or tests" (HHS, 2009, 45 CFR 46.102i).

REFERENCES

Allen, R. W., Barn, P. K., and Lanphear, B. P. 2015. "Randomized Controlled Trials in Environmental Health Research: Unethical or Underutilized?" *PLoS Medicine* 12(1): e1001775.

Brody, J. G., Morello-Frosch, R., Brown, P., Rudel, R. A., Altman, R. G., Frye, M., et al. 2007. "Improving Disclosure and Consent: 'Is it Safe?': New Ethics for Reporting Personal Exposures to Environmental Chemicals." *American Journal of Public Health* 97(9): 1547–1554.

Buchanan, D. R., and Miller, F. G. 2006. "Justice and Fairness in the Kennedy Krieger Institute Lead Paint Study: The Ethics of Public Health Research on Less Expensive, Less Effective Interventions." *American Journal of Public Health* 96(5): 781–787.

Emanuel, E., Wendler, D., and Grady, C. 2000. "What Makes Clinical Research Ethical?" *Journal of the American Medical Association* 283(20): 2701–2711.

EPA (Environmental Protection Agency). 2013. 40 CFR 26, "Protection of Human Subjects." https://www.law.cornell.edu/cfr/text/40/part-26.

Fernandez, C. V., Kodish, E., and Weijer, C. 2003. "Informing Study Participants of Research Results: An Ethical Imperative." *IRB* 25(3): 12–19.

Grimes v. Kennedy Krieger Institute, Md. Ct. App., 366 Md. 29, 782 A.2d 807 (2001).

HHS (US Department of Health and Human Services). 2009. Protection of Human Subjects. 45 CFR 46. https://www.hhs.gov/ohrp/regulations-and-policy/regulations/45-cfr-46/index.html.

HHS (US Department of Health and Human Services). 2017. "Federal Policy for the Protection of Human Subjects." *Federal Register* 82(12): 7149–7274.

Levine, C., Faden, R., Grady, C., Hammerschmidt, D., Eckenwiler, L., and Sugarman, J. 2004. "The Limitations of 'Vulnerability' as a Protection for Human Research Participants." *American Journal of Bioethics* 4(3): 44–49.

Lockwood, A. H. 2004. "Human Testing of Pesticides: Ethical and Scientific Considerations." *American Journal of Public Health* 94(11): 1908–1916.

London, L., Coggon, D., Moretto, A., Westerholm, P., Wilks, M. F., and Colosio, C. 2010. "The Ethics of Human Volunteer Studies Involving Experimental Exposure to Pesticides: Unanswered Dilemmas." *Environmental Health* 9: 50. https://ehjournal.biomedcentral.com/articles/10.1186/1476-069X-9-50.

Mastroianni, A., and Kahn, J. 2001. "Swinging on the Pendulum. Shifting Views of Justice in Human Subjects Research." *Hastings Center Report* 31(3): 21–28.

Miller, F.G., and Brody, H. 2007. "Clinical Equipoise and the Incoherence of Research Ethics." *Journal of Medicine and Philosophy* 32(2): 151–165.

Miller, P. B., and Weijer, C. 2007. "Equipoise and the Duty of Care in Clinical Research: A Philosophical Response to Our Critics." *Journal of Medicine and Philosophy* 32(2): 117–133.

National Commission (National Commission for the Protection of Human Subjects of Biomedical and Behavioral Research). 1979. *The Belmont Report* (Washington, D.C.: Department of Health, Education, and Welfare). https://www.hhs.gov/ohrp/regulations-and-policy/belmont-report/index.html.

Nelson, R. M. 2001. "Nontherapeutic Research, Minimal Risk, and the Kennedy Krieger Lead Abatement Study." *IRB* 23(6): 7–11.

NHLBI (National Heart, Lung, and Blood Institute). 2012. *What Is a Bronchoscopy?* https://www.nhlbi.nih.gov/health/health-topics/topics/bron/risks.

NRC (National Research Council). 2004. *Intentional Human Dosing Studies for EPA Regulatory Purposes: Scientific and Ethical Issues* (Washington, D.C.: National Academies Press).

OHRP (Office of Human Research Protections). 2019. "Regulations, Policy, & Posting." https://www.hhs.gov/ohrp/regulations-and-policy/index.html.

ORI (Office of Research Integrity). 2019. "Nuremberg Code: Directives for Human Experimentation."https://ori.hhs.gov/chapter-3-The-Protection-of-Human-Subjects-nuremberg-code-directives-human-experimentation.

President's Commission (President's Commission for the Study of Bioethical Issues). 2013. *Anticipate and Communicate: Ethical Management of Incidental and Secondary Findings in the Clinical, Research, and Direct-to-Consumer Contexts* (Washington, D.C.: President's Commission). https://bioethicsarchive.georgetown.edu/pcsbi/sites/default/files/FINALAnticipateCommunicate_PCSBI_0.pdf.

Resnik, D. B. 2007a. "Are the New EPA Regulations Concerning Intentional Exposure Studies with Children Overprotective?" *IRB* 29(5): 5–7.

Resnik, D. B. 2007b. "Intentional Exposure Studies of Environmental Agents on Human Subjects: Assessing Benefits and Risks." *Accountability in Research* 14(1):35–55.

Resnik, D. B. 2008. "Randomized Controlled Trials in Environmental Health Research: Ethical Issues." *Journal of Environmental Health* 70(6): 28–30.

Resnik, D. B. 2011. "Disclosure of Individualized Research Results: A Precautionary Approach." *Accountability in Research* 18(6): 382–397.

Resnik, D. B. 2012. *Environmental Health Ethics* (New York: Cambridge University Press).

Resnik, D. B. 2018. *The Ethics of Research with Human Subjects: Protecting People, Advancing Science, Promoting Trust*. Cham, Switzerland: Springer.

Resnik, D. B., and Portier, C. 2005. "Pesticide Testing on Human Subjects: Weighing Benefits and Risks." *Environmental Health Perspectives* 113(7): 813–817.

Resnik, D. B., and Wing, S. 2007. "Lessons Learned from the Children's Environmental Exposure Research Study." *American Journal of Public Health* 97(3): 414–418.

Schonfeld, T. 2013. "The Perils of Protection: Vulnerability and Women in Clinical Research." *Theoretical Medicine and Bioethics* 34(3): 189–206.

Shamoo, A. E., and Resnik, D. B. 2015. *Responsible Conduct of Research*. 3rd ed. (New York: Oxford University Press).

Spriggs, M. 2004. "Canaries in the Mines: Children, Risk, Non-therapeutic Research, and Justice." *Journal of Medical Ethics* 30(2): 176–181.

WMA (World Medical Association). 2013. Declaration of Helsinki, 2013 revision. https://www.wma.net/policies-post/wma-declaration-of-helsinki-ethical-principles-for-medical-research-involving-human-subjects/.

Wolf, S. M., Lawrenz, F. P., Nelson, C. A., Kahn, J. P., Cho, M. K., Clayton, E.W., et al. 2008. "Managing Incidental Findings in Human Subjects Research: Analysis and Recommendations." *Journal of Law, Medicine & Ethics* 36(2): 219–248.

SECTION FOURTEEN

EMERGENCY PREPAREDNESS AND RESPONSE

CHAPTER 65

AN OVERVIEW OF PUBLIC HEALTH ETHICS IN EMERGENCY PREPAREDNESS AND RESPONSE

LESLIE MELTZER HENRY

Introduction

SINCE the beginning of the twenty-first century, a growing number of large-scale events have endangered population health and challenged even the most advanced public health and health care systems. These events—whether classified as bioterrorism, such as the 2001 anthrax attacks; natural disasters, such as the 2004 Indian Ocean tsunami; industrial disasters, such as the 2010 BP Deepwater Horizon oil spill; or infectious disease outbreaks, such as Zika virus—collectively highlight human vulnerability to abrupt, unpredictable, and often uncontrollable threats. Affected populations may face imminent risk to life or health; scarce medical resources; lack of food, water, and shelter; electrical power outages; and interrupted communication networks. The urgent need to mitigate harms to population health may necessitate rapid decision-making, with incomplete or imperfect information, against a backdrop of political, economic, and social instability. These defining characteristics of public health emergencies are morally significant, not only because they reinforce the vital importance of emergency preparedness and response, but also because they present normatively complex questions about what constitutes an ethical public health emergency response (Viens and Selgelid, 2016).

Public Health Emergency Preparedness and Response Activities

Governments, institutions, and communities have prepared for and responded to public health emergencies for hundreds of years (Clements and Casani, 2016). The field of public health emergency preparedness and response, however, is relatively young (Rose et al., 2017), and efforts to address the ethical complexities arising from its practice are developing in real time (Ellis et al., 2016). Nevertheless, there is broad consensus about what public health emergency preparedness and response entails, and growing attention to the tragic choices that communities, health care providers, emergency managers, and others must confront in the emergency context.

Public health emergency preparedness and response involves taking the steps "necessary to maximize the ability" of public health and health care systems to "prevent, respond to, and recover from major events, including efforts that result in the capability to render an appropriate public health and medical response that will mitigate the effects of illness and injury, limit morbidity and mortality to the maximum extent possible, and sustain societal, economic, and political infrastructure" (DHS, 2007, sec. (2)(f)). As its definition suggests, preparedness and response is a multisector, multistep endeavor. It requires the participation, cooperation, and coordination not only of public health and health care systems, but also of other sectors, including national security agencies, humanitarian aid organizations, industries, economists, engineers, and members of the community. Each group brings important knowledge to the process, as well as particular priorities, interests, and values.

Because of the wide range of potential large-scale public health emergencies, preparedness and response activities generally follow an "all-hazards" approach (DHS, 2003; World Health Assembly, 2011). Instead of engaging in specific planning for each type of emergency, an all-hazards approach assumes that certain core functions and capacities will be required in any emergency. The process of emergency preparedness and response unfolds in four phases: mitigation, preparedness, response, and recovery. *Mitigation* takes place before an emergency event and involves assessing potential threats and present vulnerabilities in an effort to prevent either the occurrence or the impact of a large-scale public health emergency. An example of mitigation is enacting and enforcing building codes to limit structural damage during natural disasters. *Preparedness* attempts to improve the capacity of governments, institutions, and communities to respond to public health emergencies once they are underway. Establishing a strategic national stockpile of essential medicines is a form of preparedness. *Response* describes the actions taken during an emergency event to protect people, property, infrastructure, and the environment. The decision to quarantine individuals to limit the spread of an infectious disease is one type of response. *Recovery*, the final phase, describes actions that aim to return populations to normalcy as soon as possible. Reopening hospitals, restoring electricity and potable water, and offering mental health services are examples of recovery activities.

Ethical dilemmas can arise during any phase of public health emergency preparedness and response. Mitigation strategies may raise questions, for example, about the use of societal resources. How much of its budget should a city allocate to strengthening its infrastructure (e.g., buildings) against unknown and unquantifiable future natural disasters? Recognizing that emergencies often exacerbate existing patterns of social injustice, should the city focus its initial efforts on improving infrastructure in poor communities? What if better-off communities have larger populations in equal need of those improvements? Ethics does not offer quick or discrete answers to morally challenging questions that arise in the context of emergency preparedness and response. Ethical awareness and analysis can, however, illuminate the values at stake in those decisions and provide the moral language to describe and resolve situations in which values conflict.

Ethical Complexities

Events like Hurricane Katrina and the West African Ebola epidemic have graphically demonstrated that during public health emergencies, it is just as important to have policies and practices on ethics (e.g., on how to distribute scarce resources, when individual liberties can be restricted, and the scope of professional duties) as it is to have policies to minimize public health impact. Addressing those ethics issues—sometimes referred to as the three R's: rationing, restrictions, and responsibility (Wynia, 2006)—should be part of any all-hazards approach. Deliberation among diverse stakeholders about these challenges can reveal a community's values and goals, which in turn can guide decision-makers in additional, unexpected emergency situations.

Determining how to allocate scarce, life-saving resources is one of the most difficult and ethically fraught aspects of emergency preparedness and response. Regardless of whether the limited resources are medical (e.g., drugs, vaccines, ventilators, and hospital beds), structural (e.g., electricity and evacuation routes), or human (e.g., medical personnel), decisions about their distribution require prioritizing some members of the affected population over others. In confronting issues of distributive justice, decision-makers should strive for policies that are fair, steward scarce resources, and address the needs of special and at-risk populations. Fairness requires that if one group receives a more favorable distribution than others, the difference be justified by morally relevant factors, such as the priority group's importance to community survival (e.g., first responders) (IOM, 2012). Allocation schemes that treat groups differently based on morally irrelevant factors like gender or religion are, therefore, presumptively unethical. Decision-makers should also ensure that allocation policies manage limited resources prudently. Allocation criteria like "first come, first served" and random lotteries, which would provide care to some patients who are likely to die regardless of treatment, while denying care to others who might survive with treatment, fail to appropriately steward scarce resources. Lastly, every allocation policy should account for the needs of populations, which, because of social, economic, cultural, and biological factors, are especially vulnerable to harms or injustices during emergencies. Because groups that are disadvantaged or marginalized before a public health emergency are more likely to suffer poor outcomes during an emergency, planning for their needs is critical.

Several allocation schemes, each reflecting particular values, have been proposed to address the emergency distribution of scarce health care resources. One frequently articulated strategy, grounded in utilitarianism, aims to maximize net benefits, which are specified, for example, as the number of people who survive to hospital discharge (Powell, Christ, and Birkhead, 2008) or the number of adjusted life years saved (White et al., 2009). A different allocation scheme, driven by "narrow social utility" (CDC, 2011), prioritizes individuals, such as health care providers, who carry out functions essential to others' survival (HHS, 2005). Another alternative, the "fair innings" or "life cycle" approach (Emanuel and Wertheimer, 2006), takes the view that each individual ought to have equal opportunity to live through all of life's stages, and therefore prioritizes younger people to receive scarce resources. Because choosing an allocation scheme involves value-based determinations that people may disagree about, it is important that the decision-making process is itself ethical. In an emergency, resource allocation is more likely to be effective and perceived as legitimate when the planning process is transparent, inclusive, and involves open public engagement (Jennings and Arras, 2016; Daniels and Sabin, 2008).

The second ethical challenge that emergency planners should prepare for involves the tensions that can arise between protecting population health and individual liberty. The United States has a long-standing and deep tradition of protecting individual autonomy from public interference, but liberty is "not... an absolute right... at all times and in all circumstances" (*Jacobson v. Massachusetts*, 197 U.S. 11 [1905], 206). In some situations, it may be ethically justified to limit one person's liberty to prevent harm to others (Mill, [1859] 1978). In the context of an infectious disease outbreak, for example, public health interventions such as social distancing, travel restrictions, contact tracing, isolation, and quarantine, may stem the tide of new infections, but at the cost of infringing on individual liberty. Targeted individuals may also face additional burdens, including loss of privacy, stigmatization, discrimination, lost wages, and psychological stress (Wynia, 2007a). For these reasons, and because liberty-restricting interventions have historically targeted marginalized groups (e.g., the 2014 Ebola-related quarantine of the impoverished neighborhood of West Point, Liberia; see Klibanoff, 2014), there is wide consensus that decision-makers should utilize the least restrictive measure that is compatible with protecting the public's health (Presidential Commission, 2015). Whenever possible, such measures should be voluntary, but in all cases they should be implemented with due process protections, such as reasonable notice and the right to appeal.

The third moral dilemma that emergency planners should address, ideally in cooperation with professional associations, is the scope of health care workers' obligation to provide care during emergencies. Society generally expects health professionals to provide assistance as a matter of social contract or professional duty (Wynia, 2007b), and there is broad ethical agreement that providers' responsibility increases with patients' needs, providers' proximity and capability, and lack of other providers (Larkin, 2010).

Nevertheless, providers have "no duty to disaster martyrdom" (Larkin, 2010, 68), and their duty to care should be balanced against the personal risks associated with any given emergency. As the SARS and Ebola outbreaks demonstrated, health care workers exposed to infectious diseases may acquire the infection, cross-contaminate their families, and even become victims of the outbreak themselves. In addition to assuming "greater-than-ordinary" health risks (Capron, 2007, 163), providing care during emergencies may expose health care workers to legal risks, particularly when confronted with tragic choices that depart from the standard of care (Fink, 2009). For those reasons, it is essential to have an explicit agreement between emergency planners and health care workers regarding the scope of providers' responsibility. At the same time, planners should consider what society owes providers who assume personal risks to advance population health. Policies such as preferential access to countermeasures, immunity from liability under certain circumstances, and hazard pay demonstrate that emergency response is a collective undertaking.

Chapter Overviews

The chapters in the Emergency Preparedness and Response section of *The Oxford Handbook of Public Health Ethics* introduce and consider the ethical challenges associated with planning for and responding to three types of public health emergencies: biosecurity threats, natural and industrial disasters, and pandemic disease. "Biosecurity and Public Health Ethics Issues Raised by Biological Threats," by Nicholas Evans and Thomas Inglesby, examines the ethical issues associated with government efforts to prevent and mitigate serious biological threats. As a primer to biosecurity, the authors explore the moral distinction between deliberate biological attacks, which are the primary focus of the chapter, and other biological threats, such as pandemics. Because biological attacks have implications for public health and national security, ethical norms from both fields are critical in assessing government actions aimed at preventing and responding to such attacks. To account for the range of values at stake, Evans and Inglesby propose a pluralistic framework that emphasizes utility, fairness, and liberty, as well as the security of those fundamental values. They then illustrate the various ways in which those values are challenged at three critical times: before a crisis, during a crisis, and after a crisis. In the process, the authors consider circumstances, such as the allocation of scarce resources, in which two or more values are in conflict, and they suggest avenues for addressing such situations.

"Natural and Industrial Disaster Events, Public Health, and Ethics," by Elizabeth Fenton and Dan Hanfling, highlights the human vulnerability at the crux of large-scale disasters. While everyone is vulnerable to disaster events, certain subpopulations are disproportionately at risk of adverse outcomes, such as people with cognitive and physical disabilities who depend on others. Focusing on natural disasters (e.g., storms, flooding, droughts, and earthquakes) and industrial disasters (e.g., human-made or technological hazards like toxic waste and nuclear radiation), Fenton and Hanfling draw attention to "geographic vulnerability." They employ this term to describe the special vulnerability to physical hazards that people of low socioeconomic status experience as a consequence of where they live and work, as is the case for those living near a hazardous waste facility. The authors contend that those involved in emergency preparedness and response have an ethical obligation—grounded not only in the principles of social justice, equity, and reciprocity, but also as a matter of civic practice—to include all vulnerable populations in the planning process, ensure their safety during a response, and establish sufficient public health capacity to reduce systematic health disparities over the long term.

"Pandemic Disease, Public Health, and Ethics," by Maxwell Smith and Ross Upshur, discusses ethical challenges involved in planning for and responding to pandemics. Although every pandemic is different, the authors note that most pandemics pose a common set of moral dilemmas related to resource allocation, public health interventions, the scope of health care workers' duty to care, conducting research during pandemics, and global governance. Smith and Upshur examine the ethical issues that arise in each of these contexts, and consider prominent ethical frameworks developed to address these issues. Drawing on recent pandemic responses, however, they observe that the global health community remains ill-prepared for future pandemics. People living in countries with inadequate public health and health care infrastructure, for example, are especially vulnerable to pandemics. Smith and Upshur therefore urge global actors to not only strengthen outbreak capacity, but also to invest in health care systems in the worst-off countries.

Together, these chapters suggest that, in the context of public health emergencies, ethical preparedness is as important as scientific or technical preparedness. Advance planning, as Alexander Capron (2007, 174) has remarked, is "the key to an ethically responsible and appropriate" response.

References

Capron, A. 2007. "Ethical Considerations in International Preparedness Planning Efforts." In *Ethical and Legal Considerations in Mitigating Pandemic Disease: Workshop Summary*, edited by Institute of Medicine, 157–176 (Washington, D.C.: National Academies Press.

CDC (Centers for Disease Control and Prevention). 2011. *Ethical Considerations for Decision Making Regarding Allocation of Mechanical Ventilators during a Severe Influenza Pandemic or Other Public Health Emergency* (Atlanta: CDC). https://www.cdc.gov/about/pdf/advisory/ventdocument_release.pdf.

Clements, B. W., and Casani, J. A. P. 2016. *Disasters and Public Health: Planning and Response*. 2nd ed. (Oxford: Elsevier).

Daniels, N., and Sabin, J. E. 2008. *Setting Limits Fairly: Learning to Shares Resources for Health*. 2nd ed. (Oxford: Oxford University Press).

DHS (US Department of Homeland Security). 2003. *Presidential Directive/HSPD-8: National Preparedness* (Washington, D.C.: Executive Office of the President). https://www.dhs.gov/presidential-policy-directive-8-national-preparedness.

DHS (US Department of Homeland Security). 2007. *Presidential Directive/HSPD-21: Public Health and Medical Preparedness* (Washington, DC: Executive Office of the President). https://www.hsdl.org/?abstract&did=480002.

Ellis, B. A., Barrett, D. H., Arras, J. D., and Jennings, B. 2016. "Introduction." In *Emergency Ethics: Public Health Preparedness*, edited by B. Jennings, J. D. Arras, D. H. Barrett, and B. A. Ellis, ix–xxxvii (New York: Oxford University Press).

Emanuel E. J., and Wertheimer A. 2006. "Public Health: Who Should Get Influenza Vaccine When Not All Can?" *Science* 312: 854–855.

Fink, S. 2009. "The Deadly Choices at Memorial." *New York Times Magazine*, August 1. http://www.nytimes.com/2009/08/30/magazine/30doctors.html.

HHS (US Department of Health and Human Services). 2005. *HHS Pandemic Influenza Plan* (Washington, D.C.: HHS). https://www.cdc.gov/flu/pdf/professionals/hhspandemicinfluenzaplan.pdf.

IOM (Institute of Medicine). 2012. *Crisis Standards of Care: A Systems Framework for Catastrophic Disaster Response*. A Report by the Committee on Guidance for Establishing Standards of Care for Use in Disaster Situations (Washington, D.C.: National Academies Press).

Jennings, B., and Arras, J. D. 2016. "Ethical Aspects of Public Health Preparedness and Response." In *Emergency Ethics: Public Health Preparedness*, edited by B. Jennings, J. D. Arras, D. H. Barrett, and B. A. Ellis, 1–103 (New York: Oxford University Press).

Klibanoff, E. 2014. "Awful Moments in Quarantine History: Remember Typhoid Mary." National Public Radio, *Goats and Soda*, October 30. https://www.npr.org/sections/goatsandsoda/2014/10/30/360120406/awful-moments-in-quarantine-history-remember-typhoid-mary.

Larkin, G. L. 2010. "Ethical Issues in Disaster Medicine." In *Koenig and Schultz's Disaster Medicine: Comprehensive Principles and Practices*, edited by K. L. Koenig and C. H. Schultz, 62–74 (New York: Cambridge University Press).

Mill, J. S. (1859) 1978. *On Liberty*. Edited by E. Rapaport. 8th ed. (Indianapolis: Hackett).

Powell T., Christ, K. C., and Birkhead, G. S. 2008. "Allocation of Ventilators in a Public Health Disaster." *Disaster Medicine and Public Health Preparedness* 2(1): 20–26.

Presidential Commission (Presidential Commission for the Study of Bioethical Issues). 2015. *Ethics and Ebola: Public Health Planning and Response*. https://bioethicsarchive.georgetown.edu/pcsbi/sites/default/files/Ethics-and-Ebola_PCSBI_508.pdf.

Rose, D. A., Murthy, S., Brooks, J., and Bryant J. 2017. "The Evolution of Public Health Emergency Management as a Field of Practice." *American Journal of Public Health* 105(Suppl. 2): S126–S133.

Viens, A. M., and Selgelid, M. J. 2016. *Emergency Ethics*, vol. 1 (New York: Routledge).

White, D. B., Katz M. H., Luce, J. M., and Lo, B. 2009. "Who Should Receive Life Support During a Public Health Emergency? Using Ethical Principles to Improve Allocation Decisions." *Annals of Internal Medicine* 150: 132–138.

World Health Assembly. 2011. "Strengthening National Health Emergency and Disaster Management Capacities and Resilience of Health Systems." *World Health Assembly 64.10*. http://apps.who.int/gb/ebwha/pdf_files/WHA64/A64_R10-en.pdf.

Wynia, M. K. 2006. "Ethics and Public Health Emergencies: Rationing Vaccines." *American Journal of Bioethics* 6(6): 4–7.

Wynia, M. K. 2007a. "Ethics and Public Health Emergencies: Restrictions on Liberty." *American Journal of Bioethics* 7(2): 1–5.

Wynia, M. K. 2007b. "Ethics and Public Health Emergencies: Encouraging Responsibility." *American Journal of Bioethics* 7(4): 1–4.

CHAPTER 66

BIOSECURITY AND PUBLIC HEALTH ETHICS ISSUES RAISED BY BIOLOGICAL THREATS

NICHOLAS EVANS AND THOMAS INGLESBY

Introduction

The use of biological agents as a weapon of war or terror has its roots in antiquity, beginning with the use of pathogens to kill horses, which were vital resources in the age of mounted combat. The Mongols, during the siege of Caffa in 1346, purportedly pitched plague-ridden corpses over the walls of the city—attributed by some as the entry of the "black plague" into Europe (Wheelis, 2002). Contemporary concerns about bioterrorism became widespread following the discovery of letters containing *Bacillus anthracis* sent through the United States Postal Service in the fall of 2001, ultimately killing five of twenty-two people who were infected. The so-called "Amerithrax" attacks were decisive in pushing the threat of biological terrorism into the national security spotlight.

Events prior to the anthrax attacks also helped shape thinking and planning in the field. In 1984 a series of salad bars in The Dalles, Oregon, was laced with salmonella by the followers of Bhagwan Shree Rajneesh (later known as Osho). The cultists aimed to rig county elections by rendering potential voters too sick to turn out on Election Day. In the mid-1990s, the sarin gas attacks on the Tokyo subway by the Aum Shinrikyo cult killed twelve and injured hundreds. The cult had also attempted a series of biological attacks in the years leading up to the subway attacks, though none of these earlier efforts were successful (Danzig et al., 2012).

Concerns about bioterror are heightened by life sciences research that poses a "dual-use dilemma," in which ostensibly beneficial scientific research has the potential to be misused by malevolent actors, including those who would use biological weapons

(Selgelid, 2007, 36). Distinct from explicit research on bioweapons—such as the Soviet bioweapons program that worked, undetected, for decades to produce biological weapons for the former Union of Soviet Socialist Republics (USSR)—dual-use research is typically intended for beneficent purposes, such as curing disease. The possibility that twenty-first-century biotechnology could be misused has generated debate about how the benefits of biotechnology can be achieved without creating novel security threats.

For the purpose of this chapter, we define *biosecurity* as policies and actions intended to prevent the development or emergence, or mitigate the consequences, of serious biological threats—deliberate weapons, pandemics, emerging infectious diseases, or the result of major laboratory accidents. Much of this chapter focuses on the response of nation-states to deliberate biological threats, but the principles and issues related to those threats have substantial overlap and relevance for the broader range of biological threats and jurisdictions.

Principles

Biological attacks differ from pandemics, emerging infectious diseases, or accidents in one important *ethical* sense. Responses to a biological attack are governed by norms of the use of state power to defend and deter against violence by other agents (Allhoff, Evans, and Henschke, 2013; Orend, 2006), *and* by norms governing the use of state power to promote public health (Diekema, 2008; Kass, 2004). While infectious disease events—such as the 2014–2016 Ebola virus disease outbreak—may be described in terms of their threat to security (Evans, 2016), the ethics of dealing with a biological attack is distinct as a crime or act of war, and thus straddles the domains of national security and public health (Gross, 2006).

A range of ethical frameworks is consonant with an approach to public health that accounts for domestic and national security. Some frameworks are monistic, promoting a single value—such as utility or liberty (Trotter, 2007)—above all others. Others are pluralistic, conceiving of the ethics of public health as involving a trade-off among a set of plausible moral values and principles (Childress et al., 2002; Selgelid, 2009).

We endorse the latter view; further, we take the values at stake in preparing for and responding to biological threats to be utility, fairness, and liberty. By *utility*, we mean the aggregate well-being of a population, including, inter alia, efficiency, economic productivity, morbidity and mortality, and happiness. We take *fairness* to include the distribution of goods within society, and justice considerations surrounding that distribution—equality may be good for its own sake, all things considered, but we may also *owe* certain kinds of goods to others, such as health care workers who put themselves at risk on behalf of others. We understand *liberty* to broadly account for a range of negative freedoms (including rights to freedom of movement, speech, and bodily integrity) and so-called positive freedoms to welfare and education. Autonomy is a component of liberty, albeit both negative and positive: autonomy relies on freedom from coercion or unjustified interference (Beauchamp and Childress, 2001), and on having sufficient options from which to choose in making decisions (Raz, 1988).

Security plays an important role in responding to major biological threats. We take security to be "promotionally valuable": it is concerned with the promotion of utility, fairness, and liberty, and with guarding against the loss of those values (Selgelid, 2012, 36). While health security often concerns preserving lives against harm, we can also talk about the security of our institutions against injustice, or of our rights against infringement. Security is a practice (e.g., a security agency), but also a state of being (e.g., feeling secure about one's continued well-being) (Powers and Faden, 2006). Both are significant—we need the practice of security to defend against terrorism, but we also need people to, for example, feel secure that their liberties will not be violated by either terrorists or their government (Herington, 2012).

In summary, we believe the following should guide ethical action in efforts to prevent, prepare for, and respond to major biological threats: the fundamental values of utility, fairness, and liberty, and the security of these three fundamental values. Below, we elucidate how these values might guide action and where conflicts arise between these values.

Preventing, Preparing for, and Responding to Biological Threats: Ethical Issues

We can divide ethical issues associated with biosecurity and bioterrorism, broadly, into those that occur before a crisis, those that occur during a crisis (in biological terms, when cases are present), and those that occur following a crisis after cases are resolved.

Before a Crisis

Preparation is critical in responding to acts of aggression, be they armed conflict, terrorist attacks, or criminal activity (Evans, 2014). Many factors inform the probability and potential impact of major biological threats; one that bears significantly on public health ethics is the pursuit of basic scientific research that may enable or hinder a bioterror attack. Specifically, some "dual-use" research pursued in aid of public health—research that may contribute to the development of novel vaccines against potential pandemic diseases or bioterror agents, for example—may also risk the accidental or deliberate release of a dangerous pathogen. In 2011, for example, scientists reported they had created highly pathogenic avian influenza (HPAI) H5N1 viruses that were transmissible in ferrets (Herfst et al., 2012; Imai et al., 2012), which are animal models that serve as surrogates for influenza in humans (Radigan et al., 2015). The studies generated concern that such an influenza variant could accidentally or deliberately infect and harm humans and cause a deadly pandemic—wild-type avian influenza has a case fatality rate of about 53 percent (Evans, Lipsitch, and Levinson, 2015; Lipsitch and Galvani, 2014; Lipsitch and Inglesby, 2014; WHO, 2017).

The conduct and dissemination of dual-use research present a conflict between the liberty of scientists to conduct their research, and the purported public health benefits of this research, on the one hand; and the security of the public's health, on the other (Evans, 2013). Part of the tension is epistemic, because the risks and benefits that arise from the use of basic scientific research are difficult to quantify. In 2014 the US government began a deliberative process to assess the risks and benefits posed by "gain-of-function" research resulting in novel pandemic pathogens, of which the 2011 HPAI H5N1 studies are paradigm examples (NRC and IOM, 2015, 1).

While the magnitude and scope of these risks and benefits are uncertain, putative conclusions can be drawn in terms of the values at stake in dual-use research. First, the liberty of scientists is not absolute: we could envisage rare cases in which both scientific freedom and the purported benefits of research are outweighed by competing considerations. If research, for example, were reasonably expected to cause a risk of catastrophic harm in the form of a virulent and widespread disease pandemic, society should prohibit dual-use research (Evans, 2013; Selgelid, 2007).

A corollary of the above is that in cases where we can avoid the apparent dilemma between promoting public health and respecting scientific liberty, we ought to do so. For example, if research with the potential to lead to catastrophic harm could be replaced with alternative experiments that promote public health without creating additional biosecurity risks, we ought to pick this alternative over its riskier counterpart (Lipsitch and Galvani, 2014). Institutions should thus strive to fund alternate experiments that benefit public health without creating new extraordinary risks, where possible.

Beyond dilemmas posed by dual-use concerns, health security is threatened by sophisticated existing biological technologies, coupled with the ability of pandemics and emerging infectious diseases to cause widespread illness. Preparing for these scenarios requires readying resources for response to a bioterror attack—be that a local, state, national, or global community. How we ought to distribute those resources presents a series of potential conflicts between fairness and efficiency in future responses.

A Conflict between Efficiency and Substantive Justice

In an emergency such as a bioterror attack, scarce resources can be allocated according to a number of different ethical principles. Perhaps the most intuitive is distributing resources so as to maximize the expected number of lives—or, alternately, life years—saved; this may be an allocation based on prognosis of recipients of an intervention (Miller et al., 2008), or one that prioritizes the preservation of societal functioning by assigning resources such as medical countermeasures to health care workers, government officials, and operators on critical infrastructure, among others (HHS, 2005). Some have argued that a lottery is, at least in principle, the only truly fair way to assign scarce medical resources (e.g., Childress, 1970); more complex approaches to maximizing life years saved account for society's investment in individuals (and thus not necessarily prioritizing infants over young children who may have already received society's efforts in education, enculturation, and so on) (Emanuel and Wertheimer, 2006). Finally, hybrid approaches could be adopted that, for example, split efforts between life years and societal functioning.

There is no clear consensus on which of these approaches is the best. Different principles could conceivably be adopted for different resources: the Ethics Subcommittee of the Advisory Committee to the Director, Centers for Disease Control and Prevention, for example, recommended societal functioning be prioritized in case of vaccines and antivirals during pandemic influenza, as they "are predominantly used to prevent or lessen illness and thus can be useful in maintaining or restoring health for groups identified as essential for preserving the functioning of society" (CDC, 2011, 9). The group also recommended, however, that ventilators be prioritized according to a complex set of principles (including societal functioning) due to their status as "essential life-saving intervention[s]" (9).

While these principles will at times be consonant (i.e., saving life years probably also requires maintaining social functioning, at least to some degree), choosing one or a combination of principles requires trade-offs compared to other arrangements. Some of these trade-offs are a function of the conditions under which an attack occurs: allocating ventilators in a way that preserves social functioning may lead to excess deaths in cases of a bioterror attack that disproportionately targets children and the elderly, such as an attack involving the contamination of the milk supply with the botulinum toxin (Wein and Liu, 2005). Other trade-offs will arise between fairness and efficiency—the degree to which we give people a fair chance to access resources could involve a trade-off against utility, for example, if resources are not allocated to promote social function. We make no recommendation on which position ought to be favored. We do believe that the public should have systematic input into these decisions in advance of a pandemic or attack, and that, to the extent feasible, the judgments of the public should be pursued (Daugherty Biddison et al., 2014).

Conflicts between Procedural Fairness and Efficiency

Preparedness priorities are subject to reasonable disagreement, in which different parties can hold plural and conflicting values about our obligations to each other in the event of an attack or an accidental release of a virulent pathogen. Here, too, we need to ask who should be at the table when we make decisions about how to (substantively) fairly distribute pandemic preparedness resources. Many of these decisions are made at the government level using expert analysts, independent of the sphere of public deliberation. It is open question about whether this should be the case: and if the answer is "no, it shouldn't" and we ought to engage widely with the public on issues of pandemic preparedness, who should we include?

Publicizing preparedness strategies ahead of time, when based on transparent, candid, and accountable processes involving considerable public engagement, is likely to promote public trust and a sense of accountability in any future response—both of which can be in short supply in public health emergencies. While communities can come together in emergencies, recent experiences with cases of Ebola virus disease in the United States demonstrate that when government engagement is either unclear or overly optimistic, a perceived betrayal of trust or loss of control can jeopardize trust in public health authorities (Kruvand, 2016).

A caveat to this kind of engagement is in cases where engagement and publicity would undermine other kinds of work to prevent a bioterror attack from happening. Given that a deliberate adversary (not nature) would drive a bioweapons attack, there may be risks in publicizing one's preparedness strategies, depending on the specifics. At least in principle, the public health aims of a response to deliberate biological weapons use could conflict with security concerns intended to keep plans from being intentionally subverted.

During a Crisis

Our responses to a bioterror attack will have to compete, in all likelihood, with public anxiety, the realities of international politics, and the limitations of biological forensics. Disease pandemics are international events. Impulses to close borders and restrict the provision of medical aid to other communities—such as between nation-states—should be resisted. Obligations to other countries to provide access to medical countermeasures and aid are grounded in three complementary principles. First, developed countries with the means to mitigate the consequences of major biological threats—or, as some have argued, that have benefited from historical economic or political injustices (Pogge, 2008)—have a moral obligation to help countries that do not have the means to do this themselves. Second, countries that supply samples for research and manufacture of medical countermeasures—including those for defense against major biological threats such as Ebola or HPAI—may be those with little capacity to defend against these threats. Fairness, in the sense of reciprocity, obligates us to share the benefits of development with those who provide the means to defend ourselves. Finally, everyone has an interest in limiting the spread of an outbreak, whether naturally or intentionally caused. In so doing, fairness and efficiency do not conflict, as the citizens of any country have an interest in preventing an outbreak from crossing its borders.

Next, crisis communication ought to be sensitive, consistent, and transparent. In the interest of fairness, and in promoting the well-being of a community, we ought to refrain from communication that marginalizes or stigmatizes groups. Maintaining community trust, moreover, requires that consistency be maintained among different communicators, and between communication and action: when agencies and responders deviate from stated actions without justification—however well-meaning this deviation might be—community trust can be eroded. Hiding or falsifying information, particularly scientific information, can destroy trust (Kruvand, 2016; Russell, 2016).

Coercive public health measures should be deployed only when such measures are demonstrably necessary, proportionate to the expected public health gains, and are the least invasive kind of measure to achieve public health goals (both in terms of the kind of burden the measure poses and the duration of that burden). Isolation, the practice of confining an individual infected with a disease in order to protect the community, is a paradigm example of often justified liberty-limiting measures. For particularly serious contagious diseases that may occur in the setting of either natural disease outbreaks or deliberate biological weapon use, isolation is rarely an infringement on liberty because patients are so ill. It might be possible, however, for someone to be noncompliant while infectious, either while the person is sick (but not debilitated by sickness), or while recovering but still infectious. In this case, public health officials must weigh the liberty of the individual against community safety, and it should be seen as reasonable to confine individuals during the period in which they are capable of spreading a lethal infection.

Conversely, quarantine—the practice of detaining exposed individuals on the chance that they will develop a disease—is rarely justified. Quarantine is often ineffective and historically has led to individuals attempting to evade authorities, possibly spreading the disease further, but underground. Quarantine has also led to the undermining of public trust. With modern surveillance technologies, it is often possible in the right settings to closely monitor exposed individuals without restricting their liberty until they become symptomatic, and without risking others in the process. For example, during the 2014–2016 Ebola virus disease outbreak, Nigeria experienced twenty cases of the disease but controlled the outbreak using proactive contact tracing and self-monitoring of exposed individuals using cell phones, without the need for quarantine (Hills, 2016).

Quarantine might be permissible if the liberty violation is proportionate to the public health benefit, the action is necessary to curb the disease, the action itself is feasible (e.g., there is scientific justification regarding where to draw the lines around the proposed quarantine population), it is the least invasive measure available to definitively curb the spread of the disease, and the quarantined population is treated properly (i.e., their security, nutritional, social, and medical needs are taken care of by responsible government entities throughout the course of the quarantine). There might be an engineered pathogen, for example, whose spread is rapid, airborne, and whose clinical course is irreversible and terminal. In this case, quarantine of exposed individuals or communities might be justified, providing the above conditions were met.

During the response to major biological threats, there may be room for scientific advancement and the development and trial of novel therapeutics in response to the pathogens involved. The question of whether randomized controlled trials (RCTs) can proceed ethically in outbreak zones arose during the Ebola virus disease outbreaks (IOM, 2016), which at one point divided the community between those in favor of RCTs and those in favor of nonrandomized trials or compassionate use of interventions (see e.g., Rid, 2016). Similar discussion may be warranted in the aftermath of the use of biological weapons. Wherever and whenever feasible, a consistent response model and approach to clinical trials ought to be agreed upon *ahead of time* and widely implemented. If compassionate use is offered to some, while others in the same context are enrolled in RCTs as the only way to access the same medicine, this is likely to undermine public confidence.

If the safety and efficacy of an unlicensed product are uncertain, a tension arises between offering more people access to a drug and fewer logistical hurdles, and establishing a drug's causal role in patient outcomes. Trials typically occur under conditions of clinical equipoise, where there is a lack of consensus among the scientific community that an intervention is more likely than not to be beneficial, or vice versa. Because of this, appeals to the benefits of wide access may be mistaken, because while patients may be better off as a result of a novel intervention, they may also be left no better off, or even worse off, than a placebo. Moreover, appeals to the benefits of RCTs based on the *benefit to participants* must be couched carefully. Properly conducted, an RCT gives us the fastest route to knowledge of an intervention's benefits (or lack thereof), but *ex ante* claims of benefits are typically unknown (Selgelid, 2016; Burton and Loftus, 2014). As a result of this uncertainty, some have suggested that "adaptive trials" should be created that allow for changes in study design in response to new evidence of benefit or harm; this idea came to the fore during the Ebola virus disease outbreak in response to concerns about benefits to participants and access to medicines (Rid, 2016).

When trials are developed as a collaborative partnership between researchers and the community, and involve appropriate informed consent and recruitment practices (e.g., Emanuel, et al., 2004), we believe randomized clinical trials of novel therapeutics are in principle better protocols than single-arm trials—all other things being equal, we wish to avoid adding to the considerable health burden of biological disasters, and a randomized clinical trial gives us the most efficacious route to knowledge of which interventions help, and which hinder. We note, however, that responses to major biological threats can be incredibly resource-intensive and chaotic. Instigating research in the middle of such events should be approached in such a way, if at all, that it does not unduly interfere with the primary goals of a response effort.

Finally, health care workers, as professionals engaged in the promotion of the (moral) good of individual and community health, have a duty to care for the infected, even at risk to themselves (Emanuel, 1988; Evans, 2015). This duty, however, is non-absolute—it may be outweighed by particularly risky cases of disease, circumstances where a lack of resources jeopardizes health care worker safety, and excessive repeated exposure. Duty to care also invokes conditions of reciprocity: given the risks health care workers accept, we owe them protective equipment, training, and compensation for the duties they perform for society. Budgets should include "hazard pay" to reflect this added responsibility, and community engagement should be designed around providing adequate caregiving to patients in a way that shares risk.

In the course of responding to major biological threats, a tension may arise between public health and law enforcement personnel regarding procedures and priorities in responding to the health impacts of a bioterror attack, and in the prosecution of the attackers. Sample handling of dangerous pathogens has a biosafety aspect, but when samples are also potential evidence—given that all three paradigms of bioterror in the last century have been acts of domestic terrorism, and thus fall under the rubric of criminal justice—concerns of justice emerge in maintaining a chain of custody over evidence in order to ensure that potential suspects are offered a fair trial and that the criminal justice system can prosecute the guilty. Much of this tension may be, and has been, eliminated in communities where public health and law enforcement personnel train together.

After a Crisis

After a major biological threat occurs, or a disease outbreak has been controlled, the later stages of response and recovery take place. In these stages, communities should be assisted in terms of resources and personnel, in order to rebuild and replenish infrastructure. For reasons similar to those that justify helping communities that bear the brunt of the burden of disease during a crisis, we ought to assist in their redevelopment after a crisis—we are obligated because of their vulnerability, principles of fairness, and reciprocity. Redevelopment also serves to ameliorate secondary effects that may cause lasting damage to a community or region. Preventing additional illness or disability from further depleting a community's resources, stopping secondary outbreaks of other disease, and stabilizing political systems in the wake of a major outbreak would increase the likelihood of long-term security and public health in those communities. This, in turn, is beneficial to other communities and countries because disease outbreaks can be fueled and driven by communities that are the weakest links.

Conclusion

The ethics of biosecurity are generally reflective of basic strictures of biomedical and public health ethics in other emergent scenarios. At times, additional concerns unique to the maintenance of national security may conflict with the ends of public health. How we manage this conflict is complex and will depend in part on specific circumstances, as both kinds of institutions have legitimate roles, and may at times have priority over each other. Facilitating decision-making around these issues requires legal and regulatory clarity regarding powers delineated for relevant institutions. We hope that decision-makers will make these decisions—both in planning, response, and recovery—while following the ethical principles described above.

References

Allhoff, F., Evans, N. G., and Henschke, A. 2013. *Routledge Handbook of Ethics and War* (New York: Routledge).

Beauchamp, T. L., and Childress, J. F. 2001. *Principles of Biomedical Ethics*. 5th ed. (New York: Oxford University Press).

Burton, T. M., and Loftus, T. 2014. "Europeans' Plan to Do Uncontrolled Ebola Trial Draws Fire." *Wall Street Journal*, October 30. http://www.wsj.com/articles/plan-to-offer-ebola-drugs-without-clinical-trials-draws-fire-1414713563.

CDC (Centers for Disease Control and Prevention). 2011. *Ethical Considerations for Decision Making Regarding Allocation of Mechanical Ventilators during a Severe Influenza Pandemic or Other Public Health Emergency*. A Report by the Ethics Subcommittee of the Advisory Committee to the Director (Atlanta: CDC). https://www.cdc.gov/about/pdf/advisory/vent-document_release.pdf.

Childress, J. F. 1970. "Who Shall Live When Not All Can Live?" *Soundings* 53(4): 339–355.

Childress, J. F., Faden, R. R., Gaare, R. D., Gostin, L. O., Kahn, J., Bonnie, R. J., et al. 2002. "Public Health Ethics: Mapping the Terrain." *Journal of Law, Medicine & Ethics* 30(2): 170–178.

Danzig, R., Sageman, M., Leighton, T., Hough, L., Yuki, H., Kotani, R., et al. 2012. *Aum Shinrikyo*. 2nd ed. (Washington, D.C.: Center for a New American Security).

Daugherty Biddison, E. L. D., Gwon, H., Schoch-Spana, M., Cavalier, R., White, D. B., Dawson, T., et al. 2014. "The Community Speaks: Understanding Ethical Values in Allocation of Scarce Lifesaving Resources during Disasters." *Annals of the American Thoracic Society* 11(5): 777–783.

Diekema, D. S. 2008. "Public Health, Ethics, and State Compulsion." *Journal of Public Health Management and Practice* 14(4): 332–334.

Emanuel, E. J. 1988. "Do Physicians Have an Obligation to Treat Patients with AIDS?" *New England Journal of Medicine* 318(25): 1686–1690.

Emanuel, E. J., Wendler, D., Killen, J., and Grady, C. 2004. "What Makes Clinical Research in Developing Countries Ethical? The Benchmarks of Ethical Research." *Journal of Infectious Diseases* 189(5): 930–937.

Emanuel, E. J., and Wertheimer, A. 2006. "Who Should Get Influenza Vaccine When Not All Can?" *Science* 312(5775): 854–855.

Evans, N. G. 2013. "Great Expectations—Ethics, Avian Flu and the Value of Progress." *Journal of Medical Ethics* 39(4): 209–213.

Evans, N. G. 2014. "Dual-Use Decision Making: Relational and Positional Issues." *Monash Bioethics Review* 32: 268–283.

Evans, N. G. 2015. "Balancing the Duty to Treat Patients with Ebola Virus Disease with the Risks to Dialysis Personnel." *Clinical Journal of the American Society of Nephrology* 10(12): 2263–2267.

Evans, N. G. 2016. "Ebola: From Public Health Crisis to National Security Threat." In *Biological Threats in the 21st Century*, 277–292 (London: Imperial College Press).

Evans, N. G., Lipsitch, M., and Levinson, M. 2015. "The Ethics of Biosafety Considerations in Gain-of-Function Research Resulting in the Creation of Potential Pandemic Pathogens." *Journal of Medical Ethics* 41(11):901–908.

Gross, M. 2006. *Bioethics and Armed Conflict* (Cambridge, Mass.: MIT Press).

Herfst, S., Schrauwen, E. J., Linster, M., Chutinimitkul, S., de Wit, E., Munster, V. J., et al. 2012. "Airborne Transmission of Influenza A/H5N1 Virus between Ferrets." *Science* 336(6088): 1534–1541.

Herington, J. 2012. "The Concept of Security." In *Ethics and Security Aspects of Infectious Disease Control*, edited by C. Enemark and M. J. Selgelid, 7–26 (Farnham, UK: Ashgate).

HHS (US Department of Health and Human Services). 2005. *HHS Pandemic Influenza Plan* (Bethesda, Md.: HHS).

Hills, K. 2016. "Rejecting Quarantine: A Frozen-in-Time Reaction to Disease." In *Ebola's Message: Public Health and Medicine in the Twenty-First Century*, edited by N. G. Evans, T. C. Smith, and M. S. Majumder, 217–231 (Cambridge, Mass.: MIT Press).

Imai, M., Watanabe, T., Hatta, M., Das, S. C., Ozawa, M., Shinya, K., et al. 2012. "Experimental Adaptation of an Influenza H5 HA Confers Respiratory Droplet Transmission to a Reassortant H5 HA/H1N1 Virus in Ferrets." *Nature* 486(7403): 420–428.

IOM (Institute of Medicine). 2016. *Global Health Risk Framework: Research and Development of Medical Products: Workshop Summary* (Washington, D.C.: National Academies Press).

Kass, N. E. 2004. "Public Health Ethics from Foundations and Frameworks to Justice and Global Public Health." *Journal of Law, Medicine & Ethics* 32(2): 232–242.

Kruvand, M. 2016. "When Reassurance Doesn't Reassure: Reporters, Sources, and Ebola in Dallas." In *Ebola's Message: Public Health and Medicine in the Twenty-First Century*, edited by N. G. Evans, T. C. Smith, and M. S. Majumder, 157–172 (Cambridge, Mass.: MIT Press).

Lipsitch, M., and Galvani, A. P. 2014. "Ethical Alternatives to Experiments with Novel Potential Pandemic Pathogens." *PLoS Medicine* 11(5): e1001646.

Lipsitch, M., and Inglesby, T. V. 2014. "Moratorium on Research Intended to Create Novel Potential Pandemic Pathogens." *mBio* 5(6): e02366–14.

Miller, M. A., Viboud, C., Olson, D. R., Grais, R. F., Rabaa, M. A., and Simonsen, L. 2008. "Prioritization of Influenza Pandemic Vaccination to Minimize Years of Life Lost." *Journal of Infectious Diseases* 198(3): 305–311.

NRC (National Research Council), and IOM (Institute of Medicine). 2015. *Potential Risks and Benefits of Gain-of-Function Research: Summary of a Workshop* (Washington, D.C.: National Academies Press).

Orend, B. 2006. *The Morality of War* (New York: Broadview Press).

Pogge, T. W. 2008. *World Poverty and Human Rights* (New York: Polity Press).

Powers, M., and Faden, R. 2006. *Social Justice: The Moral Foundations of Public Health and Health Policy* (New York: Oxford University Press).

Radigan, K., Budinger, S., Misharin, A., and Chi, M. 2015. "Modeling Human Influenza Infection in the Laboratory." *Infection and Drug Resistance* 8: 311–320.

Raz, J. 1988. *The Morality of Freedom* (Oxford: Oxford University Press).

Rid, A. 2016. "(How) Should Experimental Vaccines and Treatments for Ebola Be Used?" In *Ebola's Message: Public Health and Medicine in the Twenty-First Century*, edited by N. G. Evans, T. C. Smith, and M. S. Majumder, 183–200 (Cambridge, Mass.: MIT Press).

Russell, C. 2016. "Risk Watch: Media Coverage of Ebola in the Digital Communication Era." In *Ebola's Message: Public Health and Medicine in the Twenty-First Century*, edited by N. G. Evans, T. C. Smith, and M. S. Majumder, 141–156 (Cambridge, Mass.: MIT Press).

Selgelid, M. J. 2007. "A Tale of Two Studies: Ethics, Bioterrorism, and the Censorship of Science." *Hastings Center Report* 37(3): 35–43.

Selgelid, M. J. 2009. "A Moderate Pluralist Approach to Public Health Policy and Ethics." *Public Health Ethics* 2(2): 195–205.

Selgelid, M. J. 2012. "The Value of Security: A Moderate Pluralist Perspective." In *Ethics and Security Aspects of Infectious Disease Control: Interdisciplinary Perspectives*, edited by C. Enemark and M. J. Selgelid, 28–38 (Farnham, UK: Ashgate).

Selgelid, Michael (2016), "The Use and Study of Unregistered Ebola Interventions: Ethics and Equipoise." In *Ebola's Message: Public Health and Medicine in the 21st Century*, edited by N. G. Evans, T. C. Smith, and M. S. Majumder, 175–182 (Cambridge, MA: MIT Press).

Trotter, G. 2007. *The Ethics of Coercion in Mass Casualty Medicine* (Baltimore, Md.: Johns Hopkins University Press).

Wein, L. M., and Liu, Y. 2005. "Analyzing a Bioterror Attack on the Food Supply: The Case of Botulinum Toxin in Milk." *Proceedings of the National Academy of Sciences* 102(28): 9984–9989.

Wheelis, M. 2002. "Biological Warfare at the 1346 Siege of Caffa." *Emerging Infectious Diseases* 8: 971–975.

WHO (World Health Organization). 2017. *Influenza at the Human-Animal Interface: Summary and Assessment, 17 May 2017 to 15 June 2017*. http://www.who.int/influenza/human_animal_interface/Influenza_Summary_IRA_HA_interface_06_15_2017.pdf?ua=1.

CHAPTER 67

NATURAL AND INDUSTRIAL DISASTER EVENTS, PUBLIC HEALTH, AND ETHICS

ELIZABETH FENTON AND DAN HANFLING

Understanding Disasters: Hazards, Vulnerability, and Risk Reduction

DISASTER events—whether large or small, contained or widespread, or the result of natural, industrial, or technological hazards—grab headlines and focus the public's attention in a way that few other life events do. Disasters call into fundamental question the ability of governments to serve their people, and they often highlight shortcomings in planning, preparedness, and response that can assume political overtones. When a disaster event occurs, lives are often lost, livelihoods are inexorably changed, and the costs, both in human and economic terms, can be devastating. This chapter describes the distinctive moral features of natural and industrial disasters and their implications for emergency preparedness and response. We highlight civic responsibility and social justice as particularly important ethical dimensions of emergency preparedness in the context of these types of disasters.

Disasters can be defined as "events that occur when significant numbers of people are exposed to extreme events to which they are vulnerable, with resulting injury and loss of life, often combined with damage to property and livelihoods" (Wisner and Adams, 2002, 10). Disasters result from the interaction of at least three factors: the exposure to a hazard, the vulnerability of the population exposed, and the capacity of the community to cope with or recover from the impact of the event (United Nations Office for Disaster Risk Reduction, 2019a). An important aspect of this definition is the distinction between disasters and hazards. A hazard is a "phenomenon that has the potential to cause disruption or damage to humans and their environment;" it is the potential for a disaster event, not the event itself (Wisner and Adams, 2002, 9). Throughout this chapter we will use the term *natural disaster* to refer to disaster events resulting from natural hazards, such as storms, flooding, drought, or earthquakes; we will use the term *industrial disaster* to refer to disaster events resulting from human-made or technological hazards, including exposures to fire, chemicals, toxic waste, and nuclear radiation. Disasters that result from infectious disease outbreaks, whether intentional or emerging, are not discussed in this chapter.

Importantly, the categories "natural" and "industrial" are not always clearly distinguishable. While the former label implies that the cause of a disaster is beyond human control, and the latter implies a clear human causal role, human actions are often implicated in causing or exacerbating so-called natural disasters. Factors such as poor resource management, urbanization, and global climate change can influence the likelihood and severity of disaster events (Wisner and Adams, 2002). Many have argued that the term *natural disaster* overlooks the critical role of human activity and vulnerability that turns an event into a disaster. O'Brien et al. (2006, 65) argue that "[h]azards may be natural in origin, but it is the way in which societies have developed that causes them to become disasters." Rather than emphasizing the origins of a disaster in a natural hazard, the emphasis should instead be placed on the social conditions that make it possible for a hazard to become a disaster (Cannon, 1994). Some argue that "there is no such thing as a natural disaster," and that all disasters are a function of the social context, such that "the difference between who lives and who dies is to a greater or lesser extent a social calculus" (Smith, 2006).

Regardless of the cause of a disaster, however, there are four phases of management that apply to all disaster events: mitigation, preparedness, response, and recovery. The intent of each of these four elements is to reduce the harm resulting from disaster events. Mitigation strategies are intended to reduce risk and address gaps in preparedness. Response efforts focus on saving lives and property, and recovery is intended to ensure that a community rebuilds better and stronger, thus promoting resilience.

Planning for disasters is also conducted in a manner that is agnostic to their root cause. The focus on commonalities in preparedness and response, rather than on preparation for every specific type of disaster imaginable, is known as an "all-hazards" approach and is at the core of national preparedness efforts in the United States and globally (DHS, 2012; WHO, 2011). The all-hazards approach recognizes that there are common processes and capabilities required to address any disaster event. It also underscores that effective disaster preparedness and response requires investment in and maintenance of a strong and reliable health and social infrastructure and the implementation of a strategy that encourages risk reduction. This platform is based upon a combination of health care and public health capabilities that aid in "supporting the nation's ability to withstand adversity, strengthening health and emergency response systems, and enhancing national health security" (HHS, 2016, 5). The ability to provide health care service delivery in the setting of a disaster is critical and requires a strong foundation for doing so, with efforts focused on continuity of services and the ability to surge medical services when they are required. In addition, a strong public health infrastructure, needed to support health care delivery, is required. Thus, the Centers for Disease Control and Prevention (CDC) notes, "Regardless of the threat, an effective public health response begins with an effective public health system with robust systems in place to conduct routine public health activities. In other words, strong state and local public health systems are the cornerstone of an effective public health response" (CDC, 2011, 2). The strength of the response lies in both the ability to provide access to and deliver health care services (diagnosis, therapeutics, and rehabilitation) to the populations in need and the maintenance and growth of public health services needed to support those efforts.

In the context of natural and industrial disasters, vulnerability involves the diminished ability of individuals or communities "to anticipate, cope with, resist and recover from the impacts of disasters" (Wisner and Adams, 2002, 13). Although everyone is vulnerable to the impact of an extreme event, disasters' predictable needs for rescue, protection, or medical intervention leave some individuals and groups within communities especially vulnerable (Jennings and Arras, 2016; Powers, 2016). Vulnerability can exist because of biological impairments, such as cognitive or physical disabilities or other medical conditions that increase dependence on others, create limitations on mobility, and make people more susceptible to adverse health outcomes. Furthermore, vulnerability can exist because of the social conditions in which people live. Poverty and lack of resources, discrimination and stigma, social isolation and marginalization, and lack of access to services such as health care or transportation all place people at greater risk of experiencing more significant losses than those in more advantaged situations (Jennings and Arras, 2016; Powers, 2016). Of particular relevance for natural and industrial disasters, vulnerability is closely tied to the physical environments in which people live. It has been described as a "general geographical law" that "marginal people are allocated to marginal places" (Wisner, 1998, 26). In the United States, Hurricane Katrina provided a profound illustration of this, as the low-lying areas of New Orleans, home to the city's poorest residents, bore the brunt of the storm's damage. The residents of those areas were geographically exposed to the greatest impact of the disaster, which was compounded by many being unable to access the basic resources, such as money and transportation, needed to protect their personal safety and evacuate. Natural disasters reveal much about the "social geography" of the impact area, where geographical vulnerability to hazards intersects with social vulnerability (Cutter, 2006).

The same can be said for industrial disasters. The environmental and health risks from industrial facilities tend to be disproportionately borne by poorer communities located near those facilities, leading to patterns of injustice in the "geographical distribution of risk" from hazards associated with industrial activities, such as chemical and toxic emissions, hazardous waste, and air pollution (Elliott et al., 2004). People and communities involved in certain occupations are also more susceptible to particular hazards, such as those working in or close to chemical facilities, miners, or forestry workers, who might be more susceptible to fires (Wisner and Adams, 2002).

The special vulnerability to natural and industrial hazards of certain individuals and groups within society creates an ethical obligation on the part of emergency planners, governmental agencies and institutions, and others involved in the development of social policies for the management of disasters to recognize, carefully consider, and plan for their needs, before, during, and after a disaster. This obligation is grounded in broader obligations of social justice to prevent or mitigate harm to others, and to do so equitably (Powers, 2016). The notion of reciprocity also grounds an obligation to ensure the safety and well-being of workers in hazardous industries, because of the higher levels of risk they assume (this is similar to the obligation to provide health care workers with a safe work environment when they are required to work during an infectious disease outbreak).

Fulfilling these obligations at the community level requires emergency planners and public health officials, as well as relevant industry representatives, to gather and have ready access to information about the number and location of particularly vulnerable and isolated groups in a community, such as legal and illegal immigrants, refugees, individuals with cognitive or physical disabilities, patients dependent upon home-based life-sustaining medical equipment, and those who are elderly, homeless, or are living in conditions of poverty. These groups will have special needs during emergencies that require careful, advance consideration. For example, those who are socially or geographically isolated might not be aware of an impending disaster or know what they should do when it strikes, those with physical impairments will need special assistance to evacuate, patients dependent on durable medical equipment such as ventilators or ventricular assist devices will require back up electrical power, and homeless persons are both more difficult to reach and less likely to participate and voice their particular needs in the planning process (Wisner, 1998). Forming an accurate picture of the diverse needs of these groups in a community requires building and sustaining trust between public health and other emergency planning officials and communities, as well as tapping into trusted and respected community networks, leaders, and organizations to understand the patterns of vulnerability within each community. Emergency planners should ensure that individuals and groups with access and functional needs are included in planning processes and given ample opportunities for meaningful participation in emergency preparedness (Jennings and Arras, 2016).[1]

More broadly, vulnerability creates obligations of justice that focus not only on the management of emergency response during and after an event, but that also penetrate the pervasive "geography of social vulnerability." A central goal of public health is to reduce health disparities and the patterns of systemic disadvantage that give rise to them. This goal is central to both emergency and non-emergency public health practice. Comprehensive emergency preparedness and response includes a moral commitment to "the prospective removal of impediments that contribute to systematic disadvantage and heightened vulnerability not experienced by the rest of society" (Powers, 2016, 151). Preparedness activities should therefore be considered broadly to involve social challenges such as urban planning and city design, housing and infrastructure improvements, access to basic health services as well as lifelines during emergencies, and effective political representation of vulnerable communities (Cutter, 2006). For any type of disaster, preparedness, response, recovery, and mitigation activities depend on well-functioning health, medical, and social systems that are established in and accessible to their communities. When present, these systems reduce the vulnerability of individuals and communities and build resilience for future disasters (Cutter, 2006). Establishing, maintaining, and supporting these systems is a broader social obligation associated with emergency planning. Without these systems firmly in place within communities, society cannot hope to meet its obligation to protect its most vulnerable members when disaster strikes (Jennings and Arras, 2016).

Because disaster risk is not equally shared across a population, the ultimate goal of emergency preparedness should be to focus on developing a culture of prevention, with an emphasis on disaster risk reduction (DRR). DRR highlights the "concept and practice of reducing disaster risks through systematic efforts to analyse and reduce the causal effects of disasters" (United Nations Office for Disaster Risk Reduction, 2019b). Disaster risk can be defined as a function of the population's vulnerability magnified by the hazards to which they are exposed, ameliorated only by existing mitigation strategies and/or coping capacity. Therefore, strategies should focus on reducing exposures to hazards and lessening the vulnerability of people and the environment that they populate.

Responsibility and Blame

Unlike war or terrorist attacks, intention to cause harm does not typically play a role in natural or industrial disasters. Natural and industrial disasters "are calamities for everyone and are wanted by no one" (Ladd, 1991, 77). Nonetheless, the notion of blame may not be identical between natural and industrial disasters.

The 1984 Bhopal industrial disaster in India, in which deadly methyl isocyanate gas was released from a Union Carbide chemical plant, resulting in thousands of deaths and hundreds of thousands of injuries, provides a useful illustration. In his analysis of moral responsibility in that case, John Ladd (1991) pointed out that the notion of responsibility is more relevant for an incident like Bhopal than for most natural disasters. In the case of natural disasters, the hazard is outside of human control and so falls outside the realm of responsibility (although, as discussed above, human activities are often heavily implicated in the extent to which an event becomes a "natural" disaster). Industrial disasters, by contrast, Ladd argued, are preventable (at least in theory), and so fall within the realm of human control, and therefore human responsibility.

In both cases, the impact of the disaster might be similar, in terms of deaths, injuries, damage to infrastructure, and communities' economic, social, and psychological well-being, but our sense of moral culpability is different. People tend to perceive industrial or "human-made" hazards as "worse" than natural hazards, even if the magnitude of their impact is the same, presumably because industrial hazards ought to be preventable.

As Jonathan Wolff (2006) points out, however, "worse" is ambiguous. It could mean that human-made hazards are more frightening, or that they are of greater moral concern. Industrial or human-made hazards might be considered worse in both of these senses, because they are more likely to be the result of morally culpable behavior—such as malice, recklessness, negligence, or incompetence—putting industrial disasters, in the mind of the public, among those that should have been preventable. The intuitive moral difference between natural and industrial disasters might then result from our sense that in industrial disasters there will be someone—an individual or collection of individuals—to blame and hold morally responsible.

Yet blame and moral responsibility are not limited to disasters resulting from hazards of human origin. In 2011, when a building collapsed in the Christchurch earthquake in New Zealand, killing 115 people, the deaths were attributed in large part to failures of specific named individuals involved in the design and construction of the building (Canterbury Earthquakes Royal Commission, 2012). Although the proximate cause of the building collapse and consequent deaths was the earthquake, responsibility for associated deaths was found to rest in human actions. Similarly, industrial disasters might not be entirely attributable to morally culpable actions. Some argue for a category of "normal accidents," which occur in systems of such complexity and "tight coupling" of processes that catastrophes are unpredictable and, to some extent, unavoidable (Perrow, 1999). In these accidents, it will likely be impossible, if not absurd, to identify someone who is at fault, someone on whom to pin the blame (though, importantly, this does not imply that such accidents or disasters are inevitable or not preventable). The operators, managers, and officials working at the Union Carbide factory in Bhopal, Ladd argues, were "just ordinary people doing their job and trying to earn a living"; their individual failures were "relatively insignificant and commonplace" (Ladd, 1991, 87). Moreover, since the scale of a disaster is in large part a function of the conditions in which people live, for which responsibility is widely distributed, any sharp distinction between natural and industrial disasters in terms of moral responsibility is difficult to sustain.

Given that some disasters resulting from natural events, such as Hurricane Katrina, and many resulting from industrial events, call for someone or something (an institution, or corporation) to take moral (or perhaps, more practically, financial) responsibility for the event, a concept of moral responsibility is needed that can operate even in the absence of a clear or direct line of fault or blame. Ladd argues that we can still satisfy our need to locate moral responsibility for such disasters by separating blame from moral responsibility—one is not required for the other. Rather than explicit fault or blameworthiness for a disaster, Ladd finds that central to the notion of responsibility in cases like Bhopal is a moral deficiency, a lack of sufficient concern for the safety and well-being of others. Whereas fault suggests "positive evil," moral deficiency suggests "a privation, something missing that ought to be there" (Ladd, 1991, 88). This shift from blame to moral deficiency both broadens the notion of responsibility beyond strict proof of fault and extends responsibility for disasters to a wider range of people and causal factors. Ladd's notion of moral responsibility complements the critical role that social vulnerability plays in creating disasters. To the extent that societies and political systems tolerate significant geographic and other forms of inequity, agents that are less intimately linked to the cause of a disaster, such as institutions responsible for housing policy or resource management, or social well-being more broadly, might share moral responsibility for their occurrence and impact.

Ethical Decision-Making and Disaster Preparedness

Since disasters share many of the same features regardless of their cause, an all-hazards approach can also be applied to preparing for and responding to the ethical challenges that are common to them. These include the fair distribution of limited resources; an awareness of the needs and vulnerabilities of particular groups within communities; appropriate restrictions on individual liberty, such as the imposition of quarantine or curfew; and the professional obligations of medical and other personnel during an emergency.

Disasters should be viewed as "special circumstances for ethical decision-making and reflection," drawing on a broader foundation of public health ethics, rather than as situations requiring their own "tailor-made ethical principles or values" (Ellis et al., 2016, xxii). Principles and values drawn from the fundamental goals of public health are as critical to emergency preparedness and response as they are to routine public health practice. These values include respect for individual liberties balanced with the protection and promotion of population health, social justice and the reduction of health inequalities, and transparency and public participation (Lee, 2012).

In defining standards of care for health professionals during catastrophic disasters, or "crisis standards of care," the US National Academy of Medicine (formerly the Institute of Medicine) also emphasizes the importance of maintaining adherence to the same ethical and professional norms that apply outside of the disaster context (IOM, 2012). Crisis standards of care provide guidance to health professionals on how to *adjust* clinical care during a disaster, since the care that clinicians are able to provide in these circumstances will likely be subject to conditions of extreme resource scarcity (including human resources). Planning for delivery of health care services under crisis conditions are predicated upon the notion that the ethical standards to which health professionals are held to account at any time remain in place, even under disaster conditions. These standards include:

- fairness and consistency in the equitable allocation of scarce resources;
- the duty of health professionals to care for individual patients, and the reciprocal duty of health care institutions to support health workers;
- the duty to steward scarce resources;
- transparency on the part of public health and emergency officials, and a willingness to engage communities actively in emergency preparedness processes;

- proportionality of restrictive public health measures, such as social distancing or quarantine; and
- accountability at all levels of the health care system (IOM, 2012).

These ethical principles of public health and clinical medicine are critical for guiding ethical decision-making in disaster preparedness and response. A distinct yet complementary approach to emergency ethics, however, focuses less on principles or a specific ethical framework for decision-making and more on the appropriate ethical orientation of emergency preparedness and response—what its goals and social goods should be (Jennings and Arras, 2016). This approach views emergency preparedness as a civic practice, one in which individual citizens participate out of a sense of membership in a community and solidarity with fellow members. This civic perspective is contrasted with a consumerist perspective, in which emergency preparedness is viewed as a specialized service or commodity that individuals purchase for protection, submitting to the instructions of experts rather than actively engaging in the planning process. One of the advantages of the civic perspective is that it emphasizes broad community participation in the planning process as an opportunity to nurture democratic values and civic virtues of responsibility, justice, and concern for others in need (Jennings and Arras, 2016).

An understanding of emergency preparedness and response as a civic practice is particularly useful and appropriate in the context of natural and industrial disasters. First, both natural and industrial disasters invoke civic obligations to invest in public safety that are borne both by corporations and public institutions, which can then be held responsible for some or all of the effects of the disaster. Industrial disasters, and some of the effects of natural disasters, might be the result, at least in part, of poor planning, lack of investment in public safety, or negligence, raising questions about the obligations of entities such as corporations and public institutions to invest in safety and infrastructure to prevent or minimize the risks of disasters.

But, like Ladd's notion of moral responsibility, which implicates large and small failures of concern for the safety and well-being of others, the civic perspective on emergency preparedness also casts a wide net in terms of who bears responsibility for preparing for and responding to disaster events. Bruce Jennings and John Arras (2016, 79) argue that although preparedness is primarily a societal and governmental responsibility, all citizens, as members of "a political community of free and equal persons, a community of reciprocal rights and obligations, a community of shared vulnerability and risk, and a community of mutual concern and respect," bear responsibility for participating in the preparedness process, to the extent that they are able. Participation is a vital instrumental good, since it helps to strengthen community bonds and tap into vital community knowledge, such as the location of particularly vulnerable individuals or groups, which can directly improve the emergency management process. But it also serves the greater goal of strengthening members' "sense of responsibility for the health and safety of themselves and their families as moral agents" (Jennings and Arras, 2016, 80). In doing so, it reinforces the moral concern for the safety and well-being of others that Ladd highlights as critical to preventing or mitigating disasters.

Second, natural and industrial disasters force all of us to confront "the deep social fissures and chronic social injustices that haunt our society" (Jennings and Arras, 2016, 24). They expose geographic and social inequities in access to highly valuable resources for mitigating personal harm from a disaster, such as finances, credit, safe housing, and social capital. Even if the effects of a disaster are distributed more or less equitably across advantaged and disadvantaged groups, those with access to greater resources will recover faster and suffer less extreme and ongoing disruption to their ordinary lives. The confluence of disasters and broader patterns of social injustice invoke social and civic obligations to prevent and mitigate harm by reducing the "pervasive forces" of social injustice that can only be compounded by disasters (Powers, 2016).

Conclusion

Natural and industrial disasters are often intuitively distinguished in moral terms by the notions of fault, blame, or responsibility. But a closer analysis of the forces that create and shape disasters reveals that culpable human actions are implicated in both. All disasters are a function of exposure to hazards and human vulnerability—often the special vulnerability of the most disadvantaged and marginalized members of society. Therefore, there is an ethical imperative to implement measures that limit the exposure to risk by reducing vulnerabilities and mitigating hazards. Preparation for natural and industrial disasters should be viewed as a civic practice, guided by civic and social obligations to participate in preparedness activities as members of a community, and to foster societal concern for the safety and well-being of others, especially the most vulnerable. Recognition of these obligations should guide ethical decision-making in preparing for and responding to natural and industrial disasters.

Note

1. Although we use the term *vulnerable* throughout this chapter to describe groups and individuals with particular needs, it is important to note that many resist the term and find that its use can be stigmatizing. For a useful discussion of this point, see Smith et al., 2010.

References

Cannon, T. 1994. "Vulnerability Analysis and the Explanation of 'Natural' Disasters." In *Disasters, Development and Environment*, edited by A. Varley (Chichester, UK: J. Wiley).

Canterbury Earthquakes Royal Commission. 2012. *Final Report*, vol. 6: *Canterbury Television Building (CTV)*. http://canterbury.royalcommission.govt.nz/Final-Report-Volume-Six-Contents.

CDC (Centers for Disease Control and Prevention). 2011. "Public Health Preparedness Capabilities: National Standards for State and Local Planning." https://www.cdc.gov/phpr/readiness/00_docs/DSLR_capabilities_July.pdf.

Cutter, S. 2006. "The Geography of Social Vulnerability: Race, Class, and Catastrophe." In *Understanding Katrina: Perspectives from the Social Sciences* (New York: Social Science Research Council). http://understandingkatrina.ssrc.org/Cutter/.

DHS (US Department of Homeland Security). 2012. "Presidential Policy Directive/PPD-8: National Preparedness." https://www.dhs.gov/presidential-policy-directive-8-national-preparedness.

Elliott, M. R., Wang, Y., Lowe, R. A., and Kleindorfer, P. R. 2004. "Environmental Justice: Frequency and Severity of US Chemical Industry Accidents and the Socioeconomic Status of Surrounding Communities." *Journal of Epidemiological and Community Health* 58(1): 24–30.

Ellis, B. A., Barrett, D. H., Arras, J. D., and Jennings, B. 2016. "Introduction." In *Emergency Ethics: Public Health Preparedness and Response*, edited by B. Jennings, J. D. Arras, D. H. Barrett, and B. A. Ellis, xvii–xxvii (Oxford: Oxford University Press).

HHS (US Department of Health and Human Services). 2016. *2017–2022 Health Care Preparedness and Response Capabilities*. Report from the Office of the Assistant Secretary for Preparedness and Response. http://www.phe.gov/Preparedness/planning/hpp/reports/Documents/2017-2022-healthcare-pr-capablities.pdf.

IOM (Institute of Medicine). 2012. *Crisis Standards of Care: A Systems Framework for Catastrophic Disaster Response* (Washington, D.C.: National Academies Press).

Jennings, B., and Arras, J. D. 2016. "Ethical Aspects of Public Health Emergency Preparedness and Response." In *Emergency Ethics: Public Health Preparedness and Response*, edited by B. Jennings, J. D. Arras, D. H. Barrett, and B. A. Ellis, 1–103 (Oxford: Oxford University Press).

Ladd, J. 1991. "Bhopal: An Essay on Moral Responsibility and Civic Virtue." *Journal of Social Philosophy* 22(1): 73–91.

Lee, L. M. 2012. "Public Health Ethics Theory: Review and Path to Convergence." *Journal of Law, Medicine & Ethics*, 40(1): 85–98.

O'Brien, G., O'Keefe, P., Rose, J., and Wisner, B. 2006. "Climate Change and Disaster Management." *Disasters* 30(1): 64–80.

Perrow, C. 1999. *Normal Accidents: Living with High-Risk Technologies* (Princeton, N.J.: Princeton University Press).

Powers, M. 2016. "Vulnerable Populations in the Context of Public Health Emergency Preparedness Planning and Response." In *Emergency Ethics: Public Health Preparedness and Response*, edited by B. Jennings, J. D. Arras, D. H. Barrett, and B. A. Ellis, 135–154 (Oxford: Oxford University Press).

Smith, M. J., Bernard, C., Rositer, K. Sahni, S., and Silva, D. 2010. "Vulnerability: A Contentious and Fluid Term." *Hastings Center Report* 40: 5–6.

Smith, N. 2006. "There's No Such Thing as a Natural Disaster." In *Understanding Katrina: Perspectives from the Social Sciences* (New York: Social Science Research Council). http://understandingkatrina.ssrc.org/Smith/.

United Nations Office for Disaster Risk Reduction. 2019a. "Terminology." https://www.unisdr.org/we/inform/terminology.

United Nations Office for Disaster Risk Reduction. 2019b. "What is Disaster Risk Reduction?" https://www.unisdr.org/who-we-are/what-is-drr.

WHO (World Health Organization). 2011. "Strengthening National Health Emergency and Disaster Management Capacities and Resilience of Health Systems—World Health Assembly 64.10." http://apps.who.int/gb/ebwha/pdf_files/WHA64/A64_R10-en.pdf.

Wisner, B. 1998. "Marginality and Vulnerability: Why the Homeless of Tokyo Don't 'Count' in Disaster Preparations." *Applied Geography* 18(1): 25–33.

Wisner, B., and Adams, J., eds. 2002. *Environmental Health in Emergencies and Disasters: A Practical Guide* (Geneva: World Health Organization).

Wolff, J. 2006. "Risk, Fear, Blame, Shame, and the Regulation of Public Safety." *Economics and Philosophy* 22: 409–427.

CHAPTER 68

PANDEMIC DISEASE, PUBLIC HEALTH, AND ETHICS

MAXWELL SMITH AND ROSS UPSHUR

Introduction

Microbes capable of infecting and causing disease in humans pose a significant and recurrent threat to public health and are a leading cause of morbidity and mortality in many parts of the world. The threat that infectious organisms pose to humans is amplified when those organisms are capable of spreading beyond a particular ecological niche or geographic region to cause infection in human populations worldwide; that is, when they have *pandemic* potential (see WHO, 2010a).

During pandemics, health needs tend to overwhelm the available human and material resources required to meet those needs. Difficult decisions must therefore be made about how, where, when, and to whom resources should be allocated. State public health authorities have the ethical and legal responsibility to protect the health of communities, and so under legitimate legal authority they may opt to use aggressive measures in an attempt to curb the spread of pandemic disease, which may challenge conventional thinking about the proper scope of the state's powers to protect and promote the public's health. Medical and public health sciences are able to provide valuable information to help inform decision-making in this context; however, science alone is insufficient. Decision-makers will be forced to consider and prioritize potentially competing ethical values.

This chapter provides an overview of the salient ethical issues involved in preparing for and responding to pandemic disease. It draws upon ethical guidance derived from prominent ethical frameworks developed to address these ethical issues, situates the discussion in terms of the global governance of pandemic disease, and concludes by discussing some pressing challenges that must be addressed if ethical reflection is to make a meaningful difference in pandemic preparedness and response.

Public Health Measures Used in Response to Pandemics

Public health officials have many tools, some legally mandated and some based on long-standing involvement with communities, that may be used to contain and curb the spread of pandemic disease. These include isolation (restricting the movement of infected and symptomatic individuals), quarantine (restricting the movement of otherwise healthy individuals exposed to an infectious disease), travel advisories and restrictions, and various other measures, such as the culling or destruction of domestic animal stock to prevent animal to human disease transmission. These may be either recommended on a voluntary basis or required by law. Public health authorities may also have legal warrant to compel medical examinations, vaccination, and other forms of medical intervention on individuals. These can be quite expansive in scope or limited to specific contexts.

Many of the measures deployed to contain and curb the spread of pandemic disease may, in turn, restrict the rights and freedoms of individuals and populations or otherwise burden individuals and communities. The use of such measures therefore highlights an ethical tension between the collective good and individual rights, and requires one to consider the extent to which individual rights and freedoms can justifiably be restricted in order to achieve intended public health goals (Segelid et al., 2009). The use of isolation and quarantine raises particularly salient ethical challenges, particularly in contexts with political and legal traditions that favor individual liberty, where an individual's freedom of movement is temporarily restricted in order to prevent the spread of disease to others. For example, during the severe acute respiratory syndrome (SARS) outbreak in Toronto, Canada, in 2002–2003, several thousand citizens were asked to remain in voluntary home quarantine for ten days. Given the potentially significant burden that these measures may have on individuals and communities, the isolation of symptomatic individuals and quarantine of their contacts should be voluntary to the greatest extent possible. Mandatory measures should only be instituted as a last resort when voluntary measures cannot reasonably be expected to succeed or when the failure to institute mandatory measures is likely to have a substantial impact on public health. In all cases, the least restrictive (i.e., least liberty-infringing) alternative should be used to achieve the public health goal (WHO, 2016).

In turn, a strong reciprocal obligation falls upon public health authorities to provide for the best possible infection control measures appropriate to each confinement context (e.g., hospitals, temporary shelters, homes) in order to protect others from infection (Viens, Bensimon, and Upshur, 2009). In addition, it is critically important to ensure safe, habitable, and humane conditions of confinement, including the provision of basic necessities (e.g., food, water, medical care) and, if feasible, psychosocial support for people who are confined (Silva and Smith, 2015). All efforts should be made to address the potential financial and employment consequences of confinement. Indeed, research indicates that the public is willing to accept the imposition of such liberty-infringing interventions provided that a clear necessity is demonstrated and reciprocal support is in place for those affected (Smith et al., 2012).

Demonstrating the effectiveness of public health measures in response to a pandemic may be difficult, because whether such measures will be employed and whether they will be effective cannot be determined in advance of substantial detailed knowledge of the dynamics of the pathogen. Factors such as the pathogen's mode of transmission, incubation period, duration of infectivity of the host, whether there is asymptomatic shedding, and survival on environmental surfaces are critical to determining both the appropriateness and effectiveness of a given public health measure (Smith and Silva, 2015). When considering whether to adopt particular public health strategies, public health officials should rely on the best available scientific evidence (WHO, 2016); however, there may be circumstances where such evidence is unavailable or where there is controversy or uncertainty regarding the evidence. In such cases, balancing the ethical tension posed by the use of restrictive public health measures is complicated by uncertainty regarding their effectiveness in achieving their intended goals. A prominent example of this complexity was manifest during the 2002–2003 SARS outbreak. Because the SARS coronavirus had not previously infected humans, information about the pathogen was unknown early in the outbreak. Until more information about the virus was known, public health authorities employed techniques such as mass quarantine, isolation, travel advisories and restrictions, and thermal screening in airports as means to stop the spread of the virus in the community (Gostin, Bayer, and Fairchild, 2003; Singer et al., 2003). There was limited empirical evidence of the effectiveness of these measures at the time they were implemented, but the use of the measures was arguably justified on the grounds of public health's mandate to protect communities from disease (Bensimon and Upshur, 2007).

It is now generally agreed that all public health measures used in response to a pandemic must accord with international human rights laws and national legal requirements (WHO, 2016). It has also been recognized that pandemics often place disproportionate burdens on populations that are more vulnerable because of biology (very young and very old), preexisting medical problems (immunocompromised, mental health issues, and multi-morbidity), or social disadvantage (stigmatized populations, minorities). The implementation of restrictive public health measures should pay special attention to protecting the interests of these vulnerable populations (Amon et al., 2006; Silva, Smith, and Upshur, 2013; Bernard, Smith, and Wagner, 2016).

Setting Priorities

Pandemics can place considerable strain on health systems, forcing decision-makers to set priorities for the allocation of available health care and public health resources at the individual level (e.g., triage of a patient to a hospital bed), the organizational level (e.g., service priorities in health care organizations), and the population level (e.g., priority groups for vaccination) (Silva et al., 2012). Many priority-setting principles intended to guide allocation decision-making during pandemics have been proposed (Daniels, 1994; Persad, Wertheimer, and Emanuel, 2009). Decision-makers must consider which principles ought to inform allocation decisions in scenarios where health needs overwhelm available resources. Ideally, priority setting exercises would occur in planning for response to expected infectious disease emergencies. The impetus behind major pandemic planning initiatives is premised on the understanding that health systems should devote resources to determining how priorities will be set in advance of emergencies so that decisions are not made on an ad hoc basis under pressure and significant time constraints.

Many priority setting principles aim to regulate or guide decisions by applying particular decision rules in order to produce favorable outcomes. Allocating resources in a way that aims to save the most lives possible is a principle of this sort, as are principles that aim to use available resources to maximize the total number of life years or quality-adjusted life years (QALYs) saved. Each of these principles, in different ways, aims to maximize benefits accrued from the allocation of available resources (Jennings and Arras, 2008; Persad, Wertheimer, and Emanuel, 2009; CDC, 2011).

These so-called maximizing principles have been criticized for not giving due consideration to the worst off or to the fair distribution of benefits and burdens (Persad, Wertheimer, and Emanuel, 2009). By contrast, some principles require the allocation of resources first to the sickest individuals or those who have had shorter lives than others (i.e., children). However, these principles generally countenance the allocation of resources to the worst off even when only minor health gains are possible, even when they come at high costs. Fairness may require that special attention be given to particular individuals or populations that are vulnerable due to biology, social disadvantage, or another form of disadvantage. Other principles prioritize those who are perceived as being instrumental to a successful pandemic response, such as health care workers and emergency services personnel (Persad, Wertheimer, and Emanuel, 2009). However, principles that take into account so-called "nonmedical" considerations have been criticized by those who argue that medical criteria (e.g., which patients are likely to benefit the most from medical treatment) ought to be the sole criteria for priority setting in this context (Rothstein, 2010). Finally, some priority setting principles aim to give individuals equal chance to benefit from available resources, either through a lottery or through a first-come, first-served system. However, these principles have been criticized for ignoring information that many believe ought to be relevant when allocating valuable, scarce resources (such as an individual's need).

Experience has shown that people, and even different nations' pandemic plans, often disagree about which of these and many other principles should be used to make fair priority setting decisions (Uscher-Pines et al., 2006). In the face of seemingly intractable disagreements on this matter, decision-makers may have to rely on a fair process to establish the legitimacy of priority setting decisions (Daniels and Sabin, 2002). The most prominent example of a procedural approach to priority setting is Daniels and Sabin's "accountability for reasonableness" priority setting framework, which outlines four procedural requirements for an ethical priority setting evaluation: "transparency about the grounds for decisions; appeals to rationales that all can accept as relevant in meeting healthcare needs fairly; . . . procedures for revising decisions in the light of challenges to them"; and a voluntary or public regulation of the process to ensure that the preceding conditions are met (Daniels, 2000, 1300). In all cases, consensus exists that the process decision-makers use to identify and set priorities for resource allocation ought to be transparent and inclusive, involving broad stakeholder engagement (WHO, 2016).

Health Care Workers' Obligations during Pandemics

Demand for health care workers' (HCWs) skills and expertise will increase during pandemics due to elevated pressures on health systems. At the same time, HCWs will be at significant risk of contracting illness during the conduct of their professional duties because of their close proximity to individuals infected with pandemic disease. As a result, an important ethical issue in this context regards the scope and limits of HCWs' obligations to provide care during a pandemic (WHO, 2016). Far from being settled, questions of HCWs' obligations to care were prominent during the human immunodeficiency virus/acquired immune deficiency syndrome (HIV/AIDS) pandemic and were renewed following the death of HCWs during the 2002–2003 SARS and 2014–2016 Ebola virus disease (EVD) outbreaks (Angoff, 1991; Ruderman et al., 2006; Yakubu et al., 2016).

HCWs are bound by an ethic of care (Ruderman et al., 2006). Therefore, obligations to the patient's well-being are generally considered to be primary. The ethical foundations of the duty to provide care can be grounded in several ethical principles, the most prominent being the principle of beneficence, which recognizes the special moral obligation on the part of HCWs to advance patients' well-being (Ruderman et al., 2006). Few challenge the position that HCWs have some degree of duty in this context (Bensimon et al., 2012). At the same time, however, HCWs have competing obligations to their families and friends, whom they may fear they will infect, in addition to obligations to themselves and to their own health. Thus, the debate surrounding HCWs' duty to care may more aptly be characterized as a question of "when and to what extent" rather than "whether or not" (Clark, 2005, 68).

Guidance from the World Health Organization (WHO) on this issue recognizes that a wide range of individuals face risk from being in close proximity to those with infectious diseases (WHO, 2016). HCWs are not necessarily unique in their exposure risks, but they do have special preexisting obligations with respect to assuming those risks (in contrast with, for example, clerical staff and sanitation workers). While the guidance does not argue for an unconstrained duty to care or set a threshold for risk, it recommends that frontline HCWs' rights and obligations be clearly established during the pre-pandemic planning period. This would ensure that all actors are aware of what can reasonably be expected if a pandemic occurs. A strong emphasis is placed on the reciprocal obligation of health systems to provide the best possible infection control modalities at the disposal of HCWs, to provide them preferential access to care should they become ill, and to consider the well-being of the families as critical to supporting HCWs. Appropriate remuneration and protection of HCWs from stigma are also regarded as important norms. In the absence of such reciprocal obligations being met, HCWs cannot legitimately be expected to assume a significant risk of harm to themselves and their families.

Research during Pandemics

In order to optimize the response to a current pandemic or improve health system performance when preventing or responding to future pandemics, there is an ethical imperative during pandemics to conduct research (WHO, 2016). In addition to improving understanding about the effectiveness of public health measures like isolation and quarantine, research conducted during pandemics is crucial in order to investigate novel medical interventions for infectious diseases that lack any effective vaccine or therapy.

Conducting research during a pandemic poses unique and significant ethical issues (WHO, 2010b). It is critical to carefully balance the need to generate new knowledge that may optimize the response to the current pandemic or improve future pandemic preparedness and response with efforts employed to actually respond to the current pandemic. Research efforts should not compromise, nor divert resources from, the public health response to a pandemic or the provision of appropriate clinical care. As in non-pandemic situations, the usual protections for human participants apply, as do standards of professional conduct. Thus, studies must be scientifically valid, add social value, and risks must be reasonable in relation to anticipated benefits (Rid and Emanuel, 2014).

Nevertheless, given the often urgent nature and acute timeline of pandemics, research ethics review boards may need to modify their standard operating procedures in order to respond to time-sensitive research proposals. Those charged with the oversight of research involving human participants should have plans in place to facilitate expedited reviews and should contemplate advance review of generic protocols for conducting research in pandemic conditions, which can be rapidly adapted and reviewed for particular contexts (Ravinetto et al., 2016).

There may be significant limitations in many countries' capacities to respond to research review, particularly in situations like the Ebola outbreak in West Africa, where there was a high volume of reviews and short time limits. This may entail a responsibility for other organizations to provide assistance to local research ethics committees to overcome these challenges. As much as possible, local researchers should be involved in the design, implementation, analysis, reporting and publication of outbreak-related research. Local researchers can help ensure that studies adequately respond to local realities and needs and that they can be implemented effectively without jeopardizing the pandemic response. Involving local researchers in international research collaborations also contributes to building long-term research capacity in affected countries and promoting the value of international equity in science (Schopper et al., 2015).

In the context of a pandemic, particularly one in which there is a dearth of evidence regarding how to optimally manage and respond, some argue that there is an ethical obligation to share preliminary research results once they are adequately quality controlled for release (Langat et al., 2011). Such information should be shared with all actors in the response, including, but not limited to, public health officials, the study participants and affected population(s), and groups involved in wider international response efforts. Scientific journals should facilitate this process by allowing researchers to publish data with immediate implications for public health without losing the opportunity for subsequent consideration for publication in a journal (Smith, 2015).

Global Health Governance during Pandemics

Pandemics, by their very nature, transcend national boundaries. Mounting an effective and rapid response to pandemics therefore necessitates not only local and national efforts but also international cooperation (WHO, 2016). It highlights the need for global solidarity and collective responsibility for preventing and tackling pandemic disease threats. Significant ethical questions exist regarding the specific obligations that individual countries have (within and beyond their borders) to prevent, prepare for, and respond to pandemics, and particularly the extent to which resource-rich nations have obligations to assist resource-poor nations in this effort. Importantly, the obligations of countries to participate in these efforts requires sustained attention to addressing the conditions that contribute to pandemics, which include global poverty and inadequate public health and primary health care infrastructures (WHO, 2016).

The International Health Regulations (IHR), a legal instrument that is binding on 196 countries, affirm and elaborate a set of obligations that countries have to one another to "prevent, protect against, control and provide a public health response to the international spread of disease" (WHO, 2005, Article 2). However, the 2014–2016 outbreak of Ebola virus disease made evident the fact that WHO member states have largely failed to implement the core capacities required under the IHR (Gostin and Friedman, 2015), which include the capacity to detect, assess, notify, and report unusual or unexpected public health events in accordance with the regulations, and provide "support to developing countries and countries with economies in transition if they so request in the building, strengthening and maintenance of the public health capacities required under the International Health Regulations" (WHO, 2005, 4). As such, without proper accountability mechanisms, the IHR may continue to fail to achieve their primary goals.

International law and pandemic plans have created a common structure and set of procedures for global cooperation in response to pandemics. However, massive inequities remain in health investment patterns, and there is little proportionality between disease burden and health spending at the global level. Progress has also been slow in improving public health practices and facilitating access to needed resources (e.g., antivirals and vaccines) in the countries most vulnerable to a pandemic. While some countries are providing public health advice and emergency response support, others are simultaneously imposing protectionist measures to isolate affected countries. As a result, poorer countries may see no alternative but to impose disproportionate measures of their own, which may include applying domestic containment strategies that breach human rights or withholding biological information and viral samples needed to track and combat infectious diseases (Thompson et al., 2015). The international community, and in particular resource-rich countries of the Organisation for Economic Co-operation and Development (OECD), has a shared responsibility to make good on legal obligations to enhance global health collaboration and moral commitments to equal human worth and dignity.

Ethical Guidance and Frameworks

Numerous ethical frameworks have been developed that aim to guide planning and decision-making for pandemic preparedness and response (see, for example, Kass, 2005; Thompson et al., 2006; CDC, 2007; WHO, 2007, 2016). No consensus ethical framework exists, but agreement largely exists on a constellation of values and considerations that ought to be considered by decision-makers in this context.

In particular, ethical frameworks for pandemic preparedness and response aim to attune decision-makers' attention to key areas where ethical issues are likely to arise so that they may, in advance, scrutinize and deliberate about the potential value conflicts that may exist in those domains. These areas largely map on to the themes discussed in this chapter up until this point.

Ethical frameworks also identify, articulate, and contextualize key ethical values and principles that ought to be considered when making decisions in these and other domains. Some values proffered in these frameworks are substantive, while others aim to enhance the ethical quality of decision-making processes. Again, many of the values articulated in these frameworks have been discussed throughout this chapter. As an example of the values enumerated in such frameworks, ten substantive values and five procedural values identified in a seminal ethical framework developed following the 2002–2003 SARS outbreak (University of Toronto Joint Centre for Bioethics Pandemic Influenza Working Group, 2005) are described in Table 68.1.

Ethical frameworks have long recognized that building and retaining public trust in public health authorities is essential for an effective pandemic response. To engender trust, the WHO has recommended that countries develop communication and social

Table 68.1 Substantive and Procedural Values to Guide Ethical Decision-Making for a Pandemic Influenza Outbreak

Substantive value	Description
Individual liberty	In a public health crisis, restrictions to individual liberty may be necessary to protect the public from serious harm. Restrictions to individual liberty should: • be proportional, necessary, and relevant; • employ the least restrictive means; and • be applied equitably.
Protection of the public from harm	To protect the public from harm, health care organizations and public health authorities may be required to take actions that impinge on individual liberty. Decision makers should: • weigh the imperative for compliance; • provide reasons for public health measures to encourage compliance; and • establish mechanisms to review decisions.
Proportionality	Proportionality requires that restrictions to individual liberty and measures taken to protect the public from harm should not exceed what is necessary to address the actual level of risk to or critical needs of the community.
Privacy	Individuals have a right to privacy in health care. In a public health crisis, it may be necessary to override this right to protect the public from serious harm.
Duty to provide care	Inherent to all codes of ethics for health care professionals is the duty to provide care and to respond to suffering. Health care providers will have to weigh demands of their professional roles against other competing obligations to their own health, and to family and friends. Moreover, health care workers will face significant challenges related to resource allocation, scope of practice, professional liability, and workplace conditions.
Reciprocity	Reciprocity requires that society support those who face a disproportionate burden in protecting the public good, and take steps to minimize burdens as much as possible. Measures to protect the public good are likely to impose a disproportionate burden on health care workers, patients, and their families.
Equity	All patients have an equal claim to receive the health care they need under normal conditions. During a pandemic, difficult decisions will need to be made about which health services to maintain and which to defer. Depending on the severity of the health crisis, this could curtail not only elective surgeries, but could also limit the provision of emergency or necessary services.
Trust	Trust is an essential component of the relationships among clinicians and patients, staff and their organizations, the public and health care providers or organizations, and among organizations within a health system. Decision makers will be confronted with the challenge of maintaining stakeholder trust while simultaneously implementing various control measures during an evolving health crisis. Trust is enhanced by upholding such process values as transparency.

(*continued*)

Table 68.1 Continued

Substantive value	Description
Solidarity	As the world learned from SARS, a pandemic influenza outbreak will require a new vision of global solidarity and a vision of solidarity among nations. A pandemic can challenge conventional ideas of national sovereignty, security or territoriality. It also requires solidarity within and among health care institutions. It calls for collaborative approaches that set aside traditional values of self-interest or territoriality among health care professionals, services, or institutions.
Stewardship	Those entrusted with governance roles should be guided by the notion of stewardship. Inherent in stewardship are the notions of trust, ethical behavior, and good decision-making. This implies that decisions regarding resources are intended to achieve the best patient health and public health outcomes given the unique circumstances of the influenza crisis.
Procedural values	**Description**
Reasonable	Decisions should be based on reasons (i.e., evidence, principles, and values) that stakeholders can agree are relevant to meeting health needs in a pandemic influenza crisis. The decisions should be made by people who are credible and accountable.
Open and transparent	The process by which decisions are made must be open to scrutiny, and the basis upon which decisions are made should be publicly accessible.
Inclusive	Decisions should be made explicitly with stakeholder views in mind, and there should be opportunities to engage stakeholders in the decision-making process.
Responsive	There should be opportunities to revisit and revise decisions as new information emerges throughout the crisis. There should be mechanisms to address disputes and complaints.
Accountable	There should be mechanisms in place to ensure that decision makers are answerable for their actions and inactions. Defense of actions and inactions should be grounded in the 14 other ethical values proposed above.

Source: University of Toronto Joint Centre for Bioethics Pandemic Influenza Working Group, 2005, 6–8.

mobilization strategies in order to inform communities about expected public health measures (WHO, 2016). Ideally, these efforts will be informed through community engagement, working with trusted leaders, and striving to be linguistically and culturally appropriate. Given that decisions during a pandemic must often be made urgently and in the context of scientific uncertainty, a significant challenge exists to provide comprehensive, timely, and balanced information that will keep communities informed on the threat's nature and evolution and on governmental policy developments, including changes in public health laws.

Ongoing Challenges: Lessons Learned

In 2014 a protracted outbreak of Ebola virus disease began in West Africa. The outbreak was devastating, as it occurred in the context of nations with poorly functioning health systems and recent history of political turmoil. There was limited spread of the disease outside of this region, but the outbreak was significant enough to warrant being declared a public health emergency of international concern under the IHR. As the outbreak was drawing to a conclusion, a commonly expressed sentiment was that it ought to serve as a "wake-up call" to improve pandemic preparedness and that there were important "lessons to be learned" (Smith and Upshur, 2015).

These sentiments reflect an acknowledgment that such outbreaks should never have occurred, and that, despite over a decade of attention to pandemic preparedness and response, the global community remains ill-prepared to prevent and respond to pandemics. Since the turn of the millennium, numerous infectious disease outbreaks and pandemics have prompted similar "wake-up calls" to improve pandemic preparedness and response, including outbreaks of SARS; H5N1, H7N9, and H1N1 influenza viruses; Middle East respiratory syndrome coronavirus (MERS-CoV); and the emergence of pathogens with antimicrobial resistance, including multidrug-resistant tuberculosis (Smith and Upshur, 2015). Taken together, these outbreaks and the recurring sentiment that they ought to serve as wake-up calls illustrate that the global health community has failed to heed the lessons of past outbreaks and pandemics.

This failure to learn affirms a defect in the collective moral attitude toward remediating the conditions that precipitate the emergence of pandemic threats. These conditions include profoundly inadequate public health and primary health care infrastructures in many countries. More fundamentally, there is an inability to recognize and accept the responsibilities that must be shared as a global community to address shared vulnerabilities to infectious diseases with pandemic potential. In practice, this translates to investment in global outbreak surveillance infrastructure as well as the strengthening of health systems in the worst-off countries (Smith and Upshur, 2015).

Ultimately, this inability to learn is an ethical failure, and ought to serve to emphasize the importance of engaging with the ethics of pandemic preparedness and response. Commitments to improving global outbreak surveillance and early outbreak warning systems (i.e., technical improvements) must therefore be matched with commitments to cultivating the ethics lessons that emerge following outbreaks and pandemics. If future actions are guided by the same values that have led to these repeated ethical failures, there should be doubt as to whether any meaningful change to pandemic preparedness and response will occur.

Conclusion

This chapter reviewed salient ethical issues associated with preparing for and responding to pandemic disease. While each pandemic has its unique characteristics, recent decades have shown that there are predictable issues that arise regarding the use of public health measures, the scope and limits of the duty to care of health care workers, setting priorities for the allocation of resources, global governance, and research ethics. Significant scholarship has evolved around each of these issues, and despite a lack of universal consensus regarding how to properly address them, numerous guidance documents exist that will aid any health system in preparing for and responding to these challenges.

As noted in response to the 2014–2016 EVD outbreak, a failure remains for these guidance documents to be accessed and used in a timely fashion that informs and shapes responses to pandemics. Part of this failure may be explained by the fact that the ethics guidance documents largely exist as stand-alone documents and are not typically integrated into operational pandemic plans. Another part of this failure may be explained by the lack of attention to ethics education in medical and public health training programs. Yet another element may be the unfamiliarity with the type of reasoning required for ethical reflection and deliberation. Indeed, more deliberative approaches may be at odds with the command and control approaches often used in emergency situations. In addition, the need for broad engagement with a range of stakeholders may be perceived as an impediment to timely action.

However, research continues to highlight the need to engage key stakeholders and communities in pandemic planning, conduct widespread and inclusive deliberation on the aforementioned ethical issues, and translate and operationalize public health ethics values and principles for pandemic preparedness and response (Garrett et al., 2011). Future efforts should be devoted to ensuring that as much of this work is done in advance of responding to an urgent situation.

References

Amon, J. J., Bond, K. C., Brahmbhatt, M. N., Buchanan, A., Capron, A. M., Cummings, D. A. T., et al. 2006. *Bellagio Statement of Principles* (Bellagio, Italy: Bellagio Group). https://www.unicef.org/avianflu/files/Bellagio_Statement.pdf.

Angoff, N. R. 1991. "Do Physicians Have an Ethical Obligation to Care for Patients with AIDS?" *Yale Journal of Biology and Medicine* 64(3): 207–246.

Bensimon, C. M., Smith, M. J., Pisarchik, D., Sahni, S., and Upshur, R. E. G. 2012. "The Duty to Care in an Influenza Pandemic: A Qualitative Study of Canadian Public Perspectives." *Social Science and Medicine* 75(12): 2425–2430.

Bensimon, C. M., and Upshur, R. E. G. 2007. "Evidence and Effectiveness in Decision Making for Quarantine." *American Journal of Public Health* 97: S44–S48.

Bernard, C. B., Smith, M. J., and Wagner, F. 2016. "Unanticipated Vulnerability: Marginalizing the Least Visible in Pandemic Planning." In *Public Health Ethics: Cases Spanning the Globe*, edited by D. H. Barrett, L. W. Ortmann, A. Dawson, C. Saenz, A. Reis, and G. Bolan, 226–230 (Cham, Switzerland: Springer International).

CDC (Centers for Disease Control and Prevention). 2007. *Ethical Guidelines in Pandemic Influenza*. A Report by the Ethics Subcommittee of the Advisory Committee to the Director (Atlanta: CDC). https://www.cdc.gov/od/science/integrity/phethics/docs/panflu_ethic_guidelines.pdf.

CDC (Centers for Disease Control and Prevention). 2011. *Ethical Considerations for Decision Making Regarding Allocation of Mechanical Ventilators during a Severe Influenza Pandemic or Other Public Health Emergency*. A Report by the Ventilator Document Workgroup, Ethics Subcommittee of the Advisory Committee to the Director (Atlanta, CDC). https://www.cdc.gov/about/pdf/advisory/ventdocument_release.pdf.

Clark, C. C., 2005. "In Harm's Way: AMA Physicians and the Duty to Treat." *Journal of Medicine and Philosophy* 30(1): 65–87.

Daniels, N. 1994. "Four Unresolved Rationing Problems: A Challenge." *Hastings Center Report* 24(4): 27–29.

Daniels, N. 2000. "Accountability for Reasonableness." *British Medical Journal* 321(7272): 1300–1301.

Daniels, N., and Sabin, J. E. 2002. *Setting Limits Fairly: Can We Learn to Share Medical Resources?* (New York: Oxford University Press).

Garrett, J. E., Vawter, D. E., Gervais, K. G., Prehn, A. W., DeBruin, D. A., Livingston, F., et al. 2011. "The Minnesota Pandemic Ethics Project: Sequenced, Robust Public Engagement Processes." *Journal of Participatory Medicine* 3. https://participatorymedicine.org/journal/evidence/research/2011/01/19/the-minnesota-pandemic-ethics-project-sequenced-robust-public-engagement-processes/.

Gostin, L. O., Bayer, R., and Fairchild, A. L. 2003. "Ethical and Legal Challenges Posed by Severe Acute Respiratory Syndrome Implications for the Control of Severe Infectious Disease Threats." *Health Law and Ethics* 290(24): 3229–3237.

Gostin, L. O., and Friedman, E. A. 2015. "A Retrospective and Prospective Analysis of the West African Ebola Virus Disease Epidemic: Robust National Health Systems at the Foundation and an Empowered WHO at the Apex." *Lancet* 385(9980): 1902–1909.

Jennings, B., and Arras, J. 2008. *Ethical Guidance for Public Health Emergency Preparedness and Response: Highlighting Ethics and Values in a Vital Public Health Service* (Atlanta: Centers for Disease Control and Prevention). https://www.cdc.gov/od/science/integrity/phethics/docs/white_paper_final_for_website_2012_4_6_12_final_for_web_508_compliant.pdf.

Kass, N. E. 2005. "An Ethics Framework for Public Health and Avian Influenza Pandemic Preparedness." *Yale Journal of Biology and Medicine* 78(5): 239–254.

Langat, P., Pisartchik, D., Silva, D., Bernard, C., Olsen, K., Smith, M., et al. 2011. "Is There a Duty to Share? Ethics of Sharing Research Data in the Context of Public Health Emergencies." *Public Health Ethics* 4(1): 4–11.

Persad, G., Wertheimer, A., and Emanuel, E. J. 2009. "Principles for Allocation of Scarce Medical Intervention." *Lancet* 373(9661): 423–431.

Ravinetto, R., Schwartz, L., Kamaara, E., Sheel, S., Segelid, M. J., Ahmad, A., et al. 2016. "Research Ethics Governance in Times of Ebola." *Public Health Ethics* 10(1): 49–61.

Rid, A., and Emanuel, E. J. 2014. "Ethical Considerations of Experimental Interventions in the Ebola Outbreak." *Lancet* 384(9957): 1896–1899.

Rothstein, M. A. 2010. "Should Health Care Providers Get Treatment Priority in an Influenza Pandemic?" *Journal of Law, Medicine & Ethics* 38(2): 412–419.

Ruderman, R., Tracy, C. S., Bensimon, C. M., Bernstein, M., Hawryluck, L., Zlotnik Shaul, R., et al. 2006. "On Pandemics and the Duty to Care: Whose Duty? Who Cares?" *BMC Medical Ethics* 7: 5.

Schopper, D., Dawson, A., Upshur, R., Ahmad, A., Jesani, A., Ravinetto, R., et al. 2015. "Innovations in Research Ethics Governance in Humanitarian Settings." *BMC Medical Ethics* 16: 10.

Segelid, M. J., McLean, A. R., Arinaminpathy, N., and Savulescu, J. 2009. "Infectious Disease Ethics: Limiting Liberty in Contexts of Contagion." *Journal of Bioethical Inquiry* 6(2): 149–152.

Silva, D. S., Gibson, J. L., Robertson, A., Bensimon, C. M., Sahni, S., Maunula, L., et al. 2012. "Priority Setting of ICU Resources in an Influenza Pandemic: A Qualitative Study of the Canadian Public's Perspectives." *BMC Public Health* 12: 241–252.

Silva, D. S., and Smith, M. J. 2015. "Limiting Rights and Freedoms in the Context of Ebola and Other Public Health Emergencies: How the Principle of Reciprocity Can Enrich the Application of the Siracusa Principles." *Health and Human Rights* 17(1): E52–57.

Silva, D. S., Smith, M. J., and Upshur R. E. G. 2013. "Disadvantaging the Disadvantaged: When Public Health Policies and Practices Negatively Affect Marginalized Populations." *Canadian Journal of Public Health* 104(5): e410–412.

Singer, P. A., Benatar, S. R., Bernstein, M., Daar, A. S., Dickens, B. M., MacRae, S. K., et al. 2003. "Ethics and SARS: Lessons from Toronto." *British Medical Journal* 327(7427): 1342–1344.

Smith, M. J. 2015. "Ethical Obligations of Researchers, Public Health Practitioners and Publishers Regarding Ownership of Scientific Data." In *Ethics in Epidemics, Emergencies and Disasters: Research, Surveillance and Patient Care* (Geneva: World Health Organization), 155–162.

Smith, M. J., Bensimon, C. M., Perez, D. F., Sahni, S. S., and Upshur, R. E. G. 2012. "Restrictive Measures in an Influenza Pandemic: A Qualitative Study of Public Perspectives." *Canadian Journal of Public Health* 103(5): 348–352.

Smith, M. J., and Silva, D. S. 2015. "Ethics for Pandemics beyond Influenza: Ebola, Drug-Resistant Tuberculosis, and Anticipating Future Ethical Challenges in Pandemic Preparedness and Response." *Monash Bioethics Review* 33(2): 130–147.

Smith, M. J., and Upshur, R. E. G. 2015. "Ebola and Learning Lessons from Moral Failures: Who Cares about Ethics?" *Public Health Ethics* 8(3): 305–318.

Thompson, A., Smith, M. J., Bensimon, C. M., McDougall, C., and Perez, D. F. 2015. " 'With Human Health It's a Global Thing': Canadian Perspectives on Ethics in the Global Governance of an Influenza Pandemic." *Journal of Bioethical Inquiry* 12(1): 115–127.

Thompson, A. K., Faith, K., Gibson, J. L., and Upshur, R. E. G. 2006. "Pandemic Influenza Preparedness: An Ethical Framework to Guide Decision-Making." *BMC Medical Ethics* 7: 12.

University of Toronto Joint Centre for Bioethics Pandemic Influenza Working Group. 2005. *Stand on Guard for Thee: Ethical Considerations in Preparedness Planning for Pandemic Influenza* (Toronto: University of Toronto Joint Centre for Bioethics). http://www.jcb.utoronto.ca/people/documents/upshur_stand_guard.pdf.

Uscher-Pines, L., Omer, S. B., Barnett, D. J., Burke, T. A., and Balicer, R. D. 2006. "Priority Setting for Pandemic Influenza: An Analysis of National Preparedness Plans." *PLoS Medicine* 3(10): e436.

Viens, A. M., Bensimon, C. M., and Upshur, R. E. G. 2009. "Your Liberty or Your Life: Reciprocity in the Use of Restrictive Measures in Contexts of Contagion." *Journal of Bioethical Inquiry* 6(2): 207–217.

WHO (World Health Organization). 2005. *International Health Regulations* (Geneva, WHO). http://apps.who.int/iris/bitstream/handle/10665/246107/9789241580496-eng.pdf;jsessionid=156F38883E450553EB8E88753D14E658?sequence=1.

WHO (World Health Organization). 2007. *Ethical Considerations in Developing a Public Health Response to Pandemic Influenza* (Geneva: WHO). http://apps.who.int/iris/bitstream/10665/70006/1/WHO_CDS_EPR_GIP_2007.2_eng.pdf?ua=1&ua=1.

WHO (World Health Organization). 2010a. "What is a Pandemic?" Health Topics, February 24 (Geneva: WHO). http://www.who.int/csr/disease/swineflu/frequently_asked_questions/pandemic/en/.

WHO (World Health Organization). 2010b. *Research Ethics in International Epidemic Response: Meeting Report* (Geneva: WHO). http://www.who.int/ethics/gip_research_ethics_.pdf.

WHO (World Health Organization). 2016. *Guidance for Managing Ethical Issues in Infectious Disease Outbreaks* (Geneva: WHO). http://apps.who.int/iris/bitstream/10665/250580/1/9789241549837-eng.pdf.

Yakubu, A., Folayan, M. O., Sani-Gwarzo, N., Nguku, P., Peterson, K., and Brown, B. 2016. "The Ebola Outbreak in Western Africa: Ethical Obligations for Care." *Journal of Medical Ethics* 42(4): 209–210.

Further Reading

Bayer, R. 1989. *Private Acts, Social Consequences: Aids and the Politics of Public Health* (New Brunswick, N.J.: Rutgers University Press).

Chalmers, C. C. 2005. "In Harm's Way: AMA Physicians and the Duty to Treat." *Journal of Medicine and Philosophy* 30(1): 65–87.

Gostin, L.O., and Lazzarini, Z. 1997. *Human Rights and Public Health in the AIDS Pandemic* (New York: Oxford University Press).

Presidential Commission (Presidential Commission for the Study of Bioethical Issues). 2015. "Ethics and Ebola: Public Health Planning and Response." https://bioethicsarchive.georgetown.edu/pcsbi/node/4637.html.

Segelid, M. 2005. "Ethics and Infectious Disease." *Bioethics* 19(3): 272–289.

SECTION FIFTEEN

PUBLIC HEALTH POLICY AND POLITICS

CHAPTER 69

AN OVERVIEW OF ETHICS, PUBLIC HEALTH POLICY, AND POLITICS

ADNAN A. HYDER AND DAVID M. BISHAI

INTRODUCTION

THE World Health Organization (WHO) is the lead agency for public health within the United Nations system, but in spite of that, or maybe because of it, the organization has come under intense scrutiny in the past decade. Concerns around the nature and type of investments in the WHO, as well as questions about the role of international health organizations and the determinants of priorities at the WHO, have been raised (Lopez, 2008; Stuckler et al., 2008). An understanding and analysis of such concerns require that the public health community prioritize critical assessments of what influences policy decisions, what determines investments for specific interventions, and how agreements are made regarding new programs in public health. International public health programs that are the focus of WHO efforts have implications for human populations, international collaborations, vulnerable segments of society, and laws across the world, and work in this space therefore invokes ethical issues that are both similar to and different from other public health actions. While there has been some attention and analysis of the ethical issues arising in this arena, they require further elaboration and reflection from those in the fields of public health, political science, bioethics, and development.

The overall goal of the Public Health Policy and Politics section of *The Oxford Handbook of Public Health Ethics* is to highlight ethical issues emerging from the work and study of politics and policy development in public health—nationally and globally. This section identifies a range of ethical dilemmas that arise in the politics of national and global public health policymaking, and also analyzes potential pathways for addressing them. It does not discuss ethical issues pertaining to the general fields of politics, political science, or development studies per se, and it does not focus on equity issues in the distribution of global resources for public health.

Infusing Ethics in Public Health Practice

By convening the authentic stakeholders involved in proposed public health efforts, informing them about shared risks, and facilitating deliberation, public health professionals can facilitate community participation in working toward acceptable public health approaches that take account of community context. In so doing, such practices will better infuse ethics into the work of public health. All too often, the initiatives and funded operations of public health fail to engage communities, preferring instead to directly provide health commodities (such as vaccines, micronutrients, bed nets, and HIV drugs) to people. The interventionist agenda crowds out an empowerment agenda, and that can perpetuate dependency, thus prompting questions about ethics. This is an important consideration for understanding the distinction between casting the mission of public health as direct service, as opposed to public health working to address unjust local institutions by creating informed and organized communities.

Power structures impact health. Those in power can be motivated by self-preservation, and power structures can therefore perpetuate the well-being of the powerful few at the expense of the health and well-being of the many who may be weak. However, a public health ethics focus can help in revealing the powerful to be myopic and short-sighted, using the analysis of "shared risks" to illuminate health threats that affect all in the population. Public health ethics offers tools and an approach to analyzing how the struggle for control of and redistribution of collective resources relates to and affects the social, natural, and built environments that impact the health of rich and poor alike.

Historically, there have always been methods in public health that use community engagement and epidemiological science to change the narrative from a political economy pitting profits against health to a communitarian realization of shared risks and shared investment in shared living spaces. Public health ethics plays a key role in the normative analysis of such tensions inherent in public health. The political economy of climate change exemplifies this perfectly. Every day, more of the rich and powerful realize that they and their children will live on a hot planet, too. This realization provides an opportunity for an understanding of shared spaces. Public health ethics can, for example, offer deliberative processes that seek to understand value systems underlying attitudes toward climate change, empirical approaches that inform decisions around climate policy, and normative ethics inquiries that demonstrate consequences of decisions taken today for the next decades.

However, public health as an action-oriented discipline must have an action-oriented ethics that moves beyond writing normative documents to more directly guiding action.

Action-oriented public health, informed by ethics, helps to guide practice that includes deliberative spaces for stakeholders where dialogue can take place, and can lead to consensus and action agreed upon by affected parties. Infusing ethics into public health practice informs and encourages efforts to convene members of affected communities and to share information and evidence about the harms and benefits of proposed public health actions. This type of ethics activism is well outside the typical professional efforts of most academic ethicists, but convening, informing, and facilitating deliberative action by those affected is standard for public health practitioners. Public health informed by ethics is critical, then, not in the sense that it dictates actions that align with principles, but because it encourages deliberations that are more likely to result in ethically informed consensus. Ensuring authentic engagement and voice for affected community members is as important as providing relevant data for their review and shared decision-making.

The practice of community convening, informing, and engagement in policy creation is, unfortunately, not reaching many communities. Thus, too many communities are not involved in the decisions being taken for their health and welfare. Sometimes public health practitioners usurp the speaking role of the community and use their own voice as experts to dictate what should be done about shared health risks, and sometimes nobody is speaking or advocating for the community. In the short run, external voices (outside the community) may be necessary to conduct advocacy; in the long run, public health professionals need to build deliberative forums into the social structure of every community to achieve appropriate consideration of ethics in public health practice. These are the types of issues at the intersection of policy, public health, and ethics highlighted in the chapters of this section.

Chapter Overviews

The four chapters in the Public Health Policy and Politics section of *The Oxford Handbook of Public Health Ethics* explore an important yet limited set of ethical issues in the analysis of politics and public health. Public health includes science-based services that emerged during the nineteenth and early twentieth centuries in response to serious health problems in countries experiencing rapid development. Gerald Bloom and Hayley MacGregor argue in "Global Development, Global Public Health, and Ethics" that the creation of scientific knowledge and the application of technological expertise to all aspects of economic and social organization provided a scientific and normative basis for changes in the role of the state. This led to an acceptance that governments have responsibilities for protecting populations against avoidable deaths and the high cost of ill health, and the ethical underpinning of this understanding reflected the social and political context in these nation-states. The construction of an ethical case for government interventions to protect public health, in turn, influenced understandings of the role of the state. Yet society does not yet have global agreement on ethical principles for complex global challenges. These principles will need to be clarified as countries build mutual agreements to address specific health issues. One cannot assume that the perspectives developed by the economically dominant countries of the last century are "universal" in this regard. An ethics of public health and development for the twenty-first century will need to emerge from a broad dialogue and process of consensus building.

In "Responsible Resource Allocation, Public Health Stewardship, and Ethics," Robert Hecht, Daniel Arias, and Carleigh Krubiner define governance as the political processes by which decisions are reached and upheld, and stewardship as the technical processes that inform those decisions. They acknowledge that these two concepts encompass a range of morally relevant considerations in public health ethics, including promoting utility, value for money, equity, accountability, and norms of distributive and procedural justice. They take a closer look at these considerations and how they enable health systems to make ethical decisions. The authors explore ethical challenges to health that arise in systems lacking good stewardship and governance. For example, decisions must be made about how limited resources are used to promote and protect public health and what governance mechanisms will guide such decisions; and health policymakers and public health practitioners have to be responsible stewards. The chapter discusses why these issues are morally important, and it raises ethical considerations relevant to ensuring the appropriate use of public resources to improve public health through good governance and stewardship.

In "The Political Economy of Public Health: Challenges for Ethics," Ted Schrecker begins to formulate a mission for public health ethics in seeking to shift the institutions that govern political economy. There are many historical examples where this happened. A leading example is the creation of public health departments dating back to the United Kingdom's Public Health Act of 1848, which started an agenda where government agents measured and proposed ways to improve population health. The political economy of health connects health consequences with "upstream" inequalities in power and resources, and with policy choices and institutional processes that instantiate, reflect, and reinforce those choices—issues best considered within the frameworks of public health ethics. Understanding these processes and their connection with institutional structures and macro-scale policies is a prerequisite for intellectually responsible discussions of public health ethics. This is because the processes in question often involve life-and-death choices made by powerful actors about third parties who may have little or no ability to influence the relevant decisions. Since these choices often do not reflect any underlying economic necessity, but rather a judgment about the relative value attached to protecting the lives and wealth of differently situated members of a society, they are a key ethics concern.

Finally, in "Incorporating Ethics in Policy Change and Health Reform," Gerard Anderson, Jeromie M. Ballreich, and Afsan Bhadelia examine the ethical considerations related to policy change and health reform and contrast ethical reasoning with policy processes. They define two broad ethical approaches for health policy: a teleological approach and a deontological approach. They then show how ethical concerns can motivate policy change and health reform, using examples from the United States,

Mexico, and India. They argue that ethics plays a key role in health policy reform. Ethics influences the policymaking process and highlights specific health policy outcomes, and ethical concerns have been part of the policy process for years. Ethics has underpinned most health policy change and reform, such as the role of the state versus the individual, the responsibility of society for the poor, and balancing not doing any harm against shifting conceptions of goodness and virtue. The policy process and ethical reasoning share many of the same attributes, and policymakers have a responsibility to embrace ethical reasoning in the process to advance better health outcomes.

Conclusion

Attention to public health ethics in the arena of policy and politics will both lead to and require greater interaction among disciplines such as bioethics, political science, and development studies. The critical topics discussed in this section of *The Oxford Handbook of Public Health Ethics* have been relatively neglected in public health and together mark an important step forward in promoting active consideration of ethics issues in the politics of public health—including the difficult issues involving the relationships of social justice, power, and community participation—within national and global public health efforts.

References

Lopez, A. 2008. "Health and Health-Research Priorities: Has WHO Got It Right?" *Lancet* 372(9649): 1525–1527. doi:10.1016/S0140-6736(08)61632-3.

Stuckler, D., King, L., Robinson, H., and McKee, M. 2008. "WHO's Budgetary Allocations and Burden of Disease: A Comparative Analysis." *Lancet* 372(9649): 1563–1669. doi:10.1016/S0140-6736(08)61656-6.

CHAPTER 70

GLOBAL DEVELOPMENT, GLOBAL PUBLIC HEALTH, AND ETHICS

GERALD BLOOM AND HAYLEY MACGREGOR

INTRODUCTION

"DEVELOPMENT" is an often used yet contested concept, with differences in opinion as to how it should be understood and what its key dimensions are. At a basic level, the process of development involves multiple changes in the way people live and support themselves and their households. The relationship between development and health is complex and involves a web of direct and indirect connections. Changes in the way people live affect their health both positively and negatively. And, sickness and early death have a significant impact on well-being and development. For example, the transition from hunter-gatherer to agricultural production, thousands of years ago, led to increases in population and the development of towns and the benefits of more settled livelihoods, but it was also associated with much greater exposure to infectious disease (Cohen, 1991; McNeil, 1977). The same applies to the movement of people across long distances, which contributed not only to economic growth, but also to recurrent pandemics of plague in Asia and Europe and the enormous mortality from infectious disease in the Western Hemisphere after Europeans invaded it.

Until recently, the response to health challenges has been evolutionary: populations gradually attained immunity through natural selection, societies evolved cultural and religious practices to reduce the risk of transmission of diseases, and states played a role in protecting public health (Porter, 1999). Jared Diamond (2006) documents the devastating impact of a society's failure to respond to health-related challenges and associated societal changes, with historical examples from Easter Island and Mayan Central America, for example, where population pressures and environmental degradation led to civil strife and violence, and eventually to a civilization's collapse.

This chapter uses the term *public health* to refer to the science-based services that initially emerged during the nineteenth and early twentieth centuries in response to serious health problems in countries experiencing rapid development (Porter, 1997). Angus Deaton (2013) argues that the creation of scientific knowledge and the application of technological expertise to all aspects of economic and social organization were important drivers of this rapid development. Increases in productivity contributed to greater consumption, improved nutrition, and better health outcomes (McKeown, 1976). Government initiatives, based on public health science, also made important contributions to health improvement. Public health, as a field of research and social practice, provided a scientific and normative basis for changes in the role of the state. It developed in a context of political mobilization and struggle, which eventually led to an acceptance that governments have responsibilities for protecting populations against avoidable deaths and the high cost of ill health (Porter, 1999). The dominant understanding of the ethics of public health and the ways that ongoing debates about government's role are framed reflect the social and political context of the nation-states where it developed.

Importantly, the distribution of the benefits and costs of development has been very unequal, and it continues to be so within societies and across the globe. Inequalities remain with respect to which "publics" of public health receive greater attention. This chapter's analysis of public health and development emphasizes the impact of development and public health actions on the people who face lives of poverty and high levels of illness. For them, the complex relationship between health and development is less likely to come out on the positive side of the balance. This has implications for debates about the ethics of public health and development at national and global levels.

Overview of Ethics of Public Health and Development

A major characteristic of development since the Industrial Revolution has been the speed and interconnected nature of changes in technology, population size, urbanization, transportation, communications, and so forth. These changes have contributed to big rises in income and consumption in places where they occurred, although the distribution of benefits has been very unequal. These shifts also exposed populations to new health risks. Many people continued to live in poverty with deleterious health effects, and in some cases they experienced a worsening in well-being and health as inequalities widened. During the early phases of the Industrial Revolution, the intensified health risks were largely associated with infectious diseases (Szreter, 1997). For example, the concentration of large numbers of poor people in rapidly growing cities was associated with periodic outbreaks of cholera. This stimulated scientific discoveries that led to the germ theory of disease and eventually to public health actions that reduced the risk of cholera and increased the safety of cities (Evans, 1990). Public health responses were primarily confined to countries that benefitted from rapid development or to defined areas of colonies. This uneven distribution of benefits from advances in public health knowledge remains apparent, and outbreaks of cholera still occur where public health systems are weak.

Public health has played an essential role in enabling societies to benefit from rapid development by helping them avoid catastrophic health outcomes. For example, the social "decision" to create large cities entailed risk, but public health knowledge and practice made it possible to reap enormous benefits from the concentration of economic and social activity. Public health science has subsequently identified many more development-related health risks, and appropriate responses to these risks have enabled societies to benefit from new technologies, while limiting possible negative health outcomes.

Both the pace and geographical spread of change have substantially increased over recent years with rapid urbanization, the global spread of industrial production, major increases in intensive animal husbandry, and growing ecological stress and climate change (Bloom et al., 2007). Rapid economic growth has enabled many to escape poverty and reap health gains, especially in Asia. The pace of change is likely to persist for as long as people seek ways to ensure that they and their offspring have a better life. Very rapid development, however, exposes people to high levels of uncertainty and risks to their health. This is reflected in contemporary anxieties about emerging infectious diseases and the consequences of environmental pollution, and in growing concerns about increases in the proportion of deaths from noncommunicable diseases. Significantly, large numbers of people have been left behind and continue to experience poverty.

Public health services can contribute to a society's management of rapid development by providing early warning of emerging problems and informing social responses to minimize health risks through preventative strategies, aimed, for example, at individual behavior or at amelioration of environmental conditions or structural inequalities (Bloom and Wolcott, 2013). In order to achieve these roles effectively, they need to be underpinned by agreed-upon social and ethical norms to guide the behavior of officials, public health practitioners, and citizens and to legitimate the use of state resources and power. In the present global context, there are large differences between countries in the formulation of ethical arguments for action on development and public health. Despite the differences, there is a need to reach agreement on a set of principles to provide a basis for global action (Pogge, 2008).

One approach for defining these principles is to agree on a core set of goods and services (including public health), access to which is recognized to be a "right" (Pogge, 2008). Deaton (2013) argues, for example, that efforts are needed to assist the many people left behind as others benefit from what he refers to as "The Great Escape." Justin Yifu Lin (2012, 234) cites his education in the Confucian tradition as the basis for his desire to "find a way of contributing to the prosperity of my country [China] so that our people would be free from the fear of poverty and hunger." Deaton and Lin emphasize the contribution of rapid economic and social development to well-being and health, but they also recognize that measures are needed to reduce the risk of deleterious health outcomes. Lin (2012) emphasizes the negative impact on large numbers of people trapped in poverty if their government fails to create the conditions for rapid development. He also refers to the sacrifices that a generation may make in investing in infrastructure, education, and research to improve the economic and health prospects of future generations. The mass movement of people to cities (in their own or another country) is another form of investment that migrants make in order to create opportunities for their descendants. It is also vital to assess likely harms to future generations from accruing debts to finance current consumption and from damage to important ecosystems (Sen, 2009).

Other analysts have focused on the complexity of social arrangements and the limited information available to planners and government decision-makers about the challenges individuals face, as well as their hopes and aspirations. This can result in serious policy mistakes (Ramalingam, 2013). Amartya Sen (2009) argues, for example, that many famines could have been avoided if policymakers had received early warning, and if they had been open to discussions on innovative strategies for addressing acute food shortages. He also argues that open and rational debates are an important mechanism for winning popular support for actions that are agreed to be in the public interest (of present and future generations). Others make a similar argument for participatory action research as a means of making known the understandings and points of view of social groups with relatively little voice in policy debates (Oswald, 2016). As the speed of change increases and the complexity of social organization grows, it is becoming increasingly important to ensure that all social groups have a voice in identifying new public health harms and in co-constructing the ethical norms that underpin public health action.

The Sustainable Development Goals (SDGs) (UN General Assembly, 2015) can be viewed as a statement of global principles of ethics and development, which have secured support from the governments of all nations. Some commentators have referred to the lack of specificity of these goals. This reflects the rudimentary nature of agreements in a rapidly changing global context. A next step toward deepening these agreements is through dialogue aimed at building mutual understanding of values underpinning actions to tackle specific global public health problems. The next sections illustrate this argument with examples of the management of rapid development and urbanization and the growing concern with antimicrobial resistance.

Management of Rapid Development and Urbanization

The benefits and harms of development have been distributed unequally within and between countries. The early political mobilizations that led to the establishment of the normative values of public health were driven by the disproportionate burden of ill health borne by the poor combined with the realization that all population groups, rich and poor, were affected when an epidemic occurred (Szreter, 1997). During the nineteenth and twentieth centuries, there was a big divergence in development and public health between countries experiencing rapid industrialization and those left behind (Pomeranz, 2000). Large proportions of the population in the latter countries experienced severe and, in some cases, worsening poverty and exclusion from the benefits of the globalizing economy. Many countries became colonies, with governments that largely reflected the interest of the metropolis and the colonialists. Public health services in these countries reflected their highly unequal social structure and concerns directed at preventing epidemics that could endanger the dominant minorities, while the health needs of the majority were, and in some cases remain, neglected.

Large structural inequalities persist within and between countries in levels of income and wealth and in exposure to health risks. This raises ethical issues concerning the distribution of benefits and harms at local, national, and global levels, and between present and future generations. These considerations need to be taken into account in the formulation of strategies for enabling rapid development and mitigating the risks that emerge.

One important aspect of rapid global development has been the movement of very large numbers of people into urban areas. This has led to the rapid growth of densely populated cities. Those cities are often characterized by striking inequalities, which translate into health inequalities. A large proportion of their residents live in low-income settlements where the risk of transmission of infections is high. This is due, among other things, to contamination of water with human waste, low-quality housing, limited infrastructure for health provision, and compromised immunity due to malnutrition and chronic disease. Residents of such settlements depend primarily on informal markets to obtain health care, often at high cost. On the other hand, access to employment in cities might also mean that households have greater resources to address episodes of ill health and access to some form of health care than might otherwise be possible in rural areas. These urban communities are likely to be important channels for the transmission of new or re-emerging infectious diseases, such as the 2014–2016 Ebola outbreak in West Africa, and of infections resistant to antibiotics. They are also likely to suffer the most from such health risks. Expanding cities, in turn, have increasingly strong transportation links with other countries through which infectious diseases can spread. At the same time, the populations of these cities face risks of chronic, noncommunicable diseases associated with a number of aspects of urban lifestyles, limited access to recreational spaces, unhealthy food environments, and exposure to environmental pollutants.

Public health services and policies can play an important role in reducing the risk of deleterious health outcomes from rapid urbanization. However, they face ethical concerns. How much should societies invest in public health surveillance as a hedge against the possibility of the rapid emergence of unexpected problems? How should public health researchers and practitioners weigh the current and anticipated future benefits of particular forms of rapid urbanization against difficult-to-quantify risks of deleterious health outcomes? This is a particularly pertinent question in societies where many people are urgently seeking ways to escape poverty and improve their lives in accordance with their understanding of the available opportunities. Who should bear the cost of delays, because of potential health risks, in measures that could provide benefits to poor people? Whose point of view should count in making these decisions? Who is responsible for action to improve urban public health? What is the role of national and city governments? What are the responsibilities of stakeholders, such as urban-based companies and extractives, that benefit from improved urban infrastructure? Are there international responsibilities? The Chinese government's Belt and Road Initiative, for example, is financing large investments in the infrastructure of several countries. They are likely to encourage urbanization and increased volumes of intercountry travel. What is China's responsibility for potential public health consequences?

Antimicrobial Resistance, Development, and Global Consensus

This section illustrates the challenge of constructing an ethics of global public health, using the example of the global response to antimicrobial resistance (AMR). AMR is a global public health crisis, said to have the potential to kill more people than climate change (Davies, 2017). The development, production, and distribution of antibiotics was a significant achievement of the second half of the twentieth century (Laxminarayan et al., 2015). It involved a combination of basic science, the organization of mass production and distribution, and the creation of institutional arrangements to enable people to use these products safely and effectively. The countries at the forefront of development integrated the arrangements for antibiotic production and use into their existing health systems. The widespread use of antibiotics is widely acknowledged to have made a large contribution to health improvements in these countries. However, it has also been associated with the emergence and spread of drug-resistant organisms.

During the last quarter of the twentieth century, access to antibiotics spread to areas where these institutional arrangements are absent or nascent. This access was stimulated by well-publicized efforts to provide access to effective treatment of common infections, often based on syndromic diagnosis and sometimes as a means of providing prophylaxis for groups of people, such as sex workers, who are at high risk of infection. It was also a result of the rapid spread of markets for drugs and medical care associated with rises in income and increases in the availability of information, including through advertising in the mass media. These developments have contributed to reductions in maternal and child mortality, for example, in Bangladesh (NIPORT, 2012). They were also associated with the further emergence of organisms resistant to antibiotics. In high-income settings, the inappropriate use of antibiotics in health care and in commercialized agriculture has continued to lead to problems of resistance.

In 2015 the WHO launched a Global Action Plan on AMR (WHO, 2015). The immediate source of pressure for action was the growing problem of antibiotic-resistant infections in hospitals and community settings in high-income countries. This is a particularly severe problem for people with immune systems that are compromised from a congenital abnormality, HIV infection, immunosuppressive treatment, or the effects of aging. In countries where entitlement to medical care is part of the social contract, the treatment of these people has become a growing problem. Despite the local nature of this manifestation of the problem, there is a growing realization that an effective response must include action in other countries and coordination at a global level.

One strategy for addressing the challenge of antibiotic resistance is to substantially increase investment in research and development of new antibiotics and other forms of antimicrobial therapy (O'Neill, 2016). In order to maximize the future benefits of investment in new antibiotics, governments and pharmaceutical companies will need to agree to limit their use to cases where existing treatments fail. This means that companies will not earn revenue from these drugs for a long time, and governments will need to finance the investment. Clear rules will be needed concerning the use of these products. But who should produce the rules—governments who are financing the investment, the governments of other countries with the capacity to produce pharmaceuticals, or all governments? The answer is important, because companies in a number of countries have the capacity to reverse-engineer new compounds and sell them at a high price. Their governments will need to prevent this. They are unlikely to do so, however, unless they have played a role in formulating the rules, and unless their health facilities have access to the new drugs. To be just, the rules will have to be understood by all. Among other things, this commitment to justice would mean making the "right" of access to antibiotic treatment of common infections a global reality in order to address the continuing excess mortality from treatable infections. Laxminarayan et al. (2016) point out that the lack of access to timely treatment of infections presently kills more people than AMR.

The existence of antibiotics is known almost universally around the world. Many populations believe that access to antibiotic treatment of common infections is an entitlement, even if they must still pay out of pocket. Indeed, there are very few places where people cannot obtain these drugs if they can afford to pay. In countries without a well-organized health sector, antibiotics are sold in unregulated markets, and studies have found high levels of antibiotic use by people using these markets (Peters and Bloom, 2012; Laxminarayan et al., 2016). Treatment efficacy, however, is frequently compromised by substandard products and the use of partial courses of treatment, affecting the quality of care and increasing the risk of antibiotic resistance. One approach to this problem would be for governments to close these markets if they had the capacity to do so. Although this may be an appropriate long-term goal, in the short run it could deny access to life-saving drugs to many people. Measures to address this problem could include investment in the development of vaccines, new combinations of existing drugs, and inexpensive diagnostic technologies. A global strategy for addressing AMR will need to balance the needs of large numbers of poor people, who rely on informal markets for antibiotics, against the needs of a subgroup of very sick people, based mostly in more affluent countries, with the aim of increasing the capacity for just and sustainable management of antibiotic use (Buckland-Merrett et al., 2016).

These arguments demonstrate the need to build a global consensus on an action plan to address AMR that should be underpinned by dialogue and agreements on what constitutes a just approach. Rules regarding, for example, the production, distribution, and use of new antibiotics will need to be widely agreed upon if they are to be enforced. Otherwise, the announcement of the development of a new product could simply create incentives to manufacture and sell it at a premium. Similarly, the understandings of the public and how the rationale for regulations is conveyed to them will strongly influence the degree to which a population accepts measures that limit access to certain antibiotics.

A global action plan will inevitably involve trade-offs between measures that benefit different population groups in each country and between countries considered to be at different levels of development. It will also involve appreciating differing understandings and perceptions by different population groups. In order to secure active consent, it will be important that the justification for the allocation of resources and for actions that limit access to antibiotics are understood to be just by all concerned parties. Actions that mostly benefit severely ill patients in better-off countries are unlikely to gain global support. A just action plan will also need to address the challenge of infectious diseases in all population groups.

The challenge of AMR also raises questions about the distribution of benefits and costs of development between generations. The residents of high-income countries have secured health benefits from antibiotics for many years, while resistance has been rare. More recently, access to antibiotics in countries with poorly organized health systems has contributed to a decrease in childhood mortality among population groups that are struggling to acquire benefits from development. However, this use of antibiotics will have a negative impact on future generations. How much risk of avoidable deaths should the present generation bear to preserve the efficacy of antibiotics? Should antibiotics be withheld from people in resource-poor countries with weak regulatory systems? Or, should the residents of rich countries, who have many opportunities to preserve their health, be asked to forgo the use of these products? Should they be withheld from residents of rich countries with severely compromised immunity?

Conclusion: Ethics of Public Health and Development for the Twenty-First Century

The examples above illustrate the kinds of challenges that public health practitioners and policymakers face in the context of rapid development and increasing globalization, where the benefits of these processes are unevenly distributed. These conditions reveal the complexity of the interaction between development and health. As the twenty-first century moves on, we can anticipate major health challenges associated with the accelerating growth of cities, the spread of industrial processes, and increasing ecological stressors. This will require large, public health responses at local, national, and global levels. However, the persistence of deep structural inequalities means that the distribution of risks and potential benefits of an intervention will have to be taken into account. As in the earlier phases of development, public health can play an important role in identifying potential health challenges, in addition to making contributions toward the design of interventions by governments and other stakeholders at local, national, and global levels to mitigate potential negative impacts. Such efforts at mitigation need to be inclusive so that those most at risk of negative health effects receive attention. This requires a public health system that is attuned to the issue of justice.

The construction of an ethics of public health that is appropriate for this era and that takes account of divergent perspectives and positions is an important task. It will take place in the context of major changes to the arrangements for global governance. The governments and private companies of large countries, such as India and China, have an increasing impact around the world. These countries are experiencing rapid development, and their governments are under pressure to create increasingly sophisticated institutions. Debates within these countries about public health and the responsibilities of national and local governments will have increasing influence on global political and ethical discourse. Global rules will also need agreement from low-income countries, since the failure and/or inability of their governments to implement basic public health measures can have a large impact on global health and on problems like AMR. This illustrates the need for an inclusive dialogue on what constitutes a just approach toward public health at a global level.

During the nineteenth and twentieth centuries, the establishment of effective national public health systems made important contributions to development. Furthermore, the construction of an ethical case for government interventions to protect public health influenced understandings of the role of the state. In the present period of rapid and globalizing change, it is important to strengthen global public health arrangements to protect against possible risks to health. One element of this endeavor will be the establishment of a normative basis for public health action that is acceptable to all actors. We do not yet have global agreement on ethical principles for complex global challenges. These principles will need to be clarified as countries build mutual agreements to address specific issues, such as AMR. We cannot assume that the perspectives developed by the economically dominant countries of the last century are "universal" in this regard. An ethics of public health and development for the twenty-first century will need to emerge from broad dialogue and the process of consensus building.

References

Bloom, G., Edstrom, J., Leach, M., Lucas, H., MacGregor, H., Standing, H. et al. 2007. "Health in a Dynamic World." STEPS Centre Working Paper 5 (Brighton, UK: STEPS Centre). https://steps-centre.org/publication/health-in-a-dynamic-world/.

Bloom, G., and Wolcott, S. 2013. "Building Institutions for Health and Health Systems in Contexts of Rapid Change." *Social Science and Medicine* 96: 216–222.

Buckland-Merrett, G., Bloom, G., Wilkinson, A., and MacGregor, H. 2016. "Towards the Just and Sustainable Use of Antibiotics." *Journal of Pharmaceutical Policy and Practice* 9(1): 31. doi:10.1186/s40545-016-0083-5.

Cohen, M. 1991. *Health and the Rise of Civilization* (New Haven, Conn.: Yale University Press).

Davies, S. 2017. "Anti-Microbial Resistance: A Cause for Collaboration." Gates Cambridge Annual Lecture on Antimicrobial Resistance. https://www.gatescambridge.org/news/antimicrobial-resistance-cause-collaboration.

Deaton, A. 2013. *The Great Escape: Health, Wealth, and the Origins of Inequality* (Princeton, N.J.: Princeton University Press).

Diamond, J. 2006. *Collapse: How Societies Choose to Fail or Survive* (London: Penguin).

Evans, R. 1990. *Death in Hamburg: Society and Politics in the Cholera Years 1830–1910* (London: Penguin).

Laxminarayan, R., Matsoso, P., Pant, S., Brower, C., Rottingen, J., Klugman, K., et al. 2015. "Access to Effective Antimicrobials: A Worldwide Challenge." *Lancet* 387 (10014): 168–175.

Laxminarayan, R., Sridhar, D., Blaser, M., Wang, M., and Woolhouse, M. 2016. "Achieving Global Targets for Antimicrobial Resistance." *Science* 353(6302): 874–875. http://science.sciencemag.org/content/early/2016/08/17/science.aaf9286.

Lin, J. Y. 2012. *The Quest for Prosperity* (Princeton, N.J.: Princeton University Press).

McKeown, T. 1976. *The Modern Rise of Population* (New York: Academic Press).

McNeil, W. 1977. *Plagues and Peoples* (Oxford: Basil Blackwell)

NIPORT (National Institute of Population Research and Training). 2012. *Bangladesh Maternal Mortality and Health Care Survey, 2010* (Dhaka, Bangladesh: NIPORT, Measure Evaluation and ICDDR, B). https://www.measureevaluation.org/resources/publications/tr-12-87.

O'Neill, J. 2016. *Tackling Drug-Resistant Infections Globally: Final Report and Recommendations* (London: Wellcome Trust and Government of UK). https://amr-review.org/sites/default/files/160518_Final%20paper_with%20cover.pdf.

Oswald, K. 2016. *Interrogating an Engaged Excellence Approach to Research.* IDS Evidence Report No. 214 (Brighton, UK: Institute of Development Studies).

Peters, D., and Bloom, G. 2012. "Developing World: Bring Order to Unregulated Health Markets." *Nature* 487: 163–165.

Pogge, T. 2008. *World Poverty and Human Rights* (Cambridge: Polity Press).

Pomeranz, K. 2000. *The Great Divergence: China, Europe and the Making of the Modern World Economy* (Princeton. N.J.: Princeton University Press).

Porter, D. 1999. *Health, Civilization and the State: A History of Public Health from Ancient to Modern Times* (Abingdon, UK: Routledge).

Porter, R. 1997. *The Greatest Benefit to Mankind: A Medical History of Humanity* (London: Harper Collins).

Ramalingam, B. 2013. *Aid on the Edge of Chaos* (Oxford: Oxford University Press).

Sen, A. 2009. *The Idea of Justice* (London: Penguin Books).

Szreter, S. 1997. "Economic Growth, Disruption, Deprivation, Disease and Death: On the Importance of Public Health for Development." *Population Development Review* 23(4): 693–728.

UN General Assembly. 2015. *Transforming Our World: the 2030 Agenda for Sustainable Development.* A/RES/70/1, adopted 21 October 2015. http://www.refworld.org/docid/57b6e3e44.html [accessed 10 April 2019]

WHO (World Health Organization). 2015. *Global Action Plan on Antimicrobial Resistance* (Geneva: WHO).

CHAPTER 71

RESPONSIBLE RESOURCE ALLOCATION, PUBLIC HEALTH STEWARDSHIP, AND ETHICS

ROBERT HECHT, DANIEL ARIAS,
AND CARLEIGH KRUBINER

Introduction

In all public health settings, the range of expressed health needs and the costs of providing services will far outstrip available public resources (Roberts et al., 2008). Decisions will thus have to be made about how limited resources are used to promote and protect public health, and about what governance mechanisms will guide such decisions. Health policymakers and public health practitioners are entrusted with the responsibility to use limited resources wisely to improve health—to be responsible *stewards* of the health system. Stewardship and governance represent critical elements of an effective health system; this chapter will discuss why they are morally important, and it will raise the ethical considerations relevant to ensuring appropriate use of public resources to improve public health through good governance and stewardship.

Defining the Terms: What Are Governance and Stewardship?

In defining governance and stewardship, it is useful to examine the origins of their root words: to *govern* and to *steward*. The word *govern* comes from Old French and Latin origins, and is derived from the nautical charge "to steer, or to pilot," as of a ship (Jessop, 1998). The word later evolved into its more contemporary definition: "to direct, rule, guide, or govern." As its etymology suggests, *governance* carries connotations of leadership and path-setting, of charting a course and faithfully navigating toward a clear direction.

By contrast, the term *steward* comes from Proto-Germanic origins, and originally described the domestic servant (the *weard*) who maintained a house or hall (the *stiġ*). The responsibilities of the steward encompassed meeting the comprehensive needs of a household and acting as its guardian (Jeavons, 1994). Historically, the word *stewardship* emerged within a theological context, later being applied to environmental movements (Saltman and Ferroussier-Davis, 2000). Today, the word retains the focus from its etymology on managing resources and maintaining the standing of an organization or entity, from a single house to an entire ecosystem.

Despite their recognized importance, universal definitions of stewardship and governance in the context of health systems remain elusive, with many sources using the terms interchangeably (Saner and Wilson, 2003; Barbazza and Tello, 2014). A selection of definitions from the relevant literature is provided in Table 71.1.

Many definitions of governance in health systems emphasize the mechanisms and institutions involved in formulating and executing decisions and policies. These definitions tend to encompass the processes by which the voices and interests of citizens are incorporated in decision-making and structures of accountability. In this way, governance appears more political than technical (Saner and Wilson, 2003): definitions of governance focus on the processes by which public authorities formulate, implement, and enforce policies concerning public health (Siddiqi et al., 2009; UNDP, 2014). Central to these definitions are the institutions—from individual stakeholders to broad systems—as well as the values and rules that structure decision-making and priority-setting.

By comparison, definitions of stewardship in health emphasize the use of intelligence and expertise to infuse and inform decision-making processes with guidance and vision (Travis et al., 2002). Many of these definitions connote elements of caution and prudence (WHO, 2000). Responsible stewards take care of resources by ensuring their effective use through informed and carefully managed processes (Carlson et al., 2015). Although definitions of stewardship also include political considerations, they emphasize the technical aspects of intelligence gathering, efficacy, and value for money. Stewardship encompasses processes that are informed by technical expertise, responsible risk management, and evidence-informed tools for implementation; within the context of public health, these are critical considerations for ensuring that public resources are being most effectively and efficiently expended toward the public's health (Kass, 1988).

For the purposes of this chapter, *governance* will refer to the political processes by which decisions are reached and upheld, and *stewardship* will refer to the technical processes that inform those decisions. This chapter argues that stewardship and governance are separate concepts, though they overlap and entwine substantially. Public

Table 71.1 Example Definitions of Governance and Stewardship in Health (emphases added)

Governance	
Siddiqi et al., 2009	"Governance comprises the complex *mechanisms, processes and institutions* through which citizens and groups *articulate their interests, mediate their differences* and *exercise their legal rights and obligations*." (2)
UNDP, 2014	"Governance processes refer to the quality of participation necessary '*to ensure that political, social and economic priorities are based on a broad consensus* in society and that the *voices of the excluded, poorest and most vulnerable are heard* in decision-making.' "(4)
	"*Accountability* is a key theme running through and underpinning many aspects of governance—both vertically, from government to people, and horizontally between parts of the state, such as the executive and the judiciary. Sustainable development will require that public officials account for actions taken in the public's name and with public resources." (4)
Stewardship	
WHO, 2000	"Governments should be 'stewards' of their national resources, maintaining and improving them for the benefit of their populations. In health, this means being ultimately responsible for the *careful management of their citizens' well-being*. Stewardship in health is *the very essence of good government*." (117)
Travis et al., 2002	"*Stewardship has similarities to the notion of public governance*, but as envisaged by WHO is more specifically focused on the state's role in *taking responsibility for the health and well-being of the population, and guiding the health system as a whole*. It influences the ways other health system functions are undertaken. In addition, it '*embeds the health system in wider society*'. In characterizing stewardship, the Report identified three broad 'tasks' of health system stewardship: *providing vision and direction* for the health system, *collecting and using intelligence*, and *exerting influence*—through regulation and other means." (1)

trust, for example, is central to many definitions of both governance and stewardship. Good governance and stewardship are dependent on the relationships between those who govern and the public who hold these leaders accountable. Agents acting on the public's behalf are entrusted with executing their duties responsibly and effectively under systems of good governance and stewardship, with accountability to the public (Gostin, 2010). This underscores the complementarity of stewardship and governance—health decision-makers are charged with responsible stewardship of the public's health and the resources to support that aim, while a number of actors and institutions can ensure that decisions and actions align with public health priorities and objectives. In a well-functioning health system, stewardship and governance should be mutually self-reinforcing.

Why Responsible Stewardship and Good Governance Are Morally Relevant

Health stewardship and governance encompass a range of morally relevant considerations found in prominent public health ethics frameworks (Lee, 2012). These include moral imperatives to build and maintain public trust, use participatory approaches to decision-making, deliver on commitments and promises, promote transparency and accountability, draw upon the evidence base, and promote efficiency to improve population health with limited resources (Childress et al., 2002; Baum et al., 2007; Lee, 2012). Furthermore, notions of good governance and stewardship—including the processes, actors, and institutional arrangements for health policymaking—closely align with theories of procedural justice (Daniels, 2013). Because many societies are pluralistic and state actors are often faced with tough trade-offs in which they will be unable to meet everyone's needs and preferences, procedural justice aims to ensure that the processes for decision-making are fair and legitimate (Daniels, 2000, 2008). One such account, Daniels's "accountability for reasonableness," proposes four conditions for health decision-making: (1) making decisions and their rationales public; (2) providing relevant and reasonable justifications for decisions, to be vetted by stakeholders; (3) mechanisms to challenge or dispute decisions; and (4) public regulation of the process to ensure it meets these conditions (Daniels, 2008). The second condition links closely with responsible stewardship and the need for decisions to be evidence-based and reasonable, while the entire account encompasses norms associated with good governance.

In contrast, the consequences of poorly stewarded resources and bad health governance have serious moral implications. Health carries special moral importance, because it is both intrinsically and instrumentally important for human well-being—and achieving a basic minimum of health is central to many accounts of social justice (Powers and Faden, 2006; Daniels, 2008; Venkatapuram, 2013). Poor stewardship of the health system will result in inefficient allocations and potentially serious opportunity costs, where alternative allocations could have yielded much greater health benefits to the population (Brock and Wikler, 2006; Krubiner and Hyder, 2014). Bad governance can lead to corruption, distortion of government budgets, and public distrust in social institutions, and it can exacerbate health inequities and social exclusion (UNDP, 1997).

Promoting Responsible Stewardship

Good governance and stewardship of public health resources are thus important components of an ethically sound health system and are essential for health policymakers to fulfill their dual remit to serve as caretaker of public resources and public health. Health policymakers must carefully consider decisions about how best to invest a limited pool of resources—financial and otherwise—to protect and promote population health.

Stewarding these resources responsibly relies on various technical inputs to realize public health objectives. An important consideration for effectively stewarding health resources is *utility*, or pursuing allocations that maximize health gains whenever possible (Marchand, Wikler, and Landesman, 1998). The principle of health maximization has long been promoted by various utilitarian theories of distributive justice (Lamont and Favor, 2014). These theories hold that the most moral action is the one that generates the greatest utility, or well-being (or happiness), for the greatest number of people. While maximizing health gains must be balanced with other ethical norms—chiefly, attention to equity—responsible stewardship entails careful consideration of which investments provide the best "value for money." Value for money takes into account the expected benefit of a health intervention against its anticipated costs. This analysis often requires quantitative costing and epidemiological impact data, making the approach reliant on data collection, statistical analysis, and methodological rigor. Cost-effectiveness analysis (CEA) is an example of such an evaluative process. Within CEA, the costs and expected outcomes of two or more interventions are compared to identify the most cost-effective intervention. This type of analysis can be helpful in identifying where constrained funds can be maximally deployed to achieve—or "purchase"—the highest quantity of health possible. Value for money analysis also ensures that public health stewards are regularly comparing and contrasting policy options against each other to determine the most efficient use of public resources, fostering a more informed and evaluative approach to policymaking through the application of decision sciences.

Utilitarian approaches, however, must be balanced with other ethical considerations, particularly those around *equity*, or eliminating avoidable differences in the health of different groups of people. While a health system should strive to improve efficiency and impact, it must also seek to foster health equity across the spectra of social, economic, and demographic groups. The implementation of universal health coverage (UHC), for example, is well understood to be an effort to promote equity of access and ensure a minimum set of basic health services for all (Rodney and Hill, 2014). Responsible stewardship motivated by equity concerns may entail, for instance, analysis of the distribution of health outcomes and of health services across household income strata and identifying measures that can make such distribution more equal, generally by redistributing benefits from those who are better off to those who are less affluent (Gwatkin, 2007).

Approaches must also *respect the autonomy* of individuals and communities—a broad principle that encompasses respect for self-rule (or self-governance) and the engagement of individuals regarding decisions that will affect them. The process by with individuals are involved in health system priority-setting and decision-making is discussed at greater length in the following section.

A concept related to value for money is *evidence-informed decision-making*, where priorities and policies are reviewed against a methodological standard such that policies that are adopted must demonstrate effectiveness and impact through empirical data.

Often, this requires a foundation of quantitative—and to some extent qualitative—data that indicates that the given policy is actually likely to achieve its stated objective; this data may be obtained from pilot studies that are subsequently scaled up, or from case studies in different settings, countries, or sectors. The use of evidence to support decision-making is critical to stewardship, since it ensures that decisions are informed by the latest and most accurate data available (WHO, 2000). Furthermore, evidence-informed approaches emphasize objectively demonstrated success across measurable and well-defined indicators, and the transparency of performance measurements allows for policymakers to clearly see and define the outcomes of health investments, expanding the foundation of available knowledge and evidence of impact.

Evidence-informed decision-making can promote value for money in health care and advance the implementation of *best practices*, another key component of stewardship. Best practices are those which have been demonstrated through successive implementation and evaluation to be the most optimal and beneficial, such that they are considered to be the standard for a given field. The dissemination of best practices supports the public health steward's responsibility to promote efficiency, effectiveness, and equity. By establishing successful strategies as a norm, the creation of best practices promotes beneficence and reduces harm. The process by which practices become accepted as standard and "best practices" is also modulated by the stewardship role of public health professionals; effective stewards of public health establish clear and accessible guidelines by which promising practices are evaluated and validated. Registries of best practices may provide searchable inventories of validated interventions, tools, and strategies, which may promote evidence-informed practices across a health system. The Cochrane Library (https://www.cochranelibrary.com/) is a prime example of a repository of best practices as well as meta-analyses of a range of detailed studies in order to identify wider patterns of "what works" and why.

Intelligence gathering through regular *monitoring and evaluation* of public health interventions may serve to continually add to knowledge surrounding evidence of impact and best practices. Interventions with monitoring and evaluation components may be more responsive to needs for course correction, enabling the adaptive use of resources to serve evolving needs. In addition, the collection of real-time data provides a component of accountability and transparency, though this is limited by the extent to which data is distributed and made public. These are all consistent with recent calls for movement toward "learning health systems" as well as a proposed ethics framework by Faden et al. (2013) that prioritizes the role of evidence generation in delivering just health care (McGinnis et al., 2013).

Ultimately, these mechanisms of good stewardship require a formal process for incorporating guidance, technical expertise, vision, and evidence-informed review into public health decision-making (see also "Health Systems Stewardship, Governance, and Accountability: Issues of Public Health Ethics," this volume). One example of these mechanisms in action is the use of national immunization technical advisory groups (NITAGs), which are independent technical committees that advise policymakers on key decisions related to immunization policies (such as whether to introduce new vaccines to the national immunization schedule). NITAGs and other health advisory bodies can provide guidance on the adoption of new policies and ensure that they are supported by up-to-date epidemiological, biomedical, and economic evidence (Duclos, 2010).

Without incorporating formal processes of technical review and analysis into public health governance, the impact of good stewardship may not be translated into good decision-making. Indeed, such decisions may be poorly supported by available evidence, inadvisable, unfeasible, or counterproductive to the public's health. Such decisions, if implemented, may corrode the public's trust that public resources are being used effectively, thus eroding the ethical values of public trust and careful management of public welfare.

It is therefore imperative that practices of good stewardship be incorporated in systems of public health decision-making, such that technical rigor informs policy and programming in a consistent and conscientious manner. Where possible, these processes should be *independent* and *autonomous* from political influence, so as to provide unbiased expertise and evaluations. These processes, moreover, should be *transparent*—with clarity on how priorities and programs are evaluated, and who is involved in determining these evaluations—and remain accountable to the public as a whole.

Promoting Good Governance

The processes by which public health decisions are made often involve compromises between individual and collective interests. Decisions on the prioritization of health resources engender decisions on who receives those resources and, consequently, who will benefit the most based on the prioritized services. These decisions are critically important: when resources are scarce, those who determine where they are allocated determine who benefits from them—and who does not.

The process by which these decisions are reached has substantial ethical implications. Ethicists have argued that decisions reached through systems of poor governance are less deserving of respect than those reached through processes with accountability, consensus-building, responsiveness, participation, transparency, rule of law, and equity (Siddiqi et al., 2009). Ethical governance must enshrine ethical principles of fairness, legitimacy, accountability, and beneficence; whether public health decisions honor and uphold these principles may be modulated by the processes by which these decisions are reached and implemented.

Given the diversity of governments, institutions, values, traditions, and systems that permeate the global field of public health, we do not propose a universal model of good public health governance. Instead, we consider the principles that should guide the robust implementation of good governance in a health system.

The ethical principles that determine whether a health system is achieving good governance are similar to those of responsible stewardship. Systems of good governance tend to be transparent, responsive, and accountable to the public, providing access to knowledge, services, and engagement in health and the health system. Good governance, however, also encompasses additional criteria that are not as closely paralleled in good stewardship: chiefly, adherence to the rule of law and the application of justice (Carlson et al., 2015).

The consistent and just application of legal frameworks is critical to establishing public trust in systems of governance. In settings where citizens hold a justiciable right to health, the enforcement of this right becomes critical in maintaining the legitimacy of the governing authority and expressing justice. More broadly, public health systems may provide strong forms of governance that ensure adequate regulation, accreditation, protection, and redress of grievances. Through these systems, citizens may engage in their health care safely, under the protection of a legal framework that will be enforced by an accountable system.

Systems of governance may also be sensitive to moral considerations of the fair distribution of benefits and burdens, or *distributive justice* (Childress et al., 2002). Good governance ensures that all citizens have fair access to public health benefits and an equitable distribution of burden and costs. Public health policies that stand to benefit a select few at a precipitous cost to the population as a whole are ethically troubling and may be indicative of governing systems that are not publicly accountable. As highlighted at the beginning of this chapter, public health interests are often many and conflicting; given limited resources, investments in one area may limit available resources in another. How can public health professionals ensure that such investments are made in ways that are legitimate, equitable, and accountable to the public they serve?

One way is to recognize that—given the breadth of stakeholders involved in and affected by public health decisions—unanimity without compromise will be impossible. To facilitate the balance of public needs and interests, a pluralistic and deliberative process of governance may be advisable (Daniels, 2000). One of the most salient forms of compromise and collaborative decision-making is that of a deliberative democratic process, whereby individuals or their representatives debate and decide on policies that will affect society as a whole.

The appeal of a democratic process of decision-making is its facilitation of debate in a public and transparent forum, an essential aspect to advancing policy within pluralistic contexts. A premise of democratic policy-shaping is that it fosters "buy-in" of affected parties; when individuals feel that they are represented in the decision-making process, affected parties becomes more enjoined to the ultimate outcome, even if it runs counter to their original position (Daniels, 2000). Even if the democratic system is not perfect, ethicists argue, the system provides a sense of *procedural justice*, or the notion that a process to allocate resources and establish priorities was executed with the participation of affected stakeholders.

Democratic decision-making for public health policy, however, is not without its challenges. A large concern is that the public may lack the expertise public health professionals possess, and thus set policies and priorities that may actually conflict with principles of stewardship, as responsibility and accountability for public health policy is shifted away from technical experts and caregivers (who may have a better sense of the needs of the health system as a whole). However, a variety of innovative ways to better engage lay audiences in complex health decision-making have emerged in recent years to improve public engagement as one input into the policymaking process (Abelson et al., 2013; Goold et al., 2005).

In addition, public health practitioners must be careful in assuring that principles of equity are maintained, and that the needs of minority groups are not eclipsed by the needs of those in the majority. This concern can be mitigated by ensuring adequate representation of marginalized and underrepresented communities and patient groups in health policy decisions, providing a broad and diverse inclusion of citizens in the political decision-making process.

The Absence of Stewardship and Governance

A failure to responsibly steward public resources and govern health systems effectively may lead to the misallocation and waste of limited resources. Rather than prioritize the use of resources by impact, cost-effectiveness, or need, poor custodians of public funds may set priorities to fulfill political or personal agendas, with little association to maximizing the public's health or serving the public's interest (Lewis, 2006). By choosing not to implement policies that demonstrate past success and/or value for money, the health sector will miss opportunities to leverage greater gains in health for greater numbers of its citizens, leading to programming that fails to target and minimize avoidable disability and death. In ethical terms, the misuse of public health resources eschews utilitarian maximization of health and happiness, prevents the minimization of harm, fails to promote public welfare, and erodes public trust in the health system at large.

One of the clearest ways that governments can fail to be responsible stewards of public resources is by ignoring scientific consensus and adopting policies that run counter to scientific evidence. A prominent example of this poor stewardship in health occurred in South Africa at the height of the human immunodeficiency virus/acquired immune deficiency syndrome (HIV/AIDS) epidemic. During the early 2000s, the government argued that HIV was not the cause of AIDS and that antiretroviral (ARV) drugs were not useful to patients. Despite widespread domestic and international outcry from the scientific and medical communities—and from civil society organizations and patients living with HIV—the government instead recommended unproven herbal remedies and declined freely donated nevirapine and grant funding from the Global Fund to treat patients with ARVs (Chigwedere et al., 2008). An estimated 330,000 lives were lost because a timely ARV treatment program was not implemented in South Africa as a result of the government's position.

Poor systems of government may concentrate decision-making authority within a small group or within a single individual, which provides tremendous authority with limited accountability. Such systems of limited accountability and concentrated power may foster decisions influenced by personal biases or, in more extreme cases, corruption, whereby public business is conducted without regard for the rule of law, transparency, and equity of access. This may erode principles of distributive and procedural justice, undermining the fairness of the health system, and delegitimizing its actions. Furthermore, with poor governance there may be an increased risk of actual harm—caused by action or inaction—against the health of the public and/or individual groups therein.

Such poorly functioning systems are anathema to the principles of ethical governance and stewardship outlined in the preceding sections, and it is hard to envision an ethical health system devoid of responsible stewardship and good governance. Where systems disregard empirical knowledge and marginalize technical expertise, public resources become decoupled from their objective to maximize public health and instead may be co-opted to serve the interests of state actors. When public officials act with self-interest rather than for collective benefit, without mechanisms to detect and prevent such action, the public health system is effectively no longer operating for the benefit of the public.

This decoupling of mission and accountability can be expected to rapidly erode public trust and confidence that public systems are operating for the public's good. This may alienate citizens from engaging in the public health system, making it increasingly difficult to implement good governance and stewardship practices in the future.

What emerges from a consideration of a public health system lacking stewardship and governance is a public health system that fails to achieve its objectives through fair processes and an adherence to core ethical principles of public health decision-making and priority-setting. Without ethical principles enshrined by good governance and good stewardship within these processes, societies endanger commitments to public accountability and responsible use of limited resources—two critical components of an ethical public health system.

References

Abelson, J., Blacksher, E. A., Li, K. K., Boesveld, S. E., and Goold, S. D. 2013 "Public Deliberation in Health Policy and Bioethics: Mapping an Emerging, Interdisciplinary Field." *Journal of Public Deliberation* 9(1): 5. http://www.publicdeliberation.net/jpd/vol9/iss1/art5.

Barbazza, E., and Tello, J. E. 2014. "A Review of Health Governance: Definitions, Dimensions and Tools to Govern." *Health Policy* 116(1): 1–11.

Baum, N. M., Gollust, S. E., Goold, S. D., and Jacobson, P. D. 2007. "Looking Ahead: Addressing Ethical Challenges in Public Health Practice" *Journal of Law, Medicine & Ethics* 35(4): 657–667.

Brock, D., and Wikler, D. 2006. "Ethical Issues in Resource Allocation, Research, and New Product Development." In *Disease Control Priorities in Developing Countries*, 2nd ed., edited by D. T. Jamison, J. G. Breman, A. R. Measham, G. Alleyne, M. Claeson, D. B. Evans, et al., 259–270 (Washington, D.C.: World Bank).

Carlson, V., Chilton, M. J., Corso, L. C., and Beitsch, L. M. 2015. "Defining the Functions of Public Health Governance." *American Journal of Public Health* 105(Suppl. 2): S159–S166.

Chigwedere, P., Seage, G. R., III, Gruskin, S., Leet, T.-H., and Essex, M. 2008. "Estimating the Lost Benefits of Antiretroviral Drug Use in South Africa." *JAIDS: Journal of Acquired Immune Deficiency Syndromes* 49(4): 410–415.

Childress, J. F., Faden, R. R., Gaare, R. D., Gostin, L. O., Kahn, J., Bonnie, R. J., et al. 2002. "Public Health Ethics: Mapping the Terrain." *Journal of Law, Medicine & Ethics* 30(2): 170–178.

Daniels, N. 2000. "Accountability for Reasonableness: Establishing a Fair Process for Priority Setting Is Easier Than Agreeing on Principles." *BMJ* 321(7272): 1300.

Daniels, N. 2008. *Just Health: Meeting Health Needs Fairly* (New York: Cambridge University Press).

Daniels, N. 2013. "Justice and Access to Health Care." In *The Stanford Encyclopedia of Philosophy*, edited by E. N. Zalta (Stanford, Calif.: Stanford University). http://plato.stanford.edu/archives/spr2013/entries/justice-healthcareaccess.

Duclos, P. 2010. "National Immunization Technical Advisory Groups (NITAGs): Guidance for Their Establishment and Strengthening." *Vaccine* 28: A18–A25.

Faden, R. R., Kass, N. E., Goodman, S. N., Pronovost, P., Tunis, S., and Beauchamp, T. L. 2013. "An Ethics Framework for a Learning Health Care System: A Departure from Traditional Research Ethics and Clinical Ethics." *Hastings Center Report* 43(Suppl. 1): S16–S27.

Goold, S. D., Biddle, A. K., Klipp, G., Hall, C. N., and Danis, M. 2005. "Choosing Healthplans All Together: A Deliberative Exercise for Allocating Limited Health Are Resources." *Journal of Health Politics, Policy and Law* 30(4): 563–602.

Gostin, L. O. 2010. "Mapping the Issues: Public Health, Law and Ethics." Georgetown Public Law Research Paper No. 10–36. In *Public Health Law and Ethics: A Reader* (New York: Milbank Memorial Fund; Berkeley: University of California Press).

Gwatkin, D. R. 2007. "10 Best Resources on . . . Health Equity." *Health Policy and Planning* 22(5): 348–351.

Jeavons, T. H. 1994. "Stewardship Revisited: Secular and Sacred Views of Governance and Management." *Nonprofit and Voluntary Sector Quarterly* 23(2): 107–122.

Jessop, B. 1998. "The Rise of Governance and the Risks of Failure: The Case of Economic Development." *International Social Science Journal* 50(155): 29–45.

Kass, H. D. 1988. "Stewardship as a Fundamental Element in Images of Public Administration." *Dialogue* 10(2): 2–48.

Krubiner, C. B., and Hyder, A. A. 2014. "A Bioethical Framework for Health Systems Activity: A Conceptual Exploration Applying 'Systems Thinking.'" *Health Systems* 3(2): 124–135.

Lamont, J., and Favor, C. 2014. "Distributive Justice." In *The Stanford Encyclopedia of Philosophy*, edited by E. N. Zalta (Stanford, Calif.: Stanford University). http://plato.stanford.edu/archives/fall2014/entries/justice-distributive.

Lee, L. M. 2012. "Public Health Ethics Theory: Review and Path to Convergence." *Journal of Law, Medicine & Ethics* 40(1): 85–98.

Lewis, M. 2006. *Governance and Corruption in Public Health Care Systems* (Washington, D.C.: Center for Global Development).

Marchand, S., Wikler, D., and Landesman, B. 1998. "Class, Health, and Justice." *Milbank Quarterly* 76(3): 449–467.

McGinnis, J. M., Stuckhardt, L., Saunders, R., and Smith, M., eds. 2013. *Best Care at Lower Cost: The Path to Continuously Learning Health Care in America* (Washington, D.C.: National Academies Press).

Powers, M., and Faden, R. 2006. *Social Justice: The Moral Foundations of Public Health and Health Policy* (New York: Oxford University Press).

Roberts, M. J., Hsiao, W., Berman, P., and Reich, M. R. 2008. *Getting Health Reform Right: A Guide to Improving Performance and Equity* (Oxford: Oxford University Press).

Rodney, A. M, and Hill, P. S. 2014. "Achieving Equity within Universal Health Coverage: A Narrative Review of Progress and Resources for Measuring Success." *International Journal for Equity in Health* 13(1): 72.

Saltman, R. B., and Ferroussier-Davis, O. 2000. "The Concept of Stewardship in Health Policy." *Bulletin of the World Health Organization* 78(6): 732–739.

Saner, M., and Wilson, J. 2003. *Stewardship, Good Governance and Ethics.* Institute on Governance Policy Brief No. 19 (Ottawa: Institute on Governance).

Siddiqi, S., Masud, T. I., Nishtar, S., Peters, D. H., Sabri, B., Bile, K. M., et al. 2009. "Framework for Assessing Governance of the Health System in Developing Countries: Gateway to Good Governance." *Health Policy* 90(1): 13–25.

Travis, P., Egger, D., Davies, P., and Mechbal, A. 2002. *Towards Better Stewardship: Concepts and Critical Issues* (Geneva: World Health Organization).

UNDP (United Nations Development Program). 1997. *Governance for Sustainable Human Development* (New York: Oxford University Press). http://hdr.undp.org/en/content/human-development-report-1997.

UNDP (United Nations Development Program). 2014. *Governance for Sustainable Development: Integrating Governance in the Post-2015 Development Framework* (New York: UNDP). http://www.undp.org/content/dam/undp/library/Democratic%20Governance/Discussion-Paper--Governance-for-Sustainable-Development.pdf.

Venkatapuram, S. 2013. "Health, Vital Goals, and Central Human Capabilities." *Bioethics* 27(5): 271–279.

WHO (World Health Organization). 2000. *The World Health Report—2000 Health Systems: Improving Performance* (Geneva: World Health Organization).

CHAPTER 72

THE POLITICAL ECONOMY OF PUBLIC HEALTH: CHALLENGES FOR ETHICS

TED SCHRECKER

Introduction: The Political Economy of Health

As an analytical approach, the political economy of health is best described by the iconoclastic epidemiologist Nancy Krieger: "[A]nalysis of causes of disease distribution requires attention to the political and economic structures, processes and power relationships that *produce* societal patterns of health, disease, and wellbeing via shaping the conditions in which people live and work" (Krieger, 2011, 168, emphasis in original; see also Birn, Pillay, and Holtz, 2017, 92–95 and chapter 7). As an illustration of the value that this perspective can add to public health ethics, consider Lisa Lee's (2017) identification of the Flint, Michigan, lead poisoning crisis (Bosman, 2016; Carmody, 2016; Osnos, 2016; Bosman, 2017) as a case study in the need for an integrative, multidisciplinary health ethics that incorporates public health and environment as well as the more familiar concerns of bio(medical) ethics.

Lee (2017, 6) argues, correctly, that "[a]n attempt to solve one problem by removing bacteria from the polluted Flint River to make it potable resulted in another—the poisoning of the economically underserved community of Flint." She does not, however, pursue such questions as *why* the community is economically underserved—a mode of inquiry that would include the history of deindustrialization in a once prosperous manufacturing center; racial segregation (Flint's population is now predominantly African American); and, more proximally, a program of shrinking public sector services and budgets that had been actively promoted by a variety of neoliberal think tanks

(MacLean, 2017, 213–215; MacLean's book, and much of the recent scholarship she cites, are essential reading for anyone wishing to take seriously the political economy of public health, especially in the US context).

The Flint case shows that the production of patterns of health and illness to which Krieger refers is more than a metaphor. For an example in the global frame of reference, a history dating back to circa 1980 connects structural adjustment conditionalities demanded by the International Monetary Fund and the World Bank in return for loans to support a restructuring of countries' external debts with rising inequality and destructive effects on health systems and social determinants of health (Kentikelenis, 2017). Several observers have connected the debilitating effects on national health systems of these conditionalities with the rapid spread of the Ebola outbreak in several African countries in 2014 (Rowden, 2014; Kentikelenis et al., 2015; Sanders, Sengupta, and Scott, 2015). Commentators differ about the motivations of those promoting such conditionalities; compare, for example, the view of the historian Ricardo Soares de Oliveira (2007, 44), writing specifically about sub-Saharan Africa, that "the goal was to debilitate the institutions and strategies that had thus far enabled the survival and prosperity of local elites and provided the structure for existing, if no longer viable, patronage systems" with the generic conclusion of a multidisciplinary panel of social scientists examining the prospects for "sustainable democracy" that "[a]n alliance of the international financial institutions, the private banks, and the Thatcher-Reagan-Kohl governments was willing to use its political and ideological power to back its ideological predilections" (Przeworski et al., 1995, 5), Whatever the operative motivations, the health consequences of structural adjustment show that understanding the relevant historical processes, institutional structures, and macro-scale policies is a prerequisite for intellectually responsible discussions of public health ethics.

Against this background, the chapter is organized around three core messages. First, and most fundamentally, public finance is a public health issue. Second, the transnational corporate role in the spread of disease, and the associated "power asymmetries" (Ottersen et al., 2014), must be taken into account in public health ethics. Third, these two observations (and others) indicate the inseparability of ethics and politics in public health. After an explication of these points, the chapter concludes with three challenges for building a public health ethics that "speaks truth about power" in an increasingly inhospitable policy environment.

Public Finance and Public Health Ethics

In the context of recent programs of fiscal austerity, in the United Kingdom in the first instance, the editor of *The Lancet* noted: "What is promoted as fiscal discipline is a political choice. A political choice that deepens the already open and bloody wounds of the poor and precarious" (Horton, 2017, 110). The choice does not, in fact, reflect any underlying economic necessity (Krugman, 2015), but rather a judgment about the relative value attached to protecting the lives and wealth of differently situated members of a society (Basu, Carney, and Kenworthy, 2017). Post-2010, a Conservative-led government expanded the Thatcher-era project of neoliberalization (Ward and England, 2007) by way of selective expenditure cutbacks that were, at this writing, on track to reduce the public sector's share of the economy to pre–World War II levels—that is, to levels that predate the establishment of the National Health Service and the institutions of the postwar welfare state (Johnson, 2014). A senior social policy scholar observed that this amounted to a "root and branch restructuring" of the United Kingdom's economy and society, of which "[t]he longer-term goal is to shrink the state, free the market and set British political economy on a new course" (Taylor-Gooby, 2012, 61). The cuts fell most heavily not only on the most vulnerable people but also on the poorest local economies (as summarized by Schrecker, 2017), which were already among the poorest regions in northern Europe (Eurostat, 2014). Notably, cutbacks in benefit levels and an aggressive and often capricious regime of benefit "sanctioning" (actual or threatened cutoffs) have been linked to rapid increases in reliance on charity food banks (Garthwaite, 2016), and—in both epidemiological studies and Parliamentary committee testimony—a rise in the prevalence of mental health problems and suicides (Mcdougall et al., 2015; Barr et al., 2016).

To reiterate: whatever the overall quantum of resources available to a government or other authoritative decision-maker, and keeping in mind that scarcity is seldom absolute in the sense that scarcities of rare earth elements or biologically compatible organ donors are absolute (Schrecker, 2013b), choices about public finance reflect assumptions or conclusions that some people's lives matter more than others' (Basu, Carney, and Kenworthy, 2017), and about why they do. This point was brought home in June 2017, when at least seventy-nine people died in a horrific fire in a London social housing tower block (Grenfell Tower). At the time of this writing, investigations were ongoing, but the use of flammable, and slightly less expensive, exterior cladding as a cost-cutting measure by contractors undertaking a refurbishment for the responsible local council (in the ultra-wealthy borough of Kensington and Chelsea) appears to have been an important factor, in turn enabled by deregulation and a lack of resources for inspection and oversight (Kirkpatrick, Hakim, and Glanz, 2017). It remains to be seen whether public revulsion in the aftermath will lead to changes in priorities. Furthermore, how that revulsion could be articulated is unclear.

Public finance is a public health issue in low- and middle-income countries (LMICs) as well. In a seeming turnaround from the legacy of structural adjustment conditionalities, universal health coverage (UHC) is now prominent on the global development policy agenda, and indeed is the topic of a target under the United Nations' 2015 Sustainable Development Goals. Although increases in development assistance will be indispensable in some countries, in many the most important prerequisite for progress toward UHC will be the ability to mobilize domestic resources more effectively through taxation (Centre on Global Health Security, 2014). This mobilization may not be politically attainable, as can be seen from the example of India—a conspicuous underachiever on health indicators relative to economically comparable countries (Drèze and Sen, 2013), yet one where a newly elected government in 2015 opted to reduce an already minimal public sector health care budget (Mudur, 2015). A similar pattern can be seen on the African continent, where, more than a decade after a 2001 commitment by African Union member countries to raise health sector spending to 15 percent of the general government budget, many countries had made only modest progress (African Union, 2013). A recent World Health Organization analysis confirms this as a general pattern, finding a recent "overall deterioration in the role of domestic public funds for health spending, especially in low-income countries" (Barroy et al., 2017, vi). Thus, the interface of public finance and public health ethics involves choices on the revenue side as well as the expenditure side. This brief description cannot do justice to the complexities of the domestic politics of health care financing, but it underscores the central importance of a health ethics focus on public finance—at least unless one regards a state of affairs in which access to health care and the prerequisites for a healthy life is proportional to a household's income or wealth as unproblematic.

In the international economic and political environment, the legacy of health systems weakened by structural adjustment has already been mentioned. A further problem, only recently recognized as consequential for health and health policy, involves the fiscally debilitating effects of capital flight (Schrecker, 2014a) and tax avoidance, which along with the desire for higher and more secure returns on investment is one of the primary motivations for capital flight (Harrington, 2016; Cobham and Jansky, 2017; Cobham, 2017). Some of the magnitudes remain contested (Forstater, 2017), but it is now clear that these processes have drained and are draining many LMIC economies of resources that—at least under favorable domestic political conditions—could have been invested in health care systems, public health programming, and efforts to address social determinants of health (for a nontechnical overview in the African context, see Ndikumana and Boyce, 2011).

An important caveat is in order at this point, given the increasing attention being paid to an approach usually described as "health in all" policies (WHO, 2015). The principle that public policy in areas that do not directly or obviously relate to health should be made with knowledge of the likely consequences for health (both positive and negative) is unexceptionable. This does not, however, imply that policies with negative consequences for health, or health inequalities, should never be adopted. As Daniel Weinstock (2015) points out, public policy is unavoidably about trade-offs among competing priorities, and it is impossible to optimize for multiple values simultaneously except as a matter of serendipity. Accepting the value of health in all policies as an approach to policy analysis does not mandate prioritizing health in all policy fields. Norms limiting the permissible negative consequences for health can be derived not only from principles of distributive justice (which admittedly represent contested terrain), but also from the norms embodied in international human rights instruments, notably those related to core obligations, progressive realization and non-retrogression (Schrecker, 2014b), but elaborating on these points would take us far beyond the scope and allowable length of this chapter.

The Corporate Role: "Vectors of Spread" for "Industrial Epidemics"?

Noncommunicable diseases (NCDs) represent most of the burden of illness in the high-income world, and their importance is rapidly increasing elsewhere. These are often inaccurately thought of as diseases of affluence, "lifestyle," or both (Ezzati et al., 2005; Glasgow and Schrecker, 2015). Alternatively, a political economy perspective foregrounds two specific phenomena. Socioeconomically patterned differences exist within societies in people's opportunities to live healthy lives. Manifestations include the unaffordability of healthy diets and the way in which housing markets in some settings segregate people on low incomes into "food deserts" (Beaulac, Kristjansson, and Cummins, 2009; Walker, Keane, and Burke, 2010; Burns, 2014). Against this background, large, mainly transnational corporations (TNCs) and their formidable investment, marketing, and lobbying resources shape both the choices available to individuals and households and the trajectory of public policies that affect health. Focusing on this dimension of public health policy, Rob Moodie and colleagues (2013, 671) have argued that the rising burden of NCDs is best explained as a congeries of "industrial epidemics" in which "the vectors of spread are not biological agents, but transnational corporations" in the tobacco, food, and drinks industries.

Comparisons with the tobacco industry are both provocative and instructive. Tobacco TNCs based in the United States and the United Kingdom are now notorious for a history of efforts to obscure or distract from scientific evidence of harm, by means ranging from selective citation to straightforward fraud (Glantz et al., 1996). They have also lobbied aggressively against public health measures, notably in expanding markets in LMICs (e.g., Egbe, Bialous, and Glantz, 2017; Boseley, 2017; Kalra et al., 2017a). Notably, recent years have also seen an intensification of the industry's efforts to shape and use the provisions of trade and investment agreements to override requirements for plain packaging and warning labels (Fooks and Gilmore, 2014), on grounds related to lost revenues or expropriation of intellectual property (Russell, Wainwright, and Mamudu, 2015; Steele et al., 2015; Eckhardt, Holden, and Callard, 2016; Roache, Gostin, and Bianco, 2016). Such efforts have so far been largely unsuccessful, but defending against them, especially at the level of trade dispute resolution, requires substantial public sector resources. In such contexts, power asymmetries between TNCs and their acolytes and governments seeking to protect public health are especially marked—as they are with regard to the tobacco industry's continued, well-resourced efforts to frustrate national implementation of the Framework Convention on Tobacco Control (Kalra et al., 2017b).

Public policy toward the tobacco industry has sometimes been characterized by what has been termed "tobacco exceptionalism," but according to one leading tobacco policy researcher, "there is little to suggest that the corporate strategies of alcohol or food corporations are inherently more conducive to positive health outcomes" (Collin, 2012, 277;

see also Freudenberg, 2014, 37–69). The motor and fossil fuel industries should almost certainly be added to this list. The strategy of "manufacturing uncertainty" with respect to scientific evidence originated with the tobacco industry, but it has since been adopted by other industrial interests, with respect not only to environmental and workplace exposures (Michaels and Monforton, 2005; Michaels, 2006; Davis, 2007, 296–434), but also to diet, perhaps most conspicuously with regard to the effects of dietary sugar, as documented in an important journalistic exposé (Taubes and Couzens, 2012). Even when such strategies are not deployed, the sheer value of resources that large corporations can devote to refining and marketing their products provides them with substantial, often unhealthy, influence on consumption patterns (Moss, 2013). This is a global concern: as barriers to trade and investment are lowered, rapid expansion of supermarket, ultra-processed food, and fast food TNCs into LMIC markets is having serious negative consequences for dietary patterns (Popkin, Adair, and Ng, 2012; Popkin and Slining, 2013; Friel et al., 2013; Monteiro et al., 2013; Freudenberg, 2014, 153–178; Popkin, 2014, 2015; Popkin and Hawkes, 2016). These portend a perfect storm in terms of future morbidity patterns and health system costs related to such NCDs as cardiovascular disease and diabetes, in addition to the obvious direct human consequences.

Such patterns are problematic because, like the tobacco industry's lobbying activities, they are a manifestation of the raw power of money to shape decisions that affect people's lives and health. This is a larger problem in democratic theory, one of several at the interface of political theory and health ethics. In addition, industry strategies distort the content of public health policy discussions by miscasting them as discussions of the strength of scientific evidence—sometimes in highly disingenuous ways—rather than of the underlying values that should guide public health policy in a context where waiting for further evidence inescapably embodies a choice to value certain outcomes and interests over others, and public health policy must accept "the inevitability of being wrong" some of the time (Jellinek, 1981). Four decades of analysis on the importance of standards of proof (choices about how much evidence is enough) in environmental policy and law have had minimal impact elsewhere in the study of population health and public health ethics (Schrecker, 2013a).

Analysis: Ethics Meets Politics in Public Health—"Choice" for Whom? From What Menu? And Who Selects the Items on the Menu?

The political economy of health foregrounds multiple economically driven power asymmetries between transnational corporate actors and others. Some of us would go beyond a focus on transnational corporations to identify a transnational capitalist class (see Sklair, 2005; Robinson, 2010; Carroll, 2014; Carroll and Sapinski, 2016, among many other sources), although the point is contested. The political economy of health thereby provides an important counterpoint to framings of public health ethics issues that focus on the extent to which policy measures represent (im)permissible restrictions on individual autonomy as manifested through consumer choice (about such matters as diet, consumption of pleasurable substances, or mode of transport). Such framings are familiar from polemics against restrictions on corporate activities that invoke the idea of the "nanny state" (Magnusson, 2015), but are also evident in more subtle form in, for example, the "intervention ladder" devised by the UK's Nuffield Council on Bioethics (Krebs et al., 2007)—a device that fails to reflect many of the nuances correctly identified in the Nuffield report's background discussion. Only two, related problems with such conceptions of choice can be identified here.

As Griffiths and West (2015, 1093) point out, the intervention ladder, organized as it is around a unidimensional conception of "liberty," embodies the presumption "that no policy can do more to promote liberty than non-intervention." A moment's reflection on this proposition in other contexts—think for example about domestic violence—suffices to show its vacuity. The implicit presumption that there are only two categories of relevant actors, the state and the individual, ignores the complex policy landscape and the role of actors such as large corporations—as well as disparities in social and economic situation—that affect what choices are available to particular individuals. The implicit, and undefended, presumption is that only state agencies are capable of choice-limiting actions or "coercion." However, as noted in the lead author's foreword to the Nuffield report: "It takes only a moment's thought to recognize that many of the 'choices' that individuals make about their lifestyle are heavily constrained as a result of policies established by central and local government, by various industries as well as by various kinds of inequality in society" (Krebs et al., 2007, v). Ignoring these dimensions in discussions of choice and autonomy is intellectually irresponsible; if state decisions about public finance shape the options available to individuals in different life situations, so too do decisions made by large corporations about such matters as investment and product line characteristics (cf., Nadel, 1976). Further, state decisions articulate the scope that such actors have to operate independently of collectively agreed-upon restrictions. Indeed, discussion of contemporary public policy that ignores corporate influence is a bit "like Frankenstein with the monster left out" (Hacker, 1973, 173).

Further, as noted in the Nuffield foreword and the extensive literature on social determinants of health, consumer choices are always constrained by a substrate of inequality. They are limited by purchasing power, which is unequally distributed, and other stratifiers related to socioeconomic position (as in the case of food deserts). Beyond this, public health ethics must interact with political theory with regard to the distinction between individual choices and collective choices about the conditions in which we may want to live and work, which, at least in idealized democratic polities, we make together. Thus, given a particular set of circumstances and life chances, we might personally want to be able to smoke at our local pub or drive home after several beers, yet also favor eliminating that option out of concern for the health of those we care about who are fellow road users or are exposed to secondhand smoke during long shifts as servers. We may want to drive to work in a single-occupancy vehicle and bring fast food home for dinner on the return journey, yet *at the same time* we might prefer a set of social arrangements that raised taxes to support functioning public transport, or at least vehicle sharing, and local tax structures that would have offered preferential rates to now-defunct local grocery stores offering healthy food choices.

The environmental law scholar Mark Sagoff (1981a, 1981b, 1981c) has made a homologous point using, as an illustration, the responses of students presented with a plan to develop a ski resort in a wilderness area. By their own account, the students would probably never visit the wilderness area and were enthusiastic about the recreational opportunities offered by the ski resort. Nevertheless, when asked whether the development proposal should proceed, the students' reaction "was unanimous, visceral and grim. All of the students believed that the Disney plan was loathsome and despicable; that the [US] Forest Service had violated a public trust by approving it; and that the values for which we stand as a nation compel us to preserve the little wilderness we have for its own sake and as an historical heritage" (Sagoff, 1981c, 284). The distinction in play is that between our preferences and values as consumers and as citizens; despite the best efforts of the acolytes of cost-benefit analysis and of public choice interpretations of political activity (MacLean, 2017), they are not reducible to one another.

Three Future Challenges

Political economy focuses on "upstream" influences on health—what Sir Michael Marmot, borrowing a phrase from Geoffrey Rose, calls "the causes of the causes" (Marmot, 2005). This formulation leaves open the question of *how far* upstream to look. In the Flint example that began the chapter, is it sufficient to examine the proximal political choices that led to the poisoning of this relatively vulnerable population—which have led to criminal charges against senior public officials (Glenza, 2017)—or is it necessary, as suggested in the introduction, to consider such structural issues as systemic racism, the nature and sources of pressures to shrink public budgets, and even the mechanisms by which revenues to support public services are raised? The author leans strongly in this latter direction, while recognizing that in many cases the "how far upstream" choice represents what Kristin Shrader-Frechette and Earl McCoy (1993, 84) refer to as methodological value judgments. Sometimes, however, the line between such judgments and scientific or explanatory incompleteness is blurred. Thus, in a critique of studies of neighborhood effects on life chances, the geographer Tom Slater (2013, 369) questioned the presumption that causal pathways run from residential location to such outcomes as escaping poverty rather than in the opposite direction: "If *where* any given individual lives affects their life chances as deeply as neighborhood effects proponents believe, it seems crucial to understand *why* that individual is living there in the first place." This means inquiring into such variables as influences on the distribution of income, and such processes as the socio-spatial sorting function performed by housing markets. It was not the white middle class that inhabited New Orleans' Lower Ninth Ward, the community most devastated by Hurricane Katrina in 2005, and least benefited by subsequent reconstruction efforts.

Such questions assume increasing importance against a background of rising inequality, in countries rich and poor alike (Bourguignon, 2015), often magnified rather than attenuated by policy choices. In the United Kingdom, the Conservative prime minister David Cameron (2009) (in)famously claimed that his government's approach to austerity would embody the principle that "we're all in this together"—a claim that was decisively refuted at the end of his first term by analysis of cumulative budget impacts (De Agostini, Hills, and Sutherland, 2015). Presciently, the editor of *New Perspectives Quarterly* observed in 1993 that "[a]lready people merely surviving in places like Bangladesh and across vast stretches of Africa are superfluous from the standpoint of the market. By and large, we don't need what they have; they can't buy what we sell"; from a public health perspective, the epidemiological worlds inhabited by these populations are in most important aspects completely different from "the archipelago of the connected classes that reside in every megacity from Bombay to São Paulo" (Gardels, 1993, 3). Even within high-income countries, barriers to replicating the "cross-class political alliance" that the historian Simon Szreter (1999) sees as having driven public health policy advances in nineteenth-century England in today's contexts are often formidable.

This is partly because, as production and finance have been reorganized across multiple national borders over the past few decades, distributional conflicts can no longer be contained and need not be resolved within national borders—a necessary precondition for settlements between labor and capital in the high-income world, many of which are now unravelling, and one reason among several to doubt that the politics of the future will be like those of the postwar past. Much ethical and policy analysis related to public health operates on the implicit and decontextualized assumption that some form, albeit rudimentary, of social contract exists between rulers and subjects. We assume that governments can be expected to care at least a little bit about the welfare of people within their national borders. However, serious consideration of the changes in social structure associated with contemporary globalization raises the prospect that even in formal democratic jurisdictions, governments and political elites may *simply not care* about the welfare of a substantial portion of their compatriots, whose command of political resources is minimal. Again, the example of Hurricane Katrina is instructive (see Hartman and Squires, 2006; Somers, 2008, 63–117).

An additional layer of complexity is introduced by the spread of "illiberal democracy" (Zakaria, 1997)—the breakdown of political accountability and the rule of law, and the simultaneous spread of authoritarianism. A founding editor of the *Journal of Democracy* has described what he calls a "democratic recession" post-2006, a turning point identified by Freedom House, with particular focus on "a class of regimes that in the last decade or so have experienced significant erosion in electoral fairness, political pluralism, and civic space for opposition and dissent, typically as a result of abusive executives intent upon concentrating their personal power and entrenching ruling-party hegemony" (Diamond, 2015). One need not look further than the lead stories of any reputable news outlet. In a growing range of contexts, it is problematic, if not fatal, for subjects to advocate for protecting their own health and to attempt to mobilize the political coalitions that drove earlier advances in public health—as shown, for example, by the work of Global Witness (2017) on the killings of activists organizing against environmental destruction. Public health ethics must come to grips with this reality, as with others, by engaging with the relevant social science, and with the relevant protagonists "on the ground."

References

African Union 2013. *Abuja +12: Shaping the Future of Health in Africa* (Geneva: UNAIDS). http://www.unaids.org/en/media/unaids/contentassets/documents/unaidspublication/2013/JC2524_Abuja_report_en.pdf.

Barr, B., Taylor-Robinson, D., Stuckler, D., Loopstra, R., Reeves, A., and Whitehead, M. 2016. "'First, Do No Harm': Are Disability Assessments Associated with Adverse Trends in Mental Health? A Longitudinal Ecological Study." *Journal of Epidemiology and Community Health* 70(4): 339–345.

Barroy, H., Vaughan, K., Tapsoba, Y., Dale, E., and Van de Maele, N. 2017. "Towards UHC: Thinking Public—Overview of Trends in Public Expenditure on Health (2000–2014)." Health Financing Working Paper No. 7 (Geneva: World Health Organization). http://www.who.int/iris/bitstream/10665/255782/1/9789241512428-eng.pdf.

Basu, S., Carney, M. A., and Kenworthy, N. J. 2017. "Ten Years after the Financial Crisis: The Long Reach of Austerity and Its Global Impacts on Health." *Social Science and Medicine* 187: 203–207.

Beaulac, J., Kristjansson, E., and Cummins, S. 2009. "A Systematic Review of Food Deserts, 1966–2007." *Preventing Chronic Disease* 6(3). http://www.cdc.gov/pcd/issues/2009/jul/08_0163.htm?s_cid=pcd63a105_e.

Birn, A.-E., Pillay, Y., and Holtz, T. 2017. *Textbook of Global Health*. 4th ed. (New York: Oxford University Press).

Boseley, S. 2017. "Threats, Bullying, Lawsuits: Tobacco Industry's Dirty War for the African Market." *Guardian*, July 12. https://www.theguardian.com/world/2017/jul/12/big-tobacco-dirty-war-africa-market.

Bosman, J. 2016. "Many Flint Residents Are Desperate to Leave, but See No Escape." *New York Times*, February 5. http://www.nytimes.com/2016/02/05/us/many-flint-residents-are-desperate-to-leave-but-see-no-escape.html.

Bosman, J. 2017. "On This Block, Worries Run Deeper than Flint's Tainted Water." *New York Times*, April 25. https://www.nytimes.com/2017/04/25/us/flint-water-blight-violence.html.

Bourguignon, F. 2015. *The Globalization of Inequality* (Princeton, N.J.: Princeton University Press).

Burns, R. 2014. "Atlanta's Food Deserts Leave Its Poorest Citizens Stranded and Struggling." *Guardian*, March 17. http://www.theguardian.com/cities/2014/mar/17/atlanta-food-deserts-stranded-struggling-survive.

Cameron, D. 2009. "Conservative Conference 2009: Full Text of David Cameron's speech." *Guardian*, October 8. https://www.theguardian.com/politics/2009/oct/08/david-cameron-speech-in-full.

Carmody, T. 2016. "How the Flint River Got So Toxic: Factories and People Have Been Dumping Sewage, Chemicals, and Road Salt in the Flint River for More than a Century." *The Verge*, February 26. http://www.theverge.com/2016/2/26/11117022/flint-michigan-water-crisis-lead-pollution-history.

Carroll, W. K. 2014. "Whither the Transnational Capitalist Class?" In *Socialist Register 2014: Registering Class*, edited by L. Panitch, G. Albo, and V. Chibber, 162–188 (London: Merlin).

Carroll, W. K., and Sapinski, J. P. 2016. "Neoliberalism and the Transnational Capitalist Class." In *The Handbook of Neoliberalism*, edited by K. Birch, J. MacLeavy, and S. Springer, 25–35 (London: Routledge).

Centre on Global Health Security Working Group on Health Financing 2014. *Shared Responsibilities for Health: A Coherent Global Framework for Health Financing*. Chatham House Report (London: Chatham House). http://www.chathamhouse.org/sites/files/chathamhouse/field/field_document/20140521HealthFinancing.pdf.

Cobham, A. 2017. "The Significance and Subversion of SDG 16.4: Multinational Tax Avoidance as IFF." Tax Justice Network, June 1. http://www.taxjustice.net/2017/06/01/subversion-sdg-16-4/.

Cobham, A., and Jansky, P. 2017. "Global Distribution of Revenue Loss from Tax Avoidance: Re-estimation and Country Results." WIDER Working Paper No. 2017/55 (Helsinki: World Institute for Development Economics Research). https://www.wider.unu.edu/sites/default/files/wp2017-55.pdf.

Collin, J. 2012. "Tobacco Control, Global Health Policy and Development: Towards Policy Coherence in Global Governance." *Tobacco Control* 21(2): 274–280.

Davis, D. L. 2007. *The Secret History of the War on Cancer* (New York: Basic Books).

De Agostini, P., Hills, J., and Sutherland, H. 2015. "Were We Really All in It Together? The Distributional Effects of the 2010–2015 UK Coalition Government's Tax-Benefit Policy Changes: An End-of-Term Update, Social Policy in a Cold Climate." Working Paper No. 22 (London: Centre for Analysis of Social Exclusion, London School of Economics and Political Science). http://sticerd.lse.ac.uk/dps/case/spcc/wp22.pdf.

Diamond, L. 2015. "Facing Up to the Democratic Recession." *Journal of Democracy* 26(1): 141–155.

Drèze, J., and Sen, A. 2013. *An Uncertain Glory: India and its Contradictions* (London: Allen Lane).

Eckhardt, J., Holden, C., and Callard, C. D. 2016. "Tobacco Control and the World Trade Organization: Mapping Member States' Positions after the Framework Convention on Tobacco Control." *Tobacco Control* 25(6): 692–698.

Egbe, C. O., Bialous, S. A., and Glantz, S. A. 2017. "Avoiding 'A Massive Spin-Off Effect in West Africa and Beyond': The Tobacco Industry Stymies Tobacco Control in Nigeria." *Nicotine and Tobacco Research* 19(7): 877–887. doi:10.1093/ntr/ntx037.

Eurostat. 2014. *GDP Per Capita in the EU in 2011: Seven Capital Regions among the Ten Most Prosperous* (Luxembourg: Eurostat). https://ec.europa.eu/eurostat/web/products-press-releases/-/1-27022014-AP.

Ezzati, M., Vander Hoorn, S., Lawes, C. M., Leach, R., James, W. P., Lopez, A. D., et al. 2005. "Rethinking the 'Diseases of Affluence' Paradigm: Global Patterns of Nutritional Risks in Relation to Economic Development." *PLoS Medicine* 2(5): e133.

Fooks, G., and Gilmore, A. B. 2014. "International Trade Law, Plain Packaging and Tobacco Industry Political Activity: The Trans-Pacific Partnership." Tobacco Control 23(1): e1–e9.

Forstater, M. 2017. "Gaps in Trade Data Do Not Equal Criminal Money Laundering." *Center for Global Development Blog*, January 6. http://www.cgdev.org/blog/gaps-trade-data-criminal-money-laundering.

Freudenberg, N. 2014. *Lethal but Legal: Corporations, Consumption, and Protecting Public Health* (New York: Oxford University Press).

Friel, S., Hattersley, L., Snowdon, W., Thow, A. M., Lobstein, T., Sanders, D., 2013. "Monitoring the Impacts of Trade Agreements on Food Environments." *Obesity Reviews* 14(Suppl. 1): 120–134.

Gardels, N. 1993. "The Post-Atlantic Capitalist Order." *New Perspectives Quarterly* 10(2): 2–3.

Garthwaite, K. 2016. *Hunger Pains: Life inside Foodbank Britain* (Bristol, UK: Policy Press).

Glantz, S. A., Slade, J., Bero, L. A., Hanauer, P., and Barnes, D. E. 1996. *The Cigarette Papers* (Berkeley: University of California Press).

Glasgow, S., and Schrecker, T. 2015. "The Double Burden of Neoliberalism? Noncommunicable Disease Policies and the Global Political Economy of Risk." *Health and Place* 34 (July): 279–286.

Glenza, J. 2017. "Flint Water Crisis: Five Officials Charged with Involuntary Manslaughter." *Guardian*, June 14. https://www.theguardian.com/us-news/2017/jun/14/flint-water-crisis-manslaughter-charges-government-officials.

Global Witness. 2017. *Defenders of the Earth* (London: Global Witness). https://www.global-witness.org/en/campaigns/environmental-activists/defenders-earth/.

Griffiths, P. E., and West, C. 2015. "A Balanced Intervention Ladder: Promoting Autonomy through Public Health Action." *Public Health* 129(8): 1092–1098.

Hacker, A. 1973. "Citizen Counteraction?" In *Corporate Power in America*, edited by R. Nader and M. Green, 171–181 (New York: Grossman).

Harrington, B. 2016. *Capital without Borders: Wealth Managers and the One Percent* (Cambridge, Mass.: Harvard University Press).

Hartman, C., and Squires, G. D. 2006. *There's No Such Thing as a Natural Disaster: Race, Class and Hurricane Katrina* (New York: Routledge).

Horton, R. 2017. "Offline: Not One Day More." *Lancet* 390(10090): 110.

Jellinek, S. D. 1981. "On the Inevitability of Being Wrong." *Annals of the New York Academy of Sciences* 363(1): 43–47.

Johnson, P. 2014. "Autumn Statement Briefing 2014: Introductory Remarks" (London: Institute for Fiscal Studies). http://www.ifs.org.uk/uploads/publications/budgets/as2014/as2014_johnson.pdf.

Kalra, A., Bansal, P., Lasseter, T., and Wilson, D. 2017a. "The Philip Morris Files, Part 2: Marlboro Country—Philip Morris Takes Aim at Young People in India, and Health Officials are Fuming." Reuters Investigates. http://www.reuters.com/investigates/special-report/pmi-india.

Kalra, A., Bansal, P., Wilson, D., and Lasseter, T. 2017b. "The Philip Morris Files, Part I: Treaty Blitz—Inside Philip Morris' Campaign to Subvert the Global Anti-smoking Treaty." Reuters Investigates. http://www.reuters.com/investigates/special-report/pmi-who-fctc/.

Kentikelenis, A. E. 2017. "Structural Adjustment and Health: A Conceptual Framework and Evidence on Pathways." *Social Science and Medicine* 187(August): 296–305.

Kentikelenis, A. E., King, L., McKee, M., and Stuckler, D. 2015. "The International Monetary Fund and the Ebola Outbreak." *Lancet Global Health* 3(2): e69–e70.

Kirkpatrick, D. D., Hakim, D, and Glanz, J. 2017. "An Accident Waiting to Happen": Blame in a Deadly London Fire." *New York Times*, June 25. https://www.nytimes.com/2017/06/24/world/europe/grenfell-tower-london-fire.html

Krebs, J. R., Ali, R., Baldwin, T., Brownsword, R., Calman, K., Godfrey, C., et al. 2007. *Public Health: Ethical Issues* (Cambridge: Nuffield Council on Bioethics). http://nuffieldbioethics.org/wp-content/uploads/2014/07/Public-health-ethical-issues.pdf.

Krieger, N. 2011. *Epidemiology and the People's Health: Theory and Context* (Oxford: Oxford University Press).

Krugman, P. 2015. "The Austerity Delusion." *Guardian*, April 29. http://www.theguardian.com/business/2015/apr/28/top-economist-attacks-tory-austerity-labours-limp-response-paul-krugman.

Lee, L. M. 2017. "A Bridge Back to the Future: Public Health Ethics, Bioethics, and Environmental Ethics." *American Journal of Bioethics* 17(9): 5–12.

MacLean, N. 2017. *Democracy in Chains: The Deep History of the Radical Right's Stealth Plan for America* (New York: Viking).

Magnusson, R. S. 2015. "Case Studies in Nanny State Name-Calling: What Can We Learn?" *Public Health* 129(8): 1074–1082.

Marmot, M. 2005. "Social Determinants of Health Inequalities." *Lancet* 365(9464): 1099–1104.

Mcdougall, G., Moriarty, S, Curtis, T, Thompson, G, and Gaze, B. J. 2015. "'My Mental Health Deteriorated Rapidly': The Real Impact of Benefit Sanctions." *Guardian*, January 27. http://www.theguardian.com/society/2015/jan/27/mental-health-benefit-sanctions-work-and-pensions-select-committee.

Michaels, D. 2006. "Manufactured Uncertainty." *Annals of the New York Academy of Sciences* 1076(1) 149–162.

Michaels, D., and Monforton, C. 2005. "Manufacturing Uncertainty: Contested Science and the Protection of the Public's Health and Environment." *American Journal of Public Health* 95(Suppl. 1): S39–S48.

Monteiro, C. A., Moubarac, J. C., Cannon, G., Ng, S. W., and Popkin, B. 2013. "Ultra-Processed Products are Becoming Dominant in the Global Food System." *Obesity Reviews* 14(S2): 21–28.

Moodie, R., Stuckler, D., Monteiro, C., Sheron, N., Neal, B., Thamarangsi, T., et al. 2013. "Profits and Pandemics: Prevention of Harmful Effects of Tobacco, Alcohol, and Ultra-processed Food and Drink Industries." *Lancet* 381(9867): 670–679.

Moss, M. 2013. *Salt, Sugar, Fat: How the Food Giants Hooked Us* (London: W.H. Allen).

Mudur, G. 2015. "Experts Question How India Will Meet Promises on Public Health after Cut in Budget for 2015–16." *British Medical Journal* 350: h1244.

Nadel, M. V. 1976. *Corporations and Political Accountability* (Lexington, Mass.: DC Heath).

Ndikumana, L., and Boyce, J. 2011. *Africa's Odious Debts: How Foreign Loans and Capital Flight Bled a Continent* (London: Zed Books).

Osnos, E. 2016. "The Crisis in Flint Goes Deeper Than the Water." *New Yorker*, January 20. http://www.newyorker.com/news/news-desk/the-crisis-in-flint-goes-deeper-than-the-water.

Ottersen, O. P., Dasgupta, J., Blouin, C., Buss, P., Chongsuvivatwong, V., Frenk, J., et al. 2014. "The Political Origins of Health Inequity: Prospects for Change." *Lancet* 383 (9917): 630–667.

Popkin, B. M. 2014. "Nutrition, Agriculture and the Global Food System in Low and Middle Income Countries." *Food Policy* 47: 91–96.

Popkin, B. M. 2015. "Nutrition Transition and the Global Diabetes Epidemic." *Current Diabetes Reports* 15(9): 1–8.

Popkin, B. M., Adair, L. S., and Ng, S. W. 2012. "Global Nutrition Transition and the Pandemic of Obesity in Developing Countries." *Nutrition Reviews* 70(1): 3–21.

Popkin, B. M., and Hawkes, C. 2016. "Sweetening of the Global Diet, Particularly Beverages: Patterns, Trends, and Policy Responses." *Lancet Diabetes and Endocrinology* 4(2) 174–186.

Popkin, B. M., and Slining, M. M. 2013. "New Dynamics in Global Obesity Facing Low- and Middle-Income Countries." *Obesity Reviews* 14(Suppl. 2): 11–20.

Przeworski, A., Bardhan, P., Bresser Pereira, L. C., Bruszt, L., Choi, J. J., Comisso, E. T., et al. 1995. *Sustainable Democracy* (Cambridge: Cambridge University Press).

Roache, S. A., Gostin, L. O., and Bianco, F. E. 2016. "Trade, Investment, and Tobacco: Philip Morris v Uruguay." *JAMA* 316 (20): 2085–2086.

Robinson, W. I. 2010. "Global Capitalism Theory and the Emergence of Transnational Elites." WIDER Working Paper No. 2010/02 (Helsinki: World Institute for Development Economics Research). http://www.wider.unu.edu/publications/working-papers/2010/en_GB/wp2010-02/_files/82825453722271811/default/2010-02.pdf.

Rowden, R. 2014. "West Africa's Financial Immune Deficiency." *Foreign Policy*, October 30. http://www.foreignpolicy.com/articles/2014/10/30/west_africas_financial_immune_deficiency_ebola_imf.

Russell, A., Wainwright, M., and Mamudu, H. 2015. "A Chilling Example? Uruguay, Philip Morris International, and WHO's Framework Convention on Tobacco Control." *Medical Anthropology Quarterly* 29(2): 256–277.

Sagoff, M. 1981a. "At the Shrine of Our Lady of Fatima, or Why Political Questions Are Not All Economic." *Arizona Law Review* 23: 1283–1298.

Sagoff, M. 1981b. "Economic Theory and Environmental Law." *Michigan Law Review* 79: 1393–1419.

Sagoff, M. 1981c. "We Have Met the Enemy and He Is Us, or, Conflict and Contradiction in Environmental Law." *Environmental Law* 12: 283–315.

Sanders, D., Sengupta, A., and Scott, V. 2015. "Ebola epidemic exposes the pathology of the global economic and political system." *International Journal of Health Services* 45(4):643–56.

Schrecker, T. 2013a. "Can Health Equity Survive Epidemiology? Standards of Proof and Social Determinants of Health." *Preventive Medicine* 57(6): 741–744.

Schrecker, T. 2013b. "Interrogating Scarcity: How to Think about 'Resource-Scarce Settings.'" *Health Policy and Planning* 28 (4): 400–409.

Schrecker, T. 2014a. "The Exterritorial Reach of Money: Global Finance and Social Determinants of Health." In *The Handbook of Global Health Policy*, edited by G. W. Brown, G. Yamey, and S. Wamala, 393–407 (New York: John Wiley).

Schrecker, T. 2014b. "Health Equity in a Globalising World: The Importance of Human Rights." In *Commonwealth Health Partnerships*, edited by A. Robertson, 18–21 (London: The Commonwealth). http://www.commonwealthhealth.org/wp-content/uploads/2014/05/2-Health-equity-Schrecker.pdf.

Schrecker, T. 2017. "Was Mackenbach Right? Towards a Practical Political Science of Redistribution and Health Inequalities." *Health and Place* 46: 293–299.

Shrader-Frechette, K. S., and McCoy, E. D. 1993. *Method in Ecology: Strategies for Conservation* (Cambridge: Cambridge University Press).

Sklair, L. 2005. "Generic Globalization, Capitalist Globalization, and Beyond: A Framework for Critical Globalization Studies." In *Critical Globalization Studies*, edited by R. P. Appelbaum and W. I. Robinson, 55–63 (London: Routledge).

Slater, T. 2013. "Your Life Chances Affect Where You Live: A Critique of the 'Cottage Industry' of Neighbourhood Effects Research." *International Journal of Urban and Regional Research* 37(2): 367–387.

Soares de Oliveira, R. 2007. *Oil and Politics in the Gulf of Guinea* (New York: Columbia University Press).

Somers, M. 2008. *Genealogies of Citizenship: Markets, Statelessness, and the Right to Have Rights* (Cambridge: Cambridge University Press).

Steele, S. L., Gilmore, A. B., McKee, M., and Stuckler, D. 2015. "The Role of Public Law-Based Litigation in Tobacco Companies' Strategies in High-Income, FCTC Ratifying Countries, 2004–14." *Journal of Public Health* 38(3): 516–521.

Szreter, S. 1999. "Rapid Economic Growth and 'the Four Ds' of Disruption, Deprivation, Disease and Death: Public Health Lessons from Nineteenth-Century Britain for Twenty-First-Century China?" *Tropical Medicine and International Health* 4(2): 146–152.

Taubes, G., and Couzens, C. K. 2012. "Big Sugar's Sweet Little Lies." *Mother Jones*, November/December. http://www.motherjones.com/environment/2012/10/sugar-industry-lies-campaign.

Taylor-Gooby, P. 2012. "Root and Branch Restructuring to Achieve Major Cuts: The Social Policy Programme of the 2010 UK Coalition Government." *Social Policy and Administration* 46(1): 61–82.

Walker, R. E., Keane, C. R., and Burke, J. G. 2010. "Disparities and Access to Healthy Food in the United States: A Review of Food Deserts Literature." *Health and Place* 16(5): 876–884.

Ward, K., and England, K. 2007. "Introduction: Reading Neoliberalization." In *Neoliberalization: States, Networks, People*, edited by K. England and K. Ward, 1–22 (Oxford: Blackwell).

Weinstock, D. M. 2015. "Health Justice after the Social Determinants of Health Revolution." *Social Theory and Health* 13(3–4): 437–453.

WHO (World Health Organization). 2015. *Health in All Policies: Training Manual* (Geneva: World Health Organization). https://www.who.int/social_determinants/publications/health-policies-manual/en/.

Zakaria, F. 1997. "The Rise of Illiberal Democracy." *Foreign Affairs* 76(6): 22–43.

CHAPTER 73

INCORPORATING ETHICS IN POLICY CHANGE AND HEALTH REFORM

GERARD ANDERSON, JEROMIE M. BALLREICH, AND AFSAN BHADELIA

Introduction

According to the World Health Organization, "[h]ealth policy refers to decisions, plans, and actions that are undertaken to achieve specific health care goals within a society" (WHO, 2019). Policy change and health reform are directed by public and private officials and promulgated in the form of laws, regulations, or organizational procedures and structures. Policymakers do not simply dictate health policy—they rely on ethical, scientific, economic, social, and political forces to guide their health policy deliberations (Brownson, Chriqui, and Stamatakis, 2009). These deliberations typically follow a policymaking process that is dictated by laws and regulations governing the policymakers.

Ethics plays a key role in health policy reform, both by influencing the policymaking process and highlighting specific health policy outcomes. In this chapter, we begin by discussing the theoretical relevance and practical impact of ethical reasoning in the policymaking process. We then provide examples of how ethical considerations are fundamental to health policy by using examples of major laws enacted in the United States, India, and Mexico. These examples are followed by a discussion of how the policymaking process operates and the similarities between ethical reasoning and the policymaking process. We illustrate the similarities using one model of the policy process and show its overlap with ethical reasoning.

Approaches in Ethical Reasoning and Their Impact on Health Policy

The deontological and teleological tenets of ethical reasoning often guide policymaking and acknowledge the implicit conflict between individual liberties and the role of the state. The teleological approach, focused on outcomes, incorporates the utilitarian tradition of moral conduct, which seeks to minimize harms and maximize benefits (Cooper, 2012). Impartiality, a tenet promoted by utilitarianism, suggests that it is important to include the preferences of all individuals when determining outcomes (Shapcott, 2010). A policymaker adopting the teleological approach is focused on the health outcomes for the entire population and is grounded by utilitarian calculations of which action will result in the best outcome for the most people. An example of applying the teleological approach to health policy is the promotion of immunizations. While there may be other reasons for promoting immunizations, emphasizing the health benefits for a population as the policy justification is an example of a teleological approach.

In contrast, a deontological approach, encompassing Kantian ethics, is grounded in moral duty and choosing the right thing to do. It is based on good will—motivation and intention to act morally for what is right—and respect for moral laws to determine the appropriate course of action (Cooper, 2012). A health policymaker following the deontological approach is concerned with a duty to align policies with specific ethical principles, such as justice or beneficence, in a way that could be independent of the population health outcomes. In practice, policymaking using a deontological approach could place extra consideration on the rights or health of minorities, persons with disabilities, and other disadvantaged populations. For example, a sense of duty might translate into crafting a policy promoting care for transgender individuals because these individuals may require specific health policies.

Deontological and teleological tenets can both be justifications for health policy. The Sustainable Development Goal (SDG) for health includes the subgoal of achieving universal health coverage in all countries. Universal health coverage may be advocated in teleological terms to expand access to care for more people, and in deontological terms to reduce health inequities (UN, 2015). Another subgoal of the SDG focuses on a subset of the population by aiming to eliminate preventable deaths of newborns and young children. This goal targets vulnerable populations, aligning with a deontological approach. Alternatively, eliminating preventable deaths of newborns and children can be viewed with teleological intent, since these health benefits can result in future economic growth benefiting the entire population.

Ethical reasoning is used as procedural guidance for various health policy reforms. A World Health Organization report, *Making Fair Choices on the Path to Universal Health Coverage*, is an example of a systematic effort to introduce ethical reasoning into policymaking. For example, the document provides three ethical rationales for achieving universal health insurance coverage—fair distribution, cost-effectiveness, and fair contribution (WHO, 2014). Fair distribution suggests health coverage policy should prioritize worse-off individuals. Cost-effectiveness suggests a promotion of fairness in the allocation of public resources. Fair contribution seeks to ensure that access cannot be limited based on an ability to pay. The report then examines critical choices concerning which services to expand first, which beneficiaries to include first, and how to structure the finances to achieve universal health coverage.

An example of ethical reasoning having a role in the policymaking process is the United States' "notice of proposed rulemaking." This mechanism is an example of the government attempting to include all perspectives and stakeholders in the policymaking process (Center for Effective Government, 2017). The notice of proposed rulemaking requires the government to notify the public of an impending regulatory change and provides the public an opportunity to comment on the regulations before the rule is finalized. While the government does not have to agree with the public comment, the government must justify its position and address the concerns of the person or entity providing the comment. This process ensures changes to regulations will consider the impact on stakeholders and weigh these against the impact on the overall population.

A Common Ethical and Policy Choice: Individual Autonomy versus the State

Ethicists and policymakers have struggled with two fundamental conflicting ideas in public health: the autonomy of the individual versus the interests of the state. Although the general aim of health policy is to simultaneously improve individual and population health, there are often conflicts. In achieving this aim, it may be necessary to impinge on the autonomy of the individual or restrict the actions of the state. Lawrence Gostin (2000, 11) characterizes the ongoing state-individual debate in public health policy by noting that the state "is compelled... to act affirmatively to promote the health of the people," but "cannot unduly invade individuals' rights in the name of the communal good." This conflict is at the center of many health policy debates and ethical concerns.

For example, consider the issue of mandatory vaccinations, whose objective is to improve population health against infectious diseases. The public health benefits of vaccination have been well documented (Andre et al., 2008; Ehreth, 2003). However, when the government mandates that an individual should be vaccinated, the government is impinging on that individual's autonomy. In this case, the argument for mandatory vaccination often prevails. However, in some circumstances the preference of the individual prevails. Policymakers need to make that trade-off in very specific circumstances.

Tobacco policy is an example of where policymakers tend to side with individual autonomy in lieu of state policies to maximize public health. Despite the enormous volume of clinical research suggesting the negative health effects of tobacco (WHO, 2011;

Frieden and Bloomberg, 2007), many governments do not ban tobacco use by adults. Rather, the government attempts to influence an individual's decision to use tobacco through public awareness campaigns, label warnings, and taxation. Banning the use of tobacco is perceived by many policymakers to impinge too much on individual autonomy, in spite of the dangers of secondhand smoke and other adverse impacts of smoking on the public.

The predominant principle that underpins the role of government in health care is the concept of the *social contract*. The idea of the social contract is that individuals within a community establish an understanding that certain freedoms and commitments to obey a government authority are exchanged for protections through the enforcement of laws to meet the "general will" and interest of society (Rousseau, 1762). Throughout history, health policy change has occurred when there was a sense that the government, through public health policy, could improve the welfare of the population after taking into account the rights of individuals.

Ethics and US Health Policy: Two Case Studies Involving Ethical Reasoning

While some policymakers view individual autonomy as paramount, for others there are strong ethical arguments for a substantial role of government in health care. Below we discuss key ethical arguments in the context of two significant US health policies over the last seventy years.

US Social Security Amendments of 1965

The 1950s was a decade of significant prosperity in the United States; however, not everyone participated in rising incomes and wealth, and by the late 1950s, a fifth of the nation was considered to be poor (Poverty in America Project, 2016). In response to these concerns over inequality, President John F. Kennedy launched the New Frontier policies in 1961. While the New Frontier platform addressed a variety of topics, ranging from science advancement to civil rights, one key concern involved "unanswered questions of poverty and surplus" (Kennedy, 1960).

One approach to address this concern was to provide adequate health insurance. At the time, the US health insurance system was based almost solely on employment, which meant few retired older Americans could afford health insurance. While President Kennedy pushed for universal coverage to address this problem, his push faced opposition from groups like the American Medical Association (AMA), which claimed the proposals would lead to socialized medicine (Dickerson, 2013). For groups like the AMA, this violated the ethical principle of individual autonomy and personal choice. It was also argued that a lack of government capability to provide health care for all would limit individual health capabilities (Sen, 1980; Nussbaum and Sen, 1993). This ethical argument over capability divides individual freedom into two aspects: one that pertains to the opportunity of the individual's "ability to achieve," and another that pertains to the "process of choice itself" (Sen, 2009, 228). Health capabilities relate to the conditions that impact health, the pursuit of good health (i.e., access to health care), and an individual's ability to make choices that can improve his or her health (Ruger, 2010). While in many countries the idea that health care is a right is a fundamental tenet, in the United States this issue is continually debated, with ethical arguments being offered to justify both positions.

While President Kennedy was unable to pass any major health reforms before his assassination, his successor, President Lyndon Johnson, was able to enact health reforms through his "Great Society" platform. In 1965 there was a recognition that health care spending was hurting many older Americans—47 percent of elderly families were impoverished and could not afford to purchase health insurance (Moon, 2006). The plight of elderly families motivated the ethical justification for the "Great Society"—a belief that a great nation did not leave elderly people behind. President Johnson's goal was to bring "equal justice to all," including eliminating poverty, eradicating disease, eliminating illiteracy, and ending bigotry.

The "Great Society," however, adopted two different approaches to health coverage policy—one approach for Medicare and a different one for Medicaid. They are based on different ethical principles, and these differences have been at the center of many ethical and policy debates over the decades. The Medicare program is government-issued insurance that provides coverage to the elderly, the disabled, and people with end-stage renal disease. People contribute to their future Medicare coverage while they are employed. The Medicaid program is government-issued insurance that covers the poor under certain conditions, but the poor are not expected to contribute to their coverage. The key ethical and financing difference between the two programs is whether the person directly contributes to funding his or her own coverage. The difference between Medicare and Medicaid has influenced much of the subsequent policy debate and reform. Internationally, some countries have adopted an entitlement approach for health insurance, while others have adopted the categorical approach.

Patient Protection and Affordable Care Act of 2010

A major US health policy change came with the Patient Protection and Affordable Care Act of 2010 (Pub. L. No. 111–148, 124 Stat. 119 [2010]), also known as the Affordable Care Act, in the United States. The law restructured the US health insurance market by mandating nearly all people purchase health insurance, prohibiting the use of preexisting conditions exclusions by health insurers, providing subsidies for poor individuals to purchase health insurance, and other health insurance reforms. It changed the economics of health care by providing income-determined financial subsidies for insurance, and these subsidies would be paid for by taxes primarily targeting the affluent. In spite of its name, the policies within the Affordable Care Act had one overarching mission—to ensure that people have access to health care and insurance. To accomplish this mission, it drew on ethical justifications in both the Medicare and Medicaid program (Cutright, 1965). It follows the Medicare principles of having people financially contribute to their own coverage. It also follows the Medicaid principles of having the more affluent population help contribute to funding for the poor. The ongoing policy debate is partially about who should be subsidized and the balance between subsidization and personal responsibility for an individual's health coverage.

While access was the overarching mission of the Affordable Care Act, policymakers recognized that affordability was impeding access, and that this was being driven by health care market failures. For policymakers, addressing the adverse selection problem in health insurance was most crucial (Handel, 2013). Adverse selection occurs when individuals purchase health insurance only when they actually need it. The people most likely to defer the purchase of health insurance are the young and healthy. Without having the young and healthy in the pool of people purchasing health insurance, insurers are unable to spread the risk, resulting in high premiums for health insurance. To counter adverse selection, the Affordable Care Act provides incentives and penalties to persuade the young and healthy to purchase health insurance. The main policy and ethical issue is whether the government should compel young and healthy people to purchase health insurance if they do not believe they need to purchase insurance. By providing incentives and penalties, the Affordable Care Act interfered with individual autonomy, but this intrusion was ethically justified by principles of beneficence and equity, since socioeconomic status should not prevent an individual from having health insurance.

While the Affordable Care Act adopted the objectives of achieving beneficence and promoting justice through equity and fairness, repeal efforts to replace the act are dominated by a desire to preserve autonomy, personal freedom, and personal responsibility. Efforts to repeal are grounded on the desire to limit government control of the health care market, because intervention is viewed as an infringement of civil liberties. This shows the ongoing tension in the United States between beneficence and justice, on the one hand, and autonomy, on the other.

Dignity in Life and Death—Amending the Narcotics and Psychotropic Substances Act of 1985

India confronted the individual autonomy versus the state debate in a very different context. In 2015, India amended its long-standing Narcotics and Psychotropic Substances Act that controlled access to opioids, including morphine for medical purposes. This act limited the availability and access to treatments commonly used in palliative care and pain control. The original 1985 act imposed major restrictions on health facilities in acquiring, storing, and dispensing opioids. The restrictions impacted licensure and policy development and limited the manufacture of opioids. This led to extended delays and, in some cases, the inability of health facilities to procure opioids. This regulatory barrier meant millions of Indians were without access to pain relief (Rajagopal and Joranson, 2007; Rajagopal and Palat, 2002).

The policy objective of the 1985 act was to advance the principle of beneficence and protect the population from illicit drug use and addiction. However, it had an unintended effect of causing immense harm to many sick people needing pain relief, directly violating a principal tenet of beneficence to do no harm. Through years of advocacy from civil society and policy champions, the 1985 act was amended. The 2015 amendment standardized regulations across India, streamlined the process of acquiring licensure by reducing bureaucratic obstacles, and changed the culture of opiophobia (Rajagopal, 2015). Policymakers in many countries have tried to balance between protecting the population from harm while allowing personal freedoms. These trade-offs require ethical considerations of beneficence, dignity, and justice.

Seguro Popular and the Right to Health: Understanding Health Reform in Mexico

Countries have adopted a number of different approaches to universal health insurance coverage. Seguro Popular is the national insurance scheme of Mexico that was established in 2003 (Knaul et al., 2012). The system was designed to respond to growing poverty and the lack of health protection among poor Mexicans, many of whom had been excluded from other social protection schemes (Frenk et al., 2006). Seguro Popular targeted vulnerable groups and sought to expand coverage over time. The system requires people receiving government assistance to undertake certain preventive health behaviors in order to continue receiving government assistance, thereby impinging on their individual autonomy.

The reform was guided by both "ideas and ideals," with the generation of evidence guiding the policy process and the choice of which preventive actions to require. The debate involved ethical deliberation over individual liberty versus a choice of additional public spending if a recipient of the financial aid got sick because he or she did not take appropriate preventive actions. (Frenk and Gómez-Dantés, 2009). The policy objective of uplifting the Mexican population from poverty and improving human development was enhanced by the adoption of health as a social right (Frenk and Gómez-Dantés, 2009). Segura Popular insures over 52 million Mexicans, providing health care with financial protection (Knaul et al., 2015).

The Relationship between the Policy Process and Ethical Reasoning

Many different models of the policy process exist (Birkland, 2014). Each model emphasizes different aspects of the policymaking process, but they all share similarities. The models are designed to help the person or the stakeholder group who is advocating a particular issue to identify the most effective policy option to present. In this way, the process is similar to what the ethicist does when conducting ethical reasoning.

Global health efforts acknowledge the need for aligning priorities based on technical, ethical, and political criteria (Roberts et al., 2004; WHO, 2010). As noted previously, the WHO published a specific report in 2014 on establishing guidelines, grounded by ethical reasoning, to aid countries as they make policy considerations on the path to achieving universal health care. The human rights framework has been championed to advance priority-setting processes to meet the SDGs, including the subgoal of achieving universal health care (Rumbold et al., 2017).

Eugene Bardach, a political scientist at the University of California-Berkeley, developed one of the most widely taught models of the policymaking process (Bardach and Patashnik, 2015). His model, known as the "eightfold path," is in the family of models that assumes that the policymaking process is rational and based on data and reasoning. It is intended to assist the person advocating for a policy change to understand what is necessary to promote change. The eight steps and respective similarities with ethical reasoning are summarized in Table 73.1 and discussed further below.

Defining the problem is perhaps the most critical step for those advocating policy change. It is essential to clearly define what is wrong with the status quo and identify opportunities for change. The policy issue has to be sufficiently important to concern the policymaker. Similarly, ethical reasoning entails a moral appraisal of the status quo and a discussion of why it violates particular ethical principles. In addition, the ethical imperative associated with the specific problem must be evident; for example, why should universal coverage in all countries be an ethical concern? Both the Bardach model and ethical reasoning recognize the importance of context in decision-making and how economic, political, and historical context can shape policy.

Assembling the evidence requires addressing why the defined problem is an important public health problem and why the status quo is unacceptable. In assembling the evidence, it is important to select evidence that appears most compelling to policymakers. There are many sources of evidence, including personal stories, analogies, surveys of best practice, and collection and analysis of primary and secondary data. It is often necessary to show why the policy change is feasible at this time, what has been tried previously, and why it has failed in the past. There also needs to be a discussion of unintended consequences with the policy recommendation. In ethical reasoning, these same principles apply, and the evidence should be ethically gathered. For example, a clinical study may provide evidence for a new medical treatment, which may have health

Table 73.1 Comparing the Policy Process with Ethical Reasoning

Policy process (Bardach model)	Ethical reasoning
1. Define the problem	Moral appraisal and identification of ethical imperatives associated with the problem
2. Assemble some evidence	Consideration of ethical implications
3. Construct the alternatives	Identification of alternatives that uphold ethical principles
4. Select the criteria	Identification of theoretical basis for evaluation
5. Project the outcomes	Determine outcomes that fulfill moral obligation on basis of theoretical basis being applied
6. Confront the trade-offs	Review trade-offs in relation to upholding of ethical principles
7. Decide	Determine actionable ethical imperative
8. Tell your story	Describe the ethical imperative and how problem violates core societal values

policy implications. However, researchers also have an obligation to conduct the study using ethical principles.

Constructing the alternatives requires the presentation of a range of policy options that could effectively address the problem. This is often very specific to the policymaker and the history of the issue. In practice, policymakers are accustomed to evaluating three or four options, including the status quo, although there are no restrictions on the number of options. In order to effect change, the advocate must select options that policymakers will actually consider, not ones that are aspirational and unlikely to be adopted. For ethicists, it is important to present alternatives that uphold a range of ethical principles. For example, one alternative may uphold individual autonomy in choice of health care, while another upholds beneficence by promoting subsidized health care.

Selecting the criteria requires the identification of criteria with which to evaluate the policy in domains of interest to the policymaker. The two most commonly used health policy criteria are cost and health impact. Policymakers focus on the cost of the various alternatives and how many people will benefit. Other criteria, such as respect, beneficence, justice, or autonomy, are potential factors. A more detailed discussion of policy criteria from an ethical perspective is included in the "benchmarks of fairness" developed by Norman Daniels (Daniels, 1996).

Projecting the outcomes requires an assessment of how each policy alternative scores with each criterion. Sometimes this is subjective, and sometimes there are models that project the outcomes. For example, the US Congressional Budget Office is required to project outcomes for each legislative proposal in the US Congress. From an ethical standpoint, an accounting of the impact of policy meets the moral duty of doing the right thing or enables a utilitarian calculation of which outcome produces the greatest good.

Confronting the trade-offs requires recognition that no policy option is likely to score highest on all criteria. For example, a policy that has the best outcomes may also be the most expensive. Ethical consideration of trade-offs will be grounded by the principle of beneficence and determining which trade-offs do no harm, or benefit-risk trade-offs. Sometimes, all policy options incur some harm to individuals.

Deciding which policy to propose can be difficult, since there is seldom universal agreement on a particular policy option and each option has strengths and weaknesses. This requires policymakers to make trade-offs (Peacock et al., 2006; Daniels and Sabin, 1998). From an ethics perspective, one perspective is to judge a priority-setting decision-making process to be fair is when the "process, decisions and rationales are accessible and relevant; and an appeals and enforcement mechanism are established" (Baltussen and Niessen, 2006).

The final step, *telling the story*, is to present the option as succinctly as possible so the policymaker can quickly recognize the importance of the problem and the proposed solution. The story is also important for ethicists, since the most compelling stories draw upon key values, and while all values may not be universally shared, certain principles, such as constitutional rights, resonate with most of society.

Conclusion

Ethical concerns have been part of the policy process for years. They also underpin most health policy change and reform, even when there is a debate on topics such as (1) the role of the state versus the role of the individual; (2) the responsibility of society for the poor and older persons; and (3) the balancing of benefits with risks to avoid doing any harm. The policy process and ethical reasoning share many of the same attributes, although the language describing them is often quite different. As noted by the World Health Organization, health policy seeks to "achieve specific health care goals within a society" (WHO, 2019), and policymakers have a responsibility to embrace ethical reasoning in the process and justification of policies to advance better health outcomes. This is the process of policy change and health reform.

References

Andre, F. E., Booy, R., Bock, H. L., Clemens, J., Datta, S. K., John, T. J., et al. 2008. "Vaccination Greatly Reduces Disease, Disability, Death and Inequity Worldwide." *Bulletin of the World Health Organization* 86(2): 140–146.

Baltussen, R., and Niessen, L. 2006. "Priority Setting of Health Interventions: The Need for Multi-Criteria Decision Analysis." *Cost Effectiveness and Resource Allocation* 4: 14, https://resource-allocation.biomedcentral.com/articles/10.1186/1478-7547-4-14.

Bardach, E., and Patashnik, E. M. 2015. *A Practical Guide for Policy Analysis: The Eightfold Path to More Effective Problem Solving* (Washington, D.C.: CQ Press).

Birkland, T. A. 2014. *An Introduction to the Policy Process: Theories, Concepts, and Models of Public Policy Making* (New York and London: Routledge).

Brownson, R. C., Chriqui, J. F., and Stamatakis, K. A. 2009. "Understanding Evidence-Based Public Health Policy." *American Journal of Public Health* 99(9): 1576–1583.

Center for Effective Government. 2017. "Regulatory Resource Center." http://www.foreffectivegov.org/node/2579.

Cooper, T. 2012. *The Responsible Administrator: An Approach to Ethics for the Administrative Role*. 6th ed. (San Francisco: Jossey-Bass).

Cutright, P. 1965. "Political Structure, Economic Development, and National Social Security Programs." *American Journal of Sociology* 70(5): 537–550.

Daniels, N. 1996. *Benchmarks of Fairness for Health Care Reform* (Oxford: Oxford University Press).

Daniels, N., and Sabin, J. 1998. "The Ethics of Accountability in Managed Care Reform." *Health Affairs* 17(5): 50–64.

Dickerson J. 2013 "Kennedy Care: Fifty Years before Obamacare, JFK Had His Own Health Care Debacle." *Slate*, November 17. http://www.slate.com/articles/news_and_politics/history/2013/11/john_f_kennedy_s_health_care_failure_jfk_and_barack_obama_s_tough_fights.html.

Ehreth, J. 2003. "The Global Value of Vaccination." *Vaccine* 21(7): 596–600.

Frenk, J., and Gómez-Dantés, O. 2009. "Ideas and Ideals: Ethical Basis of Health Reform in Mexico." *Lancet* 73(9673): 1406–1408.

Frenk, J., González-Pier, E., Gómez-Dantés, O., Lezana, M. A., and Knaul, F. M. 2006. "Comprehensive Reform to Improve Health System Performance in Mexico." *Lancet* 368(9546): 1524–1534.

Frieden, T. R., and Bloomberg, M. R. 2007. "How to Prevent 100 Million Deaths from Tobacco." *Lancet* 369(9574): 1758–1761.

Gostin, L.O. 2000. *Public Health Law: Power, Duty, Restraint* (Berkeley: University of California Press; New York: Milbank Memorial Fund).

Handel, B. R. 2013. "Adverse Selection and Inertia in Health Insurance Markets: When Nudging Hurts." *American Economic Review* 103(7): 2643–2682.

Kennedy, J. F. 1960. "The New Frontier." Democratic National Convention Nomination Acceptance Address. http://www.americanrhetoric.com/speeches/jfk1960dnc.htm.

Knaul, F. M., Bhadelia, A., Atun, R., and Frenk, J. 2015. "Achieving Effective Universal Health Coverage and Diagonal Approaches to Care for Chronic Illnesses." *Health Affairs* 34(9):1514–22.

Knaul, F.M., González-Pier, E., Gómez-Dantés, O., García-Junco, D., Arreola-Ornelas, H., Barraza-Lloréns, M., et al. 2012. "The Quest for Universal Health Coverage: Achieving Social Protection for All in Mexico." *Lancet* 380(9849): 1259–79.

Moon, M. 2006. *Medicare: A Policy Primer* (Washington, D.C.: Urban Institute Press).

Nussbaum, M., and Sen, A. 1993. *The Quality of Life* (Oxford: Clarendon Press).

Peacock, S., Ruta, D., Mitton, C., Donaldson, C., Bate, A., and Murtagh, M. 2006. "Using Economics to Set Pragmatic and Ethical Priorities." *British Medical Journal* 332(7539): 482–485.

Poverty in America Project. 2016. "The Paradox of Poverty in America." http://povertyinamerica.mit.edu/download/atlas_of_poverty_in_america_p1.pdf.

Rajagopal, M. R. 2015. "The Current Status of Palliative Care in India." *Cancer Control* 2015: 57–62. http://www.cancercontrol.info/cc2015/the-current-status-of-palliative-care-in-india/.

Rajagopal, M. R., and Joranson, D.E. 2007. "India: Opioid Availability—An Update." *Journal of Pain and Symptom Management* 33(5): 615–622.

Rajagopal, M.R., and Palat, G. 2002. "Kerala, India: Status of Cancer Pain Relief and Palliative Care." *Journal of Pain and Symptom Management* 24(2): 191–3.

Roberts, M., Hsiao, W., Berman, P., and Reich, M. 2004. *Getting Health Reform Right: A Guide to Improving Performance and Equity* (New York: Oxford University Press).

Rousseau, J. 1762. *Principes du droit politique* (Amsterdam: Chez M.M. Rey).

Ruger, J. P. 2010. "Health Capability: Conceptualization and Operationalization." *American Journal of Public Health* 100(1): 41–49.

Rumbold, B., Baker, R., Ferraz, O., Hawkes, S., Krubiner, C., Littlejohns, P., et al. 2017. "Universal Health Coverage, Priority Setting, and the Human Right to Health." *Lancet* 390(10095): 712–714.

Sen, A. 1980. "Equality of What?" In *Tanner Lectures on Human Values*, edited by S. McMurrin (Cambridge: Cambridge University Press).

Sen, A. 2009. *The Idea of Justice* (Cambridge, Mass.: Belknap Press of Harvard University Press).

Shapcott, R. 2010. *International Ethics: A Critical Introduction* (Cambridge: Polity Press).

UN (United Nations). 2015. Sustainable Development Goals. http://www.un.org/sustainabledevelopment/sustainable-development-goals/.

WHO (World Health Organization). 2010. *World Health Report 2010. Health Systems: Improving Performance* (Geneva: WHO). http://www.who.int/whr/2000/en/.

WHO (World Health Organization). 2011. *WHO Report on the Global Tobacco Epidemic 2011: Warning about the Dangers of Tobacco* (Geneva: WHO). http://www.who.int/tobacco/global_report/2011/en/.

WHO (World Health Organization). 2014. *Making Fair Choices on the Path to Universal Health Coverage: Final Report of the Consultative Group on Equity and Universal Health Coverage* (Geneva: WHO). http://www.who.int/choice/documents/making_fair_choices/en/.

WHO (World Health Organization). 2019. "Health Policy." http://www.who.int/topics/health_policy/en/.

Index

Note: Tables, Figures and Boxes are indicated by italic '*t*', '*f*', '*b*' and notes are indicated by 'n' respectively, following the page number.

C

D

E

H

M

S

T

V

W

Y

Z